W9-AUG-073

DRUGS
AND
NURSING
IMPLICATIONS

LAURA E. GOVONI Ph.D., R.N.

Formerly Professor, Graduate Division
University of Connecticut School of Nursing

JANICE E. HAYES Ph.D., R.N.

Professor and Associate Dean
University of Connecticut School of Nursing

THIRD EDITION

DRUGS AND NURSING IMPLICATIONS

APPLETON-CENTURY-CROFTS / NEW YORK

79 80 81 82 / 10 9 8 7 6 5 4 3

Prentice-Hall International, Inc., London
Prentice-Hall of Australia, Pty. Ltd., Sydney
Prentice-Hall of India Private Limited, New Delhi
Prentice-Hall of Japan, Inc., Tokyo
Prentice-Hall of Southeast Asia (Pte.) Ltd., Singapore
Whitehall Books, Ltd., Wellington, New Zealand

The use of portions of the text of the *United States Pharmacopoeia,* XVIII Revision, official September 1, 1970, is by permission received from the Board of Trustees of the United States Pharmacopoeial Convention, Inc. The said Convention is not responsible for any inaccuracy of quotation, or for any faulty or misleading implication that may arise by reason of the separation of excerpts from the original context.

Other references used by permission of the appropriate officers or councils include *The National Formulary,* XIII edition (1970), Council of American Pharmaceutical Association; *New Drugs* (1967), Secretary of the Council on Drugs of the American Medical Association; and the *British Pharmacopoeia* 1968 and *Addendum* 1969, General Medical Council.

The authors assume responsibility for inaccuracies or errors which may arise from use of these references.

Library of Congress Cataloging in Publication Data

Govoni, Laura E
    Drugs and nursing implications.

    Bibliography: p.
    Includes index.
    1. Pharmacology. 2. Nursing. I. Hayes, Janice E.,
joint author. II. Title. [DNLM: 1. Nursing care.
2. Pharmacology. QV38 G721d]
RM125.G6 1978   615'.7'024613   78–5711
ISBN 0–8385–1784–6

Cover Photogram © Martin Bough 1978
Designer: Rodelinde Albrecht

CONTENTS

PREFACE

In this completely new edition of *Drugs and Nursing Implications,* over 200 new drugs have been added, and the number of prototypes has been increased and more fully described. This edition also contains several new sections. Both format and style that students and teachers found useful in former editions have been retained, i.e., alphabetical sequence according to generic names, and use of prototypes as major sources of information about drug groups. Prototypal organization places emphasis on the fact that drugs related by chemical and structural similarities often share mechanisms of action and other pharmacologic properties. When a drug is referred to the prototype, it shares Nursing Implications, Laboratory Test Interferences, and Drug Interactions, unless otherwise noted. Differences in the congeneric and second order compounds are described briefly and include particularized nursing implications.

With each edition, our conviction grows that involvement in the total pharmacotherapeutic regimen is one of the most challenging responsibilities of the nurse. Each activity related to drug therapy is important; all aspects of safe, effective treatment beginning with the scheduling of doses and continuing through the analysis of response to the drug regimen as a base for patient teaching require the ability to integrate knowledge about pharmacodynamics into all phases of the nursing process.

Interdigitation of drug therapy with the coexisting nursing regimen requires a data bank of relevant drug information; such a resource is presented in the sections preceding nursing implications. Data about drug effects reflect increased information about what happens at the cellular and molecular levels as well as at the organ level. Information about drug entry, transport, biotransformation, and excretion has been expanded. The reader also is alerted to time factors (i.e., peak action periods, duration of effect, drug half-life) that suggest administration schedules and indicate periods of potential danger from overdose or toxicity. Sections related to limitations of drug use incorporate new knowledge about drug passage across cell membranes (passage into breast milk, across the blood–brain barrier, and the placenta), the effect of age on drug response, and the problems of multiple drug therapies. All of these sections provide clinically oriented information useful in the design of nursing-pharmacotherapeutic regimens.

When feasible, adverse reactions (allergy, sensitivity, toxicity, untoward effects) have been grouped according to body system or to clusters of reactions. All have been reported in clinical research literature and their multiplicity places a very real burden on the designer of patient care who cannot chance ignorance if drug-induced diseases or conditions are to be prevented.

New features of the third edition deal with drug interactions, drug-induced interferences with clinical tests, and pediatric dosage regimens. Information about drug interactions (already a subspecialty in pharmacology) is accumulating at a rate that creates and maintains a gap between report and validation. The full extent of patient problems directly related to drug interactions is still not clear; however, this section of the drug monograph alerts the nurse to the importance of continuous and sophisticated observation of the patient whose expected response to one drug may be altered or cancelled by another. Since interactions, usually reported by drug class and by prototypes, have been described as "almost always preventable," the significance of this new section cannot be overemphasized.*

Another new feature, the explanation of interferences with laboratory tests by selected drugs further illustrates the complexities of drug therapy. Although most changes in test results are important to the physician or nurse, some also must be made known to the patient, e.g., drug-induced color changes in urine, feces, or skin, or false positive tests for glycosuria.

Since the last edition, professional nursing responsibility and functions have continued to expand, particularly in those states where Nurse Practice Acts have been revised. These acts have either introduced or strengthened a legally protected movement toward broader decision-making activities and more independence in nursing practice. Another significant development in recent years is the increased availability of information about drugs and drug treatment to patients via lay press and visual media. Both of these forces have influenced the rationale for inclusions in the section on nursing implications in drug therapy.

Nursing implications of pharmacotherapeutics represent a synthesis of scientific information from many disciplines (medicine, nutrition, pharmacology, pathophysiology, clinical laboratory science as well as from nursing). Our experience in teaching courses in pharmacodynamics, the experiential knowledge and suggestions of colleagues in nursing and allied health sciences and of our students provided much of the data base from which nursing implications were extrapolated and made explicit. Beliefs that eventual self-care within one's own environment is an ultimate goal for all patients and that each patient has unique qualities and needs guided the design of nursing implications.

A wide variety of consequences of drug therapy and implications for nurses have been included: normal laboratory values and their alterations, new methods for drug administration, expected plasma levels of drugs, differences in drug response due to different age groups, particularities about the pathophysiological condition being treated, nutritional factors important to treatment success, and teaching plans. The latter will help the patient acquire essential information needed to provide effective safe use of the drug and to assist in the decision related to when total self-care may be assumed.

In conclusion, we have found the writing of the third edition to be a renewed education in pharmacotherapy and patient care. We can only hope that utilization of this book will help others to add to their knowledge and to appreciate the significant role of the nurse in successful drug therapy.

ACKNOWLEDGMENTS

Many individuals, including students, professional colleagues, and friends from the lay public have influenced the preparation of this edition. In

*Hansten, P: Drug Interactions, 3rd ed. Philadelphia, Lea & Febiger, 1975, p. 1.

particular we wish to express our appreciation for the expert assistance of Paul Pierpaoli whose detailed review, corrections, and suggestions provided us with a good measure of security about the substance of the manuscript. We are also grateful to Alex Cardoni and Dennis Chapron who deserve the highest praise for their efforts in providing documentation as they responded to our search for authoritative manuscript content.

We are deeply indebted to Charles Bollinger for his perceptive advice and unfailing support throughout the period of time spent in preparing the third edition. We sincerely value his friendship and continued interest. We wish also to express appreciation and thanks to Steven Abramson for his meticulous attention to the logistical details involved in completing the last draft of the manuscript. His patience and ability to coordinate final activities greatly facilitated transformation of the original copy into a printed book.

This book is dedicated to our families for providing sustained support and love even in the face of having to accommodate to changes in both life-style and living environments. We are especially indebted to Eva B. Bellini, Augusto Govoni, and Marjorie Hayes for their understanding and patience. Without their forbearance, encouragement and help this edition would not have been completed.

We gratefully acknowledge the following professional resource persons who advised us on relevant clinical applications of pharmacology in nursing: Alex Cardoni, M.S. (Pharm), Associate Clinical Professor, University of Connecticut, School of Pharmacy; Director of Drug Information Center, University of Connecticut Health Center; Cosmo Castaldi, D.M.D., Professor and Chairman, Department of Dentistry, University of Connecticut Health Center; Dennis Chapron, M.S. (Pharm), Assistant Clinical Professor, University of Connecticut, School of Pharmacy; Assistant Director of Drug Information Center, University of Connecticut Health Center; Sonya Celeste, R.N., M.S.N., Senior Nurse Clinician in Surgery, University of Connecticut Health Center; Marcia Clinton, R.N., Pediatric Nurse Practitioner, Hartford Hospital; Mary Lou Condon, R.N., B.S.N., Diabetes Nurse Clinician, Hartford Hospital; Constance Crowley, R.N., Coronary Unit, St. Francis Hospital; William J. Davis, Department Manager and Instructor in Anesthesiology, University of Connecticut Health Center; Marilyn Bellini Fall, R.N., B.S.N.; Eleanor K. Gill, Dean and Professor, School of Nursing, University of Connecticut; Christine Johnson, R.N., M.S., Master Clinician in Cardiology, Hartford Hospital; Kathleen W. Kelly, R.N., M.S., Instructor, Graduate Program in Nursing, University of Connecticut; Diane LaRochelle, R.N., M.S., Instructor, Graduate Program in Nursing, University of Connecticut; Edmund Lowrie, M.D., Director of Dialysis, Peter Bent Brigham Hospital; Assistant Professor, Harvard University; Ernestine Lowrie, R.N., Director of Clinical Services, National Medical Care, Inc.; Ann MacGillis, R.N., M.S.; Alberta Macioni, R.N., M.S., Instructor, Graduate Program in Nursing, University of Connecticut; William Mancoll, M.D., FACS, Otorhinolaryngology; Anthony Mascia, R.N., M.S. Pediatric Nurse Clinician, Maternal and Child Health Consultant, Visiting Nurse Association of Hartford; Kathleen Maxson, R.N., B.S.; Elizabeth McKinnon Mullett, R.N., Ph.D., Professor, Graduate Program in Nursing, University of Connecticut; Benjamin A. Passos, M.D., St. Joseph Nurse Hospital, Detroit, Michigan; Paul Pierpaoli, R.Ph., Director, Department of Pharmacy Services, MCV Hospitals, Richmond, Virginia; June Pierce,

x R.N., Inservice Instructor, Coronary Care Nursing, St. Raphael Hospital; Ann Powers, R.N., M.S.; Kathleen Ransom, R.N., A.D.; Marie Roberto, R.N., M.S., Associate Director, Visiting Nurse Association of Hartford; Michael A. Rossi, M.D., Chief, Cardiac Surgery, Hartford Hospital; Sandra Scantling, R.N., M.S.N., Senior Nurse Clinician in Psychiatry, University of Connecticut Health Center; Ijaz Shafi, M.D., Assistant Professor in Ophthalmology, University of Connecticut Health Center; John Shepherd, D.D.S.; Sheldon Sones, R.Ph., Director of Pharmacy Service, Mount Sinai Hospital; Irene Sopelak, R.N., Diabetes Teaching Nurse, Hartford Hospital; Helen Valentine, R.N., M.S., Assistant Director of Nursing, Manchester Hospital.

LAURA E. GOVONI
JANICE E. HAYES

DRUGS
AND
NURSING
IMPLICATIONS

ACETAMINOPHEN, U.S.P.
(ACETA, A'CENOL, ANAPAP, ANUPHEN, APAMIDE, APAP, CAPITAL, DAPA, DATRIL, DIMINDOL, FEBRIGESIC, G-1, LIQUIPRIN, NEBS, NEOPAP, PANEX, PANOFEN, PEDRIC, PHENAPHEN, PROVAL, SK-APAP, TAPAR, TEMPRA, TYLENOL, VALADOL, and others)
PARACETAMOL, B.P.

Analgesic, antipyretic

ACTIONS AND USES
p-Aminophenol (aniline) derivative and major metabolite of acetanilid and phenacetin. Analgesic and antipyretic actions approximately equivalent to those of aspirin. Unlike aspirin, it is less likely to depress prothrombin levels, does not produce gastric mucosal erosion and bleeding, has weak antiinflammatory effect, and lacks antirheumatic and uricosuric properties. Overdosage appears to be more dangerous than with aspirin because treatment is much more difficult. Produces lower incidence of methemoglobinemia, and overall toxicity is somewhat less than that of phenacetin. Produces analgesia by raising pain threshold; mechanism and locus of action uncertain. Antipyresis is produced through direct action on hypothalamic heat-regulating centers, with consequent peripheral vasodilatation and dissipation of heat. In high doses, induces synthesis of hepatic microsomal enzymes. Reported to possess antidiuretic activity. Used for temporary relief of low to moderate pain, such as simple headache, minor joint and muscle pains, neuralgia, and dysmenorrhea, and as analgesic and antipyretic in diseases accompanied by discomfort of fever, eg, common cold, flu, and other viral infections.

ABSORPTION AND FATE
Completely absorbed from GI tract and rapidly distributed to most body tissues. Peak blood levels in 30 minutes to 1 hour; plasma half-life 1 to 3 hours. Only small amounts detectable in plasma after 8 hours. Metabolized by liver microsomes. Approximately 80% of dose is excreted in urine within 24 hours as conjugated acetaminophen and other minor metabolites and about 3% as unchanged drug.

CONTRAINDICATIONS AND PRECAUTIONS
Known hypersensitivity to acetaminophen or phenacetin; children under 3 years of age; repeated administration to patients with anemia or cardiac, pulmonary, renal, or hepatic disease. Cautious use in arthritic or rheumatic conditions affecting children under 12 years of age.

ADVERSE REACTIONS
Moderate overdosage: nausea, vomiting, abdominal pain, chilliness. **Acute poisoning:** dizziness, weakness, numbness of extremities, nausea, vomiting, abdominal pain, profuse perspiration, palpitation, CNS stimulation (excitement, delirium, toxic psychosis, convulsions) followed by CNS depression, hypothermia, shock, stupor, coma. **With prolonged excessive dosage:** neutropenia, leukopenia, thrombocytopenia, pancytopenia, agranulocytosis (uncommon); methemoglobinemia:(cyanosis of skin, mucosa, fingernails; dyspnea, headache, vertigo, weakness, anginal pain, circulatory failure); sulfhemoglobinemia, GI disturbances, psychologic changes, occult bleeding (rare), hemolytic anemia (uncommon); renal and liver damage, hypoglycemic coma, cerebral edema, myocardial depression. **Hypersensitivity reactions** (laryngeal edema, mucosal lesions, erythematous or urticarial skin rash, angioneurotic edema, fever).

Oral, rectal suppository: **Adults:** 325 to 650 mg 3 or 4 times daily, if necessary; total daily dosage not to exceed 2.6 Gm. **Children** (*7 to 12 years*): 162.5 to 325 mg 3 or 4 times daily, not to exceed 1.3 Gm in 24 hours; (*3 to 6 years*): 120 mg 3 or 4 times daily, not to exceed 480 mg in 24 hours.

NURSING IMPLICATIONS

Acetaminophen is intended for temporary use only. Commercial preparations must include label warning to consult a physician for use in children under 6 years of age or for use for longer than 10 days.

Acetaminophen is a common ingredient of several OTC headache and analgesic mixtures, eg, Capron (which also contains phenacetin), Bromo Seltzer, Comeback, Contramal, Dolor, Excedrin, Medache, S-A-C, Trigesic, Vanquish.

Caution patient not to exceed recommended dosage, and point out the dangers of indiscriminate use of analgesics without medical supervision.

Most poisonings result from suicide attempts or accidental ingestion by children. Caution patient to keep drug out of reach of children.

Treatment of acute toxicity: copious gastric lavage if drug was recently ingested; activated charcoal reportedly reduces drug absorption if administered promptly. Magnesium or sodium sulfate solution instilled into stomach after lavage. Transfusion may be required.

Patient who has ingested a toxic dose should be hospitalized, because severe hepatic damage is sometimes not apparent until several days after overdosage.

Preserved in tightly covered, light-resistant containers.

LABORATORY TEST INTERFERENCES: Acetaminophen may cause false increases in urinary 5-hydroxyindoleacetic acid (5-HIAA) determinations.

DRUG INTERACTIONS: Produces slight increase (if any) in hypoprothrombinemic response to **oral anticoagulants.**

ACETAZOLAMIDE, U.S.P., B.P.
(ACETAZIDE, DIAMOX, HYDRAZOL)
ACETAZOLAMIDE, SODIUM, U.S.P.
(DIAMOX PARENTERAL SOLUTION)

Diuretic, carbonic anhydrase inhibitor, anticonvulsant

ACTIONS AND USES

Nonbacteriostatic sulfonamide derivative. Normally the enzyme carbonic anhydrase produces free hydrogen ions by facilitating intracellular hydration of CO_2 to form H^+ and HCO_3^-. H^+ exchanges with filtrate Na^+ and its counter ion HCO_3^-. Carbonic anhydrase inhibition reduces available H^+, thereby depressing Na^+ and HCO_3^- conservation mechanisms. The urine becomes alkaline, K^+ output is increased, ammonia excretion decreases, and Cl^- conservation is enhanced. After 3 or 4 days of continuous inhibition, mild metabolic acidosis may develop, with concomitant decrease in diuresis. Depresses formation of aqueous humor thereby lowering intraocular pressure; also has an anticonvulsant effect.

Used in adjunctive treatment of edema, congestive heart failure, and selected cases of petit mal epilepsy; used to reduce intracranial pressure, for relief of migraine, for chronic simple glaucoma, and preoperatively for acute angle closure glaucoma. Given occasionally in preparation for mercurial diuretics to potentiate or reinstitute their effects or to counteract the metabolic alkalosis they produce.

ABSORPTION AND FATE

Rapidly absorbed from GI tract with beginning effects in 30 minutes. Peak plasma levels are reached within 2 to 4 hours, persisting 8 to 12 hours. Sustained-release form peaks in 8 to 12 hours with duration of 18 to 24 hours. Wide distribution, with especially high concentrations in erythrocytes, pancreas, gastric mucosa, and renal cortex. About 80% of dose is excreted unchanged within 24 hours. Crosses placenta.

CONTRAINDICATIONS AND PRECAUTIONS

Sensitivity to sulfonamides; chronic pulmonary disease; renal and liver dysfunction; Addison's disease or other types of adrenocortical insufficiency; hyponatremia; hypokalemia; hyperchloremic acidosis; prolonged administration to patients with chronic noncongestive angle closure glaucoma; pregnancy. Cautious use: history of hypercalciuria, diabetes mellitus, gout.

ADVERSE REACTIONS

Mild paresthesias of face and extremities (common), fatigue, anorexia, nausea, vomiting, diarrhea, constipation, weight loss, thirst, altered taste and smell, dizziness, excitement, drowsiness, disorientation, hypokalemia, hyperchloremic acidosis, polyuria. Occasionally: hirsutism, increase or decrease in uric acid excretion, exacerbation of gout, melena, transient myopia, glycosuria, hyperglycemia, hyperuricemia, flaccid paralysis, convulsions. In common with other sulfonamides: fever, allergic manifestations, hematuria, crystalluria, hepatic dysfunction, blood dyscrasias (agranulocytosis, thrombocytopenia, hemolytic anemia, leukopenia).

ROUTE AND DOSAGE

Oral, intramuscular, intravenous: **Adults:** 250 mg to 1 Gm daily; dosage and frequency depend on condition being treated. The sodium salt for parenteral administration should be reconstituted with at least 5 ml sterile water for injection prior to use. **Pediatric** (diuretic): 5 mg/kg/24 hours. Epilepsy, glaucoma: 8 to 30 mg/kg/24 hours divided into 3 or 4 doses.

NURSING IMPLICATIONS

If necessary, regular tablet (not sustained-release form) may be softened in hot water and added to 2 teaspoonfuls of honey or syrup to disguise bitter taste. Not stable in fruit juices.

Highly alkaline pH (approximately 9.2) of the parenteral solution causes intense pain when injected intramuscularly; therefore this route is not commonly employed.

When given for diuresis, drug is generally given in the morning to avoid interference with sleep as a result of diuretic action.

Monitor intake and output for patients receiving the drug for diuresis. Failure of diuretic action may be caused by overdosage or too frequent dosing. Effectiveness as a diuretic diminishes with continuous use; therefore it is usually given on alternate days, or for 2 days followed by a day without medication.

Patient should be weighed under standard conditions before drug therapy is initiated and daily thereafter: use same scale, with same clothing, preferably in morning after voiding but before eating or defecating. Daily weight is a useful index of patient's response to diuretic action.

Advise patient to report paresthesias and drowsiness (common side effects). Note implications for ambulatory patient.

It is reported that acetazolamide may cause substantial increases in blood glucose in prediabetics and in diabetics taking insulin or oral hypoglycemic agents. Observe these patients closely for changes in antidiabetic diet or drug requirements.

Hypokalemia and severe metabolic acidosis are direct extensions of the pharmacologic actions of acetazolamide. Observe for and advise patient to report signs of hypokalemia (muscle weakness, respiratory distress, cardiac irregularities) and signs of metabolic acidosis (malaise, headache, weakness, nausea, vomiting, abdominal pain hyperpnea, dehydration).

When acetazolamide is given for diuresis, physician may order potassium supplement and potassium-rich diet (see Index).

Periodic complete blood cell counts and serum electrolyte determinations are recommended during prolonged drug therapy or during concomitant therapy with other diuretics or digitalis.

Since parenteral solution contains no preservative, its use within 24 hours of reconstitution is strongly recommended.

Stock suspensions in syrup are stable for about 1 week. Note expiration date.

Oral preparations are preserved in tightly covered, light-resistant containers.

LABORATORY TEST INTERFERENCES: False positive urinary protein determinations; falsely high values for urine urobilinogen.

DRUG INTERACTIONS: By tending to render urine alkaline, acetazolamide (and other carbonic anhydrase inhibitors) may enhance the effects of **amphetamines, procainamide, quinidine,** and **tricyclic antidepressants** by increasing their renal tubular reabsorption, and may decrease the effects of **lithium, methenamine compounds, phenobarbital,** and **salicylates** by increasing their renal excretion. Acetazolamide augments the effects of other **diuretics,** may alter response to **chlorthalidone,** and may accentuate osteomalacia induced by **phenytoin** and related drugs. Hypokalemia induced by acetazolamide may predispose patients receiving **digitalis glycosides** to digitalis toxicity, and may cause severe hypokalemia in patients receiving **amphotericin B, corticosteroids, corticosporin,** and may interfere with hypoglycemic response to **insulin** and **oral hypoglycemic agents.**

ACETOHEXAMIDE, U.S.P.
(DYMELOR)

Antidiabetic, oral hypoglycemic (Sulfonylurea)

ACTIONS AND USES

Intermediate-acting sulfonylurea that promotes increased effectiveness of endogenous insulin. Has longer action than tolbutamide (qv), but uses, precautions, and adverse reactions are similar. Also has moderate uricosuric effect, probably due to its primary metabolite, L-hydroxyhexamide.

ABSORPTION AND FATE

Rapidly absorbed from GI tract. Maximal hypoglycemic activity in 3 hours. Metabolic half-life 6 to 8 hours; duration of action 12 to 14 hours. Presumably metabolized in liver. More than 50% excreted (largely as active metabolite) in urine within 24 hours. Approximately 15% eliminated in bile.

CONTRAINDICATIONS AND PRECAUTIONS

Safe use in pregnancy or in women of childbearing age not established. Also see Tolbutamide.

Oral: 250 mg to 1.5 Gm daily. Doses higher than 1 Gm generally divided and administered before morning and evening meals. Doses in excess of 1.5 Gm not recommended.

NURSING IMPLICATIONS
Prolonged hypoglycemia may be produced in patients with any degree of renal insufficiency.
The elderly may require dosage adjustments.
See Tolbutamide.

ACETOSULFONE SODIUM
(PROMACETIN)

Antibacterial (leprostatic)

ACTIONS AND USES
Sulfone derivative similar to dapsone in actions, uses, contraindications, precautions, and adverse reactions.
ABSORPTION AND FATE
Approximately 25% absorbed from GI tract. Large portions of dose excreted in feces; some excretion in sweat, saliva, sputum, tears, and breast milk.
ROUTE AND DOSAGE
Oral: 0.5 Gm for first 2 weeks, increased by increments of 0.5 to 1.5 Gm every 2 weeks until maximum of 3 to 4 Gm daily is reached. Various dosage schedules.

NURSING IMPLICATIONS
Administer with meals to reduce incidence of gastric distress.
Treatment schedules for leprosy may be interrupted every 4 months with rest periods of 10 to 15 days.
Preserved in tightly covered, light-resistant containers.
See Dapsone.

ACETYLCHOLINE CHLORIDE
(MIOCHOL)

Miotic (cholinergic)

ACTIONS AND USES
Quaternary ammonium compound. Acts directly on postjunctional effector cells of eye; produces intense miosis by stimulating contraction of iris sphincter muscles. Contraindications to use not reported.
Used to obtain rapid and complete miosis after delivery of lens in cataract surgery, and in penetrating keratoplasty, iridectomy, and other anterior segment surgery.
ABSORPTION AND FATE
Rapidly hydrolyzed by acetylcholinesterase to choline and acetic acid. Miosis may be maintained for about 1 hour.
ADVERSE REACTIONS
With systematic absorption: hypotension, bradycardia, bronchospasm.

Intraocular instillation (1% solution): 0.5 to 2 ml (instilled gently, parallel to iris face and tangential to pupil border).

NURSING IMPLICATIONS

Immediately before use, dust cap and label should be peeled off and whole vial immersed in 70% ethanol or other sterilizing solution for 30 minutes or more. Steam or gas (eg, ethylene oxide) sterilization should not be used.

Using aseptic technique, rubber stopper is pressed down sufficiently to dislodge center rubber plug seal, thus releasing solvent (sterile water) from upper chamber. Vial should be shaken gently to dissolve and mix drug in lower chamber. (If stopper does not go down or is down, do not use vial.) Solution is drawn into dry sterile syringe with sterile new 18- to 20-gauge needle. Needle is replaced with suitable atraumatic cannula for intraocular instillation by physician.

Since solution is unstable, it should be prepared immediately before use. Discard unused portion.

Pilocarpine 2% or physostigmine 0.25% may be prescribed topically before dressing to maintain miosis.

ACETYLCYSTEINE
(MUCOMYST)

Mucolytic

ACTIONS AND USES

Derivative of the naturally occurring amino acid L-cysteine. Probably acts by disrupting disulfide linkages of mucoproteins in purulent and nonpurulent secretions, thereby lowering viscosity.

Used as adjuvant therapy in patients with abnormal, viscid, or inspissated mucous secretions in acute and chronic bronchopulmonary diseases, and in pulmonary complications of cystic fibrosis and surgery, tracheostomy, and atelectasis; used in diagnostic bronchial studies.

ABSORPTION AND FATE

Liquefaction of mucus occurs within 1 minute; maximum effects occur in 5 to 10 minutes. Most of drug appears to participate in sulfhydryl–disulfide reaction; remainder is absorbed from epithelium, deacetylated by liver to cysteine, and subsequently metabolized.

CONTRAINDICATIONS AND PRECAUTIONS

Hypersensitivity to acetylcysteine. Used with caution in patients with asthma, in the elderly, and in debilitated patients with severe respiratory insufficiency.

ADVERSE REACTIONS

Bronchospasm, nausea, rhinorrhea, burning sensation in upper passages, stomatitis, hemoptysis, fever and chills; sensitivity and sensitization (rarely).

ROUTE AND DOSAGE

Inhalation by nebulization into face mask, mouthpiece, or tracheostomy: 3 to 5 ml of 20% solution, or 6 to 10 ml of 10% solution 3 or 4 times daily. Nebulization into closed tent or croupette (10% or 20% solution). Use volume that will maintain a heavy mist for desired treatment period. Highly individualized according to equipment used. Direct instillation into tracheostomy: 1 to 2 ml of 10% or 20% solution every 1 to 4 hours. The 20% solution may be diluted to lesser concentration with either sterile normal saline or sterile water for injection.

NURSING IMPLICATIONS

Do not mix acetylcysteine with other drugs unless specifically directed to do so by physician or pharmacist.

Solutions of acetylcysteine release hydrogen sulfide and become discolored on contact with rubber and some metals (particularly iron and copper). When administering by nebulization, it is recommended that equipment made of plastic, glass, stainless steel, aluminum, chromed metal, tantalum, or other nonreactive metals be used.

Following drug administration, increased volume of respiratory tract fluid may be liberated. If patient cannot cough adequately, suction or endotracheal aspiration may be necessary to establish and maintain an open airway.

Bronchospasm is a reported side effect; it is most likely to occur in patients with asthma. If it appears, drug should be discontinued immediately; if necessary, a sympathomimetic agent (prescribed by physician) should be administered by nebulization.

When drug is administered by nebulization, compressed air should be used to provide pressure.

For maximum effect, patient should be instructed to clear his airway by coughing productively prior to aerosol administration.

With prolonged nebulization, solution may become more concentrated and impede drug delivery; therefore, after three-quarters of initial volume has been nebulized, it is recommended that the remainder be diluted with an approximately equal volume of sterile water for injection.

Intermittent aerosol treatments are commonly prescribed when patient arises, before meals, and prior to retiring at night.

Unpleasant odor of the drug (rotten-egg odor of hydrogen sulfide) and excess volume of liquefied bronchial secretions may cause nausea and possibly vomiting, particularly when face mask is used. Have suction equipment immediately available. Advise patient that the odor becomes less noticeable with continued inhalation.

Following nebulization with face mask, wash face and mask with water. The drug leaves a sticky coating.

Generally, hand bulb nebulizers are not recommended because output is too small and particle size too large.

Acetylcysteine should not be placed into the chamber of a heated (hot pot) nebulizer.

Following exposure to air, acetylcysteine solutions should be stored in refrigerator to retard oxidation; they should be used within 96 hours. Appearance of a light purple color apparently does not significantly impair its mucolytic effectiveness.

Collaborate with physician and respiratory therapist in constructing rehabilitation plan for the patient with chronic pulmonary insufficiency. Important points that should be considered include: prevention of respiratory infection; adequate hydration; maintenance of airway (eg, aerosol therapy, postural drainage, breathing exercises); improvement in ambulation through graded walking exercises and physical conditioning exercises; planned medical follow-up; occupational retraining and placement; family counseling.

(ACYLANID)

Cardiotonic, cardiac glycoside

ACTIONS AND USES
Intermediate-acting digitalis glycoside, acetyl derivative of digitoxin, prepared by enzymatic hydrolysis of lanatoside A, a glycoside of *Digitalis lanata.* Has same actions, uses, contraindications, and adverse reactions as digitalis leaf powdered (qv).

ABSORPTION AND FATE
Approximately 66% absorbed from GI tract. Onset of effects in 2 to 6 hours; peak effects in 8 to 10 hours. Action may persist 7 to 12 days. About 10% of dose excreted in urine daily as metabolites.

ROUTE AND DOSAGE
Oral (rapid digitalization): 1.6 to 2.2 mg in divided doses within 24 hours, or up to 2 mg as single dose; (slow digitalization): 1.8 to 3.2 mg over 2- to 6-day period. Maintenance: 0.1 to 0.2 mg daily.

NURSING IMPLICATIONS
During digitalization period, before administering drug check laboratory reports (know what physician regards as acceptable parameters for serum levels of potassium, magnesium, calcium). Take apical pulse for 1 full minute, noting rate, rhythm, and quality; check for signs and symptoms of acetyldigitoxin toxicity.

Preserved in tightly covered, light-resistant containers.

See Digitalis Leaf, Powdered.

ACRISORCIN, N.F.
(AKRINOL, Aminacrine Hexylresorcinate)

Fungicide

ACTIONS AND USES
Bactericidal and fungicidal agent used topically in treatment of tinea versicolor (pityriasis versicolor). Prepared from 9-aminoacridine and hexylresorcinal.

ADVERSE REACTIONS
Low order of toxicity. Blisters, erythematous vesicular eruptions, pruritus, urticaria, burning sensation, worsening of tinea versicolor.

ROUTE AND DOSAGE
Topical cream (2 mg/Gm): small quantity rubbed gently into affected areas twice daily, morning and night.

NURSING IMPLICATIONS
Night application should be preceded by a warm soapy bath, and a stiff brush should be used on lesions. Soap reduces drug effectiveness; therefore it must be completely rinsed off and skin thoroughly dried before applying the cream. Pay particular attention to friction areas.

Do not use acrisorcin near the eyes.

To avoid reinfection, towels and clothing that contact skin should be laundered after each use.

Caution patient that exposure to ultraviolet light may cause pruritus. Treatment should be discontinued if signs of irritation or sensitization occur.

Acrisorcin therapy should be continued for at least 6 weeks, even if improvement or clearing of lesions occurs. Sometimes a second or third course of therapy is required.

Since there is no reliable technique for culturing the causative organism of tinea versicolor *(Malassezia furfur)*, diagnosis and therapeutic response are determined by clinical appearance, by lesion scrapings, and by Wood's light examination of lesions.

Store drug away from heat.

ADENOSINE PHOSPHATE
(Adenosine 5-Monophosphate, A5MP, CARDIOMONE, Muscle Adenylic Acid, MY-B-DEN)

Unclassified

ACTIONS AND USES

Natural nucleotide constituent of muscle tissue essential for formation of coenzymes involved in energy transfer mechanisms, biologic oxidation, and metabolism of carbohydrates and fats. Therapeutic effect may be due in part to vasodilating action and ability to reduce tissue inflammation and edema.

Used as adjunctive therapy in treatment of stasis dermatitis, varicose ulcers, and chronic thrombophlebitis and in symptomatic treatment of acute and chronic bursitis, tendinitis, and tenosynovitis nonresponsive to other measures.

CONTRAINDICATIONS AND PRECAUTIONS

History of myocardial infarction; cerebral hemorrhage. Cautious use: patients with history of allergy.

ADVERSE REACTIONS

Epigastric discomfort, nausea, generalized flushing, dizziness, headache, diuresis, palpitation, hypotension, anaphylactoid reaction (reported following injection of sustained-action preparation): feeling of chest tightness, difficulty in breathing. Occasionally, local rash, increase in symptoms of bursitis and tendinitis, local erythema of IM site.

ROUTE AND DOSAGE

Oral (sublingual tablet): 20 to 100 mg daily. Intramuscular: not to exceed 100 mg daily. Highly individualized.

NURSING IMPLICATIONS

Patients taking the sublingual tablet should be advised to place the tablet in the buccal pouch and not to mix it with saliva, food, or liquid.

Drug should be discontinued if dyspnea or tightness in chest occurs.

Note that adenosine for intramuscular injection is available as a sodium solution and also in a repository gelatin vehicle providing sustained release.

Sustained-action preparation is administered preferably into gluteal muscle. A 20- to 22-gauge needle 1 to 1½ inches in length is recommended.

ADIPHENINE HYDROCHLORIDE
(TRASENTINE)

Antispasmodic

ACTIONS AND USES

Synthetic tertiary derivative of belladonna. Direct action on smooth muscle produces papaverinelike spasmolytic action. Also has parasympatholytic actions similar to those of atropine (qv), but reportedly lacks undesirable side effects on salivary, sweat, or GI glands, eyes, or cardiovascular system, except in large doses. Chemically related to local anesthetics, and has local anesthetic activity. Used alone or with phenobarbital in treatment of alimentary, urinary, and biliary tract spasms, side effects of radiation, and dysmenorrhea.

CONTRAINDICATIONS AND PRECAUTIONS

As for anticholinergic drugs, contraindicated in glaucoma, cardiovascular disease, pyloric obstruction, small-bowel ileus, bladder neck obstruction, prostatic hypertrophy. Safe use in pregnancy and lactation not established.

ADVERSE REACTIONS

See Atropine Sulfate.

ROUTE AND DOSAGE

Oral: 75 to 150 mg 3 times daily, 20 to 30 minutes before meals.

NURSING IMPLICATIONS

Inform patient that adiphenine should be swallowed without chewing, because of local anesthetic action.

See Atropine Sulfate.

ALBUMIN, NORMAL HUMAN SERUM, U.S.P.

(ALBUMINAR, ALBUMISOL, ALBUSPAN, ALBUTEIN, BUMINATE, PRO-BUMIN, PROSERUM)

Blood volume supporter

ACTIONS AND USES

Obtained by fractionating human blood; treated by heating to minimize risk of transmitting hepatitis B virus. Exerts approximately 80% of effective osmotic pressure of blood. Supplied in two strengths: 5% (approximately isotonic and isoosmotic with normal human plasma) and 25% (salt-poor solution), each 50 ml of which is osmotically equivalent to about 250 ml citrated plasma.

Used as blood volume expander in treatment of hypovolemic shock; used to reduce cerebral edema due to neurosurgery or anoxia. Also used in toxemia of pregnancy that fails to respond to diuretics, as adjunct in hyperbilirubinemia associated with erythroblastosis fetalis, and in treatment of hypoproteinemia, hepatic cirrhosis, and nephrosis.

ABSORPTION AND FATE

Excreted slowly by kidneys because of its high molecular weight. Effects may persist for several days.

CONTRAINDICATIONS AND PRECAUTIONS

Severe anemia, cardiac failure. Cautious use: patients with low cardiac reserve; those without albumin deficiency, patients with hepatic or renal failure or dehydration.

ADVERSE REACTIONS

Fever, chills, urticaria, rash, circulatory overload, pulmonary edema (with rapid infusion); dyspnea, change in blood pressure, pulse, respiration; nausea, vomiting, increased salivation.

ROUTE AND DOSAGE

Intravenous: volume equivalent to 25 to 75 Gm daily. Variable, depending on hemoglobin, hematocrit, and amount of pulmonary and venous congestion. No more than 250 Gm in 48 hours advised.

NURSING IMPLICATIONS

Albumin, a yellow or amber, clear, moderately viscous liquid, is supplied in two strengths: 5% and 25%.

Check expiration date on label. Solutions that show sediment or that appear turbid should not be used.

Once bottle is opened, solution should be used promptly; it contains no preservatives. Discard unused portion.

Rate of infusion will depend on patient's age, diagnosis, and general condition and on concentration of solution. Specific flow rate should be ordered by physician.

As with any oncotically active solution, infusion rate should be relatively slow. The 5% concentration is usually administered no faster than 2 to 4 ml per minute, and the 25% concentration no faster than 1 ml per minute.

Monitor blood pressure, pulse, and respiration. Frequency of readings will depend on patient's condition. Flow rate adjustments may be required to avoid too rapid a rise in blood pressure.

Observe patient closely during infusion for signs of circulatory overload (distended neck veins, pulmonary edema, shortness of breath, persistent cough, increased heart rate, sense of chest pressure). If these signs and symptoms appear, slow the infusion rate just sufficiently to keep vein open, and report immediately to physician.

Hemoglobin, hematocrit, serum protein, and electrolytes should be monitored during therapy.

Make careful observations of patients with injuries or those who have had surgery, in order to detect bleeding points that failed to bleed at lower blood pressure.

Monitor intake–output ratio and pattern. Report changes in urinary output. Osmotic effects of albumin cause mobilization of extracellular fluid and diuresis, which may persist 3 to 20 hours.

When albumin is given to patients with cerebral edema, fluids are generally withheld completely during succeeding 8 hours. Meticulous mouth care is indicated.

Serum hepatitis and interferences with blood typing or crossmatching procedures have not been reported.

Intact containers may be stored at room temperature, but not exceeding 37 C (98.6 F).

LABORATORY TEST INTERFERENCES: False rise in alkaline phosphatase levels from albumin obtained partially from pooled placental plasma (levels reportedly decline over period of 1 week).

ALLOPURINOL, U.S.P., B.P.
(ZYLOPRIM)

Antihyperuricemic, Xanthine oxidase inhibitor

ACTIONS AND USES

Selectively inhibits action of xanthine oxidase, an essential enzyme responsible for synthesis of uric acid (end product of protein metabolism). Lowers both plasma and urinary uric acid levels by inhibiting terminal step in conversion of purine ribonucleotides to uric acid; thus urate pool is decreased, resorption of tophaceous deposits begins, and hyperuricosuria is prevented. Also may inhibit hepatic microsomal enzymes. Has no analgesic, antiinflammatory, or uricosuric actions.

Used to control hyperuricemia that accompanies severe tophaceous gout and advanced renal failure. Also used prophylactically as adjunct to cytotoxic antineoplastic and radiation therapies, both of which greatly increase plasma uric acid levels by promoting nucleic acid degradation.

Approximately 80% of oral dose is absorbed. Appears in plasma in 30 to 60 minutes; peak plasma levels achieved in 2 to 6 hours. Distributed to all extracellular fluid, with exception of brain. Rapidly cleared from plasma (probable half-life less than 2 hours); small portion excreted unchanged in urine; remainder rapidly oxidized to oxypurinol (alloxanthine), which inhibits xanthine oxidase (half-life 18 to 30 hours). The metabolite is excreted slowly; therefore it may accumulate with chronic administration of allopurinol.

CONTRAINDICATIONS AND PRECAUTIONS

Hypersensitivity to allopurinol; idiopathic hemochromatosis (or those with family history), pregnant women or women of childbearing potential, nursing mothers, children (except those with hyperuricemia secondary to neoplastic disease). Cautious use: liver disease, impaired renal function.

ADVERSE REACTIONS

Idiosyncratic reaction (fever, chills, leukopenia, eosinophilia, arthralgia), pruritic maculopapular rash, exfoliative urticarial and purpural dermatitis, Stevens-Johnson syndrome, fever, acute gouty attacks, alopecia, nausea, vomiting, anorexia, diarrhea, abdominal pain, vertigo, drowsiness. Also reported: peripheral neuritis, xanthine calculi (especially in children with Lesch-Nyhan syndrome), headache, tachycardia, peptic ulceration, retinopathy, cataracts, lymphedema, adrenal insufficiency, hepatitis, jaundice, blood dyscrasias, hyperlipemia; hypersensitivity vasculitis or necrotizing angiitis (rare).

ROUTE AND DOSAGE

Oral: **Adults:** 200 to 600 mg daily. Administered twice a day if total dose is more than 300 mg. Maximum dosage 800 mg/day. **Pediatric** *6 to 10 years:* 100 mg 3 times daily; *under 6 years:* 50 mg 3 times daily. Highly individualized.

NURSING IMPLICATIONS

Generally the drug is best tolerated when taken with or immediately after meals.

Patient should be thoroughly informed about signs and symptoms to be reported. A skin rash, which may appear within 1 to 5 weeks of therapy, is the most common adverse reaction; it indicates the necessity of stopping drug therapy. The rash has been reported to appear as late as 2 years after therapy is initiated.

Aim of therapy is to lower serum urate level to about 6 mg/100 ml.

Periodic complete blood counts and liver and kidney function tests should be performed before initiating therapy, and particularly during first few months of therapy. Patients with impaired renal or hepatic function must be closely monitored.

Acute gouty attacks are most likely to occur during first 6 weeks of allopurinol therapy, possibly because of mobilization of urates from tissue deposits. Concomitant maintenance therapy with colchicine may be prescribed as prophylaxis.

Allopurinol may cause drowsiness; therefore the patient should be cautioned to avoid driving or performing other complex tasks until his reaction to the drug has been evaluated.

It is advisable to maintain fluid intake sufficient to produce urinary output of at least 2000 ml daily and to keep urine neutral or slightly alkaline. These measures are prescribed by physician.

Intake–output ratio should be monitored. Since allopurinol and metabolites are excreted only by kidneys, decreased renal function causes drug accumulation. Report diminishing volume of urinary output.

A low purine diet is not usually prescribed, but physician may advise patient to omit organ meats (eg kidney, liver) from diet and also to control or lose weight.

Therapeutic response to allopurinol is indicated by normal serum uric acid levels (usually by 7 to 10 days), gradual decrease in size of tophi, absence of new tophaceous deposits (after approximately 6 months), and relief of joint pain with increased joint mobility.

DRUG INTERACTIONS: **Ampicillin** may increase incidence of skin rash. **Probenecid** appears to reduce effect of allopurinol by enhancing renal elimination of its active metabolite. Allopurinol may increase toxicity of **azathioprine** and **mercaptomerin** unless usual dosages of these drugs are reduced 25 to 33%. Half-life of **oral anticoagulants** may be prolonged by allopurinol, possibly necessitating decrease in anticoagulant dosage. Preliminary evidence indicates that allopurinol may increase frequency of **cyclophosphamide** bone marrow depression. Manufacturer states that **iron salts** should not be given simultaneously with allopurinol (increase in hepatic iron concentration reported in animal studies). Allopurinol may enhance effect of **sulfonylurea, oral hypoglycemics. Thiazides** and other potent diuretics may increase allopurinol toxicity.

ALPHAPRODINE HYDROCHLORIDE, N.F.
(NISENTIL)

Narcotic analgesic

ACTIONS AND USES
Phenylpiperidine derivative chemically and pharmacologically similar to meperidine (qv), but with greater analgesic activity, more rapid onset of action, and shorter duration of effects.
Used for preoperative sedation, for analgesia in minor surgery, obstetrics, and diagnostic and therapeutic procedures, for relief of moderate to severe acute pains such as cardiovascular pain, and pain of renal or biliary colic.
ABSORPTION AND FATE
Following subcutaneous administration, onset of action is 5 to 10 minutes, with duration of about 2 hours. Following intravenous administration, onset of action is 1 to 2 minutes, with duration of about 30 to 60 minutes. Rapidly excreted in urine. Crosses placenta.
CONTRAINDICATIONS AND PRECAUTIONS
Hypersensitivity to the drug, chronic pain, pregnancy (except labor), final stages of labor, respiratory depression, convulsive disorders, severe CNS depression, increased intracranial pressure, myxedema, acute alcoholism, delirium tremens, hepatic insufficiency, and Addison's disease, as well as in the very elderly and the debilitated. Dosage for children under 12 years of age not established.
ADVERSE REACTIONS
Dizziness, drowsiness, sweating, urticaria, palpitation, syncope, nausea, vomiting, restlessness, confusion. Overdosage: respiratory depression, cyanosis, hypotension, pinpoint pupils, coma. Also see Meperidine.
ROUTE AND DOSAGE
Subcutaneous: 0.4 to 1.2 mg/kg. Intravenous: 0.4 to 0.6 mg/kg administered slowly. Total dose by either route should not exceed 240 mg in 24 hours.

NURSING IMPLICATIONS
Alphaprodine is reportable as a Schedule II narcotic under provisions of the federal Controlled Substances Act. Tolerance and addiction are possible with prolonged use.
Check the time last dose was given and whether physician's order is still in

effect. When used for obstetric analgesia, alphaprodine is given after cervix begins to dilate. Not given during later stages of labor, in order to avoid depression of fetal respiration.

Have readily available a narcotic antagonist (eg, levallorphan, naloxone) and resuscitation equipment when drug is administered intravenously. Possibility of respiratory depression is especially high with this route of administration.

Alphaprodine is not used for relief of chronic pain because its short duration of action would require giving it too frequently.

Chart patient's response to the drug. Evaluate continued need for this medication and suggest to physician a change to a milder analgesic when indicated.

See Meperidine Hydrochloride.

ALUMINUM ACETATE SOLUTION, U.S.P.
(ACID MANTLE, BLUBORO, BURO-SOL, BUROWETS, BUROW'S SOLUTION, DOMEBORO)

Topical astringent

ACTIONS AND USES
Mild antiseptic containing aluminum subacetate and glacial acetic acid (U.S.P.). Modified Burow's solution contains aluminum sulfate and calcium acetate.

Has antiinflammatory, antipruritic, and astringent properties, and reportedly maintains protective acidity of skin.

Used in treatment of mildly irritated or inflamed skin and mucous membranes, such as diaper rash, insect bites, poison ivy, athlete's foot, anal pruritus. Also used as astringent gargle and as irrigating solution to remove debris.

ROUTE AND DOSAGE
Topical (wet dressings) 1:10 to 1:40 solution. Astringent gargle 1:10 solution. Ointment, lotion, and cream preparations available.

NURSING IMPLICATIONS
Buro-Sol powder: 1 packet or 1 teaspoonful in 1 pint of water produces 1:15 clear Burow's solution. Domeboro or Bluboro: 1 or 2 packets in 1 pint of water produce a modified Burow's solution.

For wet dressings, solution is carefully poured on bandage every 15 to 30 minutes and continued for 4 to 8 hours. Do not cover with plastic or other occlusive material.

Keep away from eyes.

Use should be discontinued if irritation or extension of inflammatory condition appears.

The lotion must be shaken vigorously before use.

Store drug in cool place, but do not freeze.

Antacid

ACTIONS AND USES
   Has same actions, uses, contraindications, and adverse reactions as aluminum
   hydroxide gel. Appears to demonstrate greatest phosphate-binding capacity of
   all the aluminum-containing antacids. Lowers serum phosphate by binding
   dietary and gastrointestinal phosphates; thus elimination of phosphate is increased in feces and decreased in urine. In addition to use as antacid, also used
   for prophylaxis and treatment of phosphatic renal calculi and in treatment of
   hyperphosphatemia in patients with chronic renal failure.
ROUTE AND DOSAGE
   Oral (antacid): 5 to 10 ml of regular suspension, or 2 to 5 ml of extra strength
   suspension, or 1 or 2 capsules or tablets, between meals and at bedtime. For
   phosphate lowering: 10 to 30 ml of suspension or 5 to 15 ml of extra strength
   suspension, or 2 to 6 capsules or tablets, after meals and at bedtime.

NURSING IMPLICATIONS
   Shake liquid well before pouring. Tablets should be dissolved or thoroughly
      chewed for maximum effectiveness.
   Antacid dose is generally given between meals and at bedtime. For preven-
      tion of phosphate stones, mix dose in water or fruit juice; usually given
      1 hour after meals and at bedtime.
   If used to control urinary calculi, measure and record intake and output, and
      strain all urine through gauze. Since calculi may traumatize tissue, be on
      the alert for evidence of infection: fever, chills, dysuria, and hematuria.
   Physician will prescribe a high fluid intake for the patient with urinary
      calculi. The amount prescribed is highly variable. Some sources suggest
      10 or more glasses of fluid daily; some recommend daily intake in excess
      of 3000 ml; others advise sufficient liquids to produce a daily urinary
      output of 2000 to 3000 ml or more.
   Some physicians prescribe modified acid-ash diet to lower urinary pH and
      thus discourage phosphate stone formation. High-alkaline sources that
      may be restricted: milk and milk products, carbonated beverages, fruits,
      and juices (exception: cranberries, plums, and prunes are high in acid ash).
      Ascorbic acid has also been utilized as a urinary acidifier. Collaborate with
      physician and dietitian.
   Since aluminum carbonate adsorbs phosphates, excessive doses for pro-
      longed periods can lead to phosphate depletion (weakness, anorexia, mal-
      aise, bone pain, tremors, demineralization of bone, negative calcium bal-
      ance).
   Periodic determinations should be made of urinary pH and serum calcium,
      phosphates, and other electrolytes.
   Immobilization enhances urinary stasis and development of urinary calculi.
      If allowed, ambulation should be encouraged, as well as regularly sched-
      uled passive and active exercises.
   Aluminum carbonate contains approximately 5% aluminum hydroxide and
      2.4% carbon dioxide. On exposure to air, carbon dioxide is lost; therefore,
      keep container tightly covered.
   See Aluminum Hydroxide Gel for management of peptic ulcer.

(ALU-CAP, ALU-TAB, AMPHOJEL, DIALUME, NO-CO-GEL,
NUTRAJEL)

Antacid

ACTIONS AND USES
Nonsystemic antacid with ability to neutralize or reduce acidity of gastric contents without producing acid rebound. Also has some adsorbent and mild astringent properties. Forms coating on mucosa, thereby protecting it from irritating effects of hydrochloric acid. Has phosphate-binding capacity, but not as
great as that of aluminum carbonate. Some preparations contain a significant
amount of sodium.
Used for symptomatic relief of gastric hyperacidity associated with gastritis,
esophageal reflux, or hiatus hernia; used as adjunct in treatment of peptic ulcer.
ABSORPTION AND FATE
Normally not absorbed from GI tract. Gastric emptying time limits its effects
to 30 to 60 minutes. Excreted in feces, primarily as insoluble phosphates.
CONTRAINDICATIONS AND PRECAUTIONS
Sensitivity to aluminum; prolonged use of high doses in presence of low serum
phosphate; patients on low sodium diet. Cautious use: renal impairment, gastric
outlet obstruction.
ADVERSE REACTIONS
Constipation, obstipation, nausea, vomiting, intestinal obstruction, phosphate
deficiency syndrome (malaise, anorexia, generalized weakness, tremors, absent
deep tendon reflexes, mental depression, bone pain, negative Ca^{++} balance,
osteomalacia, fracture).
ROUTE AND DOSAGE
Oral (antacid): 5 to 10 ml of suspension or 1 or 2 tablets or capsules 5 or 6 times
daily, between meals and at bedtime (highly individualized). (Phosphate lowering): 40 ml after meals and at bedtime.

NURSING IMPLICATIONS
Shake liquid well before pouring.
If administered in tablet form, instruct the patient to chew the tablet until
thoroughly wetted before swallowing. For antacid use, follow with small
amount of water or milk; liquid preparation may be followed by a sip of
water.
Drug is sometimes left at the bedside if it is to be given frequently, but only
if the patient is able to assume responsibility for following a prescribed
schedule.
During the 4-to-6-week period required for healing an active peptic ulcer,
some physicians prescribe antacid 1 hour after meals, hourly between
meals, and at bedtime. Some alternate antacid and meals on a 2-hour
schedule and advise patients to take an extra antacid dose when he feels
discomfort.
The objective of ulcer therapy is not to leave the stomach empty, ie, without
food or antacid, for more than 2-hours.
Pain is used as a clinical guide for adjusting dosage. Advise patient to keep
physician informed. Pain that persists beyond 72 hours may signify serious complications such as perforation or malignancy.
When drug is administered by continuous intragastric drip, usually 1 part
antacid is diluted with 2 or 3 parts water (generally, 1500 ml is administered in 24 hours at a rate of 15 to 20 drops/minute).
Note number and consistency of stools. Intestinal obstruction from fecal

concretions has been reported. If constipation is a problem, physician may prescribe concurrent therapy with a mild cathartic antacid, such as magnesium oxide or magnesium trisilicate.

Except during acute symptomatic period, the value of strict dietary control in the management of peptic ulcer is still controversial. However, the patient and responsible family members should receive specific instructions about important dietary principles, such as these: creating a relaxed atmosphere at mealtimes; avoiding known stimulants of gastric secretion such as smoking, caffeine-containing beverages, alcohol and direct mucosal irritants such as black pepper, spices, and ulcerogenic drugs such as aspirin; recognition and control of anxiety-provoking situations and environmental factors that are irritating to the patient.

Patients with esophageal reflux or hiatus hernia are generally advised to avoid overeating, to limit fluid intake during meals, to reduce fat intake (slows gastric emptying), and to keep shoulders elevated about 30° in bed. Consult physician.

Patients receiving excessive doses of antacids for prolonged periods can develop phosphate deficiency, see Adverse Reactions. Reportedly, thiamine deficiency can occur in some patients. Phosphate depletion is usually not a problem in patients on ulcer regimen, because diet is high in phosphate.

Caution individuals who self medicate with antacids that recurring symptoms indicate need for medical investigation.

See Aluminum Carbonate Gel, Basic for management of phosphatic urinary calculi.

DRUG INTERACTIONS: Aluminum-containing antacids may inhibit GI absorption of **isoniazid** and possibly **quinidine.** Antacids containing Al, Ca, or Mg may inhibit absorption of oral **phenothiazines** and **tetracyclines** when administered simultaneously. In general, it is best not to administer other oral drugs within 1 to 2 hours of antacid ingestion.

ALUMINUM NICOTINATE
(NICALEX)

Antilipemic

ACTIONS AND USES

Chemical complex of aluminum nicotinate with added 32% niacin and 12.8% aluminum hydroxide. Antilipemic effect is dependent on niacin content. Evidence regarding mode of action is inconclusive, but its effect may be due to inhibition of coenzyme A (required for cholesterol synthesis) and enhanced hepatic cholesterol degradation. Reportedly reduces pre-β-lipoproteins (rich in triglycerides) and β-lipoproteins (approximately 50% cholesterol). Also reduces serum phospholipids and reduces serum levels of free fatty acids possibly by enhancing retention of free fatty acids in adipose tissue. Used as a source of niacin (qv) in treatment of hypercholesterolemia and all types of hyperlipoproteinemia, except type I.

ABSORPTION AND FATE

Oral preparation slowly hydrolyzed in intestinal tract to nicotinic acid and aluminum hydroxide. Following absorption, maximum blood levels of niacin are reached in 2 hours. Hepatic detoxification; excreted in urine as nicotinuric acid.

Asthma, allergies, active peptic ulcer, hepatic dysfunction, hemorrhage, severe hypotension, tuberculosis. Safe use during pregnancy, during lactation, in women of childbearing age, and in children not established. Cautious use: gout, bronchial disease, bronchospasm, gallbladder disease, past history of jaundice.

ADVERSE REACTIONS

Due chiefly to free niacin content: nausea, vomiting, anorexia, flatulence, epigastric pain, diarrhea, severe flushing, headache, pruritus, dry skin, xerostomia, keratosis nigricans, paresthesias, toxic amblyopia, hypotension, glycosuria, hyperglycemia, hyperuricemia, activation of peptic ulcer, liver dysfunction, cholestatic jaundice. Increased fibrinolysis and decreased prothrombin time reported.

ROUTE AND DOSAGE

Oral: 2 to 4 tablets (625 mg each) 3 times daily, with or after meals. Highly individualized dosage. Usually started with small doses, followed by gradual increments over time (625 mg is equivalent to 500 mg of niacin).

NURSING IMPLICATIONS

Aluminum nicotinate is generally not given simultaneously with other medications because it may decrease their absorption.

A baseline of fasting serum cholesterol and triglycerides or lipoprotein electrophoresis should be established before drug therapy is instituted.

Most side effects are due to niacin content. Flushing, pruritus, and gastrointestinal distress are usually transient, but may require dosage reduction. Advise patient to report these symptoms promptly to the physician. Persistent pruritus may signify a worsening of hypercholesterolemia.

Taking the drug with meals may help to reduce flushing and gastric irritation.

The diabetic or potential diabetic should be checked frequently for signs of decreased glucose tolerance, glycosuria, and hyperglycemia. If these are present, diet, insulin dosage, and antilipemic agent may have to be changed.

Liver function tests and blood glucose levels should be monitored at regular intervals.

Adherence to the prescribed diet is essential to successful drug therapy. Facilitate information-exchange conferences related to patient's diet-drug therapies with nutritionist, physician, patient, and a responsible family member.

Briefly, the dietary regimen adjunctive to drug therapy differs for the various types of hyperlipoproteinemia. Type II: strict low-cholesterol diet (substitute polyunsaturated for saturated fat). Type III: low-cholesterol diet; controlled protein (20% of caloric intake), fat (40%), and carbohydrate (40%). Type IV: controlled carbohydrate (45% of calories); moderately restricted cholesterol. Type V: controlled fat (30% of calories) and carbohydrate (50%); high protein; moderately restricted cholesterol.

High-cholesterol foods: egg yolk, butter, animal fats (lard, salt pork, etc), organ meats, shellfish, whole milk, and other dairy products containing fat.

Rich sources of polyunsaturated fatty acids: safflower, corn, soybean, sesame, and cottonseed oils.

Management of hyperlipemia includes reduction and maintenance of ideal body weight, because weight reduction lowers serum triglycerides. Usually the patient has been on a diet several weeks before drug therapy is instituted.

Aluminum nicotinate therapy may precipitate gout because it causes elevation of serum uric acid. Advise patient to report joint pains to physician.

A 2- to 6-week lag in therapeutic response is not unusual at onset of therapy. The ideal course of treatment should give 15% reduction of plasma cholesterol and 25% decrease in plasma triglycerides after 6 to 8 weeks of therapy.

After 6 to 8 weeks of therapy, absence of the expected fall in serum lipid levels may indicate poor absorption of drug. The physician may advise patient to chew tablets and to ingest them with a full glass of water to enhance absorption.

DRUG INTERACTIONS: The aluminum hydroxide content in aluminum nicotinate may interfere with absorption of simultaneously administered **isoniazid, phenothiazines, quinidine, tetracyclines.** It is best not to administer these drugs within 1 to 2 hours of aluminum nicotinate.

ALUMINUM PHOSPHATE GEL N.F.
(PHOSPHALJEL)

Antacid

ACTIONS AND USES

Slow-acting antacid with properties similar to those of aluminum hydroxide gel (qv), but does not increase fecal excretion of phosphate. Reported to be less efficient in equivalent doses in neutralizing gastric acid. Used as antacid in preference to aluminum hydroxide gel when a high-phosphorus diet cannot be maintained or in patients with diarrhea or pancreatic insufficiency.

ROUTE AND DOSAGE

Oral: 15 to 30 ml undiluted every 2 hours, between meals and at bedtime. For intragastric therapy, diluted 1:3 or 1:4.

NURSING IMPLICATIONS

See Aluminum Hydroxide Gel.

AMANTADINE HYDROCHLORIDE, N.F.
(SYMMETREL)

Antiparkinsonian, antiviral (prophylactic)

ACTIONS AND USES

Synthetic virostatic agent. Probably acts by inhibiting penetration of virus into host cell. Mechanism of action in Parkinson's disease not understood, but may be related to release of dopamine and other catecholamines from neuronal storage sites. Reportedly less effective than levodopa, but produces more rapid clinical response and causes fewer adverse reactions. Has virostatic action against several strains of Asian influenza.

Used in initial therapy or as adjunct to levodopa in treatment of idiopathic and postencephalitic parkinsonism and parkinsonian syndrome. Also used for prophylaxis against A_2 (Asian) influenza virus infection.

ABSORPTION AND FATE

Readily absorbed from GI tract. Maximal blood concentrations appear after 1 to 4 hours. Biologic half-life about 24 hours. Approximately 90% of dose excreted unchanged in urine. Acidification of urine increases rate of excretion.

CONTRAINDICATIONS AND PRECAUTIONS

Known hypersensitivity to amantadine; nursing mothers; safe use during pregnancy and in women of childbearing potential not established. Cautious use:

history of epilepsy or other types of seizures, congestive heart failure, peripheral edema, recurrent eczematoid dermatitis, psychoses, severe psychoneuroses, renal impairment, elderly patients with cerebral arteriosclerosis.

ADVERSE REACTIONS

Common side effects: mild indigestion, dizziness, light-headedness, orthostatic hypotension, urinary retention, nervous excitement, difficulty in concentrating, mild depression, ankle edema, livedo reticularis. Also reported: congestive heart failure, dyspnea, headache, tremors, slurred speech, lethargy, fatigue, drowsiness, ataxia, psychic disturbances (disorientation, confusion, visual hallucinations, aggressive behavior, insomnia, detachment); dry mouth, blurring or loss of vision, oculogyric episodes, anorexia, nausea, vomiting, constipation, dermatitis, convulsions (with excessive doses); leukopenia and neutropenia (rarely).

ROUTE AND DOSAGE

Oral: (Antiparkinson) **Adults**: initially, 100 mg once daily after breakfast, for 5 to 7 days; if well tolerated, additional 100 mg given after lunch. (A_2 Influenza prophylaxis): **Adults and children** *over 9 years*: 100 mg twice daily. **Children** *1 to 9 years*: 4 to 8 mg/kg up to maximum of 150 mg daily in 2 or 3 equally divided doses. Drug should be continued daily for at least 10 days following known exposure, and up to 90 days for possible repeated uncontrolled and unknown exposures to A_2 influenza.

NURSING IMPLICATIONS

Administration of last daily dose too close to retiring may produce insomnia.

Central nervous system and psychic disturbances are most likely to appear within 1 day to a few days after initiation of drug therapy, or after dosage has been increased.

Elderly patients with cerebrovascular disease or impaired renal function are more prone to develop symptoms of toxicity. Since orthostatic hypotension may be a problem, caution patient not to go to sleep in sitting position, and advise male patients to sit down to urinate, particularly at night.

Advise patient to make all position changes slowly, particularly from recumbent to upright position, and to dangle legs a few minutes before standing. Caution him to lie down immediately if he feels faint or dizzy.

Caution patient and responsible family members that drug may cause dizziness, blurred vision, drowsiness, inability to concentrate, and other changes in mental status. Therefore, activities requiring mental alertness should be avoided until patient's reaction to the drug has been evaluated.

Patients with parkinsonism may show reduction of akinesia and rigidity, but generally the drug has little effect on tremors. If significant improvement is not noted within 1 or 2 weeks, drug is usually discontinued.

Patient should remain under close medical supervision while receiving amantadine therapy. Therapeutic effectiveness of the drug sometimes wanes after a few months of treatment. Report to physician. Decision may be made to increase dosage or to discontinue drug temporarily or to use another antiparkinsonian agent.

Livedo reticularis occurs most frequently in patients receiving amantadine for parkinsonism. It is a diffuse, rose-colored mottling of skin, usually confined to lower extremities, but it may also appear on arms. Sometimes preceded by or accompanied by ankle edema. It is more noticeable when patient stands or is exposed to cold; color fades when legs are elevated. Condition may be due to abnormal capillary permeability. Generally, this side effect appears within 1 month to 1 year following initiation of drug therapy and subsides within a few weeks after drug is discontinued.

Abrupt discontinuation of amantadine therapy may precipitate parkinsonian crisis. Warn patient to adhere to established dosage regimen.

For prophylaxis against A_2 influenza, drug should be started in anticipation of contact or as soon as possible after contact with infected individuals.

DRUG INTERACTIONS: Patients receiving high dosages of anticholinergic drugs (eg, **benztropine, trihexyphenidyl,** and other antiparkinsonian agents) may have hallucinations, confusion, and other signs of excess anticholinergic activity, potentiated by amantadine.

AMBENONIUM CHLORIDE, N.F.
(MYTELASE)

Cholinergic (muscle stimulant)

ACTIONS AND USES

Synthetic quaternary compound cholinesterase inhibitor approximately 6 times more potent than neostigmine bromide, but similar with respect to uses, contraindications, and adverse reactions. Produces less severe muscarinic effects such as nausea, vomiting, abdominal pain, and diarrhea than neostigmine, and has more prolonged duration of action.

Used in symptomatic treatment of myasthenia gravis for patients who cannot tolerate neostigmine bromide or pyridostigmine bromide because of bromide sensitivity.

ROUTE AND DOSAGE

Oral: **Adults:** 5 to 25 mg 3 or 4 times a day. Highly individualized. Some patients require as much as 50 to 75 mg per dose. **Children:** initially 0.3 mg/kg/24 hours. Maintenance: 1.5 mg/kg/24 hours divided into 3 or 4 doses.

NURSING IMPLICATIONS

Atrophine sulfate should always be immediately available.

Hazards of cumulative effects and overdosage are high.

Usually medication is not required throughout the night because action is prolonged.

In most patients skeletal muscle effects persist for 4 to 8 hours after drug administration.

Early signs of overdosage include headache, weakness of muscles of neck and of chewing, and salivation. Symptoms usually start to appear in about 1 hour after drug administration.

See Neostigmine Bromide.

AMINOCAPROIC ACID, N.F., B.P.
(AMICAR)

Hemostatic (fibrinolysis inhibitor)

ACTIONS AND USES

Synthetic monaminocarboxylic acid with specific antifibrinolytic action. Acts principally by inhibiting plasminogen activator substance, and to a lesser degree by antiplasmin activity.

Used in excessive bleeding resulting from systemic hyperfibrinolysis, a pathologic condition that frequently follows heart surgery, postcaval shunt, abruptio placentae, aplastic anemia, and carcinoma of lung, prostate, cervix, and stomach. Also used in urinary fibrinolysis (usually a normal physiologic phenomenon) associated with severe trauma, anoxia, shock, surgery, or carcinoma of genitourinary system.

ABSORPTION AND FATE

Rapidly absorbed from GI tract following oral administration; peak plasma levels achieved in about 2 hours. Widely distributed through both extravascular and intravascular compartments. Readily penetrates red blood cells and other body cells; does not appear to be bound to plasma proteins. Approximately 80% of single dose eliminated within 12 hours as unmetabolized drug.

CONTRAINDICATIONS AND PRECAUTIONS

Severe renal impairment, presence of active intravascular clotting process, bleeding into body cavities, long-term use in growing children; as well as during pregnancy and in women of childbearing potential. Cautious use: cardiac, renal, or hepatic dysfunction.

ADVERSE REACTIONS

Nausea, heartburn, bloating, anorexia, abdominal cramps, diarrhea, dizziness, tinnitus, malaise, nasal stuffiness, conjunctival suffusion, headache, skin rash, pruritus, erythema, faintness, postural hypotension, diuresis, thromboses (theoretical possibility). With rapid IV infusion: hypotension, bradycardia, arrhythmias. In patients with hereditary angioneurotic edema (usually associated with large doses): elevated serum aldose and creatine phosphokinase, elevated serum potassium in patients with impaired renal function.

ROUTE AND DOSAGE

Oral, intravenous infusion (slowly): initial priming dose 4 to 5 Gm, followed by 1 to 1.25 Gm at hourly intervals for about 8 hours or until bleeding is controlled. Not to exceed 30 Gm in any 24 hours. For IV infusion, utilize usual compatible IV vehicles: eg, sterile water for injection, physiologic saline, 5% dextrose, or Ringer's solution.

NURSING IMPLICATIONS

Physician will order specific intravenous flow rate. In life-threatening situations, fresh whole blood, fibrinogen infusions, and other emergency measures may be required. (Plasma level of 0.130 mg/ml of drug is apparently necessary to inhibit systemic fibrinolysis.)

Before initiating aminocaproic acid therapy, a definite diagnosis and/or laboratory findings indicative of hyperfibrinolysis (hyperplasminemia) should be determined.

Monitor vital signs. Note and record response to aminocaproic therapy.

DRUG INTERACTIONS: Theoretical possibility of hypercoagulation with concomitant administration of **oral contraceptives**.

AMINOPHYLLINE, U.S.P., B.P.

(AMINODUR DURA-TABS, LIXAMINOL, MINI-LIX, RECTALAD-AMINOPHYLLINE, SOMOPHYLLIN, Theophylline Ethylenediamine)

Smooth-muscle relaxant (bronchodilator), xanthine

ACTIONS AND USES

Methylated xanthine salt of theophylline (qv) with effects similar to those of caffeine and theobromine. Contains approximately 85% theophylline and 15% ethylenediamine. See theophylline for actions, uses, contraindications, precautions, and adverse reactions.

ABSORPTION AND FATE

Erratic absorption rates, particularly following administration of oral tablet and rectal suppository. Therapeutic levels achieved in 1 to 1½ hours (uncoated oral tablet), 3 to 7 hours (sustained-release tablet), 2 to 4 hours (rectal suppository), 30 to 60 minutes (retention enema). Half-life variable due to differences in rates of metabolism and distribution of drug. Levels persist 6 to 12 hours. Retention enema produces blood levels comparable to those with IV administration. Metabolized in liver and excreted by kidneys, primarily as metabolites. Crosses placenta; secreted in breast milk.

CONTRAINDICATIONS AND PRECAUTIONS

Hypersensitivity to xanthine preparations. Cautious use: severe hypertension, and in infants and young children. See Theophylline.

ROUTE AND DOSAGE

Adults: Oral: 100 to 250 mg at 6- to 8-hour intervals. Intramuscular (infrequently used): 500 mg, as required. Intravenous (loading dose): 5.6 mg/kg over 30 minutes; maintenance: up to 0.9 mg/kg/hour by continuous infusion. Rectal (suppository or solution): 250 to 500 mg 1 to 3 times daily. **Children**: 3.5 to 5 mg/kg at 6-hour intervals.

NURSING IMPLICATIONS

Some patients may require around-the-clock dosage schedule.

Side effects are generally related to elevated theophylline serum levels.

Absorption may be delayed but is not reduced by presence of food in stomach. GI symptoms may be relieved by administering oral drug with or immediately following a meal or food. Lowering of dosage may be necessary, and in some cases discontinuation of therapy may be indicated.

There is no evidence that preparations containing antacids appreciably reduce incidence of gastrointestinal side effects. While enteric-coated tablets are efficient in this respect, they may impair drug absorption.

Rectally administered preparations are generally ordered when the patient cannot tolerate the drug orally. Drug absorption is enhanced if rectum is free of feces; therefore, if possible, schedule drug administration in relation to patient's evacuation time.

Since peristaltic activity is stimulated reflexly by presence of food in stomach, patient may experience less difficulty in retaining rectal medication if it can be given before a meal. Also advise patient to remain recumbent for 15 to 20 minutes or until defecation reflex subsides.

High incidence of toxicity is associated with rectal suppository use because of erratic rate of absorption. Children in contrast to adults absorb drug more quickly by rectum.

Children appear to be more susceptible than adults to the CNS stimulating effects of xanthines.

When a change is made from one route of administration to another observe patient closely until dosage is regulated.

Intramuscular route is generally avoided because injection causes intense prolonged pain. Note that intravenous and intramuscular preparations are not interchangeable.

Patients receiving parenteral aminophylline should be closely observed for signs of hypotension, arrhythmias, and convulsions.

Monitor vital signs; measure and record intake and output. Improvements in quality and rate of pulse and respiration, as well as diuresis, are expected clinical effects.

Dizziness is a relatively common side effect, particularly in the elderly. Take necessary safety precautions and forewarn patient of this possibility.

Many popular over-the-counter remedies for treatment of asthma contain ephedrine in combination with various salts of theophylline. Caution patient to take only those medications approved by his physician.

Store suppositories at temperature not exceeding 8 C (46 F).

Do not use aminophylline solutions if crystals are present.

See Theophylline.

AMINOSALICYLATE CALCIUM, U.S.P.
(PARASAL CALCIUM, PAS CALCIUM, TEEBACIN CALCIUM)
AMINOSALICYLATE POTASSIUM
(TEEBACIN KALIUM)
AMINOSALICYLATE SODIUM
(PAMISYL SODIUM, PARASAL SODIUM, PAS SODIUM, TEEBACIN)
AMINOSALICYLIC ACID, N.F.
(PAMISYL, Para-aminosalicylic Acid, PARASAL, PAS, TEEBACIN
ACID)

Antibacterial (tuberculostatic)

ACTIONS AND USES

Aminosalicylic acid and its salts are highly specific bacteriostatic agents that suppress growth and multiplication of *Mycobacterium tuberculosis.* Despite close chemical relationship to salicylic acid, pharmacodynamics are not similar. Apparently do not produce syndrome of salicylism. Aminosalicylic acid has been shown to reduce serum cholesterol, but mechanism of this effect has not been established. The incidence of GI disturbances and crystalluria is reportedly greater with aminosalicylic acid than with its salts.

Used in combination with streptomycin or isoniazid or both in treatment of pulmonary and extrapulmonary tuberculosis to delay emergence of strains resistant to these drugs.

ABSORPTION AND FATE

Readily and almost completely absorbed from GI tract, producing maximal blood concentrations within 1½ to 2 hours. Well distributed to most tissues and body fluids, except cerebrospinal fluid; rapidly penetrates caseous tissue. Blood levels negligible after 4 to 5 hours because renal excretion is rapid. Approximately 80% eliminated in urine within first 7 to 10 hours, in part as free drug and as acetylated compounds. Scant amounts excreted in bile, milk, and tracheobronchial and exocrine secretions.

CONTRAINDICATIONS AND PRECAUTIONS

Hypersensitivity to aminosalicylates or to compounds containing para-aminophenyl groups (eg, sulfonamides, certain hair dyes); use of the potassium salt in patients with hyperkalemia or renal impairment; use of the sodium salt in patients on sodium restriction or known or impending congestive failure. Cautious use: impaired renal and hepatic function, blood dyscrasias, goiter, gastric ulcer.

ADVERSE REACTIONS

GI: anorexia, nausea, vomiting, epigastric pain and burning, abdominal distress, diarrhea, peptic ulceration, gastric hemorrhage. **Hypersensitivity**: high temperature with intermittent spiking, or low-grade fever, generalized malaise, joint pain, sore throat, skin eruptions, syndrome resembling infectious mononucleosis, neurologic manifestations. **Hematologic reactions:** (leukopenia, agranulocytosis, eosinophilia, lymphocytosis, thrombocytopenia, acute hemolytic anemia), Loeffler's syndrome (lung tissue changes, fever, cough, breathlessness). **Other:** renal irritation, crystalluria, metabolic acidosis (especially in children), hypokalemia, pancreatitis (elevated serum amylase levels), glycosuria, jaundice, acute hepatitis (prothrombinemia), goiter with or without myxedema, vasculitis, possibility of impaired intestinal absorption of vitamin B_{12} and development of megaloblastic anemia. With long-term administration: decreased serum PBI and 24-hour ^{131}I uptake.

ROUTE AND DOSAGE

Oral: **Adults**: 8 to 15 Gm daily in 2 to 4 divided doses. Highly individualized.
Pediatric: 200 to 300 mg/kg daily in divided doses.

NURSING IMPLICATIONS

Check expiration date on label before giving drug.

Administer with or immediately following meals to reduce irritative gastric effects. Physician may order an antacid to be given concomitantly. Generally, GI side effects disappear after a few days of therapy. However, if they persist it may be necessary to reduce dosage or interrupt therapy for several days and then start with lower doses, or it may be necessary to terminate therapy.

Aminosalicylic acid is mildly sour to the taste, and it sometimes leaves a bitter aftertaste that may be relieved by sugarless gum or candy.

Appropriate bacterial susceptibility tests should be performed before therapy begins and periodically thereafter to detect bacterial resistance. Also, sputum smears and cultures and blood cell counts should be performed regularly throughout therapy.

Intake and output should be monitored. High concentrations of the drug are excreted in urine, and this can cause crystalluria and hematuria. Keeping urine neutral or alkaline with adjunctive drugs (such as absorbable antacids) or diet therapy (ie, high intake of fruits and fruit juices, with the exception of cranberry, plum, or prune) and high fluid intake can reduce the risk of crystalluria. These measures are to be used only if prescribed by physician.

Reportedly may cause discoloration of urine (color change not described).

Hypersensitivity reactions may occur after a few days, but generally they appear between the second and seventh weeks of drug therapy, most commonly in the fourth or fifth week.

Monitor temperature. Abrupt onset of fever, particularly during the early weeks of therapy, and a clinical picture resembling that of infectious mononucleosis (malaise, fatigue, generalized lymphadenopathy, splenomegaly, sore throat), as well as minor complaints of pruritus, joint pains, and headache, are strongly suggestive of hypersensitivity; these symptoms should be reported promptly. Continued administration of drug in the presence of hypersensitivity reactions can lead to hepatic damage, pancreatitis, and nephritis.

Check weight semiweekly under standard conditions.

Therapeutic response to drug therapy is indicated by a feeling of well-being, improved appetite, weight gain, reduced fever, lessening of fatigue, decreased cough and sputum, improved chest x-rays, and negative sputum cultures.

Generally, chemotherapy is continued for about 2 years. Patient and responsible family members must understand signs and symptoms of drug toxicity, the importance of developing a daily routine for taking tuberculostatic drugs, and the need for remaining under close medical supervision to detect covert adverse drug effects. Point out that resistant strains develop more rapidly when drug regimen is interrupted.

A brownish or purplish discoloration of the drug signifies decomposition. If this occurs, discard drug.

Aminosalicylic acid is an unstable drug that is affected by time, heat, air, and moisture. Store in tight, light-resistant containers in a cool, dry place. Solutions of aminosalicylate salts generally should be used within 24 hours.

LABORATORY TEST INTERFERENCES: Interferes with urine urobilinogen determinations; possibility of false positive test results reported for certain urinary protein and VMA determinations, and for copper sulfur reagents, ie, Benedict's solution (but not with glucose oxidase reagents, eg, Tes-Tape, Clinistix).

DRUG INTERACTIONS: **Ammonium chloride** and **ascorbic acid** render urine acid and therefore increase the possibility of aminosalicylic acid crystalluria. **Diphenhydramine** and **rifampin** may impair GI absorption of aminosalicylic acid; space administrations as far apart as possible. **Para-aminobenzoic acid (PABA)** may inhibit antimicrobial activity of aminosalicylic acid; concomitant administration is usually avoided. **Probenecid, phenytoin, salicylates** (limited evidence), and **sulfinpyrazole** may increase aminosalicylic acid blood levels (inhibit renal excretion). Aminosalicylic acid may enhance excretion of **oral anticoagulants**, and may decrease absorption of **vitamin B$_{12}$.**

AMITRIPTYLINE HYDROCHLORIDE, U.S.P., B.P.
(ELAVIL, ENDEP)

Tricyclic antidepressant

ACTIONS AND USES
Structurally and pharmacologically related to imipramine (qv); they have similar actions, uses, contraindications, and adverse reactions. Reported to be superior to imipramine in severe depressions and in patients over 50 years of age; has greater sedative effect than imipramine.
CONTRAINDICATIONS AND PRECAUTIONS
Safe use in children under 12 years of age not established. See Imipramine.
ROUTE AND DOSAGE
Oral, intramuscular: 10 to 25 mg 2 to 4 times a day. Highly individualized. Adolescents, elderly patients, and outpatients usually given lower dosage range. Hospitalized patients may be given up to 300 mg daily in divided doses.

NURSING IMPLICATIONS
Sedative action may be apparent before antidepressant effect is noted. Full therapeutic effect may not develop until after 30 days of therapy.
Dosage increases, if required, should be made in late afternoon or at bedtime because of drug sedative action.
In depressed patients with insomnia, the side effect of drowsiness may be put to therapeutic use by scheduling a dose of the drug at bedtime. Discuss with physician.
The elderly may require dosage adjustments. Monitor these patients with this possibility in mind.
Caution patient to avoid driving and other hazardous tasks.
In rare instances amitriptyline may impart a blue-green color to urine.
See Imipramine Hydrochloride.

AMMONIUM CHLORIDE, N.F., B.P.

Systemic acidifier, diuretic, expectorant

ACTIONS AND USES
Acid-forming property is due to conversion of ammonium ion (NH$_4$$^+$) to urea in liver with release of H$^+$ and Cl$^-$. Chloride anions displace bicarbonate, producing acidosis that causes temporary (1 to 2 days) secondary excretion of Na$^+$ and hence diuresis. Potassium excretion also increases, but to a lesser extent. Tolerance to diuretic effects occurs by compensatory mechanisms, including renal excretion of H$^+$ and K$^+$ cations and formation of ammonia by renal cells, with recovery of corresponding amounts of sodium ions. Also has mild expectorant action; presumably decreases viscosity and increases volume of sputum reflexly by gastric irritation.
Used to augment effects of mercurial diuretics and to correct hypochloremic

alkalosis produced by these compounds. Limited use as a primary diuretic. Used to lower urinary pH as an aid in excretion of certain basic drugs and lead in cases of lead poisoning. A common ingredient in cough mixtures.

ABSORPTION AND FATE

Complete absorption occurs in 3 to 6 hours (enteric-coated tablet absorption is erratic). Metabolized in body to form HCl and urea. Primarily excreted in urine; 1% to 3% excreted in feces.

CONTRAINDICATIONS AND PRECAUTIONS

Renal, hepatic, and pulmonary insufficiency. Used with caution in cardiac edema.

ADVERSE REACTIONS

GI: irritation (nausea, vomiting, anorexia, diarrhea). Metabolic acidosis: nausea, vomiting, increased rate and depth of respirations (Kussmaul breathing), thirst, weakness, flushed face, full bounding pulse, lethargy, progressive drowsiness, mental confusion, excitement alternating with coma. Also reported: skin rash, headache, calcium deficiency, tetany, hyperreflexia, hypokalemia, hyperglycemia, glycosuria, increased urinary magnesium excretion, decreased urine urobilinogen. With rapid IV administration: bradycardia, irregular respiration, ammonia toxicity.

ROUTE AND DOSAGE

Oral: **Adults**: 0.3 to 1 Gm every 2 to 4 hours. Intravenous infusion: **Adults and Pediatrics**: 10 ml/kg of 2.14% solution. Administration rate always less than 2 ml/minute. Highly individualized. Has been given by hypodermoclysis in infants and young children.

NURSING IMPLICATIONS

GI side effects may be minimized by administration of enteric-coated tablets (however absorption of this form is unpredictable), and by giving drug immediately after meals.

Carbon dioxide combining power and serum electrolytes should be monitored prior to IV infusions of ammonium chloride and periodically during oral drug therapy to determine dosage and to avoid serious acidosis.

Urinary pH may also be used as a guide for therapy (normal range 4.8 to 7.8).

Note rate and depth of respirations. Shortness of breath and increased ventilation at rest are signs of acidosis (see Adverse Reactions). Intravenous sodium bicarbonate or sodium lactate may be used to treat severe acidosis.

Report change in intake–output ratio. Because of compensatory mechanisms the diuretic effect of ammonium chloride lasts only 1 or 2 days. Most effective as a diuretic when administered in intermittent 3- or 4-day courses followed by a rest period of a few days.

In the elderly, vigorous diuresis may precipitate renal insufficiency, urinary retention in males with prostatic hypertrophy, incontinence in both sexes, and acute Na^+ and K^+ depletion. Report signs of weakness and confusion and changes in voiding pattern and comfort.

Check urine specific gravity of the older person on diuretics; elevation accompanying even mild diuresis is suggestive of renal insufficiency.

When used as an expectorant, do not give enteric-coated tablets since expectorant activity is believed to be due to reflex gastric irritation. Administer drug in liquid or tablet form with full glass of water. Fluids help to stimulate respiratory tract fluid, thereby decreasing viscosity of bronchial secretions.

DRUG INTERACTIONS: Ammonium chloride renders urine acidic, thereby increasing the possibility of **aminosalicylic acid** crystalluria, increased plasma **salicylate** levels (in patients on high salicylate doses), and systemic acidosis with **spironolactone**. Ammonium chloride may decrease effect of **amphetamines** and **tricyclic antidepressants** by reducing their tubular reabsorption.

(AMYTAL)
AMOBARBITAL SODIUM, U.S.P.
(AMYTAL SODIUM)
AMYLOBARBITONE SODIUM, B.P.

Sedative, hypnotic

ACTIONS AND USES
Intermediate-acting barbiturate with actions, uses, contraindications, and precautions similar to those of phenobarbital (qv).
Used in treatment of insomnia and to relieve preoperative anxiety. Also used parenterally to control status epilepticus or acute convulsive episodes and agitated behavior, as well as in narcoanalysis and narcotherapy.

ABSORPTION AND FATE
Onset of action within 1 hour following oral administration; duration of action approximately 6 to 8 hours. Intravenous administration: onset of effects within 5 minutes; duration about 3 to 6 hours. Inactivated in liver by hydroxylation. Excreted in urine primarily as inactive metabolites.

ROUTE AND DOSAGE
Oral intramuscular, intravenous: **Adults** (Sedation): 30 to 50 mg 2 to 3 times daily. (Hypnotic): 100 to 200 mg. Highly individualized. **Pediatric**: 3 to 6 mg/kg/24 hours divided into 3 doses.

NURSING IMPLICATIONS
Prolonged use may lead to tolerance and dependence. Classified as a schedule II drug under federal Controlled Substances Act.
Parenteral solution is prepared with sterile water for injection. After adding diluent, rotate vial to facilitate solution. Do not shake vial. If solution is not absolutely clear after 5 minutes, do not use.
Amobarbital sodium hydrolyzes in dry form or in solution when exposed to air. No more than 30 minutes should elapse from time ampul is opened until drug is injected.
Intramuscular injection should be made deep in a large muscle mass, such as the gluteus maximus. Superficial injections are painful and can cause sterile abscesses or sloughing.
No more than 5 ml should be injected IM into any one site.
Intravenous amobarbital sodium is given only to hospitalized patients under close supervision. Large intravenous doses, or too rapid intravenous injection, may cause apnea and hypotension. Blood pressure, pulse, and respiration should be monitored during injection and for several hours after injection.
Rate of absorption is increased if drug is taken orally on an empty stomach. Caution patient not to take alcoholic beverages.
See Phenobarbital.

AMODIAQUINE HYDROCHLORIDE, U.S.P., B.P.
(CAMOQUIN)

Antimalarial, plasmocide

ACTIONS AND USES
4-aminoquinoline derivative similar to chloroquine in actions, uses, contraindications, and adverse reactions.

Used for suppressive prophylaxis and clinical cure of *Plasmodium ovale, P. malariae, P. vivax,* and *P. falciparum.* Used alone, amodiaquine provides causal prophylaxis and radical cure of *P. falciparum* malaria, but it must be used with a secondary tissue schizonticide to exert the same effects on *P. vivax, P. malariae,* and *P. ovale.* Has been used for *Giardia lamblia* and extraintestinal amebiasis.

CONTRAINDICATIONS AND PRECAUTIONS

Used with extreme caution in severe gastrointestinal, neurologic, or blood disorders. See Chloroquine.

ADVERSE REACTIONS

Nausea, vomiting, diarrhea, lethargy. With prolonged use: corneal deposits, pigmentary reactions (melanosis), polyneuritis, toxic psychosis, blood dyscrasias (leukopenia, pancytopenia, fatal agranulocytosis), toxic hepatitis. See Chloroquine.

ROUTE AND DOSAGE

Oral (For acute attack): **Adults:** 600 mg initially, followed by 300 mg 6 hours later and 300 mg at 24 and 48 hours. **Children:**10 mg/kg divided into 3 doses at 12-hour intervals. Not to exceed adult dosage. (Suppressive prophylaxis): **Adults:** 300 to 400 mg once weekly, on the same day of each week. **Children:** 5 mg/kg once weekly.

NURSING IMPLICATIONS

GI side effects may be minimized by giving the drug with meals.

If no improvement in acute symptoms is noted after 48 hours of therapy in patients with falciparum malaria, treatment with another antimalarial agent is usually instituted.

Bluish gray pigmentation of fingernails, skin, and hard palate has occurred in patients receiving weekly antimalarial doses over prolonged periods. The reaction disappears slowly (4 to 9 months) after drug is discontinued.

Children are especially sensitive to 4-aminoquinoline compounds and therefore should be closely monitored.

For prophylaxis, travelers should be advised how soon to begin taking the drug before entering a malarious area and how long to continue taking it after leaving the area.

See Chloroquine.

AMOXICILLIN
(AMOXIL, LAROTID, POLYMOX)

Antibacterial (antibiotic)

ACTIONS AND USES

Semisynthetic analogue of ampicillin with a broad spectrum of antibacterial activity similar to that of penicillin G (qv). Reported to cause fewer GI side effects than oral forms of ampicillin. Inactivated by penicillinase.

Used in treatment of genitourinary tract infections caused by *Escherichia coli, Proteus mirabilis,* or *Streptococcus faecalis;* used for acute uncomplicated gonorrhea; for infections of ears, respiratory tract, skin, and soft tissue caused by streptococci and non-penicillinase-producing staphylococci; and for *Haemophilus influenzae* infection. Commercially available only in oral dosage form; therefore not indicated for initial treatment of life-threatening infections.

ABSORPTION AND FATE

Rapidly absorbed following oral administration. Resists inactivation by gastric acid. Diffuses into most tissues and body fluids, except brain and spinal fluid, unless meninges are inflamed. Measurable serum levels are still present 6 hours following single 250 mg dose. Approximately 20% is protein-bound. Half-life is approximately 1 hour. About 60% of dose is excreted in urine as intact amoxicillin and penicillinoic acid.

CONTRAINDICATIONS AND PRECAUTIONS

Hypersensitivity to penicillins or cephalosporins. Safe use during pregnancy not established. Used with caution, if at all, in patients with history of asthma or allergies.

ADVERSE REACTIONS

As with other penicillins: nausea, vomiting, diarrhea, hypersensitivity reactions, anemia, thrombocytopenic purpura, eosinophilia, leukopenia, agranulocytosis, superinfections.

ROUTE AND DOSAGE

Oral: **Adults and Children** *weighing 20 kg or more*: 250 to 500 mg every 8 hours. For gonorrhea: **Adults**: 3 Gm as single dose. **Children** *weighing under 20 kg*: 20 to 40 mg/kg/day in divided doses every 8 hours.

NURSING IMPLICATIONS

Serum levels not significantly affected by food; therefore amoxicillin may be given without regard to meals.

Therapy may be instituted prior to obtaining results of bacteriologic and susceptibility tests.

Periodic assessment of renal, hepatic, and hematopoietic functions should be made during prolonged drug therapy.

Patient in whom syphilitic lesion is suspected should have dark-field examination before receiving amoxicillin, as well as monthly serologic tests for a minimum of 4 months.

When amoxicillin is used to treat urinary tract infections, frequent bacteriologic and clinical evaluations are recommended.

For most infections, treatment is continued for a minimum of 48 to 72 hours beyond the time patient appears asymptomatic or evidence of bacterial eradication is obtained.

It is recommended that patients with hemolytic streptococcal infections receive at least 10 days of treatment to prevent occurrence of acute rheumatic fever or glomerulonephritis.

Any unused portion of reconstituted oral suspension should be discarded after 7 days at room temperature, or after 14 days if refrigerated. Shake well before pouring.

See Penicillin G Potassium.

AMPHETAMINE SULFATE, N.F., B.P. (BENZEDRINE)

Central stimulant

ACTIONS AND USES

Synthetic sympathomimetic amine (noncatecholamine) of the phenylisopropamine type with α- and β-adrenergic activity. Chemically and pharmacologically related to ephedrine. Marked stimulant effect on CNS is thought to be due to action on cortex and possibly reticular activating system. Increases synaptic release of norepinephrine and dopamine in brain and impairs their reuptake in nerve endings. CNS stimulation results in marked analeptic effect, diminished sense of fatigue, alertness, wakefulness, and elevation of mood. Peripheral actions produce mydriasis without cycloplegia, nasal decongestion, weak bronchodilator and respiratory stimulation, increased blood pressure, and decreased urinary bladder tone coupled with sphincter constriction. Anorexigenic effect is thought to result from direct inhibitory action on lateral hypothalamic appetite area and possibly from drug-induced loss of acuity of smell and taste, as well as mood elevation.

Used as adjunct in certain depressive reactions characterized by apathy and psychomotor retardation, postencephalitic parkinsonism, narcolepsy, minimal brain dysfunction (MBD), and respiratory depression; used as short-term adjunct to control exogenous obesity. Also has been used in treatment of persistent hiccups, urinary incontinence, and nocturnal enuresis.

ABSORPTION AND FATE

Rapid absorption and distribution to all tissues. Duration of effect: 4 to 24 hours following oral administration. High concentration in brain and cerebrospinal fluid results from rapid passage across blood–brain barrier. Some deamination and conjugation probably occurs in liver. Appears in urine within 3 hours following oral administration; approximately 50% of drug is excreted by kidneys. Acidic urine enhances excretion.

CONTRAINDICATIONS AND PRECAUTIONS

Hypersensitivity to sympathomimetic amines, history of drug abuse, hyperthyroidism, severe agitation, endogenous depression, renal disease, diabetes mellitus, hypertension, angina pectoris or other cardiovascular disorders, glaucoma, arteriosclerotic parkinsonism. Not used as anorexic in children under 12 years of age or in MBD for children under 3 years. Not used during pregnancy; not used in conjunction with or for 14 days following cessation of MAO inhibitors. Cautious use: elderly, debilitated, or asthenic patients; anorexia, insomnia, psychopathic personality, history of suicidal tendencies.

ADVERSE REACTIONS

Dry mouth, metallic taste, nausea, anorexia, constipation or diarrhea, mydriasis, difficulty in micturition, agitation, dizziness, nervousness, restlessness, insomnia, palpitation, tachycardia. With high doses: elevated blood pressure or hypotension, syncope, dyspnea, anginal pain, cardiac arrhythmias, fatigue, chills, mental depression, disorientation, hallucinations, compulsive behavior, hyperreflexia, severe headache, convulsions, respiratory failure. Also reported: aplastic anemia and pancytopenia (with prolonged use), impotence, changes in libido, urticaria. Chronic intoxication: severe dermatoses, marked insomnia, irritability, hyperactivity, personality changes, psychosis.

ROUTE AND DOSAGE

Oral: **Adults**: 5 to 60 mg per day in divided doses. Sustained-release form: 15 to 30 mg daily. **Children** 3 to 5 years: 2.5 mg daily; 6 to 12 years: 5 mg daily; 12 years and older: 10 mg daily. Doses may be raised at weekly intervals in increments equal to initial dose until optimum response is achieved.

NURSING IMPLICATIONS

To avoid insomnia, last dose should be administered no later than 6 hours before retiring.

When used as an anorexigenic, drug is generally administered ½ to 1 hour before meals. Sustained-release form is given once daily in the morning.

Since tolerance (tachyphylaxis) to the anorexigenic and mood-elevating effects commonly occurs within a few weeks, continuous weight reduction cannot be achieved without additional dietary restriction. A structured weight reduction program should be planned in collaboration with physician, dietitian, patient, and responsible family members.

In patients with diabetes mellitus, insulin requirements may be altered in association with use of amphetamines and the concomitant dietary regimen.

In a state of fatigue, amphetamine exerts a stimulating effect that masks the feeling of being tired. After the exhilarating effect has disappeared there is usually greater fatigue and depression than before, and a longer period of rest is needed. Therefore, inform the patient that amphetamine does not obviate the need for planned rest, and caution him that the drug may impair his ability to engage in hazardous activities such as operating a car or machinery.

Following prolonged administration of high doses, the drug should be withdrawn gradually. Abrupt withdrawal may result in lethargy, profound depression, or other psychotic manifestations that may persist for several weeks.

Response to the drug is more variable in children than in adults. Acute toxicity has occurred over a wide range of dosage.

Addiction potential is controversial. Most authorities seem to agree that long-term therapy is unlikely to produce addiction and that habituation or psychic dependence is caused by psychologic factors rather than by pharmacologic action. Pronounced tolerance develops with repeated use.

Lay terms used for amphetamines include pep pills, wake-ups, and bennies, among others.

Amphetamines have a high abuse potential because of their excitatory and euphoric effects.

Classified as Schedule II drug under the federal Controlled Substances Act.

Amphetamine sulfate injection should be protected from light.

DRUG INTERACTIONS: Amphetamines are potentiated by **acetazolamide**, and **sodium bicarbonate,** (increase renal tubular reabsorption of **amphetamines**) and antagonized by **haloperidol, lithium carbonate** (based on limited studies), and **reserpine, phenothiazines** (inhibit uptake of amphetamines). Amphetamines may enhance toxicity of **furazolidone, MAO inhibitors, propoxyphene**, and **tricyclic antidepressants**, and may decrease the antihypertensive effect of **guanethidine** and **methyldopa**.

AMPHOTERICIN B, U.S.P.
(FUNGIZONE)
AMPHOTERICIN, B.P.

Antifungal, antibiotic

ACTIONS AND USES

Fungistatic antibiotic produced by *Streptomyces nodosus.* Probably exerts antifungal activity by binding sterols in fungus cell membrane, with resultant change in membrane permeability, thus allowing leakage of K^+ and other intracellular constituents.

Used intravenously for a wide spectrum of potentially fatal systemic fungal infections, including blastomycosis, coccidioidomycosis, cryptococcosis, disseminated candidiasis, histoplasmosis, and others. Not effective against bacteria, rickettsiae, or viruses. Used topically for cutaneous and mucocutaneous infections caused by *Candida albicans.*

ABSORPTION AND FATE

After IV injection, approximately 90% is bound to serum proteins and 10% is in serum. Elimination half-life is about 24 hours. Excreted slowly by kidneys, over 7-day period; cumulative urinary excretion of a single dose is around 40%. Can be detected in blood and urine up to 4 weeks after discontinuation of therapy.

CONTRAINDICATIONS AND PRECAUTIONS

Hypersensitivity to amphotericin B; renal impairment; concomitant administration of corticosteroids, other nephrotoxic antibiotics, and antineoplastic agents. Safe use during pregnancy not established.

Intravenous therapy: fever, chills, headache, malaise, anorexia, weight loss, nausea, vomiting, epigastric cramps, diarrhea, hemorrhagic gastroenteritis with melena; myalgia, arthralgia, muscle weakness (from hypokalemia), peripheral neuropathies, thrombophlebitis, febrile reactions, maculopapular rash, transient vertigo, tinnitus, hearing loss, blurred vision, diplopia, normochromic normocytic anemia, convulsions. With large doses over prolonged periods: hypokalemia, hypomagnesemia, proteinuria, nephrotoxicity, bacterial superinfection. Rarely: anaphylactoid reaction, hypertension or hypotension, cardiac disturbances including ventricular fibrillation and cardiac arrest, coagulation defects, thrombocytopenia, leukopenia, agranulocytosis, eosinophilia, Coombs-positive hemolytic anemia, elevated CPK, acute liver failure. **Topical therapy:** dry skin, erythema, pruritus, burning sensation. Rarely: allergic contact dermatitis.

ROUTE AND DOSAGE

Intravenous infusion: initially 0.25 mg/kg body weight daily. Dosage gradually increased to 1 mg/kg/day as tolerance permits. Up to 1.5 mg/kg/day may be given with alternate-day therapy. Topical (3% cream, lotion, ointment): applied by rubbing well into affected area 2 to 4 times a day.

NURSING IMPLICATIONS

Keep dry powder refrigerated and protected from exposure to light. Solution for IV infusion should be used promptly after preparation and protected from light during administration (aluminum foil is useful). Refer to package insert for diluents and recommended pH.

Prior to systemic therapy, diagnosis is confirmed by positive cultures or histologic studies.

Amphotericin B is administered IV only to hospitalized patients or to those under close clinical supervision who have confirmed diagnoses of progressive, potentially fatal fungal infections susceptible to the drug.

Several months of therapy are usually required to assure adequate response and to prevent relapse.

Check with physician regarding IV flow rate. Generally the drug is administered slowly over a 6-hour period. If a reaction occurs, interrupt therapy and report promptly to physician.

Monitor vital signs. Febrile reactions usually appear about 1 to 2 hours after start of IV infusion and subside within 4 hours after it is discontinued.

Monitor intake and output. Report immediately any change in intake–output ratio or the appearance of oliguria, hematuria, sediment, or cloudy urine. Renal damage is usually reversible if the drug is discontinued when the first signs of renal dysfunction appear.

During therapy, blood counts, serum electrolyte determinations, and renal function tests are advised at least weekly. If blood urea nitrogen exceeds 40 mg/dl, if nonprotein nitrogen exceeds 100 mg/dl, or if serum creatinine exceeds 3 mg/dl, the physician may reduce dosage or discontinue the drug until renal function improves.

The drug is irritating to venous endothelium and may cause local inflammatory reaction or thrombosis at the injection site, particulary if extravasation occurs.

Be on the alert for signs of hypokalemia: anorexia, drowsiness, muscle weakness, hypoactive reflexes, paresthesias.

The drug is potentially ototoxic. Report immediately any evidence of hearing loss or complaints of tinnitus, or dizziness.

Topical cream discolors the skin minimally. Generally, lotion and cream do not stain skin when thoroughly rubbed into lesion, but they may stain nail lesions.

To remove cream or lotion from fabric, wash with soap and water; ointment

may be removed from fabric with a standard cleaning fluid.
Drug should be withdrawn immediately if signs of hypersensitivity or irritation appear.

DRUG INTERACTIONS: **Corticosteroids** may enhance potassium depletion caused by amphotericin B. Amphotericin-induced potassium depletion may increase toxicity of **digitalis glycosides,** may enhance the effect of **curariform muscle relaxants,** and decrease adrenocortical responsiveness to **corticotropin.**

AMPICILLIN, U.S.P., B.P.
(ALPEN, AMCILL, OMNIPEN, PEN A, PENBRITIN, PENSYN, POLYCILLIN, PRINCIPEN, TOTACILLIN, SK-AMPICILLIN)
AMPICILLIN SODIUM
(ALPEN-N, AMCILL-S, OMNIPEN-N, PEN A/N, PENBRITIN-S, PENSYN-N, POLYCILLIN-N, PRINCIPEN/N, SK-AMPICILLIN-N, TOTALCILLIN-N)

Antibacterial, antibiotic

ACTIONS AND USES

Broad-spectrum semisynthetic penicillin derived from 6-aminopenicillanic acid. Bactericidal action similar to that of penicillin G potassium. Active against Gram-negative organisms including *Escherichia coli, Neisseria gonorrhoeae, Haemophilus influenzae, N. meningitidis, Proteus mirabilis, Salmonella,* and *Shigella.* Also effective against Gram-positive organisms (eg, α- and β-hemolytic streptococci, *Diplococcus pneumoniae,* enterococci, and non-penicillinase-producing staphylococci). Inactivated by penicillinase.
Used in infections of respiratory, gastrointestinal, and genitourinary tracts and infections of skin and soft tissues; used in bacterial meningitis and otitis media. Used parenterally only in treatment of moderately severe to severe infections. Available as the trihydrate, as anhydrous ampicillin, and as the sodium salt.

ABSORPTION AND FATE

Approximately 30% to 60% of oral dose absorbed from GI tract. Peak serum concentrations following administration occur as follows: within 2 hours, oral route; within 1 hour, IM route; within 5 minutes, IV route. About 20% bound to plasma proteins. Diffuses into most body tissues and fluids; high concentrations in cerebrospinal fluid only when meninges are inflamed. Detectable in blood for about 8 hours after oral dose and IM dose, and for 6 hours after IV. Appears to be partially inactivated by liver; excreted in high concentrations in urine and bile. Crosses placenta and appears in breast milk.

CONTRAINDICATIONS AND PRECAUTIONS

Hypersensitivity to penicillin derivatives, cephalosporins, or other allergens. Safe use during pregnancy not established. Cautious use: liver and renal disease. Because of high incidence of ampicillin rash, also used with caution in infectious mononucleosis, hyperuricemia, and lymphatic leukemia.

ADVERSE REACTIONS

Nausea, vomiting, diarrhea, abdominal pain, superinfections (black, furry tongue and foul-smelling diarrhea, glossitis, stomatitis); impaired hepatic function. Hypersensitivity reactions: drug fever, urticaria, maculopapular rash, eosinophilia, thrombocytopenia, leukopenia, agranulocytosis. Rarely: interstitial nephritis (hematuria, proteinuria, pyuria, azotemia), anaphylactoid reaction. Following parenteral administration: severe pain (IM), phlebitis (IV). Also see Penicillin G Potassium.

Oral, intramuscular, intravenous: **Adults** (Respiratory tract and soft tissue infections): 250 to 500 mg every 6 hours. **Children**: 25 to 50 mg/kg/day in equally divided doses at 6 to 8 hour intervals. (Uncomplicated gonorrhea) **Adults**: 3.5 Gm together with 1 Gm probenecid, orally. (Septicemia and bacterial meningitis) **Adults and Children**: 50 to 200 mg/kg daily in divided doses every 3 to 4 hours.

NURSING IMPLICATIONS

A careful history should be taken before therapy begins to determine previous hypersensitivity reactions.

As a guide to therapy, the invading organism should be cultured and tested for sensitivity.

Although ampicillin may be given with meals, maximum absorption is achieved if taken on an empty stomach, 1 hour before or 2 hours after meals.

Chewable tablets should be thoroughly masticated before being swallowed.

Ampicillin is acid-labile; therefore oral preparations added to acidic beverages, such as tomato juice or fruit juices, should not be allowed to stand for any length of time. Also, concomitant ingestion of large amounts of such fluids should be avoided.

Shake oral suspension well before pouring. Suspensions are stable for 7 days at room temperature and for 14 days under refrigeration.

Following reconstitution, ampicillin sodium solutions for IM or direct IV injection are stable for about 1 hour. Stability of IV infusion depends on diluent used. Consult product information.

Contact dermatitis occurs frequently; therefore those who handle the drug repeatedly are advised to wear plastic gloves.

Skin eruptions occur fairly commonly in patients on ampicillin therapy. The rash may be maculopapular (also called ampicillin rash) or urticarial. It may spread to various parts of the body, but it has a tendency to involve light-exposed or pressure areas, eg, knees, elbows, palms, soles.

Inspect skin daily, and advise the home patient to do the same. Rash may appear after onset of therapy, or it may be delayed for as long as 3 weeks. Report to physician if it occurs.

Periodic assessments of renal, hepatic, and hematopoietic functions are advised during prolonged therapy.

Frequent bacteriologic and clinical evaluations are necessary in treatment of chronic urinary tract and intestinal infections. It may be necessary to continue appraisals for several months after cessation of therapy.

Treatment with ampicillin for most infections is usually continued 48 to 72 hours beyond the time the patient becomes asymptomatic or evidence of bacterial eradication has been obtained. A minimum of 10 days treatment is recommended for infections with group A β-hemolytic streptococci to prevent occurrence of rheumatic fever or acute glomerulonephritis.

Since it is not known whether ampicillin can abort preclinical syphilis, patients with gonorrhea and suspected primary lesions of syphilis should have dark-field examinations before receiving ampicillin therapy and monthly serologic tests for a minimum of 4 months. Cultures of endocervical and anal canals are advised, in order to test for cure of gonorrhea in female patients.

Also see Penicillin G Potassium.

LABORATORY TEST INTERFERENCES: Ampicillin IM may produce elevated CPK levels as a result of skeletal muscle injury.

DRUG INTERACTIONS: Reportedly, **allopurinol** predisposes some patients receiving ampicillin to development of skin rash. Also see Penicillin G Potassium.

AMYL NITRITE, N.F.

Vasodilator

ACTIONS AND USES
Short-acting vasodilator and smooth muscle relaxant with actions, contraindications, and adverse reactions similar to those of nitroglycerin.
Used for prompt, symptomatic relief of angina pectoris and renal and gallbladder colic. Repeated inhalations are administered as immediate treatment of cyanide poisoning to induce formation of methemoglobin, which forms a nontoxic complex with cyanide ion.
ABSORPTION AND FATE
Rapidly absorbed from mucous membranes and lungs. Onset of action, 10 to 30 seconds; duration, 3 to 5 minutes. Excreted by kidney.
ROUTE AND DOSAGE
Inhalation: 0.18 ml or 0.3 ml as required.

NURSING IMPLICATIONS

Amyl nitrite is available in 0.18-ml and 0.3-ml pearls (thin, friable glass ampuls enveloped with woven fabric cover). To prepare for administration, wrap ampul in gauze or cloth and crush between fingers.
Inform patient that drug has a strongly ethereal and fruity odor.
Syncope, due to a sudden drop in systolic blood pressure, sometimes follows amyl nitrite inhalation; therefore, have patient seated or lying down when administering drug. If syncope occurs, have patient breathe deeply and move legs and ankles to facilitate venous return and increase cerebral blood flow.
After administration of drug, note length of time required for pain to subside; monitor vital signs until they are normal. Rapid pulse, which usually lasts for a brief period, is an expected baroreceptor response to the fall in blood pressure produced by the nitrite ion.
Amyl nitrite is volatile and highly flammable and should not be used where its vapors may be ignited.
Tolerance may develop with repeated use over prolonged periods.
Generally, if continued therapy is indicated, a less expensive vasodilator such as nitroglycerin may be prescribed.
See Nitroglycerin.

ANILERIDINE HYDROCHLORIDE, N.F.
(LERITINE HYDROCHLORIDE)
ANILERIDINE PHOSPHATE, N.F.
(LERITINE PHOSPHATE INJECTION)

Narcotic analgesic

ACTIONS AND USES
Phenylpiperidine derivative reported to have a range of 2 to 12 times the analgesic potency of meperidine (qv). As compared with meperidine, anileridine produces less constipation or no constipation; it may have less sedative action, and it causes more frequent nausea and vomiting; respiratory depressant effects are less, but longer in duration. Unlike meperidine, it does not release histamine, and it has some antitussive action. In very large doses anileridine substitutes

completely for morphine in morphine-dependent patients. May produce dependence of morphine type; euphoria is uncommon.

Used for relief of moderate to severe pain, for relief of anxiety in patients with dyspnea associated with acute left ventricular failure, for preoperative sedation, as supplement to anesthesia, and for analgesia during labor.

ABSORPTION AND FATE

Readily absorbed from all sites. Onset of action within 15 minutes following parenteral administration. Analgesic effects of IV dose last 1 hour; IM, 2 hours; subcutaneous and oral, 4 hours. Metabolized chiefly in liver; excreted primarily in urine as metabolites and unchanged drug.

CONTRAINDICATIONS AND PRECAUTIONS

Respiratory edema caused by chemical respiratory irritant; children 12 years or younger; pregnancy, shock, head injuries, and conditions associated with increased intracranial pressure. Used with caution in patients receiving other CNS depressants. Also see Meperidine.

ADVERSE REACTIONS

See Meperidine.

ROUTE AND DOSAGE

Oral: 25 to 50 mg every 4 to 6 hours, if necessary. Subcutaneous, intramuscular, 25 to 50 mg every 4 to 6 hours, if necessary (not to exceed 200 mg in 24-hour period). Intravenous, 10 mg injected slowly. Dosage range generally lower for elderly, debilitated, and very young patients.

NURSING IMPLICATIONS

In evaluating patient's need for the drug, note that indications for its administration for pain include signs similar to those of toxicity: restlessness, excitement, and nervousness.

Respiratory and circulatory depression are likely to appear in the very young and the elderly, as well as when the IV preparation is given too rapidly or when anileridine is administered concomitantly with other respiratory depressants.

Check rate and depth of respiration before administering drug and again during peak plasma levels (1 to 2 hours). Severe respiratory depression may be overlooked, since tidal volume rather than respiratory rate may be affected. Withhold drug and report to physician if respiration is shallow.

Carefully aspirate before subcutaneous and intramuscular administration in order to avoid intravenous injection. Sudden intravenous injection of a dose larger than 10 mg may result in hypotension, apnea, and cardiac arrest.

Subcutaneous administration is more likely to produce local irritation than the intramuscular route.

A narcotic antagonist (eg, naloxone) and facilities for oxygen administration and control of respiration should be available if anileridine is being given intravenously.

Sudden discontinuation of long-term therapy may initiate withdrawal symptoms similar to the meperidine pattern.

Ambulatory patients should be warned to avoid driving or other hazardous activities while under the effects of the drug.

Anileridine is reportable as a narcotic under provisions of Schedule II of the federal Controlled Substances Act.

Anileridine shares with narcotic analgesics toxic potential for addiction and abuse. Usual precautions of narcotic therapy should be followed: evaluation of need, careful monitoring of response, record-keeping, and reporting.

Protect drug from light.

See Meperidine Hydrochloride.

 LABORATORY TEST INTERFERENCES: May produce false positive VMA (Gitlow method).

ANISINDIONE, N.F.
(MIRADON)

Anticoagulant

ACTIONS AND USES

Long-acting indandione derivative. Similar to coumarin anticoagulants in actions, uses, contraindications, precautions, and adverse reactions, but with potentially greater spectrum of adverse effects. See Warfarin.

ABSORPTION AND FATE

Readily absorbed from GI tract. Peak prothrombin time effect in 48 to 72 hours; effects may persist up to 3 days after cessation of therapy. Considerable differences in individual absorption and metabolism rates. Almost completely bound to plasma proteins. Metabolized by liver. Excreted primarily in urine as metabolites. Crosses placenta and may pass into breast milk.

ADVERSE REACTIONS

Potential for agranulocytosis, jaundice, nephropathy, diarrhea, urticaria, fever. Also see Warfarin.

ROUTE AND DOSAGE

Oral: initially, 300 mg on first day, 200 mg on second day, 100 mg on third day. Maintenance: 25 to 250 mg daily. Dosages based on prothrombin time determinations and clinical findings.

NURSING IMPLICATIONS

During period of dosage adjustment, prothrombin time results should be checked daily by physician, and a dose order should be obtained.

When patient is controlled on maintenance dose, prothrombin times may be prescribed semiweekly, weekly, or at 2- to 4-week intervals, depending on uniformity of patient's response.

Periodic blood studies and liver function tests advised for patients on prolonged therapy. Urine should be checked regularly for albumin and blood.

Advise patient to report immediately the onset of fever, chills, sore throat or mouth, marked fatigue, jaundice, or any other unusual signs or symptons.

Metabolites of anisindione may impart a harmless red orange color to alkaline urine. Alert patient to this possibility. Acidification of urine causes color to disappear (preliminary test for differentiating it from hematuria).

See Warfarin.

ANTHRALIN, U.S.P.
(ANTHRA-DERM, LASAN POMADE)
DITHRANOL, B.P.

Antipsoriatic

ACTIONS AND USES

Similar to chrysarobin in physical properties, but reported to be effective in lower concentrations, less irritating to skin and kidney, and less prone to discolor skin and clothing.

Used in treatment of psoriasis, ringworm infections, and other chronic dermatoses.

ABSORPTION AND FATE
Absorbed from skin and excreted partly as chrysophanic acid and unchanged drug.

CONTRAINDICATIONS AND PRECAUTIONS
Renal disease; applications to acute eruptions or where inflammation is present or to face, scalp, genitalia, or intertriginous areas.

ADVERSE REACTIONS
Renal irritation (casts, albuminuria), erythema of adjacent normal skin, pustular folliculitis, temporary staining of skin and hair.

ROUTE AND DOSAGE
Usually weakest concentration is first employed, and strength is then increased according to patient's tolerance and response. Topical (ointment, oil, liquid) 0.1% to 0.4%. Lasan pomade (manufacturer's directions): massage into scalp at bedtime and remove in morning with tar shampoo.

NURSING IMPLICATIONS

Consult physician about procedure for cleansing skin before applying medication. Ointments and oils do not permit evaporation from skin surfaces; with continued applications, without intermittent cleansing, moisture and desquamated epidermis are trapped and may cause maceration.

Some physicians recommend removing anthralin ointment with mineral and a tub bath after 4 to 8 hours and to follow with controlled exposure to ultraviolet light, once or twice a day.

Care must be taken when applying medication to avoid normal skin, acute eruptions, or inflamed skin. Wear a finger cot or plastic glove or use a tongue depressor to apply the preparation, and wash hands thoroughly after completing treatment.

Nonocclusive bandages may be used. Stockinette may help to keep anthralin off normal skin. It is also used effectively to cover limbs and trunk to avoid staining outer clothing.

Avoid getting anthralin into the eyes. The drug is a powerful ocular irritant and can cause severe conjunctivitis and corneal opacities.

For excessive scalp scaliness, physician may prescribe warm olive oil massage and hot wet towel turban to head prior to shampoo. After shampoo, scale removal can be facilitated by use of fine tooth comb through hair.

Since some patients are hypersensitive to anthralin, it is advisable to make a preliminary test for sensitivity on a small area of skin. It is reported that red-haired individuals may be particularly sensitive to the drug.

Treatment should be discontinued if skin irritation or pustular folliculitis occurs. Folliculitis is most likely to appear in hairy areas.

Weekly urine tests are recommended to determine evidence of renal irritation.

Anthralin may impart a temporary yellowish brown discoloration to skin, hair, and alkaline urine. It may also stain clothing.

Salicylic acid ointment (4 to 5%) has been prescribed by some physicians to peel off pigment left by medication.

Anthralin therapy is generally continued for 2 to 4 weeks.

Psychologic effects of psoriasis on the patient and family members can be especially severe. Direct relationship between stressful situations and flares of psoriasis has been emphasized by some investigators.

Preserved in tightly covered containers, protected from light.

ANTIHEMOPHILIC FACTOR (HUMAN), U.S.P.
(AHF, AHG, Factor VIII, FACTORATE, HEMOFIL, HUMAFAC, KOATE, PROFILATE)

Antihemophilic

ACTIONS AND USES
Stable lyophilized concentrate of human antihemophilic factor obtained from fresh normal human plasma. Antihemophilic factor is essential in the body for conversion of prothrombin to thrombin in blood clotting and for maintaining effective hemostasis.
Used in treatment of hemophilia A when deficiency of factor VIII has been demonstrated, as well as in patients with acquired circulating factor VIII inhibitors.
ABSORPTION AND FATE
Following intravenous administration, rapidly cleared from plasma. Half-life reported to range from 4 to 24 hours. Does not readily cross placenta.
ADVERSE REACTIONS
Headache, flushing, tachycardia, paresthesias, nausea, vomiting, back pains, fever, urticaria, hypotension, clouding or loss of consciousness, disturbed vision, feeling of chest constriction, viral hepatitis, jaundice; intravascular hemolysis (when large volumes given to patients of blood group A, B, or AB).
ROUTE AND DOSAGE
Intravenous: Dosages are highly individualized according to weight of patient, severity of bleeding, and coagulation studies.

NURSING IMPLICATIONS
Expiration date should be checked carefully.
Concentrate and diluent bottles should be warmed to room temperature before reconstitution.
Following the addition of diluent to the vial, rotate gently until concentrate is completely dissolved. Vial should not be shaken vigorously. Administer within 2 hours after reconstitution. Do not refrigerate after reconstitution as precipitation may occur.
Check vital signs before IV administration and monitor following drug injection.
Bear in mind that the preparation may contain the causative agents of homologous serum hepatitis.
Unopened vials should be stored in refrigerator until ready for use.

ANTIMONY POTASSIUM TARTRATE, U.S.P., B.P.
(TARTAR EMETIC)

Antischistosomal

ACTIONS AND USES
Trivalent antimony compound chemically similar to arsenic. Precise parasiticidal action not known. Powerful emetic action due to irritation of gastric mucosa, but in toxic doses emesis is also produced by stimulation of chemoreceptor trigger zone in medulla.
Used primarily in treatment of *Schistosoma japonicum*. Used also for granuloma inguinale and mycosis fungoides. Because of toxicity, use as an emetic and expectorant has largely been replaced by other drugs.

ABSORPTION AND FATE

Rapidly bound to erythrocytes following intravenous administration. Slow renal excretion. Following a single dose, 10% may be recovered in urine within 24 hours, and about 30% within 1 week. Still detectable in urine for about 100 days after drug is discontinued.

CONTRAINDICATIONS AND PRECAUTIONS

Renal, hepatic, or cardiac insufficiency; febrile conditions other than those caused by *Schistosoma;* concomitant administration of other heavy metals; antiemetics (may mask warning symptoms of nausea and vomiting).

ADVERSE REACTIONS

Cough (common), nausea, vomiting, diarrhea, abdominal colic, headache, facial edema, skin rash, diaphoresis, pneumonia, dyspnea, apnea, depressed hepatic function, jaundice, hepatitis, albuminuria, phlebitis (IV site), joint and muscle pain, acute arthritis, fever, chills, vertigo, syncope, shock syndrome, EKG changes, marked bradycardia, cardiac standstill, anaphylactoid response, thrombocytopenic purpura, hemolytic anemia.

ROUTE AND DOSAGE

Intravenous: initial dose of 40 mg repeated every 2 days, with dose increase of 20 mg until 140 mg is reached; then 140 mg every other day to a total of 2 Gm. Administer slowly through fine needle. Usually given as 0.5% to 1% solution in sterile water for injection, normal saline, or saline-dextrose solution.

NURSING IMPLICATIONS

Preparation is administered by a physician and is usually given 2 hours after a light meal.

Paroxysms of coughing occur in most patients following intravenous injection, but they usually subside within a few minutes.

Patient must be closely observed while receiving this toxic drug. Margin between toxicity and therapeutic safety is narrow. Have the antidote dimercaprol (BAL) immediately available.

Following injection, patient should remain recumbent for 1 hour or longer if necessary. Monitor vital signs.

Drug is a powerful tissue irritant; extravasation into perivascular tissues can cause necrosis. Observe injection sites.

Instruct patient to refrain from vigorous exercise during drug therapy. Many patients show EKG changes; these may persist for 2 months after treatment is completed. These changes are apparently not associated with permanent cardiac injury.

Nausea and vomiting may indicate hepatotoxicity and should be reported promptly.

Joint and muscle pain and bradycardia occur most commonly near end of a course of treatment. Vital signs should be monitored during entire course of therapy.

Depressed hepatic function is not uncommon during drug therapy and may persist for several months after cessation of treatment. Periodic hepatic function tests should be performed.

APOMORPHINE HYDROCHLORIDE, B.P., N.F.

Emetic

ACTIONS AND USES

Prepared by treating morphine with dilute hydrochloric acid. Retains ability to produce CNS excitation and depression. Stimulant action on chemoreceptor trigger zone is markedly increased. Depresses medullary center that controls respiration and vasomotor tone and stimulates salivation. Elevates plasma levels of human growth hormone and reduces serum prolactin levels by stimulating dopamine receptors. Reduces tremor and rigidity in parkinsonism. Has sedative and hypnotic action in small nonemetic doses.

Primary therapeutic use is to produce emesis, particularly after oral ingestion of poisons.

ABSORPTION AND FATE

Vomiting occurs within 15 minutes following SC injection; sedative effect occurs within a few minutes and persists about 2 hours.

CONTRAINDICATIONS AND PRECAUTIONS

Hypersensitivity to morphine derivatives; after ingestion of corrosive substances or petroleum distillates; inebriated patients; shock; in narcosis due to alcohol, barbiturates, opiates, and other CNS depressants. Cautious use: children, elderly and debilitated patients, cardiac decompensation.

ADVERSE REACTIONS

Salivation, lacrimation, perspiration, weakness, dizziness, drowsiness, orthostatic hypotension, fainting; CNS stimulation (euphoria, restlessness, tremors, polypnea); respiratory depression (with large doses). Overdosage: violent and persistent vomiting, retching, CNS depression, muscular weakness, irregular and rapid respirations, tachycardia, coma, acute circulatory failure, reversible renal damage.

ROUTE AND DOSAGE

Subcutaneous: **Adults and Children**: 0.07 to 0.1 mg/kg in one dose. Do not repeat.

NURSING IMPLICATIONS

Physicians may give the adult patient 200 to 300 ml of water or preferably evaporated milk immediately before injection to induce more efficient emesis. Smaller amounts of liquid are recommended for the small child. Emetic effect may be enhanced by gently bouncing the child.

Vomiting occurs in about 5 minutes and may be preceded by salivation and nausea. When vomiting ceases, patient usually falls into a profound sleep.

Some physicians recommend giving activated charcoal before apomorphine or follow apomorphine with activated charcoal after vomiting is completed.

Monitor vital signs closely for at least 2 hours after drug administration.

Have on hand equipment for gastric lavage, suction, respiratory assistance, naloxone (narcotic antagonist), and atropine (for treatment of cardiac depression).

Classified as Schedule II drug under federal Controlled Substances Act.

Apomorphine deteriorates with age and on exposure to light and air. Solutions that are green or brown or otherwise discolored or that contain a precipitate should not be used. Note expiration date of prepared solutions of apomorphine.

AROMATIC AMMONIA SPIRIT, N.F.

Respiratory inhalant

ACTIONS AND USES

Stimulates respiratory and vasomotor centers in medulla reflexly by peripheral irritation of sensory receptors in nasal membrane, mucosa of esophagus, and fundus of stomach. Also acts as an antacid and carminative.

ROUTE AND DOSAGE

Inhalation of vapors as required. Oral: 2 to 4 ml well diluted with water.

NURSING IMPLICATIONS
For inhalation, also available in single dose glass vials (pearls) covered with woven fabric. Wrap in gauze or cloth and crush between fingers.
Preserved in tight, light-resistant containers in a cool place.

ASCORBATE SODIUM, U.S.P.
(CENOLATE, CEVITA, C-JECT, LIQUI-CEE)
ASCORBIC ACID, U.S.P.
(ASCOR, ASCORBICAP, BEST C, C-LONG, CEBID, CECON, CEMILL, CETANE, CEVALIN, CEVI-BID, CE-VI-SOL, Cevitamic Acid, SARO-C, Vitamin C)

Antiscorbutic vitamin

ACTIONS AND USES
Naturally occurring water-soluble vitamin essential for synthesis and maintenance of collagen and intercellular ground substance and thus for adequate wound healing. Powerful antioxidant essential to many enzymatic activities. Functions in carbohydrate metabolism, and in the conversion of folic acid (folacin) to folinic acid (leucovorin), the metabolism of phenylalanine and tyrosine, the reduction of plasma transferrin to liver ferritin, the formation of serotonin, and in maintenance of vascular tone.
Specific therapeutic use: prophylaxis and treatment of scurvy. Also used to enhance intestinal absorption of iron, for treatment of methemoglobinemia, to promote tissue healing, and in a wide variety of malnutrition, deficiency, and hemorrhagic states.

ABSORPTION AND FATE
Readily absorbed following oral or parenteral administration; distributed to all body tissues, with highest concentrations in glandular tissue. Limited body storage. Excess amounts excreted chiefly in urine.

CONTRAINDICATIONS AND PRECAUTIONS
Use of ascorbate sodium in patients on sodium restriction.
Cautious use: excessive doses in patients with glucose-6-phosphate dehydrogenase (G6PD) deficiency, patients prone to gout and crystalluria, and during pregnancy.

ADVERSE REACTIONS
Hemolytic anemia in certain patients with deficiency of G6PD; decreased urine urobilinogen excretion. With excessive oral doses: diarrhea, high acidification of urine, and possibly crystalluria. IV administration: mild soreness at injection site; dizziness and temporary faintness with rapid administration.

ROUTE AND DOSAGE
Oral, parenteral (therapeutic): **Adults**: 300 mg to 1 Gm or more daily in divided doses; (prophylactic): 50 to 150 mg daily in divided doses. **Infants** (therapeutic): 100 to 300 mg daily; (prophylactic): 30 mg daily, in divided doses.

NURSING IMPLICATIONS
Minimum daily requirement of vitamin C to prevent scurvy is 10 mg. Recommended adult daily dietary allowance is 45 mg; during pregnancy, 60 mg; during lactation, 80 mg; for children 4 to 6 years: 40 mg.
Vitamin C requirements are significantly increased in conditions that elevate metabolic rate, eg, hyperthyroidism, fever, infection, burns and other severe trauma, postoperative states, and neoplastic disease.
Infants fed on cow's milk alone require supplemental vitamin C. A daily dose of 35 mg has been recommended for infants during first week of life if

formula contains 2 to 3 times the amount of protein found in human milk.

Smokers appear to oxidize and excrete ascorbic acid at a greater rate than nonsmokers; therefore they require a higher intake of the vitamin.

Subclinical vitamin C deficiency may exist in persons who subsist on diets low in fruits and vegetables; particularly vulnerable are the indigent, the elderly, food faddists, alcoholics, patients on restricted therapeutic diets, and those receiving prolonged intravenous fluids without adequate supplementation.

Symptoms of vitamin C deficiency include general debility, pallor, anorexia, sensitivity to touch, limb and joint pain, follicular hyperkeratosis, easy bruising, petechiae, bloody diarrhea, delayed wound healing, loosening of teeth, and sensitive, swollen, bleeding gums.

Most fruits and vegetables contain vitamin C, but the highest levels are found in citrus fruits, strawberries, guava, leafy vegetables, cantaloupes, tomatoes, potatoes, green peppers, and parsley. A 6-ounce glass of juice from the fruit of the acerola tree or Puerto Rican cherry yields about 8650 mg of vitamin C, approximately 85 times as much as an equal amount of orange juice.

Further studies are needed to determine the true value of ascorbic acid in the prevention of atherosclerosis and in the prophylaxis or treatment of the common cold.

Vitamin C is easily oxidized when exposed to air, light, and heat. Large losses can occur from storage of fruit juices in uncovered containers, from prolonged cooking, from addition of sodium bicarbonate to foods, and from contact with copper and iron utensils.

LABORATORY TEST INTERFERENCES: False negative results for urine glucose when glucose oxidase methods are used (eg, Clinitest, Tes-Tape; apparently less likely with Diastix). Reportedly, false negative results may be avoided by dipping only a portion of the test patch and by taking reading in area wet by diffusion or at margin of wet and dry tape. Patients taking high doses of vitamin C may show false positive results using Benedict's solution or Clinitest tablets. False increase: serum uric acid determinations when not done by enzymatic methods. Interference with urinary steroid (17-hydroxycorticosteroids) determinations by modified Reddy-Jenkin-Thorn procedure. Possibility of false positive tests for occult blood in stool.

DRUG INTERACTIONS: Large doses of ascorbic acid or its salts may increase possibility of crystalluria with **aminosalicylic acid** and **sulfonamides** and may enhance the effects of **salicylates** by increasing their renal tubular reabsorption; and may decrease the effects of **amphetamines** and **tricyclic antidepressants** by decreasing their renal tubular reabsorption.

ASPIRIN, U.S.P., B.P.

(Acetylsalicylic Acid, A.S.A., ASPERGUM, DECAPRIN, ECOTRIN)

Analgesic, antipyretic, antirheumatic

ACTIONS AND USES

Salicylate with antipyretic, analgesic, antiinflammatory, antirheumatoid effects. Precise mechanisms of action not clear. Fever reduced by action on hypothalamus and possibly by interference with formation and release of leukocytic pyrogen. Heat loss increased by vasodilation of skin blood vessels and capillaries, increased cutaneous blood flow, and marked sweating. Suggested mechanisms of analgesic action include interference with pain reception or transmission at peripheral chemoreceptors, change in water balance to reduce edema, selective depression of CNS at subcortical level, placebo effect. Antiinflammatory and antirheumatoid actions possibly due to reduction of capillary permeability or to inhibited synthesis of prostaglandins E_2 and E_{2a}. Inhibits platelet aggregation and, in large doses, reduces plasma prothrombin levels. Urinary excretion of urates is enhanced by large doses of aspirin; paradoxically, urate excretion is decreased with small doses. Has hypocholesterolemic and hypoglycemic activity in large doses.

Used to relieve circumscribed and widespread pain of low to moderate intensity. Relieves headache and other discomforts of common cold, reduces fever in selected febrile conditions, and acts as analgesic and antiinflammatory agent in palliative treatment of arthritic diseases. Largely replaced as a uricosuric by other agents.

ABSORPTION AND FATE

Rapidly absorbed from stomach and intestinal tract. Rate of absorption dependent on drug preparation, gastric emptying time, pH of absorptive area. Coadministration of alkaline salt modifies solubility and increases absorption rate and renal clearance. Detectable in plasma 30 minutes after administration; peak plasma level in 1 to 2 hours, maintained 4 to 6 hours. Rapid distribution to most body fluids (including saliva, synovial fluid) and tissues, including brain and skeletal muscle. Metabolized chiefly by liver microsomes. Circadian excretion rhythm has been reported. At low doses 50% of dose is excreted in 2 to 4 hours (high doses, 15 to 30 hours) in urine as salicylic acid and conjugates. Prolonged action and cumulative effects occur with kidney and liver dysfunction. Crosses placenta and may be excreted in breast milk.

CONTRAINDICATIONS AND PRECAUTIONS

Salicylate sensitivity, history or existence of gastric ulcer, hemorrhage, erosive gastritis, bleeding disorders, vitamin K deficiency, anemia or predisposition to anemia, infants under 1 year of age. Cautious use: aural diseases, asthma, nasal polyps, allergies, children with fever combined with dehydration; G6PD deficiency, Hodgkin's disease, acute severe carditis, patients undergoing surgery.

ADVERSE REACTIONS

Occasionally, nausea, vomiting, GI bleeding, heartburn, skin eruptions, hypoglycemia, hypoprothrombinemia, and sensitivity (aspirin triad: vasomotor rhinitis, asthma, nasal polyps). **Mild intoxication** (large doses and/or prolonged therapy): salicylism (mental confusion, nausea, vomiting, occasional diarrhea, hyperventilation, high-pitched tinnitus, deafness, headache, dizziness, dimmed vision, fever, flushing, sweating, thirst, tachycardia, lassitude, drowsiness); anorexia, decreased protein-bound iodine (PBI), increased plasma prothrombin time, prolonged bleeding time, iron-deficiency anemia, thrombocytopenic purpura (rare), and elevations in serum amylase, SGOT, SGPT, and serum CO_2. **Marked intoxication**: respiratory alkalosis, metabolic acidosis, nephropathy, ketosis, hyponatremia, hypokalemia, acute pancreatitis, hepatotoxicity, CNS stimulation (salicylic jag: resembles alcoholic inebriation, but without euphoria), delirium, coma, oliguria, death.

ROUTE AND DOSAGE

Oral, rectal suppository: **Adults**: 325 to 650 mg (5 to 10 grains) every 3 to 4 hours if necessary. (Antiinflammatory): 2.6 to 7.8 Gm daily in divided doses. **Children**: 65 mg/kg/24 hours in divided doses every 6 hours.

NURSING IMPLICATIONS

May be administered with food, milk, antacids (if prescribed), or with full glass of water to reduce GI side effects.

Dyspepsia sometimes eliminated simply by changing brand of aspirin.

Fairly constant salicylate plasma levels can usually be maintained by 4- to 6-hour spacing of therapeutic doses. Impress on the patient the importance of adhering to scheduled rather than prn dosage if antiinflammatory effect is to be maintained.

In treatment of acute rheumatic fever the physician may prescribe daily dose increases of 1 or 2 tablets per day until therapeutic response occurs or until tinnitus supervenes (sign of early toxicity). Warn patient that this symptom indicates the need for change in dosage. Tinnitus is often eliminated after a dosage reduction of as little as 325 mg (5 grains).

Patients receiving repetitious or large doses of aspirin should be advised to observe for petechiae, bleeding gums, gastric bleeding (melena), and to maintain adequate fluid intake to prevent salicylate crystalluria (consult physician). Periodic hemoglobin and prothrombin tests are indicated. Inform patient that urine may be green-brown in color (due to high salicylate and related metabolite levels).

Schedule physical therapy or planned exercise at least 30 minutes after a therapeutic dose of aspirin, in order to keep discomfort at a minimum.

Aspirin in chewing gum has no local effect; relief of sore throat or toothache is a systemic response.

Prolonged use of high doses can lead to iron-deficiency anemia, especially in women. Average fecal blood loss in normal individuals is 0.5 ml/day. Average blood loss with daily use of several aspirin tablets may be as much as 4 to 5 ml. In 10% of patients on chronic high dosage, blood loss may reach 80 ml/day. Periodic stool examinations for melena is an important diagnostic measure.

Accidental ingestion of salicylates is one of the most common causes of poisoning in young children. Caution patient to keep drug out of reach of children.

Children on high doses of aspirin are particularly prone to develop hypoglycemia. The child diabetic must be monitored carefully for indicated need of insulin adjustment.

Patients with asthma and nasal polyps demonstrate a high frequency of salicylate sensitivity. Caution patient to read labels of all over-the-counter drugs. There are over 500 aspirin-containing compounds.

Hearing loss (dose-related) is generally characterized by bilateral symmetric loss of 30 to 40 decibels. Usually the loss is completely reversible within 7 to 10 days after withdrawal of aspirin.

No guarantee on the basis of previous safety in taking aspirin can be assumed. Subsequent sensitivity to salicylates, especially aspirin, is not uncommon.

Salicylate intoxication requires prompt emesis or gastric lavage, intensive supportive therapy, including fluids and electrolytes, blood transfusion, artificial ventilation, and oxygen. Hemodialysis in adults, peritoneal dialysis in children, and exchange transfusions in infants may be required.

Reduction of fever with aspirin may obscure patient's illness; self-medication for this purpose without medical supervision should be discouraged.

All brands of aspirin must pass the U.S.P. standard disintegration test (5 minutes). Brands differ in the binder used and moisture content of product. Extensive studies suggest that inexpensive aspirin is as effective as the more expensive preparations.

Most aspirin tablets develop a hard external shell with age. While this does not change the active ingredient, it does increase disintegration time and thus delays the onset of therapeutic action.

Available evidence fails to indicate that buffered aspirin tablets produce faster analgesia or less irritating effects than plain aspirin; however, buffering does increase rate of dissolution and thus may reduce gastric bleeding.

When compared with plain aspirin, buffered aspirin in effervescent preparations (eg, Alka-Seltzer) has a more rapid rate of absorption, results in a higher plasma level of salicylate, and causes less gastric irritation and bleeding. However, repeated use causes alkaline urine and subsequent decrease in plasma levels. Additionally, it has a high sodium content (contains sodium bicarbonate and sodium citrate).

A.P.C., an over-the-counter combination of aspirin, phenacetin, and caffeine, is the most frequently used mixture of analgesic drugs; well-controlled clinical studies have proved that the combination of drugs is no better than aspirin alone.

At room temperature, aspirin tablets exposed to moisture, heat, and air may rapidly hydrolyze. Hydrolysis products may be detectable by an acetic odor. Discard the entire bottle of such tablets.

Store aspirin tablets in airtight containers.

LABORATORY TEST INTERFERENCES: Possibility of interference with urinary 5-hydroxyindoleacetic acid (fluorescent method), VMA, ketones (Gerhardt method), and PSP excretion, as well as a false increase in uric acid determinations (enzymatic method). In patients on moderate to large doses (eg, 2.4 to 5 Gm/day), false negative tests for urine glucose by glucose oxidase methods (eg, Clinistix, Tes-Tape) and false positive results with Clinitest may occur.

DRUG INTERACTIONS: Possibility of increased plasma salicylate concentrations with **para-aminobenzoic acid** and drugs that acidify urine (eg, **ammonium chloride, ascorbic acid**). **Alcohol** and **corticosteroids** may increase the incidence of GI ulceration and bleeding; corticosteroids may increase serum salicylate levels. Salicylates may increase **aminosalicylic acid** toxicity. **Phenylbutazone** inhibits uricosuric effects of large salicylate doses. Large doses of salicylates may enhance hypoprothrombinemic effects of **anticoagulants** and may increase plasma levels of **indomethacin, methotrexate, penicillin, phenytoin**, and **sulfonamides**. Salicylates enhance hypoglycemic response to **sulfonurea antidiabetic agents** and inhibit uricosuric effect of **probenecid** and **sulfinpyrazone**.

ATROPINE SULFATE, U.S.P., N.F., B.P.
(BUF-OPTO ATROPINE, ISOPTO ATROPINE)

Anticholinergic, mydriatic

ACTIONS AND USES

Tertiary amine derived from *Atropa belladonna.* Forms strong drug-receptor complex at cholinergic postganglionic receptor sites in smooth muscle, cardiac muscle, and exocrine glands, thereby blocking action of acetylcholine. Also interferes with action of acetylcholine in CNS and antagonizes action of 5-hydroxytryptamine (serotonin) and histamine. Blocks vagal impulses to heart with resulting acceleration of heart rate, increased cardiac output, and shortened P-R interval. Causes vasodilation of small blood vessels; has little effect on blood pressure. Produces selective depression of CNS to relieve rigidity and tremor of Parkinson's syndrome. Therapeutic doses increase respiration; large or toxic doses cause CNS stimulation. Reduces amplitude, tone, and frequency of smooth-muscle contractions; decreases sweating, lacrimation, and salivation, as well as bronchial mucus, gastric, and pancreatic secretions. Increases tone of urinary bladder sphincter. Systemic and local administrations produce mydriasis and cycloplegia.

Used in symptomatic treatment of peptic ulcer, pylorospasm, spasm of intestinal and biliary tracts, ureteral spasm, enuresis, Parkinson's syndrome, dysmenorrhea, anterior uveitis, iritis, and refraction. Also used to suppress salivation and perspiration, and to control respiratory tract secretions in infections, allergies, and during surgery. Used to counteract bradycardia induced by propranolol and organophosphorous insecticides, as antidote for Amanita mushroom poisoning, and as temporary measure to relieve carotid sinus hypersensitivity or heart block in selected patients with early myocardial infarction.

ABSORPTION AND FATE

Action begins in 1 to 2 hours and persists for about 4 hours. Well absorbed from all administration sites and widely distributed; crosses blood–brain and placental barriers. About 50% of dose rapidly excreted in urine within 4 hours, and remainder within 24 hours as unchanged drug and metabolites. Traces appear in breast milk.

CONTRAINDICATIONS AND PRECAUTIONS

Hypersensitivity, synechiae, glaucoma, parotitis, prostatic hypertrophy, paralytic ileus, pyloric stenosis, severe ulcerative colitis, tachycardia, arteriosclerosis, cardiac insufficiency and failure, chronic lung disease, asthma, myasthenia gravis, nursing mothers. Cautious use: hypertension, elderly and debilitated patients, children under 6 years of age.

ADVERSE REACTIONS

Xerostomia with thirst and dysphagia; bronchial plugging; headache, blurred vision, photophobia, mydriasis, cycloplegia, increased intraocular pressure, eye pain, dry and flushed skin, anhydrosis (atropine fever), drowsiness, vomiting, dizziness, lightheadedness, tachycardia, palpitation, urinary hesitancy or retention, constipation, paralytic ileus, allergic reactions. Excessive or toxic doses: rash (face and upper trunk), hypertension, restlessness, excitement, disorientation, delirium, hallucinations, hyperthermia, respiratory depression, death. Prolonged ophthalmic use: follicular conjunctivitis, edema, dermatitis.

ROUTE AND DOSAGE

Oral, subcutaneous, intramuscular, intravenous: **Adults**: 0.4 mg to 0.6 mg may be repeated every 4 to 6 hours. **Children**: 0.01 mg/kg may be repeated every 4 to 6 hours. Ophthalmic: ointment, solution (0.125 to 3%). Dosage adjusted to severity of condition.

NURSING IMPLICATIONS

Oral atrophine is usually given 30 minutes before meals.

Following parenteral administration, postural hypotension may occur if the patient ambulates too soon after drug is given.

Smaller doses of atropine are indicated for the elderly because of associated stress of atropine-produced tachycardia and because of the danger of mydriasis and increased intraocular pressure in this glaucoma-prone age group.

Atropine produces a weaker mydriatic effects in blacks.

Monitor vital signs. Be alert to changes in quality and rate of pulse and respiration. Initial paradoxic bradycardia following IV atropine may last 1 to 2 minutes.

If patient's mouth is dry, sugar-free chewing gum or hard candy may afford some relief. Reduction of dosage may be necessary.

Atropine may contribute to the problem of urinary retention. On initiation of therapy, establish a baseline of 24-hour urinary output, and monitor daily output thereafter; this is especially important in older patients and in patients who have had surgery. Have patient void before giving drug.

Increased fluid intake and increased bulk in the diet may help to overcome constipating effects of atropine.

Inform patient that drug may increase risk of heat stroke by suppressing perspiration (heat loss) and therefore to avoid excessive heat.

Advise patient to avoid hazardous activities if blurred vision, dizziness or drowsiness occur.

Intraocular tension should be determined before and during therapy with ophthalmic preparations.

Suggested technique for administering eye preparations: Instill drop of solution or ribbon of ointment into lower conjunctival fornix. Once drug is introduced, direct patient to close lids, without squeezing, while gentle pressure is applied to lacrimal duct for 1 minute. This method obstructs drug flow into lacrimal duct and thus helps to prevent systemic absorption.

Ophthalmic preparations should be discontinued if eye pain, conjunctivitis, palpitation, rapid pulse, or dizziness occurs.

Frequent and continued use of eye preparations, as well as overdosage, can produce peripheral symptoms of atropine toxicity.

Mydriatic action following topical application reaches a maximum in ½ hour and may persist 10 days; cycloplegia follows more slowly over 1 to 2 hours and may last as long as 5 days. Instruct patient to prepare for impaired acuity and to protect eyes by wearing dark glasses during drug action period.

Children with mongolism react more quickly and for longer periods of time than do normal children when a drop of atropine is placed in the eye.

Studies reveal that over one-half of atropine deaths have resulted from systemic absorption following ocular administration and have been in infants and children.

Pilocarpine and physostigmine are physiologic antidotes for atropine poisoning.

Protected in light-resistant containers.

DRUG INTERACTIONS: Possibility of additive anticholinergic effects with **MAO inhibitors, procainamide** (theoretically possible), and **quinidine.**

ATTAPULGITE, ACTIVATED
(CLAYSORB, QUINTESS)

Antidiarrheal

ACTIONS AND USES
Inert clay composed primarily of hydrous magnesium oxide. Claimed to be superior to kaolin as absorbent and adsorbent of certain alkaloids, bacteria, enteroviruses, and toxins. No adverse effects or known contraindications have been reported.

Used for symptomatic treatment of uncomplicated diarrhea.

ABSORPTION AND FATE
Not absorbed from GI tract.

ROUTE AND DOSAGE
Oral: initially, 2 to 4 Gm. Subsequent doses: 500 mg to 1 Gm after each bowel movement until diarrhea is controlled.

NURSING IMPLICATIONS
Prolonged use may interfere with intestinal absorption of nutrients and may cause constipation.

Replacement of fluids and electrolytes is a part of diarrhea therapy.

Attapulgite is a common ingredient of several commercially available antidiarrheal mixtures.

See Paregoric for patient teaching.

(Gold Thioglucose, SOLGANAL)

Antirheumatic

ACTIONS AND USES
   Water-soluble organic nonionizable preparation of approximately 50% gold. Mechanism of action unknown; major effect is reduction of inflammatory process in early arthritic disease, with no effect on reparative processes. Therapeutic usefulness restricted to treatment of active rheumatoid arthritis and nondisseminated lupus erythematosus.
ABSORPTION AND FATE
   Slow absorption from site of injection, with wide distribution to soft tissues, especially liver, spleen, kidneys, and skin. About 20% eliminated slowly in urine and feces; 80% remains in tissues for long periods. Cumulative effects easily result.
CONTRAINDICATIONS AND PRECAUTIONS
   Actinotherapy, severe diabetes, pregnancy, renal or hepatic insufficiency, marked hypertension, heart failure, tuberculosis, agranulocytic angina or its history, hemorrhagic diathesis, abnormalities of hematopoietic system, recent radiation therapy, urticaria, eczema, colitis.
ADVERSE REACTIONS
   Minor or moderate transient toxicity in nearly one-half of patients on chrysotherapy. Mucous membrane lesions (stomatitis, glossitis, vaginitis, gold bronchitis), erythema, pruritus, rash, exfoliative dermatitis, pigmentation (chrysiasis), Stevens-Johnson syndrome, aplastic anemia, agranulocytosis, thrombocytopenia, hemorrhagic diathesis, leukopenia, eosinophilia, headache, gastritis, diarrhea, colic, toxic hepatitis, acute yellow atrophy, polyneuritis.
ROUTE AND DOSAGE
   Intramuscular (suspension in sesame oil): **Adults**: 10 to 25 mg weekly for 3 weeks followed by 50 mg weekly until a total of 0.8 to 1 Gm is reached. Maintenance: 25 to 50 mg every 3 to 4 weeks. **Children** *6 to 12 years*: one-fourth of adult dose governed chiefly by body weight.

NURSING IMPLICATIONS
Hold vial horizontally and shake thoroughly to suspend active material. Heating vial to body temperature facilitates withdrawing medication. Needle and syringe must be dry. Inject solution deep into gluteal muscle. An 18-gauge 1½-inch needle is recommended (for obese patients, 2-inch needle may be used).
Patient should remain recumbent for ½ hour after injection to overcome possible dizziness.
Examination and interview of patient before each injection are essential to detect earliest signs of gold toxicity (pruritus, sore mouth, indigestion, dermatitis, jaundice).
During early treatment phase a urinalysis should be done prior to each injection to detect presence of proteinuria and microscopic hematuria; both are early signs of nephropathy and indicate the need to discontinue therapy.
Complete blood counts and urinalyses should be performed every 2 weeks throughout therapy.
Pruritus is usually a first sign of gold toxicity. Combination of pruritus and fine morbilliform rash, often on neck and extremities, may necessitate discontinuation of treatment. Occasionally rash disappears spontaneously in several days. Caution patient to avoid exposure to sunlight.
Persistent dermatitis may require vigorous treatment with steroids or penicil-

lamine therapy to prevent scratching and attendant inflammatory reaction.

Some patients develop a gray-to-blue pigmentation of mucous membranes and light-exposed skin areas.

Toxic effects are not always dose-related and may persist for months after termination of drug treatment.

A metallic taste frequently precedes painful ulceration of mouth.

Treatment of stomatitis: Use soft tooth brush or gauze-covered finger to clean teeth after meals. Rinse mouth frequently with warm water or warm tea. Sometimes hydrogen peroxide 1:1 is ordered (solution should be made immediately before use). Avoid commercial mouth rinses, hard or dry food, and fruit juices high in citric acid, as well as smoking and alcohol. Meticulous nonirritating mouth hygiene is essential.

Epistaxis, gum bleeding, and petechiae are signs of hematopoietic system toxicity and call for immediate termination of aurothioglucose.

Instruct patient to report promptly early signs of infection that may indicate onset of agranulocytosis: overpowering weakness, malaise, chills, fever, sore mouth or throat, dysphagia.

Inform any patient with arthritis who is on intermittent therapy that the number of aspirin tablets taken for analgesia is an important indication of diminishing response to gold therapy. The physician will want to know about this when deciding the time to begin another regimen of gold.

After a course of gold therapy most patients with rheumatoid arthritis are better for as long as a year. Patients who respond positively may be given another series of injections in a year.

Resumption of therapy after drug discontinuation because of toxicity should be gradual and well monitored.

Specific antidote for severe reaction to aurothioglucose is dimercaprol (BAL).

Stored in tight, light-resistant container at room temperature.

AZATHIOPRINE, U.S.P., B.P.
(IMURAN)

Antineoplastic, immunosuppressive

ACTIONS AND USES

Antimetabolite and cytotoxic purine antagonist. Converted in vivo to mercaptopurine (qv). Precise mechanism of action not determined. Appears to interfere with nucleic acid synthesis in proliferating cells; also thought to inhibit coenzyme function. Produces severe and irreversible immunosuppression; maximum effectiveness occurs during induction period of antibody response.

Principal use is as adjunctive agent to prevent rejection of renal homotransplant. Use for immunologic conditions other than kidney transplant is investigational.

ABSORPTION AND FATE

See Mercaptopurine.

CONTRAINDICATIONS AND PRECAUTIONS

Hypersensitivity to drug, clinically active infection, pregnancy, women of childbearing potential. Cautious use: impaired kidney and liver function.

ADVERSE REACTIONS

Serum sickness, infection, pancreatitis, toxic hepatitis, muscle wasting, arthralgia, retinopathy, Raynaud's disease, alopecia, pulmonary edema, oral lesions, rash. See Mercaptopurine.

Oral, intravenous (highly individualized on basis of clinical response and hematopoietic toxicity): initially, 3 to 5 mg/kg body weight daily; maintenance 1 to 2 mg/kg/day.

NURSING IMPLICATIONS

IV preparation usually given during first 24 to 96 hours after renal homotransplantation. A shift to oral preparation is made as soon as patient can tolerate it.

Azathioprine therapy is usually instituted 1 to 5 days before kidney transplantation.

Dosage is adjusted to maintain homograft without producing toxicity. If WBC count descends to 3000/mm³ the drug is discontinued.

Close medical supervision both in and out of hospital is necessary during therapy. The patient should understand toxicity potential, as well as expected benefits.

Azathioprine dosage is reduced by approximately one-fourth to one-third when allopurinol is given concurrently.

Kidney clearance of drug should be monitored to prevent accumulation. Surveillance of intake–output ratio is crucial. Up to a twofold increase in toxicity is possible in anephric or anuric patients.

Complete blood counts (including platelets) and liver and kidney function tests should be performed at least weekly (more frequently during initiation of therapy) for first 4 to 6 weeks and every 2 to 3 weeks theraf-ter.

Thrombocytopenia occurs less commonly than leukopenia; however, be alert to signs of abnormal bleeding (purpura, melena, epistaxis, hemoptysis, hematemesis).

If hepatic dysfunction occurs (clay-colored stools, dark urine, pruritus, yellow skin and sclera) report promptly. Another antineoplastic agent may be substituted.

Clinical effects of azathioprine appear within 2 to 4 days of administration.

Bland foods in small amounts with antiemetic drugs help diminish nausea and vomiting. Decreased fruit juice intake may reduce diarrhea. Consult physician.

Intercurrent infection is a constant hazard of immunosuppressive therapy. Warn patient to avoid contact with persons with colds or other infections and to report signs of impending infection (coryza, fever, sore throat, malaise). Personal hygiene should be scrupulous. Azathioprine dosage may be reduced until the infection is controlled by appropriate therapy.

Hospitalized patient may be on reverse isolation; explain significance to patient and family.

Patients should be advised to practice birth control during azathioprine therapy and for 4 months after discontinuation.

Preserved in tightly closed, light-resistant containers.

Also see Mercaptopurine.

DRUG INTERACTIONS: **Allopurinol** impairs conversion to inactive products; therefore it increases azathioprine toxicity.

BACITRACIN, U.S.P., B.P.
(BACIGUENT)

Antibacterial, antibiotic

ACTIONS AND USES
Polypeptide antibiotic containing a thiazolidine ring structure. Derived from cultures of *Bacillus subtilis.* Precise mechanism of action not known; appears to interfere with function of bacterial cell membrane by suppressing cell-wall and protein synthesis. Spectrum of antibacterial activity similar to that of penicillin. Bactericidal against many Gram-positive organisms including streptococci, staphylococci, pneumococci, corynebacteria, and clostridia. Also active against gonococci and meningococci; ineffective against most Gram-negative organisms. Has neuromuscular blocking action.

Used for treatment of infections due to susceptible organisms. Parenteral therapy restricted to infants with staphylococcal pneumonia and empyema due to susceptible organisms where adequate laboratory facilities and constant supervision are available.

ABSORPTION AND FATE
Following intramuscular injection, rapidly and completely absorbed. Maximal bactericidal plasma concentrations in 1 to 2 hours, with duration of action 6 to 8 hours. Widely distributed in body and in ascitic and pleural fluids. Only traces in cerebrospinal fluid, unless meninges are inflamed. Slow renal excretion; 10% to 40% of single dose excreted within 24 hours.

CONTRAINDICATIONS AND PRECAUTIONS
Previous hypersensitivity or toxic reaction to bacitracin; impaired renal function.

ADVERSE REACTIONS
Systemic effects: anorexia, nausea, vomiting, diarrhea, tinnitus, peculiar taste sensations, nephrotoxicity: frequent urination, oliguria, anuria, albuminuria, cylinduria, hematuria, increased blood urea nitrogen (BUN), uremia. Hypersensitivity reactions (urticaria, skin rashes, tightness of chest, hypotension). Also reported: pain and inflammation at injection site, superinfection, neuromuscular weakness.

ROUTE AND DOSAGE
Intramuscular: **Infants** *under 2.5 kg:* 900 units/kg/24 hours in 2 or 3 divided doses; **Infants** *over 2.5 kg:* 1000 units/kg/24 hours in 2 or 3 divided doses. Topical: ointment (500 units/Gm) applied in thin layer to cleansed area 2 or 3 times a day, or as solution containing 250 to 1000 units/ml applied as wet dressing. Ophthalmic ointment (500 units/Gm).

NURSING IMPLICATIONS
Before systemic therapy is begun, determinations should be made of BUN and nonprotein nitrogen (NPN), and urine should be examined for albumin, casts, and cellular elements. Blood and urine values are monitored throughout therapy. Use for longer than 12 days not advised.

Parenteral solution should be dissolved in sodium chloride injection containing 2% procaine hydrochloride, since injections are painful. Concentration should be not less than 5000 units/ml nor more than 10,000 units/ml. Consult physician.

Monitor intake and output during parenteral therapy. Fluids should be forced to reduce possibility of renal toxicity. If fluid intake is inadequate and/or urinary output decreases, report to physician.

Inspect urine for turbidity and hematuria, and be on the alert for other signs and symptoms of urinary tract dysfunction.

As with other antibiotics, prolonged use of bacitracin may result in overgrowth of nonsusceptible organisms, especially *Candida albicans*.

Topical application can cause systemic effects if applied to large denuded areas.

Consult physician for guidelines for cleansing skin before reapplications of bacitracin.

Bacitracin solutions are stable for 1 week if refrigerated; deterioration occurs at room temperature.

DRUG INTERACTIONS: Manufacturer's warning: concurrent use of other nephrotoxic drugs, particularly **kanamycin, neomycin, polymyxin B, polymyxin E (colistin), streptomycin,** and **viomycin,** should be avoided. Bacitracin may enhance respiratory depression or prolong neuromuscular blockade in patients receiving **ether** and related anesthetics, and **tubocurarine** or other neuromuscular depressants.

BELLADONNA EXTRACT, N.F.
BELLADONNA TINCTURE, B.P., U.S.P.

Anticholinergic

ACTIONS AND USES

Prepared from *Atropa belladonna*. Similar to atropine in actions, precautions, and adverse reactions.

Used as adjuvant to control hypermotility associated with gastric, duodenal, or intestinal ulcers and to control hyperirritability or spasm in pylorospasm, spastic constipation, ulcerative colitis, and spasms of urinary tract. Commercially available in combination with phenobarbital.

ROUTE AND DOSAGE

Oral (belladonna extract): 15 mg 3 times a day; (belladonna tincture): 0.6 to 1 ml 3 or 4 times a day

NURSING IMPLICATIONS

When given for gastrointestinal hypermotility, these drugs are usually administered 30 to 60 minutes before meals.

Preserved in tight, light-resistant containers away from excessive heat.

See Atropine Sulfate.

BENDROFLUMETHIAZIDE, N.F.
(NATURETIN)
BENDROFLUAZIDE, B.P.

Diuretic (thiazide), antihypertensive

ACTIONS AND USES

Benzothiadiazine (thiazide) derivative. Similar to chlorothiazide (qv) in pharmacologic actions, uses, contraindications, precautions, and adverse reactions, but with longer duration of action. Does not appreciably alter serum electrolyte concentrations at recommended doses. Commercially available in fixed combination with potassium chloride (Naturetin W-K) and with rauwolfia serpentina and potassium chloride (Rautrax-N), and with rauwolfia serpentina alone (Rauzide).

Onset of diuretic effect in 1 to 2 hours; peaks between 6 and 12 hours and lasts 18 to 24 hours. See Chlorothiazide.

ROUTE AND DOSAGE

Oral (diuretic): initially 5 mg daily; may be increased to 20 mg daily as a single dose or in 2 divided doses. Maintenance at 2.5 to 5 mg daily or on alternate days; (antihypertensive): initially 5 to 20 mg daily, with maintenance at 2.5 to 15 mg daily. Highly individualized according to patient's requirements and response.

NURSING IMPLICATIONS

Long-acting diuretics are administered preferably in the morning to avoid nocturia and thus interruption of patient's sleep.

See Chlorothiazide.

BENOXINATE HYDROCHLORIDE, N.F. (DORSACAINE)

Anesthetic (topical)

ACTIONS AND USES

Benzoic acid ester chemically related to procaine. Exerts surface anesthesia of short duration and has slight bacteriostatic properties. Instillation into eye does not change size of pupil, reaction to light, or accommodation. Reportedly, prolonged use does not produce local or systemic toxicity.

Used for its short-acting local anesthetic effect in minor ophthalmologic procedures such as tonometry, gonioscopy, or removal of foreign bodies from cornea or for short operative procedures on cornea or conjunctiva.

CONTRAINDICATIONS AND PRECAUTIONS

Cautious use: patients with known allergies, cardiac disease, hyperthyroidism, open lesions.

ADVERSE REACTIONS

Occasionally: temporary stinging, burning, conjunctival erythema. Rarely: allergic corneal reaction. Prolonged use: corneal opacity with vision loss.

ROUTE AND DOSAGE

Topical instillation: 0.4% ophthalmic solution. For tonometry and other minor procedures: 1 or 2 drops in single instillations prior to procedure. Deep ophthalmic anesthesia: 2 drops at 90-second intervals for 3 instillations.

NURSING IMPLICATIONS

One drop instilled into conjunctival sac allows tonometry, gonioscopy or removal of foreign body within 60 seconds.

Three instillations at 90-second intervals produce sufficient anesthesia for short corneal and conjunctival procedures.

Protective eye patch is recommended following procedure.

Corneal reflex is fully restored in about 1 hour.

Caution patient to avoid touching eyes while protective reflexes are blocked.

BENZALKONIUM CHLORIDE, U.S.P., B.P. (ZEPHIRAN)

Antiinfective, topical

ACTIONS AND USES

Quaternary ammonium cationic surface-active agent. Solutions have low surface tension and demonstrate detergent, deodorant, keratolytic, wetting, and emulsifying actions. Bactericidal or bacteriostatic, depending on concentration. Probably acts by inhibiting bacterial respiration and glycolysis or by enzyme inactivation. Effective against Gram-positive and Gram-negative organisms, fungi, and protozoa, eg, *Trichomonas vaginalis*. Generally not active against spore-forming bacteria and viruses.

Used in appropriate dilutions for antisepsis of skin, mucous membranes, superficial injuries, and infected wounds, for irrigation of eye and body cavities, and to preserve sterility of instruments and utensils.

CONTRAINDICATIONS AND PRECAUTIONS

Use in occlusive dressings, casts, and anal or vaginal packs not advised. Used with caution for irrigation of body cavities.

ADVERSE REACTIONS

Few or no toxic effects in recommended dilutions. Erythema from long periods of contact or with higher concentrations; hypersensitivity (rarely). Systemic toxicity: nausea, vomiting, muscle weakness, restlessness, apprehension, confusion, dyspnea, cyanosis, collapse, convulsions, coma, respiratory paralysis.

ROUTE AND DOSAGE

Topical: aqueous solution, 1:40,000 to 1:750. Tinted or untinted tincture or spray: 1:750.

NURSING IMPLICATIONS

Action of cationic detergents is antagonized by organic matter, anionic compounds such as soaps and soap substitutes (eg, pHisoHex, pHisoderm), hard water, and certain chemicals (see list of incompatible substances below).

If red-tinted tincture turns yellow on application to patient's skin, there is usually a soap residue. Rinse skin thoroughly and dry it; then reapply the antiseptic.

Benzalkonium chloride solutions must be prepared, stored, and used correctly to achieve and maintain antiseptic action. Significant inactivation and contamination may occur with misuse.

The correct diluent for irrigating body cavities is sterile water for injection; for other irrigations fresh sterile distilled water is used. Tap water may contain metallic ions and organic matter that reduce antibacterial potency of benzalkonium chloride; therefore it should not be used.

For preoperative skin preparation, follow use of soap with thorough rinsing, first with water, then with 70% alcohol, before applying benzalkonium chloride. Avoid pooling and thus prolonged contact of solution with skin.

The tincture and spray preparations contain flammable solvents; they should not be used near an open flame or cautery. Keep away from eyes.

If solution stronger than 1:3000 enters the eyes, irrigate immediately and repeatedly with water, then see a physician promptly.

Solutions used on denuded skin or inflamed or irritated tissues should be more dilute than those used on normal tissue.

Do not reuse solutions in which porous materials such as gauze, applicators, cotton, plastic, or rubber have soaked. These materials adsorb benzalkonium chloride and thus reduce its concentration.

Cationic detergents are unreliable substitutes for heat sterilization of surgical instruments; however, they are sometimes used to preserve established sterility of instruments.

Prolonged contact of metal with benzalkonium chloride will result in corrosion unless antirust tablets are added to the solution. A prepared solution for instrument sterilization is available from pharmacy. The solution should be changed at least once a week.

Recommended treatment of accidental ingestion: immediate administration of several glasses of mild soap solution, milk, or egg whites beaten in water, followed by gastric lavage with mild soap solution. Avoid alcohol, as it promotes gastric absorption.

Substances potentially incompatible with benzalkonium chloride solutions: aluminum, caramel, citrates, fluorescein, iodine, kaolin, lanolin, nitrates, peroxide, pine oil, potassium permanganate, silver nitrate, zinc oxide, zinc sulfate, yellow oxide of mercury.

Stored in airtight containers, protected from light.

BENZESTROL, N.F.
(OCTOFOLLIN)

Estrogen

ACTIONS AND USES
Synthetic estrogen with actions, uses, contraindications, and adverse reactions similar to those of estradiol (qv).
ROUTE AND DOSAGE
Oral: 1 to 2 mg daily.

NURSING IMPLICATIONS
See Estradiol.

BENZOCAINE, N.F., B.P.
(AMERICAINE, AEROCAINE, BENZOCOL, BURNTAME, Ethyl Aminobenzoate, HURRICAINE, SOLARCAINE, UROLOCAINE, and others)

Anesthetic (topical)

ACTIONS AND USES
Ethyl ester of para-aminobenzoic acid. Produces anesthesia by inhibiting conduction of nerve impulses from sensory nerves. Differs from procaine in having low solubility; therefore it is slowly absorbed and has prolonged duration of action.
Used as local anesthetic to relieve pruritus and also surface pain of intact and abraded skin and mucous membranes.
CONTRAINDICATIONS AND PRECAUTIONS
Hypersensitivity to benzocaine; infants under 1 year of age. Safe use in women of childbearing potential or during pregnancy not established. Cautious use: history of drug sensitivities; severly traumatized mucosa; sepsis in region of application.
ADVERSE REACTIONS
Low toxicity. Sensitization in susceptible patients and when applied repeatedly or over extensive areas. Methemoglobinemia reported in infants with suppository form.
ROUTE AND DOSAGE
Topical: 0.5% to 20%. Available as ointment, rectal suppository, spray solution, and troches.

NURSING IMPLICATIONS
Before administration of hemorrhoidal ointment or suppository, thoroughly clean and dry rectal area. Usually administered morning and evening and after each bowel movement.

Otic preparation should be warmed by placing container in warm water bath. Have patient lying with affected side up. Instill drops along side of auditory canal to prevent air pocket. Advise patient to remain on affected side several minutes.

Indiscriminate use of anesthetic ear drops may mask symptoms of fulminating middle ear infection.

Avoid contact of all preparations with eyes, and be careful not to inhale mist when spray form is used.

Most local anesthetics are potentially sensitizing. The medication should be discontinued if the condition being treated worsens or if signs of sensitivity occur.

Bear in mind that use on oral mucosa may interfere with second stage (pharyngeal) of swallowing. If possible, foods and liquids should be withheld for about 1 hour to prevent possible aspiration.

BENZONATATE, N.F.
(TESSALON)

Antitussive

ACTIONS AND USES

Nonnarcotic antitussive chemically related to tetracaine. Antitussive activity reported to be as effective as that of codeine. Apparently inhibits cough reflex at afferent endings of vagus nerve and suppresses transmission of cough reflex at level of medulla. Also believed to exert selective topical anesthetic action on pulmonary stretch receptors, thus relieving sensation of tightness of chest. More effective in treatment of nonproductive cough than cough associated with copious sputum.

Used to decrease frequency and intensity of cough in acute and chronic respiratory conditions. Also used in bronchoscopy, thoracentesis, and other procedures when coughing must be avoided.

ABSORPTION AND FATE

Action begins within 15 to 30 minutes and lasts 3 to 8 hours.

CONTRAINDICATIONS AND PRECAUTIONS

Hypersensitivity to benzonate or related compounds. Safe use during pregnancy and lactation not established.

ADVERSE REACTIONS

Low incidence: nasal congestion, chilly sensation, burning sensation of eyes, drowsiness, skin rash, pruritus, numbness in chest, vertigo, dizziness, constipation, nausea, headache, transitory rise in blood pressure, hypersensitivity reactions (rarely). Overdosage: CNS stimulation (restlessness, tremors, convulsions).

ROUTE AND DOSAGE

Oral: **Adults and Children** *over 10 years:* 100 mg 3 times a day, as required. If necessary, up to 600 mg daily may be given.

NURSING IMPLICATIONS

Instruct patient to avoid chewing oral preparation or allowing it to dissolve in mouth. If it dissolves, it produces local anesthesia of oral mucosa.

Antitussive agents are used selectively. Suppression of cough and gag reflex in the immediate postoperative period may lead to aspiration and development of atelectasis and pneumonitis.

Objective of treatment with an antitussive agent is to reduce overactive nonproductive coughing, not to suppress the cough completely.

Observe character and frequency of coughing and volume and quality of sputum. Keep physician informed.

Changing the patient's position at least hourly helps to prevent pooling of lung secretions. Concomitant deep breathing exercises may stimulate productive coughing.

The following measures may provide relief of nonproductive cough: limitation on talking, no smoking, adequate fluid intake, maintenance of environmental humidity, and use of sugarless hard candy to increase flow of saliva (a normal protective demulcent to pharyngeal mucosa).

Stored in airtight containers, protected from light.

BENZPHETAMINE HYDROCHLORIDE, N.F. (DIDREX)

Anorexiant

ACTIONS AND USES

Sympathomimetic amine with actions similar to those of amphetamine (qv). Anorexigenic effect thought to be secondary to CNS stimulation.

Used as short-term adjunct in management of exogenous obesity.

ABSORPTION AND FATE

Following oral administration, readily absorbed from GI tract; effects persist for about 4 hours.

CONTRAINDICATIONS AND PRECAUTIONS

Known hypersensitivity to sympathomimetic amines, advanced arteriosclerosis, symptomatic cardiovascular disease, hypertension, hyperthyroidism, agitated states, history of drug abuse, children under 12 years of age. Safe use during pregnancy or in women of childbearing potential not established. Also see Amphetamine.

ADVERSE REACTIONS

Low incidence: restlessness, dizziness, insomnia, sweating, xerostomia, nausea, vomiting, diarrhea, tremor, palpitation, tachycardia, headache, elevated blood pressure, urticaria and other allergic skin reactions, change in libido. Chronic intoxication: marked insomnia, irritability, hyperactivity, personality changes, psychosis, severe dermatoses. See Amphetamine.

ROUTE AND DOSAGE

Oral: 25 to 50 mg 1 to 3 times daily.

NURSING IMPLICATIONS

Administering drug before meals may serve as a reminder of the need for self-discipline during mealtime. A single daily dose is given, preferably mid-morning or mid-afternoon, according to patient's eating habits.

To avoid insomnia, the last dose should be scheduled no later than 6 hours before patient retires.

For maximal results, drug therapy should be used as part of a plan that includes reeducation with respect to eating habits, nutritional needs, and resolution of underlying psychologic factors.

Anorexigenic effects are temporary, seldom lasting more than a few weeks; tolerance may occur. Therefore long-term use is not indicated.

The possibility of psychic dependence should be borne in mind.

Classified as Schedule IV drug under the Federal Controlled Substances Act.

Preserved in tight, light-resistant containers.

See Amphetamine Sulfate.

(EMETE-CON)

Antiemetic

ACTIONS AND USES

Benzoquinolizine amide similar to phenothiazines in ability to depress conditioned avoidance behavior; also like antihistamine antiemetics; but chemically unrelated to both. Mechanism of antiemetic action unknown, but believed to be by depression of chemoreceptor trigger zone. Also thought to have some reserpinelike antiserotonin activity.

Used for prevention and treatment of nausea and vomiting associated with anesthesia and surgery.

ABSORPTION AND FATE

Rapidly and completely absorbed. Onset of antiemetic action within 15 minutes, with duration of 3 to 4 hours. Peak blood levels achieved in about 30 minutes. Distributed throughout body tissues, with highest concentrations in liver and kidneys. Approximately 58% protein-bound; half-life is about 40 minutes. Rapidly metabolized in liver; excreted in urine and feces primarily as metabolites. Less than 10% of dose is excreted in urine as unchanged drug.

CONTRAINDICATIONS AND PRECAUTIONS

Hypersensitivity to the drug; intravenous administration to patients with cardiovascular disease or to those receiving preanesthetic and/or concomitant cardiovascular drugs. Safe use during pregnancy and in children not established. Cautious use and low doses in elderly and debilitated patients.

ADVERSE REACTIONS

CNS: drowsiness (common), insomnia, headache, excitement, restlessness, nervousness. **Autonomic:** xerostomia, blurred vision, sweating, shivering, flushing, hiccups. **GI**: anorexia, nausea, vomiting, abdominal cramps. **Cardiovascular** (particularly following IV): sudden increase in blood pressure, hypotension, dizziness, atrial fibrillation, premature artrial and ventricular contractions. Others reported: allergic reactions (urticaria, skin rash, pyrexia, chills); extrapyramidal symptoms (in large doses): tremors, twitching, rigidity, hypersalivation, weakness, motor restlessness, fatigue.

ROUTE AND DOSAGE

Intramuscular (preferred route): 50 mg (0.5 mg/kg to 1 mg/kg). First dose may be repeated in 1 hour; subsequent doses every 3 or 4 hours, if necessary. Intravenous: 25 mg (0.2 to 0.4 mg/kg) (reconstituted with 2.2 ml sterile water for injection) administered at rate not exceeding 1 ml per 0.5 to 1 minute. Subsequent doses given intramuscularly, if necessary.

NURSING IMPLICATIONS

IM injection should be made into a large muscle. Aspirate carefully to avoid inadvertent intravascular injection.

When prescribed for prophylaxis of nausea and vomiting associated with anesthesia, benzquinamide should be administered at least 15 minutes prior to expected emergence from anesthesia.

Drowsiness is a common side effect.

In common with other antiemetics, benzquinamide may mask signs and symptoms of overdosage from other drugs and obscure diagnosis of conditions associated with nausea.

Reconstituted solutions maintain potency for 14 days at room temperature. Do not refrigerate.

Preserved in light-resistant containers.

BENZTHIAZIDE, N.F.
(AQUAPRES, AQUASEC, AQUASTAT, AQUATAG, EXNA, HYDREX, HY-DRINE, LEMAZIDE, MARAZIDE, PROAQUA, RID-EMA, ROLA-BENZ, S-AQUA, URAZIDE)

Diuretic (thiazide), antihypertensive

ACTIONS AND USES

Benzothiadiazine (thiazide) derivative. Similar to chlorothiazide in actions, uses, contraindications, precautions, and adverse reactions, but reported to be approximately 10 times as potent on a weight basis.

ABSORPTION AND FATE

Onset of diuretic effect in 2 hours; peaks in 4 to 6 hours and persists 12 to 18 hours. Distribution and fate assumed to be similar to those of other thiazides. See Chlorothiazide.

ROUTE AND DOSAGE

Oral: **Adults:** 50 to 150 mg daily. Highly individualized. Preferably given in 2 doses when 100 mg or more daily is prescribed or when given for treatment of hypertension. Maintenance (hypertension): determined by patient's blood pressure response Some patients require up to 200 mg daily in 2 or 3 divided doses. **Children:** 1 to 4 mg/kg daily in 3 divided doses.

NURSING IMPLICATIONS

Physician will rely on accurate observations and recordings to determine patient's minimal effective dosage level.
See Chlorothiazide.

BENZTROPINE MESYLATE, U.S.P., B.P.
(COGENTIN)

Antiparkinsonian

ACTIONS AND USES

Synthetic centrally acting anticholinergic drug that resembles atropine and diphenhydramine in chemical structure. Exhibits anticholinergic, antihistaminic, and local anesthetic properties. Suppresses tremor and rigidity by action on basal ganglia.

Used in symptomatic treatment of all types of parkinsonism (arteriosclerotic, idiopathic, postencephaletic) and to relieve extrapyramidal symptoms associated with phenothiazines, reserpine, and other drugs. Commonly used as supplement with trihexyphenidyl or dopa therapy.

ABSORPTION AND FATE

Onset of action following IM and IV injections occurs within 15 minutes; onset occurs about 1 hour following oral administration. Effects may persist 8 hours or more.

CONTRAINDICATIONS AND PRECAUTIONS

Children under 3 years of age. Cautious use: in older children and in patients with poor mental outlook. Also see Atropine.

ADVERSE REACTIONS

Nausea, vomiting. **Atropinelike side effects:** xerostomia, blurred vision, mydriasis, anhidrosis, palpitation, constipation, paralytic ileus, dysuria. **Antihistaminic effect:** sedation, dizziness, paresthesia. In high doses: CNS depression, preceded or followed by stimulation, mental confusion, toxic psychosis, muscular weakness, ataxia. Also see Atropine.

ROUTE AND DOSAGE

Oral, intramuscular, intravenous: 0.5 to 6 mg daily. Dosage scheduling highly individualized according to patient's requirements and response. (Generally, low doses are given to patients with arteriosclerotic parkinsonism, the elderly, and thin patients.)

NURSING IMPLICATIONS

Patients with arteriosclerotic or idiopathic parkinsonism generally experience greatest relief by taking benztropine at bedtime. Younger patients with postencephalitic parkinsonism usually require more frequent scheduling.

Physician will rely on accurate observations and reporting to establish patient's optimum dosage level and frequency of scheduling.

Effects of benztropine are cumulative; therefore therapeutic effects may not be evident until 2 or 3 days after drug is started. Drug therapy is usually initiated at low doses, with subsequent increments of 0.5 mg made at 5- or 6-day intervals, if necessary.

Appearance of intermittent constipation, abdominal pain and distention may herald onset of paralytic ileus. Monitor patient for these symptoms.

Caution patient of possibility of drowsiness and blurred vision, and advise against operating vehicles or machinery requiring alertness until reaction to the drug has been evaluated by physician. Supervision of ambulation and bedsides may be indicated.

Appearance of intermittent constipation, abdominal pain, and distention may herald onset of paralytic ileus. Monitor patient for these symptoms.

Most of the atropinelike side effects of benztropine are controlled by adjustment of dosage. However, severe reactions such as signs and symptoms of CNS depression or excitement generally require interruption of drug therapy.

Administration of drug after meals may help to prevent gastric irritation.

Mouth dryness may be relieved by rinsing mouth with water or by sugarless gum or hard candy.

Anhidrosis, especially in hot weather, may require dose adjustments because of possibility of heat stroke.

Therapeutic effect is evidenced by lessening of rigidity, drooling (sialorrhea), and oculogyric crises and by improvement in gait, balance, and posture. Usually, tremors are not appreciably relieved.

Abrupt withdrawal of antiparkinson medications may precipitate parkinsonian crisis.

Preserved in tightly covered, light-resistant container

Also see Atropine Sulfate.

DRUG INTERACTIONS: In common with other anticholinergic antiparkinson agents, possibility exists that benztropine may decrease therapeutic effectiveness and also aggravate extrapyramidal symptoms induced by **haloperidol** and other **butyrophenones, chlorpromazine** and other **phenothiazines,** and **methotrimeprazine.** Anticholinergic side effects may be potentiated by **amantadine, MAO inhibitors, procainamide, quinidine** (additive vagal blocking action), and **tricyclic antidepressants.** Benztropine may decrease effect of **levodopa** by delaying gastric emptying.

(ALCOPARA)

Anthelmintic

ACTIONS AND USES
  Quaternary ammonium compound that produces contracture of nematode muscles. Appears to act as myoneural blocking agent and may also inhibit glucose transport system and aerobic glycolysis in parasite worm.
  Used in treatment of hookworm infestations *(Ancylostoma duodenale, Necator americanus)* and in mixed hookworm and roundworm *(Ascaris lumbricoides)* infections.
ABSORPTION AND FATE
  Poorly absorbed from GI tract. Absorbed drug is excreted in urine within 24 hours.
CONTRAINDICATIONS AND PRECAUTIONS
  Safe use during pregnancy not established. Cautious use: hypertension, hepatic, renal, or cardiac disease, children younger than 1 year of age.
ADVERSE REACTIONS
  Low toxicity, nausea, vomiting, dizziness, giddiness, abdominal cramps, diarrhea, headache; temporary but marked fall in blood pressure.
ROUTE AND DOSAGE
  Oral: Hookworm *(Ancylostoma duodenale):* **Adults and children** *over 22 kg:* 2.5 Gm twice daily for 1 day; dose may be repeated in a few days, if necessary. **Children** *under 22 kg:* ½ dosage. Hookworm *(Necator americanus)* **Adults and Children** *over 22 kg:* 2.5 Gm twice daily for 3 days. **Children** *under 22 kg:* ½ dosage.

NURSING IMPLICATIONS
Corrective and supportive measures should be instituted before drug therapy in patients with debilitation, anemia, electrolyte imbalance, and dehydration.
No purgation is required before or after drug therapy.
Given preferably on an empty stomach; food is then withheld for another 2 hours to prevent vomiting.
Bephenium has a bitter taste when mixed with water. More palatable when mixed with milk or chocolate milk, flavored syrup, orange juice, or a carbonated beverage just before administration.
Alcohol may reduce effects of bephenium. Advise patient not to drink alcoholic beverages for at least 24 hours before and after a dose is given.
Stools should be examined for ova and adult worms at 2- or 3-week intervals after a course of treatment. If ova are found, patient may be given another course of therapy.
Hookworm is acquired by penetration of skin of feet and ankles by larvae present in contaminated soil, and possibly by contaminated water and hand-to-mouth transmission. Roundworm is contracted by ingestion of embryonated ova.
Prevention of reinfection depends on the patient and the family gaining an understanding of the life cycle of the worm, the vectors and fomites of transmission, sanitary disposal of fecal material, personal hygiene, the importance of washing the hands, and hygienic handling of foods.
A careful diet history should be elicited to determine adequacy of diet. Supportive diet therapy may be indicated in some patients.
Hospital patients should have their own toilet facilities. Advise home patient to scrub toilet seat with soap and water after each use.

64 BETAMETHASONE, N.F., B.P.
(CELESTONE)
BETAMETHASONE BENZOATE
(BENISONE, FLUROBATE)
BETAMETHASONE DIPROPIONATE
(DIPROSONE)
BETAMETHASONE VALERATE, N.F., B.P.
(VALISONE)

Adrenocortical steroid

ACTIONS AND USES

Long-acting glucocorticoid steroid with minor mineralocorticoid properties. With exception of Addison's disease and salt-losing forms of adrenocortical syndromes, it has the same indications for use as hydrocortisone (qv). Also used in topical management of pruritus erythema and swelling associated with dermatoses, and some lesions of psoriasis. For absorption, fate, contraindications, and adverse reactions, see Hydrocortisone.

ROUTE AND DOSAGE

Oral: 0.6 to 7.2 mg daily. Intramuscular: initially 0.5 to 9 mg daily; maintenance highly individualized on basis of patient response and condition being treated. Intraarticular: 1.5 to 9 mg depending on size of joint. Topical (cream, lotion, gel, ointment, spray): applied to affected area 2 or 3 times daily.

NURSING IMPLICATIONS

Betamethasone acetate is combined with betamethasone sodium phosphate as Celestone Soluspan and used for intraarticular, intramuscular, and intralesional injection. Response follows in 3 hours and persists for 1 to 4 weeks.

Since mineralocorticoid properties are minimal, diet supplements of potassium and restriction of sodium are usually unnecessary during short-term therapy with betamethasone.

Absorption following use of aerosol preparation (Valisone) equals that of oral and parenteral administration. Avoid inhaling drug. Do not spray mucous membranes or external ear canal.

Special points about aerosol administration: hold container upright or inverted; spray no more than 3 seconds and at a distance of no less than 6 inches. Do not apply to area that is to be covered by occlusive dressing.

Carefully and routinely note condition of skin to which topical betamethasone has been applied. Report evidence of limited response or intercurrent infection which may necessitate adjunctive treatment with an appropriate antifungal or antibacterial agent.

Advise patient to avoid exposing areas treated with topical glucocorticoid to sunlight. Severe burns have been reported, especially when occlusive dressings are used.

Keep betamethasone aerosol container out of reach of children.

See Hydrocortisone.

(MYOTONACHOL, URECHOLINE)

Cholinergic

ACTIONS AND USES
Produces effects similar to those of acetylcholine, acting directly on effector cells innervated by cholinergic system. Unlike acetylcholine, it is not hydrolyzed by cholinesterase; thus it has more prolonged activity in the body. Exerts minimal effects on cardiovascular system, and has little effect on autonomic ganglia, skeletal muscles, neuromuscular junction, sweat glands, salivary glands, and eyes. Actions are primarily muscarinic and appear to be selective on GI tract and urinary bladder. Increases tone, and peristaltic activity of esophagus, stomach and intestines; contracts detrusor muscle of urinary bladder, usually sufficiently to initiate micturition.

Used in treatment of acute postoperative and postpartum nonobstructive (functional) urinary retention, and for neurogenic atony of urinary bladder with retention. Has been used in selected cases of adynamic ileus secondary to toxic states, postoperative abdominal distention, gastric atony and retention and as diagnostic test for pancreatic enzymatic function.

ABSORPTION AND FATE
Following oral administration, onset of action occurs within 30 to 90 minutes (5 to 15 minutes after SC injection). Effects persist about 1 hour after oral and up to 2 hours after SC administration.

CONTRAINDICATIONS AND PRECAUTIONS
Obstructive pulmonary disease, asthma, hyperthyroid states, urinary bladder surgery, cystitis, urinary bladder neck or intestinal obstruction, peptic ulcer, recent GI surgery, peritonitis, marked vagotonia, pronounced vasomotor instability, severe bradycardia, hypotension or hypertension, coronary artery diseases, recent myocardial infarction, epilepsy, parkinsonism, pregnancy.

ADVERSE REACTIONS
Flushing of skin, sweating, salivation, abdominal cramps, diarrhea, borborygmi, incontinence, nausea, vomiting, belching, malaise, headache, substernal pain, asthmatic attack, transient fall in blood pressure. Hypersensitivity, or when given inadvertently IV or IM: fall in blood pressure, reflex tachycardia, severe abdominal cramps, bloody diarrhea, shock, sudden cardiac arrest.

ROUTE AND DOSAGE
Oral: 5 to 30 mg 3 or 4 times daily. Subcutaneous: 2.5 to 5 mg 3 or 4 times daily, as required. Highly individualized.

NURSING IMPLICATIONS
To determine minimum effective oral dose, physician may prescribe an initial test dose of 5 to 10 mg and a repeat of same dose at hourly intervals to a maximum of 30 mg, unless satisfactory response or disturbing side effects intervene.

To determine minimum effective subcutaneous dose, physician may prescribe an initial test dose of 2.5 mg and a repeat of the same dose at 15- to 30-minute intervals to a maximum of 4 doses, unless satisfactory response or disturbing side effects intervene.

Sterile solution of bethanechol is intended for subcutaneous use only. After inserting needle, aspirate carefully before injecting drug to avoid inadvertent entry into a blood vessel. Severe symptoms of cholinergic stimulation may occur if it is given IM or IV (see Adverse Reactions).

Observe for and report early signs of overdosage: salivation, sweating, flushing, abdominal cramps, nausea.

Syringe containing 0.6 mg of atropine sulfate (antidote) should be ready for instant use to abolish severe side effects. Specific directions for administering antidote should be prescribed by physician.

Monitor blood pressure and pulse when bethanechol is given subcutaneously or in high oral doses.

Bethanechol should be given on an empty stomach in order to prevent nausea and vomiting.

When bethanechol is administered to relieve urinary retention or abdominal distention, a bedpan or urinal should be readily available to the patient. It may be necessary to insert a rectal tube to facilitate passage of flatus.

Monitor intake and output. Observe patient's response to bethanechol, and report any failure of the drug to relieve the particular condition for which it was prescribed.

DRUG INTERACTIONS: Bethanechol, in common with other cholinergic drugs, may be antagonized by **atropine, procainamide, quinidine, epinephrine** and other **sympathomimetic agents.** Concurrent administration of **ganglionic blocking agents** may cause critical fall in blood pressure. Bethanechol toxicity may be potentiated by other **cholinergic drugs** and **anticholinesterase agents** (eq, **neostigmine**).

BIPERIDEN HYDROCHLORIDE, N.F.
(AKINETON HYDROCHLORIDE)
BIPERIDEN LACTATE, N.F.
(AKINETON LACTATE)

Anticholinergic, antiparkinsonian

ACTIONS AND USES

Analogue of trihexyphenidyl, with actions, uses, contraindications, and adverse reactions similar to those of atropine (qv). Drying effects are reported to be relatively weak compared with atropine.

Used in all forms of parkinsonism, but appears to be more effective in postencephalitic and idiopathic parkinsonism than in arteriosclerotic type.

ROUTE AND DOSAGE

Oral (biperiden hydrochloride): 2 mg 1 to 4 times daily. Intramuscular and intravenous (biperiden lactate): 2 mg injected slowly; may be repeated every half hour until resolution of symptoms, but not more than 4 doses per 24-hour period.

NURSING IMPLICATIONS

GI disturbances may be alleviated by administering drug with or after meals.

Dryness of mouth and blurred vision are common side effects and may be relieved or eliminated by dosage reduction.

Postural hypotension, disturbances of coordination, and temporary euphoria may occur when drug is administered parenterally, particularly after IV injection. Monitor blood pressure and pulse and supervise ambulation.

It is reported that certain susceptible patients may manifest mental confusion, drowsiness, dizziness, agitation, hematuria (rarely), and decrease in urinary flow. Report these symptoms immediately.

In patients with severe parkinsonism, tremors may increase as spasticity is relieved.

Patients on prolonged therapy can develop tolerance; an increase in dosage may be required.

Preserved in tightly closed, light-resistant containers.

See Atropine Sulfate.

BISACODYL, N.F., B.P.
(BICOL, BISCO-LAX, BON-O-LAX, DULCOLAX, FLEET BISACODYL, THERALAX, LAXADAN SUPULES)

Stimulant cathartic

ACTIONS AND USES
Synthetic contact or stimulant cathartic structurally related to phenolphthalein. Directly stimulates sensory nerve endings in colonic mucosa to produce parasympathetic reflexes resulting in increased peristalsis and evacuation of large intestine.

Used to relieve constipation and for evacuation of colon before surgery, endoscopy, and radiologic examination.

ABSORPTION AND FATE
Acts within 6 to 12 hours following oral administration; acts 15 to 60 minutes after insertion of rectal suppository. Approximately 5% absorbed from GI tract and excreted in urine as glucuronide. Rectal absorption appears to be negligible.

CONTRAINDICATIONS AND PRECAUTIONS
Acute surgical abdomen, abdominal cramps, intestinal obstruction, fecal impaction; use of rectal suppository in presence of anal or rectal fissures, ulcerated hemorrhoids, proctitis.

ADVERSE REACTIONS
Systemic effects not reported. Occasionally: mild cramping, nausea, vertigo, diarrhea. Rectal burning and mild pruritus following use of suppositories for several weeks.

ROUTE AND DOSAGE
Oral: 10 to 15 mg (up to 30 mg may be given in preparation for special procedures). Rectal suppository: 10 mg.

NURSING IMPLICATIONS
In view of action time, administer oral drug in the evening or before breakfast.

Tablets are enteric coated; therefore, to avoid gastric irritation, they should not be cut, crushed, or chewed.

Advise patient not to take tablets within 1 hour of antacids or milk. These substances may cause dissolution of enteric coating, with release of drug and resultant gastric irritation.

Evaluate patient's need for continued use of bisacodyl. Cathartic use may become habitual and tends to reinforce neurotic preoccupation with bowels.

Patients with hypertension and cardiovascular disease should be cautioned to avoid excessive straining (Valsalva maneuver) during defecation. Straining causes concurrent rises in intrathoracic and venous pressures, momentarily interfering with free flow of blood out of heart. When patient stops straining, blood is quickly propelled through the heart; this may result in tachycardia and even cardiac arrest in susceptible patients.

Widespread abuse of OTC cathartics is evidence of the need for public education concerning their proper use.

The aim in treatment of constipation is to relieve the cause.

Functional constipation can be corrected by regularity of meals, addition of bulk and fiber to diet: raw and cooked vegetables and fruits, natural laxative fruits such as plums, prunes, and rhubarb, whole-grain breads and cereals. Some physicians recommend 4 to 6 tablespoonsful of whole bran taken directly or added to cereals or stewed fruits. Other important measures include adequate fluid intake (8 to 10 glasses), exercise, unhurried defecation, and regular defecation time. Duodenocolic and defecation reflexes are most active after meals, especially breakfast.

Bisacodyl tablets and suppositories are preserved in tight containers at temperatures not exceeding 30 C (86 F).

BISMUTH SUBCARBONATE, U.S.P.
(Basic Bismuth Carbonate)

Antidiarrheal, topical protectant

ACTIONS AND USES
Relatively insoluble compound with protective, adsorbent, astringent, and weak antacid properties. Reported to assist in removing gas, toxins, bacteria, and viruses by adsorption.

Used in treatment of diarrhea, enteritis, dysentery, and ulcerations of bowel. Available in combination with paregoric. Sometimes used topically as protectant for skin.

ABSORPTION AND FATE
Only slightly absorbed following oral use; excreted in feces.

ROUTE AND DOSAGE
Oral: 0.5 to 4 Gm. Topical: lotion, ointment.

NURSING IMPLICATIONS
Preserved in tightly closed, light-resistant containers.
See Paregoric for management of patient with diarrhea.

BISMUTH SUBSALICYLATE
(Basic Bismuth Salicylate)
BISMUTH SALICYLATE, B.P.

Treponemicide

ACTIONS AND USES
Basic salt of bismuth used in treatment of syphilis in patients sensitized to penicillin. Also has been used in treatment of yaws and occasionally as suppressant for discoid lupus erythematosus.

ABSORPTION AND FATE
Slowly and irregularly absorbed following IM injection. Excreted slowly, primarily by kidneys.

CONTRAINDICATIONS AND PRECAUTIONS
Renal disease, early or active syphilis.

ADVERSE REACTIONS
Ulcerative stomatitis, GI disturbances, headache, depression, albuminuria, renal failure.

ROUTE AND DOSAGE
Intramuscular: 100 to 200 mg weekly for 8 to 10 weeks.

NURSING IMPLICATIONS
Shake IM preparation thoroughly (suspended in oil) before a dose is withdrawn.

Inject deep into outer upper quadrant of gluteus maximus. Aspirate carefully to make sure needle is not in a blood vessel. IV injection can cause oil embolism.

Early symptoms of toxicity relate to mouth, digestive system, and kidneys: salivation, foul breath, bismuth deposition (black patches on soft palate and inner surfaces of cheeks, bismuth gum line), anorexia, nausea, vomiting, diarrhea, abdominal pain, albuminuria. Advise patient to report all signs and symptoms.

Inspect mouth daily, and maintain meticulous mouth hygiene. Encourage patient to brush teeth with soft tooth brush and to rinse mouth thoroughly after each meal.

Urine should be examined for albumin and bacteria before therapy is initiated and periodically thereafter. Adequate fluid intake should be maintained.

Protect drug from light.

BLEOMYCIN SULFATE
(BLENOXANE, BLM)

Antineoplastic

ACTIONS AND USES
Mixture of cytotoxic glycopeptide antibiotics from a strain of *Streptomyces verticillus*. By poorly understood mechanism, blocks incorporation of thymidine into DNA molecule, thereby interfering with DNA, RNA, and protein synthesis. Causes minimal immunosuppression and myelosuppression, but has unusual mucocutaneous and pulmonary toxicity.

Used as palliative treatment and/or adjuvant to surgery and radiation therapy of lymphomas, squamous cell carcinomas, testicular carcinoma, and other selected malignancies; used intrapleurally to prevent pleural fluid accumulation. Used investigationally in mycosis fungoides, as supplement to MOPP regimen.

ABSORPTION AND FATE
Absorbed systemically following parenteral administration; appears to concentrate in skin and lungs; trace amounts in brain, kidney, spleen, liver, and heart. Metabolic fate poorly understood; 20% to 40% excreted in urine as active drug.

CONTRAINDICATIONS AND PRECAUTIONS
Bleomycin sensitivity, pregnancy, women of childbearing age. Cautious use: renal or pulmonary impairment of nonmalignant origin.

ADVERSE REACTIONS
Dermatologic (over 50% of patients): stomatitis, oral ulceration, alopecia, hyperpigmentation, hyperkeratosis, ichthyosis, peeling, bleeding, pruritic erythema, vesiculation, nail changes, hypoesthesia progressing to hyperesthesia, paresthesias. **Pulmonary** (dose- and age-related): interstitial pneumonitis, fibrosis. **GI:** nausea, vomiting, anorexia, weight loss. **Hematopoietic** (rare): thrombocytopenia, leukopenia, mild anemia. Other: chills, hyperpyrexia, headache, hypotension, prolonged cardiorespiratory collapse, exacerbation of rheumatoid arthritis, cystitis, anaphylactoid reaction, pain at tumor site, and renal, hepatic, and CNS toxicity.

ROUTE AND DOSAGE

Dose and schedule highly individualized. Routes employed: intraarterial, intramuscular, intrapleural, intravenous, subcutaneous. Usual dosage for intramuscular or intravenous: 0.25 to 0.50 units/Gm body weight once or twice a week; maintenance: 1 unit daily or 5 units weekly. When the total of all doses reaches 400 units, bleomycin must be given with extreme caution.

NURSING IMPLICATIONS

Expiration date of commercially available sterile powder is 18 months from date of manufacture. Solutions reconstituted with sodium chloride or 5% dextrose injection are stable at room temperature for 24 hours. Discard unused solutions.

Used only under constant supervision by personnel experienced in cancer chemotherapy.

IV and intraarterial injections should be administered slowly over a 10-minute period.

Renal, pulmonary, CNS, hepatic, and hematopoietic functions should be monitored throughout therapy period.

Monitor blood test reports. If leukopenia and thrombocytopenia occur (infrequent), nadirs are usually reached 12 to 14 days after beginning of therapy.

Chest x-rays should be taken every 1 to 2 weeks to monitor lung changes.

Bleomycin pneumonitis (the most serious toxic effect) occurs most frequently in patients over 70 years of age, or when the total of all doses approaches 400 units. Early signs: dyspnea, fine rales, nonproductive cough, decreased pulmonary function, sore throat. If pulmonary fibrosis is present, drug will be discontinued.

Chest auscultation for rales once or twice a day is indicated. Report to physician if patient develops a cough, dyspnea, or rales.

Mucocutaneous toxicity (dose-related) usually develops in second or third week of treatment. Hypoesthesias, urticaria, and tender swollen hands (early symptoms) should be reported promptly. Therapy may be discontinued.

Prevent erythema or abrasions over pressure areas by frequent observation, scheduled skin care, and programmed mobility.

Inform patient that hyperpigmentation may occur in areas subject to friction and pressure, skin folds, nail cuticles, scars, and intramuscular sites.

Febrile reactions usually lessen with continued use of drug, but they may recur sporadically. Salicylates are usually not effective; tepid sponge baths may provide relief.

Anaphylactoid reactions (hypotension, fever, chills, mental confusion, wheezing) frequently occur several hours after first or second dose, especially in patients with lymphoma; they are sometimes fatal. Usually a test dose of 2 units or less of bleomycin is given to these patients for the first 2 doses; then if no acute reaction occurs, regular dosage schedule begins.

Fastidious mouth care is indicated if stomatitis and dysphagia occur. See Mechlorethamine for mouth care.

Check weight at regular intervals under standard conditions.

One member of the ABVD, BACOP combination chemotherapeutic regimens.

(Citrated Whole Blood)
WHOLE HUMAN BLOOD, B.P.

Blood replenisher

ACTIONS AND USES
Drawn aseptically from healthy human donor, with citrate ion or heparin added as anticoagulant.
Used for transfusion to replace red blood cells, clotting factors, and blood protein and to restore or maintain circulating blood volume.

ADVERSE REACTIONS
Hemolytic reaction (incompatibility): chills, fever, headache, apprehension, pain (substernal, flank, abdominal, and infusion-site), hemoglobinemia, hemoglobinuria, oliguria, jaundice, dyspnea, hypotension, vascular collapse. **Allergic reaction**: pruritus, urticarial rash, bronchospasm. **Febrile (bacterial) reaction**: malaise, headache, hyperpyrexia, fall in blood pressure, dry and flushed skin (red shock). **Circulatory overload**: cough, dyspnea, hemoptysis, edema, congestive heart failure. **Citrate overload** (with massive transfusion): acidosis, calcium deficiency, hyperkalemia, arrhythmias, coagulation defects.

ROUTE AND DOSAGE
Intravenous: 500 ml (1 unit), repeated as necessary.

NURSING IMPLICATIONS

If possible, baseline TPR and blood pressure should be established before transfusion begins.

Note expiration date of whole blood (typing and cross matching required). Also, carefully check label to confirm blood group and Rh factor against those of patient; check whether test for Australia antigen (hepatitis-associated antigen, HAA) was done. If blood is cloudy, contains gas bubbles or particulate matter, or is abnormal in color, it should not be used.

Most hemolytic reactions result from carelessness in checking blood and patient's identity.

Physician will prescribe specific IV flow rate. Generally, blood is started at 20 drops/minute for the first 10 minutes. If no reaction occurs, flow rate is increased to 60 to 70 drops/minute (rate varies).

Flow rates slower than usual are used for patients with heart disease and severe anemia and for the elderly.

Check flow rate frequently. Change in height of bed or in position of extremity during transfusion may alter flow rate.

Patient should be under constant surveillance. Reactions may occur during infusion of first 50 to 100 ml of blood or up to 96 hours after transfusion. Sensitivity reactions may develop after 10 days or more. See Adverse Reactions.

Monitor vital signs every ½ to 1 hour during transfusion, or more frequently if indicated.

If a reaction occurs, stop transfusion immediately and notify physician and laboratory. Follow institutional policy for reporting transfusion reactions. Generally, the blood remaining in the container, with tubing attached, and a sample of the patient's blood are sent immediately to laboratory for antibody screening, direct Coombs test, and sensitivity and repeat cross-matching procedures. Urine specimen is also sent to determine presence of free hemoglobin (indication of intravascular hemolysis). Monitor vital signs, and intake and output.

Bear in mind that anesthetized patients receiving whole blood are unable to complain of early symptoms of hemolytic reaction (e.g., pain in back, chest, abdomen, or injection site). Critical signs may be elevated temperature and falling blood pressure.

Patients with Hodgkin's disease, various lymphomas, and liver disease appear to be particularly prone to febrile reactions.

Administration set (tubing and filter) should be changed if another unit of blood is to be given (filter usually clogs after administration of 1 unit of blood).

Dextrose should not be administered with blood, as it causes clumping of red blood cells. If glucose is to follow transfusion, tubing should first be flushed with normal saline.

Whole blood carries risk of homologous serum hepatitis, malaria, and syphilis (freshly drawn blood). Serum hepatitis develops within a period of 50 to 180 days posttransfusion.

Whole blood should be stored at a temperature between 1 C and 10 C (held constant within range of 2 degrees).

BORIC ACID, N.F., B.P.
(Boracic Acid, BOROFAX)

Antiinfective (local)

ACTIONS AND USES
Weak acid with questionably effective fungistatic and bacteriostatic properties. Used externally for various minor conditions of eye, ear, skin, and mucous membranes.

CONTRAINDICATIONS AND PRECAUTIONS
Application to abraded or denuded surfaces or granulating tissue; preparation of nipples for nursing; for irrigation of closed body cavities.

ADVERSE REACTIONS
From absorption or accidental ingestion: nausea, vomiting, diarrhea, abdominal pain, muscular weakness, hypothermia, headache, restlessness, skin eruptions, kidney damage, tachycardia, dyspnea, circulatory collapse, delirium, convulsions, coma.

ROUTE AND DOSAGE
Topical: aqueous solution, powder (2% to 4%), topical ointment (5%).

NURSING IMPLICATIONS

Boric acid should be applied only to intact skin. Applications to abraded skin or open wounds has caused fatal poisoning in infants. Deaths from accidental ingestion have also been reported.

The Subcommittee on Accidental Poisoning of the American Academy of Pediatrics has recommended that boric acid be eliminated from newborn nurseries in all hospitals.

Applications should not be made over large areas or for prolonged periods, in order to avoid possibility of absorption.

Because of danger of contamination, boric acid solution should be used as soon as reconstituted. Label container clearly as to contents.

Use sterile boric acid solution for application to eyes.

BROMELAINS
(ANANASE)

Enzyme

ACTIONS AND USES
Mixture of proteolytic enzymes derived from pineapple plant. Thought to exert antiinflammatory effect in traumatic states by aiding digestion of fibrin and increasing permeability of venules and lymphatics.
Used as adjunctive in treatment of soft-tissue inflammation and edema associated with trauma, surgery (eg, episiotomy), cellulitis, furunculosis, and ulceration. Effectiveness is equivocal and has not been clearly established in clinical studies.

CONTRAINDICATIONS AND PRECAUTIONS
Known hypersensitivity to pineapple or its products, patients with abnormal blood clotting mechanisms, severe hepatic or renal disease, systemic infection. Safe use during pregnancy or in children 12 years of age or younger not established. Cautious use, if at all, in patients receiving anticoagulant therapy.

ADVERSE REACTIONS
Low incidence: nausea, vomiting, mild diarrhea, sensitivity reactions (rash, urticaria, pruritus). Rare: hypofibrinogenemia, menorrhagia, metrorrhagia.

ROUTE AND DOSAGE
Oral: initially 100,000 units 4 times daily; maintenance 50,000 units 3 or 4 times daily, or 100,000 units 2 times daily.

NURSING IMPLICATIONS
Drug should be discontinued if signs of sensitivity appear.
Instruct patient to use medication only for acute episode prescribed by physician.

BROMISOVALUM, N.F.
(BROMURAL)

Central depressant (sedative, hypnotic)

ACTIONS AND USES
Monoureide obtained from interaction of urea with a bromide. Has mild CNS depressant action.
Used as daytime sedative in anxiety and excitability states and as quick-acting hypnotic for insomnia or early morning wakefulness.

ABSORPTION AND FATE
Acts rapidly; duration of action 3 to 5 hours. Uniformly distributed in brain and other body tissues. Converted in body to urea and free bromide. Excreted in urine.

CONTRAINDICATIONS AND PRECAUTIONS
Sensitivity to bromides.

ADVERSE REACTIONS
Large doses: drowsiness. **Overdosage:** narcosis, respiratory depression, bromism: headache, drowsiness, dysarthria, acneiform skin rash, psychotic behavior, depressed or absent deep tendon reflexes.

ROUTE AND DOSAGE
Oral (sedative): 325 mg every 3 to 4 hours; (hypnotic): 650 to 975 mg at bedtime or on waking.

NURSING IMPLICATIONS
Evaluate patient's continued need for this drug; bromisovalum may be habit-forming.
Chronic use can result in bromide toxicity.

BROMODIPHENHYDRAMINE HYDROCHLORIDE, N.F. (AMBODRYL)

Antihistaminic

ACTIONS AND USES
Ethanolamine derivative similar to diphenhydramine in actions, uses, contraindications, precautions, and adverse reactions.
ROUTE AND DOSAGE
Oral: 25 mg 3 times daily; up to 150 mg daily may be required.

NURSING IMPLICATIONS
Caution patient that alcohol, tranquilizers, sedatives, or hypnotics may have additive effects.
Because of possibility of drowsiness and blurred vision, advise patient not to operate motor vehicle or machinery or perform tasks requiring skill and alertness.
Patients undergoing long-term antihistaminic therapy should have periodic blood counts.
See Diphenhydramine Hydrochloride.

BROMPHENIRAMINE MALEATE, N.F. (DIMETANE, ROLABROMOPHEN, VELTANE)

Antihistaminic

ACTIONS AND USES
Propylamine (alkylamine) antihistaminic similar to chlorpheniramine (qv) in actions, uses, contraindications, and adverse reactions. Reportedly produces less sedative effect than chlorpheniramine.
Used for symptomatic treatment of allergic manifestations. Also used in various cough mixtures and antihistamine-decongestant cold formulations.
ROUTE AND DOSAGE
Oral: 4 to 8 mg 3 or 4 times daily or 8 to 12 mg of sustained action form every 8 to 12 hours. Subcutaneous, intramuscular, intravenous: 5 to 20 mg (not to exceed 40 mg in 24-hour period). **Pediatric:** 0.5 mg/kg/24 hours divided into 3 or 4 doses.

NURSING IMPLICATIONS
The brompheniramine injection containing 100 mg/ml is not recommended for IV use since it contains a preservative.
Drowsiness, sweating, transient hypotension, and syncope may follow IV administration. Patient should be recumbent while receiving injection, and his reaction to drug should be evaluated.
Blood counts should be performed in patients receiving long-term therapy, in order to preclude possibility of blood dyscrasias.
Preserved in tightly covered, light-resistant containers.
See Chlorpheniramine Maleate.

(BUCLADIN-S SOFTABS, SOFTRAN)

Antianxiety agent (minor tranquilizer), antivertigo agent

ACTIONS AND USES
Piperazine derivative of diphenylmethane structurally and pharmacologically related to other cyclizine compounds. In common with similar compounds, exhibits mild CNS depressant, anticholinergic, antispasmodic, antiemetic, and local anesthetic effects in addition to antihistaminic activity.
Used in management of mild anxiety states and to alleviate nausea, vomiting, and vertigo associated with motion sickness, labyrinthitis, and Meniere's syndrome.

ABSORPTION AND FATE
Duration of action 12 to 24 hours. Metabolic fate unknown.

CONTRAINDICATIONS AND PRECAUTIONS
Safe use during pregnancy and for children not established.

ADVERSE REACTIONS
Drowsiness, dizziness, headache, insomnia, nervousness, dry mouth, mild hypotension, anorexia, nausea, vomiting.

ROUTE AND DOSAGE
Oral: 25 to 50 mg 1 to 3 times daily at 4- to 6-hour intervals.

NURSING IMPLICATIONS
Bucladin-S Softabs may be chewed, swallowed whole, or allowed to dissolve in the mouth.

When used to prevent motion sickness, buclizine should be taken at least 30 minutes before beginning travel.

Warn patient of possibility of pronounced sedative effect, and caution against driving a car or operating machinery or other activities requiring mental alertness.

Psychic dependence and addiction have not been reported, but they should be borne in mind when drug is administered for tranquilizing effect, particularly in patients who may abuse its use. Watch to see that patient takes drug and does not hoard it.

Abrupt withdrawal of buclizine after extended use with large doses may cause sudden reversal of an improved state or may cause paradoxic reactions.

See Hydroxyzine Hydrochloride.

BUSULFAN, U.S.P., B.P.
(MYLERAN)

Antineoplastic

ACTIONS AND USES
Potent cytotoxic alkylating agent. Mechanism of action not clear, but appears to cause chromosome alterations, thereby inhibiting DNA, RNA, and protein synthesis. Depresses myelopoiesis, but has little effect on lymphocytes and platelets. Has minimal immunosuppressive activity. In large doses it may cause irreversible bone marrow damage (evident in 4 to 6 months) and thrombocytopenia. Does not appreciably extend survival time.
Used in palliative treatment of chronic myelocytic leukemia for patients no longer responsive to radiation therapy or to previously tried antineoplastics.

ABSORPTION AND FATE

Rapidly absorbed from GI tract and reportedly metabolized extensively. Slowly excreted in urine; 10% to 50% of a dose excreted as metabolites within 24 hours.

CONTRAINDICATIONS AND PRECAUTIONS

Recent irradiation or administration of other antineoplastics, neutrophilia, thrombocytopenia, first trimester of pregnancy. Safe use during lactation not established. Cautious use: late pregnancy, men and women in childbearing years.

ADVERSE REACTIONS

Major toxic effects are related to myelosuppression: thrombocytopenia, leukopenia, anemia, agranulocytosis (rare), pancytopenia. Also hyperuricemia, renal stones, uric acid nephropathy, gynecomastia (occasionally), testicular atrophy, impotence, sterility, amenorrhea. Nausea, vomiting, diarrhea, cheilosis, glossitis, anhidrosis, alopecia, muscular weakness. With long-term or excessive therapy: splenomegaly, cataracts (rare), Addisonlike syndrome (melanoderma, fatigue, confusion, weight loss), pulmonary fibrosis ("busulfan lung").

ROUTE AND DOSAGE

Oral: **Adults:** 4 to 8 mg daily until maximal clinical and hematologic improvement is obtained. Dosage highly individualized. Maintenance (for patients who cannot maintain a remission): 2 mg/week to 4 mg/day. **Pediatric:** 60 to 120 μg/kg daily.

NURSING IMPLICATIONS

Establish data base with flow chart, recording initial vital signs and weight.

Complete blood counts, including thrombocyte levels, are taken not less than weekly throughout therapy.

Weigh patient at least weekly. A slow but steady change in weight should be communicated to physician.

Therapy is continued until leukocyte count falls to 10,000/mm³ in adults, and to about 20,000/mm³ in children (figures vary with physicians). Initial remissions last 2 months to many months. Subsequent remissions are usually shorter.

During remission, patient should be examined at monthly intervals. As WBC returns to around 50,000/mm³, symptoms of chronic myelogenous leukemia recur, and drug therapy is resumed.

Remissions are characterized by increased appetite and sense of well-being within a few days after therapy begins. Leukocyte reduction in second or third week is followed by regression of splenomegaly and increase in hemoglobin.

Monitor intake–output ratio and pattern. Patient is susceptible to hyperuricemia because of extensive purine destruction; therefore adequate hydration should be maintained (consult physician). Allopurinol (qv) may be prescribed during therapy with busulfan to reduce incidence of uric acid deposition.

Make daily inspection of skin, oral membranes, and sites used for blood specimens for abnormal bleeding due to thrombocytopenia. Ecchymotic or petechial bleeding or epistaxis should be reported promptly.

Advise patient to report immediately the onset of cough, fever, dyspnea. Pulmonary fibrosis and infections are possible complications of long-term therapy.

Amenorrhea may not be apparent for 4 to 6 months, but it is an expected effect.

Discuss possibility of alopecia with patient so that plans for temporary cosmetic substitution can be made. Advise patient to brush hair gently and no more than is necessary.

See Mechlorethamine for nursing care of stomatitis and cheilosis.

Preserved in tightly capped, light-resistant containers.

(BBS, BUTAL, BUTALAN, BUTAZEM, BUTICAPS, BUTISOL SODIUM, BUTTE, SARISOL)

Sedative, hypnotic

ACTIONS AND USES
Intermediate-acting barbiturate. Similar to phenobarbital (qv) in actions, contraindications, and adverse reactions.
Used as hypnotic in treatment of simple insomnia, as sedative for relief of anxiety, and to provide sedation preoperatively.

ABSORPTION AND FATE
Onset of action occurs in 30 to 45 minutes; duration of action is 5 to 6 hours. Metabolized in liver. Excreted in urine primarily as metabolites; 1% to 2% excreted as unchanged drug.

ROUTE AND DOSAGE
Oral (sedative): **Adults**: 15 to 30 mg 3 or 4 times a day; (hypnotic): 50 to 100 mg. **Children**: 6 mg/kg/24 hours divided into 3 doses. Highly individualized.

NURSING IMPLICATIONS
Elderly patients sometimes react with morbid excitement. Bedsides may be advisable.
Tolerance and dependence may develop with prolonged use. Following long-term use, drug should be withdrawn slowly to avoid precipitating withdrawal symptoms.
Subject to control under federal Controlled Substances Act as Schedule III drug.
See Phenobarbital.

BUTAPERAZINE MALEATE
(REPOISE)

Antipsychotic (major tranquilizer)

ACTIONS AND USES
Piperazine phenothiazine derivative similar to chlorpromazine (qv) in actions, contraindications, toxicity, and uses. More active than chlorpromazine in extrapyramidal effects and antiemetic action; produces less severe sedative and hypotensive effects.
Used for management of manifestations of psychotic disorders.

ROUTE AND DOSAGE
Oral: initially, 5 to 10 mg 3 times a day; increased by increments of 5 to 10 mg every few days until desired psychotherapeutic response is obtained. Dosage not to exceed 100 mg daily. Maintenance: usually one-fourth to one-half the dosage required during acute phase.

NURSING IMPLICATIONS
Physician may prescribe less than usual dosages for elderly and debilitated patients to reduce possibility of extrapyramidal effects.
Dosage should be adjusted weekly during early treatment program.
Report onset of extrapyramidal manifestations. Dosage reduction and/or

introduction of an antiparkinsonian agent may be necessary.

Butaperazine may impair mental and physical abilities, especially during early therapy. Caution patient to avoid driving a vehicle or other hazardous activities until his reaction to the drug is known.

See Chlorpromazine.

CAFFEINE, U.S.P.
(NODOZ, STIM TABS TIREND, VIVARIN)
CAFFEINE AND SODIUM BENZOATE, U.S.P.
CITRATED CAFFEINE, NF.

Central stimulant (analeptic), xanthine

ACTIONS AND USES

Trimethyl xanthine with actions similar to those of other xanthines. Capable of stimulating all parts of CNS in descending fashion, depending on dosage. Small doses improve psychic and sensory awareness and allay drowsiness and fatigue by stimulating cerebral cortex. Higher doses produce stimulation of medullary, respiratory, vasomotor, and vagal centers. Toxic doses result in convulsions. Relaxes smooth muscle, especially of bronchi, and causes dilatation of coronary, pulmonary, and general system blood vessels by direct action on vascular musculature. Increases contractile force of heart and cardiac output by direct stimulation of myocardium. Also has diuretic action, but less than that produced by other xanthines (theobromine and theophylline). Ability to relieve headache is thought to be due to mild cerebral vasoconstriction action and possibly to increased vascular tone.

Used parenterally as respiratory stimulant in treatment of mild to moderate respiratory depression, particularly that due to alcohol, barbiturates, morphine, and electric shock. Also has been used to relieve headache caused by spinal puncture. Used orally as an aid in staying awake and to restore mental alertness.

ABSORPTION AND FATE

Readily absorbed following injection and rapidly demethylated and oxidized in body. Approximately 17% protein-bound. Excreted in urine; about 10% excreted as unchanged drug.

CONTRAINDICATIONS AND PRECAUTIONS

Hypersensitivity to caffeine, deep respiratory depression, acute myocardial infarction, gastric ulcer.

ADVERSE REACTIONS

With large doses: restlessness, irritability, agitation, nervousness, insomnia, headache, tinnitus, scintillating scotomata, nausea, vomiting, epigastric discomfort, gastric irritation (oral form), hematemesis, elevation of blood glucose (in diabetic patients), tingling of face, flushing, palpitation, tachycardia or bradycardia, ventricular ectopic beats, hypotension, tachypnea, marked diuresis, hyperexcitability, delirium, twitching, tremors, clonic convulsions, respiratory arrest.

ROUTE AND DOSAGE

Oral: 65 to 250 mg. Intramuscular, intravenous (Caffeine and sodium benzoate): 250 to 500 mg, repeated in 4 hours if necessary. (Single dose not to exceed 1 Gm.)

NURSING IMPLICATIONS

Caffeine and sodium benzoate should be administered slowly.

Overdosage may be treated with short-acting barbiturate such as pentobarbital sodium.

Monitor vital signs closely. Large doses may cause intensification rather than reversal of severe drug-induced depressions.

Children are more susceptible than adults to the effects of caffeine and other xanthines.

An average cup of coffee prepared by drip, percolation, or vacuum methods contains approximately 100 to 150 mg of caffeine; instant coffee contains 80 to 100 mg/cup; decaffeinated coffee contains 1 to 6 mg/cup. Tea may contain 43 to 110 mg/cup; 12 ounces of cola contains 35 to 55 mg.

Caffeine-containing beverages are contraindicated in patients with ulcers because caffeine stimulates gastric secretions. Patients who insist on drinking coffee should be advised to drink it with meals, well diluted with milk.

Patients with diabetes should be advised that caffeine may impair glucose tolerance.

Habituation to alerting effects and tolerance to insomnia and diuretic action of caffeine are easily established.

Caffeine is a component of many OTC analgesic mixtures containing aspirin and/or phenacetin because of its apparent ability to enhance the effects of these agents. Anacin contains 400 mg aspirin and 32.5 mg caffeine; A.P.C. contains 227 mg aspirin, 162 mg phenacetin, and 32 mg caffeine; Empirin compound contains 227 mg aspirin, 162 mg phenacetin, and 32 mg caffeine.

Caffeine appears to be synergistic with ergotamine (vasoconstrictive effect) and is used for vasoconstriction in treatment of migraine (eg, Cafergot).

There is some evidence that headache, dizziness, and nervousness may result from excessive use of coffee, as well as from abrupt withdrawal of coffee in heavy users.

LABORATORY TEST INTERFERENCES: Caffeine reportedly may interfere with determinations of urinary 5-HIAA.

DRUG INTERACTIONS: In excessive amounts, caffeine may decrease the effect of **anticoagulants** (by increasing plasma prothrombin and factor V), and may contribute to the production of hypertensive crisis in pateints receiving **MAO inhibitors.**

CALAMINE LOTION, U.S.P., B.P.
PHENOLATED CALAMINE LOTION, U.S.P.

Protectant (topical)

ACTIONS AND USES

Contains calamine, zinc oxide, glycerin, bentonite magma, and calcium hydroxide solution. Phenolated calamine lotion also contains liquefied phenol 1%. Both preparations are soothing and protective and have mildly antiseptic and astringent properties. Phenolated calamine provides antipruritic effect by anesthetic action on sensory nerve endings.

Calamine lotion is used for temporary relief of minor skin irritations such as insect bites, poison ivy, sunburn, and prickly heat. Phenolated calamine lotion is used for temporary relief of itching and discomfort of allergic skin reactions and other minor skin disorders.

ROUTE AND DOSAGE

Topical: patted on involved skin area 3 to 5 times a day, or as needed.

NURSING IMPLICATIONS

Shake lotion well before using.

It is advisable to remove the lotion at least once daily by gently cleansing the affected area with a mild soap and water; rinse and dry throughly. Consult physician about specific procedure.

Do not use near eyes.

Prolonged use may cause excessive drying and may aggravate itching.

If irritation develops, lotion should be discontinued.

Calamine is an ingredient in several OTC skin preparations: eg, Caladryl (calamine and diphenhydramine [Benadryl]); Dome-Paste (medicated bandage impregnated with zinc oxide, calamine, and gelatin).

CALCITONIN
(CALCIMAR)

Antihypercalcemic

ACTIONS AND USES

Synthetically prepared polypeptide hormone; dosage expressed in Medical Research Council (MRC) units. Acts on bones and kidneys to produce effects opposed to those of parathyroid hormone, thus lowering serum calcium and alkaline phosphatase levels. In patients with generalized Paget's disease, inhibits osteoclastic bone resorption and reportedly may induce new bone formation by increasing osteoblastic activity. Also promotes renal excretion of calcium and phosphate by blocking tubular reabsorption. Appears to have regulatory function in the release or catabolism of gastrin and pancreatic enzymes. Short-term administration causes decrease in volume and acidity of gastric juice. Following chronic administration in about half of patients, neutralizing antibodies to calcitonin are formed, with subsequent loss of therapeutic effects.

Used in treatment of symptomatic Paget's disease of the bone (osteitis deformans) and investigationally in short-term treatment of hypercalcemia.

ABSORPTION AND FATE

Following IM or subcutaneous injection, action begins within 15 minutes, peaks in 4 hours, and persists 8 to 24 hours. Rapidly metabolized, primarily in kidneys, but also in blood and peripheral tissues. Excreted as inactive metabolites in urine.

CONTRAINDICATIONS AND PRECAUTIONS

Clinical allergy to calcitonin or to gelatin (diluent); lactation, pregnancy; in children.

ADVERSE REACTIONS

Transient nausea with or without vomiting (reversible with continued therapy); local inflammatory reaction at injection site; swelling, tingling, and tenderness of hands; facial flushing; unusual taste sensation; headache; diarrhea; skin rash and urticaria; diuresis (during first few days of calcitonin administration); calcitonin antibody formation; hypersensitivity (systemic) reaction; hypocalcemic tetany (theoretical possibility).

ROUTE AND DOSAGE

Subcutaneous, intramuscular: initially 100 MRC units daily.

NURSING IMPLICATIONS

Solution is reconstituted with volume of supplied diluent (gelatin) so that volume of dose to be administered is approximately 0.5 ml. Solubilization requires 2 or 3 minutes of gentle agitation.

Reconstituted solution that has been refrigerated should be warmed in the hands or allowed to stand at room temperature for about 15 to 30 minutes to facilitate withdrawal of dose.

A skin test is usually done prior to initiation of therapy. The appearance of more than mild erythema or wheal formation 15 minutes after intracutaneous injection of calcitonin constitutes a positive response.

Drug effect is monitored by evaluation of symptoms and periodic measurement of serum alkaline phosphatase and 24-hour urinary hydroxyproline levels.

If biochemical or clinical relapse occurs, patient compliance and calcitonin antibody titer should be evaluated.

Test for antibody titer: After overnight fasting, serum calcium is determined prior to IM administration of calcitonin. Patient eats usual breakfast. At 3 and 6 hours post injection, additional blood samples are drawn. Findings: a decrease of 0.3 mg/dl or less constitutes inadequate response to calcitonin. If hypocalcemic action of calcitonin is lost, further treatment is rarely effective.

Biochemical relapse (hypercalcemia) is suspected if the following symptoms present: deep bone and flank pain, renal calculi, polyuria, anorexia, nausea, vomiting, thirst, constipation, muscle hypotonicity, pathologic fracture, bradycardia, lethargy, psychosis, coma.

Periodically check the sterile technique of the patient who has been taught self-administration of calcitonin.

Teach the patient the importance of maintaining drug administration even though symptoms have been ameliorated.

Reconstituted solution is stable for up to 2 weeks if refrigerated. In a dry state calcitonin is stable at room temperature.

CALCIUM ASCORBATE
(CALSCORBATE)

Antiscorbutic vitamin

ACTIONS AND USES
Used for parenteral vitamin C therapy (each 5-ml ampul provides the equivalent of 413 mg ascorbic acid).

CONTRAINDICATIONS AND PRECAUTIONS
Contraindicated in patients receiving digitalis, since it may precipitate cardiac arrhythmias (elevated serum calcium increases digitalis toxicity); SC administration.

ROUTE AND DOSAGE
Intramuscular (deep), intravenous (slow): 5 to 10 ml; may be repeated daily or twice weekly as needed.

NURSING IMPLICATIONS
IM injections should be made deep, preferably in upper outer quadrant of buttock. Subcutaneous administration is specifically contraindicated.

Too rapid IV administration may result in temporary faintness or dizziness.
See Ascorbic Acid.

CALCIUM CARBASPIRIN
(Calcium Acetylsalicylate Carbamide, CALURIN)

Analgesic

ACTIONS AND USES
Complex salt of urea with soluble calcium salt of aspirin. Similar to aspirin (qv) in actions, uses, contraindications, and adverse reactions. Claimed to be more soluble than aspirin and less irritating to gastric mucosa.

Oral: **Adults**: 300 to 600 mg every 4 hours. **Children** *6 to 12 years*: 300 mg every 4 hours; *3 to 6 years*: 150 mg every 4 hours.

NURSING IMPLICATIONS
See Aspirin.

CALCIUM CARBONATE, PRECIPITATED, U.S.P., B.P.
(AMITONE, DICARBOSIL, MALLAMINT, Precipitated Chalk, TITRALAC, TUMS)

Antacid, oral calcium

ACTIONS AND USES
Reportedly regarded as antacid of choice by many physicians because of its rapid action, high neutralizing capacity, relatively prolonged duration of action, and low cost. Classified as a nonsystemic antacid, since it tends not to cause systemic alkalosis. Acid rebound may follow occasional use or high doses (eg, 4 Gm), possibly by local action of calcium ion in intestines. Liberation of carbon dioxide in stomach causes belching in some patients. Contains 400 mg (20 mEq) of calcium per gram.
Used for symptomatic relief of hyperacidity associated with peptic ulcer and for relief of transient symptoms of acid indigestion, heartburn, sour stomach, peptic esophagitis, and hiatal hernia. Also used as calcium supplement when calcium intake may be inadequate, as in childhood and adolescence, during pregnancy, lactation, and postmenopause, in the aged, and in treatment and prophylaxis of mild calcium deficiency states.
ABSORPTION AND FATE
Reacts with gastric acid to form calcium chloride, carbon dioxide, and water. Converted in part to soluble calcium salts that are absorbed from intestines; about 73% to 85% is reconverted to insoluble calcium chloride, phosphate, and calcium soaps and is excreted in feces.
CONTRAINDICATIONS AND PRECAUTIONS
Renal dysfunction, renal calculi, GI hemorrhage, dehydration, hypochloremic alkalosis.
ADVERSE REACTIONS
Constipation (common), rebound hyperacidity, nausea, eructation, flatulence. With prolonged high doses: hypercalcemia with alkalosis, hypercalciuria, hypomagnesemia, hypophosphatemia (when phosphate intake is low), renal calculi, renal dysfunction, GI hemorrhage, fecal concretions, milk-alkali syndrome.
ROUTE AND DOSAGE
Oral (antacid): 1 Gm 4 to 6 times daily. (Calcium supplement): 1 to 2 Gm 3 times daily. Dosage should not exceed 8 Gm/day.

NURSING IMPLICATIONS
When used as antacid, taken between meals (eg, 1 hour after meals) and at bedtime. When used as calcium supplement, taken with meals.
Available in tablet and powder form. For maximum effectiveness, tablet should be chewed before swallowing, or allowed to dissolve in mouth; follow with water. Powder form is dispersed in water or may be sprinkled on food if taken as calcium supplement..
Frequently combined or alternated with magnesium antacid to avoid disruption of bowel routine.
Chronic usage of calcium carbonate together with foods high in vitamin D

(such as milk) can cause milk-alkali syndrome: distaste for food, headache, confusion, nausea, vomiting, abdominal pain, hypercalcemia, hypercalciuria, soft tissue calcification (calcinosis), hyperphosphatemia, renal insufficiency, metabolic alkalosis.

Weekly serum and urine calcium determinations (see Index for Sulkowitch test) are recommended in patients receiving high doses for prolonged periods.

Observe for signs and symptoms of hypercalcemia in patients receiving high doses: nausea, vomiting, anorexia, abdominal pain, constipation, nocturia, polyuria, thirst, cloudy memory, confusion, loss of muscle tone, muscle and joint pain, psychosis.

Recommended daily allowance (RDA) of calcium for infants ½ to 1 year is 540 mg, for children and adults 800 mg; during pregnancy, lactation, and adolescence (ages 11 to 18) RDA is 1.2 Gm.

See Aluminum Hydroxide Gel for management of patient with peptic ulcer.

DRUG INTERACTIONS: Calcium enhances actions of **digitalis glycosides** and decreases GI absorption of oral tetracyclines (simultaneous use with tetracyclines not recommended).

CALCIUM CHLORIDE, U.S.P., B.P.

Calcium replenisher

ACTIONS AND USES

Actions, uses, contraindications, precautions, and adverse reactions similar to those of calcium gluconate (qv). More potent than calcium gluconate and more irritating to tissues. Also acts as acidifying diuretic by providing excess chloride ions that produce acidosis and temporary (1 to 2 days) diuresis secondary to excretion of sodium.

CONTRAINDICATIONS AND PRECAUTIONS

Presence of ventricular fibrillation, injection into myocardial or other tissue. Cautious use: patients receiving digitalis glycosides, renal insufficiency, history of renal stone formation.

ROUTE AND DOSAGE

Oral: **Adults**: 1 to 2 Gm, 3 or 4 times a day. **Children**: 300 mg/kg daily of 2% solution in divided doses every 6 hours. Intravenous: 500 mg to 1 Gm (5 to 10 ml) of 5% solution injected slowly. IV injection should be made with small-bore needle into a large vein to minimize venous irritation and undesirable reactions. IV infusion rate not to exceed 0.5 to 1 ml/min. For cardiac resuscitation (intraventricular): 200 to 400 mg.

NURSING IMPLICATIONS

Each gram provides 272 mg (13.6 mEq) of calcium.

Monitor vital signs and flow rate and observe patient closely when administered by IV infusion.

IV injection may be accompanied by cutaneous burning sensation and peripheral vasodilation, with moderate fall in blood pressure. Advise ambulatory patient to remain in bed following injection for ½ to 1 hour, depending on response.

Extravasation must be avoided during IV injection, since necrosis can result.

Calcium chloride should never be given subcutaneously or IM or by gavage, as it is a tissue irritant.

Oral preparation is better utilized if given 1 to 1½ hours after meals. Since it is irritating to GI tract, it should be administered in a demulcent vehicle such as milk.
See Calcium Gluconate.

CALCIUM GLUCONATE, U.S.P., B.P.

Calcium replenisher

ACTIONS AND USES
Calcium is an essential element for regulating the excitation threshold of nerves and muscles, for blood clotting mechanisms, for cardiac function (rhythm, tonicity, contractility), for maintenance of body skeleton and teeth; it may play a role in maintaining structural and functional integrity of cell membranes and capillaries. Calcium gluconate acts like digitalis on heart, increasing the tone of cardiac muscle and the force of systolic contractions (positive inotropic effect). Used to treat negative calcium balance, as in neonatal tetany, hypoparathyroidism, vitamin D deficiency, alkalosis, and intestinal malabsorption states. Also used to overcome cardiac toxicity of potassium, for cardiopulmonary resuscitation, to prevent hypocalcemia during exchange transfusion, and as antidote for magnesium sulfate, acute symptoms of lead colic, sensitivity reactions, and insect bites or stings. May be used to maintain normal calcium balance during pregnancy, lactation, and childhood growth period.

ABSORPTION AND FATE
Cardiac response to IV injection is immediate and lasts 1 to 2 hours. Following oral administration, approximately one-third of dose is absorbed, primarily from proximal segments of small bowel. Vitamin D probably increases active component of calcium transport from gut lumen. Largely excreted unchanged in urine and feces; small amounts also excreted in pancreatic juice, saliva, urine, and breast milk.

CONTRAINDICATIONS AND PRECAUTIONS
Cautious use: patients receiving digitalis glycosides, renal insufficiency, history of lithiasis.

ADVERSE REACTIONS
Constipation (oral preparation), hypercalcemia: anorexia, nausea, vomiting, abdominal pain, constipation, ileus, somnolence, fatigue, headache, decreased excitability of muscles and nerves, pathologic fractures, muscle and joint pain, excessive thirst, nocturia, polyuria, azotemia, mental confusion, psychosis, renal calculi, bradycardia and other arrhythmias. With rapid IV injection: tingling sensations, calcium (chalky) taste, sense of oppression or "heat waves," cardiac arrest. Tissue irritation, necrosis following IM administration or IV extravasation.

ROUTE AND DOSAGE
Adults: Oral: 1 to 5 Gm 3 times a day. Intravenous: 5 to 20 ml daily of 10% solution given slowly at rate not exceeding 0.5 ml/minute. **Children:** 500 mg/kg/day in divided doses.

NURSING IMPLICATIONS
Each gram contains 90 mg (4.5 mEq) of calcium.
Physician will prescribe specific IV flow rate. High concentrations of calcium suddenly reaching the heart can cause fatal cardiac arrest.
During IV administration, ECG is monitored to detect evidence of hypercalcemia: prolonged Q-T interval associated with inverted T wave.
Direct IV injection may be accompanied by cutaneous burning sensations and peripheral vasodilatation, with moderate fall in blood pressure. Pa-

tient should be advised to remain in bed for ½ to 1 hour following injection, depending on response.

Oral calcium preparations are best utilized when administered 1 to 1½ hours after meals. Calcium gluconate is reported to be nonirritating to GI mucosa.

Therapeutic effects in treatment of tetany (hypocalcemia) are evaluated by amelioration of neuromuscular hyperexcitability: paresthesias (numbness and tingling of fingers, toes, and lips), skeletal muscle spasms, twitching of facial muscles, intestinal hypermotility and colic, carpopedal spasm, laryngospasm, convulsions, and cardiac arrhythmias.

Latent tetany may be detected by Chvostek's and Trousseau's signs.

Chvostek's sign: Tap facial nerve (cranial nerve VII) just below temple where it emerges. Hyperirritability of nerve manifested by twitching of facial muscles is a positive sign of tetany.

Trousseau's sign: Apply sphygmomanometer cuff to upper arm and inflate until radial pulse is obliterated and keep inflated for about 3 minutes. The ischemia produced increases excitability of peripheral nerves and causes spasms of lower arm and hand muscles (carpal spasm) if tetany exists. Alternative method: Grasp patient's wrist firmly enough to constrict circulation for a few minutes.

If patient has hypocalcemia or if it is suspected, padded side rails are advisable. Also, have on hand mouth gag, airway, and suction apparatus.

Sulkowitch's test (may be performed at home by patient or family member) is a simple test for urinary calcium, which gives an approximate index of serum calcium level. To rule out hypercalcemia (hypercalciuria), examine early morning specimen, since excretion is lowest at this time. For hypocalcemia, take urine sample after a meal, when Ca excretion is maximal. Results (qualitative): fine white cloud (normal), clear solution (decreased serum calcium), heavy precipitate (excessive serum calcium).

To facilitate intestinal absorption of calcium gluconate, physician may prescribe reduced phosphate intake (milk and other dairy products) or simultaneous administration of aluminum hydroxide, which forms insoluble phosphate salts. Other dietary substances that may be restricted because they interfere with calcium absorption include oxalic acid (eg, in spinach, rhubarb) and phytic acid (in bran, whole cereals).

In sustained therapy, frequent determinations should be made of calcium and phosphorus (tend to vary inversely). Normal serum calcium is 9 to 10.6 mg/dl; normal serum inorganic phosphorus is 3 to 4.5 mg/dl.

RDA of calcium for infants ½ to 1 year is 540 mg; for children and adults 800 mg/day; for pregnant and lactating women, and during adolescence 1200 mg/day. Milk products are best sources of calcium (and phosphorus); dark green leafy vegetables such as kale, broccoli, and mustard or turnip greens, as well as sardines, clams, and oysters, are good sources.

LABORATORY TEST INTERFERENCES: IV calcium gluconate may cause false decreases in serum and urine magnesium (by Titan yellow method) and transient elevations of plasma 11-hydroxycorticosteroid levels by Glenn-Nelson technique.

DRUG INTERACTIONS: Calcium gluconate and other Ca containing drugs enhance the inotropic and toxic effects of **digitalis glycosides** and may precipitate cardiac arrhythmias. Calcium complexes **tetracyclines** and thus decreases their effect. The 2 drugs should not be given at the same time orally nor should they be mixed for parenteral administration.

Calcium replenisher

ACTIONS AND USES
Contains approximately 13% calcium. Similar to calcium gluconate (qv) in actions, uses, contraindications, and adverse reactions.
ROUTE AND DOSAGE
Oral: 1 to 5 Gm 3 times a day, with meals.

NURSING IMPLICATIONS
Contains 130 mg (6.5 mEq) of calcium per gram.
Tablets or powder can be dissolved in hot water; then add cool water to patient's taste.
Hospital pharmacy may prepare calcium lactate solution on request.
See Calcium Gluconate.

CALCIUM PANTOTHENATE, U.S.P.
(Dextro-Calcium Pantothenate, PANTHOLIN)

Enzyme cofactor vitamin

ACTIONS AND USES
Calcium salt of pantothenic acid readily converted to the acid in vivo. Pantothenic acid, a member of the B-complex group, is precursor of coenzyme A. Coenzyme A functions in a variety of metabolic reactions involving transfer of acetyl groups, and is associated with release of energy from carbohydrates and the biosynthesis and degradation of fatty acids, sterols, and steroid hormones. Widely employed in conjunction with other B vitamins and in multiple vitamin preparations as nutritional supplement. Its use for gray hair and in treatment of alopecia has not been successful.
ROUTE AND DOSAGE
Oral: 10 to 50 mg daily.

NURSING IMPLICATIONS
Minimum daily requirement not established, but estimates of 5 to 10 mg have been made.
No human deficiency syndrome identified. Presumed signs of pantothenic acid deficiency include neurologic disturbances (burning feet and other paresthesias, steppage gait), muscle and abdominal cramps, nausea, adrenocortical hypofunction (defective water excretion, sensitivity to insulin), dermatoses, weakness, fatigue, insomnia, cardiovascular instability, mood changes, psychoses.
Pantothenic acid is widely distributed in animal and vegetable foods. Especially good sources: liver, kidney, muscle tissue, egg yolk, wheat bran, rice bran, dry milk, peanuts.

CALUSTERONE
(METHOSARB)

Antineoplastic

ACTIONS AND USES
Synthetic steroid structurally and pharmacologically related to testosterone. Appears to protect neoplastic cell surface from growth stimulation of progesterone, estradiol-17β and related steroids. Androgenic effects are minimal and mild. Stimulates platelet production.
Used in palliative management of inoperable or disseminated carcinoma of breast in postmenopausal women, when hormone therapy is indicated.
ABSORPTION AND FATE
Well absorbed from GI tract. Distribution, metabolism, and excretion data not determined.
CONTRAINDICATIONS AND PRECAUTIONS
Premenopausal women; prostate or breast malignancy in men; pregnancy. Cautious use: renal or cardiac disease predisposing to edema.
ADVERSE REACTIONS
Virilization (hirsutism, deepening of voice, acne, facial hair growth, increased oiliness of skin, mild scalp hair loss, clitoral enlargement); fever, nausea, vomiting, edema, cholestatic jaundice, intensified pain (during osseous flare), mild increases in BSP retention and SGOT levels.
ROUTE AND DOSAGE
Oral: 50 mg 4 times daily. (Dose range: 150 to 300 mg/day.)

NURSING IMPLICATIONS
Protracted vomiting necessitates stopping drug.
Monitor intake–output ratio and pattern; report significant or gradual change.
Weigh patient under standard conditions at regular intervals. Check dependent areas for objective signs of edema; if edema is evident, diuretic therapy may be required.
Hepatic function tests, determinations of serum calcium and alkaline phosphatase levels and physical examination should be performed routinely throughout therapy.
Slight rise in alkaline phosphatase level (normal 1.5 to 4.5 units/dl, Bodansky) after initiation of treatment reflects improvement in osseous lesions; marked elevation may indicate extensive liver metastasis.
Hypercalcemia (normal serum calcium: 9 to 10.6 mg/dl) usually is most prominent during active remission of bony metastases.
Inspect sclera, skin, and soft palate frequently for jaundice. Instruct patient to report dark urine or clay-colored stools. Dosage may need to be adjusted if these signs appears.
In order to evaluate patient's response to calusterone, therapy should be continued for a minimum of 3 months unless there is active progression of the disease.

DRUG INTERACTIONS: Calusterone may increase the effects of **oral anticoagulants**.

CAPREOMYCIN SULFATE
(CAPASTAT SULFATE)

Antibacterial (tuberculostatic)

ACTIONS AND USES

Polypeptide antibiotic derived from *Streptomyces capreolus*. Similar to viomycin in structure and action mechanism; classified as secondary antitubercular agent: Active in vitro against human strains of *Mycobacterium tuberculosis*. Frequent cross-resistance occurs between capreomycin and viomycin and occasionally between capreomycin and both kanamycin and neomycin. Capable of producing neuromuscular blockade in large doses.

Used in conjunction with appropriate antitubercular drugs in treatment of pulmonary tuberculosis when primary agents (aminosalicylic acid, isoniazid, and streptomycin) cannot be tolerated or when causative organism has become resistant.

ABSORPTION AND FATE

Following IM injection of 1-Gm dose, peak drug serum levels of approximately 30 μg/ml are produced in 1 to 2 hours. Serum levels fall rapidly; 52% is excreted within 12 hours (if renal function is normal). Low concentrations present after 24 hours. Excreted unchanged, primarily in urine.

CONTRAINDICATIONS AND PRECAUTIONS

Hypersensitivity to capreomycin; simultaneous administration of streptomycin, viomycin. Safe use during pregnancy or in infants and children not established. Extreme caution, if used at all, in patients receiving other potentially ototoxic or nephrotoxic drugs, as well as in patients with renal insufficiency, auditory impairment, history of allergies (especially to drugs), and preexisting liver disease.

ADVERSE REACTIONS

Nephrotoxicity: elevated BUN and NPN, abnormal urine sediment, hematuria, pyuria, albuminuria, depressed PSP excretion, tubular necrosis. **Ototoxicity**: hearing loss, tinnitus, vertigo. **Hematologic**: leukocytosis, leukopenia, eosinophilia. **Hypersensitivity**: urticaria, maculopapular rash associated with febrile reaction. Other: hypokalemia; decreased BSP excretion; pain, induration, excessive bleeding, and sterile abscess at injection site; headache; muscle weakness.

ROUTE AND DOSAGE

Intramuscular: 1 Gm daily (not to exceed 20 mg/kg body weight per day) given for 60 to 120 days, followed by 1 Gm 2 or 3 times weekly.

NURSING IMPLICATIONS

IM injections should be made deep into large muscle mass. Superficial injections are more painful and are associated with sterile abscess. Observe injection sites for signs of excessive bleeding or inflammation.

Capreomycin is reconstituted by adding isotonic sodium chloride injection or sterile water for injection to vial; allow 2 to 3 minutes for drug to dissolve completely. See manufacturer's directions for volume of diluent.

After reconstitution, solution may be stored 48 hours at room temperature and up to 14 days under refrigeration. Solution may acquire pale straw color and darken with time, but this is not associated with loss of potency or toxicity.

The following determinations used as guidelines for therapy should be performed before drug is started and at regular intervals during therapy: (1) appropriate bacterial susceptibility tests; (2) audiometric measurements and tests of vestibular function; (3) renal function studies (weekly); (4) liver function tests; (5) serum potassium levels.

Monitor intake and output. Report immediately to physician any change in

output or intake-output ratio, any unusual appearance of urine, or elevation of BUN above 30 mg/dl.

Instruct patient to report any change in hearing or disturbance of balance.
Capreomycin can cause injury to both auditory and vestibular portions
of cranial nerve VIII. These effects are sometimes reversible if drug is
withdrawn promptly when first signs appear.

Patient and responsible family members should be completely informed
about adverse reactions; they should be urged to report immediately the
appearance of any unusual symptom, regardless how vague it may seem.

CARBACHOL, U.S.P., B.P.
(CARBACEL, ISOPTO CARBACHOL, MISTURA C, MIOSTAT INTRAOCULAR SOLUTION)

Cholinergic (ophthalmic)

ACTIONS AND USES

Potent synthetic choline ester similar to acetylcholine in pharmacologic properties. Not rapidly inactivated by cholinesterase, and therefore its actions are more
prolonged than those of acetylcholine; also more potent and longer-acting than
pilocarpine. Acts directly on neuroeffectors of circular pupillary constrictor and
ciliary muscles, producing miosis and spasms of accommodation, thus facilitating drainage from arterior chamber and lowered intraocular pressure. Usually
prepared with wetting agent such as benzalkonium chloride to enhance corneal
penetration.

Used intraocularly to produce pupillary miosis during ocular surgery. Used
topically to reduce intraocular pressure in open-angle or narrow-angle glaucoma, particularly when patient has become intolerant of or resistant to pilocarpine.

ABSORPTION AND FATE

Miotic action lasts 4 to 8 hours after topical application.

CONTRAINDICATIONS AND PRECAUTIONS

Known hypersensitivity, corneal abrasions, acute iritis. Cautious use: acute
cardiac failure, bronchial asthma, peptic ulcer, GI spasms, obstructive ileus,
hyperthyroidism, urinary tract obstruction, Parkinson's disease.

ADVERSE REACTIONS

Headache, brow and eye pain, conjunctival hyperemia. Systemic absorption:
sweating, flushing, ciliary spasm, abdominal cramps, increased peristalsis, diarrhea, contractions of urinary bladder, transient fall in blood pressure with reflex
tachycardia, asthma.

ROUTE AND DOSAGE

Topical ophthalmic: 1 or 2 drops of 0.75% to 3% solution instilled into lower
conjunctival sac 2 or 3 times daily. Intraocular (administered by physician):
0.01% intraocular solution.

NURSING IMPLICATIONS

Frequent administration of potent eye preparations presents the danger of
systemic absorption if drug is allowed to drain into lacrimal system.
Application of gentle pressure to nasolacrimal duct immediately after
drop is instilled and before patient closes his eyes prevents entry of drug
into nasopharynx and general circulation.

Instill into conjunctival sac of lower lid. Patient may blot lid with sterile
cotton ball or gauze, but advise him not to rub or squeeze lids together.

Frequency and strength of drops are determined by patient's response and
tolerance.

Eye drops are sterile and therefore should be handled so as to avoid contamination.

The patient with glaucoma should remain under medical supervision for periodic tonometer measurements, since he usually will require miotics for the rest of his life. The patient must understand that even in the absence of symptoms progressive ocular damage can occur unless he receives appropriate treatment.

Intraocular carbachol (eg, Miostat) is intended for single-dose intraocular use only (administered by physician). Unused portions should be discarded.

CARBAMAZEPINE, U.S.P., B.P.
(TEGRETOL)

Anticonvulsant, specific analgesic

ACTIONS AND USES

Structurally related to tricyclic antidepressants; anticonvulsant properties appear qualitatively similar to those of phenytoin (diphenylhydantoin). Like phenytoin, provides relief in trigeminal neuralgia by reducing synaptic transmission within trigeminal nucleus. Also has sedative, anticholinergic, antidepressant, muscle relaxant, and neuromuscular transmission inhibitory actions.

Used as anticonvulsant in treatment of grand mal and psychomotor epilepsy and mixed seizures in patients who have not responded satisfactorily to other agents, and for symptomatic treatment of trigeminal neuralgia (tic douloureux) and glossopharyngeal neuralgia.

ABSORPTION AND FATE

Slowly absorbed from GI tract. Peak serum levels in 2 to 8 hours; wide distribution. Serum half-life thought to be between 14 and 29 hours. Induces liver microsomal enzymes and thus may accelerate its own metabolism and that of concomitantly administered drugs. Excreted in urine as the glucuronide, and less than 1% as unchanged drug. Crosses placenta and may appear in breast milk.

CONTRAINDICATIONS AND PRECAUTIONS

Hypersensitivity to carbamazepine and to tricyclic compounds; history of myelosuppression or hematologic reaction to other drugs; increased intraocular pressure; disseminated lupus erythematosus; cardiac, hepatic, renal, or urinary tract disease; hypertension; nursing mothers. Safe use in women of childbearing potential and during pregnancy not established. Cautious use in the elderly.

ADVERSE REACTIONS

Hematologic: aplastic anemia, leukopenia, leukocytosis, agranulocytosis, eosinophilia, thrombocytopenia, purpura. **Hepatic**: abnormal liver function tests, cholestatic and hepatocellular jaundice. **GU and renal**: urinary frequency and retention, oliguria, impotence, albuminuria, glycosuria, elevated blood urea nitrogen (BUN). **Nervous and musculoskeletal systems**: dizziness, vertigo, drowsiness, disturbances of coordination, ataxia, confusion, headache, fatigue, tinnitus, abnormal hearing acuity, speech difficulty, involuntary movements, peripheral neuritis, paresthesias, visual hallucinations, activation of latent psychosis, mental depression with agitation and talkativeness, myalgia, arthralgia. **Dermatologic**: skin rashes, urticaria, Stevens-Johnson syndrome, photosensitivity reactions, altered skin pigmentation, exfoliative dermatitis, alopecia. **GI**: nausea, vomiting, anorexia, abdominal pain, diarrhea, constipation, dry mouth and pharynx, glossitis, stomatitis. **Cardiovascular**: congestive heart failure, aggravation of coronary artery disease and hypertension, hypotension, syncope, arrhythmias, edema, thrombophlebitis. **Eyes**: lens opacities, conjunctivitis, blurred vision, transient diplopia, oculomotor disturbances, nystagmus, mydriasis. Other: fever, chills, lymphadenopathy, diaphoresis, hyponatremia.

Oral (epilepsy): initially 200 mg 2 times a day, increased gradually to t.i.d. or q.i.d. regimen until best results are obtained; (trigeminal neuralgia): initially 100 mg twice a day, with meals; thereafter, dose is increased gradually by 100-mg increments every 12 hours until pain is relieved or side effects occur. Usual daily maintenance dose is 200 to 800 mg. Generally, maximum dosage not to exceed 1200 mg/day. Highly individualized.

NURSING IMPLICATIONS

Prior to initiation of carbamazepine therapy, the following procedures for eliciting baseline data are recommended: (1) detailed health history; (2) physical examination, including ophthalmoscopy (slit lamp, fundoscopy, tonometry) and ECG; (3) laboratory studies: complete blood counts including platelets, reticulocytes, and serum iron, liver function tests, and complete urinalysis and BUN determinations.

Blood counts (see above) should be repeated weekly during first 3 months of therapy and monthly thereafter for at least 2 to 3 years. Other tests listed above should be performed at regular intervals during drug treatment. Abnormal findings signal the need for dose reduction or drug withdrawal.

Physician will rely on accurate observation and reporting to determine lowest effective dosage level.

In general, therapy should be discontinued if any of the following signs of myelosuppression occur: erythrocyte count less than 4,000,000/mm^3, HCT less than 32%, Hgb less than 11 Gm/dl, leukocyte count less than 4,000/mm^3, platelet count less than 100,000/mm^3, reticulocyte count less than 20,000/mm^3, serum iron greater than 150 μg/dl.

Monitor intake–output ratio and vital signs during period of dosage adjustment. Report oliguria, changes in intake–output ratio, and changes in blood pressure or pulse patterns.

The pain of tic douloureux is so excruciating that it has driven some patients to suicide. Learn from the patient what provokes attacks. Common triggering stimuli include drafts, shaving, washing face, talking, chewing, hot or cold fluids or foods, and jarring the bed.

Home patients and responsible family members should be instructed to withhold drug and notify physician immediately if adverse reactions occur.

Since dizziness, drowsiness, and ataxia are common side effects, warn patient to avoid hazardous tasks requiring mental alertness and physical coordination.

Impress on the patient and family the importance of remaining under close medical supervision throughout therapy.

Confusion and agitation may be aggravated in the elderly; therefore bedsides and supervision of ambulation may be indicated.

At least every 3 months throughout therapy it is recommended that physician attempt dosage reduction or termination of drug therapy, if possible, in patients with trigeminal neuralgia. Some patients develop tolerance to the effects of carbamazepine.

In patients with epilepsy, abrupt withdrawal of any anticonvulsant drug may precipitate seizures or even status epilepticus.

LABORATORY TEST INTERFERENCES: Possibility of falsely decreased urinary steroid values: Zimmerman reactions for 17-hydroxycorticosterone and 17-ketosteroids (based on limited studies).

DRUG INTERACTIONS: Concomitant administration of **MAO inhibitors** and carbamazepine, or administration within 14 days of each other, is contraindicated. Concomitant use of carbamazepine and **digitalis glycosides** may result in bradycardia. **Phenobarbitol** may stimulate carbamazepine metabolism and result in lower plasma levels. By causing microsomal enzyme induction, carbamazepine may reduce the effects of **oral anticoagulants, antiepilepsy agents** (eg, **phenobarbital, phenytoin**), and **doxycycline.**

CARBARSONE, N.F.

Antiamebic

ACTIONS AND USES
Pentavalent organic arsenical containing 28.5% arsenic. Acts primarily in intestinal lumen against amebic intestinal trophozoites of *Entamoeba histolytica,* the source of cysts.
Used alone or in combination with other amebicides in treatment of acute and chronic intestinal amebiasis.

ABSORPTION AND FATE
Readily absorbed from GI tract. Presumed to be reduced in body to trivalent derivative, carbarsone oxide. Accumulates in tissues; slowly excreted by kidneys.

CONTRAINDICATIONS AND PRECAUTIONS
Hypersensitivity or intolerance to arsenic compounds, amebic hepatitis or other liver disease, kidney disease, contraction of visual or color fields or other visual disturbances.

ADVERSE REACTIONS
Nausea, vomiting, increased diarrhea, epigastric burning, abdominal cramps, weight loss, sore throat, ulcerations of mucous membranes, agranulocytosis, splenomegaly, hepatitis, hepatomegaly, neuritis, skin rashes, pruritus. Edema of ankles, knees, and wrists; polyuria, kidney damage, retinal edema, visual disturbances, hemorrhagic encephalitis; shock, coma, and convulsions.

ROUTE AND DOSAGE
Adults: Oral: 250 mg 2 or 3 times daily for 10 days. Course of therapy repeated if necessary after rest interval of 10 to 14 days. Rectal (as retention enema): 2 Gm dissolved in 200 ml warm 2% sodium bicarbonate solution, administered every other night for 5 doses. **Children:** average total dose over a 10-day period is about 75 mg/kg.

NURSING IMPLICATIONS
For children, it will be necessary to divide contents of a capsule and give in half a glass of milk, orange juice, in jelly, or some other food, or in a small volume of sodium bicarbonate solution 1%, if allowed.
Liver function tests are advised before initiation of carbarsone therapy and periodically during treatment.
Regular and careful inspection of skin, vision testing, and palpation of liver and spleen should be done during therapy.
Monitor intake and output. Amebiasis may produce liquid stools containing blood and mucus. Keep physician informed of number, frequency, and character of stools.
Low-residue diet may be prescribed, and patient is usually advised to limit physical activities during treatment period.
Because drug is excreted slowly, a rest period of 10 to 14 days must follow each 10-day course of therapy before starting another course, in order to prevent accumulation and toxicity.
At the first appearance of adverse reaction, drug should be discontinued.
Instruct patient and responsible family members to report immediately ag-

gravation of symptoms already present or appearance of any unusual signs or symptoms, even after therapy has been discontinued.

Carbarsone retention enema is generally ordered if patient has deep ulcers of lower colon.

The retention enema is instilled after a cleansing enema (after a delay sufficient that the urge to defecate has passed). Oral dose should be omitted when retention enema is given. A sedative may be prescribed to help patient retain medication.

Stools should be examined daily for amebic cysts. Presence of cysts indicates the need for an additional course of therapy.

If enema is to be given to obtain stool specimen, normal saline or tap water should be used. Hypertonic solutions may alter appearance of amebae.

Stool specimen should be delivered promptly to laboratory for incubation. Characteristic movements of parasites are seen only when specimen is warm.

Microscopic examination should be made of feces of other household members, supplemented by search for source of infection and mode of transmission.

Amebic cysts are transmitted by water, vegetables (especially those served raw), and flies, and by hand-to-mouth transfer of fresh feces and by soiled hands of food handlers. In teaching the patient, emphasize personal hygiene, particularly sanitary disposal of feces, hand washing after defecation and before eating, and risks of eating raw foods.

Isolation is not required, but patient must be excluded from preparing, processing, and serving foods until treatment is completed.

Beginning 1 week after completion of therapy, stools should be examined for cysts on 3 alternate days and at monthly intervals for about 3 months to assure that amebae have been eliminated.

Have on hand the antidote dimercaprol (BAL), a chelating agent and specific antiarsenical.

CARBAZOCHROME SALICYLATE
(ADRENOSEM SALICYLATE)

Antihemorrhagic

ACTIONS AND USES

Adrenochrome semicarbazone compound with sodium salicylate. Reportedly capable of controlling capillary permeability, fragility, bleeding, and oozing without affecting blood clotting time, prothrombin time, or vitamin K level. Mechanism of action not understood. Has no sympathomimetic action; not effective in massive hemorrhage or arterial bleeding.

Has been used preoperatively (prophylaxis) and therapeutically to control bleeding caused by increased capillary permeability, as in epistaxis, tonsillectomy, idiopathic purpura, retinal hemorrhage, and hereditary telangiectasia.

ABSORPTION AND FATE

Completely oxidized in body and eliminated within 12 hours.

CONTRAINDICATIONS AND PRECAUTIONS

Sensitivity to carbazochrome or salicylates, or other known allergies. Safe use during pregnancy and in women of childbearing potential not established.

ADVERSE REACTIONS

Toxicity is minimal. Transient stinging sensation at injection site.

ROUTE AND DOSAGE

Preoperative (prophylactic): **Adults and Children** *over 12 years*: 10 mg IM the evening before operation; 10 mg IM with on-call medication; **Children** *under 12* *years*: 5 mg. Postoperative: **Adults and Children** *over 12 years*: 5 to 10 mg IM or orally every 2 hours as indicated; **Children** *under 12 years*: 5 mg.

NURSING IMPLICATIONS
Sensitization to the salicylate component may develop with repeated use. Advise patient to report the onset of skin rash, swelling of eyelids or face, difficulty in breathing, tinnitus.

DRUG INTERACTIONS: Inhibited by **antihistamines** (they should be discontinued 48 hours before initiation of carbazochrome therapy).

CARBENICILLIN DISODIUM, U.S.P.
(GEOPEN, PYOPEN)

Antibacterial, antibiotic

ACTIONS AND USES
Semisynthetic benzylpenicillin derived from penicillin G potassium, but differing in range of antibacterial activity. Primarily indicated in Gram-negative infections. Particularly effective against *Pseudomonas aeruginosa, Proteus* (especially indole-positive strains), susceptible strains of *Escherichia coli,* and *Neisseria gonorrhoeae.* Inactivated by penicillinase.
Used in treatment of septicemia, gonorrhea, and urinary, respiratory, intraocular, soft-tissue, and systemic infections. Sometimes used for mixed Gram-negative and Gram-positive infections caused by susceptible organisms. May be used in conjunction with gentamicin in treatment of *Pseudomonas* infections.

ABSORPTION AND FATE
Peak serum concentrations reached 1 to 2 hours following IM injection; low or absent by 6 hours. Blood levels are higher following IV administration, but decrease more rapidly. Serum half-life is approximately 1 hour; it may be prolonged to 10 to 15 hours in renal impairment. Widely distributed in body tissues; about 50% is bound to plasma proteins. Generally, 60% to 90% of dose is excreted in urine within 6 to 8 hours.

CONTRAINDICATIONS AND PRECAUTIONS
Hypersensitivity to penicillins or cephalosporins; history of allergies, asthma, hay fever. Safe use during pregnancy not established. Cautious use: renal and hepatic disease; patients on sodium restriction.

ADVERSE REACTIONS
Nausea, vomiting, unpleasant taste (following rapid IV), neurotoxicity, hemorrhagic manifestations, pain and induration at IM site, thrombophlebitis (IV), neuromuscular irritability (high doses), allergic symptoms (skin rash, pruritus, urticaria, eosinophilia), anaphylactic reactions, hemolytic anemia, neutropenia, thrombocytopenia, leukopenia, hypokalemic alkalosis. Altered laboratory values: elevations of SGOT, SGPT, alkaline phosphatase, bilirubin, and lactic dehydrogenase; elevated CPK levels (following IM, probably due to muscle injury).

ROUTE AND DOSAGE
Intramuscular: **Adults:** 1 to 2 Gm every 4 to 6 hours. Intravenous: 6 to 30 Gm daily in divided doses or by continuous infusion. Highly individualized according to severity of infection. Recommended maximum dose is 40 Gm/day. Lower dosage for patients with impaired renal function. See manufacturer's directions for dilutions. **Pediatric:** 50 to 250 mg/kg/24 hours divided into 4 to 6 doses IV or IM.

NURSING IMPLICATIONS

Culture and sensitivity tests should be performed before initiation of drug therapy and at regular intervals during therapy in order to monitor effectiveness of drug and detect possible emergence of resistant organisms.

If drug is given by infusion, physician should prescribe specific flow rate.

IM injections should not exceed 2 Gm per individual injection site. Administer injection well into body of large muscle. Gluteus maximus or mid-lateral thigh for adults, and mid-lateral thigh for children are preferred sites. Aspirate carefully to prevent inadvertent injection into blood vessel. Rotate injection sites.

Local reactions (without epinephrine) at IM sites may be minimized by reconstituting drug with 0.5% lidocaine hydrochloride or bacteriostatic water for injection containing 0.9% benzyl alcohol. Consult physician.

Monitor intake and output. Patients with impaired renal function are particularly susceptible to nephrotoxicity, neurotoxicity, and hemorrhagic manifestations.

Bleeding tendencies result from inhibition of platelet aggregation and may occur 12 to 24 hours after therapy is initiated. Watch for frank bleeding, purpura, easy bruising, ecchymoses, petechiae.

Clotting time and prothrombin time determinations should be made at regular intervals.

During prolonged therapy, periodic assessments of hepatic, renal, and hematopoietic functions and determinations of serum electrolytes, SGOT, SGPT, alkaline phosphatase, bilirubin, and lactic dehydrogenase are advised.

Serum electrolytes and cardiac status should be closely monitored in patients on sodium restriction. (Each gram of drug contains 4.7 mEq of sodium.)

Patients treated for gonorrhea who are suspected of having syphilitic lesions should have dark-field examinations before drug therapy and at monthly intervals thereafter for a minimum of 4 months.

As with other penicillins, superinfection by nonsusceptible organisms may result from prolonged use of carbenicillin disodium.

After reconstitution, solutions should be used within 24 hours if kept at room temperature and within 72 hours if refrigerated.

Carbenicillin and gentamicin should not be mixed in the same infusion fluid.

See Penicillin G Potassium for drug interactions.

CARBENICILLIN INDANYL SODIUM
(GEOCILLIN)

Antibacterial

ACTIONS AND USES

Semisynthetic penicillin and indanyl ester of carbenicillin prepared for oral use, with similar actions, contraindications, and adverse reactions.

Used in treatment of acute and chronic infections of upper and lower urinary tract caused by susceptible strains of *E. coli, Enterobacter, Enterococci, Proteus,* and *Pseudomonas* species.

ABSORPTION AND FATE

Acid-stable and well absorbed from GI tract. Peak serum levels attained in 1 hour. Not detectable in serum after 6 hours. Rapidly excreted unchanged in urine.

CONTRAINDICATIONS AND PRECAUTIONS

Safe use in children and during pregnancy not established. Also see Carbenicillin Disodium.

ADVERSE REACTIONS

Flatulence, dryness of mouth, unpleasant taste, furry tongue, vaginitis, abdominal cramps. Also see Carbenicillin, Disodium.

ROUTE AND DOSAGE

Oral: 382 to 764 mg 4 times daily.

NURSING IMPLICATIONS

Protect tablets from moisture, and store at temperature not exceeding 30 C (86 F).

See Carbenicillin Disodium.

CARBETAPENTANE CITRATE, N.F.
(TOCLASE)

Antitussive

ACTIONS AND USES

Structurally related to caramiphen and local anesthetics. Exerts atropinelike action and appears to depress cough reflex by selective action on medullary center. Also exhibits local anesthetic and antihistaminic effects. Used to control nonproductive cough.

ADVERSE REACTIONS

Dryness of mouth and throat, sensation of chest tightness, slight respiratory depression, allergic dermatitis, nausea, dizziness, drowsiness (rarely).

ROUTE AND DOSAGE

Oral: **Adults and children** *over 12 years:* 15 to 30 mg 3 or 4 times daily. **Children** *4 to 12 years:* up to 30 mg/24 hours. *2 to 4 years:* up to 15 mg/24 hours. Divided into 3 or 4 doses.

NURSING IMPLICATIONS

See Benzonate for patient teaching point.

CARBIDOPA/LEVODOPA
(SINEMET)

Antiparkinsonian

ACTION AND USES

Carbidopa, a hydrazine derivative of methyldopa, is a peripheral dopa decarboxylase inhibitor. When levodopa is given alone, large doses must be administered to compensate for peripheral decarboxylation in order to provide adequate amounts of dopamine at appropriate sites in the corpus striatum. Carbidopa prevents peripheral decarboxylation of levodopa and thereby makes more levodopa available for transport to the brain. Carbidopa does not cross blood–brain barrier and therefore does not affect metabolism of levodopa within the brain. Addition of carbidopa reduces amount of levodopa required by about 75%, since levodopa plasma levels and plasma half-life are increased. Although incidence of nausea and vomiting associated with levodopa is decreased, adverse CNS effects (eg, dykinesias) may occur at lower dosages and sooner with carbidopa/levodopa combination than with levodopa alone.

Carbidopa also prevents the inhibitory effect of pyridoxine (vitamin B_6) on levodopa. Indications for use are as for levodopa (qv).

Hypersensitivity to carbidopa or levodopa, narrow-angle glaucoma. Also see Levodopa.

ADVERSE REACTIONS

Involuntary movements, mental disturbances and depression, nausea, orthostatic hypotension. Also see Levodopa.

ROUTE AND DOSAGE

Highly individualized. Oral (*patients not receiving levodopa*): initially 1 tablet containing 10 mg carbidopa and 100 mg levodopa (10/100 mixture) 3 times daily, increased by 1 tablet every day or every other day up to 6 tablets daily; if further titration is necessary, 1 tablet of the 25/250 mixture 3 times a day is substituted; may be increased by one-half tablet to 1 tablet every day or every other day, if needed; (*patients receiving levodopa*): initially 1 tablet of the 25/250 mixture 3 or 4 times daily, or 1 tablet of the 10/100 mixture 3 or 4 times daily in patients who require less than 1.5 Gm of levodopa; dosage adjustments made as necessary by adding or omitting one-half or 1 tablet per day.

NURSING IMPLICATIONS

Carbidopa/levodopa is usually initiated with a morning dose after patient has been without levodopa for at least 8 hours.

Patients who have been taking levodopa must be carefully instructed regarding continuation or discontinuation of levodopa as prescribed by physician

Monitor patient closely during dosage adjustment period. Both therapeutic and adverse effects appear more rapidly than with use of levodopa alone.

Observe for and report immediately the onset of CNS side effects such as choreiform, dystonic, and other involuntary movements. Dosage reduction may be required. Blepharospasm (involuntary winking) is a useful early sign of excessive dosage.

Orthostatic hypotension with weakness, dizziness, and faintness can occur. Observe necessary safety precautions.

See nursing implications for levodopa. Drug interactions are the same as those for levodopa, with exception of the statement regarding pyridoxine. Pyridoxine does not reverse the action of the carbidopa/levodopa combination.

CARBINOXAMINE MALEATE, N.F.
(CLISTIN)

Antihistaminic

ACTIONS AND USES

Ethanolamine derivative similar to diphenhydramine (qv) in actions, contraindications, and adverse reactions.

Used in symptomatic treatment of bronchial asthma and other allergic disorders.

ABSORPTION AND FATE

Completely absorbed from GI tract. Onset of action in 30 to 60 minutes, with duration of 4 to 6 hours. Degraded in liver; excreted in urine in inactive form.

ADVERSE REACTIONS

Low incidence of drowsiness, GI distress, dizziness, dryness of mouth.

ROUTE AND DOSAGE

Oral: **Adults:** 4 to 8 mg 3 or 4 times daily. Repeat-action tablets: 8 or 12 mg at 12-hour intervals. **Children** *over 6 years:* 4 mg 3 or 4 times daily. *3 to 6 years:* 2 to 4 mg 3 or 4 times/day. *1 to 3 years:* 2 mg 3 or 4 times/day.

NURSING IMPLICATIONS
Tolerance usually develops to sedative effects. Caution patient to avoid
driving or other activities requiring mental alertness, until his response to
drug has been evaluated.
Stored in tightly covered, light-resistant containers.
See Diphenhydramine Hydrochloride.

CARISOPRODOL
(RELA, SOMA)

Skeletal muscle relaxant

ACTIONS AND USES
Propanediol derivative monocarbamate with central depressant action. Modifies
pain perception centrally without affecting peripheral pain reflexes or withdrawal reflexes. Relaxes abnormal tension of skeletal muscles by selective
blocking action on multisynaptic pathways in spinal cord and possibly by
sedative effect. Has antipyretic properties and weak anticholinergic action.
Used for muscle spasm, stiffness, and pain in a variety of musculoskeletal
disorders and to relieve spasticity and rigidity in cerebral palsy.

ABSORPTION AND FATE
Rapidly absorbed from GI tract. Effects usually appear within 30 minutes and
persist 4 to 6 hours. Metabolized by liver and excreted by kidney. Concentration
in breast milk is two to four times that in plasma.

CONTRAINDICATIONS AND PRECAUTIONS
Hypersensitivity to carisoprodol and related compounds (eg, meprobamate,
tybamate); porphyria; children under 12 years of age; nursing mothers. Safe use
during pregnancy not established. Cautious use: compromised liver or kidney
function, addiction-prone individuals.

ADVERSE REACTIONS
Low incidence of toxicity. **CNS:** drowsiness, vertigo, ataxia, tremor, headache,
irritability, depressive reactions, syncope, insomnia. **Allergic or idiosyncratic
reactions:** skin rash, erythema multiforme, pruritus, eosinophilia, asthma, fever,
extreme weakness, dizziness, transient quadriplegia, angioneurotic edema,
smarting eyes, temporary loss of vision, diplopia, mydriasis, euphoria, confusion, agitation, disorientation, dysarthria, anaphylactic shock. **GI:** nausea, vomiting, hiccups. **Cardiovascular:** tachycardia, postural hypotension, facial flushing.

ROUTE AND DOSAGE
Oral: 350 mg 4 times daily.

NURSING IMPLICATIONS
Last dose should be taken at bedtime.
Drowsiness is a common side effect and may require reduction in dosage.
Advise patient to avoid activities requiring mental alertness and physical
coordination until his response to the drug has been evaluated.
Allergic or idiosyncratic reactions generally occur within the period from the
first to the fourth dose in patients taking the drug for the first time.
Symptoms usually subside after several hours; they are treated by sup-
portive and symptomatic measures.
Carisoprodol is used as an adjunct to rest and physical therapy modalities.
Caution patient not to take alcohol, other CNS depressants, or psychotropic
drugs.
Advise patient to discontinue drug and notify physician if skin rash, di-

plopia, dizziness, or other unusual signs or symptoms appear.

There are some indications that psychologic dependence may occur with long-term use.

Withdrawal symptoms may occur with abrupt termination of drug following prolonged use of doses higher than those recommended: abdominal cramps, insomnia, chilliness, headache, nausea.

CARMUSTINE
(BCNU, BiCNU)

Antineoplastic

ACTIONS AND USES

Highly lipid-soluble nitrosurea with alkylating properties especially against rapidly proliferating cell populations. Following intracellular biotransformation, carmustine produces cross-linking with DNA strands, thereby blocking DNA, RNA, and protein synthesis. Not cross-reactive with respect to resistance to other alkylating agents. Causes delayed myelosuppression.

Used in Hodgkin's disease and other lymphomas and meningeal leukemia. Also used in treatment of primary and metastatic tumors of brain, breast, and GI tract and in bronchogenic and renal cell carcinomas.

ABSORPTION AND FATE

Intestinal absorption is rapid, but IV route is used because of rapid tissue uptake and metabolism; disappears from plasma in 5 minutes. Degraded in liver; 70% of unchanged drug appears in urine within 96 hours, but protein-bound active metabolites persist in plasma for a long time, thus explaining delayed bone marrow toxicity. Entry into cerebrospinal fluid is rapid.

CONTRAINDICATIONS AND PRECAUTIONS

Myelosuppression, hepatic and renal insufficiency, pregnancy.

ADVERSE REACTIONS

Nausea, vomiting, diarrhea, hepatic and renal damage (occasional); leukopenia, thrombocytopenia, burning and pain along infusion vein, flushing, dyspnea, esophagitis, CNS toxicity.

ROUTE AND DOSAGE

Intravenous: 150 to 200 mg/m^2 as single dose; repeated in 6 weeks.

NURSING IMPLICATIONS

Slow infusion and adequate dilution will reduce pain of administration. Frequently check rate of flow set by physician.

Nadirs of leukocyte and thrombocyte counts may not be reached for 6 weeks following drug administration. Blood studies are continued following infusion, at weekly intervals.

Carmustine is not a vesicant, but it can cause burning discomfort even in the absence of extravasation. Instruct patient to report burning sensation immediately. Infusion will be discontinued and restarted in another site.

Nausea and vomiting may occur 2 to 6 hours after administration. In second and subsequent treatments, if drug-induced vomiting is a problem, consult physician about antiemetic to be given before next infusion.

Instruct patient to inform physician promptly about onset of sore throat, weakness, fever, infection of any kind, or abnormal bleeding (ecchymosis, epistaxis, petechiae, hematemesis, melena).

Be alert to signs of hepatic toxicity (jaundice, dark urine, pruritus, clay-colored stools) and renal insufficiency (dysuria, oliguria, hematuria).

Infection prevention during period of leukopenia is imperative. Screen con-

tacts to prevent exposure of patient to colds or infection.
Check temperature daily. Avoid use of rectal thermometer to prevent injury to mucosa. An elevation in temperature requires medical attention.
Antibiotics and red cell and platelet transfusions may be given to control infections during periods of drug-induced leukopenia and thrombocytopenia.

CARPHENAZINE MALEATE, N.F.
(PROKETAZINE)

Antipsychotic (major tranquilizer)

ACTIONS AND USES
Relatively short-acting piperazine phenothiazine derivative. Similar to chlorpromazine in actions, uses, contraindications, and toxicity. More active than chlorpromazine in producing extrapyramidal effects. See Chlorpromazine.

ROUTE AND DOSAGE
Oral: 12.5 to 25 mg 2 or 3 times daily. Dosage may be increased by 12.5 to 25 mg/day at 4- to 7-day intervals until optimum effect is obtained. Maximum dosage not to exceed 400 mg daily.

NURSING IMPLICATIONS
Physician may prescribe less than usual dosages for elderly and debilitated patients in order to reduce the possibility of extrapyramidal effects.
Carphenazine concentrate may be administered in fruit juice.
Preserved in airtight, light-resistant containers.
See Chlorpromazine.

CASCARA SAGRADA, U.S.P., N.F.
(BILEO SECRIN, CAS-EVAC, Cascara Fluidextract Aromatic, Cascara Sagrada Fluidextract)

Stimulant cathartic

ACTIONS AND USES
Anthraquinone cathartic obtained from bark of buckhorn tree *(Rhamnus purshiana)*. Acts principally in large intestine. Following partial absorption, reaches large intestine indirectly via bloodstream and partly by direct passage through small intestine. Causes propulsive movements of colon by direct chemical irritation.
Used for temporary relief of constipation and to prevent straining at stool in various disease conditions.

ABSORPTION AND FATE
Active principles absorbed in small intestine and conveyed directly or by bloodstream to large intestine. Acts in 6 to 8 hours. Excreted into breast milk.

CONTRAINDICATIONS AND PRECAUTIONS
Nausea, vomiting, abdominal pain, fecal impaction; GI bleeding, ulcerations; appendicitis, gastroenteritis, intestinal obstruction, nursing mothers.

ADVERSE REACTIONS
Large doses: anorexia, nausea, griping, abnormally loose stools, hypokalemia, impaired glucose tolerance, calcium deficiency. Chronic use: constipation rebound.

Oral (tablet): 300 mg; fluidextract: 1 ml; aromatic fluidextract: 5 ml.

NURSING IMPLICATIONS
A single dose taken before retiring usually results in evacuation of soft stool 8 to 12 hours later.

Frequent or prolonged use of irritant cathartics disrupts normal reflex activity of colon and rectum and can result in drug dependence for evacuation.

Constipation, which is especially common in the elderly, may result from poor eating habits, inadequate fluid intake, lack of exercise, or habitual use of cathartics based on the erroneous notion that autointoxication will result if bowels are not evacuated daily.

Evaluate patient's need for continued use of drug.

Prolonged ingestion of anthraquinone cathartics can cause benign melanotic pigmentation of rectal mucosa and may impart a reddish hue to alkaline urine and a yellowish brown color to acid urine.

Preserved in tightly covered, light-resistant containers. Avoid exposure to direct sunlight and excessive heat.

See Bisacodyl for other patient teaching points.

LABORATORY TEST INTERFERENCES: Possibility of interference with PSP excretion test because of urine discoloration.

DRUG INTERACTIONS: Cathartics in large doses may result in decreased absorption of **vitamin K** and/or **oral anticoagulants,** by increasing speed of contents through intestinal tract.

CASTOR OIL, U.S.P., B.P.
(ALPHAMUL, NEOLOID, Oleum Ricini)

Stimulant cathartic

ACTIONS AND USES
Obtained from the seeds of *Ricinus communis.* Hydrolyzed in small intestine to glycerol and ricinoleic acid, a local irritant. Stimulates motor activity in small intestine and inhibits antiperistalsis in colon, thus preventing normal fluid absorption from intestinal contents. Rapid evacuation of copious liquid or semiliquid stools follows, with little or no colic.

Used to prepare abdomen for radiographic examination of colon and kidneys and to evacuate irritants and poisons from intestinal tract. Rarely used to relieve constipation. Also applied locally to skin as emollient and protectant and to conjunctiva (sterile) to alleviate irritation caused by the presence of a foreign body.

ABSORPTION AND FATE
Poorly absorbed. Acts in 2 to 6 hours. Excreted into breast milk.

CONTRAINDICATIONS AND PRECAUTIONS
Hypersensitivity to castor bean; dehydration; fecal impaction; abdominal pain; appendicitis, GI bleeding, ulcerations, perforation, obstruction; pregnancy; nursing mothers; menstruation.

ADVERSE REACTIONS
Severe purgation, nausea, vomiting, abdominal cramps, dehydration, electrolyte imbalance, rebound constipation.

Oral: **Adults:** castor oil, U.S.P., 15 to 60 ml. **Children:** 5 to 15 ml. **Infants:** 1 to 5 ml.

NURSING IMPLICATIONS
More active if taken on empty stomach. Since castor oil is a fat, it may retard gastric emptying time.

Action begins in 2 to 6 hours, depending on dose. Time the administration so as not to interfere with patient's sleep.

Castor oil has objectionable odor, taste, and consistency. It may be made more palatable by mixing it with a glass of cold fruit juice or carbonated beverage if allowed.

Emulsified forms are reported to be less disagreeable to taste. Castor oil is also available in capsule form.

Inform patient that castor oil causes complete emptying of intestinal contents, and therefore normal evacuation may be delayed for 1 day or more.

Preserved in tightly covered containers. Avoid exposure to excessive light.

CEFAZOLIN SODIUM
(ANCEF, KEFZOL)

Antibacterial

ACTIONS AND USES
Semisynthetic cephalosporin broad-spectrum antibiotic. Similar to cephalothin (qv) in actions, uses, contraindications, precautions, and adverse reactions. Reported to be less irritating to tissue and less nephrotoxic than cephalothin. Appears to be less resistant to cephalosporinases than other cephalosporins. Recommended by USPHS Center for Disease Control as alternative therapy for uncomplicated gonorrhea in pregnant patients allergic to penicillin.

ABSORPTION AND FATE
Peak serum concentrations in 5 minutes following IV injection; average half-life 1.4 to 2.2 hours. Concentrations in gallbladder and bile may exceed those in serum. Approximately 74% to 86% bound to plasma proteins. Excreted unchanged in urine. Approximately 56% to 89% excreted within 6 hours, 80% to 100% within 24 hours (slow excretion in patients with renal impairment). Readily crosses placenta. Excreted in small amounts in breast milk.

ADVERSE REACTIONS
Nausea, vomiting, anorexia, diarrhea, oral candidiasis. Also see Cephalothin.

ROUTE AND DOSAGE
Intramuscular, intravenous: **Adults:** 250 mg to 1 Gm every 6 to 8 hours; as much as 6 Gm/day in severe infections. Highly individualized. For treatment of gonorrhea: 2 Gm IM with 1 Gm of probenecid. **Children** *over 1 month*: 25 to 50 mg/kg/day divided into 3 or 4 equal doses.

NURSING IMPLICATIONS
IM injections should be made deep into large muscle mass. Pain on injection is infrequent. Rotate injection sites.

Reconstituted solutions are stable for 24 hours at room temperature and for 96 hours if stored under refrigeration. (After reconstitution, shake well until drug is entirely dissolved.)

For urinary sugar determinations, use Tes-Tape or Clinistix and not Clinitest, or Benedict's Solution.

Although clinical evidence of renal damage has not been reported, precautions outlined for cephalothin should be observed.
See Cephalothin Sodium.

CEPHALEXIN MONOHYDRATE
(KEFLEX)

Antibacterial

ACTIONS AND USES
Semisynthetic cephalosporin broad-spectrum antibiotic similar to cephalothin (qv), but generally less potent.
Used as follow-up oral therapy in patients initially treated with parenteral cephalosporins. Some clinicians recommend that it be reserved for treatment of urinary tract infections due to susceptible *Klebsiella* organisms resistant to other oral antibacterials.

ABSORPTION AND FATE
Stable in stomach acid; rapidly and almost completely absorbed following oral administration. (Absorption may be reduced in patients with pernicious anemia or obstructive jaundice.) Peak serum level of 9 μg/ml in 1 hour. Measurable levels persist for 6 hours. Higher and more prolonged blood levels in patients with renal insufficiency. Widely distributed to body fluids, with highest concentrations in kidneys. About 6% to 15% bound to plasma proteins. Serum half-life 0.6 to 1.2 hours. Within 8 hours over 90% of dose is excreted in urine as unchanged drug. May cross placenta; appears in breast milk.

CONTRAINDICATIONS AND PRECAUTIONS
Hypersensitivity to cephalosporins. Cautious use: history of penicillin or other drug allergy. See Cephalothin.

ADVERSE REACTIONS
Diarrhea, nausea, vomiting, abdominal pain, anal and genital pruritus, vulvovaginitis, dizziness, headache, fatigue, slightly elevated SGPT and SGOT. Also see Cephalothin.

ROUTE AND DOSAGE
Oral: **Adults:** 250 to 500 mg every 6 hours (usual dose range 1 to 4 Gm daily in divided doses). **Children** *over 1 month:* 25 to 50 mg/kg/day in 4 equally divided doses.

NURSING IMPLICATIONS
Cephalexin is not destroyed by gastric acid, but peak blood levels are slightly lower and delayed when it is administered with food. However, the total amount of drug absorbed is unchanged.

After reconstitution, cephalexin oral suspension should be refrigerated; unused portions should be discarded 14 days after preparation. Keep tightly covered; shake well before using.

For urinary sugar determinations, use Tes-Tape or Clinistix and not Clinitest or Benedict's Solution.

See Cephalothin, Sodium.

(KAFOCIN)

Antibacterial

ACTIONS AND USES
Semisynthetic cephalosporin broad-spectrum antibiotic similar to cephalothin (qv). Reportedly associated with highest incidence of severe GI side effects, and produces lower serum levels than other cephalosporins.
Used in treatment of acute and chronic urinary tract infections caused by susceptible strains of uropathogens. Generally not used for treatment of infections in other locations.

ABSORPTION AND FATE
Stable in gastric acid. Peak serum levels are reached within 2 hours; higher and more prolonged levels in patients with renal insufficiency. Thought to have similar distribution in body as other cephalosporins. Up to 30% bound to plasma proteins; serum half-life is 90 minutes. Excreted almost entirely in urine as active desacetyl derivative. About 20% to 25% of 500-mg dose is excreted within 8 hours.

CONTRAINDICATIONS AND PRECAUTIONS
Hypersensitivity to cephalosporins. Cautious use: history of penicillin or other drug allergy; impaired renal function; history of peptic ulcer. Also see Cephalothin.

ADVERSE REACTIONS
Diarrhea, constipation, abdominal pain, nausea, vomiting, GI bleeding, severe enterocolitis, malaise, fever, chills, headache, dizziness, vertigo, mental confusion. Also see Cephalothin.

ROUTE AND DOSAGE
Oral: **Adults:** 250 to 500 mg 4 times daily. **Children** *over 1 year:* 25 to 50 mg/kg/day in divided doses.

NURSING IMPLICATIONS
Diarrhea is the most frequent side effect. If it is severe and persistent, cessation of therapy may be necessary.
Cephaloglycin is not destroyed by gastric acid, but peak blood levels are slightly lower and delayed when it is administered with food. However, total amount of drug absorbed is not affected.
Renal function studies and careful clinical observations of renal status and effects of drug therapy should be made during cephaloglycin therapy.
For urinary sugar determinations, use Tes-Tape or Clinistix and not Clinitest or Benedict's Solution.
See Cephalothin Sodium.

CEPHALORIDINE
(LORIDINE)

Antibacterial

ACTIONS AND USES
Semisynthetic cephalosporin broad-spectrum antibiotic. Similar to cephalothin (qv). Causes less pain on IM injection than cephalothin. Reported to be the most nephrotoxic of the cephalosporins, and not as resistant to the action of cephalosporinases as are other cephalosporins.

Peak blood levels in 30 minutes following IM dose. In contrast to cephalothin, measurable levels persist 12 hours or more. Widely distributed to body fluids and tissues, with highest concentrations in kidney; 0 to 31% bound to serum proteins. Serum half-life is 40 to 108 minutes. Minimal hepatic degradation. Excreted unchanged in urine. Most excreted in first 6 hours; about 75% of dose excreted in 24 hours. Readily crosses placenta.

CONTRAINDICATIONS AND PRECAUTIONS

Hypersensitivity to cephalosporins; shock, oliguria, azotemia, concomitant use of nephrotoxic drugs. Cautious use: history of penicillin or other drug allergy. Also see Cephalothin.

ADVERSE REACTIONS

Hallucinations, nystagmus, transient elevations of prothrombin time, agranulocytosis, proximal renal tubular necrosis. Also see Cephalothin.

ROUTE AND DOSAGE

Intramuscular, intravenous: **Adults:** 250 mg to 1 Gm 2 to 4 times a day at equally spaced intervals. Daily dosage not to exceed 4 Gm (reduced dosage employed in patients known to have or suspected of having renal impairment). **Children** *over 1 month;* 30 to 50 mg/kg/day in divided doses.

NURSING IMPLICATIONS

Renal studies and appropriate culture and susceptibility tests should be performed prior to initiation of therapy.

Nephrotoxicity is dose-related. Serum cephaloridine concentrations should be kept below 75 μg/ml.

Renal function studies should be performed regularly during treatment (urine protein, cells, and casts, BUN, serum creatinine), particularly in patients receiving more than 2 Gm/day.

Report falling urinary output or change in intake–output ratio.

IM injections are usually made into large muscle mass such as gluteus or lateral aspect of thigh.

Pale straw color of fresh solutions has no effect on potency.

If necessary, aqueous solutions may be stored 96 hours under refrigeration; thereafter, discard unused portion.

If crystals form, warm vial in the hand while agitating solution until it becomes clear.

Protect cephaloridine from light.

For urinary sugar determinations, use Tes-Tape or Clinistix and not Clinitest or Benedict's Solution.

See Cephalothin, Sodium.

CEPHALOTHIN SODIUM, U.S.P, B.P.
(KEFLIN)

Antibacterial

ACTIONS AND USES

Semisynthetic derivative of cephalosporin C, a substance produced by the fungus *Cephalosporium acremonium*. Structurally and pharmacologically related to penicillins. Inhibits synthesis of bacterial cell wall; has broad antibacterial spectrum. Primarily bactericidal but also bacteriostatic against most Gram-positive organisms including penicillinase-producing staphylococci and some Gram-negative strains. *Pseudomonas serratia,* and most indole-positive *Proteus* and motile *Enterobacter* species are resistant. Most resistant of the cephalosporins to cephalosporinases (inactivating enzyme produced by certain bacteria).

Used in treatment of severe infections of respiratory and urinary tracts, bones, joints, and soft tissue.

ABSORPTION AND FATE

Peak serum levels of 10 μg/ml 30 minutes following IM injection of 500-mg dose; 30 μg/ml in 15 minutes following 1-Gm IV dose. Widely distributed to body tissues and fluids, except brain and cerebrospinal fluid (unless inflamed). Serum half-life is 30 to 60 mintues; 65% to 79% bound to plasma proteins. Partly deacetylated in liver. About 60% to 70% of dose is excreted by kidneys within 6 hours, largely as unchanged drug and active desacetyl metabolite. Readily crosses placenta; low concentrations in breast milk.

CONTRAINDICATIONS AND PRECAUTIONS

Hypersensitivity to cephalosporin antibiotics. Safe use during pregnancy and in infants under 1 year of age not determined. Cautious use: history of allergies, hypersensitivity to penicillins (possibility of cross-allergenicity), impaired renal function.

ADVERSE REACTIONS

Nausea, vomiting, diarrhea, superinfections. **Local reactions:** pain, induration, slough, abscess (IM site), thrombophlebitis (IV site). **Hypersensitivity:** maculopapular rash, urticaria, vulvar pruritus, serum-sickness-like reactions, anaphylactic shock, eosinophilia, drug fever. **Renal:** nephrotoxicity (rarely). **Hematologic:** neutropenia, leukopenia, thrombocytopenia, hemolytic anemia, direct positive Coombs test (particularly patients with azotemia). **Hepatic:** transient rise in SGOT, SGPT, and alkaline phosphatase; increased plasma thymol turbidity and increased serum bilirubin.

ROUTE AND DOSAGE

Intramuscular, intravenous: **Adults:** 500 mg to 1 Gm every 4 to 6 hours (usual dose range 2 to 8 Gm daily). Intraperitoneal: up to 6 mg/100 ml of dialysis fluid. **Children** *over 1 year:* 100 mg/kg/day in divided doses.

NURSING IMPLICATIONS

Culture and susceptibility studies should be performed prior to and during therapy. Therapy may be started pending test results.

A careful drug history should be elicited before therapy in order to determine previous hypersensitivity to cephalosporin antibiotics and penicillins and other drug allergies.

Physicians generally prefer other cephalosporins for IM injection because cephalothin causes intense pain and induration. However, if cephalothin IM is prescribed, administer injection deep into large muscle mass such as gluteus or lateral aspect of thigh. Rotate injection sites.

Observe IV sites for evidence of inflammatory reaction. IV infusions of doses larger than 6 Gm/day for more than 3 days may be associated with thrombophlebitis.

Report falling urinary output or change in intake–output ratio. Patients with renal dysfunction and those receiving high doses in the presence of dehydration are particularly susceptible to nephrotoxic reactions.

When renal function is reduced, dosage is based on creatinine clearance values.

Periodic hematologic studies and evaluations of renal and hepatic functions are recommended in patients receiving high doses and during prolonged therapy.

Immediately report signs and symptoms of hypersensitivity reaction. If it occurs, drug should be discontinued.

Superinfections caused by emergence of nonsusceptible organisms may occur, particularly during prolonged use of cephalosporins. Mouth, vagina, and anus are susceptible areas; meticulous hygiene is indicated. Appropriate cultures should be taken if superinfection is suspected.

Drug treatment for all infections should be continued at least 48 to 72 hours after patient becomes asymptomatic or after evidence of bacterial eradication is obtained.

In infections caused by β-hemolytic streptococci, therapy should be continued at least 10 days in order to prevent the occurrence of rheumatic fever or glomerulonephritis.

Kept at room temperature, reconstituted solutions for IM injection should be administered within 12 hours. Refrigeration protects potency for 96 hours after reconstitution.

Slight discoloration of solution does not affect potency.

Crystallization may occur. To redissolve crystals, warm to room temperature with constant agitation.

IV infusions should be started within 12 hours and completed within 24 hours of preparation.

LABORATORY TEST INTERFERENCES: Cephalosporins cause confusing black-brown or green-brown color or false positive urine glucose determinations with copper reduction reagents such as Benedict's, Fehling's, and Clinitest. Tests based on enzymatic glucose oxidase reactions, such as Clinistix and Tes-Tape, are not affected. False positive urinary protein (sulfosalicylic acid method); falsely elevated urinary 17-ketosteroids (Zimmerman reaction); false positive direct Coombs' test reported.

DRUG INTERACTIONS: Increased possibility of nephrotoxicity with concomitant use of cephalosporins and **aminoglycoside antibiotics, colistin, ethacrynic acid, furosemide, polymyxin B, probenecid,** or **sulfinpyrazone.** Cephalosporins may increase the effect of **oral anticoagulants.**

CEPHAPIRIN SODIUM
(CEFADYL)

Antibacterial

ACTIONS AND USES
Semisynthetic cephalosporin broad-spectrum antibiotic similar to cephalothin in actions, uses, contraindications, precautions, and adverse reactions. Reported to cause less tissue irritation and to be less nephrotoxic than either cephalothin or cephaloridine.

ABSORPTION AND FATE
Peak serum levels in 30 minutes following IM injection and in 5 minutes following IV administration. Average serum half-life is 21 to 47 minutes; 44% to 50% bound to serum proteins. Excreted in urine; 70% of administered dose excreted within 6 hours as active desacetyl metabolite and unchanged drug. Crosses placenta; excreted in breast milk.

ROUTE AND DOSAGE
Intramuscular, intravenous: **Adults:** 500 mg to 1 Gm every 4 to 6 hours. **Children** *over 3 months:* 40 to 80 mg/kg/24 hours in 4 equally divided doses.

NURSING IMPLICATIONS
IM injections should be made deep into large muscle mass. Rotate injection sites.

Although clinical evidence of renal damage has not been reported, the precautions outlined for cephalothin should be observed.

For urinary sugar determinations, use Tes-Tape or Clinistix and not Clinitest or Benedict's Solution.
See Cephalothin Sodium.

CEPHRADINE
(ANSPOR, VELOSEF)

Antibacterial

ACTIONS AND USES
Semisynthetic cephalosporin broad-spectrum antibiotic similar to cephalothin (qv). Oral preparation is used primarily as follow-up to parenteral cephalosporin therapy and in treatment of urinary tract infections due to susceptible *Klebsiella* organisms resistant to other antibacterials.

ABSORPTION AND FATE
Well absorbed from GI tract. Peak serum levels obtained within 1 hour. Serum half-life 1 to 2 hours. Up to 20% bound to plasma proteins. High urine concentrations. Approximately 57% to 95% excreted unchanged in urine within 6 hours. Crosses placenta; excreted in breast milk.

CONTRAINDICATIONS AND PRECAUTIONS:
Hypersensitivity to cephalosporins. Cautious use: history of penicillin or other drug allergy.

ADVERSE REACTIONS
Glossitis, nausea, vomiting, diarrhea or loose stools, abdominal pain, heartburn, dizziness, tightness in chest, candidal vaginitis. See also Cephalothin.

ROUTE AND DOSAGE
Adults: Oral: 250 to 500 mg every 6 hours or 500 mg to 1 Gm every 12 hours. Intramuscular, intravenous: 500 mg to 1 Gm 4 times daily; not to exceed 8 Gm/day. **Children** *over 9 months:* Oral: 25 to 100 mg/kg/day in 4 equally divided doses every 6 to 12 hours. Not to exceed 4 Gm/day. Intramuscular, intravenous: *over 1 year:* 50 to 100 mg/kg/day in 4 equally divided doses. Not to exceed daily adult dose.

NURSING IMPLICATIONS
Culture and sensitivity tests and renal function studies should be performed prior to and during drug therapy. Recommended dosage schedule in patients with reduced renal function is lower than usual and is based on creatinine clearance determinations.

To minimize pain and induration of IM site, inject deep into large muscle mass such as gluteus or lateral aspect of thigh. Sterile abscess has been reported to occur with subcutaneous injection.

Cephradine may be given without regard to meals, as it is not destroyed by gastric acid; however, the presence of food may delay absorption.

Following reconstitution, IM or direct IV solutions should be used within 2 hours at room temperature; with refrigeration (5 C), potency is retained 24 hours. Reconstituted solutions may vary in color from light straw to yellow; this does not affect potency.

Continuous or intermittent IV infusion solutions retain potency for 10 hours at room temperature or 48 hours when refrigerated at 5 C. Prolonged infusions should be replaced every 10 hours with freshly prepared solution.

Protect solutions from concentrated light or direct sunlight.

For urinary sugar determinations, use Tes-Tape or Clinistix and not Clinitest or Benedict's Solution.

See Cephalothin, Sodium.

(CEEPRYN, CĒPACOL)

Topical antiinfective

ACTIONS AND USES
Cationic quaternary ammonium surfactant related to benzalkonium chloride (qv). Bactericidal and bacteriostatic against a wide variety of Gram-positive and Gram-negative nonsporulating bacteria and against some fungi, including *Candida albicans* and *Trichomonas vaginalis*. Also has emulsifying and wetting properties; its surface tension is about half that of water.

Used for antisepsis of minor skin wounds, to stimulate salivation for relief of dryness and minor mouth and throat irritations.

ROUTE AND DOSAGE
Topical: minor wounds and preoperative preparation of skin (1:1000); mucous membranes (1:10,000 to 1:4000). Oral lozenge (1:1500): allow to dissolve slowly in mouth; used as needed. Mouthwash, gargle: (1:2000).

NURSING IMPLICATIONS

Drug activity is decreased by soaps and soap substitutes, hard water, lipids, serum, tissue fluids, and other organic matter.

Rubber goods and catgut may fade in color when immersed in cetylpyridinium chloride solution, but they are not otherwise affected.

Color markings on clinical thermometers may be removed if they are allowed to remain in a solution of the drug.

Caution patient to keep drug out of reach of children. Poisoning after oral ingestion has been reported.

See Benzalkonium Chloride.

CHARCOAL, ACTIVATED, U.S.P.
(Activated Carbon, Adsorbent Charcoal, CHARCODOTE, Medicinal Charcoal, DARCO 60)

Antidote (general purpose), adsorbent

ACTIONS AND USES
Residue from destructive distillation of various organic substances, treated to increase adsorptive power (referred to as activation). Activated charcoal is a chemically inert, odorless, tasteless, fine black powder with wide spectrum of adsorptive activity. Does not adsorb cyanide and is reportedly ineffective in poisonings due to ethanol, methanol, ferrous sulfate, caustic alkalis, and mineral acids. Used as general-purpose emergency antidote in treatment of certain oral poisonings. Has been used to adsorb intestinal gases in treatment of dyspepsia, flatulence, and distention, but its value in these conditions is not established. Sometimes used topically as deodorant for foul-smelling wounds and ulcers. Used investigationally in uremia to adsorb various waste products from GI tract.

ABSORPTION AND FATE
Not absorbed from GI tract, and not metabolized. Excreted in feces.

ROUTE AND DOSAGE
Oral (acute poisoning): 5 to 50 Gm (in general, dose should be 5 to 10 times estimated weight of ingested poison; larger doses are necessary if food is present in stomach); (GI disturbances): 600 mg to 5 Gm.

NURSING IMPLICATIONS

Activated charcoal tablets or granules are less effective than powder form; therefore they are not recommended in treatment of acute poisoning.

Most effective when administered during early management of acute poisoning (preferably within 30 minutes after ingestion of poison), but even late administration may be of benefit.

In an emergency, dose may be approximated by stirring sufficient activated charcoal into tap water to make a slurry with consistency of thick soup.

Activated charcoal may be swallowed or used as the gastric lavage fluid. It is not a substitute for lavage.

If necessary, palatability may be improved by adding small amount of concentrated fruit juice or chocolate powder (reportedly, these agents do not significantly alter adsorptive activity).

Many physicians recommend that vomiting first be induced by ipecac syrup or apomorphine. Apomorphine may be given before or following activated charcoal, but ipecac must be administered before, because activated charcoal will adsorb ipecac and thus reduce its effectiveness.

So-called universal antidote (2 parts activated charcoal, 1 part magnesium oxide, 1 part tannic acid) is reportedly inferior to activated charcoal used alone.

Burnt toast is not a form of activated charcoal and is not a useful antidote in management of acute poisonings.

Activated charcoal will color feces black.

Stored in tightly covered glass or metal containers.

CHLORAL BETAINE, N.F., B.P.
(BETA-CHLOR, Chloral Hydrate Betaine)

Sedative, hypnotic

ACTIONS AND USES

Crystalline complex containing one molecule of betaine for each molecule of chloral hydrate formulated in tasteless stable tablets. Liberates chloral hydrate after ingestion. Reportedly produces less undesirable GI effects than chloral hydrate. Actions, uses, contraindications, precautions, and potential for adverse reactions as for chloral hydrate.

ROUTE AND DOSAGE

Oral: 1 or 2 tablets 60 to 90 minutes before surgery or 15 to 30 minutes before bedtime. (Each 870 mg. tablet contains the equivalent of 500 mg chloral hydrate.)

NURSING IMPLICATIONS

Preserved in tightly covered, light-resistant containers.

See Chloral Hydrate.

CHLORAL HYDRATE, U.S.P., B.P.
(AQUACHLORAL, COHIDRATE, FELSULES, H. S. NEED, KESSODRATE, NOCTEC, ORADRATE, RECTULES, SOMNOS)

Sedative, hypnotic

ACTIONS AND USES

Produces "physiologic sleep" by mild cerebral depression with no suppression of REM sleep and little or no hangover. Principal action thought to be due in part to trichloroethanol, its reduction product. The oldest chloral derivative and still regarded as a relatively safe, effective, and inexpensive sedative-hypnotic.

Used in management of insomnia, for nocturnal sedation (especially in the young and the elderly), and for preoperative and postoperative sedation. Has little or no analgesic action. May cause enzyme induction and displace certain drugs from protein binding sites.

ABSORPTION AND FATE

Readily absorbed following oral or rectal administration. Hypnotic dose produces sleep within 1 hour, lasting 4 to 8 hours. Rapidly reduced in body to active trichloroethanol and distributed to all tissues. Variable amount oxidized to trichloroacetic acid in liver and kidney; this, together with free trichloroethanol and its glucuronide, is excreted in urine in 24 to 48 hours. Small portion excreted in feces via bile. Crosses placenta and may appear in breast milk.

CONTRAINDICATIONS AND PRECAUTIONS

Known hypersensitivity to drug, severe hepatitis, renal and cardiac disease, esophagitis, gastritis, gastric or duodenal ulcers, nursing mothers. Cautious use: pregnancy, asthma, history of or proneness to drug dependence.

ADVERSE REACTIONS

Large doses: nausea, vomiting, gastric irritation, increased peristalsis, esophageal stricture, reduced urinary output, paradoxic excitement, disorientation, delirium, paranoid reactions, marked cutaneous vasodilation, pinpoint pupils, myocardial depression, arrhythmias, hypotension, depressed respiration, hypotension, hypothermia, coma, anesthesia. Chronic use: skin eruptions, severe gastritis, renal and hepatic damage, sudden death.

ROUTE AND DOSAGE

Oral, rectal suppository, retention enema: **Adults:** (sedative): 250 mg 3 times a day after meals; (hypnotic): 500 mg to 1 Gm 15 to 30 minutes before bedtime. Generally, single dose or total daily dosage should not exceed 2 Gm. **Pediatric** (sedative): 25 mg/kg/24 hours divided into 3 or 4 doses; (hypnotic): 50 mg/kg with a maximun of 1 Gm.

NURSING IMPLICATIONS

Chloral hydrate is not intended for relief of pain. When used alone it may cause excitement and delirium in presence of pain.

Corrosive to skin and mucous membranes unless well diluted. Has an aromatic, pungent odor and bitter, pungent taste; these may be minimized by use of the capsule form or by dilution of liquid preparations in chilled fluids.

To minimize gastric irritation, administer drug after meals. Capsules and aqueous solutions should be taken with full glass of water, fruit juice, or ginger ale. Syrups or elixirs are administered in half a glass of same liquids.

Suppository form: moisten suppository and the inserting finger with water only.

For retention enema, drug is dissolved in 120 to 150 ml olive oil or other bland oil.

When used rectally, observe skin area around anus for irritation.

Prolonged use can lead to tolerance, physical dependence, and addiction. Sudden withdrawal from dependent patients may produce delirium, mania, or convulsions.

Allergic skin reactions may occur within several hours or as long as 10 days after drug administration.

Caution patient to avoid concomitant use of alcoholic beverages. The acute poisoning that occurs from the combination of chloral hydrate and alcohol (Mickey Finn or knockout drops) produces vasodilation, with flushing, headache, tachycardia, and hypotension.

Inform patient that activities requiring mental alertness or physical dexterity should be avoided while under the influence of chloral hydrate.

Evaluate patient's response to chloral hydrate and his continued need for the drug.

Habituation may be minimized by evaluating and treating the basic cause or
causes of insomnia.
Classified as Schedule IV drug under the federal Controlled Substances Act.
Solutions are preserved in tightly covered, light-resistant containers. Store
capsule at room temperature away from heat, and store suppositories in
refrigerator.

LABORATORY TEST INTERFERENCES: False positive results for urinary glucose with Fehling's and Benedict's solutions, but not with Clinitest (except
possibly in large doses) or glucose oxidase method (eg, Clinistix, Tes-Tape, and
the like). Possible interference with fluorometric test for urine catecholamines
and urinary steroid determinations by certain methods.

DRUG INTERACTIONS: The sedative action of chloral hydrate is potentiated
by **alcohol, barbiturates, tranquilizers,** and other **CNS depressants.** Chloral
hydrate may potentiate effects of **warfarin,** or other **oral anticoagulants,** and
cause flushing, diaphoresis, and BP changes in patients receiving IV **furosemide.**

CHLORAMBUCIL, U.S.P., B.P.
(LEUKERAN)

Antineoplastic

ACTIONS AND USES
Aromatic derivative of alkylating agent mechlorethamine (qv). Slowest acting
and least toxic nitrogen mustard in clinical use. Damages dividing cells and
mature lymphocytes.
Myelosuppressive properties are moderate, develop gradually, and are com-
pletely reversible.
Used in treatment of chronic lymphocytic leukemia, and malignant lymphomas
(including lymphosarcoma and Hodgkin's disease) as single agent or in combi-
nation with other antineoplastics.
ABSORPTION AND FATE
Adequate reliable absorbtion from oral administration.
Information about metabolism, fate, and excretion incomplete.
CONTRAINDICATIONS AND PRECAUTIONS
First trimester of pregnancy; use during first 4 weeks after myelosuppression by
radiation or chemotherapy; bone marrow infiltration with lymphomatous tis-
sue. See Mechlorethamine.
ADVERSE REACTIONS
Relatively infrequent: nausea, anorexia, and vomiting; with large doses: irrev-
ersible myelosuppression (rare): neutropenia.
See Mechlorethamine.
ROUTE AND DOSAGE
Oral: 0.1 to 0.2 mg/kg/body weight daily for 3 to 6 weeks as required (Average:
4 to 10 mg/day). Dosage and schedule individualized according to response of
patient. Maintenance: 0.03 mg/kg/day up to 0.1 mg/day.

NURSING IMPLICATIONS
Entire daily dose may be given at once. If given before breakfast or at
bedtime, nausea and vomiting may be controlled.
An abrupt fall in WBC calls for reduction in chlorambucil dosage.
Clinical improvement is usually apparent by third week.

CBC, hemoglobin, differential counts, and spleen size should be checked at least every two weeks during treatment.

A slowly progressive lymphopenia that may develop during treatment is reversible at end of therapy; however, neutropenia may continue 8 to 10 days after the last dose.

During maintenance therapy, physician may interrupt occasionally drug schedule in order to determine if patient is in remission.

Preserved in air-tight, light-resistant containers, in a cool place.

See Mechlorethamine.

CHLORAMPHENICOL, U.S.P., B.P.
(AMPHICOL, CHLOROMYCETIN, CHLOROPTIC, ECONOCHLOR, KEMICETINE, MYCHEL, OPHTHOCHLOR, PARAXIN)

Antibacterial, antirickettsial

ACTIONS AND USES

Broad-spectrum antibiotic formerly derived from *Streptomyces venezuelae,* now produced synthetically. Principally bacteriostatic on a wide variety of Gram-negative and Gram-positive bacteria. Acts by interfering with protein synthesis of bacterial ribosomes.

Used only in severe infections when other antibiotics are ineffective or are contraindicated. Effective against *Salmonella typhi* and other *Salmonella* species, *Haemophilus influenzae,* Rocky Mountain spotted fever and other rickettsiae, the lymphogranuloma-psittacosis group, and various Gram-negative bacteria. Also used in cystic fibrosis regimens and used topically for infections of skin, eyes, and external auditory canal.

ABSORPTION AND FATE

Readily and almost completely absorbed from GI tract. Peak plasma levels in about 2 hours; disappears after 12 to 18 hours. Half-life about 4 hours. Approximately 60% bound to plasma proteins. Widely distributed in body, with highest concentrations in liver and kidney and lowest in cerebrospinal fluid. Measurable levels in pleural and ascitic fluid, saliva, and aqueous and vitreous humor. Conjugates with glucuronic acid in liver, then is rapidly excreted in urine along with some free drug; 80% to 92% of dose is excreted within 24 hours. Minimal excretion in feces. Readily crosses placenta and may appear in breast milk.

CONTRAINDICATIONS AND PRECAUTIONS

Treatment of minor infections, prophylactic use; concomitant therapy with drugs that produce bone marrow depression. Safe use during pregnancy and lactation not established. Cautious use: impaired hepatic or renal function, premenopausal women, nursing mothers, premature and full-term infants, children.

ADVERSE REACTIONS

Bone marrow depression (dose-related and reversible): reticulocytosis, leukopenia, granulocytopenia, anemia; (non-dose-related and irreversible): agranulocytosis, aplastic anemia, paroxysmal nocturnal hemoglobinuria, pancytopenia, leukemia. **GI:** nausea, vomiting, diarrhea, enterocolitis, unpleasant taste, dryness of mouth. **Neurotoxicity:** headache, mental depression, confusion, delirium, optic neuritis, digital paresthesias, peripheral neuritis. **Hypersensitivity:** fever; macular and vesicular rashes; hemorrhages of skin, mucosal and serosal surfaces of mouth, intestines, and bladder; angioedema; urticaria; anaphylaxis; Herxheimer-like reaction. **Gray syndrome** (prematures and newborns): abdominal distension, vomiting, pallid cyanosis, blotchy skin, vasomotor collapse, irregular respiration, hypothermia, death. Other: jaundice, hypoprothrombinemia, superinfections.

Oral, intravenous: **Adults, Children, and Infants** *over 2 weeks:* 50 mg/kg body weight daily in equally divided doses, every 6 hours; up to 100 mg/kg/day for exceptionally severe infection. **Infants** *up to 2 weeks* and **Children** *with immature metabolic function*: 25 mg/kg/day in 4 equally divided doses at 6 hour intervals. Topical: cream (1%). Ophthalmic ointment (1%); ophthalmic solution (0.5%): administered every 3 to 6 hours (during day and night for first 48 hours); therapy continued for at least 48 hours after eye appears normal. Otic solution (0.5%): 2 or 3 drops into ear 3 times daily.

NURSING IMPLICATIONS

Generally patient is hospitalized during chloramphenicol therapy to facilitate laboratory tests and close observations.

Bacterial culture and sensitivity tests are essential and may be performed concurrently with initiation of therapy and periodically thereafter.

Baseline leukocyte, differential, hematocrit, and reticulocyte cell counts are recommended prior to initiation of therapy and at 48-hour intervals during therapy and periodically during follow-up period (bone marrow depression has occurred weeks or months following therapy).

Check temperature at least every 4 hours. Usually chloramphenicol is discontinued if temperature remains normal for 48 hours.

Some authorities recommend that treatment for typhoid be continued 8 to 10 days after patient becomes afebrile in order to lessen the possibility of relapse.

Drug therapy should be promptly terminated if abnormal blood findings intervene.

Close observation of the patient is crucial, since blood studies are unreliable predictors of irreversible bone marrow depression. Report immediately sore throat, fever, fatigue, petechiae, ecchymosis, or any other suspect sign or symptom.

Non-dose-related irreversible bone marrow depression may appear weeks or months after drug therapy is terminated. Counsel patient to report immediately any unusual signs or symptoms to his physician.

Possibility of bone marrow depression is greater in patients with impaired hepatic or renal function, infants and other children, and premenopausal women. Chloramphenicol blood levels should be closely monitored (desired concentration between 5 and 20 μg/ml).

Watch for signs and symptoms of superinfection by nonsusceptible organisms: stomatitis, glossitis with or without black tongue, perianal irritation or itching, vaginal discharge, elevated temperature, diarrhea.

Frequent determinations of serum glucose are recommended in patients receiving oral antidiabetic agents (see Drug Interactions).

Avoid warming chloramphenicol solutions (eg, otic solution) above body temperature in order to prevent loss of potency.

Ophthalmic solution should be protected from light.

LABORATORY TEST INTERFERENCES: Possibility of false positive results for urinary glucose by copper reduction methods (eg, Benedict's solution, Clinitest). Chloramphenicol may interfere with urinary steroid (17-OHCS) determinations.

DRUG INTERACTIONS: Chloramphenicol may potentiate the effects of **oral anticoagulants**, oral **antidiabetic agents** (possibility of severe hypoglycemia), **methotrexates**, and **phenytoin**. By interfering with erythrocyte maturation, chloramphenicol may reduce response to **cyanocobalamin (vitamin B$_{12}$)**, **folic acid**, and **iron**.

CHLORAMPHENICOL PALMITATE, U.S.P.
(CHLOROMYCETIN PALMITATE)

Antibacterial, antirickettsial

ACTIONS AND USES
Actions, uses, contraindications, precautions, and adverse reactions as for chloramphenicol (qv). Oral suspension is hydrolyzed in GI tract and absorbed as free chloramphenicol.
ROUTE AND DOSAGE
Oral: 50 to 100 mg/kg body weight in equally divided doses every 6 hours.

NURSING IMPLICATIONS
See Chloramphenicol.

CHLORAMPHENICOL SODIUM SUCCINATE, U.S.P.
(CHLOROMYCETIN SODIUM SUCCINATE, MYCHEL-S)

Antibacterial, antirickettsial

ACTIONS AND USES
Actions, uses, contraindications, precautions, and adverse reactions as for chloramphenicol (qv). This is the preferred form for IV administration, particularly in children, because of its high solubility.
ROUTE AND DOSAGE
Intravenous (as 10% solution): 50 to 100 mg/kg body weight in equally divided doses every 6 hours. Injected over period of at least 1 minute. Prepared by adding 10 ml sterile water for injection or 5% dextrose for injection to each 1 Gm.

NURSING IMPLICATIONS
Intended for IV use only.
Inform patient that bitter taste may occur 15 to 20 seconds after IV injection, lasting 2 to 3 minutes.
Reconstituted solutions are stable for 30 days at room temperature.
A slight change in color reportedly does not indicate loss of potency, but cloudy solutions should not be used.
See Chloramphenicol.

CHLORCYCLIZINE HYDROCHLORIDE, N.F., B.P.
(DI-PARALENE, PERAZIL)

Antihistaminic, antiemetic

ACTIONS AND USES
Long-acting piperazine derivative structurally and pharmacologically related to other cyclizine compounds. Advantages claimed for chlorcyclizine are prolonged action and low incidence of side effects, however symptomatic relief may be erratic.

Onset of action in 1 to 2 hours, with effects lasting 8 to 24 hours.
CONTRAINDICATIONS AND PRECAUTIONS
During pregnancy and in women of childbearing potential.
ROUTE AND DOSAGE
Oral: **Adults:** 50 mg once or twice daily (may be given up to 4 times a day).
Children: 1.5 mg/kg/24 hours divided into 2 doses.

NURSING IMPLICATIONS
Patients performing tasks requiring coordination and mental alertness should
be forewarned that drowsiness may occur.
Preserved in tightly covered, light-resistant containers.
See Hydroxyzine Hydrochloride.

CHLORDIAZEPOXIDE, N.F.
(LIBRITABS)
CHLORDIAZEPOXIDE HYDROCHLORIDE, U.S.P., B.P.
(CHLORDIAZACHEL, J-LIBERTY, LIBRIUM, SEREEN, SK-LYGEN, TENAX)

Antianxiety agent (minor tranquilizer)

ACTIONS AND USES
Benzodiazepine derivative related to diazepam and oxazepam. Exerts depressant
effects on subcortical levels of CNS, and in high doses, on the cortex. Calming
effect thought to be due to action on the limbic system. Produces mild sedative,
anticonvulsant, and skeletal muscle relaxant effects and has weak appetite-
stimulating and analgesic actions. Therapeutic dosages do not produce ganglionic
blockade or reduce affective responses as do phenothiazines and reserpine.
Used for relief of various anxiety and tension states, preoperative apprehension
and anxiety, and withdrawal symptoms of acute alcoholism. Not effective in
long-term management of chronic schizophrenia or other psychoses.
ABSORPTION AND FATE
Well absorbed from GI tract. Peak plasma levels occur about 2 hours after oral
administration, 15 to 30 minutes after IM, and 3 to 30 minutes after IV. Plasma
half-life of single oral dose is about 24 hours. Metabolized in liver and slowly
excreted, primarily in urine and small amount in feces. Urinary excretion continues for several days after last dose. Crosses placenta; excreted in breast milk.
CONTRAINDICATIONS AND PRECAUTIONS
Hypersensitivity to chlordiazepoxide, narrow-angle glaucoma, prostatic hypertrophy, shock, comatose states, psychoses, pregnancy, nursing mothers; oral use
in children under 6 years of age; parenteral use in children under 12 years of
age. Cautious use: anxiety states associated with impending depression, history
of impaired hepatic or renal function; addiction-prone individuals, allergic dermatoses, blood dyscrasias, in the elderly, debilitated patients, and children.
ADVERSE REACTIONS
Frequent: drowsiness, dizziness, ataxia, irritability, confusion, lethargy, fatigue,
constipation. Others reported: changes in salivation, pain at injection site,
changes in EEG patterns, blurred vision, nystagmus, diplopia, voracious appetite, vivid dreams, nausea, headache, extrapyramidal symptoms, urinary frequency, menstrual irregularities, changes in libido, failure to ejaculate, orthostatic hypotension, tachycardia, vertigo, syncope, tinnitus, depression, delirium,
photosensitivity, skin rashes, edema, blood dyscrasias, jaundice, acute hepatic
necrosis. Overdosage: somnolence, confusion, diminished reflexes, paradoxic
excitation, depressed respiration, coma.

Adults: Oral: 5 to 25 mg 2 to 4 times a day. Intramuscular, intravenous: 25 to 50 mg repeated in 4 to 6 hours, if necessary (not to exceed 300 mg daily). Lower dosage range recommended for elderly and debilitated patients. **Children** *over 6 years:* Oral: 5 mg 2 to 4 times daily.

NURSING IMPLICATIONS

Most signs and symptoms associated with chlordiazepoxide therapy are dose-related. Physician will rely on accurate observations and reporting of patient's response to drug to determine lowest effective maintenance dose.

Drug therapy is not a substitute for sensitive, thoughtful, and unhurried communication with the patient to explore and understand his concerns, anxieties, and tensions.

Parenteral drug should be prepared immediately before use; unused portions should be discarded, because the drug is unstable in solution. Chlordiazepoxide should not be mixed with other drugs. See package insert.

Add diluent slowly to avoid bubble formation and agitate ampoule gently until drug is completely dissolved.

Use only special IM diluent for IM administration (do not use diluent if it is opalescent or hazy). Administer drug slowly deep into upper outer quadrant of gluteus.

For IV injection, sterile physiologic saline or sterile water for injection is a suitable diluent. Chlordiazepoxide should not be administered by IV infusion because of its instability in solution.

Orthostatic hypotension and tachycardia occur more frequently with parenteral administration. Patient should remain in bed at least 3 hours after IM or IV injection; observe closely for adverse reactions. Monitor vital signs.

Since chlordiazepoxide is excreted slowly, a cumulative effect may occur, particularly during the first several days of drug therapy.

Adverse reactions such as drowsiness, syncope, ataxia, confusion, constipation, and urinary retention are dose-related and are more likely to occur in elderly and debilitated patients, even at lower dosage ranges. Supervision of ambulation is indicated, and possibly bedsides.

Monitor intake and output until drug dosage is stabilized.

Patients who complain of gastric distress may obtain relief by taking the drug with or immediately after meals or with milk.

Paradoxic reactions (euphoria, excitement, stimulation, disturbed sleep patterns, acute rage, depression) may occur during the first few weeks of therapy in psychiatric patients and in hyperactive and aggressive children receiving chlordiazepoxide. Suicidal tendencies may be manifested in anxiety states accompanied by depression. Observe necessary protective precautions.

Occurrences of sore throat or mouth, upper respiratory infection, fever, and malaise should alert one to the possibility of agranulocytosis. Total and differential WBC counts should be ordered immediately, and reverse precautions should be instituted.

Periodic blood cell counts and liver function tests are recommended during prolonged therapy.

Advise patient to avoid excessive sunlight. Photosensitivity has been reported.

Warn ambulatory patient that sedation may occur during early therapy and that activities requiring mental alertness and precision such as driving a car and operating machinery should be avoided until his reaction to the drug has been evaluated.

Caution patient against drinking alcoholic beverages (see Drug Interactions).

Advise patient to take chlordiazepoxide specifically as prescribed and to take no other drugs without his physician's advice.

Inform patient that cigarette smoking may impair therapeutic effectiveness of chlordiazepoxide.

Psychic and physical dependence may occur in patients receiving large doses for protracted periods. Chlordiazepoxide is classified as a Schedule IV drug under the federal Controlled Substances Act.

Abrupt discontinuation of drug has precipitated withdrawal reactions in patients receiving high doses for at least a month. Symptoms may include restlessness, abdominal and muscle cramps, tremors, insomnia, vomiting, anorexia, profuse sweating, psychomotor activity, and delirium. Convulsions may occur 1 week after drug has been terminated because of slow elimination.

If patient becomes pregnant during therapy or intends to become pregnant advise her to communicate with physician about desirability of discontinuing therapy.

Chlordiazepoxide is stored in tight, light-resistant containers.

LABORATORY TEST INTERFERENCES: False positive or spuriously high readings: SGOT, SGPT, serum bilirubin, serum creatinine (equivocal reports), urinary 17-ketosteroids (equivocal reports). False negative or spuriously low readings: uptake of radiopharmaceuticals (equivocal reports).

DRUG INTERACTIONS: Potentiation of CNS depressant effects may occur with concomitant administration of chlordiazepoxide and other benzodiazepines with **alcohol,** (impairment of psychomotor skills and coordination may occur even 10 hours after last dose of a benzodiazepine); **general anesthetic, barbiturates, narcotics, sedatives,** and **tricyclic antidepressants** (also additive atropine-like effects). Benzodiazepines may enhance toxicity of **phenytoin** (diphenylhydantoin), and may block therapeutic response to **levodopa.**

CHLOROQUINE HYDROCHLORIDE, U.S.P.
(ARALEN HYDROCHLORIDE)
CHLOROQUINE PHOSPHATE, U.S.P., B.P.
(ARALEN PHOSPHATE)

Antimalarial (plasmocide), antiamebic

ACTIONS AND USES

Synthetic 4-aminoquinoline derivative. Antimalarial activity is believed to be based on ability to form complexes with DNA of parasite, thereby inhibiting replication and transcription to RNA and nucleic acid synthesis. Highly active against erythrocytic forms of plasmodia, providing suppressive prophylaxis and clinical cure. Also has amebicidal activity, antiinflammatory action, and quinidinelike effect on heart.

Used for suppressive treatment and acute attacks of malaria caused by *Plasmodium malariae, P. ovale, P. vivax,* and susceptible forms of *P. falciparum* and in treatment of extraintestinal amebiasis. Concomitant therapy with an 8-aminoquinoline is necessary for radical cure of vivax and malarias. Has been used in treatment of giardiasis, discoid lupus erythematosus, as alternative to quinidine in treatment of cardiac arrhythmias; and in rheumatoid arthritis not controlled by other less toxic drugs.

ABSORPTION AND FATE

Rapidly absorbed following oral administration. Maximum plasma concentration in 1 to 2 hours. Approximately 55% bound to plasma proteins. High concentrations in liver, kidney, lung, brain, spinal cord and erythrocytes. Partially metabolized in liver. Excreted slowly in urine as metabolites and free drug; 8% excreted unchanged in feces. Urinary excretion increased by acidification and decreased by alkalinization of urine. Small amounts of drug detectable in urine for weeks, months, and occasionally years after therapy discontinued. Crosses placenta.

CONTRAINDICATIONS AND PRECAUTIONS

Hypersensitivity to 4-aminoquinoline, psoriatic arthritis, porphyria, presence of retinal or visual field changes, long-term therapy in children, during pregnancy and in women of childbearing potential, concomitant use of hepatotoxic drugs or drugs known to cause dermatitis (eg., phenylbutazone, gold compounds). Cautious use: impaired hepatic function, alcoholism, patients with glucose-6-phosphate dehydrogenase deficiency, infants and children, hematologic, gastrointestinal, and neurologic disorders.

ADVERSE REACTIONS

Mild transient headache, pruritus, skin eruptions, anorexia, nausea, vomiting, diarrhea, abdominal cramps, visual disturbances, slight weight loss, fatigue, psychic stimulation, psychoses, nightmares, hypotension, ECG changes (rarely). Prolonged therapy: corneal and retinal damage, vertigo, tinnitus, reduced hearing, auditory nerve damage, skeletal muscle weakness, reduced or absent reflexes, gray pigmentation (skin, nails, and mucous membranes), bleaching of hair and patchy alopecia (reversible), various dermatoses, desquamation, lymphedema of hands and arms, blood dyscrasias (leukopenia, aplastic anemia, thrombocytopenia, agranulocytosis, pancytopenia). Overdosage: shock, cardiac arrhythmias, convulsions, respiratory and cardiac arrest, sudden death (infants and children).

ROUTE AND DOSAGE

Dosage is often expressed or calculated in terms of chloroquine base. Each 500-mg tablet is equivalent to 300 mg of base; 1 ml (50 mg) of parenteral solution is equivalent to 40 mg of base.

Acute malarial attack: **Adults:** Oral (chloroquine phosphate): 1 Gm initially, followed by 500 mg 6 hours later, then 500 mg daily for 2 consecutive days. Intramuscular (chloroquine hydrochloride): 4 to 5 ml (160 to 200 mg base) initially, repeated in 6 hours if necessary. Not to exceed 800 mg base in first 24 hours. **Children:** Oral: initially, 10 mg (base)/kg followed by 5 mg (base)/kg 6 hours later and for 2 consecutive days. Intramuscular: 5 mg (base)/kg; may be repeated in 6 hours.

Malarial suppression: **Adults and children** *over 8 years:* Oral: 500 mg weekly on same day each week. *4 to 8 years:* 250 mg weekly; *1 to 4 years:* 125 mg weekly; *younger than 1 year:* 62 mg weekly.

Extraintestinal amebiasis: Oral: 1 Gm daily for 2 days, then 500 mg daily for at least 2 to 3 weeks. Intramuscular: 200 to 250 mg daily (oral therapy resumed as soon as possible).

Discoid lupus: initially, 250 mg twice daily for 1 or 2 weeks; maintenance: 250 mg daily.

Rheumatoid arthritis: 250 mg daily, usually as a single dose with evening meal.

NURSING IMPLICATIONS

GI side effects may be minimized by administering oral drug before or after meals.

Aspirate carefully before injecting drug IM in order to avoid inadvertent intravascular injection. IV injection may produce quinidinelike effects on heart.

Complete blood cell counts are advised prior to initiation of therapy and periodically thereafter in patients on long-term therapy.

Baseline and regularly scheduled ophthalmoscopic examinations, including slit lamp, fundus, and visual fields, should be performed.

Retinopathy (generally irreversible) can be progressive even after termination of therapy. Patient may be asymptomatic or may complain of night blindness, scotomata, visual field changes, blurred vision, or difficulty in focusing. Advise patient to report visual symptoms promptly.

Use of dark glasses in sunlight or bright light may reduce risk of ocular damage.

Patients on long-term therapy should be questioned regularly about skeletal muscle weakness, and periodic tests should be made of muscle strength and deep tendon reflexes. Positive signs are indications to terminate therapy.

If possible, suppressive therapy should begin 2 weeks before exposure and should be continued for 8 weeks after leaving endemic area.

Therapeutic effects in rheumatoid arthritis do not generally occur until after several weeks of therapy, and maximal benefit may not occur until 6 months to 1 year of therapy. Chloroquine is usually discontinued if no objective improvement occurs within 6 months.

Caution patient to keep chloroquine out of reach of children; a number of fatalities have been reported following accidental ingestion.

Inform patient that chloroquine may cause rusty yellow or brown discoloration of urine.

CHLOROTHIAZIDE, U.S.P., B.P.
(DIURIL, RO-CHLOROZIDE)
CHLOROTHIAZIDE, SODIUM, N.F.
(DIURIL SODIUM)

Diuretic (thiazide), antihypertensive

ACTIONS AND USES

Benzothiadiazine (thiazide) diuretic chemically related to sulfonamides. Enhances excretion of sodium, chloride, and water by interfering with tubular reabsorption of sodium; promotes potassium loss and bicarbonate excretion and increases uric acid excretion. Initially, blood pressure is lowered by decreased cardiac output and plasma volume; continued antihypertensive effect is postulated to result from direct arteriolar dilation and decreased extracellular sodium. May induce hyperglycemia in diabetes mellitus and prediabetic states by suppressing pancreatic insulin release by unknown mechanism. Causes paradoxic antidiuretic effect in diabetes insipidus.

Used adjunctively to manage edema associated with congestive heart failure, hepatic cirrhosis, renal dysfunction, corticosteroid and estrogen therapy, and toxemia of pregnancy. Used alone in mild hypertension or with other antihypertensives to permit lower dosage and to reduce unpleasant side effects. Also used for palliative reduction of polyuria in diabetes insipidus.

ABSORPTION AND FATE

Diuretic response following oral administration occurs in 2 hours and peaks in 4 hours, with duration of 6 to 12 hours. Following IV injection, onset of diuresis occurs in 15 minutes, with maximal effect in 30 minutes and duration of 2 to 4 hours. Distributed throughout extracellular fluid; concentrates in renal tissues. Readily crosses placenta; appears in breast milk. Excreted in urine unchanged within 3 to 6 hours.

CONTRAINDICATIONS AND PRECAUTIONS

Hypersensitivity to thiazides or sulfonamides; anuria, oliguria, increasing azotemia, hypokalemia, IV use in infants and children; hazardous potential in women of childbearing age, during pregnancy, and in nursing mothers. Cautious use: history of allergy, bronchial asthma, impaired renal or hepatic function, or gout; diabetes mellitus; lupus erythematosus; advanced arteriosclerosis; elderly or debilitated patients.

ADVERSE REACTIONS

GI: nausea, vomiting, anorexia, heartburn, diarrhea, constipation, abdominal cramps, sialadenitis. **CNS**: dizziness, vertigo, headache, paresthesias, yellow vision. **Hypersensitivity**: urticaria, purpura, photosensitivity, skin rashes, fever, necrotizing vasculitis with hematuria (rare), respiratory distress, anaphylactic reactions. **Cardiovascular**: orthostatic hypotension. **Hematologic** (rare): leukopenia, agranulocytosis, thrombocytopenia, aplastic anemia. Other: transient blurred vision, dehydration, hyponatremia, hypokalemia, metabolic alkalosis, hypomagnesemia, hyperglycemia, glycosuria, hyperuricemia, gout, jaundice, rise in blood ammonia level, acute pancreatitis, vascular thrombosis, and parathyroid pathology with hypercalcemia and hypophosphatemia (rarely).

ROUTE AND DOSAGE

Oral, intravenous: **Adults** (Edema): 0.5 to 1 Gm once or twice daily, or on alternate days, or 3 to 5 days each week. (Antihypertensive): oral form only: **Adults**: initially 0.5 Gm twice daily, with maintenance dosage determined by blood pressure response (some patients may require up to 2 Gm daily in divided doses). **Pediatric**: Oral: 20 mg/kg/day divided in 2 doses.

NURSING IMPLICATIONS

Baseline and periodic determinations should be made of blood count, serum electrolytes, CO_2, BUN, creatinine, uric acid, and blood sugar. For patients on maintenance doses, some physicians suggest repeat determinations every 6 to 8 weeks until stable and at least every 6 months thereafter.

Schedule doses to avoid nocturia and interrupted sleep. Administer oral drug after food intake to prevent gastric irritation.

Observe injection sites. Extravasation during IV administration can cause severe tissue irritation.

Explain to patient that he will be urinating greater amounts and more frequently than usual. With continued therapy, refractoriness to diuretic action may develop, but not to hypotensive effects.

Monitor intake–output ratio. Excessive diuresis or oliguria may cause electrolyte imbalance and necessitate dosage adjustment.

Establish baseline weight prior to initiation of therapy. Weigh patient at the same time each morning under standard conditions. Consult physician about acceptable range of weight change.

Blood pressure should be closely monitored during early drug therapy. Physician may want initial measurements for patients with hypertension taken in standing, sitting, and lying positions to evaluate drug effects.

Consistency in technique and readings is essential. Some physicians advocate taking blood pressures in the arm with the higher reading (if one is higher), taking supine blood pressure after patient has been reclining for 10 minutes, and taking standing blood pressure after patient stands for 3 minutes. Consult physician.

To avoid orthostatic hypotension, instruct patient to change position slowly and to avoid standing still, hot showers or baths, sunbathing, and strenuous exercises. Physician may prescribe elastic stockings and firm girdle to augment circulation from extremities.

Skin and mucous membranes should be inspected daily for evidence of petechiae in patients receiving large doses and those on prolonged therapy.

Patients on digitalis therapy should be observed closely for signs and symptoms of hypokalemia. Even moderate reduction in serum potassium can precipitate digitalis intoxication in these patients.

Warning signs and symptoms of electrolyte imbalance from whatever cause include anorexia, nausea, vomiting, thirst, dryness of mouth, excessive diuresis, oliguria, weakness, fatigue, dizziness, drowsiness, restlessness, and muscle cramps.

Electrolyte imbalance is most likely to develop in patients with edema, in the elderly and debilitated, and after loss of body fluids (vomiting, diarrhea, paracentesis, GI drainage, excessive sweating).

Specifically, signs and symptoms of hypokalemia include anorexia, nausea, vomiting, circumoral numbness or other paresthesias, mental confusion, irritability, drowsiness, muscle weakness, paralytic ileus, abdominal distention, hypoactive reflexes, polyuria, hypotension, dyspnea, and cardiac arrthymias.

Hypokalemia is rarely severe in most patients on prolonged therapy if the daily diet contains liberal amounts of foods high in potassium (eg., bananas, oranges, grapefruit, prune juice, canned apricots, potatoes). Many other foods are rich in potassium but are also high in sodium.

Thiazide therapy can cause hyperglycemia and glycosuria in diabetic and diabetic-prone individuals. Dosage adjustment of antidiabetic drugs may be required.

Thiazides should be discontinued 48 hours before elective surgery because they may reduce arterial responsiveness to pressor amines (eg, norepinephrine, levarterenol) and augment the paralyzing action of tubocurarine.

Thiazides can interfere with uric acid excretion, and thus they may precipitate acute gout in susceptible patients. Report onset of joint pain or limited motion.

Weight control is an important adjunct to hypertension therapy, and the patient should be advised to avoid excess coffee and tea and to stop smoking, if possible. Some patients may require a diet tailored to correct lipid abnormalities. Collaborate with physician and dietitian.

Strict sodium restriction is not usually prescribed; however, foods high in sodium content should be avoided, and the physician may advise the patient not to add salt to food. The physician may allow a salt substitute (see Index), provided the patient has no renal problems.

Discharge instructions (written and verbal) for patients on continuing thiazide therapy should include the following: dosage regimen; drug action; symptoms to report; importance of compliance in preventing complications of hypertension; when and how to weigh and keep weight record; diet restrictions, if any; moderate exercise plan; follow-up plans. Some physicians want the patient to be taught to take his own blood pressure at home and even at his job.

Unused reconstituted IV solutions may be stored at room temperature up to 24 hours. Use only clear solutions.

LABORATORY TEST INTERFERENCES: Thiazides may cause false negative results in tyramine, phentolamine (Regitine), and probably histamine test for pheochromocytoma; false increase in BSP retention test, and may interfere with urinary steroid determinations (modification of Glenn-Nelson Technique).

DRUG INTERACTIONS: Absorption of thiazides may be inhibited by **cholestyramine** (schedule as far apart as possible). There may be potentiation of orthostatic hypotension when thiazides are administered concomitantly with **alcohol, barbiturates, narcotics,** other **CNS depressants,** and other **antihypertensive agents.** Thiazides may antagonize the hypoprothrombinemic effects of **oral anticoagulants** and the hypoglycemic effects of **antidiabetic drugs;** increase responsiveness to **curare derivatives** and **gallamine;** enhance hyperglycemia, hypotension, and hyperuricemia with **diazoxide;** enhance potassium loss with **corticosteroids** and **digitalis** (with resulting digitalis toxicity); and may decrease excretion of **amphetamines** and **quinidine**, with possible toxicity.

CHLOROTRIANISENE, N.F., B.P.
(TACE)

Estrogen

ACTIONS AND USES
Nonesteroidal synthetic estrogenic compound derived from diethylstilbestrol. Following metabolism in liver, estrogenic activity becomes more potent. Stored in fat tissue; released slowly to give delayed onset and prolonged duration of action. Effect may persist for some time after therapy is discontinued.
Used in treatment of postpartum breast engorgement, in treatment of inoperable progressing prostatic cancer, and as replacement therapy in estrogen deficiency. See Estradiol.
CONTRAINDICATIONS AND PRECAUTIONS
Patients suspected of having estrogen-dependent carcinoma. Cautious use: renal dysfunction, borderline decompensation. See Estradiol.
ADVERSE REACTIONS
Long-term use: endometrial hyperplasia and breakthrough bleeding, gynecomastia, reduced potency (male), urticaria. Also see Estradiol.
ROUTE AND DOSAGE
Oral: *Prostatic cancer or replacement therapy*: 12 to 25 mg daily. Highly individualized dosage. *Breast engorgement*: 12 mg 4 times daily for 7 days or 50 mg every 6 hours for 6 doses; the first dose is given within 8 hours of delivery.

NURSING IMPLICATIONS
Capsules should be stored in well-closed container and protected from excessive heat or cold or humidity higher than 50%.
See Estradiol.

CHLORPHENIRAMINE MALEATE, U.S.P., N.F., B.P.
(ALLERBID TYMCAPS, AL-R, ANTAGONATE, CHLORAMATE UNICELLES, CHLORMENE, CHLORTAB, CHLOR-TRIMETON, CIRAMINE, COSEA, HISTASPAN, HISTEX, TELDRIN)

Antihistaminic

ACTIONS AND USES
Propylamine (alkylamine) antihistamine. Produces less sedation than other antihistamines, but side effects involving CNS stimulation may be more common. Competes for histamine receptor sites on effector cells, thus blocking the histamine action that promotes capillary permeability and edema formation and the constrictive action on respiratory, gastrointestinal, and vascular smooth muscles. Has antiemetic, antitussive, anticholinergic, and local anesthetic actions.
Used for symptomatic relief of various uncomplicated allergic conditions; to prevent transfusion reactions and drug reactions in susceptible patients; and used as adjunct to epinephrine and other standard measures in anaphylactic reactions.
ABSORPTION AND FATE
Onset of action following oral administration occurs in 20 to 60 minutes; duration 3 to 6 hours. Detoxified in liver. Metabolites and some free drug excreted in urine.

Hypersensitivity to antihistamines of similar structure; lower respiratory tract symptoms (including asthma), narrow-angle glaucoma, prostatic hypertrophy, bladder neck obstruction, GI obstruction or stenosis, pregnancy, nursing mothers, premature and newborn infants, patients receiving MAO inhibitors. Cautious use: convulsive disorders, increased intraocular pressure, hyperthyroidism, cardiovasular disease, hypertension, diabetes mellitus, history of asthma.

ADVERSE REACTIONS

Low incidence of side effects. **CNS:** sedation, dizziness, vertigo, tinnitus, fatigue, disturbed coordination, tingling, heaviness, weakness of hands, tremors, euphoria, nervousness, restlessness, insomnia. **Overdosage** (especially in children): hallucinations, excitement, fever, ataxia, athetosis, convulsions, coma, cardiovascular collapse. **Atropinelike effects:** dryness of mouth, nose, and throat, thickened bronchial secretions, wheezing, sensation of chest tightness, blurred vision, diplopia, headache, urinary frequency or retention, dysuria, palpitation, tachycardia, mild hypotension or hypertension. **GI:** epigastric distress, anorexia, nausea, vomiting, constipation or diarrhea. **Hypersensitivity:** skin rash, urticaria, photosensitization, anaphylactic shock. **Hematologic:** leukopenia, agranulocytosis, hemolytic anemia. Other (following parenteral administration): transitory stinging or burning at injection site, sweating, pallor, transient hypotension.

ROUTE AND DOSAGE

Adults: Oral: 2 to 4 mg 3 or 4 times daily. Repeat-action preparations: 8 or 12 mg once daily or every 8 to 12 hours. Subcutaneous, intramuscular, and intravenous: 5 to 20 mg. Maximum 40 mg/24 hours. **Children** *6 to 12 years:* Oral: ½ adult dose; *2 to 6 years:* 1 mg 3 or 4 times daily.

NURSING IMPLICATIONS

In patients receiving antihistamines for allergic manifestations, a careful history should be taken to reveal any change from the usual patterns: recently ingested foods and drugs, social or emotional stresses.

Only solutions without preservatives should be given IV.

For prevention of transfusion reaction, chlorpheniramine *without preservatives* may be added directly to stored blood.

If patient manifests any reaction following parenteral administration, drug should be discontinued. (Exception: patient may experience transitory stinging sensation that rarely lasts longer than a few minutes.

Although drowsiness is rarely a problem, caution the patient to avoid operating motor vehicles or engaging in hazardous activities until drug response has been determined.

Also caution patient that antihistamines have additive effects with alcohol and other CNS depressants (hypnotics, sedatives, tranquilizers).

Patients on prolonged therapy should have periodic blood cell counts.

Antihistamines have no therapeutic effect on the common cold. Their continued popularity, despite their having been debunked as cold cures, apparently stems from the comfort afforded by their drying effect. Patients with cough should be advised that this drying action may cause thickened bronchial secretions, thus making expectoration difficult.

Chlorpheniramine (Chlor-Trimeton) is sold over the counter and is a common ingredient with a sympathomimetic agent and other drugs in many so-called cold remedies (eg, Allerest, Contac, Coricidin "D," Dristan, Duadacin, Romilar, Sinarest, and others).

Caution patient to store antihistamines out of reach of children. Fatalities have been reported.

Antihistamines should be discontinued prior to skin testing procedures for allergy, since they may obscure otherwise positive reactions.

Patients with allergies should be advised to carry at all times medical identification jewelry or card indicating his specific allergy and his and the physician's name, address, and telephone number.

Preserved in tight, light-resistant containers.

DRUG INTERACTIONS: **Tricyclic antidepressants** may prolong and intensify the anticholinergic (drying) effects of antihistamines. Concurrent use of antihistamine, and any CNS depressant may enhance CNS depression (drowsiness, impaired psychomotor ability) caused by either drug.

CHLORPHENOXAMINE HYDROCHLORIDE
(PHENOXENE)

Antiparkinsonian agent, skeletal muscle relaxant

ACTIONS AND USES
Diphenhydramine derivative with antihistamic and peripheral anticholinergic properties. Similar actions, contraindications, precautions, and adverse reactions same as for diphenhydramine. Mode of action in parkinsonism is obscure, but believed to depress motor nerve centers in brain stem and spinal cord. Also a mild euphoriant.
Used as adjunct in symptomatic treatment of all types of parkinsonism.
ABSORPTION AND FATE
Onset of action in about 30 minutes; duration of action 4 to 6 hours.
ROUTE AND DOSAGE
Oral: initially 50 mg 3 times a day. Dosage gradually increased to 100 mg 2 to 4 times daily, if needed.

NURSING IMPLICATIONS
Incidence of GI side effects is less if drug is administered after meals, with milk.
Chlorphenoxamine may reduce muscular rigidity and sweating and improve gait, but it has little effect on tremor.
Caution patient to avoid driving or other potentially hazardous activities until his reaction to drug is known.
Tolerance to chlorphenoxamine may develop after continuous use over a period of several months.
See Diphenhydramine Hydrochloride.

CHLORPHENTERMINE HYDROCHLORIDE
(ORASATE, PRE-SATE)

Anorexiant

ACTIONS AND USES
Amphetamine congener, with actions, contraindications, precautions, and adverse reactions similar to those of amphetamine (qv). Reportedly produces fewer side effects attributable to CNS stimulation than amphetamine.
Used as temporary adjunct in treatment of exogenous obesity.
ABSORPTION AND FATE
Peak levels occur in 2 to 4 hours. Excreted primarily in urine.

Cardiovascular disease, including arrhythmias; children under 12 years of age. Safe use during pregnancy and in women of childbearing potential not established. Cautious use: hypertension.

ADVERSE REACTIONS

Dry mouth, insomnia, sedation, drowsiness, dizziness, unpleasant taste, diarrhea, restlessness, nervousness, elevated blood pressure, tachycardia, palpitation. Also see Amphetamine Sulfate.

ROUTE AND DOSAGE

Oral: 65 mg (slow-release tablet) daily.

NURSING IMPLICATIONS

Administered after first meal of the day.

Blood pressure should be monitored in patients with hypertension.

Inform patient of the possibility of drowsiness and dizziness, and caution against potentially hazardous activities such as driving a motor vehicle or operating machinery until his reaction to the drug is known.

Since tolerance to anorexigenic action often develops within a few weeks, therapy is usually discontinued at that time.

Habituation or addiction may result from long-term use, especially with large doses. Classified as Schedule III drug under federal Controlled Substances Act.

Chlorphentermine is used as an adjunct in a regimen of weight reduction that includes reeducation with respect to eating habits, an appropriate exercise program, and psychologic support.

See Amphetamine Sulfate.

CHLORPROMAZINE, U.S.P.
CHLORPROMAZINE HYDROCHLORIDE, U.S.P., B.P.
(CHLOR-PZ, KLORAZINE, LARGACTIL, PROMACHEL, PROMACHLOR, PROMAPAR, PROMAZ, SONAZINE, THORAZINE)

Antipsychotic (major tranquilizer), antiemetic

ACTIONS AND USES

Dimethylamine derivative of phenothiazine with actions at all levels of CNS. Depresses subcortical CNS; produces psychotrophic effects, sedation, antiemesis, and possibly suppression of cough reflex. Inhibition of hypothalamus may affect temperature-regulating mechanism and release of pituitary tropic hormones. Also capable of releasing melanocyte-stimulating hormone and has central skeletal motor effects, α-adrenergic blocking and adrenergic potentiating activities. Produces cholinergic blocking effect; has antiserotonin, antihistaminic, and antipruritic actions and quinidinelike effect on heart.

Used in management of acute and chronic psychoses including schizophrenia and manic phase of manic–depressive illness. Also used to control excessive anxiety and agitation prior to surgery, as well as in cancer, certain neuroses, and mild alcohol withdrawal; used in management of severe nausea and vomiting and intractable hiccups and as adjunct in treatment of tetanus and acute intermittent porphyria.

ABSORPTION AND FATE

Well absorbed after parenteral administration; erratic absorption following oral doses. Readily distributed to all body tissues; unevenly distributed to brain. High concentrations in lungs and keratin structures. Plasma levels peak rapidly following IM; duration of action 3 to 4 hours. Peak plasma levels in 1½ to 3 hours following oral administration; duration of action 4 to 6 hours. IM plasma levels about three or four times as high as those achieved by equivalent oral doses. Plasma half-life less than 6 hours. Metabolized in liver; excreted in urine and feces. Urinary excretion of metabolites over 24-hour period accounts for less than one-third of single administered dose. Following discontinuation of drug after chronic use, patient continues to excrete metabolites for 6 weeks to 6 months. Crosses placenta.

CONTRAINDICATIONS AND PRECAUTIONS

Hypersensitivity to phenothiazine derivatives; chronic alcoholism, bone marrow depression, brain damage, comatose states, myasthenia gravis, prostatic hypertrophy, history of glaucoma; acute and chronic respiratory infections, particularly in children, Reye's syndrome. Safe use during pregnancy and lactation and in children younger than 6 months of age not established. Cautious use: history of convulsive disorders, diabetes, hypertensive disease, peptic ulcer, cardiovascular disease, impaired hepatic function, patients exposed to extreme heat or organophosphate insecticides.

ADVERSE REACTIONS

Sedation, dizziness, syncope, faintness, orthostatic hypotension, palpitation, reflex tachycardia. **Autonomic reactions:** oral syndrome (dry mouth; redness, vesicles, or patches in mouth; white or black hairy tongue; loosened dentures, stomatitis, cheilosis), blurred vision, mydriasis (or miosis), constipation, adynamic ileus, urinary retention (or diuresis), delayed ejaculation. **Extrapyramidal:** parkinsonism, dystonia, akathisia, tardive dyskinesia. **Endocrinologic:** menstrual irregularities, gynecomastia, galactorrhea, reduced libido, increased appetite, weight gain, edema, glycosuria, hyperglycemia or hypoglycemia. **Hypersensitivity:** cholestatic jaundice, blood dyscrasias (agranulocytosis, pancytopenia); dermatologic: urticaria, petechiae, exfoliative dermatitis, photosensitivity (erythema on exposure to sunlight, gray to purplish brown discoloration of exposed skin), anaphylactoid reactions. **Ophthalmologic:** pigmentary retinopathy, opacities in lens and cornea. Other reported: ECG alterations (Q- and T-wave distortions), sudden death, reactivation of psychotic symptoms, reduced REM sleep, bizarre dreams, cerebral edema, grand mal seizures, aggravation of peptic ulcer, heat prostration, hyperpyrexia, respiratory depression.

ROUTE AND DOSAGE

Adults: Oral, intramuscular, intravenous: 25 mg to 1 Gm daily in divided doses. Rectal (suppository): 50 to 100 mg every 6 to 8 hours, as necessary. Dosages by all routes highly individualized. **Children:** Oral : 2 mg/kg/24 hours divided into 4 to 6 doses.

NURSING IMPLICATIONS

Before initiating treatment with phenothiazine derivatives, baseline evaluations should be made of blood pressure in standing and recumbent positions. Complete blood counts, liver function tests, urinalysis, ECG (in patients over 50 years of age), and ophthalmoscopic examinations are recommended before and periodically during prolonged therapy.

Suicide attempt is a constant possibility in the depressed patient, particularly when he is improving. Watch to see that drug is swallowed and not hoarded. In some cases it may be advisable to put patient on a liquid chlorpromazine preparation.

Many side effects associated with phenothiazine therapy are dose-related; others involve individual sensitivity. The physician will rely on accurate observations and early reporting of the patient's responses to prevent serious adverse reactions and to determine dose spacing and lowest effective dose level.

Hypotensive reactions, dizziness, and sedation are common during the first few weeks of therapy, particularly in patients receiving large oral doses or in the elderly when drug is administered parenterally. Patients usually develop tolerance to these side effects; however, lower doses or longer intervals between doses may be required.

In titrating initial dosages, blood pressure and respirations (rate and quality) should be taken before administering the drug and between doses.

Elastic stockings and elevation of legs when sitting may minimize hypotensive effect (discuss with physician). Supervise ambulation. Instruct patient to make gradual changes to all positions, especially from recumbent to upright posture, and to dangle legs over bed a few minutes before ambulating. Caution against standing still for prolonged periods and advise against hot showers or baths, because the resulting vasodilatation may potentiate hypotensive effects.

The patient should remain recumbent for at least 1 hour after parenteral administration and should be observed closely. Hypotensive reactions may require the head-low position with legs raised and pressor drugs such as levarterenol or phenylephrine. Epinephrine and other pressor agents are contraindicated because they may cause paradoxic further lowering of blood pressure.

IM preparations should be administered slowly and deep into upper outer quadrant of buttock; massage injection site well. Avoid subcutaneous injection, as it may produce tissue irritation. If irritation is a problem, consult physician about advisability of diluting medication with normal saline for injection or with 2% procaine. Rotate injection sites.

Avoid drug contact with skin, eyes, and clothing. Contact dermatitis has been reported. Personnel who handle injectable preparation frequently should use plastic gloves; susceptible individuals are advised to wear masks.

A specific flow rate should be ordered when patient is receiving drug by IV infusion. Monitor blood pressure closely.

Since chlorpromazine reduces REM sleep, it is usually not used for nighttime sedation in patients with audio or visual hallucinations.

Be on the alert for appearance of extrapyramidal side effects. These reactions can be life-threatening if not promptly treated by dose reduction or termination of therapy and possibly antiparkinsonian drugs. Pediatric patients with severe dehydration and acute infection, the elderly, and women appear to be particularly susceptible.

Extrapyramidal side effects: Parkinsonism (masklike facies, tremors at rest, muscular rigidity, weakness of motor function, pill-rolling motion) occurs most frequently in women, dehydrated patients, and the elderly of both sexes. Dystonia (increased muscle tone and spasm) and dyskinesia (abrupt onset of involuntary rhythmic movements such as tics, as well as jaw pain, dysphagia, dysphasia, stiff neck, opisthotonos, and oculogyric crises) mimic symptoms of meningitis; generally occur during first few days or weeks of therapy and appear most frequently in men and children. Akathisia (involuntary motor restlessness, inability to sit still or sleep) occurs most frequently in women and is often misdiagnosed as anxiety. Tardive dyskinesia (involuntary rhythmic, bizarre movements of face, jaw, mouth, and tongue and sometimes extremities) appears most commonly in women and the elderly. May be irreversible. An early sign of tardive dyskinesia is a fine wormlike movement of the tongue. Prompt recognition and cessation of drug therapy may prevent progression of symptoms. Condition usually subsides within 6 months after drug is discontinued. Antiparkinsonian drugs appear to aggravate symptoms.

Monitor dietary and fluid intake and urinary and fecal output. Urinary retention, diuresis, constipation, fecal impaction, and adynamic ileus are possible complications of drug therapy. The combination of depression and drug therapy usually causes constipation; an increase of fluid intake and dietary roughage, if allowed, may help.

Patients continuing the drug at home should be advised which laxative to take, if needed. Many over-the-counter formulations contain anticholinergic drugs such as atropine or scopolamine that can precipitate adynamic ileus. Patients receiving combination therapy of a phenothiazine, an antiparkinsonian agent, and a tricyclic antidepressant are particularly susceptible.

Inform patient that the drug may impart a pink, red, or red brown color to urine.

Based on the hypothesis that inspissation of bile is the mechanism of jaundice, it has been suggested that maintaining a high fluid intake may reduce the incidence of jaundice. Discuss with physician.

Chlolestatic jaundice occurs more frequently in women, usually between the second and fourth weeks; it is generally reversible if drug is withdrawn. It may begin with abrupt fever, grippelike symptoms, and abdominal discomfort, followed in about 1 week by jaundice. Pruritus, usually an early symptom of jaundice, may not be present because of the antipruritic effect of phenothiazines. Bilirubin and urobilinogen determinations are indicated with onset of symptoms.

An elevated temperature associated with sore mouth or throat, upper respiratory infection, fatigue, and weakness may be early manifestations of agranulocytosis. It is most likely to occur within the first 4 to 10 weeks of therapy, particularly in women and in the elderly.

Patients with diabetes who are receiving large doses of chlorpromazine should be watched carefully for loss of diabetes control. Urine and blood glucose should be checked regularly.

Since chlorpromazine may affect the temperature-regulating mechanism, heed and report the patient's complaint of feeling cold. Applying a blanket next to the body may help. Hot-water bottles and other heating devices are not recommended because phenothiazines tend to depress conditioned avoidance responses.

Hyperthermia, heat prostration, and photosensitivity reactions occur most frequently in patients on moderate to high doses for extended periods. Caution patient to avoid exposure to sun and heat.

Dryness of mouth and loosening of dentures may be relieved by frequent sips of water or by rinsing mouth with water. Sugarless candy or chewing gum may also help to stimulate salivary flow (regular gum or candy contains sucrose which is a good culture medium for *Candida* and also can lead to dental caries).

Oral candidiasis occurs frequently in patients receiving chlorpromazine therapy; emphasize meticulous oral hygiene. Overuse of antiseptic mouthwashes can change mouth flora and therefore should be avoided. See oral syndrome under Adverse Reactions.

Be alert to complaints of diminished visual acuity, reduced night vision, photophobia, and a perceived brownish discoloration of objects. Deposits may occur on cornea and lens and in extreme cases can impair vision.

Bear in mind that phenothiazines have an antiemetic effect that may obscure the signs of overdosage of other drugs or other causes of nausea and vomiting.

The therapeutic effects of phenothiazine therapy include the following: emotional and psychomotor quieting in excited, hyperactive patients; reduction of paranoidal symptoms, hallucinations, delusions, fears, and hostility; stimulation of withdrawn patients; organization of thought and behavior.

Abrupt withdrawal of drug, especially after prolonged therapy with large doses, can cause gastritis, nausea, vomiting, rhinorrhea, dizziness, tremulousness, insomnia, and exacerbation of psychotic states; therefore drug must be withdrawn gradually over a period of several weeks.

Inform and reassure the patient that side effects are reversible with prompt dosage adjustment or discontinuation of drug. Advise him to report unusual signs or symptoms without delay.

Chlorpromazine may impair mental and physical abilities, especially during the first few days of therapy. Caution the patient against driving a car or engaging in other activities requiring precision, mental alertness, and motor coordination until drug response has been evaluated by the physician.

Warn the patient to avoid any medication not specifically prescribed by his physician.

Some patients do not manifest improvement until after 7 or 8 weeks of therapy; therefore they may not realize the importance of medication compliance. Stress the necessity of continuing the prescribed medication regimen and the need for follow-up care to determine whether the maintenance dosage requires adjustment or discontinuation.

Preserved in tightly covered, light-resistant containers. Slight yellowing of parenteral preparation does not alter potency; if otherwise colored or markedly discolored solutions should be discarded.

Phenothiazine derivatives form incompatible admixtures with many drugs; therefore, consult pharmacist for guidance.

Do not mix solutions without a specific directive from physician.

LABORATORY TEST INTERFERENCES: Phenothiazines may affect the results of tests for urinary catecholamines (Pisano method), urine ketones (Gerhardt ferric chloride test), and ^{131}I uptake (increased). There may be false positive results for urobilinogen (Ehrlich's reagent), urine bilirubin (Bili-Labstix), and pregnancy tests (some may be falsely negative). False decreases in urinary 5-HIAA (nitrosonaphthol reagent) and urinary steroids may occur.

DRUG INTERACTIONS: **Antacids** and **attapulgite** may inhibit absorption of oral phenothiazines; space dosing so that mixing in GI tract is minimized. Effect may be increased by **estrogens** and by **MAO inhibitors.** Prolonged use of **phenobarbital** may decrease effects of chlorpromazine and possibly other phenothiazines. **Piperazine** may exaggerate phenothiazine-induced extrapyramidal effects. **Thiazide diuretics** may potentiate hypotensive effect of phenothiazines. Enhanced CNS depression may occur with concomitant use of phenothiazines and: **alcohol** (in excessive amounts), **anesthetic** and **preanesthetic agents, barbituates,** and **procarbazine.** Phenothiazines may decrease therapeutic effects of: **amphetamines** (mutally antagonistic), **antidiabetic agents,** and **anticonvulsants,** eg, **phenytoin** (diphenylhydantoin). In general, phenothiazines potentiate the effects of **antihypertensive agents** including **propranolol;** however, chlorpromazine may inhibit hypotensive effects of **guanethidine** and may cause paradoxical hypertensive response with **methyldopa.** Phenothiazine-induced extrapyramidal effects may be intensified by **atropinelike antiparkinson agents** and these agents may intensify anticholinergic effects of phenothiazines. **Epinephrine** may cause paradoxical lowering of blood pressure, and **stimulants** such as **picrotoxin** may produce convulsions in phenothiazine overdosage. Phenothiazines may decrease effects of **levodopa** (effect of either drug is reduced); may cause additive hyperglycemia with **lithium carbonate;** may produce additive cardiac depression with **quinidine;** and may enhance neuromuscular blockade of **succinylcholine.**

Oral hypoglycemic

ACTIONS AND USES

Longest-acting sulfonylurea compound, structurally and pharmacologically related to tolbutamide (qv). Although a sulfonamide derivative, it has no antibacterial activity. Lowers blood sugar by stimulating beta cells in pancreas to release endogenous insulin. May potentiate available antidiuretic hormone, a property not shared by other sulfonylureas. Has longer duration of action and about six times the potency of tolbutamide, as well as a higher incidence of side effects.

Used in treatment of maturity-onset diabetes mellitus. Also used in treatment of mild to moderate diabetes insipidus in patients with partial posterior pituitary deficiency.

ABSORPTION AND FATE

Promptly and completely absorbed from intestinal tract after oral ingestion. Wide distribution in extracellular fluid compartment. Action begins in 1 hour; peaks in 3 to 6 hours, with duration of about 72 hours. Half-life averages 36 hours. Plasma levels become stabilized 5 to 7 days after initiation of therapy; therefore, undue accumulation in blood does not occur during prolonged therapy. Recent studies indicate that as much as 80% may be metabolized. Slow renal excretion. Approximately 20% excreted in urine as unchanged drug; 80% to 90% of single oral dose excreted within 96 hours.

CONTRAINDICATIONS AND PRECAUTIONS

Juvenile diabetes, diabetes complicated by severe infection, acidosis, or severe renal, hepatic, or thyroid dysfunction. Cautious use: elderly patients, congestive heart failure. Also see Tolbutamide.

ADVERSE REACTIONS

Diarrhea, GI distress, potentiation of antidiuretic hormone (infrequent), cholestatic jaundice (rare), photosensitivity, hypoglycemia with mild CNS symptoms; agranulocytosis and positive direct Coombs' test (rare), disulfiramlike reaction to alcohol. Also see Tolbutamide.

ROUTE AND DOSAGE

Oral: initially 100 to 250 mg daily (elderly patient: 100 to 125 mg daily); maintenance 100 to 500 mg daily. Maintenance doses in excess of 750 mg are not recommended.

NURSING IMPLICATIONS

Chlorpropamide is generally prescribed as a single dose each morning with breakfast.

To alleviate GI symptoms, total daily drug requirement may be prescribed in two doses instead of one.

Patients who become hypoglycemic should be closely monitered for 3 to 5 days because of prolonged drug action. Hypoglycemia is controlled by administration of glucose.

With long-acting hypoglycemic agents, mild CNS symptoms of hypoglycemia predominate, while others may go unnoticed or may simply be tolerated (eg, abnormalities in sleep pattern, frequent nightmares, night sweats, morning headache). The patient and responsible family members should be alerted to the necessity of reporting all symptoms promptly to the physician.

If, prior to transfer to chlorpropamide, the patient required less than 40 units of insulin daily, the insulin may be withdrawn abruptly at the beginning of oral hypoglycemic therapy. If more than 40 units/day were needed, the insulin dose should be reduced by 50% for the first few transition days. Further adjustment is individualized.

It is not uncommon for hypoglycemia to occur during the period of transition from insulin to an oral hypoglycemic preparation; the patient will require close medical supervision for 3 to 5 days. Urine tests for ketone bodies and sugar should be done at least 3 times daily. Test abnormalities or any signs and symptoms should be reported promptly to the physician.

The more severe toxic effects, jaundice and granulocytopenia, are often preceded by skin eruptions, malaise, fever, or photosensitivity. Immediately report these symptoms to the physician. A change to another hypoglycemic may be indicated.

Instruct the controlled diabetic patient on chlorpropamide to monitor his weight and to be aware of his intake–output ratio and pattern. Infrequently this drug produces an antidiuretic effect, with resulting severe hyponatremia, edema, and water intoxication. Thus, if fluid intake far exceeds output and edema develops (weight gain), the patient should report to his physician. The most noticeable early symptoms may include mental confusion, drowsiness, and lethargy. If not treated promptly, overt psychotic behavior, coma, grand mal convulsions, irreversible neurologic damage, and death may occur.

Because the elderly generally have decreased renal function, close medical supervision is essential. Maintenance dosage of chlorpropamide is particularly hard to establish.

The patient and responsible family members should be instructed about the importance of exercise, strict adherence to diet and weight control, personal hygiene, avoidance of infection, and how and when to test for glycosuria and ketonuria as significant adjuncts to drug therapy.

Chronic mild hypoglycemia (which can be overlooked) increases the incidence of diabetes mellitus complications.

The patient on chlorpropamide needs to know how to administer insulin, because it is standard therapy in times of stress (severe trauma, infection, surgery). Also teach him how to recognize and counteract impending hypoglycemia (feeling of hunger and weakness, lightheadedness, sweating, tachycardia, anxiety, numbness, tremor, headache).

In accidental ingestion of this drug, complete elimination does not occur for 3 to 5 days. The patient should be hospitalized for close observation.

Alcohol intolerance may occur in up to 30% of patients receiving normal doses of chlorpropamide. Disulfiram-like reaction (facial flushing, pounding headache, feeling of breathlessness, tachycardia) occurs within 2 to 3 minutes, peaks in 15 to 20 minutes, and may last 1 to 4 hours. Caution the patient about this reaction.

Also see Tolbutamide.

CHLORPROTHIXENE, N.F.
(TARACTAN)

Antipsychotic (major tranquilizer)

ACTIONS AND USES

Thioxanthene derivative structurally and pharmacologically related to chlorpromazine (qv) and other phenothiazine derivatives, and to thiothixene. Has sedative, adrenolytic, antihistaminic, antiemetic, anticholinergic, and possibly uricosuric activity. Appears to be more effective in management of acute schizophrenia than chronic schizophrenia. See Chlorpromazine.

ABSORPTION AND FATE

Onset of effects occurs 10 to 30 minutes following IM administration. Presumably metabolized in liver and excreted in urine and feces as unchanged drug and its sulfoxide metabolite.

CONTRAINDICATIONS AND PRECAUTIONS

Hypersensitivity to thioxanthene and phenothiazine derivatives, circulatory collapse, congestive heart failure, coronary artery disease, cerebral vascular disorders, comatose states. Safe use not established for following situations: pregnancy, lactation, women of childbearing potential, children younger than 6 years of age, parenteral use in those under 12 years of age. See Chlorpromazine.

ADVERSE REACTIONS

Drowsiness, lethargy, dizziness, orthostatic hypotension, tachycardia, dry mouth, constipation, ocular disturbances, photosensitivity. Potentially, it has the same toxicity as phenothiazine derivatives. See Chlorpromazine.

ROUTE AND DOSAGE

Adults and children *over 12 years:* Oral, intramuscular: 25 to 50 mg 3 to 4 times daily (up to 600 mg/day). Elderly and debilitated patients: 10 to 25 mg 3 or 4 times daily. **Children** *over 6 years:* Oral: 10 to 25 mg 3 to 4 times daily.

NURSING IMPLICATIONS

Palatability of the commercial oral preparation may be improved by mixing it with milk, fruit juice, water, or carbonated beverage.

Since postural hypotension may occur in some patients, IM injection should be given with patient recumbent. Observe patient for signs of weakness or dizziness.

Observe patient closely when changeover from parenteral to oral doses are made.

Caution patient to avoid excessive exposure to sunlight.

See Chlorpromazine.

LABORATORY TEST INTERFERENCES: Chlorprothixene may cause false positive **urine bilirubin** test.

DRUG INTERACTIONS: Observe all precautions associated with phenothiazine therapy.

CHLORTHALIDONE, U.S.P., B.P. (HYGROTON)

Diuretic, antihypertensive

ACTIONS AND USES

Phthalimidine derivative of benzenesulfonamide. Structurally and pharmacologically related to thiazides, with similar actions, uses, contraindications, precautions, and adverse reactions. More slowly absorbed than chlorothiazide, and has longer duration of action.

ABSORPTION AND FATE

Onset of diuretic effect in 2 hours; peaks in 6 to 18 hours; duration 48 to 72 hours. About 90% bound primarily in or to red blood cells. Half-life 54 hours. Excreted unchanged in urine.

CONTRAINDICATIONS AND PRECAUTIONS

Hypersensitivity to sulfonamides. See Chlorothiazide.

Oral: **Adults**: initially 50 to 100 mg daily (maximum 200 mg/day). Alternatively, 100 mg every other day or 3 times weekly. Maintenance level adjusted according to individual patient's response and requirements. **Children**: initially, 3 mg/kg as single dose repeated 3 times weekly; maintenance dose adjusted to need.

NURSING IMPLICATIONS
Administration as single dose in the morning with food is recommended. See Chlorothiazide.

CHOLECALCIFEROL, U.S.P.
(Activated 7-Dehydrocholesterol, Vitamin D₃)
ERGOCALCIFEROL, U.S.P.
(Calciferol, DELTALIN, DRISDOL, GELTABS, Oleovitamin D, Vitamin D₂)

Antirachitic vitamin

ACTIONS AND USES
The term vitamin D encompasses two related fat-soluble substances (sterols) which are converted to ergocalciferol (vitamin D_2) and cholecalciferol (vitamin D_3), respectively, under the influence of ultraviolet light. Each has essentially equal antirachitic potency. Vitamin D increases blood calcium and phosphate ion levels by enhancing their intestinal absorption and promoting renal tubular resorption of phosphate. Stimulates development of osteoclasts and prolongs their life span, promotes mineral resorption by bones; functions in magnesium metabolism and in maintenance of normal parathyroid activity.
Used in treatment of refractory rickets (vitamin-D-resistant rickets), infantile tetany, osteomalacia (adult rickets), hypoparathyroidism; and in prophylaxis and treatment of nutritional rickets. Also has been used in Fanconi's syndrome and, with varying clinical results, in lupus vulgaris and psoriasis.
ABSORPTION AND FATE
Readily absorbed from GI tract (reduced absorption in intestinal malabsorption syndrome, hepatic or biliary dysfunction). Most of drug appears first in lymph, then concentrates rapidly in liver. Inert until hydroxylated in liver and kidney to active metabolites (12 to 24 hours after administration). About one-half of oral dose excreted via bile in feces; small amounts excreted slowly in urine. Stored chiefly in liver and to lesser extent in skin, brain, spleen, and bones. Has cumulative action.
CONTRAINDICATIONS AND PRECAUTIONS
Hypersensitivity to vitamin D, hypervitaminosis D, hypercalcemia, hyperphosphatemia, renal osteodystrophy with hyperphosphatemia, malabsorption syndrome, decreased renal function. Cautious use: patients with coronary disease, arteriosclerosis (especially in the elderly). Safety of amounts in excess of 400 IU daily in pregnancy not established.
ADVERSE REACTIONS
Vitamin D toxicity (hypervitaminosis D) is reversible if medication is withdrawn promptly. Initially, hypercalcemia with drowsiness, fatigue, lassitude, anorexia, nausea, vomiting, diarrhea, constipation, profuse sweating, vague aches, and stiffness; later, anemia, metastatic calcification (kidneys, blood vessels, myocardium, lungs, skin). Nephrotoxicity: polyuria, polydipsia, nocturia, casts, albuminuria, hematuria, hypertension, mild acidosis, convulsions, renal failure. Infants and children: mental retardation, increased mineralization of bone, and decline in linear growth rate (dwarfism). Altered laboratory values: elevated serum and urine calcium, protein, and inorganic phosphate determinations; decreased alkaline phosphatase, and elevated NPN.

Oral (*prophylactic against rickets*): 400 units daily. *Treatment of nutritional rickets*: 1000 to 4000 units daily. *Vitamin-D-resistant rickets*: 12,000 to 500,000 units daily. *Hypoparathyroidism*: 50,000 to 200,000 units (generally, plus 4 Gm of calcium lactate, administered 6 times a day). Highly individualized dosages.

NURSING IMPLICATIONS

Patients receiving therapeutic doses of vitamin D must remain under close medical supervision. The margin of safety between therapeutic and toxic doses is extremely narrow.

Therapeutic dosages are based on consideration of dietary and drug sources of vitamin D, calcium, and phosphate; adjustments are made according to clinical response.

When high therapeutic doses are used, progress is followed by frequent determinations (every 2 weeks or more frequently) of serum calcium, phosphates, and urea, and urine determinations of calcium (Sulkowitch test, see Index), casts, albumin, and red blood cells. Blood calcium concentration is generally kept between 9 and 10 mg/dl. Normal vitamin D blood levels range from 50 to 135 IU/dl.

Indiscriminate use of vitamin D is hazardous because of its cumulative action. Several weeks are required before the hypercalcemia and hypercalciuria that accompany overdosage are cleared.

Treatment of vitamin D toxicity consists of prompt discontinuation of the vitamin, a low-calcium diet, generous fluid intake, acidification of urine (to prevent calculus formation and enhance urinary excretion of calcium), and general symptomatic and supportive treatment.

Most foods contain little or no vitamin D. High concentrations are found in liver oil from cod, burbot, and halibut. Other good sources include salmon, sardines, herring, egg yolk, fortified milk, butter, and margarine. Most milk in the U.S. is fortified with 400 units of vitamin D per quart. Patients receiving therapeutic doses of cholecalciferol should be informed regarding allowable intake of these foods.

Advise patient not to take mineral oil because it may interfere with absorption of vitamin D and other fat-soluble vitamins.

Vitamin D supplements are generally not required by the healthy individual who has access to sunlight and fortified food sources. The RDA of vitamin D for infants, children, adults under 22 years of age, and during pregnancy and lactation is 400 units. There is no RDA for adults over 22 years (except during pregnancy and lactation), but intake should not exceed 400 units.

More than 85% of calcium is stored in bone and teeth during the last trimester of pregnancy; thus prematures require therapeutic doses of vitamin D.

Preserved in tightly covered, light-resistant containers.

LABORATORY TEST INTERFERENCES: Vitamin D may interfere with serum cholesterol measurements.

DRUG INTERACTIONS: Long-term, high-dose **barbiturate** anticonvulsant therapy may decrease the effects of vitamin D. **Cholestyramine** may interfere with absorption of vitamin D. **Phenytoin** (Diphenylhydantoin) increases the metabolic inactivation of vitamin D and decreases its half-life in body, resulting in hypocalcemia, osteomalacia, or rickets.

(CUEMID, QUESTRAN)

Ion-exchange resin, bile-acid-sequestering agent

ACTIONS AND USES

Quaternary ammonium anion-exchange resin. Adsorbs and combines with intestinal bile salts to form an insoluble, nonabsorbable complex that is excreted in feces. As a result, bile salts are continually (but not entirely) prevented from reentry to the enterohepatic circulation. Increased fecal loss of bile acids leads to increased oxidation of cholesterol to bile acids, lowered plasma cholesterol, decreased plasma low-density (beta) lipoproteins, and relief of pruritus of cholestatic origin. Serum triglyceride levels may increase or remain unchanged. Ability to bind digitoxin in GI tract is the basis for its use in digitoxin intoxication. Since it sequesters bile acids, it may interfere with absorption of calcium and with normal fat absorption and including the absorption of fat-soluble vitamins A, D, E, and K. The effects of drug-induced lowering of serum cholesterol and other lipid levels on morbidity and mortality due to atherosclerosis or coronary heart disease have not been determined.

Used primarily for relief of pruritus associated with biliary stasis. Also used as adjunct to dietary therapy in management of primary type II hyperlipoproteinemia (pure hypercholesterolemia) and in treatment of acute toxicity of digitoxin.

ABSORPTION AND FATE

Not absorbed from GI tract. Excreted in feces as insoluble complex.

CONTRAINDICATIONS AND PRECAUTIONS

Complete biliary obstruction, hypersensitivity. Safe use during pregnancy and lactation not established. Cautious use: steatorrhea, impaired renal function.

ADVERSE REACTIONS

Constipation (may be severe), intestinal impaction, abdominal pain and distention, flatulence, nausea, vomiting, diarrhea, heartburn, anorexia, steatorrhea, vitamin A, D, E, and K deficiencies, hypoprothrombinemia, bleeding tendencies, rash and irritation (skin, tongue, perianal area), hyperchloremic acidosis in children, osteoporosis. Others reported but not necessarily drug-related: pancreatitis, rectal pain, hiccups, sour taste, claudication, xanthomata, arteritis, chest pain, backache, joint pain, vertigo, headache, anxiety, syncope, tinnitus, drowsiness, paresthesias, uveitis, arcus juvenilis, hematuria, dysuria, diuresis, weight changes, swollen glands, increased libido, calcification on biliary tree.

ROUTE AND DOSAGE

Oral: **Adults**: 4 Gm 3 or 4 times daily before meals (dose titrated to patient's needs). **Pediatric**: dosage not established. **Children** *over 6 years* have been given 80 mg/kg 3 times daily.

NURSING IMPLICATIONS

Cholestyramine is buff colored and has a slight aminelike odor and a disagreeable taste; in solution its consistency is sandy or gritty.

Always dissolve cholestyramine before administration, as it is irritating to mucous membranes and may cause esophageal impaction if administered in dry form.

Water, highly flavored liquids, carbonated drinks, thin soups, pulpy fruits with high moisture content (applesauce, crushed pineapple) disguise the taste somewhat. If diluent is carbonated, use a large glass and stir slowly; small drug particles release CO_2 rapidly and cause excessive foaming.

Place contents of one pack or one level scoopful of cholestyramine on surface of 4 to 6 fluid ounces of preferred vehicle. Permit drug to hydrate by standing without stirring 1 to 2 minutes, twirling glass occasionally; then stir until suspension is uniform. After ingestion of preparation, rinse glass with small amount liquid and have patient drink remainder to ensure taking entire dose.

A trial of diet therapy and weight reduction is usually instituted before starting resin treatment.

Baseline serum cholesterol and triglyceride levels will be established at beginning of therapy and determined at intervals during treatment.

With dosage higher than 24 Gm, side effects increase.

Supplemental water-miscible or parenteral vitamins A, D, and E and parenteral K should be taken during long-term therapy with cholestyramine.

Preexisting constipation should be evaluated before starting treatment, since it may be worsened by the drug, particularly in elderly patients and women and when dose is high (24 Gm or more). Instruct patient to report change in normal elimination pattern promptly to physician.

High-bulk diet (bran, fruit, raw vegetables) with adequate fluid intake is an essential adjunct to cholestyramine treatment. Consult physician.

If constipation becomes a problem, dosage may be lowered or temporarily interrupted. A stool softener is frequently ordered, especially if patient has heart disease. Occasionally this side effect necessitates withdrawal of the drug.

Encourage patient to continue taking the drug even though it may be distasteful. Usually GI side effects subside after first month of drug therapy.

When other oral drugs are being given during cholestyramine therapy, it is recommended that they be administered at least 1 hour before or 4 to 6 hours after the resin to avoid interference with their absorption.

Chronic use can cause increased bleeding tendency. Patient should be alert to early symptoms of hypoprothrombinemia (petechiae, ecchymoses, abnormal bleeding from mucous membranes, tarry stools) and report their occurrence promptly. Usually, parenteral vitamin K preparation will reverse the symptoms.

Relief of pruritus is an individual response, but therapy is usually continued at least 2 weeks before final evaluation. With improvement, dosage is lowered (withdrawal of drug may result in increased serum bile acid and return of pruritus).

DRUG INTERACTIONS: Cholestyramine may interfere with absorption of: **oral anticoagulants, digitalis, glycosides, iron preparations, thiazide diuretics, phenylbutazone, thyroid hormones.**

CHOLINE SALICYLATE
(ARTHROPAN)

Analgesic, antipyretic, antirheumatic

ACTIONS AND USES

Choline salt of salicylic acid supplied commercially as a stable liquid salicylate preparation. Reported to have analgesic, antiinflammatory, and antipyretic effectiveness equal to that of aspirin, but with more rapid absorption, greater tolerance, and less gastric damage and erosion.

Indicated in those conditions for which oral salicylates are usually recommended (see Aspirin). May be indicated for patients who have difficulty swallowing tablets or capsules; patients who show gastric intolerance to aspirin; and for patients who should avoid sodium-containing salicylates.

ABSORPTION AND FATE
Rapidly absorbed from GI tract. Peak blood levels occur in 10 to 30 minutes. Distribution and fate as for aspirin.
CONTRAINDICATIONS AND PRECAUTIONS
Salicylate sensitivity. Also see Aspirin.
ADVERSE REACTIONS
Nausea, vomiting. High doses: tinnitus, deafness, dizziness, sweating, mental confusion, hyperventilation, hepatotoxicity. Also see Aspirin.
ROUTE AND DOSAGE
Oral: **Adults and children** *over 12 years*: 870 mg repeated every 3 or 4 hours, if necessary, but not more than 6 times in one day. Each 5 ml contains 870 mg; equivalent to 650 mg (10 grains) of aspirin.

NURSING IMPLICATIONS
Although the preparation is mint flavored, the taste is objectionable to some patients. May be mixed with fruit juices, carbonated beverages, or water. See Aspirin.

CHORIONIC GONADOTROPIN, U.S.P.
(ANDROID-HCG, ANTUITRIN-S, A.P.L., CHOREX, FOLLUTEIN, GONADEX, LIBIGEN, PREGNYL, STEMUTROLIN)

Gonad-stimulating principle

ACTIONS AND USES
Purified preparation of gonadotropic glycoprotein hormone extracted from gravid human urine, with actions nearly identical to those of pituitary luteinizing hormone. Promotes production of gonadal steroid hormones by stimulating the interstitial cells of testes (Leydig cells) to produce androgen and the corpus luteum of ovaries to produce progesterone. In women of childbearing age with normally functioning ovaries, it causes ovulation of follicles stimulated by follicle-stimulating hormone and promotes corpus luteum development.
Used in treatment of cryptorchidism not due to anatomic obstruction and male hypogonadism secondary to pituitary failure. Also used in conjunction with menotropins to induce ovulation and pregnancy in infertile women in whom the cause of anovulation is secondary.
ABSORPTION AND FATE
Following IM administration, peak levels are attained in 6 hours. Biphasic clearance from blood, followed by concentration in testes or ovaries. Serum half-life 8 and 24 hours for fast and slow components, respectively. From 10% to 12% excreted in urine in 24 hours; detectable amounts appear in urine for as long as 3 to 4 days.
CONTRAINDICATIONS AND PRECAUTIONS
Known hypersensitivity to the drug, hypertrophy or tumor of pituitary, androgen-dependent neoplasms, precocious puberty. Cautious use: epilepsy, migraine, asthma, cardiac or renal disease.
ADVERSE REACTIONS
Headache, irritability, restlessness, depression, fatigue, gynecomastia, edema, sexual precocity in prepubertal patients, pain at site of injection; increased urinary steroid excretion.
ROUTE AND DOSAGE
Potency expressed in U.S.P. units; 1500 units are equal to 1 mg of drug; 1 U.S.P. unit equals 1 international unit (IU) of the WHO. Intramuscular: dosage highly individualized.

NURSING IMPLICATIONS

Following reconstitution (diluent furnished by manufacturer), solution is stable 1 to 3 months when refrigerated.

Weight should be monitored during therapy as a clue to edema development. Dosage reduction is indicated if edema develops.

Vaginal bleeding during treatment of corpus luteum deficiency should be reported; drug will be discontinued.

Patients with prepubertal cryptorchism should be advised to report immediately to physician if signs of precocius puberty occur.

Although this drug has been used to treat obesity, reportedly it has no known effect on fat mobilization, appetite, or body fat distribution.

CLINDAMYCIN HYDROCHLORIDE, U.S.P.
(CLEOCIN HYDROCHLORIDE)
CLINDAMYCIN PALMITATE HYDROCHLORIDE, N.F.
(CLEOCIN PEDIATRIC)
CLINDAMYCIN PHOSPHATE, N.F.
(CLEOCIN PHOSPHATE)

Antibacterial

ACTIONS AND USES

Semisynthetic derivative of lincomycin, with which it shares neuromuscular blocking properties; has actions, uses, contraindications, precautions, and adverse reactions similar to those of lincomycin. Reported to have greater degree of antibacterial activity in vitro, better absorption, and lower incidence of GI side effects than lincomycin. Particularly effective in treatment of serious infections caused by susceptible strains of anaerobic streptococci, *Bacteroides* (especially *B. fragilis*), *Fusobacterium,* and *Actinomyces israelii.*

ABSORPTION AND FATE

Almost complete (90%) absorption following oral administration. Peak plasma concentrations within 45 minutes following 150-mg oral dose; effective levels persist 6 hours. Following IM injection, peak levels within 3 hours; effective levels persist 8 to 12 hours. Widely distributed to body fluids and tissues, including saliva and bone. No significant concentrations in cerebrospinal fluid, even when meninges are inflamed. About 90% protein-bound. Average biologic half-life 2.4 hours. Most of drug is inactivated by metabolism. Excreted in urine, bile, and feces as bioactive and inactive metabolites and about 10% unchanged drug. Readily crosses placenta and may appear in breast milk.

CONTRAINDICATIONS AND PRECAUTIONS

History of hypersensitivity to clindamycin or lincomycin. Safe use during pregnancy not established. Not recommended for infants younger than 1 month of age. Cautious use: history of GI disease, renal disease; atopic individuals. Also see Lincomycin.

ADVERSE REACTIONS

Severe colitis, sometimes fatal. Also reported: pain, induration, sterile abscess at IM site, elevated creatine phosphokinase (CPK) levels following IM use, thrombophlebitis (IV site), eosinophilia, hyperbilirubinemia. See Lincomycin.

ROUTE AND DOSAGE

Oral: **Adults**: 150 to 450 mg every 6 hours. **Pediatric** *over 1 month:* 8 to 20 mg/kg/day divided into 3 or 4 equal doses. Intramuscular, intravenous (clindamycin phosphate): **Adults**: 600 mg to 2700 mg daily in 2, 3, or 4 equally divided doses. Not more than 1200 mg should be administered by IV infusion in a 1-hour period. **Pediatric** *over 1 month*: 15 to 40 mg/kg/day divided into 3 or 4 equal doses. All dosages individualized according to severity of infection and **141** renal status.

NURSING IMPLICATIONS

Absorption of oral clindamycin is not significantly affected by food, although peak serum levels may be delayed.

Note expiration date of oral solution; retains potency for 14 days at room temperature. Do not refrigerate as chilling causes thickening and thus makes pouring difficult.

Deep IM injection is recommended to minimize complications of administration. Rotate injection sites.

Single IM doses should not exceed 600 mg.

Colitis and pseudomembranous colitis have been associated with both oral and parenteral clindamycin. Report immediately the onset of diarrhea, passage of tarry or bloody stools or mucus, abdominal cramps, or ileus. Symptoms may appear up to several weeks following cessation of therapy.

During prolonged therapy, periodic liver and kidney function tests and blood cell counts are recommended.

Serum clindamycin levels are monitored during high-dose therapy, particularly in patients with renal or hepatic disease.

See Lincomycin.

CLOFIBRATE, N.F.
(ATROMID-S)

Antihyperlipidemic

ACTIONS AND USES

Aryloxisobutyric acid derivative structurally unrelated to other antilipemic agents. Reduces very low-density lipoproteins (VLDL) rich in triglycerides to a greater extent than low-density lipoproteins (LDL) rich in cholesterol. Mechanism of action is unclear; it appears to inhibit cholesterol biosynthesis prior to mevalonate formation and transfer of triglycerides from liver to serum. Interferes with binding of free fatty acids to albumin and increases fecal excretion of neutral sterols. Its ability to cause regression of xanthomatous lesions is thought to be due to mobilization of cholesterol from tissue. Clofibrate does not alter the seasonal variation of serum cholesterol (peak elevations occur in midwinter and late summer and decrease in fall and spring). Reportedly reduces serum fibrinogen levels and platelet adhesiveness and has significant SIADH-like activity (syndrome of inappropriate antidiuretic hormone). The effects of drug-induced lowering of serum cholesterol and other lipids on morbidity and mortality due to atherosclerosis or coronary heart disease have not been determined.

Used as adjunct to appropriate dietary regulation and other measures for reduction of serum lipids in patients with hypercholesterolemia and/or hypertriglyceridema. Also used in treatment of xanthoma tuberosum associated with hyperlipidemia. Reportedly useful in treatment of diabetes insipidus.

ABSORPTION AND FATE

Completely absorbed from intestines. Measurable serum levels attained in 3 to 24 hours. Rapidly hydrolyzed by serum enzymes to free acid which is extensively bound to plasma proteins. Major fraction bound to plasma proteins and well distributed to extracellular sites. Half-life 10 to 14 hours. Excreted almost entirely in urine, primarily as glucuronide conjugate.

Impaired renal or hepatic function, primary biliary cirrhosis, pregnancy, nursing mothers. Safe use in children not established. Cautious use: history of jaundice or hepatic disease, peptic ulcer, gout, patients receiving hypoglycemic agents or oral anticoagulants.

ADVERSE REACTIONS

GI: nausea (common), vomiting, loose stools, flatulence, bloating, abdominal distress, gastritis, polyphagia, weight gain or loss, stomatitis, hepatomegaly. **Musculoskeletal**: flulike symptoms, myositis, arthralgia. **Neurologic**: fatigue, weakness, drowsiness, dizziness, headache. **Hematologic**: leukopenia, anemia, eosinophilia, agranulocytosis, potentiation of anticoagulant effect. **Genitourinary**: impotence, decreased libido, renal dysfunction (dysuria, hematuria, proteinuria, decreased urinary output). **Cardiovascular**: increase or decrease in angina, congestive failure, arrhythmias. **Dermatologic**: swelling and phlebitis at xanthoma sites, dry skin, dry and brittle hair, alopecia, allergy, urticaria, pruritus. **Hepatic**: abnormal liver function tests: increased transaminase (SGOT and SGPT), increased BSP retention, increased thymol turbidity. **Also reported** (direct relationship to drug action not known): peptic ulcer, GI hemorrhage, hypoglycemia, tremor, diaphoresis, systemic lupus erythematosus, rheumatoid arthritis, thrombocytopenic purpura, gynecomastia, blurred vision, acute gout (rare).

ROUTE AND DOSAGE

Oral: 500 mg 4 times daily.

NURSING IMPLICATIONS

Clofibrate is indicated as adjunctive therapy, but only when an appropriate dietary regimen of weight control, and other measures have been tried and have proved unsuccessful.

Before initiation of therapy a complete health history should be obtained, including physical examination and appropriate laboratory determinations and personal, family, and dietary history.

Serum cholesterol and triglyceride levels should be determined initially and evaluated every 2 weeks during first few months of therapy, and then at monthly intervals.

Frequent serum transaminase and other liver tests are advocated, as well as periodic complete blood counts, renal function tests, and determinations of plasma and urine steroid levels, serum electrolyte levels and blood sugar. (Clofibrate is associated with malabsorption of iron, electrolytes, sugar, and Vitamin B_{12}.)

Clofibrate should be withdrawn if serum transaminase or other liver function tests show a steady rise or are otherwise abnormal.

Patients receiving oral hypoglycemic agents should be observed for excessive hypoglycemic activity.

Flulike symptoms (malaise, muscle soreness, aching, weakness) should be reported promptly to the physician.

Therapeutic response is indicated by reduction of lipid level; this generally occurs during the first or second month of therapy. Rebound may occur in second or third month, followed by a further decrease.

Clofibrate is generally withdrawn after 3 months if the response is not adequate. When used for xanthoma, therapy may be continued even up to 1 year, provided that there is some reduction in size of lesions.

Since hyperlipoproteinemia is frequently genetically determined, family members of the patient, especially children, should be screened for abnormal lipid levels.

Reduction to ideal weight, correction of sedentary habits, and control of smoking are applicable to all patients with hyperlipoproteinemia.

Preserved in closed, light-resistant containers.

Concomitant use of clofibrate and **furosemide** may result in higher free levels of both drugs. It has been proposed that clofibrate may prolong the half-life of **oral hypoglycemic agents.**

CLOMIPHENE CITRATE, U.S.P.
(CLOMID)

Gonad-stimulating principle

ACTIONS AND USES
Nonsteroid compound (structurally related to chlorotrianisene) used to induce ovulation in anovulatory women. Has both estrogenic and antiestrogenic properties, but its mechanism of action is not clear. Appears to stimulate release of pituitary gonadotropins, and may act directly on the biosynthesis of ovarian hormones. Ineffective in the presence of panhypopituitarism or ovarian failure. A single ovulation is induced by a single course of therapy; normal ovulatory function does not usually resume after treatment or after pregnancy.
Used for treating disorders of ovulation in appropriately selected women desiring pregnancy.
ABSORPTION AND FATE
Readily absorbed from GI tract. Detoxified in liver; 50% of dose is excreted in feces after 5 days; the remaining metabolites and drug are excreted from enterohepatic pool or are stored in body fat for later release.
CONTRAINDICATIONS AND PRECAUTIONS
Pregnancy, hepatic disease, history of hepatic dysfunction; abnormal and unexplained bleeding, ovarian cyst. Cautious use: enlarged ovaries, pelvic discomfort, sensitivity to pituitary gonadotropins.
ADVERSE REACTIONS
Early abortion, multiple births, congenital abnormalities, hydatidiform mole, mild hot flushes, abdominal symptoms and pelvic discomfort (distention, bloating, constipation, pain related to mittelschmerz, heavy menses, ovarian enlargement); visual disturbances (short duration): transient blurring, diplopia, scotomata, photophobia, phosphenes, decreased visual acuity (rare). Also reported: nausea, vomiting, increased appetite and weight gain, urinary frequency, polyuria, dermatologic conditions (rash, urticaria, allergic dermatitis), breast discomfort, nervous tension, depression, headache, restlessness, insomnia, dizziness, fatigue, alopecia (reversible).
ROUTE AND DOSAGE
Oral: 50 mg daily for 5 days; if menses and ovulation occur, subsequent course is started on fifth day of cycle. Failure to ovulate in first course is criterion for increasing dosage to 100 mg daily for 5 days starting as early as 30 days after previous course. Total dose during a single course should not exceed 600 mg.

NURSING IMPLICATIONS
Patient who is going to respond usually ovulates after first course of therapy (within 5 to 14 days).
Three courses of therapy are usually considered an adequate clinical trial before the patient is considered a so-called clomiphene failure.
Tests of liver function are usually performed before therapy begins. If they are abnormal, therapy generally will not be started.
Encourage patient to establish a flow chart for recording weight and basal temperatures to determine day of ovulation.
Multiple pregnancies and the incidence of side effects are expected to increase at the higher dose of 100 mg/day.

Although congenital defects have been described in children resulting from clomiphene pregnancies, the incidence reportedly is no greater than in the general population.

Visual symptoms apparently due to intensification and prolongation of afterimages are accentuated on exposure to a more brightly lit environment. If they occur, clomiphene should be discontinued and a complete ophthalmologic evaluation carried out.

Because of the possibility of lightheadedness and visual disturbances, the patient should be cautioned against performing hazardous tasks requiring mental alertness and physical coordination, especially in an environment with variable lighting.

Hot flushes resembling those of menopause disappear when the drug is discontinued.

CLONIDINE HYDROCHLORIDE
(CATAPRES)

Antihypertensive

ACTIONS AND USES

Imidazoline derivative chemically related to tolazoline. Stimulates α-adrenergic receptors in CNS to produce inhibition of sympathetic vasomotor centers. Central effects result in reduced peripheral sympathetic nervous system activity, reduction in systolic and diastolic blood pressure and bradycardia. Orthostatic effects tend to be mild and infrequent. Initial dose is followed by enhanced tubular reabsorption of sodium and chloride; after 3 to 4 days sodium retention is reversed and natriuresis occurs. Other possible effects: decreased urinary excretion of catecholamines, inhibition of centrally induced salivation, decreased GI secretions and motility, decreased intraocular pressure, prolonged circulation time and inhibition of renin release from kidneys.

Used in treatment of hypertension alone or with diuretic or other antihypertensive agents. Has been used investigationally in management of acute hypertensive crises, as prophylaxis for migraine, and in treatment of dysmenorrhea and menopausal flushing.

ABSORPTION AND FATE

Well absorbed from GI tract. Plasma drug level peaks in 3 to 5 hours; plasma half-life 12 to 30 hours (25 to 37 hours in patients with impaired renal function). Believed to be widely distributed in body tissues. Metabolized in liver; 65% of dose is excreted by kidneys as unchanged drug and metabolites, and about 20% is excreted through enterohepatic route in feces. Approximately 85% of single dose is eliminated within 72 hours; excretion completed after 5 days. Crosses blood–brain barrier.

CONTRAINDICATIONS AND PRECAUTIONS

Safe use during pregnancy and in women of childbearing potential and children not established. Cautious use: severe coronary insufficiency, recent myocardial infarction, cerebrovascular disease, chronic renal failure, Raynaud's disease, thromboangiitis obliterans, history of mental depression.

ADVERSE REACTIONS

Most frequent: dry mouth (transient), drowsiness, sedation, constipation, dizziness, headache, weakness, fatigue, slight transient bradycardia. **GI and metabolic**: anorexia, nausea, vomiting, parotid pain, mild transient abnormalities in liver function tests, hepatitis without icterus (possible), hyperbilirubinemia, transient elevation of blood glucose, weight gain (sodium retention). **Cardiovascular**: postural hypotension (mild), Raynaud's phenomenon, congestive heart failure, ECG changes, bradycardia, palpitation, flushes. **CNS**: vivid dreams, nightmares, insomnia, behavior changes, nervousness, restlessness, anxiety, mental depression. **Dermatologic**: rash, angioneurotic edema, urticaria, pruritus, thinning of hair. **Genitourinary**: impotence, urinary retention. Other: dry, itchy, and burning eyes, dry nasal mucosa, pallor, increased sensitivity to alcohol, ophthalmologic changes (possible), weakly positive Coombs' test, elevated serum CPK, gynecomastia.

ROUTE AND DOSAGE

Oral: initially 0.1 mg twice daily; increments of 0.1 or 0.2 mg per day may be made until desired response is achieved. Maintenance: 0.2 to 0.8 mg daily in divided doses. (Studies have indicated that 2.4 mg is the maximun effective daily dose.)

NURSING IMPLICATIONS

Consult physician regarding schedule of blood pressure determinations. Hypotensive response begins within 30 to 60 minutes after drug administration. Maximun decrease in blood pressure occurs in 2 to 4 hours. Antihypertensive effect lasts approximately 6 to 8 hours.

Last dose is commonly administered immediately before retiring to ensure overnight blood pressure control.

Side effects that occur most frequently (see Adverse Reactions) tend to diminish with continued therapy, or they may be relieved by dosage reduction.

Although postural hypotension occurs infrequently, advise patient to make position changes slowly, particularly from recumbent to upright position, and to dangle legs a few minutes before standing. Caution him to lie down immediately if he feels faint.

Monitor intake and output during period of dosage adjustment. Report change in intake–output ratio or change in voiding pattern.

Determine weight daily. Patients not receiving a concomitant diuretic agent may gain weight, particularly during first 3 or 4 days of therapy, because of marked reduction in sodium and chloride excretion. Consult physician regarding allowable sodium intake.

Patients with histories of mental depression require close supervision, as they may be subject to further depressive episodes.

Tolerance may develop in some patients. Physician may increase dosage or prescribe concomitant administration of a diuretic to enhance antihypertensive response.

Inform the patient of the possible sedative effect and caution against potentially hazardous activities such as operating machinery or driving.

If drug is to be discontinued, it is withdrawn over a period of 2 to 4 days. Abrupt withdrawal, particularly after long-term therapy, may result in restlessness and headache 2 to 3 hours after a missed dose and a significant increase in blood pressure within 8 to 24 hours. Other symptoms associated with sudden withdrawal include anxiety, sweating, palpitation, increased heart rate, insomnia, tremors, muscle and stomach pain, and salivation; rarely, hypertensive encephalopathy and death may ensue.

It is recommended that patient be monitored for at least one month after clonidine is withdrawn.

Warn the patient of the danger of missing a dose or stopping the drug without consulting his physician.

Periodic eye examination is advised (based on animal studies).

DRUG INTERACTIONS: Clonidine may enhance CNS depressant effects of **alcohol, barbiturates,** other **sedatives,** and **tranquilizers.** Possibility of additive bradycardic effect with drugs that increase heart rate such as **digitalis glycosides, guanethidine,** and **propanolol. Tricyclic antidepressants** may block antihypertensive effects of clonidine.

CLORAZEPATE DIPOTASSIUM
(TRANXENE)

Antianxiety agent (minor tranquilizer)

ACTIONS AND USES
  Benzodiazepine psychotherapeutic agent with actions, uses, contraindications, precautions, and adverse reactions qualitatively similar to those of chlordiazepoxide and other benzodiazepines. Has been used investigationally in the management of petit mal, akinetic, and myoclonic seizures refractory to other drugs.
ABSORPTION AND FATE
  Decarboxylated in stomach to nordiazepam and absorbed as this metabolite. Metabolite reaches peak serum levels in about 1 hour; antianxiety action may persist about 24 hours. Half-life approximately 48 hours. Nordiazepam is metabolized in liver. About 83% of dose is excreted in urine, and small amount in feces, within 10 days.
CONTRAINDICATIONS AND PRECAUTIONS
  Hypersensitivity to clorazepate; acute narrow-angle glaucoma; nursing mothers; pregnancy. Also see Chlordiazepoxide.
ROUTE AND DOSAGE
  Oral: 15 to 60 mg daily in divided doses adjusted to patient response. Elderly patients: 7.5 to 15 mg daily. Sustained-action tablet: 22.5 mg once daily.

> **NURSING IMPLICATIONS**
> Caution patient to avoid potentially hazardous activities until his reaction to drug is known.
> Drowsiness, a common side effect, is more likely to occur at initiation of therapy and with dosage increments.
> Effectiveness of clorazepate for long-term use (more than 4 months) has not been determined. Usefulness of drug should be periodically reassessed.
> Classified as Schedule IV drug under the federal Controlled Substances Act.
> See Chlordiazepoxide.

CLOXACILLIN, SODIUM, U.S.P., B.P.
(CLOXAPEN, TEGOPEN)

Antibacterial

ACTIONS AND USES
  Semisynthetic, monohydrated salt of isoxazolyl penicillin. Resistant to inactivation by penicillinase. Mechanism of antibacterial action as for penicillin G potassium
  Used primarily in treatment of mild to moderate infections caused by penicillinase-producing staphylococci, but may also be used to initiate therapy in suspected staphylococcal infections pending culture and sensitivity results.
ABSORPTION AND FATE
  Peak serum levels within 1 hour; effective levels maintained 4 to 6 hours after single dose. Distributed throughout body, with highest concentrations in kidneys and liver; 90% to 95% protein-bound. Half-life 30 to 60 minutes. Excreted primarily in urine as active metabolite and intact drug; also significant hepatic elimination through bile. Crosses placenta.
CONTRAINDICATIONS AND PRECAUTIONS
  Hypersensitivity to penicillins or cephalosporins. Safe use during pregnancy and in neonates not established. Cautious use: history of allergies, asthma.

Nausea, vomiting, flatulence, diarrhea, pruritus, urticaria, wheezing, drug fever. Generally well tolerated, but same potential as for other penicillins. See Penicillin G Potassium.

ROUTE AND DOSAGE

Oral: **Adults and children** *weighing 20 kg or more*: 250 to 500 mg or more every 6 hours. **Children** *weighing less than 20 kg*: 50 to 100 mg/kg/day in equally divided doses every 6 hours.

NURSING IMPLICATIONS

Careful inquiry should be made concerning previous hypersensitivity reactions to penicillins, cephalosporins, and other allergens.

Administer at least 1 or 2 hours before meals (preferably) or 2 hours after meals. Food reduces absorption.

Periodic assessments of renal, hepatic, and hematopoietic function should be made in patients on prolonged therapy.

Reconstituted oral solution is stable for 14 days if refrigerated. Shake well before pouring.

See Penicillin G Potassium.

LABORATORY TEST INTERFERENCES: Possible interference with urinary steroid determinations.

See Penicillin G Potassium.

COCAINE, N.F.
COCAINE HYDROCHLORIDE, U.S.P., B.P.

Topical anesthetic

ACTIONS AND USES

Alkaloid obtained from leaves of *Erythroxylon coca*. Topical application blocks nerve conduction and produces surface anesthesia accompanied by local vasoconstriction. Exerts adrenergic effect by potentiating action of endogenous (and injected) epinephrine and norepinephrine. Systemic absorption produces descending CNS stimulation.

Used for surface anesthesia of ear, nose, throat, rectum, and vagina.

ABSORPTION AND FATE

Readily absorbed through mucous membranes. Onset of action within 1 minute, with duration up to 2 hours, depending on dose and concentration used. Slowly detoxified by liver. Excreted primarily in urine as metabolites and some unchanged drug.

CONTRAINDICATIONS AND PRECAUTIONS

Systemic or ophthalmic use; sepsis in region of proposed application. Safe use in women of childbearing potential or during pregnancy not established. Cautious use: history of drug sensitivities, history of drug abuse.

ADVERSE REACTIONS

Perforated nasal septum (prolonged application); clouding, pitting, and ulceration of cornea (direct application). Systemic absorption: euphoria, excitement, restlessness, tremors, hyperreflexia, convulsions, chills, fever, nausea, vomiting, abdominal pain, mydriasis, exophthalmos, formication, marked rise of blood pressure, tachycardia, ventricular fibrillation, tachypnea, respiratory failure. Hypersensitivity reactions.

Topical: 1% or 2% solution.

NURSING IMPLICATIONS
Administration of a test dose has been suggested.

When used for anesthesia of throat, cocaine may interfere with pharyngeal stage of swallowing. Give nothing by mouth until sensation returns.

Continued use can result in addiction and tolerance. Classified as Schedule II drug under the Controlled Substances Act.

Cocaine has been abused for its cortical stimulant effect. Addicts take cocaine as snuff ("snow") or by injection mixed with morphine or other opiates ("speedball"). Other names applied by drug abusers: "girl," "student," "C," and "coke."

Preserved in tightly closed, light-resistant containers.

CODEINE, N.F.
(Methylmorphine)
CODEINE PHOSPHATE, U.S.P., B.P.
CODEINE SULFATE, N.F.

Narcotic analgesic, antitussive

ACTIONS AND USES
Phenaenthrene derivative of opium made by methylation of morphine. Similar to morphine in actions, uses, contraindications, precautions, and adverse reactions. Not as potent as morphine and has shorter duration of action; thus produces less severe adverse reactions. In equianalgesic doses parenteral codeine produces similar degree of respiratory depression.

Used for symptomatic relief of mild to moderately severe pain, when relief cannot be obtained by nonnarcotic analgesics, and to suppress nonproductive cough. Commonly used in antitussive mixtures and in combination with aspirin and/or phenacetin for additive analgesic effect.

ABSORPTION AND FATE
Following oral or parenteral administration, onset of action occurs in 5 to 10 minutes and peaks in 3 minutes to 1 hour; duration of action 4 to 6 hours. Metabolized primarily in liver. Excreted chiefly in urine as norcodeine and free and conjugated morphine. Negligible amounts of codeine and metabolites excreted in feces. Crosses placenta and appears in breast milk.

ROUTE AND DOSAGE
Oral, subcutaneous, intramuscular (*analgesic*): **Adults**: 15 to 60 mg 4 times a day. **Children**: 3 mg/kg/day divided into 6 doses. Oral (*antitussive*): **Adults**: 8 to 20 mg every 3 to 4 hours if necessary. **Children**: 1 to 1.5 mg/kg/day divided into 6 doses.

NURSING IMPLICATIONS
Narcotics should not be administered routinely. Patient's individual need for medication should be evaluated before administration.

Record relief of pain and duration of analgesia.

Treatment of cough is directed toward decreasing frequency and intensity of cough without eliminating protective cough reflex.

Excessive nonproductive cough tends to be self-perpetuating because it causes irritation of pharyngeal and tracheal mucosa.

Inform patient that unnecessary cough may be lessened by voluntary re-

straint and by avoiding irritants such as smoking, dust, fumes, and other
air pollutants. Humidification of ambient air may provide some relief.

Locally acting sialagogues, eg, hard candy (sugarless), may help to relieve
cough due to irritation of pharyngeal mucosa.

Adequate hydration (at least 1500 to 1800 ml/day) may help to liquefy
sputum.

Terpin hydrate and codeine, N.F., contains 10 mg of codeine in 5 ml.

Although codeine has less abuse liability than morphine, dependence is a
major unwanted effect.

Classified as a Schedule II drug under the federal Controlled Substances Act.
Combination capsule formulations containing codeine are included under
Schedule III; combination liquid or syrup preparations are classified under
Schedule V.

Preserved in tight, light-resistant containers.

See Morphine Sulfate.

COLCHICINE, U.S.P., B.P.

Gout suppressant

ACTIONS AND USES

Alkaloid of the autumn crocus *Colchicum autumnale* with antimitotic and indirect
antiinflammatory properties. Binds to microtubular protein, thereby arresting
spindle formation in metaphase and interfering with movement of mobile cells.
Selective action in gouty arthritis related to inhibition of leukocyte migration
and phagocytosis in gouty joints. Lactic acid produced by phagocytosis is reduced, and crystal deposition fostered by acid pH is decreased. Colchicine is
nonanalgesic and nonuricosuric. Direct action on bone marrow produces temporary leukopenia replaced by leukocytosis. Tends to increase fecal excretion of
Na, K, fat, nitrogen, and carotene; in large doses may interfere with absorption
of vitamin B.

Used prophylactically for recurrent gouty arthritis and as specific for acute gout,
either as single agent or in combination with a uricosuric such as probenecid or
allopurinol. Colchicine and derivatives have been used investigationally in
treatment of sarcoid arthritis, leukemia, adenocarcinoma, acute calcific tendinitis, familial Mediterranean fever, and mycosis fungoides and in experimental
study of normal and abnormal cell division.

ABSORPTION AND FATE

Following oral administration, absorbed from GI tract and partially metabolized
in liver. Plasma half-life 20 minutes; metabolites and active drug recycled to
intestinal tract via biliary and intestinal secretions. Plasma levels decline 1 to 2
hours after administration, then increase due to recyling. High concentrations
appear in kidney, liver, spleen, and intestinal tract. Drug concentrations in
leukocytes may persist 9 days after single IV dose. Partly deacetylated in liver.
Metabolites and active drug excreted primarily in feces; 10% to 20% (variable)
excreted in urine.

CONTRAINDICATIONS AND PRECAUTIONS

Hypersensitivity; serious GI, renal, hepatic, or cardiac disease; subcutaneous or
intramuscular use. Cautious use: elderly and debilitated patients, early manifestations of GI, renal, or cardiac disease.

ADVERSE REACTIONS

Nausea, vomiting, diarrhea, abdominal pain. With IV extravasation: pain, tissue
necrosis, thrombophlebitis, severe neutropenia. **Overdosage**: severe GI symptoms, steatorrhea, hemorrhagic gastroenteritis, paralytic ileus, burning sensa-

tion (throat, stomach, skin), extensive vascular damage, shock, renal damage (hematuria, oliguria), bladder spasm, hepatomegaly (elevated SGOT and SGPT), marked muscular weakness, ascending CNS paralysis, fever, delirium, convulsions, respiratory depression, bone marrow depression (agranulocytosis, temporary leukopenia followed by leukocytosis, thrombocytopenia, aplastic anemia), peripheral neuritis, alopecia, urticaria, dermatitis, purpura, malabsorption syndrome, hypothyroidism.

ROUTE AND DOSAGE

Oral (*acute gouty attack*): initially 1 to 1.2 mg, followed by 0.5 or 0.6 mg every hour, or 1 to 1.2 mg every 2 hours until pain is relieved or GI symptoms appear. Oral (*prophylaxis*) mild to moderate cases: 0.5 or 0.6 mg 3 or more times weekly; *severe cases*: 0.5 to 1.8 mg daily. Intravenous (*acute gouty attack*): initially 1 to 3 mg; may be followed by 0.5 mg every 6 hours until satisfactory response is obtained or GI symptoms intervene. Intravenous (*prophylaxis*): 0.5 to 1 mg once or twice daily.

NURSING IMPLICATIONS

Baseline and periodic determinations of serum uric acid are advised, as well as complete blood count, including hemoglobin. Normal serum uric acid is approximately 2.1 to 7.8 mg/dl (males), 2.0 to 6.4 mg/dl (females).

Gastric irritation may be reduced if oral colchicine is taken immediately before, with, or after meals.

IV preparation: needle should be discarded after withdrawing solution from vial and replaced with fresh sterile needle for injection procedure to avoid tissue irritation.

Side effects (dose-related) are most likely to occur during the initial course of treatment. A latent period of several hours between drug administration and onset of toxic symptoms is usual.

Early signs of toxicity include weakness, abdominal discomfort, anorexia, nausea, vomiting, and diarrhea, regardless of administration route. Report to physician. Drug is generally discontinued until symptoms subside, then reinstituted.

Monitor intake and output (during acute gouty attack). High fluid intake promotes urate excretion and reduces danger of crystal formation in kidneys and ureters; intake is usually prescribed to maintain urinary output of at least 2000 ml/day.

Since acute gout can be precipitated by even minor surgical procedures, the patient is usually given colchicine 0.6 mg 3 times daily for 3 days before and 3 days after surgery.

To avoid cumulative toxicity, a given course of colchicine therapy for acute gout is generally not repeated within 3 days.

During acute attack, weight-bearing and heat to involved joint should be avoided. Mobilization is permitted when joint is no longer painful. Physical therapy and self-help devices may be indicated for patients with residual disability.

Gout commonly affects the great toe, the instep, the ankle, and the knee. However, wrist, finger, or elbow may be affected with recurrent attacks.

Therapeutic response: articular pain and swelling generally subside within 8 to 12 hours and usually disappear in 24 to 72 hours.

Patients taking colchicine at home should be advised to withhold drug and report to the physician the onset of GI symptoms or signs of bone marrow depression (sore throat, bleeding gums, sore mouth, fever, fatigue, malaise).

Long-term dietary management for patients with gout includes gradual weight reduction for obese patients (no more than 2 to 2½ pounds/week). Sudden weight loss can precipitate gouty attack. Physician may prescribe a diet high in carbohydrate, with moderate protein and low fat. Some advise increased intake of alkaline ash foods (most fruits and vegetables, with the exceptions of corn, lentils, plums, prunes, cranberries).

During an acute gouty attack a purine-restricted diet is prescribed by some physicians as a supplement to drug therapy. Others merely advise patients to omit organ meats such as liver and kidney. A strict low-purine diet is unpleasant for most patients since it contains almost no meat; it is seldom prescribed today. Foods high in purine content include wild game, organ meats, goose, anchovies, herring, sardines, mackerel, scallops, broth, meat extracts, gravy. Foods containing moderate amounts of purines include other meats, fish, seafood, fowl, asparagus, spinach, peas, and dried legumes.

In addition to diet prescription, a teaching plan for patients with chronic gout should include the following points: nature and volume of fluid intake; how to test urine pH with nitrazine paper (marked urinary acidity tends to occur during acute gout); importance of early recognition of prodromal symptoms to abort or reduce severity of acute attack (mood changes, diuresis, local pruritus or discomfort in the to-be-affected joint); importance of keeping drug at hand at all times; prescribed regimen to be initiated when prodromal symptoms appear. Confer with physician for specific guidelines.

Fermented beverages such as beer, ale, and wine may precipitate gouty attack and therefore should be avoided. The physician may allow distilled alcoholic beverages in moderation; apparently they have little influence on the gouty process.

Colchicine is available in combination with probenecid, eg, Colbenemid, Robenecid with colchicine.

Preserved in tight, light-resistant containers.

LABORATORY TEST INTERFERENCES: Possible interference with urinary steroid (17-OHCS) determinations when done by modifications of Reddy Jenkins-Thorn procedure.

COLISTIMETHATE SODIUM, U.S.P.
(COLY-MYCIN M)

Antibacterial

ACTIONS AND USES

Polymyxin antibiotic, colistin derivative with neuromuscular blocking action. Similar to polymycin B in structure and actions. Antibacterial activity and overall toxicity are less, but nephrotoxic potential is almost identical with that of polymycin B (qv). Complete cross-resistance and cross-sensitivity to polymycin B reported.

Used primarily in treatment of acute and chronic urinary tract infections caused by susceptible strains of *Pseudomonas aeruginosa* and other Gram-negative organisms resistant to other antibiotics.

ABSORPTION AND FATE

Peak plasma concentrations within 1 to 2 hours following IM injection; detectable for 8 to 12 hours. Peak serum levels following IV dose occur within 10 minutes; they are higher, but they decline more rapidly. Serum half-life 2 to 3 hours. No distribution to cerebrospinal fluid, even when meninges are inflamed. About 66% to 75% of dose is excreted in urine within 24 hours, primarily as active metabolite. Crosses placenta.

Hypersensitivity to colistin antibiotics. Safe use in pregnancy not established. Cautious use: impaired renal function, myasthenia gravis, concomitant use of drugs that potentiate neuromuscular blocking effect (aminoglycoside antibiotics, colistins, anticholinesterases, curariform muscle relaxants, ether, sodium citrate), nephrotoxic and ototoxic drugs.

ADVERSE REACTIONS

Respiratory arrest following IM injection. **Neurotoxicity**: circumoral, lingual, and peripheral paresthesias and numbness; visual and speech disturbances, impaired hearing, ataxia, dizziness, vertigo, neuromuscular blockade (generalized muscle weakness, dyspnea, respiratory depression or paralysis). **Hypersensitivity**: drug fever, pruritus, urticaria, dermatoses. **Nephrotoxicity**: albuminuria, cylinduria, azotemia. Others: GI disturbances, pain at IM site, agranulocytosis, leukopenia, superinfections.

ROUTE AND DOSAGE

Intramuscular, intravenous: **Adults and children**: 1.5 to 5 mg/kg body weight daily divided into 2 to 4 doses. Maximum daily dose should not exceed 5 mg/kg body weight in patients with normal renal function. Lower doses in patients with impaired renal functions.

NURSING IMPLICATIONS

Respiratory arrest has been reported following IM administration. Resuscitative equipment, oxygen, and IV calcium chloride should be immediately available. Report promptly restlessness or dyspnea.

IM injection should be made deep into upper outer quadrant of buttock. Patient may complain of pain at injection site. Rotate sites.

Culture and sensitivity tests are essential to determine susceptibility of causative organisms.

Baseline renal function tests should be performed prior to therapy; frequent monitoring of renal function and serum drug levels is advisable during therapy. Impaired renal function increases the possibility of apnea and neuromuscular blockade.

Monitor intake and output. Decrease in urine output or change in intake–output ratio, and rising BUN, serum creatinine, and serum drug levels (without dosage increase) are indications of renal toxicity. If they occur, withhold drug and report to physician. (Normal BUN: 8 to 18 mg/dl serum creatinine: 0.6 to 1.2 mg/dl.)

Be alert to changes in speech and hearing, visual changes, drowsiness, dizziness, and paresthesias and report them to the physician. Symptoms may be alleviated by reduction of dosage. Supervision of ambulation may be indicated.

Transient paresthesias usually respond to reduction in dosage. Report promptly.

Because of the possibility of transient neurologic disturbances, caution the ambulatory patient to avoid operating vehicles or other activities requiring mental alertness and coordination while on drug therapy.

IV infusion rate is prescribed by physician. (Rate of 5 to 6 mg/hour is recommended for patients with normal renal function.)

Infusion solution should be freshly prepared and used within 24 hours.

Store unopened vials at room temperature. Reconstituted solution may be stored in refrigerator or at room temperature; discard within 7 days.

Postoperative patients who have received curariform muscle relaxants, ether, or sodium citrate should be closely monitored for signs of neuromuscular blockade (delayed recovery, muscle weakness, depressed respiration).

Also see Polymyxin B Sulfate.

COLISTIN SULFATE, N.F.
(COLY-MYCIN S)

Antibacterial

ACTIONS AND USES
  Polymyxin antibiotic derived from *Bacillus polymyxa* var. *colistinus.* Bactericidal against most Gram-negative enteric pathogens especially *E. coli* and *Shigella* (but not *Proteus*).
  Used in treatment of diarrhea in infants and children, caused by susceptible organisms. Available in fixed combination with hydrocortisone and neomycin (Coly-Mycin S Otic) for treatment of superficial infections of auditory canal.
ABSORPTION AND FATE
  May be slightly absorbed from GI tract (degree of absorption in infants is unpredictable).
CONTRAINDICATIONS AND PRECAUTIONS
  Hypersensitivity to colistin derivatives. See Colistimethate Sodium.
ADVERSE REACTIONS
  Not reported within recommended dosage range, but potential as for colistimethate sodium (qv).
ROUTE AND DOSAGE
  Oral: 5 to 15 mg/kg/day in 3 divided doses.

NURSING IMPLICATIONS
Renal function should be assessed prior to initiation of therapy.
To prepare oral suspension: reconstitute with 37 ml of distilled water. Add one-half of the diluent, replace cap, and shake vigorously. Then add remaining diluent and repeat shaking.
Following reconstitution, solution is stable for 2 weeks when kept in a cool place. Unopened bottles may be stored at controlled room temperature 59 to 86 F (15 to 30 C).
See Colistimethate Sodium.

CORTICOTROPIN INJECTION, U.S.P.
(ACTH, ACTHAR)
REPOSITORY CORTICOTROPIN INJECTION, U.S.P., B.P.
(ACTH GEL, CORTICOTROPIN GEL, CORTIGEL, CORTROPHIN GEL, DEPO-ACTH, H.P. ACTHAR GEL)
STERILE CORTICOTROPIN ZINC HYDROXIDE SUSPENSION, U.S.P., B.P.
(CORTROPHIN ZINC)

Adrenocorticotropic hormone, glucocorticoid

ACTIONS AND USES
  Polypeptide (39 amino acids in molecule) derived from anterior pituitary of certain domesticated animals. Stimulates functioning adrenal gland to secrete all of its hormones, including cortisone and cortisol (hydrocortisone). Therapeutic effects appear more rapidly than do those of cortisone (qv). Decreases further release of corticotropin by inhibiting secretion of corticotropin releasing factor. Used for diagnostic test of adrenocortical function (Thorn ACTH test), for

treatment of panhypopituitarism, as adjunct to colchicine treatment of acute gouty arthritis, and to control idiopathic hypoglycemia. May be used to stimulate the functioning adrenal cortex to produce and secrete adrenocortical hormones; however, corticosteroid therapy is considered the treatment of choice.

ABSORPTION AND FATE

Rapid utilization (within 6 hours) following injection; half-life less than 20 minutes (the repository preparation activity persists 18 to 24 hours). Binds to plasma proteins and concentrates in several tissues, including adrenal cortex, kidneys, and placenta; some appears in urine.

CONTRAINDICATIONS AND PRECAUTIONS

Sensitivity to proteins of porcine origin; IV use except for diagnostic testing. Also see Hydrocortisone.

ADVERSE REACTIONS

Hypersensitivity. See Hydrocortisone.

ROUTE AND DOSAGE

Corticotropin injection: 20 units 4 times daily, subcutaneous or IM. *For diagnostic purposes*, given IV: 10 to 25 units dissolved in 500 ml of 5% dextrose injection. Repository corticotropin injection: 40 to 80 units every 24 to 72 hours, subcutaneous or IM. Corticotropin zinc hydroxide: 10 to 160 units once or twice daily, given IM only.

NURSING IMPLICATIONS

Skin testing is recommended prior to treatment in patients with suspected sensitivity to proteins of porcine origin.

Reconstitute corticotropin injection at time of use by dissolving in sterile water for injection or NaCl injection.

Refrigerate reconstituted solution. Discard unused portion after 24 hours.

Repository forms of corticotropin should not be given IV.

The zinc preparation is also a repository form and is intended for IM use only. Inject deep into gluteal muscle.

Observe for and report immediately the onset of psychic manifestations: euphoria, insomnia, mood swings, depression, personality changes, frank psychosis.

For the Thorn ACTH test, corticotropin injection labeled specifically for IV use is given by IV drip over an 8-hour period. Best results are obtained when test is done on 2 successive days. Plasma cortisol or urinary 17-hydroxycorticosteroids levels are determined; elevated values indicate a functional adrenal cortex and pituitary or hypothalamic dysfunction. In primary adrenocortical insufficiency, no increase in adrenal steroids occurs.

Normal plasma cortisol: 8 AM to 10 AM: 5 to 25 μg/dl. Normal 17-OH (males): 5.5 to 14.5 mg/24 hours; (females): 4.9 to 12.9 mg/24 hours. After corticotropin injection, the normal response is a two- to fourfold response.

A low-sodium, high-potassium, high-protein diet is effective in minimizing the edema caused by overstimulation of the adrenal cortex by corticotropin. Facilitate information-exchange conferences related to patient's diet–drug therapies with nutritionist, physician, patient, and responsible family member.

Administration of the hormone at high dosage levels should be tapered rather than suddenly withdrawn. A 2- to 5-day period of adrenal cortical hypofunction follows discontinuation of corticotropin.

Also see Hydrocortisone.

CORTISONE ACETATE, U.S.P., B.P.
(CORTOGEN ACETATE, CORTONE ACETATE, Kendall's Compound E)

Adrenocortical steroid, glucocorticoid

ACTIONS AND USES

Short-acting synthetic steroid with prominent glucocorticoid actions and, in high doses, mineralocorticoid properties. Therapeutic activity depends on in vivo conversion to hydrocortisone (qv), with which it shares uses, absorption, fate, contraindications, and adverse reactions.

ROUTE AND DOSAGE

Highly individualized. **Adults**: Oral, intramuscular: initially 100 to 300 mg daily; dose reduced by periodic decrements of 10 to 12.5 mg daily to lowest effective dose. Topical: suspension, 0.5% to 2.5%; ointment, 1.5%. **Children**: Oral: 0.7 mg/kg/24 hours; intramuscular: one-third to one-half oral dose.

NURSING IMPLICATIONS

A mineralocorticoid and salt (NaCl) are usually given with cortisone as treatment of Addison's disease.

Opthalmic ointment is particularly useful when an eye pad is required or for appilcation at night as adjunctive treatment with daytime ophthalmic suspension.

See Hydrocortisone.

COSYNTROPIN
(CORTROSYN)

Adrenocorticotropic hormone

ACTIONS AND USES

Synthetic polypeptide; structure is identical to that of ACTH in the first 24 of the 39 amino acids in naturally occurring ACTH. Exhibits full adrenocortical stimulation activity and less severe antigenic or allergic reactions than corticotropin.

Used as an aid in diagnosis of adrenocortical insufficiency. Has been used in treatment of long-term chronic inflammatory and degenerative disorders.

ABSORPTION AND FATE

Following IV administration to normal individual, plasma cortisol levels begin to rise within 5 minutes; they double in 15 to 30 minutes and reach a maximum in about 1 hour. Plasma levels remain elevated at least 4 hours after injection. Biologic half-life less than 30 minutes. Metabolic fate unknown.

CONTRAINDICATIONS AND PRECAUTIONS

Known hypersensitivity to cosyntropin; preexisting allergic diseases; hydrocortisone on day of testing.

ADVERSE REACTIONS

Hypersensitivity, including pruritus and flushing.

ROUTE AND DOSAGE

Intramuscular, intravenous injection or infusion: dosage range is 0.125 to 0.75 mg. Highly individualized.

NURSING IMPLICATIONS

Reconstituted with 0.9% sodium chloride injection. Remains stable 48 hours if refrigerated. Infusion solutions should be used within 12 hours if stored at room temperature.

Cosyntropin test of adrenocortical function: baseline plasma cortisol level is determined before test (normal: 8 AM to 10 AM: 5 to 25 μg/dl; 4 PM to 6 PM: 2 to 18 μg/dl.) and repeated 30 to 60 minutes after injection of 0.25 mg cosyntropin. Normal response is approximately double that of basal cortisol level; if a subnormal value is obtained, the patient is assumed to have adrenocortical insufficiency. To distinguish between adrenal and pituitary dysfunction, cosyntropin (0.25 mg) may be infused over a 4- to 8-hour period, with plasma cortisol level (adrenal response) being measured at end of infusion.

Patient should be closely observed for evidence of allergic response.

CROMOLYN SODIUM
(AARANE, DSCG, INTAL)
SODIUM CROMOGLYCATE, B.P.

Antiasthmatic (prophylactic)

ACTIONS AND USES

Synthetic drug with local effect on pulmonary mast cells. Inhibits release of histamine and slow-reacting substance of anaphylaxis (SRS-A) from sensitized mast cells after antigen–antibody union has taken place. Has no direct bronchodilator, antihistaminic, or antiinflammatory properties.

Used prophylactically as adjunct in management of severe perennial bronchial asthma. Of no value in acute asthmatic attack, especially status asthmaticus.

ABSORPTION AND FATE

Peak plasma concentrations within 15 minutes, half-life, 80 minutes. Following inhalation, about 8% of dose reaching lungs is readily absorbed into systemic circulation. Excreted unchanged in bile and urine in approximately equal amounts. Elimination half-life 80 minutes. Small amounts exhaled; portions swallowed are excreted in feces.

CONTRAINDICATIONS AND PRECAUTIONS

Previous hypersensitivity to cromolyn; children younger than 5 years of age. Safe use during pregnancy not established. Cautious use: renal or hepatic dysfunction, long-term use.

ADVERSE REACTIONS

Irritated throat and trachea, cough, hoarseness, nasal congestion, bronchospasm, nausea. Allergic reactions: contact dermatitis, erythema, urticaria, angioedema, eosinophilic pneumonia, polymyositis, anaphylaxis (rare). Nephrotoxicity (systemic absorption).

ROUTE AND DOSAGE

Inhalation: **Adults and children** *5 years or older*: contents of one capsule inhaled 4 times daily at regular intervals, using special accompanying inhaler. Each capsule (for inhalation only) contains 20 mg cromolyn in lactose powder vehicle.

NURSING IMPLICATIONS

Pulmonary function test recommended prior to initiation of therapy. (Candidates for therapy must have a significant bronchodilator-reversible component to their airway obstruction.)

Patient should receive detailed instructions for loading the inhaler and administering preparation (see manufacturer's instructions). Therapeutic effect is dependent on proper scheduling and use of inhaler.

Advise patient to clear as much mucus as possible before using inhaler.

Caution patient not to exhale into inhaler, because moisture from breath will interfere with its proper operation. Also inform patient that capsule is intended for inhalation only and is ineffective if swallowed.

Exacerbation of asthmatic symptoms may occur in patients receiving cromolyn during corticosteroid withdrawal. The same is true of patients on maintenance steroid therapy when cromolyn is withdrawn. Close supervision is required.

Instruct patient to pay careful attention to general health and to protect himself against colds and flu.

Some physicians advise against sudden discontinuation of cromolyn and recommend reducing the dosage gradually over period of 1 week.

Drug should be discontinued if allergic reactions appear.

Therapeutic effects are generally noted after 2 to 4 weeks of therapy: reduced number of asthmatic attacks; decreased cough, sputum, wheezing, and breathlessness; decreased requirement for concomitant drug therapy.

Protect cromolyn from moisture and heat.

CROTAMITON, N.F., B.P.
(EURAX)

Antipruritic, scabicide

ACTIONS AND USES

Used for eradication of scabies *(Sarcoptes scabiei)* and for symptomatic treatment of pruritus.

CONTRAINDICATIONS AND PRECAUTIONS

Should not be applied to acutely inflamed skin, raw or weeping surfaces, eyes, or mouth or used by patients with history of previous sensitivity to crotamiton.

ADVERSE REACTIONS

Skin irritation, erythema, sensation of warmth, allergic sensitization.

ROUTE AND DOSAGE

Topical: 10% in vanishing cream base.

NURSING IMPLICATIONS

Preliminary bathing of skin is not essential, but if it is done, the skin must be thoroughly dry before applying medication.

Treatment for scabies: Massage medication into skin on all parts of body from chin downward, paying particular attention to folds and creases. A second application 24 hours later is advised. Clothing and bedding should be changed the next morning. Cleansing bath should follow 48 hours after last application.

Treatment for pruritus: Massage medication gently into affected areas until it is completely absorbed. Repeat as needed (usually effective for 6 to 10 hours).

Instruct the patient to discontinue medication and report to his physician if irritation or sensitization develops.

See Gamma Benzene Hexachloride for additional points on scabies management.

(BERUBIGEN, BETALIN 12, B-TWELVE, COBEX, CRYSTIMIN, DODEX, KAYBOVITE, PERNAVIT, REDISOL, RUBESOL, RUBRAMIN PC, SYTOBEX, Vitamin B_{12}, VI-TWEL)

Hematopoietic vitamin

ACTIONS AND USES

Vitamin B_{12} is a cobalt-containing substance produced by *Streptomyces griseus* (chief source) or obtained from liver. Essential for normal growth, cell reproduction, nucleoprotein and myelin synthesis, and believed to be involved in protein and carbohydrate metabolism. Also acts as coenzyme in various biologic reactions. Stimulates reticulocytes and together with folic acid is involved in formation of oxyribonucleotides from ribonucleotides.

Used in treatment of pernicious anemia and other macrocytic and megaloblastic anemias caused by malabsorption of vitamin B_{12} (eg, tropical and nontropical sprue; GI pathology, dysfunction, or surgery; fish tapeworm). Used in vitamin B_{12} deficiency caused by increased physiologic requirements or inadequate dietary intake; used in vitamin B_{12} absorption (Schilling) test.

ABSORPTION AND FATE

Intestinal absorption requires presence of gastric intrinsic factor (lacking in pernicious anemia), which binds vitamin B_{12} and protects it from GI microorganisms. Absorbed from ileum in presence of calcium and bound to plasma proteins. With large oral doses, some absorption by diffusion. Converted in tissues to active coenzymes methylcobalamin and deoxyadenosylcobalamin. Small injected doses almost completely retained; urinary loss increases with doses exceeding 50 μg. Negligible amounts excreted via bile and feces. Widely distributed in most tissues. Principal storage site is in liver; also stored in kidneys and adrenals. Crosses placenta.

CONTRAINDICATIONS AND PRECAUTIONS

History of sensitivity to vitamin B_{12} or cobalamins, or cobalt; hereditary optic nerve atrophy, indiscriminate use in folic acid deficiency.

ADVERSE REACTIONS

Mild transient diarrhea, itching, rash, flushing, feeling of swelling of body, peripheral vascular thrombosis, pulmonary edema, congestive heart failure, hypokalemia, sudden death. Severe optic nerve atrophy (in patients with Leber's disease), anaphylactic shock. Also reported: unmasking of polycythemia vera with correction of vitamin B_{12} deficiency.

ROUTE AND DOSAGE

Vitamin B_{12} deficiency: Intramuscular, deep subcutaneous: **Adults**: 30 μg daily for 5 to 10 days; maintenance: 100 to 200 μg monthly. **Children**: 100 μg doses to total of 1 to 5 mg over 2 or more weeks; maintenance: 60 μg/month. *Nutritional supplement*: Oral: 1 to 25 μg/day. *Schilling test*: 1000-μg flushing dose IM.

NURSING IMPLICATIONS

Prior to initiation of therapy, reticulocyte plasma count and vitamin B_{12} and folic acid levels should be determined; these should be repeated between 5 and 7 days after start of therapy. In some cases bone marrow studies, tests for gastric free acid, and GI series will be performed.

A careful history of previous sensitivities should be obtained. An intradermal test dose is recommended in patients suspected of being sensitive to cyanocobalamin.

Potassium levels should be monitored during the first 48 hours in patients with Addisonian pernicious anemia or megaloblastic anemia, with supplementation if necessary. Conversion to normal erythropoiesis increases erythrocyte potassium requirement and can result in fatal hypokalemia in these patients.

Monitor vital sign is patients receiving parenteral cyanocobalamin, and be alert to symptoms of pulmonary edema which generally occur early in therapy.

A complete diet history should be taken for all patients receiving cyanocobalamin to identify and correct poor dietary habits. Single deficiency of one vitamin is rare; generally patients will have multiple vitamin deficiency. Collaborate with physician, dietitian, patient, and responsible family member in planning for diet teaching.

The Schilling test for pernicious anemia measures vitamin B_{12} absorption: Patient fasts 12 hours and drinks no water 4 hours before test. Radioactive $^{57}Co-B_{12}$ (0.5 to 1.0 μg) is given by mouth; 2 hours later urine sample is collected and discarded, and an IM flushing dose (1000 μg) of nonradioactive B_{12} is administered. Urine is accurately collected for a 24-hour period, and radioactivity is measured. Impaired absorption: less than 5% urinary excretion (normal is 7% to 30%).

Parenteral therapy is the preferred treatment for patients with pernicious anemia, since oral administration is unreliable. In the presence of neurologic complications, prolonged inadequate oral therapy may lead to permanent spinal cord damage. However, oral therapy may be used when the condition is mild and is without neurologic signs, or in rare patients who are sensitive to the parenteral form or who refuse it.

Oral preparations mixed with fruit juices should be administered promptly; ascorbic acid affects the stability of vitamin B_{12}.

Bowel regularity is essential for consistent absorption of oral preparations.

Administration of oral vitamin B_{12} with meals increases its absorption presumably by stimulating production of intrinsic factor.

Therapeutic response to drug therapy is usually dramatic, occurring within 48 hours. Effectiveness is measured by laboratory values and improvement of manifestations of vitamin B_{12} deficiency: fatigue, GI symptoms, glossitis, distaste for meat, dyspnea on exertion, palpitation, nervous system degeneration (paresthesias, loss of vibratory and position sense and deep reflexes, incoordination), mental aberrations, anosmia, visual disturbances.

Characteristically, reticulocyte concentration rises in 3 to 4 days, peaks in 5 to 8 days, and then gradually declines as erythrocyte count and hemoglobin rise to normal levels (in 4 to 6 weeks).

Instruct patient to notify physician if an intercurrent disease or infection occurs. Increase in cyanocobalamin dosage may be required.

Patients with mild peripheral neurologic defects may respond to concomitant physical therapy. Usually, demonstrable neurologic damage is considered irreversible if there is no improvement after 1 to 1½ years of adequate therapy. Severe vitamin B_{12} deficiency that is allowed to progress 3 months or longer may cause permanent degenerative lesions of spinal cord; this is generally observed when folic acid is used as the sole hematopoietic agent.

It is imperative for the patient with pernicious anemia to understand that he must continue parenteral drug therapy throughout his life to prevent irreversible neurologic damage.

Follow-up with oral therapeutic multivitamin preparation (containing 15 μg of vitamin B_{12}) daily for 1 month is recommended for patients with normal intestinal absorption.

The minimum effective daily requirement of vitamin B_{12} for adults is 0.1 μg. The RDA for adults and children over 11 years is 3 μg; during pregnancy and lactation 4 μg; infants 0.3 μg. The average diet in most western countries supplies 5 to 30 μg.

Dietary deficiency of vitamin B_{12} alone is rare; however, it has been observed in vegetarians and their breast-fed infants. Rich food sources: organ

meats, clams, oysters; good sources: egg yolk, crabs, salmon, sardines, muscle meat, milk and dairy products.
Preserved in light-resistant containers.

LABORATORY TEST INTERFERENCES: Most antibiotics, methotrexate, and pyrimethamine may produce invalid diagnostic blood assays for **folic acid** and **vitamin B$_{12}$**.

DRUG INTERACTIONS: Absorption of oral vitamin B$_{12}$ may be decreased by **alcohol** (excessive intake), **aminosalicylic acid, anticonvulsants, ascorbic acid** (large doses ingested within 1 hour of vitamin B$_{12}$), **cobalt irradiation** of small bowel, **colchicine, neomycin. Chloramphenicol** interferes with erythrocyte maturation and thus may cause poor therapeutic response to vitamin B$_{12}$ therapy. Vitamin B$_{12}$ absorption is increased by **prednisone**.

CYCLANDELATE
(CYCLOSPASMOL)

Vasodilator

ACTIONS AND USES
Produces vasodilation by exerting papaverinelike relaxation of peripheral vascular smooth muscle by direct action. Principle effect is on smooth muscle tissue. Has no significant adrenergic stimulating or blocking actions.
Used as adjunctive therapy in arteriosclerosis obliterans, intermittent claudication, thrombophlebitis, nocturnal leg cramps, and Raynaud's phenomenon and in selected cases of ischemic cerebral vascular disease.
ABSORPTION AND FATE
Readily absorbed from GI tract. Effects appear in 15 minutes, with maximum response in about 1 to 1½ hours. Duration of action approximately 3 to 4 hours.
CONTRAINDICATIONS AND PRECAUTIONS
Known hypersensitivity to cyclandelate. Safe use during pregnancy or in women of childbearing potential not established. Extreme caution in obliterative coronary artery disease or cerebral vascular disease, bleeding tendencies, active bleeding, glaucoma.
ADVERSE REACTIONS
Reported to be relatively nontoxic. Infrequent: dizziness, flushing, sweating, tingling, tachycardia, weakness, headache, GI disturbances (heartburn, eructation, pain).
ROUTE AND DOSAGE
Oral: initially 200 to 400 mg 4 times daily, before meals and at bedtime. Once clinical response has occurred, dosage may be reduced by 200 mg decrements to maintenance dosage of 400 to 800 mg/day in 2 to 4 divided doses.

NURSING IMPLICATIONS
GI distress may be relieved by taking medication with meals or an antacid (if prescribed).
Some patients experience flushing, headaches, and tachycardia during the first week of therapy, requiring dosage reduction.
Patient should be informed that improvement usually occurs gradually and that prolonged therapy may be necessary.
Therapeutic effect on peripheral circulation may be manifested by a slight

rise in skin temperature, by the ability to walk longer distances without discomfort, and by lessened pain.

Meticulous hygiene is an important adjunct in treatment of peripheral vascular problems.

CYCLIZINE HYDROCHLORIDE, U.S.P., B.P.
(MAREZINE HYDROCHLORIDE)
CYCLIZINE LACTATE
(MAREZINE LACTATE)

Antihistamine, antiemetic

ACTIONS AND USES

Piperazine derivative of diphenylmethane structurally and pharmacologically related to cyclizine compounds (eg, buclizine, hydroxyzine). In common with these agents, it exhibits CNS depression and anticholinergic, antispasmodic, local anesthetic, and antihistaminic activity. Has prominent depressant action on labyrinthine excitability and on conduction in vestibular-cerebellar pathways, thus producing marked antimotion and antiemetic effect.

Used chiefly for prevention and treatment of motion sickness and postoperative nausea and vomiting.

ABSORPTION AND FATE

Rapid onset of action, with duration of 4 to 6 hours. Metabolic fate unknown.

CONTRAINDICATIONS AND PRECAUTIONS

Pregnancy, women of childbearing potential, nursing mothers, children under 6 years of age. Cautious use: glaucoma, prostatic hypertrophy, obstructive disease of GU or GI tracts, glaucoma.

ADVERSE REACTIONS

Low incidence of drowsiness, dizziness, dryness of mouth, blurred vision, fatigue, urticaria, drug rash. Usually with high doses: nausea, vomiting, anorexia, tinnitus, palpitation, tachycardia, hypotension, constipation, urinary problems, hyperexcitability, hallucinations, cholestatic jaundice..

ROUTE AND DOSAGE

Oral: 50 mg every 4 to 6 hours; not to exceed 200 mg daily. Rectal suppository: 100 mg every 4 to 6 hours. Intramuscular: 50 mg every 4 to 6 hours. **Children** *6 to 10 years*: One-half the adult dose.

NURSING IMPLICATIONS

Forewarn the patient about the side effects of drowsiness and dizziness and advise him not to drive a car or engage in other hazardous activities until his reaction to the drug is known.

Caution the patient that the sedative action may be additive to that of alcohol, barbiturates, and narcotic analgesic and other CNS depressants.

Recommended dosage when used to prevent motion sickness: 1 tablet (50 mg) ½ hour before anticipated departure, repeated in 4 to 6 hours if required. No more than 4 tablets should be taken in 1 day. For succeeding days of travel, 50 mg 3 or 4 times daily before meals. Continued administration after first 2 or 3 days of extended travel may be unnecessary.

For prophylaxis of postoperative nausea and vomiting, cyclizine is usually prescribed with preoperative medication or is administered 20 to 30 minutes before expected termination of surgery.

Preserved in tight, light-resistant containers.

DRUG INTERACTIONS: Cyclizine may have additive effects with **alcohol, barbituates, CNS depressants** (ie, hypnotics, sedatives, tranquilizers. and antianxiety agents).

CYCLOPHOSPHAMIDE, U.S.P., B.P.
(CTX, CYTOXAN)

Antineoplastic, immunosuppressive

ACTIONS AND USES

Nitrogen mustard alkylating agent structurally related to mechlorethamine. Cytotoxicity depends on its hepatic conversion to an active nitrogen mustard that causes chromosomal cross-linking of DNA strands, thereby blocking synthesis of DNA, RNA, and protein. Has a pronounced immunosuppressant action and it may lower blood sugar concentrations. Advantages over other nitrogen mustards include oral effectiveness and the possibility of giving fractional doses over long periods of time.

Use is generally confined to nonterminal stages of neoplastic disease including lymphosarcomas and bronchogenic carcinoma. Additionally, used in treatment of acute lymphoblastic leukemia of childhood, multiple myeloma, and neuroblastoma; one member of the BACOP, CHOP, CMFOP, COMA, COP combination chemotherapeutic regimens. Investigative uses include control of organ rejection after transplantation and use in nonneoplastic disorders associated with altered immune reactivity.

ABSORPTION AND FATE

Completely absorbed from GI tract. Disappears rapidly from plasma, with peak concentration 1 hour after oral dose. Activated intracellularly. Eliminated from body very slowly. Excretion in urine as metabolites, and up to 14% unchanged drug. Excreted in breast milk.

CONTRAINDICATIONS AND PRECAUTIONS

Pregnancy, lactation, men and women in childbearing years, serious infections, myelosuppression. Cautious use: history of treatment by x-ray or other cytotoxic agents, hepatic and renal dysfunction, diabetes mellitus, recent history of steroid therapy.

ADVERSE REACTIONS

Myelosuppression: leukopenia, thrombocytopenia, anemia, thrombophlebitis, pulmonary emboli. **Dermatologic**: alopecia, transverse ridging and darkening of nails and skin, nonspecific dermatitis. **GI**: nausea, vomiting, mucositis, anorexia, hepatotoxicity, weight loss, diarrhea. **Genitourinary**: sterile hemorrhagic and nonhemorrhagic cystitis, bladder fibrosis, nephrotoxicity, gonadal suppression (amenorrhea, azoospermia, possibly irreversible). **Pulmonary**: interstitial pulmonary fibrosis. Other: transient dizziness, fatigue, blurred vision, confusion, fever, syndrome of inappropriate antidiuretic hormone secretion (SIADH), dilutional hyponatremia with weight gain, severe hyperkalemia, hypoglycemia.

ROUTE AND DOSAGE

Intravenous: initially 2 to 3 mg/kg body weight daily for at least 6 days. Drug is then withdrawn until maximum leukopenia develops (to 1500/mm^3). When count begins to increase, treatment at same dosage is resumed. Ordinarily, leukopenia of 3000/mm^3 to 5000/mm^3 can be maintained without complication. Oral: 50 to 200 mg/day. Occasionally, oral and IV routes are used simultaneously.

NURSING IMPLICATIONS

Following reconstitution allow solution to stand until clear before administration; given within 3 to 4 hours after preparation. Avoid inhaling or exposing skin to drug particles during preparation.

Reconstituted solution should be used within 24 hours if stored at room temperature or within 6 days if stored under refrigeration.

Usually, extravasation does not cause local irritation, unlike other nitrogen mustards.

Administer oral drug on empty stomach. Nausea and vomiting are usually controlled by antiemetic medication given before this drug.

Oral liquid preparations should be stored under refrigeration and used within 14 days.

Total WBC and thrombocyte counts are determined at least twice a week (when on maintenance regimen). Periodic determinations of liver and kidney functions, serum electrolytes, and blood sugar should be made.

Thrombocytopenia is rare, but if thrombocyte counts are 100,000/mm³ or lower, watch for signs of abnormal bleeding. If count continues to descend or if symptoms are manifest, drug will be discontinued.

Marked leukopenia is the most serious side effect. Nadir usually occurs 2 days after first dose, but may be as late as 1 month after series of several daily doses. Leukopenia usually reverses 7 to 14 days after therapy is discontinued. Has been fatal.

Check leukocyte count values. During severe leukopenic period, protect the patient from infection and trauma and from visitors and medical personnel who have colds or other infections.

The immunosuppressive property of cyclophosphamide makes the patient particularly susceptible to varicella-zoster infections (chicken pox, herpes zoster).

Anorexia should not be ignored. Plan with patient, dietitian, and physician a nutritional regimen, especially for leukopenic period.

Report any sign of overgrowth with opportunistic organisms (black furry tongue, foul-smelling stools). Drug will be discontinued with corroboration of infections.

Untreated stomatitis is not only uncomfortable, it also interferes with drinking and eating. See Mechlorethamine for nursing implications.

Diarrhea may signal onset of hyperkalemia, particularly if accompanied by colic and skeletal muscle weakness. These symptoms warrant prompt reporting to physician.

Promptly report hematuria or dysuria. Drug schedule is usually interrupted and fluids are forced.

Intake–output ratio should be monitored carefully. Since drug is a chemical irritant, fluid intake is generally increased to prevent renal irritation. Paradoxically, in patients with SIADH (a rare side effect) fluid intake may be restricted. Consult physician.

When fluid intake is to be pushed, encourage the patient to start increased intake early in the day to reduce night voiding.

Since patients are usually well hydrated during therapy, watch for symptoms of dilutional hyponatremia (water intoxication): lethargy, confusion, stupor, coma, neuromuscular hyperexcitability with muscular twitching, normal or increased skin turgor and blood pressure, convulsions.

Monitor vital signs. Report fever, dyspnea, and nonproductive cough. Pulmonary toxicity is not usual, but it should be sought at onset to assure appropriate treatment in the already debilitated patient.

Record body weight at least weekly (basis for dose determination). Alert physician to sudden change or slow, steady weight gain or loss over a period of time that appears inconsistent with caloric intake.

Observe and report signs of hepatotoxicity (frothy dark urine, clay-colored stools, jaundice, pruritus). These are most apt to appear in the patient with liver dysfunction prior to institution of cyclophosphamide therapy.

High doses may induce blurred vision and confused orientation. Supervision of ambulation and bedsides may be required, especially in the elderly.

Because of mutagenic potential, adequate means of contraception are desirable during cyclophosphamide therapy.

Alopecia occurs in 20% to 30% of patients on cyclophosphamide therapy. Discuss the possibility with the patient early in therapy. Hair loss may be noted 3 weeks after therapy begins; regrowth (may differ in texture and color) usually starts 5 to 6 weeks after drug is withheld and may occur while patient is on maintenance doses. This side effect, related as it is to sexuality and self-image, requires much understanding. Help the patient to plan for cosmetic substitution if desired.

Amenorrhea may last up to 1 year after cessation of therapy in approximately 50% of women receiving cyclophosphamide (due to lack of follicular maturation).

Consult physician about plans for disclosure of diagnosis, prognosis, and particulars about treatment so that discussions with patient and family are supportive and nonconflicting.

DRUG INTERACTIONS: Concomitant use with **allopurinol** may increase the incidence of bone marrow depression. Enhanced cyclophosphamide toxicity reportedly may result from concomitant **barbiturate** administration. **Corticosteroids** may inhibit microsomal activation of cyclophosphamide; if dosage of corticosteroids is reduced or discontinued, cyclophosphamide may also have to be reduced. **Succinylcholine** is to be administered with caution; cyclophosphamide decreases pseudocholinesterase levels (the latter metabolizes succinylcholine).

CYCLOSERINE, U.S.P., B.P.
(SEROMYCIN)

Antibacterial (tuberculostatic)

ACTIONS AND USES

Broad-spectrum antibiotic derived from strains of *Streptomyces orchidaceus.* Inhibits cell wall synthesis in susceptible strains of Gram-positive and Gram-negative bacteria and in *Mycobacterium tuberculosis.*

Used in conjunction with other tuberculostatic drugs in treatment of active pulmonary and extrapulmonary tuberculosis (including renal disease) when primary agents (streptomycin, isoniazid, aminosalicylic acid) have failed. Also used in treatment of acute urinary infections caused by *Enterobacter* and *Escherichia coli* that are unresponsive to conventional treatment.

ABSORPTION AND FATE

Readily absorbed from GI tract, with peak serum levels in 4 to 8 hours. Concentrations in cerebrospinal and pleural fluid approximately the same as plasma levels. Also diffuses into ascitic fluid, bile, sputum, and lymph tissues. About 50% of drug is eliminated unchanged in urine in 12 hours; 65% recoverable in active form over 72 hours. Crosses placenta and may appear in breast milk.

CONTRAINDICATIONS AND PRECAUTIONS

Hypersensitivity to cycloserine, epilepsy, depression, severe anxiety, history of psychoses, severe renal insufficiency, chronic alcoholism. Safe use during pregnancy and safe pediatric use not established.

Neurotoxicity: drowsiness, anxiety, headache, tremors, myoclonic jerking, convulsions, vertigo, visual disturbances, speech difficulties (dysarthria), loss of memory, confusion, psychoses (possibly with suicidal tendencies), character changes, hyperirritability, aggression, hyperreflexia, paresthesias, paresis, dyskinesias. Allergic dermatitis; elevated serum transaminases (especially patients with preexisting liver disease); occasionally, vitamin B_{12} and/or folic acid deficiency, megaloblastic or sideroblastic anemia.

ROUTE AND DOSAGE

Oral: initially 250 mg twice daily at 12-hour intervals for first 2 weeks. Usual dosage: 500 mg to 1 Gm daily in divided doses, monitored by blood levels. Daily dosage should not exceed 1 Gm.

NURSING IMPLICATIONS

Culture and bacterial susceptibility tests should be done prior to initiation of therapy and periodically thereafter to detect possible bacterial resistance.

Monitoring of drug blood levels, hematologic and liver function, and renal clearance is advised.

Maintenance of drug blood level below 30 μg/ml considerably reduces incidence of neurotoxicity. Possibility of neurotoxicity increases when dose is 500 mg or more, when renal clearance is inadequate, or when patient shows signs suggestive of toxicity. Drug blood levels should be determined at least weekly in these patients.

Neurotoxic effects generally appear within first 2 weeks of therapy and disappear after drug is discontinued. Be alert to early signs of neurotoxicity: drowsiness, confusion, headache, anxiety, tremors, paresthesias, behavior changes.

Drug should be discontinued or dosage reduced if symptoms of neurotoxicity or allergy develop.

Bedsides and supervision of ambulation may be required.

Advise patient to avoid potentially hazardous tasks such as driving until his reaction to cycloserine has been determined.

Caution patient to avoid alcoholic beverages. Ingestion of alcohol increases the risk of convulsive seizures.

Cycloserine overdosage is treated with pyridoxine, 300 mg or more daily, and anticonvulsants for seizure control, and symptomatic and supportive therapy such as gastric lavage, oxygen, artificial respiration, measures for shock, and maintenance of body temperature.

DRUG INTERACTIONS: Concurrent administration of **ethionamide** reportedly potentiates neurotoxic effects of cycloserine.

CYCLOTHIAZIDE, N.F.
(ANHYDRON)

Diuretic, antihypertensive

ACTIONS AND USES

Benzothiadiazine (thiazide) derivative. Similar to chlorothiazide (qv) in actions, uses, contraindications, precautions, and adverse reactions, but is effective in smaller doses and produces more prolonged effects.

Onset of diuretic effect occurs within 6 hours and peaks in 7 to 12 hours; duration 18 to 24 hours. Presumed to be distributed and excreted similarly to other thiazides. See Chlorothiazide.

ROUTE AND DOSAGE

Adults: Oral (*Edema*): initially 1 to 2 mg daily; maintenance 1 to 2 mg on alternate days or 2 or 3 times weekly. (*Hypertension*): 2 mg 1 to 3 times daily. Highly individualized according to patient's requirements and response. **Children**: 0.02 to 0.04 mg/kg/24 hours divided into 2 doses.

NURSING IMPLICATIONS

Preferably given early in the morning in patients with edema so that diuresis occurs predominantly during day to avoid disturbing patient's sleep.

Intake–output ratio and daily weight are important indicators of response to diuretic therapy.

Observe patient for signs of fluid and electrolyte imbalance.

See Chlorothiazide.

CYPROHEPTADINE HYDROCHLORIDE, N.F., B.P. (PERIACTIN)

Antihistaminic, antipruritic

ACTIONS AND USES

Potent antihistaminic. Structurally similar to phenothiazine antihistaminic drugs. Mechanism of action is uncertain. Produces mild central depression and weak peripheral anticholinergic effects and has significant antipruritic, local anesthetic, and antiserotonin activity. Also stimulates appetite, perhaps by activation of hypothalamic appetite-regulating center. Shares uses, contraindications, precautions, and adverse reactions of antihistamines. See Diphenhydramine.

Used for symptomatic relief of various allergic conditions, including hay fever, vasomotor rhinitis, allergic conjunctivitis, pruritus of allergic dermatoses, and to ameliorate drug, blood, and plasma reactions. Also used in treatment of anaphylactoid reactions as adjunct to epinephrine and other standard measures, after acute symptoms have been controlled. Its use as appetite stimulant in children has been questioned.

ABSORPTION AND FATE

Duration of action approximately 4 to 6 hours.

CONTRAINDICATIONS AND PRECAUTIONS

Elderly and debilitated patients, patients predisposed to urinary retention; glaucoma. Also see Diphenhydramine.

ADVERSE REACTIONS

Drowsiness (common), dizziness, faintness, headache, jitteriness, disturbed coordination, dry mouth, nose, and throat, urinary frequency, retention, and difficult urination, skin rash, nausea, epigastric distress, appetite stimulation, weight gain accompanied in children by increased rate of growth. Rarely, CNS stimulation (agitation, confusion, visual hallucinations, ataxia, especially in children), transient decrease in fasting blood sugar level, increased serum amylase level. Also see Diphenhydramine.

ROUTE AND DOSAGE

Adults: Oral: 4 mg 3 or 4 times daily. Therapeutic dose range is 4 to 20 mg/day. Total daily dose should not exceed 0.5 mg/kg. **Children**: approximately 0.25 mg/kg/24 hours divided into 3 or 4 doses. **Children**: *2 to 6 years*: not to exceed 12 mg daily; *7 to 14 years*: not to exceed 16 mg daily.

NURSING IMPLICATIONS

In some patients the sedative effect disappears spontaneously after 3 or 4 days of drug administration.

Warn the patient to avoid any activities requiring mental alertness and physical coordination, such as driving a car, until his reaction to the drug is known.

Patient should know that cyproheptadine may increase and prolong the effects of alcohol, barbiturates, narcotic analgesics, tranquilizers, and other CNS depressants.

See Diphenhydramine Hydrochloride.

CYTARABINE
(ARA-C, CYTOSAR, Cytosine Arabinoside)

Antineoplastic

ACTIONS AND USES

Antimetabolite and pyrimidine analogue. Interferes with DNA synthesis by blocking conversion of cytidine to deoxycytidine; also may be incorporated into RNA molecule. Has strong myelosuppressive and immunosuppressive properties.

Used primarily to induce of remission in acute granulocytic leukemia in adults and secondarily to treat other acute leukemias in adults and children. Also used investigationally in treatment of solid tumors, lymphomas, and Hodgkin's disease with equivocal results. One member of the COAP, COMA combination chemotherapeutic regimens.

ABSORPTION AND FATE

Incompletely absorbed from GI tract. After IV dose, drug is rapidly cleared from blood (5 to 20 minutes). Metabolized in liver and perhaps in kidneys. Crosses blood–brain barrier. Excreted in urine.

CONTRAINDICATIONS AND PRECAUTIONS

Known hypersensitivity to cytarabine, drug-induced myelosuppression, infants, during pregnancy, women of childbearing age. Cautious use: impaired renal or hepatic function, gout, previous therapy with cytotoxic drug or irradiation.

ADVERSE REACTIONS

Hematologic: myelosuppression (reversible): leukopenia, thrombocytopenia, anemia, megaloblastosis, reduced reticulocytes (rare). **GI**: nausea, vomiting, stomatitis, esophagitis, anorexia, diarrhea, abdominal pain, hemorrhage. **Integument**: freckling, rash, keratitis, alopecia (rare), skin ulcerations. Other: weight loss, sore throat, fever, dizziness; cellulitis, thrombophlebitis and pain at injection site; hepatic dysfunction, jaundice, urinary retention, transient hyperuricemia, chest pain, conjunctivitis, neuritis, joint pain, lethargy, confusion.

ROUTE AND DOSAGE

Intravenous (direct): initially 2 mg/kg/day for 10 days; in the absence of remission or toxicity, increased to 4 mg/kg/day and continued to toxicity or remission. Continuous IV infusion: initially 0.5 mg/kg/day increased to 2 mg/kg/day in the absence of toxicity or remission. Highly individualized dose and schedule. Maintenance (subcutaneous): 1 mg/kg body weight at weekly or semiweekly intervals.

NURSING IMPLICATIONS

Store cytarabine in refrigerator until reconstituted. The 100-mg and 500-mg vials are reconstituted with 5 ml and 10 ml, respectively, of bacteriostatic water for injection, containing benzyl alcohol 0.9%. Reconstituted solution may be stored at room temperature no more than 48 hours. Solutions with a slight haze should be discarded.

Toxicity necessitating dosage alterations almost always occurs. Report adverse reactions immediately.

Leukocyte and platelet counts should be evaluated daily during initial therapy. Blood uric acid and hepatic function tests should be performed at regular intervals during therapy.

Monitor blood reports for indicated adaptations of drug and nursing regimens.

When large IV doses are given rapidly, nausea and vomiting of several hours duration may follow.

Noncontinuous dosage schedules may permit the patient to tolerate larger amounts of drug.

Hyperuricemia due to excessive cell destruction may accompany cytarabine therapy. (Normal serum uric acid is 2 to 7 mg/dl). A uricosuric agent such as allopurinol may be prescribed.

To reduce potential for urate stone formation, fluids are forced in excess of 2 liters if possible. Consult physician.

Monitor intake-output ratio and pattern.

During the granulocytic period, development of usual signs of inflammation may be inhibited. Monitor temperature. Be alert to the most subtle signs especially low grade fever and report promptly.

When platelets decrease below 50,000/mm^3 and polymorphonuclear granulocytes are under 1000/mm^3 the drug is discontinued. The blood cell count usually continues to fall for 5 to 7 days after therapy has been interrupted. If indicated, therapy is restarted when definite signs of bone marrow recovery occur.

Equipment and facilities for treatment of myelosuppressive emergencies (hemorrhage, granulocytopenia, and other impaired body defenses) should be at hand at all times.

See Mechlorethamine for the nursing implications of stomatitis.

DACARBAZINE
(DIC, DTIC-DOME, IMIDAZOLE CARBOXAMIDE)

Antineoplastic

ACTIONS AND USES
  Cytotoxic triazine with alkylating properties. Interferes with DNA, RNA, and protein synthesis in rapidly proliferating cells. Has minimal myelosuppressive action.
  Used in treatment of metastatic malignant melanoma. Has been used investigationally in Hodgkin's disease, various sarcomas, and neuroblastoma.
ABSORPTION AND FATE
  Only slightly bound to plasma proteins; plasma half-life about 35 minutes. Probably localizes in liver; 30% to 46% of dose secreted by renal tubule within 6 hours as unchanged drug and metabolite in approximately equal amounts.
CONTRAINDICATIONS AND PRECAUTIONS
  Hypersensitivity to dacarbazine. Safe use in pregnancy not established.
ADVERSE REACTIONS
  GI symptoms (most frequent): anorexia, nausea, vomiting. Hematologic depression: leukopenia and thrombocytopenia, mild anemia; influenzalike syndrome; alopecia; facial flushing and paresthesia; hepatotoxicity; abnormal renal function tests; confusion, lethargy, blurred vision, headache, seizures; erythematosus, macular or papular rash; severe pain and tissue damage following extravasation of dacarbazine.
ROUTE AND DOSAGE
  Intravenous: 2 to 4.5 mg/kg daily for 10 days; repeated at 4-week intervals. Alternatively, 250 mg/M²/day for 5 days; repeated at 3-week intervals if necessary.

NURSING IMPLICATIONS
Preferably should be administered to patients who are hospitalized, since close observation and frequent determination of hematologic status are required during and after therapy.
WBC, RBC, and platelet counts should be determined prior to and at regular intervals during therapy.
Inspect administraion sites. Apply ice compresses if extravasation occurs.
Hematopoietic toxicity usually appears 2 to 4 weeks after last dose. Generally a leukocyte count of less than 3000/mm³ and a platelet count of less than 100,000/mm³ require suspension or cessation of therapy.
Leukopenia and thrombocytopenia may be severe enough to cause death.
GI symptoms reportedly appear in over 90% of patients. Symptoms usually appear within 1 hour after initial dose and may persist up to 12 hours. Most patients develop tolerance to these effects after the first 1 or 2 days. If vomiting persists, discontinuation of therapy with dacarbazine may be necessary.
Monitor intake-output ratio and pattern and daily temperature. Report even a slight elevation of temperature.
Consult physician regarding oral intake. Restriction of foods and fluids for 4 to 6 hours prior to treatment may reduce incidence of vomiting and diarrhea. However, some physicians recommend good hydration to within 1 hour of drug administration to avoid dehydration from vomiting.
Influenzalike syndrome (fever, myalgia, malaise) may occur during or even

a week after treatment with dacarbazine and may last 7 to 21 days. Symptoms may recur with successive treatments.

Any solution remaining in the vial may be stored at 4 C for up to 72 hours; at 20 C the solution is not stable for more than 8 hours.

Protect dacarbazine powder from light.

DACTINOMYCIN, U.S.P.
(Actinomycin D, COSMEGEN)

Antineoplastic

ACTIONS AND USES

Potent cytotoxic antibiotic derived from mixture of actinomycins produced by *Streptomyces parvullus*. Complexes with DNA, thereby inhibiting DNA-directed RNA synthesis. Also interferes with protein synthesis and mitosis in rapidly proliferating neoplastic and normal cells. Causes delayed myelosuppression; has low therapeutic index.

Used in short courses, alone or in combined modalities with surgery or radiation, to produce remissions in patients with Wilms' tumor, embryonal rhabdomyosarcoma, and carcinoma of testes and uterus (embryonal, teratocarcinoma, choriosarcoma). All other uses are experimental.

ABSORPTION AND FATE

Very little active drug is detected in plasma 2 to 5 minutes after IV injection. Animal studies suggest that the drug concentrates in liver, spleen, and kidneys. About 50% of dose is excreted unchanged in bile and 10% in urine.

CONTRAINDICATIONS AND PRECAUTIONS

Chicken pox, patients of childbearing age, pregnancy, infants under 6 months of age, impairment of kidney, liver, or bone marrow function.

ADVERSE REACTIONS

Hematopoietic: anemia (including aplastic anemia), agranulocytosis, leukopenia, thrombocytopenia, pancytopenia, reticulopenia. **GI**: cheilitis, ulcerative stomatitis, esophagitis, dysphagia, pharyngitis, proctitis, anorexia, nausea, vomiting, abdominal pain, diarrhea, GI ulceration. **Dermatologic**: acne, reactivation of latent skin effects over previously irradiated areas, alopecia (reversible). Other: malaise, fatigue, lethargy, myalgia, epistaxis, anaphylactoid reaction, hypocalcemia, transient increase in uric acid excretion, thrombophlebitis, necrosis and sloughing at site of extravasation.

ROUTE AND DOSAGE

Intravenous: **Adults**: 0.5 mg daily for a maximum of 5 days, or single weekly doses of 2 mg for 3 weeks. **Children**: 15 µg/kg (up to maximum of 0.5 mg) daily for 5 days. Second course (both adults and children) may be given after at least 2 weeks have elapsed, provided all signs of toxicity have disappeared. Dose and schedule are highly individualized on basis of patient's tolerance, size and location of neoplasm, and concomitant therapy.

NURSING IMPLICATIONS

Dactinomycin is reconstituted by adding only sterile water for injection (without preservative); other solvents may cause precipitation. Protect from light and heat.

Once reconstituted, dactinomycin may be added directly to infusion solution of dextrose injection 5% or sodium chloride injection, or it may be injected into tubing of running IV infusion.

Since there is no preservative in the solution, discard any unused portion prepared for injection.

Particular care should be taken to avoid extravasation. Dactinomycin is extremely corrosive to tissue; if extravasation occurs, stop infusion immediately and report to physician. Prompt institution of local treatment such as cold packs may help to prevent thrombophlebitis and necrosis.

If direct IV injection is given, the two-needle technique is used to prevent tissue irritation: the needle used to withdraw dose from vial after reconstitution is discarded; a fresh sterile needle is used for direct injection into vein.

Nausea and vomiting usually occur a few hours after drug administration and are generally controlled by antiemetic drug.

Frequent determinations of renal, hepatic, and bone marrow function are advised. White blood cell counts should be performed daily and platelet counts every 3 days to detect hematopoietic depression. Check laboratory values for indicated adaptations to nursing care.

Monitor temperature and inspect oral membranes daily. See Mechlorethamine for nursing care of stomatitis.

Be alert to signs of agranulocytosis, which may develop abruptly (especially when dactinomycin and radiation are combined): extreme weakness and fatigue, sore throat, stomatitis, fever, chills. Report to physician. Antibiotic therapy, reverse precautions, and cessation of the antineoplastic are indicated.

Dactinomycin reactivates the latent skin effects of previous irradiation, causing recurrence of erythema, desquamation, and pigmentation; it also intensifies the erythema of concurrent irradiation treatment. Therapy is generally continued despite the occurrence of these side effects. Increased incidences of GI toxicity and bone marrow depression are reported in these patients.

The combination of stomatitis and diarrhea with leukopenia or thrombocytopenia usually requires prompt interruption of therapy until drug toxicity subsides.

Severe, sometimes fatal, toxic effects occur with high frequency in patients receiving dactinomycin. Effects usually appear 2 to 4 days after a course of therapy is stopped and may reach maximal severity 1 to 2 weeks following discontinuation of therapy. Monitoring of laboratory values and clinical condition should continue during this period.

DANAZOL
(DANOCRINE)

Androgen, anterior pituitary suppressant

ACTIONS AND USES

Synthetic androgen derivative of alpha-ethinyl testosterone with dose-related mild androgenic properties. Exerts no estrogenic or progestational activity. Suppresses pituitary output of follicle-stimulating hormone and luteinizing hormone, resulting in anovulation and amenorrhea. Interrupts progress and pain of endometriosis by causing atrophy and involution of both normal and ectopic endometrial tissue. Has no effect on large endometriomas or on anatomic deformities associated with pain of dysmenorrhea.

Used for palliative treatment of endometriosis when alternative hormonal therapy is ineffective, contraindicated, or intolerable. Reportedly has restored fertility in female made infertile by mild to moderate endometriosis.

ABSORPTION AND FATE

Metabolized to 2-hydroxymethylethisterone, which attains plasma levels 5 to 10 times higher than that of unchanged drug. Distribution and elimination data not available.

Pregnancy, nursing mothers, undiagnosed abnormal genital bleeding; impaired renal, cardiac, or hepatic function. Cautious use: migraine headache, epilepsy. Also see Testosterone.

ADVERSE REACTIONS

Androgenic side effects (virilization): acneiform lesions, oily skin and hair, edema, weight gain, clitoral enlargement, mild hirsutism, deepening of voice, increased hoarseness, decrease in breast size. **Hypoestrogenic effects**: flushing; sweating; emotional lability; nervousness; vaginitis with itching, drying, burning, or bleeding; amenorrhea. Causal relationship of danazol to the following reactions has been neither confirmed nor refuted. **Allergic**: skin rashes, nasal congestion. **CNS**: dizziness, headache, sleep disorders, fatigue, tremor, paresthesias in extremities (rare), irritability, visual disturbances, changes in appetite, chills. **GI**: gastroenteritis; rarely, nausea, vomiting, and constipation. **Musculoskeletal**: muscle cramps or spasms in back, neck, or legs. **Genitourinary**: hematuria (rare). **Other**: hair loss, decreased libido, elevated blood pressure, pelvic pain, conjunctival edema, possibility of cholestatic jaundice.

ROUTE AND DOSAGE

Oral: **400 mg** twice daily for 3 to 6 months. Started during menstruation or if pregnancy test is negative. Therapy may be extended 9 months if necessary. If symptoms recur after termination of therapy, drug can be reinstituted.

NURSING IMPLICATIONS

Inform patient that drug-induced amenorrhea (due to anovulation) is reversible. Ovulation and cyclic bleeding usually return within 60 to 90 days after therapeutic regimen is discontinued. Advise patient that potential for conception may also be restored at that time.

Because danazol may cause fluid retention, patients with epilepsy or migraine should be observed closely during therapy.

Although the side effects usually disappear when drug therapy is terminated, continue to observe patient for signs of virilization (sometimes irreversible).

Danzol is very expensive.

Also see Testosterone.

DANTHRON, N.F.
(CHRYSAZIN, DORBANE, MODANE)

Stimulant, cathartic

ACTIONS AND USES

Synthetic anthraquinone irritant cathartic. Similar to natural anthraquinone cathartics, eg, Cascara Sagroda (qv) in pharmacologic properties, uses, adverse reactions, contraindications, and precautions. Siutable for patients on low sodium diets. Also available in combination with diocytl sodium sulfosuccinate for fecal softening effect.

ABSORPTION AND FATE

Acts about 8 to 12 hours following administration. May impart laxative properties to breast milk.

ROUTE AND DOSAGE

Oral: **37.5 to 150 mg.**

NURSING IMPLICATIONS

Administration of danthron shortly after the evening meal usually produces evacuation of a soft stool the next morning.

Prolonged use may lead to dependence.
Pink to red coloration of urine is harmless and usually indicates that urine
is alkaline,
See Cascara Sagrada.

LABORATORY TEST INTERFERENCES: Danthron can cause apparent increase in **urinary PSP excretion.**

DAPSONE, U.S.P., B.P.
(AVLOSULFON, DDS, Diaminodiphenyl Sulfone)

Antibacterial (leprostatic)

ACTIONS AND USES
Sulfone derivative chemically related to sulfonamides, with bacteriostatic rather than bactericidal action. Greatest area of clinical use in leprosy (Hansen's disease). Causes fragmentation of bacilli in lesions by unknown mechanism and is thought to increase resistance of host.
Used in treatment of all types of leprosy. Has been used to control symptoms of dermatitis herpetiformis.
ABSORPTION AND FATE
Almost completely absorbed from GI tract. Peak plasma levels in 4 to 8 hours. Distributed to all body tissues, with high concentrations in kidney and liver. About 50% bound to plasma proteins. Approximately 85% of dose is excreted slowly in urine, primarily as water-soluble metabolites, with some free drug; a small percentage is excreted in feces. Traces may be found in blood 8 to 12 days after single 200-mg dose and for 35 days following discontinuation of repeated doses. Excreted in breast milk.
CONTRAINDICATIONS AND PRECAUTIONS
Hypersensitivity to sulfones, advanced amyloidosis of kidneys, pregnancy. Cautious use: chronic renal, hepatic, pulmonary, or cardiovascular disease, refractory anemias, albuminuria.
ADVERSE REACTIONS
GI: anorexia, nausea, vomiting, abdominal colic. **Neurologic:** headache, dizziness, lethargy, malaise, insomnia, tinnitus, blurred vision, peripheral neuropathy (especially thumbs), paresthesias, muscle weakness; neuralgic pain. **Erythema nodosum leprosum** (lepra reaction): malaise, fever, painful indurations of skin and mucosa, arthralgia, lymphadenitis, orchitis, iritis, swelling of hands and feet, hepatomegaly. **Hematologic:** methemoglobinemia (common), hemolytic-type anemia, leukopenia, agranulocytosis, aplastic anemia, and pancytopenia (infrequent). **Sensitivity reactions:** generalized and diffuse maculopapular eruptions, hypermelanotic macules (fixed eruptions), drug fever, allergic rhinitis. Other: tachycardia, hepatitis, hematuria, proteinuria, psychosis.
ROUTE AND DOSAGE
Oral: **Adult:** *Spaced Regimen:* (*lepromatous leprosy*): initially 25 mg twice weekly increased every 4th week by increments of 25 mg up to 100 mg twice weekly. Weeks (17 to 20): 100 mg 3 times/week; (21 to 24): 100 mg 4 times/week. (*Tuberculoid and dimorphous leprosy*): Similar regimen but dosage should not exceed 200 mg/week in tuberculoid leprosy, and 300 mg/week in dimorphous leprosy. **Children:** ¼ to ½ the adult dosage. *Daily Regimen:* 10 to 15 mg daily for 6 days a week. Dose is increased gradually to maximum in about 4 to 6 months. Total weekly dosage for each regimen should be the same.

NURSING IMPLICATIONS

Complete blood counts are performed prior to initiation of therapy, weekly during the first few weeks of therapy, and at monthly intervals thereafter. Periodic determinations of dapsone blood levels are also recommended.

Mild decrease in hemoglobin level may occur during the first few weeks of therapy. If hemoglobin falls below 9 Gm/dl, the dosage should be reduced or the drug temporarily discontinued.

Drug therapy is usually terminated if RBC count falls below 2.5 million/mm³ or remains persistently low after 6 weeks of therapy, or if leukocyte count falls below 5000/mm³.

Monitor temperature during first few weeks of therapy. If fever is frequent or severe, dosage should be reduced or therapy interrupted.

Lepra reaction is believed to be a response to circulating antigens from disintegrating *Mycobacterium leprae* and not a specific drug reaction. It may also be precipitated by infection, fever, vaccinations, or stress. Dosage adjustment or temporary interruption of therapy may be required.

Suspect methemoglobinemia if patient appears cyanotic and mucous membranes have brownish hue. Report to physician. Usually, discontinuation of therapy is not required unless anoxemia is present.

Generalized allergic skin reactions occur most frequently before the tenth week of therapy and are usually associated with increase in dosage. Therapy should be terminated. Interruption of therapy is usually not necessary for hypermelanotic, macular-type dermatitis, which may develop 1 week to 1 year after treatment begins.

Because of cumulative effects, scheduled rest periods from sulfone therapy are necessary to avoid toxicity. Dapsone blood levels of 0.1 to 1 mg/dl reflect safe dosage.

Therapeutic effects may not appear until after 3 to 6 months of therapy. Skin lesions respond well; recovery from nerve involvement is usually limited.

Deformities such as contractures may be prevented by physical therapy and application of casts. Other disfigurements may necessitate reconstructive surgery.

Lepromatous eye lesions sometimes develop or progress during treatment, since the drug does not appreciably penetrate ocular tissues.

Optimum duration of therapy has not been determined. Some authorities recommend continuing treatment for lepromatous leprosy 1 or 2 years following negative skin smears; others recommend maintenance therapy for life. For the tuberculoid type, treatment may be continued for 2 years after disease is clinically quiescent.

Scheduled follow-up is critical to detection of possible relapse. Examination of close contacts at 6- to 12-month intervals for at least 10 years is recommended.

Although a small amount of drug is excreted in breast milk, no harm to breast-fed infants has been reported. Blue color of infant will disappear.

Preserved in tightly covered, light-resistant containers. Drug discoloration apparently does not indicate a chemical change.

DRUG INTERACTIONS: **Probenecid** and **sulfinpyrazone** may cause elevated dapsone blood levels (by inhibiting renal excretion of dapsone).

DEANOL ACETAMIDOBENZOATE
(DEANER)

CNS stimulant

ACTIONS AND USES
  Tertiary amine thought to be an acetylcholine precursor. Crosses blood–brain barrier and then is converted to acetylcholine intracerebrally. Effects similar to those of amphetamine, but in therapeutic doses does not depress appetite or cause jitteriness.
  Used to relieve a variety of ill-defined symptoms such as chronic fatigue, neurasthenia, mild neurotic depression, and chronic headache. Also has been used for hyperkinetic behavior and learning problems in children.

ABSORPTION AND FATE
  Absorbed adequately from GI tract. Effects of mild stimulation develop slowly over period of days to weeks.

CONTRAINDICATIONS AND PRECAUTIONS
  Convulsive states.

ADVERSE REACTIONS
  Low toxicity: occipital headache (early in therapy); tenseness (neck, masseter, and quadriceps muscles), irritability, restlessness, fatigue, insomnia, transient rash, pruritus, weight loss, constipation, postural hypotension (rarely).

ROUTE AND DOSAGE
  Oral: initially 300 mg daily in single dose or divided doses. Maintenance: 25 to 100 mg daily. Highly individualized.

NURSING IMPLICATIONS

Generally administered in the morning when prescribed as a single dose.

Three or more weeks of therapy may be required before maximum effects are apparent. Actions appear to be cumulative.

Note that some adverse reactions may be similar to the indications for using the drug.

Most side effects disappear with continued treatment.

DECAMETHONIUM BROMIDE, N.F.
(C-10, SYNCURINE)

Skeletal muscle relaxant

ACTIONS AND USES
  Synthetic depolarizing neuromuscular blocking agent. Similar to succinylcholine (qv) in actions, uses, contraindications, precautions, and adverse reactions. Unlike succinylcholine, it does not cause a rise in intraocular pressure, it is minimally affected by pseudocholinesterase levels, and its histamine-releasing properties are less. Occasionally, effects are unpredictable, and abrupt cessation of neuromuscular blockade or paralysis of respiratory muscles may occur with no effect on abdominal muscles.
  Used as adjunct to general anesthesia and to reduce intensity of muscular contractions in electroshock therapy.

ABSORPTION AND FATE
  Muscle relaxation occurs within 2 minutes; maximal effect in 3 to 6 minutes, with duration of about 15 minutes. Does not readily cross placenta. No apparent metabolic degradation. Approximately 80% to 90% of dose is excreted as unchanged drug within 24 hours.

CONTRAINDICATIONS AND PRECAUTIONS
  Hypersensitivity to decamethonium or to bromides. Safe use in women of childbearing potential or during pregnancy not established. Cautious use: in the

elderly and very young; impaired renal function, patients recently digitalized, patients with fractures or muscle spasms; concomitant use of aminoglycoside antibiotics; surgery in lithotomy position. Also see Succinylcholine.

ADVERSE REACTIONS

Profound and prolonged muscle relaxation, respiratory depression, apnea, arrhythmias, rise or fall in blood pressure, hyperthermia, excessive salivation, postoperative muscle pain. Also see Succinylcholine.

ROUTE AND DOSAGE

Intravenous: range: 0.5 to 3 mg at rate not exceeding 1 mg/minute. *Electroshock therapy*: 1.5 to 1.75 mg given over 1 to 2 minute period. *Anesthesia*: initially 2 to 2.5 mg. Supplemental doses of 0.5 to 1 mg at 10- to 30-minute intervals, or 2 to 2.5 mg at 30- to 40-minute intervals as required, up to 3 doses.

NURSING IMPLICATIONS

Facilities must be immediately available to correct respiratory obstruction or arrest.

Tachyphylaxis occurs with repeated doses.

See Succinylcholine Chloride.

DEFEROXAMINE MESYLATE, U.S.P.
(DESFERAL)
DESFERRIOXAMINE MESYLATE, B.P.

Chelating agent, antidote (to iron poisoning)

ACTIONS AND USES

Chelating agent isolated from *Streptomyces pilosus* with specific affinity for ferric ion and low affinity for calcium. Binds ferric ions to form ferrioxamine complex, a stable water-soluble chelate readily excreted by kidneys. Main effect is removal of iron from ferritin, hemosiderin, and transferrin. Does not affect hemoglobin or cytochromes or increase excretion of electrolytes and other trace elements. Has histamine-releasing properties when administered rapidly by IV route. Theoretically, 100 mg of deferoxamine can chelate 8.5 mg of iron.

Used as adjunct in treatment of acute iron intoxication. Has been used in management of hemochromatosis and hemosiderosis secondary to increased iron storage, such as follows transfusion, dietary, and medicinal iron overload and hemolytic anemias (eg, thalassemia, sickle cell anemia).

ABSORPTION AND FATE

Rapidly forms nontoxic complex with iron (complex is dialyzable). Metabolized primarily by plasma enzymes by unknown mechanism. Excreted rapidly in urine as iron chelate and unchanged drug.

CONTRAINDICATIONS AND PRECAUTIONS

Severe renal disease, anuria, pregnancy, women of childbearing potential. Cautious use: history of pyelonephritis.

ADVERSE REACTIONS

Pain and induration at injection site; generalized erythema, urticaria, pruritus, fever, hypotension, shock (most commonly with rapid IV injection). Long-term therapy particularly: allergic-type reactions (pruritus, urticaria, rash, anaphylactoid reactions), blurred vision, cataracts, abdominal discomfort, diarrhea, leg cramps, tachycardia, fever, exacerbation of pyelonephritis.

ROUTE AND DOSAGE

Intramuscular (preferred route), intravenous infusion: **Adults and Children**: 1 Gm followed by 500 mg at 4-hour intervals for 2 doses. Depending on clinical response, subsequent doses of 500 mg every 4 to 12 hours. Reconstituted by adding 2 ml sterile water for injection to 500-mg ampul. For IV infusion,

Ringer's lactate solution. Not more than 6 Gm in 24 hours advised.

NURSING IMPLICATIONS
Baseline tests of kidney function should be performed.
Make certain that drug is completely dissolved before withdrawing from ampul.
Physician will prescribe specific infusion flow rate (should not exceed 15 mg/kg of body weight per hour). Monitor vital signs.
Monitor intake–output ratio. Report any change. Observe stools for blood (iron intoxication frequently causes necrosis of GI tract).
Deferoxamine is used as adjunct to standard treatment for acute iron intoxication: emesis with syrup of ipecac, gastric lavage with 5% sodium bicarbonate, suction and maintenance of airway, control of shock (IV fluids, blood, oxygen, vasopressors), correction of acidosis.
Deferoxamine chelate imparts a characteristic reddish color to urine (presumptive evidence of elevated serum iron and indication for further therapy).
Periodic ophthalmoscopic examinations advisable for patients on prolonged therapy.
Solutions reconstituted with sterile water may be stored at room temperature for not longer than 1 week.

DEHYDROCHOLIC ACID, N.F.
(CHOLAN-DH, DECHOLIN, NEOCHOLAN)
DEHYDROCHOLATE SODIUM INJECTION, N.F.
(DECHOLIN SODIUM)

Hydrocholeretic, diagnostic aid (circulation time)

ACTIONS AND USES
Unconjugated oxidized acid made synthetically from cholonic acids (chiefly cholic acid) found in natural bile. Increases volume and flow of low-viscosity water-diluted bile by hydrocholeretic action and thus facilitates biliary tract drainage. Doubtful effect on production of bile salts. Probably much less effective than natural bile salts in lowering surface tension and hence emulsification or in promoting absorption of fats or fat-soluble vitamins.
Used as adjunct, primarily for flushing action, in management of chronic and recurring biliary tract disorders; and used prophylactically following biliary tract surgery; used to promote T-tube drainage. Sodium salt also used for cholecystography and cholangiography and for diagnostic determination of arm-to-tongue circulation time in selected patients. Oral drug has also been used for temporary relief of constipation, with questionable efficacy.
ABSORPTION AND FATE
Oral drug absorbed from intestines; enters liver from portal circulation and reenters intestinal tract via bile ducts and is excreted in feces.
CONTRAINDICATIONS AND PRECAUTIONS
Cholelithiasis, jaundice, marked hepatic insufficiency, complete obstruction of common or hepatic bile ducts, GI or GU tracts; use as diuretic, critically or terminally ill patients, use for constipation in presence of nausea and abdominal pain. Cautious use: history of asthma or allergy, prostatic hypertrophy, acute hepatitis, acute yellow atrophy of liver, children under 6 years of age, the elderly.
ADVERSE REACTIONS
Associated with intravenous use: abdominal discomfort, nausea, vomiting, diarrhea, headache, fainting, dyspnea, fever, chills, sweating, hypotension, tachy-

cardia, erythema, pruritus, urticaria, anaphylactoid reactions, persistent local inflammation following extravasation of IV injection.

ROUTE AND DOSAGE

Oral (dehydrocholic acid): 250 to 500 mg 2 or 3 times a day. Intravenous (sodium dehydrocholate): *for hydrocholeretic effect*, 5 to 10 ml of 20% solution on the first day; 10 ml on second and third days; *for circulation time*, 3 to 5 ml of 20% solution injected rapidly into cubital vein.

NURSING IMPLICATIONS

IV preparation is administered by physician.

Skin tests are advised prior to IV administration for patients with history of allergy or asthma.

Warm moist compresses may help to reduce inflammatory reaction of IV site.

Oral drug is administered with or after meals.

Arm-to-tongue circulation time test: Patient is usually advised to fast for 3 hours prior to the test and to rest in bed 30 minutes before injection is made. Explain procedure to patient.

To determine circulation time: Patient should be supine with antecubital fossa at level of right atrium. For most accurate results a 15-second wait is recommended after releasing tourniquet before injecting drug. The time from the beginning of injection to perception of bitter taste is measured in seconds (normal: 8 to 16 seconds).

Circulation time is prolonged in shock, myxedema, polycythemia vera, congestive heart failure, complete atrioventricular block and other cardiac conditions, and shortened in hyperthyroidism, anemia, beriberi, and congenital cardiac anomalies.

IV therapy should be replaced by oral therapy as soon as possible.

Therapy usually is discontinued if no clinical improvement is noted within 4 to 6 weeks.

LABORATORY TEST INTERFERENCES: Dehydrocholic acid may interfere with hepatic uptake or biliary excretion of **bromsulphalein**.

DEMECARIUM BROMIDE, N.F.
(HUMORSOL)

Cholinergic (ophthalmic)

ACTIONS AND USES

Potent, long-acting quaternary ammonium compound. Action attributed to reversible cholinesterase inhibition, which permits accumulation of anticholinesterase at neuromuscular junctions. Local application to conjunctiva produces constriction of iris sphincter and ciliary muscle; intraocular pressure is thereby reduced by facilitated aqueous humor outflow. Also enhances resorption of aqueous humor by increasing permeability and dilation of conjunctival vessels. Indirectly decreases activity of extraocular muscles of convergence.

Used infrequently because of toxicity. Clinical indications include open-angle glaucoma; selected cases of glaucoma due to synechial formation; following iridectomy; and management of accommodative esotropia (convergent strabismus) when less potent miotics have failed. Carbonic anhydrase inhibitor may be used concomitantly to enhance action.

ABSORPTION AND FATE

Absorbed through conjunctiva and intact skin. Miosis begins within 1 hour and reaches maximum in 2 to 4 hours. Reduction of intraocular pressure occurs in

12 hours and is maximal in 24 hours. Residual miosis and decreased intraocular pressure may persist 7 days or more following single instillation.

CONTRAINDICATIONS AND PRECAUTIONS

Narrow-angle glaucoma, history of retinal detachment, ocular hypertension accompanied by inflammation, bronchial asthma, spastic GI conditions, peptic ulcer, marked vagotonia, pronounced bradycardia or hypotension, recent myocardial infarction, parkinsonism, epilepsy. Safe use in pregnancy not established. Cautious use: myasthenia gravis.

ADVERSE REACTIONS

Stinging, burning, lacrimation, ciliary spasm with eye and brow pain, frontal headache, increased myopia with visual blurring, twitching of eyelids, conjunctival and ciliary hyperemia, iris cysts (particularly in children following prolonged use), activation of latent iritis or uveitis, retinal detachment (occasionally), conjunctival thickening and obstruction of nasolacrimal canals (prolonged use), lens opacity, contact dermatitis. Systemic effects (parasympathetic stimulation): nausea, vomiting, abdominal pain, diarrhea, urinary frequency or incontinence, excessive salivation, profuse sweating, flushing, muscular weakness, paresthesias, bronchospasm, hypotension, bradycardia, depression of serum cholinesterase and erythrocytes.

ROUTE AND DOSAGE

Topical: **Adults** (*glaucoma*): 1 drop of 0.125% solution twice weekly to 2 drops of 0.25% solution twice daily. Intervals determined by intraocular pressure evaluations. **Children** (accommodative esotropia): 1 drop of 0.125% solution instilled into each eye daily for 2 or 3 weeks, then 1 drop every 2 days for 3 to 4 weeks. Highly individualized dosages.

NURSING IMPLICATIONS

Demecarium bromide is a dangerous drug capable of producing cumulative systemic effects. It is essential to adhere precisely to prescribed drug concentration, dosage schedule, and technique of administration. Closely observe patient during initial period.

Usually gonioscopy (examination of angle) is performed before therapy is started in patients with glaucoma.

The first instillation will be made by physician. Since a transient paradoxic increase in intraocular pressure may occur initially, tonometer readings should be made at least hourly for 3 or 4 hours after first instillation.

Procedure for instilling eye drop to minimize overflow of solution into nasal and pharyngeal spaces, and possibly systemic absorption: After drop is instilled into lower conjunctival sac, have patient keep lids apart until gentle pressure can be applied to inner angle of eye against nose (nasolacrimal duct). Maintain pressure for 1 or 2 minutes. Instruct patient to avoid squeezing lids together. Blot excess medication with a clean tissue. Wash hands immediately after administration.

Avoid prolonged contact of drug with skin. If solution contacts skin, wash promptly with large volumes of water.

Maintain sterility of dropper. If it becomes contaminated it should be sterilized before being returned to bottle.

Supervise ambulation. Inform patient that difficulty in accommodating to degree of light, blurred distant vision (ciliary or accommodative spasm), and miosis with dimmed vision and eyelid twitching may persist for a week or more. He should avoid performing hazardous activities until these side effects have disappeared.

Physician may prescribe schedule so that drug is instilled at bedtime in order to minimize disturbing visual effects.

Pain in affected eye is more intense with accommodative effort to near objects and with exposure to light. These effects appear more frequently in younger patients than in older patients.

Advise patient to report promptly to the physician the onset of excessive salivation, diaphoresis, urinary incontinence, diarrhea, or muscle weakness. Drug should be discontinued.

Patients receiving demecarium should remain under constant medical supervision. Tolerance may develop with prolonged use. Patient should be examined for lenticular opacities at intervals of 6 months or less.

In the event of systemic toxicity, atropine sulfate is used as antidote. Artificial respiration, oxygen, and other supportive measures may be necessary.

Caution patient of possible added systemic effects from skin contact or inhalation of organophosphate-type insecticides or pesticides, while receiving demecarium.

Preserved in tight, light-resistant containers.

DEMECLOCYCLINE, N.F.
(DECLOMYCIN, DEMETHYLCHLORTETRACYCLINE, DMCT)
DEMECLOCYCLINE HYDROCHLORIDE, N.F.
(DECLOMYCIN HYDROCHLORIDE)

Antibacterial

ACTIONS AND USES

Tetracycline antibiotic isolated from mutant strain of *Streptomyces aureofaciens.* Similar to other tetracycline antibiotics in actions, uses, contraindications, precautions, and adverse reactions. Excreted more slowly than other tetracyclines.

ABSORPTION AND FATE

Peak serum concentrations within 3 to 6 hours; effective serum levels may persist 48 to 72 hours after last dose. About 40% to 50% is bound to serum proteins. Concentrates in liver and is excreted in bile. Enterohepatic cycle maintains serum levels and delays ultimate removal. Approximately 38% of dose is excreted in urine and feces in 24 hours.

ADVERSE REACTIONS

Phototoxicity (from sun exposure), erythematous eruptions, edema, increased pigmentation of skin and nails, loosening or softening of nails (onycholysis), GI disturbances, superinfections, blood dyscrasias, acute renal failure (in patients with Laennec's cirrhosis. Following long-term therapy: diabetes insipidus syndrome. Also see Tetracycline.

ROUTE AND DOSAGE

Oral: **Adults:** 150 mg 4 times a day or 300 mg 2 times a day. Usually given at 6-hour intervals. Reduced dosage in patients with renal impairment. **Children**: 3 to 6 mg/kg/day divided into 2 to 4 doses.

NURSING IMPLICATIONS

Check expiration date before administering drug. Renal damage (Fanconi syndrome) and death have resulted from use of outdated tetracyclines.

Since food interferes with absorption, administer demeclocycline not less than 1 hour before nor sooner than 2 hours after meals.

Demeclocycline absorption may also be impaired by milk or other calcium-containing foods, iron salts, antacids, and sodium bicarbonate.

For most infections, therapy is usually continued 24 to 48 hours after fever and other symptoms have subsided. Exception: therapy for at least 10 days is recommended for streptococcal infections.

If drug therapy is prolonged, determinations of serum drug levels are recommended.

Caution patient to avoid exposure to sunlight or ultraviolet light during treatment and for several weeks after treatment so as to prevent severe burns (phototoxic reaction).

Demeclocycline should be discontinued at first evidence of erythema.

Monitor intake–output ratio in patients on prolonged therapy. Some patients develop diabetes insipidus syndrome (polydipsia, polyuria, weakness). It is usually dose-related and is reversible with discontinuation of therapy.

Expiration dates vary from 1 to 5 years following date of manufacture, depending on formulation.

Preserved in tight, light-resistant containers.

See Tetracycline Hydrochloride.

DESERPIDINE
(HARMONYL)

Antihypertensive

ACTIONS AND USES

Rauwolfia alkaloid almost identical to reserpine (qv) in actions, contraindications, precautions, and adverse reactions. Used in treatment of mild essential hypertension and as adjunctive therapy with other antihypertensive agents in the more severe forms. Also used for relief of symptoms in agitated psychotic states, eg, schizophrenia in patients unable to tolerate phenothiazines or in patients who also require antihypertensive medication.

ROUTE AND DOSAGE

Oral (hypertension): initially 0.75 to 1 mg daily in divided doses; maintenance 0.25 mg daily. Psychiatric disorders: initially 0.5 mg daily (range 0.1 to 1 mg). Dosage adjusted according to patient's response.

NURSING IMPLICATIONS

Since the full effect of deserpidine may not be produced before 10 to 14 days of therapy in patients being treated for hypertension, dosage adjustments should not be made more frequently.

See Reserpine.

DESIPRAMINE HYDROCHLORIDE, N.F., B.P.
(NORPRAMIN, PERTOFRANE)

Antidepressant

ACTIONS AND USES

Tricyclic antidepressant. Active desmethyl metabolite of imipramine (qv), with similar pharmacologic actions, uses, contraindications, and adverse reactions. Some studies report that it has a somewhat faster onset of action than imipramine and that side effects occur less frequently; however, it has the same potential for toxicity as imipramine.

Indicated for relief of depressive symptoms. Endogenous depressions are more likely to be alleviated than other types of depression.

ABSORPTION AND FATE

Well absorbed following oral administration. Detoxified in liver. Approximately 70% of drug is excreted in urine. See Imipramine.

Prostatic hypertrophy, glaucoma, recent myocardial infarction, epilepsy. Safe use in pediatric age group not established. Also see Imipramine.

ADVERSE REACTIONS

Dry mouth, blurred vision, mydriasis, constipation, urinary retention, drowsiness, sweating, dizziness, orthostatic hypotension, tremors, peculiar taste sensation, photosensitivity. Also see imipramine.

ROUTE AND DOSAGE

Oral: 25 to 50 mg 3 times a day, increased if necessary after 7 to 10 days to maximum of 200 mg daily; maintenance: 50 to 100 mg/day. Highly individualized. Lower dosage range recommended for adolescents, elderly patients, and outpatients.

NURSING IMPLICATIONS

Doses are carefully titrated to reduce possibility of severe side effects.

Monitor blood pressure during initial phase of therapy. Desipramine is especially noted to cause postural hypotension.

Caution patient to make all position changes slowly particularly from recumbent to upright position. Also advise him to dangle legs for a few minutes before ambulating, and to lie down immediately if he feels weak or faint.

Warn patient to avoid potentially hazardous activities such as driving until his reaction to drug is known.

Desipramine may cause photosensitization. Warn patient to avoid excessive exposure to sunlight or ultraviolet light.

The earliest manifestation of antidepressant action consists primarily of psychomotor activity, generally within the first week or more of therapy. Observe necessary environmental precautions.

Full treatment benefit is seldom attained before end of second week of therapy.

In some patients, for unknown reasons, therapeutic effectiveness of desipramine declines after 2 to 6 weeks of therapy. Keep physician informed of patient's progress.

If therapeutic effectiveness is not noted after 3 weeks of therapy, it is unlikely that continued administration will be of benefit.

See Imipramine Hydrochloride.

DESLANOSIDE, N.F.
(CEDILANID-D, Desacetyl-lanatoside C)

Cardiotonic

ACTIONS AND USES

Rapid-acting cardiotonic glycoside obtained by alkaline hydrolysis of lanatoside C, a glycoside of *Digitalis lanata*. Shares actions, contraindications, and adverse reactions of digitalis leaf, powdered (qv).

Used parenterally for rapid digitalizing effect in emergency treatment of acute pulmonary edema and supraventricular arrhythmias.

ABSORPTION AND FATE

Onset of action in 5 to 30 minutes following IV or IM dose; peak effect in 1 to 4 hours. Action usually regresses over 16 to 36 hours, but may persist for 5 days. Approximately 20% excreted daily in urine.

ROUTE AND DOSAGE

Intramuscular (digitalization): 1.6 mg (8 ml) divided into 0.8-mg (4-ml) portions and injected in each of two sites. Intravenous: 1.6 mg as single injection or divided into two injections.

NURSING IMPLICATIONS
Maintenance therapy with an oral digitalis glycoside is preferred and may
  be instituted within 12 hours after digitalization with deslanoside.
Deslanoside should be protected from light.
See Digitalis Leaf, Powdered.

DESOXYCORTICOSTERONE ACETATE, U.S.P. (AND PELLETS, N.F.)
(DCA, DOCA ACETATE, PERCORTEN ACETATE, SYNCORT, and others)
DESOXYCORTICOSTERONE PIVALATE, N.F.
(PERCORTEN PIVALATE)
DEOXYCORTONE, B.P.

Adrenocortical steroid (salt-regulating)

ACTIONS AND USES
  Potent synthetic mineralocorticoid. Major action reflected by increased retention of sodium and water and increased excretion of potassium apparently due
  to altered patterns of renal tubular reabsorption. Therapeutic dose produces
  correction of electrolyte imbalance, hypertension, and expanded blood volume,
  leading to increased cardiac output and decreased nitrogen retention. Also promotes fat and glucose absorption from GI tract. Lacks glucocorticoid properties
  of hydrocortisone. Has no effect on inflammatory process, skin pigmentation,
  allergy, hypoglycemic tendency, or circulating eosins or on the ability to excrete
  excess water or to withstand stress.
  Used only in conjunction with other supplementary measures (glucocorticoids,
  glucose, control of infection and fluid and electrolytes) as partial replacement
  therapy for primary and secondary adrenocortical insufficiency in Addison's
  disease; also used for treatment of salt-losing adrenogenital syndrome. Newer
  drugs are replacing it.
ABSORPTION AND FATE
  Following parenteral administration binds to serum proteins. Diffuses into tissue fluids, including cerebrospinal fluid. Hepatic metabolism is followed by
  excretion in urine.
CONTRAINDICATIONS AND PRECAUTIONS
  Hypersensitivity to components; hypertension; cardiac disease; glucose tolerance test (patient with Addison's disease); particularly IV (may cause severe
  hypoglycemia). Safe use during pregnancy or lactation not established. Cautious
  use: Addison's disease.
ADVERSE REACTIONS
  Generalized edema, hypokalemia, frontal or occipital headaches, pulmonary
  congestion, hypertension; cardiac arrhythmias, enlargement, failure; arthralgia,
  tendon contractures, muscle weakness with ascending paralysis, hypersensitivity, irritation at site of pellet implant.
ROUTE AND DOSAGE
  Intramuscular (pivalate repository): 25 to 100 mg every 4 weeks. (acetate in
  sesame oil): 1 to 5 mg daily. Subcutaneous implantation: one pellet implanted
  for each 0.5 mg of the daily injected maintenance dose (each pellet contains 125
  mg desoxycorticosterone).

NURSING IMPLICATIONS

For IM injection of desoxycorticosterone acetate: Withdraw oily solution into syringe with a 19-gauge needle, then change to a 23-gauge needle of sufficient length for IM injection procedure. Inject deep into upper outer quadrant of buttock; alternate injection sites. When it is not feasible to use lower extremity, preferably given subcutaneously into upper extremity.

Desoxycorticosterone pivalate should be administered no more than once a month. Dose is determined after daily requirement for maintenance has been established with the acetate formulation. Inject through a 20-gauge needle into upper outer quadrant of buttock.

Infrascapular region is most frequently used area for pellet implant. As many as 15 may be inserted in a single incision.

Sodium intake may or may not require regulation, depending on individual needs and clinical situation. In general, a high intake of salt accelerates loss of K and retention of Na. Teach the patient that salt intake is a significant regulator of drug efficacy. Signs of edema should be reported immediately.

Alert patient to signs of potassium depletion (associated with high sodium intake): muscle weakness, paresthesias, circumoral numbness; fatigue, anorexia, nausea, mental depression, polyuria, delirium, diminished reflexes, arrhythmias, cardiac failure, ileus, ECG changes.

Establish baseline and continuing data regarding blood pressure, intake–output ratio and pattern, and weight. Start flow chart as reference for planning individual patient care indicated by drug response. During period of dosage adjustment, blood pressure should be checked every 4 to 6 hours and weight at least every other day.

The patient maintained on pellets should be instructed to weigh himself under standard conditions every other day and to keep a record for the physician. He should understand the significance of weight changes and other symptoms of overdosage and underdosage.

Signs of overdosage: psychosis, excess weight gain, pulmonary edema, congestive heart failure, ravenous appetite, severe insomnia, increase in blood pressure. Signs of insufficient dosage: loss of weight, anorexia, nausea, vomiting, diarrhea, muscular weakness, increased fatigue.

Implant dosage (highly individualized) is based on the maintenance dosage established during 2 to 3 months with desoxycorticosterone acetate injection.

Signs of insufficient pellet-supplied dosage may begin about 8 months after implant and should be reported promptly to the physician. Daily supplementary injections of desoxycorticosterone may be necessary for the next 4 to 6 weeks until the maintenance dose is reestablished. Reimplantation then follows.

Caution the patient with a pellet implant to notify his physician if he anticipates vacationing in a climate warmer than that of his home environment or if he anticipates a change of work to heavy physical labor in the heat (both changes may produce salt loss through excess sweating). Dose reevaluation may be necessary.

Intercurrent infection, trauma, or unexpected stress of any kind should be reported promptly by the patient on maintenance therapy. A supplementary rapid-acting corticosteroid before, during, and after the stressful situation may be ordered, as well as other measures such as change in amount of salt intake (tablet or diet).

After the initial postoperative period of healing following pellet implantation, promptly report soreness or inflammation over implant site.

Drug is not withdrawn from a patient undergoing major surgery if he has been on long-term therapy, but the surgeon should be aware of the history. Advise the patient to wear or carry medical identification card or jewelry stating drug being used and physician's identity.

Pellets are preserved in tight containers suitable for maintaining sterile contents. Injectable forms are preserved in light-resistant containers.

The patient with insufficiency may become hypoglycemic during the dose regulation period if he is without food more than 4 to 5 hours. Schedule laboratory tests so as to prevent long periods without nourishment.

DEXAMETHASONE, N.F., B.P.
(AEROSEB-D, DECADERM, DECADRON, DECASPRAY, DERONIL, DEXAMETH, DEXONE, GAMMACORTEN, HEXADROL, MAXIDEX)
DEXAMETHASONE ACETATE
(DECADRON-LA)
DEXAMETHASONE SODIUM PHOSPHATE, N.F.
(DECADRON PHOSPHATE, DEKSONE, DEXASONE PHOSPHATE, DEZONE, HEXADROL PHOSPHATE)

Adrenocortical steroid (glucocorticoid)

ACTIONS AND USES

Long-acting synthetic adrenocorticoid with intense antiinflammatory activity. Rarely causes sodium and water retention; may promote potassium and nitrogen loss and exacerbation of glycosuria in diabetic patient. See Hydrocortisone for uses, absorption, and fate.

CONTRAINDICATIONS AND PRECAUTIONS

Systemic fungal infection, acute infections, positive sputum culture of *Candida albicans,* viral diseases, ocular herpes simplex and tuberculosis of eye, perforated ear drum (otic use).

ADVERSE REACTIONS

Following aerosol therapy: nasal irritation and dryness, epistaxis rebound congestion, bronchial asthma, anosomia, perforation of nasal septum. Also see Hydrocortisone.

ROUTE AND DOSAGE

Oral: (Dexamethasone) 1.5 to 4.5 mg daily (massive doses as high as 15 mg may be given for certain conditions). Intramuscular, intralesional, intraarticular, soft tissue: Dexamethasone Acetate; Dexamethasone Sodium Phosphate. Intravenous: Dexamethasone Sodium Phosphate. Doses highly individualized according to condition being treated and patient's observed response. Topical: solutions, creams, gels, ointments of various strengths. Ophthalmic: 0.1% solution; 0.05% ointment. Intranasal: aerosol (each metered spray delivers 0.084 mg dexamethasone): 2 or 3 sprays in each nostril 2 or 3 times daily.

NURSING IMPLICATIONS

Dexamethasone sodium phosphate with lidocaine should not be administered intravenously.

Effects of local injections persist about 24 hours. Injections may be repeated from once every 3 days to once every 3 weeks.

Diuresis may follow transfer from another steroid preparation to dexamethasone.

Repository acetate (for IM or local injection only) is a white suspension that settles on standing; mild shaking will resuspend the drug. Protect from heat.

Systemic effect of dexamethasone may follow topical, intralesional, or intraarticular use, particularly with long-term use and high dosage.

Caution patient on prolonged therapy not to use over-the-counter medications unless the physician has approved.

Ophthalmic preparations: Warn patient to consult physician promptly and to interrupt treatment with ophthalmic preparation if changes in visual acuity or diminished visual fields occur. Frequent measurement of intraocular pressure, slit-lamp microscopy, and examination of optic nerve head should accompany long-term therapy with ophthalmic formulation. An eye pad may be used with ointment to enhance effect of drug on corneal surface.

Ophthalmic solution may also be used for treatment of inflammatory condition of the external auditory meatus. Consult physician regarding preparation of aural canal before instillation of medication. If gauze wick is used, it should be kept moist with medication while in place and removed after 12 to 24 hours. Treatment may be repeated by specific order.

Observe eyelids and eye surfaces being treated with solution or ointment. If evidence of irritation develops, stop the treatment and consult physician.

Aerosol preparations: Theoretically, 12 sprays of aerosol will deliver 1.0 mg dexamethasone. No more than 12 sprays daily; therefore the order should be specific as to number of sprays for each nostril, for each administration.

Hypoadrenalism can be induced with chronic use of aerosol preparation; thus the duration of treatment period should be understood by the patient in order to prevent overdosage.

To administer drug, hold aerosol container upright approximately 6 inches from area being treated. Shake well before spraying. Usual dosage regimen: spray each 4-inch square of affected area for 1 to 2 seconds, 2 or 3 times daily.

If spray is to be applied about the face, the eyes should be protected, and spray should not be inhaled. If eyes are accidentally exposed to the aerosol, wash eyes thoroughly with water and contact physician at once.

Dexamethasone suppression test is a screening test for Cushing's syndrome and a test to distinguish adrenal tumors from adrenal hyperplasia.

Also see Hydrocortisone.

DEXBROMPHENIRAMINE MALEATE, N.F. (DISOMER)

Antihistaminic

ACTIONS AND USES

Propylamine (alkylamine) histamine antagonist and dextro isomer of brompheniramine. Shares actions, uses, contraindications, precautions, and adverse reactions of other antihistamines. See chlorpheniramine.

ABSORPTION AND FATE

Repeat-action tablet: one-half of quantity is rapidly released from outer layer following ingestion; remainder is released 3 to 6 hours later.

CONTRAINDICATIONS AND PRECAUTIONS

History of hypersensitivity to antihistamines. Safe use during pregnancy not established. Also see chlorpheniramine.

ADVERSE REACTIONS

Hypersensitivity reactions (skin rash, urticaria, hypotension, thrombocytopenia), drowsiness, dizziness, dry mouth, diplopia, headache, nausea. Also see chlorpheniramine.

Oral: 2 to 4 mg every 6 to 8 hours. Repeat-action tablet: one tablet (6 mg) in morning and one at bedtime; 6 mg every 8 hours may be required.

NURSING IMPLICATIONS
Alert patient to the possibility of drowsiness. Caution him to avoid potentially hazardous activities until his reaction to the drug has been determined.

Included in antihistaminic-decongestant combinations, eg, Disophrol, Drixoral.

Preserved in tight, light-resistant containers.

See chlorpheniramine.

DEXPANTHENOL
(ILOPAN, INTRAPAN, PANTHENOL, PANTHODERM, D-PANTOTHENYL ALCOHOL)

Cholinergic

ACTIONS AND USES

Alcohol analogue of the coenzyme vitamin, pantothenic acid, to which it is readily converted. A member of the B-complex group and precursor of coenzyme A, which is essential to normal epithelial function and biosynthesis of fatty acids, amino acids, and acetylcholine. Use in treatment of postoperative distention or delayed intestinal motility is based on the presumption that these conditions result from stress and/or antibiotic-induced alterations in pantothenic acid metabolism. Topical application reportedly relieves itching and may aid healing of skin lesions by stimulating epithelialization and granulation. Also has antibacterial activity.

Used in prevention or treatment of postoperative abdominal distention, intestinal atony and paralytic ileus. Also has been used to reduce ototoxicity in streptomycin and salicylate overdosage. Used topically in treatment of minor skin lesions.

ABSORPTION AND FATE

Well absorbed; very little is metabolized in body. Excreted as pantothenic acid, mostly in urine; small amount excreted in feces.

CONTRAINDICATIONS AND PRECAUTIONS

Hemophilia, ileus due to mechanical obstruction.

ADVERSE REACTIONS

Generally well tolerated. Rare: allergic manifestations, diarrhea.

ROUTE AND DOSAGE

Intramuscular: 250 to 500 mg repeated in 2 hours, then at 4- to 6-hour intervals, if necessary. Intravenous: 500 mg mixed with IV infusion solutions such as glucose or lactated Ringer's and administered by slow infusion. Topical: (2% cream or lotion): applied directly to affected area once or twice daily, or more often as needed.

NURSING IMPLICATIONS
Dexpanthenol may prolong bleeding time in some patients.

Report immediately any evidence of allergic reaction; drug should be discontinued.

Therapeutic results may not be obtained in patients with hypokalemia.

DRUG INTERACTIONS: Concomitant use of dexpanthenol with **antibiotics, narcotics,** and **barbiturates** have caused allergic reactions in some patients (mechanism unknown). Concomitant use with **succinylcholine** or other **skeletal muscle relaxants** may cause respiratory embarrassment.

DEXTRAN 40
(GENTRAN 40, L.M.D., RHEOMACRODEX)

Plasma volume expander, blood flow adjuvant

ACTIONS AND USES

Low-molecular-weight polymer of glucose (average molecular weight is approximately 40,000; range 10,000 to 90,000). As a hypertonic colloidal solution, produces immediate and short-lived expansion of plasma volume by drawing fluid from interstitial to intravascular spaces. Cardiovascular response to volume expansion includes increased blood pressure, pulse, central venous pressures, cardiac output, venous return to heart, and diuresis, and decreased heart rate, peripheral resistance, and blood viscosity. In addition to plasma volume expansion, it improves microcirculation, possibly by decreasing blood viscosity (lower hematocrit) and by retarding rouleaux formation and RBC sludging that may accompany shock.

Used in adjunctive treatment of shock or impending shock caused by hemorrhage, burns, surgery, or other trauma. It should not replace other forms of therapy known to be of value in treatment of shock. Also used as priming fluid or as additive to other primers in pump oxygenators during extracorporeal circulation.

ABSORPTION AND FATE

Produces rapid expansion of plasma volume, generally 1 to 2 times the volume of dextran 40 infused, within minutes after end of infusion; gradually reverses over succeeding 12 hours, depending on renal clearance rate. About 70% is excreted in urine within 24 hours. Dextran molecules of higher molecular weights (50,000 d or greater) are degraded to glucose and metabolized to carbon dioxide and water. Small amounts are also excreted in GI tract and eliminated in feces.

CONTRAINDICATIONS AND PRECAUTIONS

Hypersensitivity to dextran, renal failure, hypervolemic conditions, severe congestive heart failure, thrombocytopenia, hypofibrinogenemia or other marked hemostatic defects. Safe use during pregnancy and in women of childbearing age not established. Cautious use: active hemorrhage, severe dehydration, chronic liver disease, impaired renal function, patients susceptible to pulmonary edema or congestive heart failure.

ADVERSE REACTIONS

Allergic reactions: mild urticarial reactions; severe anaphylactoid reactions (rare): nasal congestion, wheezing, tightness in chest, hypotension, nausea, vomiting, fever, arthralgia, cardiac arrest. Renal tubule vacuolization (osmotic nephrosis), stasis, and blocking; renal failure; increased SGOT and SGPT (specific connection with dextran not established). **With high doses:** prolonged bleeding and coagulation times, decreased hematocrit and plasma protein levels, pulmonary edema.

ROUTE AND DOSAGE

Available as 10% dextran 40 in 5% dextrose or in 0.9% sodium chloride. Intravenous infusion *(adjunctive therapy for shock):* total dosage during first 24 hours should not exceed 20 ml/kg body weight. First 500 ml may be administered rapidly (over 15 to 30 minutes), with repeated doses given more slowly. Succeeding doses for maximum of 4 additional days should not exceed 10

ml/kg/day. (*Priming fluid for extracorporeal circulation:* dosage varies with volume of
pump oxygenator): generally 10 to 20 ml/kg added to perfusion circuit.

NURSING IMPLICATIONS

Not to be confused with dextran 70 or other dextrans.

Use only if seal is intact, vacuum is detectable, and solution is absolutely clear.

When stored for long periods, dextran flakes may form. To dissolve flakes, place bottle in warm water bath until solution clears.

Baseline hematocrit should be taken prior to initiation of dextran and after administration (dextran usually lowers hematocrit). Notify physician if hematocrit is depressed below 30 vol%.

If blood is to be administered, a cross-match specimen should be drawn prior to dextran infusion (see Laboratory Test Interferences).

Specific flow rate should be prescribed by physician.

Allergic reactions are most likely to occur during the first few minutes of administration in patients not previously exposed to dextran. Observe patient closely. Therapy should be terminated at the first sign of a reaction. Other means of sustaining circulation should be immediately available. Have on hand resuscitative equipment, parenteral epinephrine, and antihistamines.

When dextran 40 is administered by rapid infusion, monitoring of central venous pressure is advised as an estimate of blood volume status. Normal CVP: 5 to 10 cm H_2O.

Observe patient for clinical signs of circulatory overload (shortness of breath, wheezing, coughing, marked increase in pulse and respiratory rate, sensation of chest pressure).

In patients for whom sodium restriction is indicated, it should be noted that 500 ml of dextran 40 in 0.9% normal saline contains 77 mEq of both sodium and chloride.

Monitor pulse, blood pressure, and urine output every 5 to 15 minutes for the first hour and hourly thereafter while indicated. Report oliguria or anuria or lack of improvement of urinary output (dextran usually causes an increase in urinary output).

Check urine specific gravity at regular intervals (normal: 1.005 to 1.025).Renal excretion of dextran produces minor elevations of urine viscosity and specific gravity in patients with adequate urine flow, but marked elevations occur in patients with diminished urine flow. Low urine specific gravity may signify failure of renal dextran clearance and is an indication for discontinuing therapy.

In poorly hydrated patients dextran may attract water from extravascular spaces and cause dehydration (elevated temperature, dry skin and mucous membranes, scant urinary output, specific gravity) above 1.030, elevated Hgb.

Transient prolongation of bleeding time and interference with normal blood coagulation may occur when high doses are administered. Patients who have had major surgery or trauma are particularly susceptible to increased blood loss.

Hepatitis virus is not transmitted by dextran.

When blood samples are drawn for study, notify laboratory that patient has received dextran. See Laboratory Test Interferences.

Dextran should be stored at a constant temperature, preferably 25 C (77F) to prevent crystallization. Once opened, unused portion should be discarded because dextran contains no preservative.

Compatibility of dextran with added solutions or medications not established.

LABORATORY TEST INTERFERENCES: Dextran may cause false increases in **blood glucose** values (ortho-toluidine methods or determinations employing sulfuric or acetic acid hydrolysis). Possibility of false increases in **urinary protein** determinations (Lowry method), **bilirubin** assays (when alcohol is used), and **total protein assays** (biuret reagent). May interfere with **blood typing** and **cross-matching** procedures when proteolytic enzyme techniques are used (saline agglutination and indirect antiglobulin methods reportedly not affected).

DEXTRAN 70
(MACRODEX)
DEXTRAN 75
(GENTRAN 75)

Plasma volume expander

ACTIONS AND USES
High-molecular-weight polymers of glucose. Dextran 70 has an average molecular weight of 70,000; that of dextran 75 is 75,000 (molecular weight range for both: 20,000 to 200,000). Colloidal properties approximate those of serum albumin. They differ from dextran 40 in molecular weight, and have less effect on rouleaux formation and sludging of red blood cells and less severe adverse reactions.
Used primarily for emergency treatment of hypovolemic shock or impending shock caused by hemorrhage, burns, surgery, or other trauma. Intended for emergency treatment only when whole blood or blood products are not available or when haste precludes cross matching of blood.

ABSORPTION AND FATE
Produces plasma volume expansion slightly in excess of volume infused, approximately 1 hour after infusion; decreases over succeeding 24 hours, depending on renal clearance rate. Dextran molecules with molecular weights less than 50,000 are excreted by kidneys (approximately 40% of dose within 24 hours in patients with normal renal function). Molecules with molecular weights of 50,000 or greater are slowly degraded to dextrose and eliminated as carbon dioxide and water.

CONTRAINDICATIONS AND PRECAUTIONS
Known hypersensitivity to dextran, severe bleeding disorders, severe congestive failure, renal failure. See Dextran 40.

ADVERSE REACTIONS
Allergic reactions, severe and fatal anaphylactoid reaction, lowered plasma protein levels (high doses). Also see Dextran 40.

ROUTE AND DOSAGE
Intravenous infusion: 500 ml. Total daily dosage should not exceed 20 ml/kg body weight during first 24 hours. If therapy continues beyond 24 hours, total daily dosage should not exceed 10 ml/kg body weight.

NURSING IMPLICATIONS
Use only if seal is intact, vacuum is detectable, and solution is absolutely clear.
Specific flow rate should be prescribed by physician. (For emergency treatment of shock, rate of administration for first 500 ml may be 20 to 40 ml/minute. In normovolemic patients flow rate should not exceed 4 ml/minute.)
Bleeding time may be temporarily prolonged in patients receiving more than 1000 ml of dextran 70 or 75.

Patient should be closely observed during first few minutes of infusion for evidence of allergic or anaphylactoid reactions. Severe reactions occasionally have resulted in fatalities.
See Dextran 40.

DEXTROAMPHETAMINE HYDROCHLORIDE
(DARO)
DEXTROAMPHETAMINE SULFATE, U.S.P.
(DEXAMPEX, DEXEDRINE, FERNDEX)
DEXTROAMPHETAMINE TANNATE
(OBOTAN)

Central stimulant

ACTIONS AND USES
Dextroamphetamine is the dextrorotatory isomer of amphetamine (qv), with which it shares actions, uses, contraindications, precautions, and adverse reactions. On a weight basis, has less pronounced action on cardiovascular and peripheral nervous systems and is a more potent appetite suppressant. CNS stimulating effect approximately twice that of racemic amphetamine.
Used primarily as adjunct in short-term treatment of exogenous obesity, narcolepsy, and minimal brain dysfunction in children (ie, hyperkinetic behavior disorders).
ADVERSE REACTIONS
Drug effect on laboratory values: significant elevations in plasma corticosteroids (increase greater in evening than in morning), increased urinary epinephrine excretion during first 3 hours after drug administration. See Amphetamine.
ROUTE AND DOSAGE
Oral: **Adults** (*anorexiant*): 2.5 to 10 mg 1 to 3 times a day. Sustained-release form: 1 or 2 capsules daily. *Narcolepsy*: 5 to 60 mg/day in divided doses. **Children**: 2 to 15 mg/day divided into 3 doses or as a single dose of sustained release form.

NURSING IMPLICATIONS
Administered 30 to 60 minutes before meals for treatment of obesity. Long-acting form is administered in the morning.
Tolerance to anorexigenic effects may develop after a few weeks.
To avoid insomnia, administer last dose no later than 6 hours before patient retires.
Classified as Schedule II drug under Controlled Substances Act. High abuse potential in common with other amphetamines.
Dextroamphetamine is a constituent of several combination preparations, eg, Amphaplex, Delcobese, Dexamyl, Eskatrol.
See Amphetamine Sulphate

DEXTROMETHORPHAN HYDROBROMIDE, N.F., B.P.
(CONGESPIRIN, COUGH SYRUP, DORMETHAN, PINETUSS DM, ROMILAR, TUSSADE, and others)

Antitussive

ACTIONS AND USES
Nonnarcotic derivative of levorphanol. Chemically related to morphine, but without its hypnotic or analgesic effect and capacity to cause tolerance or

addiction. Controls cough spasms by depressing cough center in medulla. Does not depress respiration or inhibit ciliary action. Antitussive activity comparable to that of codeine and is less likely than codeine to cause constipation.

Used for temporary relief of cough spasms in nonproductive coughs due to colds, pertussis, and influenza.

ABSORPTION AND FATE

Antitussive action begins in 15 to 30 minutes and lasts 3 to 6 hours.

CONTRAINDICATIONS AND PRECAUTIONS

Sensitivity, children under 2 years of age, concomitant use of MAO inhibitors. Cautious use: productive cough.

ADVERSE REACTIONS

Rare: dizziness, drowsiness, GI upset.

ROUTE AND DOSAGE

Oral: **Adults:** 10 to 20 mg every 4 hours or 30 mg every 6 to 8 hours. **Children** *6 to 12 years*: 5 to 10 mg every 4 hours or 15 mg every 6 to 8 hours; *2 to 6 years*: 2.5 to 5 mg every 4 hours or 7.5 mg every 6 to 8 hours.

NURSING IMPLICATIONS

Soothing local effect of the syrup is enhanced if it is administered undiluted and not immediately followed by water.

Excessive, nonproductive cough tends to be self-perpetuating because it causes irritation of pharyngeal and tracheal mucosa.

Unnecessary cough may be lessened by voluntary restraint and by avoiding irritants such as smoking, dust, fumes, and other air pollutants. Humidification of ambient air may provide some relief.

Locally acting sialagogues (eg, hard candy) may help to relieve cough produced by irritation of pharyngeal mucosa.

Treatment is directed toward decreasing the frequency and intensity of cough without completely eliminating protective cough reflex.

Dextromethorphan may be purchased over the counter. Persons who self-medicate should be advised that symptom suppression does not mean cure of the underlying problem. Any cough persisting longer than 1 week or 10 days should be medically diagnosed.

DRUG INTERACTIONS: Concurrent administration of dextromethorphan and **MAO inhibitors** may result in CNS excitation and depression leading to death.

DEXTROTHYROXINE SODIUM, N.F.
(CHOLOXIN, *D*-Thyroxine)

Anticholesteremic

ACTIONS AND USES

Sodium salt of dextrorotatory isomer of thyroxine. In both euthyroids and hypothyroids, it reduces serum cholesterol levels in hyperlipidemia; triglycerides, alpha- and beta-lipoproteins may also be lowered from previously elevated levels. By means of an unclear mechanism, liver is stimulated to increase catabolism and excretion of cholesterol without significantly increasing BMR, or affecting cholesterol synthesis. Greatest decrease in serum cholesterol occurs in patients with highest baseline concentrations, with maximum therapeutic effects in 1 or 2 months. Has little effect on elevated pre-beta-lipoprotein levels. Margin between effective and toxic doses is narrow.

Used to treat hypothyroidism in patients with cardiac disease unable to tolerate other types of thyroid medication; as adjunct to diet and other measures to lower serum cholesterol concentrations in type II hyper-beta-lipoproteinemia in euthyroid patients with no evidence of cardiac disease. It has not been determined whether drug-induced lowering of serum cholesterol or other lipids has beneficial, detrimental, or no effects on morbidity or mortality due to atherosclerosis or coronary heart disease.

ABSORPTION AND FATE

Absorbed from GI tract. Loosely bound to plasma proteins; metabolized in liver. Rapidly excreted in urine and feces in approximately equal amounts as intact drug and metabolites. Small amounts excreted in breast milk.

CONTRAINDICATIONS AND PRECAUTIONS

In euthyroids: known organic heart disease including angina pectoris; arrhythmias, decompensated or borderline compensated cardiac states; history of myocardial infarction or congestive heart failure; rheumatic heart disease, hypertension, advanced liver or kidney disease, history of iodism; pregnancy, nursing mothers; at least 2 weeks prior to elective surgery. Cautious use: hypothyroid patients with concomitant coronary artery disease; women of childbearing age with familial hypercholesterolemia; diabetes mellitus.

ADVERSE REACTIONS

Low incidence in euthyroid patients without cardiac disease; higher in hypothyroid patients, especially if organic heart disease is present. **Cardiovascular**: angina pectoris, cardiac arrhythmia, ECG evidence of ischemic myocardial changes, increase in heart size; myocardial infarction (relationship to drug effect not known). **Signs of hypermetabolism**: nervousness, weakness, lid lag, insomnia, tremors, twitching, intolerance to heat, hyperpyrexia, flushing, sweating, palpitation, tachycardia, weight loss, altered taste sensation, anorexia, nausea, vomiting, diarrhea, constipation, menstrual irregularities, exophthalmos. **Iodism**: acneiform rash, pruritus, coryza, conjunctivitis, stomatitis, brassy taste, laryngitis, bronchitis. Other: dizziness, tinnitus, vertigo, diuresis, peripheral edema, malaise, fatigue, headache, hoarseness, visual disturbances, retinopathy, changes in libido, hair loss, psychic changes, paresthesias, muscle pain, various subjective complaints; gallstones and cholestatic jaundice (causal relationship not established), increased blood sugar levels (diabetic patients), elevated PBI, depressed I^{131} uptake, worsening of peripheral vascular disease, changes in intellectual functioning.

ROUTE AND DOSAGE

Oral: **Adults:** initially 1 or 2 mg daily, increased in 1- or 2-mg increments at intervals of not less than 1 month to a maximum level of 4 to 8 mg daily, if indicated. **Children:** initially approximately 0.05 mg/kg daily, increased by 0.05-mg/kg daily at monthly intervals. Recommended maximal daily dose is 4 mg, if indicated.

NURSING IMPLICATIONS

Goal of therapy in hypercholesterolemia is to prevent further atherosclerosis, not merely to lower serum lipids. Encourage patient to adhere to diet regimen, an important adjunct to therapeutic plan.

Before initiation of therapy, a complete health history (personal, family, dietary) as well as physical examination and appropriate laboratory studies should be obtained.

Since hyperlipoproteinemia is frequently genetically determined, family members of patient, especially children 5 years and older, should be screened for abnormal lipid values to permit early treatment if indicated.

Serum lipids should be determined initially and evaluated at monthly intervals during therapy. Patient should be on a normal diet for several days prior to the test.

Cholesterol and triglyceride values are age-related: average normal total cholesterol is 150 to 250 mg/dl; triglycerides, 10 to 190 mg/dl.

Initial decrease in cholesterol levels may not occur until 2 weeks to 1 month after initiation of therapy. Maximum decrease usually occurs during second or third month of therapy.

Elevation of serum protein-bound iodine (PBI) levels in patients receiving dextrothyroxine is evidence of drug absorption and transport rather than hypermetabolism. A PBI range of 10 to 25 μg/dl in treated patients is common (Normal: 4 to 8 μg/dl).

Patients with diabetes should be closely monitored. Dosage adjustment of antidiabetic agent may be required on initiation and on withdrawal of dextrothyroxine. Advise patients to report diminishing control of diabetes (glycosuria, hyperglycemic episode, polydipsia, diuresis).

Patients with cardiac disease should be observed closely during dose adjustment period and seen at frequent intervals throughout therapy.

No more than 4 mg/day dextrothyroxine should be given to a patient already receiving digitalis because of danger of additive effects on oxygen requirements of myocardium.

Report immediately new signs and symptoms of cardiac disease or increased decompensation in the borderline compensated patient, eg, dyspnea, pain on exercise, nocturnal cough, increased use of nitroglycerin to relieve angina, edema, palpitation, arrhythmias. Dosage should be reduced or drug discontinued.

Teratogenic studies have been inconclusive; thus strict birth control measures are advised for the woman of childbearing potential receiving dextrothyroxine.

Advise patient to report promptly the onset of iodism (see Adverse Reactions). If iodism is developing, the drug will be withdrawn.

Drug therapy in children with familial hypercholesterolemia should continue only if a significant serum cholesterol lowering effect is achieved.

DRUG INTERACTIONS: Patients treated concurrently with **oral anticoagulants** and dextrothyroxine may require reduction in anticoagulant dosage within 1 to 4 weeks after initiation of dextrothyroxine therapy. Close monitoring of prothrombin time is required. Dextrothyroxine may elevate blood glucose in diabetic patients, with resulting increased requirement for **antidiabetic drugs. Cholestyramine** may significantly decrease absorption of dextrothyroxine when used concurrently; administration should be spaced as far apart as possible (optimally 5 hours).

DIAZEPAM, U.S.P., B.P.
(VALIUM)

Antianxiety agent (minor tranquilizer), anticonvulsant, skeletal muscle relaxant

ACTIONS AND USES

Benzodiazepine derivative related to chlordiazepoxide. Reportedly superior to chlordiazepoxide in antianxiety and anticonvulsant activity, with somewhat shorter duration of action. Like chlordiazepoxide, appears to act at limbic and subcortical levels of CNS, producing sedative, skeletal muscle relaxant, and anticonvulsant effects. May produce transient retrograde amnesia when administered IV.

Used in psychoneurotic reactions manifested by tension and anxiety alone or with depressive symptoms or agitation; and to allay anxiety and tension prior to surgery, cardioversion, and endoscopic procedures; and to alleviate acute withdrawal symptoms of alcoholism. Used as adjunct for relief of skeletal muscle spasm accompanying neurologic disorders such as cerebral palsy and paraplegia or caused by local pathology. Also used adjunctively in status epilepticus, severe recurrent convulsive seizures, and tetanus.

ABSORPTION AND FATE

Onset of action in 30 to 60 minutes after oral administration and in 15 to 30 minutes after IM injection. More rapid onset following IV injection; effects may persist up to 3 hours.

Following absorption from GI tract, peak plasma concentrations occur in 2 to 4 hours. Metabolized in liver and excreted as metabolites in urine and small amount in feces. One portion excreted rapidly (half-life 7 to 10 hours); remaining portion excreted slowly (half-life 2 to 8 days). Crosses placenta and appears in breast milk.

CONTRAINDICATIONS AND PRECAUTIONS

Hypersensitivity to diazepam, use of injectable form in infants under 30 days of age or tablet form in children under 6 months of age, acute-angle glaucoma, shock, coma, psychoses, acute alcoholic intoxication with depressed vital signs. Safe use during pregnancy and lactation and in women of childbearing age not established. Cautious use: peroral endoscopic procedures, impaired hepatic or renal function, addiction-prone individuals. Injectable diazepam used with extreme caution in the elderly, the very ill, and patients with limited pulmonary reserve.

ADVERSE REACTIONS

CNS: drowsiness (common), fatigue, ataxia, confusion, dizziness, vertigo, amnesia, increase in vivid dreams, headache, slurred speech, syncope, tremor, muscle weakness. **Cardiovascular**: bradycardia, hypotension, tachycardia, edema, cardiovascular collapse. **Eyes**: blurred vision, diplopia, nystagmus. **GI**: nausea, constipation, changes in salivation. **Genitourinary**: incontinence, urinary retention, changes in libido. **Other**: skin rashes, urticaria, hiccups, coughing, throat and chest pain, laryngospasm (peroral endoscopic procedures); menstrual irregularities, neutropenia, hepatic dysfunction including jaundice; pain following IM injection; local irritation, thrombosis, phlebitis at IV site. With rapid IV, respiratory depression, apnea, cardiac arrest. Paradoxic reactions in psychiatric patients.

ROUTE AND DOSAGE

Adults: Oral: 2 to 10 mg 2 to 4 times a day. Intramuscular, intravenous (preferred): 2 to 10 mg repeated in 3 to 4 hours if necessary. IV injection rate should not exceed 5 mg (1 ml) per minute. Small veins such as on dorsum of hand or wrist should not be used because of danger of extravasation. Doses highly individualized for all routes. Lower dosage ranges recommended for elderly and debilitated patients. **Pediatric**: Oral: *Over 6 months*: initially 1 to 2.5 mg 3 or 4 times daily. Intramuscular, intravenous: *Over 30 days of age*: 1 to 2 mg every 3 to 4 hours if necessary.

NURSING IMPLICATIONS

Most adverse signs and symptoms associated with diazepam therapy are dose-related. Physician will rely on accurate observations and reporting of patient's response to the drug to determine lowest effective maintenance dose.

Drug therapy for tension and anxiety is not a substitute for sensitive, thoughtful, and unhurried communication with the patient to explore and to understand his concerns and feelings.

IM administration should be made deep into large muscle mass. Aspirate carefully before injecting drug to avoid inadvertent intraarterial administration. Inject slowly.

When given parenterally, hypotension, muscular weakness, tachycardia, and
respiratory depression may occur, particularly if alcohol, barbiturates, or
narcotics are used concomitantly. Observe patient closely and monitor
vital signs. Resuscitative equipment should be readily available.

Although they are infrequent, paradoxic reactions have been reported in
psychiatric patients. Reactions may be secondary to relief of anxiety; they
usually appear in first 2 weeks of therapy. Be on the alert for such symptoms as excitement, anxiety, acute rage, depression, hallucinations, increased muscle spasticity, and sleep disturbances. If symptoms occur, drug
should be discontinued.

Bear in mind that suicidal tendencies may be present in anxiety states accompanied by depression. Observe necessary preventive precautions.

Adverse reactions such as drowsiness, fatigue, ataxia, constipation, and urinary retention are more likely to occur in the elderly and debilitated or
in those receiving larger doses. Dosage adjustment may be necessary.
Supervision of ambulation is advisable, and possibly bedsides. Monitor
intake and output until drug dosage is stabilized.

Warn the ambulatory patient that sedation may occur during early therapy
and that he should avoid activities requiring mental alertness and precision, such as driving a car and operating machinery, until his reaction to
the drug has been evaluated.

Also caution the patient and family that alcoholic beverages, barbiturates,
and other sedative-hypnotics may augment CNS depression. Stress the
importance of taking diazepam specifically as prescribed and the potential
danger of introducing other drugs without the physician's advice.

Female patients should be advised that if they become pregnant during
therapy or intend to become pregnant they should communicate with
their physician regarding desirability of discontinuing drug.

Periodic blood cell counts and liver function tests are recommended during
prolonged therapy.

Reportedly, the pharmacologic effects of diazepam are decreased among
smokers.

Psychic and physical dependence may occur in patients on long-term high-
dosage therapy, in those with histories of alcohol or drug addiction, or in
those whose histories suggest self-medication.

Close supervision should be maintained over the amount and duration of use
of antianxiety drugs.

Abrupt drug withdrawal may produce reactions in patients on high dosages for extended periods (vomiting, sweating, abdominal and muscle cramps, tremor, convulsions). Symptoms may persist for several
weeks.

Diazepam is classified as a Schedule IV drug under the federal Controlled
Substances Act.

Do not mix or dilute parenteral diazepam with other solutions or drugs, and
do not add it to IV fluids.

Preserved in tight, light-resistant containers.

DRUG INTERACTIONS: Concurrent ingestion of diazepam and **alcohol** may
intensify the CNS depressant effect of each drug. Potentiation of CNS depression reportedly may also occur with **antihistamines, sedatives, narcotics,
MAO inhibitors, phenothiazines,** and **tricyclic antidepressants** (concomitant
use not contraindicated, but dosage adjustments may be required). Diazepam
may block therapeutic effect in some patients stabilized on **levodopa**; and may
increase the effects of **phenytoin** (diphenylhydantoin) when given concurrently. Patients receiving diazepam and **gallamine triethiodide** (and possibly
other nondepolarizing neuromuscular blocking agents, eg, **pancuronium, suc-**

DIAZOXIDE, U.S.P.
(HYPERSTAT I.V., PROGLYCEM)

Antihypertensive, glucose elevating agent

ACTIONS AND USES

Rapid-acting benzothiadiazine (thiazide) nondiuretic hypotensive agent. In contrast to thiazide diuretics, it causes sodium and water retention and decreased urinary output, probably because of increased proximal tubular reabsorption of sodium and decreased glomerular filtration rate. Like thiazide diuretics, it produces hyperglycemia by inhibiting pancreatic insulin secretion and by catecholamine-induced glycogenesis. Reduces peripheral vascular resistance and blood pressure by direct vasodilatory effect on peripheral arteriolar smooth muscles, perhaps by direct competition for calcium receptor sites. Hypotensive effect may be accompanied by increased heart rate, cardiac output, and renal blood flow. May also inhibit ureteral and gastrointestinal motility, as well as uterine contractions; may cause an increase in renin secretion and a decrease in plasma free fatty acid levels.

Used intravenously for emergency lowering of blood pressure in hospitalized patients with malignant hypertension, particularly when associated with renal impairment. Not effective in pheochromocytoma. Used orally in treatment of various diagnosed hypoglycemic states due to hyperinsulinism when other medical treatment or surgical management has been unsuccessful or is not feasible.

ABSORPTION AND FATE

Rapid IV injection of 300-mg bolus dose produces fall in blood pressure in 30 to 60 seconds, with maximal effect within 5 minutes and duration 2 to 12 hours or longer. Following oral administration, hyperglycemic effect begins within 1 hour and may last up to 8 hours if renal function is normal. Plasma half-life (limited data): 24 to 36 hours in adults, 9.5 to 24 hours in children. Highly bound (about 90%) to plasma albumin; may displace other substances or drugs also bound to proteins. Average plasma half-life approximately 28 hours. Crosses placenta and appears in breast milk. Slowly excreted in urine.

CONTRAINDICATIONS AND PRECAUTIONS

Hypersensitivity to thiazides; eclampsia; aortic coarctation; A-V shunt. Safe use during pregnancy and in nursing mothers and use of parenteral drug in children not established. Use of oral diazoxide for functional hypoglycemia or in presence of increased bilirubin in newborns. Cautious use: diabetes mellitus, impaired cerebral or cardiac circulation, impaired renal function, patients taking corticosteroids or estrogen-progestogen combinations, history of gout.

ADVERSE REACTIONS

GI: nausea, vomiting, diarrhea, constipation, ileus, anorexia, transient loss of taste, parotid swelling. **Ophthalmic**: blurred vision, transient cataracts, subconjunctival hemorrhage, ring scotoma, diplopia, lacrimation. **Dermatologic**: skin rash, monilial dermatitis, herpes, hypertrichosis (especially in children), loss of scalp hair, hirsutism. **Neurologic**: headache, polyneuritis, sleepiness, euphoria, anxiety, cerebral ischemia, paresthesias, extrapyramidal signs. **Cardiovascular**: palpitations, arrhythmias, flushing, hypotension with lightheadedness, dizziness, myocardial ischemia. **Other**: sensitivity reactions; impaired renal and hepatic function; chest and back pain, muscle cramps; acute pancreatitis; advance in bone age (children); sodium and water retention, hyperglycemia, glycosuria, diabetic ketoacidosis and coma; thrombocytopenia (with or without purpura), transient neutropenia; galactorrhea; decrease in hemoglobin, hematocrit, or IgG; decreased PAH excretion; elevated serum uric acid and free fatty acid levels.

ROUTE AND DOSAGE

Treatment of hypertension: Intravenous: **Adults only**: 300 mg administered undiluted over 30 seconds or less. Additional dose if no response within 30 minutes. Subsequent doses at 4- to 24-hour intervals depending on patient's response. *Treatment of hypoglycemia*: Oral: **Adults and children**: 3 to 8 mg/kg divided into 2 or 3 equal doses every 8 or 12 hours. **Infants and newborns**: Oral: 8 to 15 mg/kg divided into 2 or 3 equal doses every 8 or 12 hours. Highly individualized.

NURSING IMPLICATIONS

Treatment of hypertension (intravenous preparation):

Blood glucose, serum electrolytes, and complete blood counts should be determined at start of therapy and regularly thereafter in patients receiving multiple doses.

Patient should be recumbent while receiving IV diazoxide and should remain in bed for at least 30 minutes following administration.

Monitor blood pressure closely until stabilized, then hourly for balance of drug effect. In ambulatory patients, blood pressure measurement should be made with patient in standing position, before ending surveillance.

Since diazoxide causes sodium and water retention, a diuretic is generally prescribed in patients receiving multiple doses for treatment of hypertension to avoid congestive heart failure and drug resistance and to maximize hypotensive effect.

When a diuretic is administered in conjunction with IV diazoxide, patient should remain recumbent 8 to 10 hours because of possible additive hypotensive effect.

Intake and output should be monitored. Report promptly any change in intake–output ratio, constipation, abdominal distension, or absence of bowel sounds.

If feasible, daily weight provides another objective measure of fluid retention or mobilization.

Observe patient closely for signs and symptoms of congestive heart failure (distended neck veins, rales at bases of lungs, dyspnea, orthopnea, cough, fatigue, weakness, dependent edema).

Diazoxide may cause hyperglycemia and glycosuria in diabetic and diabetic-prone individuals. Dosage adjustment of antidiabetic drugs may be required. Closely monitor urine for sugar.

Check intravenous injection sites daily. Extravasation of medication into subcutaneous or intramuscular tissues can cause severe inflammatory reaction.

Treatment of hypoglycemia (oral preparation):

During initial therapy, patient should be closely supervised, with blood glucose, serum electrolytes, and clinical response being carefully monitored until condition stabilizes satisfactorily on minimum dosage. Blood glucose level should be determined periodically thereafter to evaluate need of dosage adjustment. Serum electrolyte levels should be evaluated in patient with impaired renal function.

In contrast to IV administration of diazoxide, oral administration does not usually produce marked effects on blood pressure. However, periodic measurements of blood pressure and other vital signs should be made.

Monitor intake–output ratio and weight. Diazoxide promotes sodium and water retention, most commonly in young infants and in adults, and may precipitate congestive failure in patients with compromised cardiac reserve.

Patients on prolonged therapy should be taught to monitor urine for sugar and ketones, especially during stress conditions, and instructed to report abnormal findings to physician. Hyperglycemia may require reduction in dosage or treatment with hypoglycemic agent to avoid progression to ketoacidosis.

Ketoacidosis and hyperosmolar coma have been reported in patients treated with recommended doses, usually during an intercurrent illness. Insulin therapy and restoration of fluid and electrolyte balance are usually effective if instituted promptly. Prolonged surveillance is essential because of long half-life of diazoxide (approximately 30 hours). In the event of overdosage, surveillance as long as 7 days may be required.

Lanugo type hirsutism (mainly on forehead, back, limbs) occurs frequently and is most common in children and women (reversible with discontinuation of drug).

In some patients, higher diazoxide levels are attained with liquid than with capsule formulation. Dosage may require adjustment if patient is changed from one formulation to another.

Diazoxide is discontinued if not effective in 2 or 3 weeks.

Protect diazoxide from light, heat, and freezing. Suspension formula should be shaken well before use.

DRUG INTERACTIONS: Concomitant administration of **thiazide diuretics** may intensify hyperglycemic and hyperuricemic effects of diazoxide. Antihypertensive effect of drug may be enhanced when administered with **antihypertensive agents** or other drugs that cause elevated blood pressure. Possibility of altered anticoagulant effect when diazoxide is started or stopped in patient receiving **oral anticoagulants.**

DICHLORPHENAMIDE, U.S.P., B.P.
(DARANIDE, ORATROL)

Carbonic anhydrase inhibitor

ACTIONS AND USES

Nonbacteriostatic sulfonamide derivative similar to acetazolamide, but with more prolonged action. Contraindications, precautions, and adverse reactions as for acetazolamide (qv).

Used in adjunctive treatment of open-angle (chronic simple) glaucoma or secondary glaucoma and preoperatively in acute-angle closure glaucoma when delay of surgery is desired in order to lower intraocular pressure. Commonly used in conjunction with a miotic.

ABSORPTION AND FATE

Onset of action within 1 hour; peaks in 2 to 4 hours and lasts 6 to 12 hours.

ROUTE AND DOSAGE

Oral: initially 100 to 200 mg, followed by 100 mg every 12 hours until desired response is obtained; maintenance 25 to 50 mg 1 to 3 times daily.

NURSING IMPLICATIONS
See Acetazolamide.

(DYCILL, DYNAPEN, PATHOCIL, VERACILLIN)

Antibacterial

ACTIONS AND USES

Semisynthetic penicillinase-resistant isoxazolyl penicillin. Mechanism of antibacterial action as for penicillin G potassium. Blood levels claimed to be higher than those attained by equivalent doses of other oral penicillins and comparable to those attained with similar IM doses of penicillin G potassium.

Used primarily in treatment of infections caused by penicillinase-producing staphylococci, but may also be used to initiate therapy in suspected staphylococcal infection pending culture and sensitivity results.

ABSORPTION AND FATE

Peak plasma concentrations in 1 hour; effective level maintained 4 to 6 hours. About 90% to 95% protein-bound. Excreted primarily in urine; small amounts eliminated by liver through bile. Crosses placenta.

CONTRAINDICATIONS AND PRECAUTIONS

Hypersensitivity to penicillins or cephalosporins. Safe use during pregnancy and in neonates not established. Cautious use: history of allergies, asthma.

ADVERSE REACTIONS

Nausea, vomiting, flatulence, diarrhea, pruritus, urticaria, wheezing. Generally well tolerated, but same potential for adverse effects as other penicillins. See Penicillin G Potassium.

ROUTE AND DOSAGE

Oral: **Adults and children** *weighing 40 kg or more*: 125 to 250 mg or higher every 6 hours. **Children** *under 40 kg*: 12.5 to 25 mg/kg/day or higher in equally divided doses every 6 hours.

NURSING IMPLICATIONS

Careful inquiry should be made concerning previous hypersensitivity reactions to penicillins, cephalosporins, and other allergens.

Administer 1 or 2 hours before meals (preferably) or 2 hours after meals. Food reduces absorption.

Periodic assessments of renal, hepatic, and hematopoietic functions should be made in patients on prolonged therapy.

Reconstituted oral suspension is stable for 14 days under refrigeration. Shake well before using.

See Penicillin G Potassium.

DICUMAROL, U.S.P.
(DICOUMAROL, DICOUMARIN, Bishydroxycoumarin)

Anticoagulant

ACTIONS AND USES

Long-acting coumarin derivative. Similar to other drugs of this series in actions, uses, contraindications, precautions, and adverse reactions. See Warfarin.

ABSORPTION AND FATE

Slowly and incompletely absorbed from GI tract. Onset of action in 1 to 2 days; peak effect 3 to 5 days; duration 2 to 10 days. Excreted in urine largely as metabolites; small amounts excreted in stool as unchanged drug. Crosses placenta and enters breast milk.

Oral: initially 200 to 300 mg; maintenance 25 to 200 mg daily. Dosages based on prothrombin time determinations and clinical findings.

NURSING IMPLICATIONS

During period of dosage adjustment, prothrombin time results should be checked daily by physician, and dose order should be obtained. Follow hospital policies regarding administration of anticoagulants.

When patient is controlled on maintenance dose, prothrombin times may be checked semiweekly, weekly, or at 2- to 4-week intervals, depending on stability of patient's response.

See Warfarin.

DICYCLOMINE HYDROCHLORIDE, U.S.P.
(BENTYL, DIBENT, DYSPAS, OR-TYL)

Anticholinergic

ACTIONS AND USES

Synthetic antispasmodic agent. Effect on smooth muscle appears to be more musculotropic than anticholinergic; thus atropinelike side effects are generally slight with average dosage. Does not produce ganglionic blockade or reduce gastric secretions. Relieves smooth-muscle spasm in GI and biliary tracts, uterus, and ureters. Exhibits local anesthetic properties.

Used adjunctively in treatment of irritable bowel syndrome, neurogenic bowel disturbances, and infant colic. There are varied opinions about its value in treatment of peptic ulcer because of uncertainty as to its specific action.

ABSORPTION AND FATE

Readily absorbed after oral or parenteral administration. Almost completely metabolized and eliminated in urine; small percentage excreted as unchanged drug.

CONTRAINDICATIONS AND PRECAUTIONS

Obstructive diseases of GU and GI tracts, paralytic ileus, intestinal atony, biliary tract disease, unstable cardiovascular status, severe ulcerative colitis, toxic megacolon, myasthenia gravis. Cautious use: glaucoma, prostatic hypertrophy, autonomic neuropathy, ulcerative colitis, hyperthyroidism, coronary heart disease, congestive heart failure, arrhythmias, hypertension, hiatal hernia associated with esophageal reflux.

ADVERSE REACTIONS

Transient dizziness, brief euphoria, bloated feeling. Atropinelike side effects are usually minimal with average doses, but may be prominent with large doses. Overdosage: curarelike effect. See Atropine Sulfate.

ROUTE AND DOSAGE

Adults: Oral: 10 to 20 mg 3 or 4 times daily. **Children:** 10 mg 3 or 4 times daily. **Infants:** 5 mg 3 or 4 times daily (oral liquid formulation may be diulted with equal volume of water). **Adults:** Intramuscular: 20 mg every 4 to 6 hours.

NURSING IMPLICATIONS

Since dicyclomine may produce drowsiness and blurred vision, caution the patient to avoid activities requiring mental alertness, such as operating a motor vehicle or dangerous machinery, until his reaction to the drug is known.

Instruct the patient to report changes in urinary volume or pattern.

See Atropine Sulfate.

(DV, ESTRAGUARD, SYNESTROL)

Estrogen

ACTIONS AND USES

Synthetic nonsteroidal estrogen structurally related to diethylstilbestrol. Shares actions of estradiol (qv).

Used for treatment of atrophic vaginitis and related disorders, for postpartum breast engorgement, and for palliative treatment of advanced carcinoma of female breast and prostatic carcinoma. Also used for habitual and threatened abortion, menopausal symptoms, and uterine bleeding. See Estradiol.

ABSORPTION, FATE, CONTRAINDICATIONS, PRECAUTIONS, AND ADVERSE REACTIONS

See Estradiol.

ROUTE AND DOSAGE

Oral (tablets): 0.1 to 1.5 mg daily. (Dose may be as high as 15 mg daily for treatment of mammary and prostatic carcinoma.) Topical (vaginal cream 0.01%): 1 or 2 applicatorsful daily for 1 to 2 weeks. Dosage then reduced to half of initial dose for another 1- or 2-week period. Topical (foam, 0.01% dienestrol in an oil-in-water emulsion in aerosol): 1 to 2 applicatorsful daily for 2 weeks, then reduce to half initial dose for another 1 to 2 weeks. Vaginal suppository (0.7 mg): 1 or 2 daily. All dosage regimens highly individualized.

NURSING IMPLICATIONS

Dienestrol absorption through vaginal mucosa (use of cream, foam, or suppository) is possible; overdosage may stimulate bleeding in menopausal women. Advise patient to follow directions carefully and not to overdose.

The initial dose given to control uterine bleeding (5 to 20 mg 4 times daily) is continued until bleeding is controlled. Dose is then reduced (5 to 15 mg daily for 25 days). If withdrawal bleeding does not occur within 2 to 8 days after last dose, or if bleeding is profuse, 5 to 10 mg daily will be continued for an additional 25 days.

Sudden discontinuation of drug may cause breast tenderness and withdrawal bleeding in some women. Instruct patient to consult physician should these symptoms occur.

Protect all formulations from light.

See Estradiol.

DIETHYLPROPION HYDROCHLORIDE, N.F.
(D.E.P.-75, NU-DISPOZ, RO-DIET, TENUATE, TEPANIL, WEH-LESS TIMECELLES)

Anorexiant

ACTIONS AND USES

Sympathomimetic amine (adrenergic) similar to amphetamine (qv) in action. Lower incidence of amphetamine-type adverse effects, but also less effective as anorexiant. Anorexigenic effect probably secondary to CNS stimulation.

Used solely in management of exogenous obesity as short-term (a few weeks) adjunct in a regimen of weight reduction based on caloric restriction.

ABSORPTION AND FATE

Readily absorbed from GI tract. Effects persist about 4 hours; however, bioavailability of controlled-release formulations may not be uniform. Excreted in urine.

Known hypersensitivity or idiosyncrasy to sympathomimetic amines, severe hypertension, advanced arteriosclerosis, symptomatic cardiovascular disease, hyperthyroidism, glaucoma, agitated states, history of drug abuse, during or within 14 days following use of MAO inhibitors, concomitant use of CNS stimulants. Safe use during pregnancy and in children under 12 years of age not established. Cautious use: hypertension, arrhythmias, symptomatic cardiovascular disease, epilepsy.

ADVERSE REACTIONS

Muscle pain, dyspnea, hair loss, polyuria, dysuria, increased sweating, insomnia, gynecomastia, menstrual irregularities, psychoses, bone marrow depression, increase in convulsive episodes in patients with epilepsy. Also see Amphetamine.

ROUTE AND DOSAGE

Oral: 25 mg 3 times daily, 1 hour before meals. Alternatively, controlled-release preparation: 75 mg daily in midmorning.

NURSING IMPLICATIONS

Additional dose sometimes prescribed in midevening to control nighttime hunger. Rarely causes insomnia except in high doses.

Controlled-release formulations should be swallowed whole and not chewed.

Anorexigenic effect seldom lasts more than a few weeks. If tolerance develops, drug should be discontinued.

Classified as Schedule IV drug under the federal Controlled Substances Act. Drugs related to amphetamines are frequently misused by emotionally unstable individuals.

Since dizziness, drowsiness, and sedation may occur, caution the patient to avoid operating machinery or driving a car or other hazardous activities.

See Amphetamine Sulfate.

DIETHYLSTILBESTROL, U.S.P.

(ACNESTROL, CYREN A, DES, DICORVIN, DOMESTROL, FONATOL, PALESTROL, STILBESTROL)

Estrogen

ACTIONS AND USES

Reportedly the most potent nonsteroidal synthetic estrogen compound. Has strong teratogenic potential; may cause vaginal or cervical cancer in offspring if mother is treated with diethylstilbestrol during pregnancy. Interferes with implantation of fertilized ovum in uterus by unclear mechanism; does not terminate pregnancy. Suppresses lactation. Excessive or prolonged use may inhibit anterior pituitary secretions. Basis for use in treatment of acne vulgaris is to help counteract stimulative effect of a relative or actual excess of androgen on sebaceous glands and hair follicles.

Used in treatment of estrogen deficiency states, including menopausal symptoms, postmenopausal and senile vulvovaginitis, atrophic vaginitis, pruritus vulvae, and prostatic carcinoma. Combined with methyltestosterone in several formulations for additive effects. Topical applications possibly effective in treatment of cystic-type acne vulgaris, oily skin, and premenstrual acnegenic exacerbations.

See Estradiol.

CONTRAINDICATIONS AND PRECAUTIONS

Hypersensitivity to any components; use as postcoital contraceptive; malignancies or precarcinomatous lesions (vagina, vulva, or breasts), pregnancy, blood clotting disorders, hepatic dysfunction, undiagnosed vaginal bleeding. Also see Estradiol.

ADVERSE REACTIONS

Nausea and vomiting (major side effects), thromboembolic disease. Prolonged use: gynecomastia, nipple pigmentation, testicular atrophy, loss of libido (in males), uterine bleeding, porphyria cutanea tarda, increased incidence of deaths from cardiovascular disorders in males reported. Also see Estradiol.

ROUTE AND DOSAGE

Oral: 0.1 to 15 mg daily. Highly individualized. Topical (lotion, 0.7 mg/Gm): applied 1 or 2 times daily. Vaginal suppository (0.1 to 1 mg): up to 1 mg daily for 10 to 14 days, along with oral dose; maintenance dose (without oral supplement) 1 to 5 mg weekly.

NURSING IMPLICATIONS

Cyclic therapy consisting of 3 weeks on diethylstilbestrol followed by 1 week rest period is the usual regimen for prolonged treatment of menopausal symptoms.

Nausea and vomiting are common in the menopausal group of patients receiving 1 mg or more daily. Men and nonpregnant women reportedly do not usually manifest nausea, even when doses are 3 to 5 mg daily.

Reassure the male patient that drug-induced loss of libido and development of feminine characteristics will disappear with termination of therapy.

Women should have breasts and pelvic organs examined before treatment begins and at intervals throughout therapy. Teach the patient how to examine her own breasts, and encourage her to do so on a regular monthly basis. Urge her to keep check-up appointments.

A pregnancy test is advised before the patient is started on therapy.

If the patient who has been taking diethylstilbestrol becomes pregnant, she should be advised to give serious thought to having an abortion because of the teratogenic potential.

Liver, adrenal, or thyroid function tests may be affected by estrogen therapy and should not be performed until drug has been discontinued for 2 months.

Advise the patient to report to physician promptly sudden weight gain or any soreness or tenderness in an extremity. Teach patient Homan's sign: pain in back of knee or calf when foot is forcibly dorsiflexed (early sign of venous thrombosis).

External applications of diethylstilbestrol and derivatives usually cause little or no systemic absorption, unless used excessively or for long periods of time.

The lotion should not be applied to denuded or abraded skin or to the eyes. Shake container well before application to disperse active agent evenly. Apply thin film with light massaging to affected area. Advise the patient not to continue therapy with lotion beyond the point that improvement is evident. Also advise the patient to discontinue use and consult the physician if any reaction indicating sensitivity is observed.

Store suppositories in refrigerator.

Also see Estradiol.

DIETHYLSTILBESTROL DIPHOSPHATE, U.S.P.
(STILPHOSTROL)

Estrogen

ACTIONS AND USES
Nonsteroidal synthetic estrogen with same actions, uses, absorption, fate, contraindications, and precautions as estradiol (qv). Exerts significant cytolytic action in treatment of prostatic carcinoma. Well tolerated in large doses; side effects are considerably less severe than those of diethylstilbestrol.
Used in advanced stages of prostatic cancer, especially when tolerance to other estrogenic regimens has developed.

ADVERSE REACTIONS
Nausea, vomiting, dizziness. Temporary: burning and local pain in perineal and sacral regions and at metastasis sites, abdominal cramps, gynecomastia, anemia, increased prothrombin time. See Estradiol.

ROUTE AND DOSAGE
Oral: initially 50 mg 3 times daily; increased to 200 mg or more 3 times daily, depending on patient's tolerance. Intravenous: on first day 0.5 Gm; on subsequent 5 days (or longer) 1 Gm. Dose is dissolved in 300 mg saline or 5% dextrose administered slowly at prescribed rate of flow. Maintenance 0.25 to 0.5 Gm given IV or orally once or twice weekly.

NURSING IMPLICATIONS
IV flow rate is usually adjusted so that after the first 10 to 15 minutes at 20 to 30 drops/minute the subsequent rate permits remainder to be administered in 1-hour period.
Patients should be lying down during infusion in order to reduce the incidence of dizziness.
See Estradiol.

DIGITALIS (LEAF, POWDERED), N.F.
(DIGIFORTIS, DIGITORA, PIL-DIGIS)

Cardiotonic, cardiac (or digitalis) glycoside

ACTIONS AND USES
Prepared from dried leaves of *Digitalis purpurea*. Consists primarily of three glycosides: gitalin, gitoxin, and digitoxin (which is responsible for most of its pharmacologic action). Mechanism of action unknown, but studies suggest that glycosides affect ATPases that promote passage of calcium, sodium, and potassium ions across sarcolemma. Chief effect is increased force of contraction by direct action on myocardium (positive inotropic effect). In the failing heart it increases stroke volume and cardiac output, reduces residual diastolic volume, decreases heart size, improves systemic and pulmonary circulation, and results in diuresis and reduction of venous pressures. Heart rate is slowed by direct action and by vagal action (negative chronotropic effect). Bases for use in supraventricular tachyarrhythmias include reflex vagal stimulation, depression of impulse formation at sinoatrial (S-A) node, and decreased conduction rate through atrioventricular (A-V) nodal and bundle tissues (negative dromotropic effect).
Used in treatment and prophylaxis of congestive heart failure and supraventricular tachycardias (atrial fibrillation, atrial flutter, paroxysmal atrial tachycardia).

Action begins in 2 to 4 hours, peaks in 12 to 24 hours, and diminishes over next 48 to 72 hours. Some activity persists 2 to 3 weeks. Binds to plasma proteins. Wide body distribution, with high concentrations in myocardium, intestines, liver, and kidney. Metabolized by liver; unchanged drug and metabolites excreted slowly in urine. Crosses placenta and may appear in breast milk.

CONTRAINDICATIONS AND PRECAUTIONS

Hypersensitivity to digitalis preparations; full digitalizing doses to patients on long-acting digitalis preparations during preceding 2 weeks or digoxin within 1 week; ventricular tachycardia, severe myocarditis, heart failure (from thyrotoxicosis, diphtheria, or shock), use in treatment of obesity. Cautious use: hypothyroidism, impaired renal or hepatic function, hypokalemia, hypercalcemia, acute myocardial infarction, Stokes-Adams Syndrome, hypersensitive carotid sinus, chronic constrictive pericarditis, idiopathic hypertrophic subaortic stenosis, severe pulmonary disease, myxedema, elderly or debilitated patients, pregnant women or nursing mothers, premature and immature infants, children with rheumatic carditis.

ADVERSE REACTIONS

GI: anorexia, nausea, vomiting, salivation, diarrhea, abdominal pain, bowel necrosis (rare). **CNS**: extreme fatigue, mental depression, lethargy, apathy, headache, drowsiness or insomnia, mood changes, restlessness, disorientation, confusion, nightmares, agitation, delirium, hallucinations, convulsions (rare), facial and lumbar neuralgia, paresthesias of hands and feet, generalized weakness. **Ophthalmologic**: disturbed color perception (objects appear yellow or green or, less frequently, red, brown, or blue), hazy vision, flickering dots, halos on dark objects, diplopia, amblyopia, scotomata, retrobulbar and optic neuritis. **Cardiac** (all types of arrhythmias and all grades of impaired conduction possible): ectopic beats (most common): premature ventricular contractions (PVCs) including multifocal PVCs, bigeminy and trigeminy, premature nodal and atrial contractions; paroxysmal atrial tachycardia with A-V block, sinus bradycardia, S-A block, and S-A arrest; ventricular tachycardia; ventricular fibrillation; thromboembolism (particularly in atrial fibrillation with congestive failure). **Hypersensitivity**: pruritus, urticaria, facial edema, fever, joint tenderness, eosinophilia, thrombocytopenia. Other: gynecomastia (uncommon).

ROUTE AND DOSAGE

Oral digitalization: 1.5 Gm divided into 4 equal parts and administered every 4 to 6 hours; *maintenance* 100 mg daily. Highly individualized according to individual requirements.

NURSING IMPLICATIONS

Read label carefully. Digitalis glycosides have similar names, but they differ widely in strengths and dosages.

Be familiar with the patient's baseline data (vital signs, quality of peripheral pulses, clinical symptoms, serum electrolytes) as a foundation for making sensitive assessments.

For dosage regulation the physician will rely on accurate observations and prompt reporting of signs and symptoms of toxicity and therapeutic response. Digitalis is cumulative in action.

ECG, determinations of serum electrolytes, and liver and kidney function tests should be performed prior to and periodically during digitalis glycoside therapy.

The following guidelines are especially important during the digitalization period and whenever dosage regimen is altered. Before administering digitalis preparation: (1) check laboratory reports (know what the physician regards as acceptable parameters for serum levels of digitalis, potassium, magnesium, and calcium; (2) take apical pulse 1 full minute, noting rate, rhythm, and quality (if patient is on ECG monitor, look for changes in rhythm); (3) check for signs and symptoms of toxicity.

Although a fall in ventricular rate to 60/minute in adults, 70/minute in children, is used as one criterion for withholding medication and reporting to physician, actually any change in pulse rate or rhythm should be interpreted as a sign of digitalis intoxication and should be reported (eg, a sudden increase or decrease in rate, irregular rhythm, regularization of a chronic irregular pulse).

The physician may prescribe apical-radial pulse determinations in patients with atrial fibrillation to determine pulse deficit (apical pulse minus radial pulse).

Digitalis may cause nausea and vomiting by local or central effects. Administration of drug after meals may relieve gastric distress due to local irritation but not that due to stimulation of vomiting center (toxicity).

Intake–output ratio and daily weight are excellent indicators of fluid mobilization or retention. Weigh the patient each day under standard conditions (before breakfast and defecation, after voiding, same scale, similar type clothes).

Report any changes in weight and intake–output ratio. Weight gain in excess of 1 or 2 pounds/day usually indicates fluid retention (1 pint of fluid = 1 pound). Digitalis dosage decrease is indicated in diminished renal function.

Infants and the elderly appear to be more sensitive to the actions of digitalis glycosides. Incidence of toxicity is high in these groups. Monitor these patients closely.

A dose of digitalis that was once tolerated may produce toxicity if the patient is experiencing conditions that sensitize the myocardium to cardiotonic glycosides (eg, hypokalemia, hypomagnesemia, hypercalcemia, hypoxia due to pulmonary abnormalities).

Manifestations of hypokalemia: anorexia, paresthesias, drowsiness, mental depression, polyuria, cardiac irritability with PVCs, hypoperistalsis, weakness of large muscle group, hypoactive reflexes, postural hypotension, dyspnea.

Intracellular potassium depletion may be induced by concomitant administration of insulin, diuretics that increase potassium excretion, corticosteroids, or large amounts of ingested carbohydrates or infused glucose (may cause intracellular shift of potassium, with resultant decrease in serum potassium); or it may result from prolonged nasogastric suction, diarrhea, or persistent vomiting (also see Drug Interactions).

The margin between therapeutic effect and toxic effect is extremely narrow. Report any of these early indications of digitalis intoxication: fatigue, weakness, anorexia, salivation, nausea, vomiting, diarrhea, mental depression, apathy, headache, visual disturbances, facial neuralgia, premature ventricular beats (may be experienced in some patients as palpitation, choking sensation, sinking feeling in pit of stomach, precordial pain, dizziness, faintness), CNS manifestations: confusion, anxiety, hallucinations (particularly in the elderly).

In children, cardiac arrhythmias are the more reliable signs of toxicity. Vomiting, diarrhea, neurologic and visual disturbances are rare as initial signs.

In patients with atrial fibrillation, slowing of ventricular rate may be used as a guide in digitalization. Generally the patient is considered digitalized when the apical rate is reduced between 60 and 80 beats/minute at rest and 80 to 100 beats/minute with exertion. These patients tend to tolerate large doses of digitalis; however, with resumption of sinus rhythm the same digitalis level may produce serious arrhythmias.

Therapeutic response to digitalis in congestive heart failure: relief of nausea, vomiting, anorexia, weakness, and fatigue; diuresis, with relief of dyspnea, productive cough, distended neck veins, rales, and edema; improved pulse rate and rhythm; improved peripheral pulses; increased tolerance to mild exertion. Persistence of symptoms may indicate underdigitalization.

Since most patients on digitalis glycosides will continue therapy for a lifetime, it is important to design a comprehensive teaching plan in collaboration with physician, patient, and responsible family members. Instructions (verbal and written) should cover these points: the medical problem; drug action and dosage regimen; how to keep record of drug administration by check of calender; how and when to take pulse eg, before taking digitalis and again around time of peak drug action; (omit if it causes anxiety); reportable signs and symptoms; daily weight (some physicians advise reporting weight gain of more than 3 to 5 pounds/week); diet and fluid restrictions, if any; graduated physical activity program; follow-up plans; VNA referral.

Rigid sodium restriction generally is not required except in severe forms of congestive failure. However, the physician will usually prescribe reduction of salt intake. The average American diet contains approximately 6 to 10 Gm of sodium chloride per day. This amount can be reduced 50% by eliminating salt-rich foods and not adding salt to served foods (1 teaspoon of salt contains 2.3 Gm sodium).

Salt substitutes should be prescribed only by a physician. The main ingredient is potassium chloride, eg, Co-Salt, Diasal, Neocurtasal. Not advised for patients with impaired renal function, since they tend to retain potassium.

Foods high in sodium content include the following: luncheon meats; canned, salted, or smoked meats and fish; "instant" or "quick" cooked foods; bouillon; soy sauce; Chinese foods (high in monosodium glutamate); processed cheese and cheese spreads; salted snack foods. Over-the-counter drugs high in sodium: Alka-Seltzer, Bisodol, Bromo Seltzer, Fizrin, Sal Hepatica, Fleet enema.

In communities where drinking water is high in sodium, patient should be advised to use bottled water.

Licorice in large quantities can induce salt and water retention, hypokalemia, hypertension, paresthesias, and symptoms of congestive failure. (Licorice contains glycyrrhizic acid, which resembles mineralocorticoids in chemical structure.)

Attention should also be directed to the caloric content of the diet; the physician may advise weight loss to reduce myocardial work load. If diet restrictions are prescribed, collaborate with physician, dietitian, patient, and family members.

Pamphlets supplied by the American Heart Association (contact local chapter) are excellent teaching aides. Free copies are available for professional and lay use.

Digitalis preparations are preserved in tightly covered, light-resistant containers.

DRUG INTERACTIONS: Possibility of underdigitalization when oral digitalis glycosides are given concomitantly with **barbiturates** (increase hepatic breakdown) **cholestyramine resin** (drug binding), **neomycin** (inhibits absorption), **phenylbutazone,** and **phenytoin** (increase hepatic breakdown); these drugs and digitalis should be spaced as far apart as possible. Absorption of an oral digitalis glycoside may be delayed by **antacids, antidiarrheals,** and **cathartics;** space them accordingly. There is increased possibility of cardiac arrhythmias with concomitant use of **sympathomimetic amines,** parenteral **calcium salts, reserpine** (possibly other rauwolfia alkaloids), **succinylcholine,** and **thyroid prepa-**

rations. Propranolol may potentiate digitalis-induced bradycardia. Digitalis toxicity may be enhanced by drugs that cause electrolyte loss: **amphotericin B** (K loss), **glucose infusions** in large amounts (K loss), **thiazides,** and other **potent diuretics** (loss of K, Ca, and Mg).

DIGITOXIN, U.S.P., B.P.
(CRYSTODIGIN, DE-TONE, DIGITALINE NATIVELLE, PURODIGIN)

Cardiotonic

ACTIONS AND USES
Long-acting glycoside of *Digitalis purpurea.* Has same actions, uses, precautions, and adverse reactions as digitalis (qv). Has slowest onset of action, slowest peak-effect time, and longest half-life of all digitalis glycosides. Therefore it is generally preferred for maintenance therapy rather than for rapid digitalization in emergency situations.

ABSORPTION AND FATE
Onset of action following IV administration occurs in ½ to 2 hours; maximum effect occurs at 4 to 12 hours; half-life is 5 to 7 days. Almost completely absorbed following oral administration; effects are noticeable in 2 to 4 hours and peak in 12 to 24 hours. Action begins to regress in 2 or 3 days; almost completely absent in 2 to 3 weeks, although ECG effects may persist 6 weeks after single dose. About 97% protein-bound. Primarily metabolized by liver to inactive metabolites (92%) and to digoxin and other active metabolites (8%), which are excreted in urine. Small amounts of inactive metabolites are excreted in bile and feces. Active metabolites may persist in urine 4 to 12 weeks. Only 11.4% of total body store is eliminated daily.

CONTRAINDICATIONS AND PRECAUTIONS
Full digitalizing doses in patients who have received digitalis preparations during preceding 3 weeks. Also see Digitalis.

ADVERSE REACTIONS
Thrombocytopenic purpura (rarely). Also see Digitalis.

ROUTE AND DOSAGE
Oral, intravenous, and intramuscular: *total digitalizing dose:* **Adults:** 1.2 to 1.6 mg; **children** *1 month to 2 years:* 0.033 mg/kg; *2 to 5 years:* 0.024 mg/kg; *5 to 12 years:* 0.022 mg/kg. For both adults and children: initially 30% to 50% of total digitalizing dose is followed by ⅛ to ⅓ of total dose at 3 to 6-hour intervals. Maintenance: **Adults and Children** *12 years and older:* 0.05 to 0.2 mg daily; most common dose is 0.15 mg daily; *under 12 years:* V_{10} of total digitalizing dose.

NURSING IMPLICATIONS
Not to be confused with digoxin or other digitalis glycosides.
Dosage must be carefully titrated. Close observation of patient, ECG monitoring, and determinations of serum digitoxin levels are essential to avoid toxicity. Serum digitoxin levels exceeding 25 mg/ml support clinical diagnosis of toxicity.
The following guidelines are especially important during digitalization period or whenever dosage regimen is altered. Before administering digitoxin: (1) check laboratory reports if available (know what the physician regards as acceptable parameters for serum levels of digitoxin, potassium, magnesium, and calcium); (2) take apical pulse for 1 full minute, noting rate, rhythm, and quality (if patient is on ECG monitor, look for changes in rhythm); (3) check for signs and symptoms of digitoxin toxicity (see Digitalis).

Digitoxin is rarely given by the IM route because it may cause painful local reaction. If prescribed, inject deep into gluteal muscle.

Digitoxin is slowly eliminated; it has the greatest cumulative effects of all cardiotonic glycosides.

Symptoms of toxicity must be reported immediately.

Teach the patient the importance of taking the drug at the same time each day to avoid forgetting. Taking an extra dose of digitoxin poses more danger than omitting a dose.

Stored in airtight containers protected from light.

See Digitalis.

DIGOXIN, U.S.P., B.P.
(LANOXIN, MASOXIN, SK-DIGOXIN)

Cardiotonic

ACTIONS AND USES

Glycoside of *Digitalis lanata.* Shares actions, uses, contraindications, and adverse reactions of digitalis and other cardiotonic glycosides. Its action is more prompt and less prolonged than that of digitalis and digitoxin. Also, it is less likely to give rise to cumulative effects because it is more readily absorbed and exchanged in the body and is rather rapidly excreted in urine.

Used for rapid digitalization and for maintenance therapy.

ABSORPTION AND FATE

Absorption of oral liquid preparation is virtually complete (80% to 90%); absorption of oral tablets varies (50% to 85%). Onset of effects occurs in 1 hour; effects develop fully in 3 to 6 hours and may last 2 to 6 days. Action following IV dose begins within 15 minutes and peaks in 1 to 5 hours; action regresses in 8 to 10 hours and is almost entirely absent in 2 to 6 days. Half-life 33 to 46 hours. Approximately 23% protein-bound. Erratic absorption patterns following IM injection; effects may occur later than with equivalent oral doses. Only 14% eliminated by hepatic metabolism; 80% of dose excreted via kidneys by glomerular filtration, primarily as unchanged drug. Small amounts excreted in feces.

CONTRAINDICATIONS AND PRECAUTIONS

Full digitalizing dose not given if patient has received digoxin during previous week or if slowly excreted cardiotonic glycoside has been given during previous 2 weeks.

See Digitalis.

ADVERSE REACTIONS

Elevated creatine phosphokinase following IM administration. See Digitalis.

ROUTE AND DOSAGE

Adults and Children *10 years and over:* Total digitalizing dose: Oral: 2 to 3 mg in divided doses. Intravenous: 1 to 1.5 mg; Intramuscular: 1 to 2 mg. Digitalization schedules are highly individualized. Maintenance: 0.125 to 0.5 mg daily.

Pediatric: Total digitalizing dose: Oral, intramuscular: *premature and newborns up to 2 weeks:* 44 to 66 μg/kg; *2 weeks to 2 years:* 66 to 88 μg/kg; *2 to 10 years:* 44 to 66 μg/kg. Administered in divided doses. Intravenous (*Premature and newborns up to 2 weeks:* 22 to 44 μg/kg; *2 weeks to 2 years:* 44 to 66 μg/kg; *2 to 10 years:* 22 to 44 μg/kg. Administered in divided doses. Maintenance: 20% to 30% of total digitalizing dose daily.

NURSING IMPLICATIONS

Not to be confused with digitoxin.

Dosage must be carefully titrated by close observation of patient, ECG monitoring, determinations of serum digoxin levels, renal and hepatic status. The following guidelines are especially important during digitalization period or whenever dosage regimen is altered. Before administering digoxin: (1) check laboratory reports; (know what the physician regards as acceptable parameters for serum levels of digoxin, potassium, magnesium, and calcium); (2) take apical pulse for 1 full minute, noting rate, rhythm, and quality; (if patient is on ECG monitor, look for changes in rhythm); (3) check for signs and symptoms of digoxin toxicity. (See Digitalis).

Serum digoxin levels are currently used as aid in individualizing dosage levels in order to avoid toxicity and to confirm suspected toxicity. Therapeutic levels 0.8 to 2 ng/ml.

The IM route is infrequently used because injection causes intense pain that may last for several days; it is also associated with erratic absorption patterns.

If prescribed, make IM injection deep into large muscle mass and follow by firm massage. No more than 0.5 mg should be injected into a single IM site.

Infiltration of parenteral drug into subcutaneous tissue can cause local irritation and sloughing.

Administration of oral digoxin with meals affects its rate of absorption, and thus peak concentration times may be delayed; however, the extent of absorption is not affected.

Alterations of digoxin absorption may occur in patients with bowel hypermotility secondary to laxative use and in patients with malabsorption syndrome.

Monitor intake and output. Patients with renal insufficiency must be closely monitored. Report any change in intake–output ratio. Creatinine clearance may be used to determine the need for dosage adjustment (renal excretion of digoxin is reduced in proprotion to creatinine clearance). Normal creatinine clearance: 123 ± 16 ml/minute (males); 97 ± 10 ml/minute (female).

Preserved in airtight containers protected from light.

Also see Digitalis.

DIHYDROERGOTAMINE MESYLATE, N.F.
(D.H.E. 45)

Analgesic (migraine-specific), antiadrenergic

ACTIONS AND USES

α-Adrenergic blocking agent and dihydrogenated ergot alkaloid with direct constricting effect on smooth muscle of peripheral and cranial blood vessels. Has somewhat weaker vasoconstrictor action than ergotamine (qv), but greater adrenergic blocking activity. Toxicity potential is about one-tenth that of parent drug. Lacks uterine stimulating action in therapeutic dose. Offers no advantage if equipotent doses are compared with ergotamine.

Used to prevent or abort vascular headache (eg, migraine or histaminic cephalalgia) when rapid control is desired or other routes are not feasible.

ABSORPTION AND FATE

Onset of action in 15 to 30 minutes following IM injection, persisting 3 to 4 hours.

CONTRAINDICATIONS AND PRECAUTIONS

History of hypersensitivity to ergot preparations; presence of peripheral vascular disease, coronary heart disease, hypertension, peptic ulcer, impaired hepatic or renal function, sepsis, pregnancy. Also see Ergotamine.

Numbness and tingling in fingers and toes, muscle pains and weakness of legs, precordial distress and pain, transient tachycardia or bradycardia, nausea, vomiting, localized edema and itching; ergotism (excessive doses). See Ergotamine.

ROUTE AND DOSAGE

Intramuscular: 1 ml repeated at 1-hour intervals to a total of 3 ml. Intravenous: 1 or 2 ml maximum.

NURSING IMPLICATIONS

Drug is given at first warning of migraine headache. Optimum results are obtained by titrating the doses required to give relief for several headaches to determine the minimal effective dose. This dose is used for subsequent attacks.

Onset of action after IM injection is delayed about 20 minutes; therefore, when more rapid relief is required, the IV route is prescribed.

Protect ampuls from heat and light. Discard ampul if solution becomes discolored.

See Ergotamine Tartrate.

DIHYDROTACHYSTEROL, U.S.P., B.P. (A.T. 10, HYTAKEROL)

Antihypocalcemic

ACTIONS AND USES

Pharmacologic actions similar to those of both ergocalciferol (vitamin D_2) and parathyroid hormone. In contrast with ergocalciferol, dihydrotachysterol has weak antirachitic activity and shorter duration of action, but in equivalent high doses it is more effective in mobilization of calcium from bone. Elevates serum calcium concentration by increasing intestinal absorption of calcium and possibly by enhancing urinary excretion of inorganic phosphate. Phosphaturia induced by this drug is accompanied by mobilization of calcium and phosphate from bone. Also reported to increase intestinal absorption of sodium, potassium, and magnesium.

Used in treatment of hypocalcemia associated with hypoparathyroidism, both postoperative and idiopathic, and in treatment of pseudohypoparathyroidism. Often administered in conjunction with calcium salts. Also used in treatment of vitamin-D-resistant rickets, frequently in conjunction with oral phosphate salts.

ABSORPTION AND FATE

Maximum hypercalcemic effects occur within 2 weeks (within 1 week following loading doses). Following withdrawal, calcium blood levels decrease markedly within 4 or 5 days; hypercalcemic effects can persist up to 1 month. Metabolized by liver; major metabolite is 40% more active than parent drug. Probably secreted into bile and excreted in feces as active and inactive metabolites. Reported to be excreted in breast milk.

CONTRAINDICATIONS AND PRECAUTIONS

Sensitivity to vitamin D; hypercalcemia and hypocalcemia associated with renal insufficiency and hyperphosphatemia; renal stones, hypervitaminosis D, nursing mothers. Safe use during pregnancy not established.

ADVERSE REACTIONS

Overdosage: symptoms of hypercalcemia (anorexia, constipation, nausea, vomiting, ileus, abdominal pain, nocturia, polyuria, thirst, dehydration, neuromuscular disturbances, psychosis, renal calculi). See Ergocalciferol.

Oral: initially 0.8 to 2.4 mg once daily for several days; maintenance 0.2 to 1 mg daily as required for normal serum calcium levels (this dose may be supplemented with 10 to 15 Gm of calcium lactate or gluconate by mouth daily).

NURSING IMPLICATIONS

Careful monitoring of serum and urinary calcium levels is essential. The margin between a therapeutic dose and a dose causing hypercalcemia is very small. Serum calcium level should be maintained between 9 and 10.6 mg/dl.

Adequate calcium is necessary for clinical response to dihydrotachysterol therapy. Consult physician regarding allowable dietary intake of calcium.

Patients receiving thiazide diuretics concurrently with dihydrotachysterol may be predisposed to the development of hypercalcemia.

Withhold drug if symptoms of hypercalcemia appear (see Adverse Reactions) and report to physician.

Dihydrotachysterol is not intended for prophylactic use.

Preserved in tightly closed, light-resistant containers. Do not store capsules in refrigerator, because they may crack and leak drug.

See Cholecalciferol.

DIHYDROXYALUMINUM AMINOACETATE, N.F.
(ALZINOX, HYPERACID, ROBALATE)

Antacid

ACTIONS AND USES

Nonsystemic antacid similar to aluminum hydroxide gel (qv) in actions, uses, contraindications, precautions, and adverse reactions. In dried form it is reported to have greater neutralizing capacity than dried aluminum hydroxide gel, but the liquid preparation is not as effective.

ROUTE AND DOSAGE

Oral: 500 mg to 1 Gm 4 times a day, after meals and at bedtime. Available as tablets, magma, or suspension form.

NURSING IMPLICATIONS

Drug is usually administered 1 or 2 hours after meals and on retiring to control gastric hyperacidity.

Tablets should be chewed thoroughly before swallowing and preferably followed by a small quantity of water.

Prolonged administration may produce constipation; therefore, the physician may prescribe alternation with magnesium antacids, which tend to have a cathartic effect.

DRUG INTERACTIONS: Aluminum-containing antacids may complex with and thus reduce absorption of **tetracycline** derivatives when administered concomitantly. Also see Aluminum Hydroxide Gel.

DIMENHYDRINATE, U.S.P., B.P.
(DIMEN, DIMENEST, DRAMALIN, DRAMAMINE, ELDODRAM,
HYDRATE, NAUZINE, REIDAMINE)

Antihistaminic, antiemic, antivertigo

ACTIONS AND USES
Ethanolamine derivative and chlorotheophylline salt of diphenhydramine (qv), with which it shares similar properties. Precise mode of antinauseant action not known, but thought to be due to ability to inhibit cholinergic stimulation in vestibular and associated neural pathways.

Used chiefly in prevention and treatment of motion sickness. Also has been used in management of vertigo, nausea, and vomiting associated with radiation sickness, labyrinthitis, Meniere's syndrome, stapedectomy, anesthesia, and various medications.

ABSORPTION AND FATE
Duration of action approximately 4 to 6 hours. Also see Diphenhydramine.

CONTRAINDICATIONS AND PRECAUTIONS
Narrow-angle glaucoma, prostatic hypertrophy. Cautious use: convulsive disorders.

ADVERSE REACTIONS
Drowsiness, headache, blurred vision, incoordination, palpitation, dizziness, hypotension. Less frequently: anorexia, constipation or diarrhea, urinary frequency, dysuria. Also see Diphenhydramine.

ROUTE AND DOSAGE
Adults: Oral: 50 to 100 mg every 4 hours. Intramuscular, intravenous: 50 mg. For intravenous use, each 50 mg (1 ml) should be diluted in 10 ml of 0.9% sodium chloride injection; rate of administration, 2 minutes for each 50 mg. Rectal suppository: 100 mg once or twice daily. **Children:** Oral, rectal, intramuscular: 1.25 mg/kg 4 times daily up to maximum of 300 mg daily. IV dosage not established for children.

NURSING IMPLICATIONS
High incidence of drowsiness; this is often a desirable reaction for some patients. Bedsides and supervision of ambulation may be advisable. Caution ambulatory patient not to operate automobile or dangerous machinery until drowsiness has passed.

To prevent motion sickness, dimenhydrinate should be taken 30 minutes before departure and should be repeated before meals and upon retiring.

To prevent radiation sickness, drug is usually administered 30 to 60 minutes before treatment, then repeated 1.5 hours after treatment and again in 3 hours.

Tolerance to CNS depressant effects usually occurs after a few days of therapy. Some decrease in antiemetic action may result with prolonged use.

Avoid mixing parenteral preparation with other drugs. Dimenhydrinate is incompatible with many solutions.

DRUG INTERACTIONS: Dimenhydrinate may mask ototoxic symptoms associated with **aminoglycoside antibiotics.** Enhanced CNS depression (drowsiness) may occur when antihistamines are used concurrently with **barbiturates** and **other CNS depressants.**
Also see Diphenhydramine Hydrochloride.

Chelating agent, antidote (heavy metal)

ACTIONS AND USES
Dithiol compound originally developed as antidote for Lewisite, an arsenic-containing chemical warfare agent. Combines with ions of various heavy metals to form relatively stable, nontoxic, soluble complexes called chelates (mercaptides), which can be excreted; inhibition of sulfhydryl enzymes by toxic metals is thus prevented. May also reactivate affected enzymes, but most effective when administered prior to enzyme damage.
Used in treatment of acute poisoning by arsenic, gold, and mercury. Also has been used as adjunct to edetate calcium disodium in treatment of lead encephalopathy and as adjunct to penicillamine to increase rate of copper excretion in Wilson's disease.

ABSORPTION AND FATE
Peak blood levels in 30 to 60 minutes. Distributed mainly in intercellular spaces. Short half-life; metabolic degradation and urinary excretion essentially complete within 4 hours.

CONTRAINDICATIONS AND PRECAUTIONS
Hepatic insufficiency (with exception of postarsenical jaundice); pregnancy; severe renal insufficiency; concurrent iron therapy; treatment of poisoning due to cadmium, iron, selenium, and uranium. Cautious use: hypertension.

ADVERSE REACTIONS
Listed in approximate order of frequency, high doses are associated with: elevated blood pressure, tachycardia, nausea, vomiting, headache; burning sensation of lips, mouth, throat; feeling of constriction and pain in throat, chest, or hands; conjunctivitis, lacrimation, rhinorrhea, blepharospasm, salivation, paresthesias, burning sensation in penis, sweating, abdominal pain; local pain, sterile abscess at injection site; anxiety, weakness, restlessness, reduction in polymorphonuclear leukocytes; transient fever (in children). Toxic doses: tremors, convulsions, shock, metabolic acidosis with elevated serum lactate levels.

ROUTE AND DOSAGE
Intramuscular (mild arsenic or gold poisoning): 2.5 mg/kg body weight 4 times a day for first 2 days, 2 times on third day, then once daily for 10 days; (severe arsenic or gold poisoning): 3 mg/kg body weight every 4 hours for first 2 days, then 4 times a day on third day, then twice daily thereafter for 10 days; (mercury poisoning): initially 5 mg/kg body weight, followed by 2.5 mg/kg 1 or 2 times daily for 10 days. (BAL in oil: each 1 ml contains 100 mg dimercaprol.)

NURSING IMPLICATIONS
Since irreversible tissue damage may occur quickly, particularly in mercury poisoning, dimercaprol therapy must be initiated as soon as possible (within 1 or 2 hours) after ingestion.
Usual emergency treatment for the particular poison should be carried out, as well as maintenance of body heat, fluids, electrolytes, and other supportive measures.
Administered only by deep IM injection. Local pain, gluteal abscess, and skin sensitization reported. Rotate injection sites and observe daily.
Monitor vital signs. Elevations of systolic and diastolic blood pressures accompanied by tachycardia frequently occur within a few minutes following injection and may remain elevated up to 2 hours. Degree of elevation is roughly proportional to dose administered.
Fever occurs in approximately 30% of children receiving treatment and may persist throughout therapy (reaction is apparently peculiar to children).

Intake and output should be monitored. Potentially nephrotoxic. Report
oliguria or change in intake–output ratio. If renal insufficiency develops,
drug should be discontinued or used with extreme caution, since toxic
serum concentrations may result.

Urine should be kept alkaline to reduce possibility of renal damage during
elimination of dimercaprol chelate. In acid medium, chelate rapidly dis-
sociates and releases bound metal.

Daily urine examinations should be made for albumin, blood, casts, and pH.
Blood and urinary levels of the metal serve as guides for dosage adjustments.

Minor adverse reactions usually reach maximum 15 to 20 minutes after drug
administration and generally subside in 30 to 90 minutes. Antihistamine
is sometimes administered to relieve symptoms.

Contact of drug with skin may produce erythema, edema, dermatitis. Handle
with caution.

Dimercaprol may impart an unpleasant garliclike odor to patient's breath.

LABORATORY TEST INTERFERENCES: I[131] thyroidal uptake values may be
decreased if test is done during or immediately following dimercaprol therapy.

DRUG INTERACTIONS: Dimercaprol forms toxic complexes with **iron, cadmium, selenium,** and **uranium.**

DINOPROST TROMETHAMINE
(PGF$_{2\alpha}$, PROSTIN F$_2$ ALPHA)

Oxytocic, prostaglandin

ACTIONS AND USES

Salt of naturally occurring compound in the prostaglandin F series. Abortifa-
cient that imitates and augments contractions of gravid uterus, not just at term
as is the case with oxytocics and ergot alkaloids, but throughout pregnancy.
Contractions usually sufficient to evacuate uterus, but drug-induced abortion
may be incomplete. Increases intestinal motility (cause of several troublesome
side effects), and constricts arteries and veins, usually without affecting blood
pressure. May precipitate asthma. Intraamniotic instillation appears to be more
effective than intraamniotic injection of hypertonic saline in induced abortion.
Used to terminate second-trimester pregnancy, often in conjunction with dilation and curettage or suction curettement to assure complete abortion.

ABSORPTION AND FATE

Following intraamniotic administration, drug slowly diffuses into maternal
bloodstream. Half-life in amniotic fluid 3 to 6 hours; in plasma, less than 1
minute; maximum plasma levels occur about 2 hours after administration.
Widely distributed in maternal and fetal bodies; concentrated in fetal liver and
rapidly metabolized in maternal lungs and liver. Metabolites completely excreted in 24 hours in urine, with about 5% excreted in feces.

CONTRAINDICATIONS AND PRECAUTIONS

Hypersensitivity, acute pelvic inflammatory disease. Cautious use: patients with
history of asthma, glaucoma, hypertension, cardiovascular disease, history of
epilepsy; concomitant administration with IV oxytocin.

ADVERSE REACTIONS

Nausea, vomiting, diarrhea, abdominal cramps, uterine pain. Other (occur in
2.7% to 0.1% of patients, in decreasing order of frequency): epigastric, substernal, leg, or shoulder pains; bradycardia; headache; flushing; bachache; dizziness;

dyspnea; chills; endometritis; coughing; wheezing; grand mal convulsion; paresthesias; burning sensation in eye or breast; breast pain; diplopia; hiccough; hypertension; hyperventilation; bronchospasm; hematuria, polydipsia; urinary problems; uterine rupture; vasovagal symptoms; second-degree heart block.

ROUTE AND DOSAGE

Intraamniotic sac injection: 40 mg (8 ml). If abortion process has not been established or completed within 24 hours and if membranes are intact, patient is given additional 10 to 40 mg (2 to 8 ml).

NURSING IMPLICATIONS

Dinoprost ampuls should be stored at 2 C to 8 C and should be discarded 24 months following date of manufacture.

Drug should be used only by qualified personnel in an agency with facilities that are immediately available for intensive care and surgery.

One milliliter of amniotic fluid is withdrawn at time of transabdominal tap to determine if blood is present. If not, dinoprost is slowly injected into amniotic sac. The first milliliter is injected very slowly via a transabdominal intraamniotic catheter while observing patient for signs of sensitivity or adverse reactions. If none appears, remainder of dose is given over next 5 minutes. If the abortion process has not been established within 24 hours (and in the presence of intact membranes), additional 10 to 40 mg may be administered.

Patient should be well aware of benefits and risks of dinoprost-induced abortion.

A complete medical history and physical examination should be performed before starting therapy with dinoprost.

Instruct the patient to empty her bladder before the transabdominal tap.

Before each dose is given, a vaginal exam should be performed to insure that the catheter has not prolapsed into the vagina.

The drug is not injected if there is a bloody tap.

Monitor blood pressure, pulse, respirations, and uterine activity following drug administration. Report significant signs: pulse and blood pressure changes may signal hemorrhage; hypertonic uterine contractions can promote hemorrhage and cervical trauma. Blood transfusions may be necessary.

Promptly report vasovagal symptoms (pallor, nausea, vomiting, bradycardia, rapid fall in arterial blood pressure). Instruct patient to remain in recumbent position.

Inadvertent administration of drug into maternal bloodstream causes syndrome of vasoconstriction, tachycardia, and vasovagal effects.

The primipara may experience cervical perforation, particularly if oxytocin has been given with dinoprost and when cervix is poorly dilated, if at all.

Examine the patient post abortion for possibility of incomplete abortion and cervical trauma (may be symptomless).

Lactation of several days' duration may occur following successful termination of pregnancy.

Does not seem to affect integrity of fetal-placental unit; thus, a live-born fetus may be delivered, particularly if abortion is accomplished at end of second trimester.

If drug fails to terminate pregnancy, another method is usually employed; animal studies have suggested a teratogenic potential in prostaglandins.

When procedure to abort is unsuccessful, hypertonic saline may be utilized after cessation of uterine contractions.

Avoid administering aspirin or any compound with aspirin to patient receiving dinoprost.

DRUG INTERACTIONS: **Aspirin** reportedly increases the time interval between dinoprost administration and abortion.

DIOCTYL SODIUM SULFOSUCCINATE, U.S.P., B.P.
(BU-LAX, COLACE, COMFOLAX, DILAX, DIOMEDICONE, DISONATE, DIOSUCCIN, DOCTATE, DOSS 300, DOXINATE, DSS, LAXINATE, MODANE SOFT CAPSULES, PROVILAX, PARLAX)

Stool softener, surfactant

ACTIONS AND USES
Anionic surface-active agent with emulsifying and wetting properties. Lowers surface tension, permitting water and fats to penetrate and soften stools for easier passage.
Used in treatment of constipation associated with hard, dry stools; used for painful anorectal conditions and in cardiac or other patients who should avoid straining during defecation.
CONTRAINDICATIONS AND PRECAUTIONS
Atonic constipation, nausea, vomiting, abdominal pain, fecal impaction, intestinal obstruction or perforation, concomitant use of mineral oil (theoretical possibility of systemic absorption of mineral oil).
ADVERSE REACTIONS
Rare: occasional mild abdominal cramps.
ROUTE AND DOSAGE
Oral: **Adults and children** *over 12 years:* 50 to 200 mg; *6 to 12 years:* 40 to 120 mg; *3 to 6 years:* 20 to 60 mg; *under 3 years:* 10 to 40 mg. High doses recommended for initial therapy, then adjusted according to individual response. Rectal: 50 to 100 mg (5 to 10 ml of solution added to retention or flushing enema). Available as capsule, tablet, syrup, and solution.

NURSING IMPLICATIONS
Oral solutions may be administered in one-half glass of milk or fruit juice to mask taste.
Effect on stools is usually apparent 1 to 3 days after first dose.
Should not be administered for prolonged periods in treatment of constipation in lieu of proper dietary management or other treatment of underlying causes. See Bisacodyl.
Dioctyl sodium sulfosuccinate is available in combination with peristaltic stimulants when laxative as well as fecal softening action is desired, eg, with casanthranol (Peri-Colace), with senna fruit (Senokap DSS), and with phenolphthalein (Novalax).

DIPHENHYDRAMINE HYDROCHLORIDE, U.S.P., B.P.
(BAX, BENADRYL, FENYLHIST, HYREXIN, ROHYDRA, VALDRENE, WEHDRYL)

Antihistaminic

ACTIONS AND USES
Ethanolamine (aminoalkyl ether) antihistamine with significant anticholinergic (antispasmodic) activity. High incidence of drowsiness, but GI side effects are minor. Like other antihistamines, competes for histamine receptor sites on effec-

tor cells, thus blocking the histamine action that promotes capillary permeability and edema formation and constriction of respiratory, GI, and vascular smooth muscle. Does not inhibit gastric secretion, but has antiemetic effect. Also has antitussive and some local anesthetic actions.

Used for symptomatic relief of various allergic conditions and to treat or prevent motion sickness and reactions to blood or plasma in susceptible patients. Also used in anaphylaxis as adjunct to epinephrine and other standard measures and after acute symptoms have been controlled and in treatment of parkinsonism and intractable insomnia. Incorporated in elixirs and syrups and other antihistaminic-decongestant preparations to relieve symptoms of coughs due to colds or allergies.

ABSORPTION AND FATE

Readily absorbed from GI tract; peak activity in about 1 hour; duration 4 to 6 hours. Metabolized primarily by liver; some degradation by lung and kidney. Excreted in urine within 24 hours, chiefly as metabolites; small portion may be excreted as unchanged drug.

CONTRAINDICATIONS AND PRECAUTIONS

Hypersensitivity to antihistamines of similar structure, lower respiratory tract symptoms (including asthma), narrow-angle glaucoma, prostatic hypertrophy, bladder neck obstruction, GI obstruction or stenosis, pregnancy, nursing mothers, prematures and newborns, patients receiving MAO inhibitors. Cautious use: history of asthma, convulsive disorders, increased intraocular pressure, hyperthyroidism, hypertension, cardiovascular disease, diabetes mellitus.

ADVERSE REACTIONS

CNS (common): drowsiness, dizziness, tinnitus, vertigo, fatigue, disturbed coordination, tingling, heaviness and weakness of hands, tremors, euphoria, nervousness, restlessness, insomnia. **Overdosage** (especially in children): hallucinations, excitement, fever, ataxia, athetosis, convulsions, coma, cardiovascular collapse, dryness (mouth, nose, and throat), thickened bronchial secretions, wheezing, sensation of chest tightness, blurred vision, diplopia, headache, urinary frequency or retention, dysuria, palpitation, tachycardia, mild hypotension or hypertension. **GI:** epigastric distress, anorexia, nausea, vomiting, constipation or diarrhea. **Hypersensitivity:** skin rash, urticaria, photosensitivity, anaphylactic shock. **Hematologic:** leukopenia, agranulocytosis, hemolytic anemia.

ROUTE AND DOSAGE

Adults: Oral, intramuscular, intravenous: 25 to 50 mg 3 or 4 times a day. Maximum daily parenteral dosage is 400 mg. **Children:** Oral, IV, IM: 5 mg/kg/24 hours in 4 divided doses as required.

NURSING IMPLICATIONS

In patients taking diphenhydramine for allergic manifestations, a careful history should be taken that includes change from usual pattern of recently ingested foods and drugs, as well as social or emotional stress.

Administer IM deep into large muscle mass. Avoid perivascular or subcutaneous injections of the drug because of its irritating effects. Hypersensitivity reactions (including anaphylactic shock) are more likely to occur with parenteral injections than with oral administration.

GI side effects may be lessened by administration of drug with meals or with milk.

When used for motion sickness, the first dose is given 30 minutes before exposure to motion. For duration of exposure it is given before meals and on retiring.

Drowsiness, the principal side effect, is most prominent during the first few days of therapy and often disappears with continued therapy. Bedsides and supervision of ambulation may be advisable for some patients.

Patients with blood pressure problems receiving the drug parenterally should be closely observed, with blood pressure being monitored.

Caution the patient against activities requiring alertness and coordination until drug response has been evaluated.

Warn the patient about possible additive CNS depressant effects with concurrent use of alcohol and other CNS depressants (such as sedatives, hypnotics, and tranquilizers) while taking antihistamines.

Urge the patient on continuing therapy to report any unusual signs or symptoms to his physician. Most mild reactions can be alleviated by decreasing dosage; however, a change to another preparation may be necessary.

Patients receiving long-term therapy should have periodic blood cell counts.

When elixir or syrup formulations are used for relief of cough, bear in mind that the drug has an atropinelike drying effect (thickened bronchial secretions) that may make expectoration difficult.

Antihistamines have no therapeutic effect on the common cold. Their continued popularity, despite their being debunked as cures for the common cold, apparently stems from their drying effect.

Antihistamines should be discontinued prior to skin testing procedures for allergy, since they may obscure otherwise positive reactions.

Caution the patient to store antihistamines out of reach of children. Fatalities have been reported.

Caladryl (1% cream or lotion) contains diphenhydramine in a calamine base. Topical applications carry great risk of skin sensitization.

Patients with allergies should be advised to carry medical information card or jewelry indicating type allergy, medication, his and physician's name, address, and telephone number.

Preserved in tight, light-resistant containers.

DRUG INTERACTIONS: Concurrent administration of antihistamines and **barbituates** may enhance CNS depression caused by either drug. **MAO inhibitors** prolong and intensify the anticholinergic (drying) effects of antihistamines and can cause severe hypertension.

DIPHENIDOL HYDROCHLORIDE
(VONTROL)

Antiemetic, antivertigo

ACTIONS AND USES

Agent with strong antivertigo and antiemetic effects. Mechanism of action is unknown; it appears to have direct depressant action on labyrinthine excitability and on conduction in vestibular-cerebellar pathways and possibly depressant action in CTZ in medulla. Also exhibits weak anticholinergic, CNS depressant, and antihistaminic activity.

Used in management of nausea and vomiting associated with infectious diseases, malignancies, radiation sickness, antineoplastic therapy, general anesthesia; management of vertigo in motion sickness; labyrinthitis, following middle and inner ear surgery; Meniere's disease.

ABSORPTION AND FATE

Onset of action within 30 to 45 minutes after oral administration and within 15 minutes after IM or IV injection. Duration of action 3 to 6 hours. Readily metabolized in liver; approximately 90% excreted in urine.

CONTRAINDICATIONS AND PRECAUTIONS

Known hypersensitivity to diphenidol; anuria; hypotension; use of diphenidol in infants under 6 months of age or in those weighing less than 12 kg; IV use in children of any age; use in patients with history of sinus tachycardia. Safe use during pregnancy or lactation or in women of childbearing potential not established. Cautious use: glaucoma, pyloric stenosis, pylorospasm, prostatic hypertrophy, other obstructive lesions of GI tract or genitourinary tract.

ADVERSE REACTIONS

Auditory and visual hallucinations, disorientation, confusion; drowsiness, overstimulation, depression, sleep disturbances, dry mouth, nausea, indigestion, blurred vision. Rarely: dizziness, skin rash, malaise, headache, heartburn, mild jaundice; slight transient lowering of blood pressure.

ROUTE AND DOSAGE

Adults: Oral, rectal suppository: 25 to 50 mg every 4 hours as needed. Intramuscular: initially 20 to 40 mg; 20-mg dose repeated after 1 hour if symptoms persist; thereafter, 20 to 40 mg every 4 hours as needed. Intravenous: initially 20 mg (injected directly or through venoclysis already in operation); repeated after 1 hour if symptoms persist; thereafter, by other routes. Maximum 300 mg/24 hrs. **Children** (for nausea and vomiting only): Oral, rectal suppository: 0.4 mg/lb; total dose in 24 hours should not exceed 2.5 mg/lb. Intramuscular: 0.2 mg/lb; total IM dose in 24 hours should not exceed 1.5 mg/lb. Children's doses usually not given more often than every 4 hours; however, if symptoms persist after first dose, physician may order repeat dose after 1 hour.

NURSING IMPLICATIONS

Diphenidol may cause hallucinations, disorientation, or confusion. For this reason, use is limited to hospitalized patients or to patients under comparable close, professional supervision.

Notify physician of side effects. Auditory and visual hallucinations, disorientation, and confusion usually occur within 3 days after initiation of drug therapy and usually subside spontaneously within 3 days after drug is discontinued. Observe appropriate safety precautions.

IM administration should be deep. Subcutaneous (and perivenous) infiltration is specifically contraindicated.

Monitor intake and output. Report oliguria or change in intake-output ratio.

Monitor blood pressure when diphenidol is given by parenteral routes.

Because of possible drowsiness and dizziness, caution patient against performing hazardous activities requiring mental alertness and physical coordination. Supervision of ambulation may be indicated.

Blood dyscrasias have not been reported, but since diphenidol is a comparatively new drug, manufacturer recommends regularly scheduled blood studies.

Bear in mind that antiemetic effect of diphenidol may obscure signs of overdosage of concomitant drug therapy or underlying pathology.

There is a possibility of additive effects with concurrent administration of CNS depressants.

DIPHENOXYLATE HYDROCHLORIDE AND ATROPINE SULFATE SOLUTION (AND TABLETS) U.S.P., B.P.

(LOMOTIL)

Antiperistaltic

ACTIONS AND USES

Synthetic narcotic and phenylpiperidine analog structurally related to meperidine. Commercially available only with atropine sulfate added to discourage deliberate overdosage. Diphenoxylate acts on smooth muscles of intestinal tract, inhibiting motility and excessive propulsion. Has little or no analgesic activity or risk of dependence, except in high doses.

Used as adjunct in symptomatic management of diarrhea.

ABSORPTION AND FATE

Well absorbed after oral administration; onset of action within 45 to 60 minutes, with duration of 3 to 4 hours. Peak plasma levels reached in 2 hours; plasma half-life 2.5 hours. Rapidly metabolized to active metabolite diphenoxylic acid (plasma half-life 4.4 hours) and inactive metabolites. Excreted slowly, primarily in feces via bile; small amounts eliminated in urine. Appears in breast milk.

CONTRAINDICATIONS AND PRECAUTIONS

Hypersensitivity to diphenoxylate or atropine; severe dehydration or electrolyte imbalance, advanced liver disease, glaucoma, jaundice, children less than 2 years of age. Safe use during pregnancy or lactation or in women of childbearing potential not established. Cautious use: abnormal liver function tests; patients receiving addicting drugs, addiction-prone individuals or whose history suggests drug abuse; ulcerative colitis; young children (particularly in patients with Down's syndrome). Also see Atropine Sulfate.

ADVERSE REACTIONS

Nausea, vomiting, anorexia, sedation, dizziness, lethargy, abdominal discomfort or distention, paralytic ileus, toxic megacolon, headache; pruritus, angioneurotic edema, giant urticaria; tachycardia, numbness of extremities, blurred vision, dry mouth, swelling of gums, restlessness, euphoria, mental depression, weakness, general malaise. Overdosage: atropine side effects (see Atropine Sulfate); drowsiness, hypotonia, loss of reflexes, nystagmus, miosis, urinary retention, flushing, fever, seizures, respiratory depression, coma.

ROUTE AND DOSAGE

Adults: Oral: initially 5 mg 3 or 4 times a day. Commercial tablet (Lomotil) contains 2.5 mg diphenoxylate hydrochloride with 0.025 mg atropine sulfate; liquid preparation contains same amount per 5 ml. **Children:** *2 to 5 years:* 4 ml t.i.d.; *5 to 8 years:* 4 ml q.i.d.; *8 to 12 years:* 4 ml 5 times daily. Dosage may be reduced to as low as one-quarter dose as soon as symptoms are controlled.

NURSING IMPLICATIONS

A careful history usually points to the source of acute diarrhea.

Use only the plastic calibrated dropper supplied by manufacturer for measuring liquid preparation.

Report signs of atropinism (dry mouth, flushing, hyperthermia, tachycardia, urinary retention); may occur even with recommended doses in children, particularly those with Down's syndrome.

Dehydration, particularly in younger children, may further influence variability of response to diphenoxylate and predispose patient to delayed toxic effects.

Drug should be withheld in presence of severe dehydration or electrolyte imbalance until appropriate corrective therapy has been initiated.

Magnitudes of fluid and electrolyte deficits can be estimated by observing skin turgor and texture, as well as appearance of tongue and mucous membranes, eyeball tension (sunken in dehydration), temperature, blood pressure, pulse, and muscle strength.

Further gross calculations of fluid loss can be made by careful measurements of body weight and intake and output. Note frequency, color, odor, and consistency of stools and presence of blood, pus, mucus, or other foreign matter.

Observe for and report abdominal distention. In ulcerative colitis, diphenoxylate-induced delay of intestinal motility has been reported to cause toxic megacolon; may also result in fluid retention in colon, thus further aggravating dehydration and electrolyte imbalance. Distention is an ominous sign in patient with ulcerative colitis.

Consult physician regarding management of oral fluids and electrolytes. For acute diarrhea, food is generally withheld 24 hours to reduce bowel stimulation, or restricted to only clear liquids such as broth, bouillon, weak tea, ginger ale, gelatin. Ice-cold liquids, milk and milk products, and concentrated sweets are usually avoided. Bland diet is then added as tolerated, gradually progressing to normal diet.

Counsel patient to take medication only as directed by physician.

Caution patients to keep drug out of reach of children. Fatalities have been reported.

Overdosage treatment: gastric lavage is effective even several hours after drug ingestion. Facilities for resuscitation and a narcotic antagonist (eg, naloxone) should be readily available. Respiratory depression may occur 25 to 30 hours after overdose; therefore, extend the period of observation over at least 48 hours.

Addiction to diphenoxylate is theoretically possible at high dosages and prolonged use. Classified as schedule V drug under federal Controlled Substances Act.

DRUG INTERACTIONS: Concomitant use of **MAO inhibitors** with diphenoxylate may in theory precipitate hypertensive crisis. Diphenoxylate may potentiate action of **alcohol, barbiturates,** and **tranquilizers.** Patient should be observed closely if these are used concomitantly.

DIPYRIDAMOLE
(PERSANTINE)

Vasodilator (coronary)

ACTIONS AND USES

Non-nitrate coronary vasodilator with many properties similar to those of papaverine. Increases oxygen saturation in coronary sinus without coincident elevation in myocardial oxygen consumption. Also increases coronary blood flow, decreases coronary vascular resistance, and reportedly promotes development of collateral circulation in the diseased heart. May block ADP-induced platelet aggregation.

Used for long-term management of chronic angina pectoris, but not useful for preventing or relieving acute anginal attacks. Also used in treatment regimen following myocardial infarction. Investigational uses include trials with aspirin and with oral anticoagulants in thromboembolic disorders.

ABSORPTION AND FATE

Readily absorbed from GI tract. Concentrates in liver; mainly excreted in feces as intact drug or as glucuronide.

CONTRAINDICATIONS AND PRECAUTIONS

Hypotension, acute myocardial infarction.

ADVERSE REACTIONS

Minimal and transient: gastric distress, headache, dizziness, faintness, weakness, hypotension, aggravation of angina pectoris (rarely), peripheral vasodilation, skin rash.

ROUTE AND DOSAGE

Oral: 50 mg 3 times daily.

NURSING IMPLICATIONS
Administer at least 1 hour before meals.
Counsel patient to notify physician of any side effects.

Clinical response may not be evident before second or third month of continuous therapy.

Expected therapeutic effects: reduced frequency or elimination of anginal episodes, improved exercise tolerance, reduced requirement for nitrates.

DRUG INTERACTIONS: Dipyridamole increases the danger of hemorrhage in patients receiving heparin.

DIPYRONE
(DIMETHONE, K-PYRONE, Methampyrone, NARONE, PYRAL, PYRILGIN, PYRO, PYRODYN, PYROTYNE)

Antipyretic

ACTIONS AND USES

Synthetic pyrazolone derivative of aminopyrine. Produces antipyresis by acting on hypothalamus; heat dissipation is increased as result of vasodilation and increased peripheral blood flow. Also has analgesic properties.

Used only for treatment of intractable fever that is unresponsive to adequate trial with other drugs and measures.

ABSORPTION AND FATE

Readily and completely absorbed from GI tract. Onset of action within 20 to 45 minutes. Metabolized by liver; excreted in urine.

CONTRAINDICATIONS AND PRECAUTIONS

During menstruation; liver disease; history of intolerance or reaction to aminopyrine, antipyrine, or dipyrone; concomitant use of chlorpromazine and dipyrone. Safe use during pregnancy and for nursing mothers and women of child-bearing potential not established. Cautious use: blood dyscrasias, prothrombin deficiency.

ADVERSE REACTIONS

Nausea, vomiting, epigastric discomfort, GI bleeding, edema, tremor, pain and irritation at injection site, anuria, aggravation of prothrombin deficiency, allergic reactions (skin eruptions, angioneurotic edema, asthma), agranulocytosis, aplastic and hemolytic anemia, thrombocytopenic purpura. Toxic doses: CNS stimulation followed by depression, hyperventilation (with respiratory alkalosis and metabolic acidosis).

ROUTE AND DOSAGE

Oral, intramuscular, intravenous: **Adults:** 500 mg to 1 Gm. Single dose should not exceed 1 Gm, and maximum daily dosage should not exceed 3 Gm. **Children:** 250 to 500 mg per dose, repeated in 3 to 4 hours if necessary. Not to exceed 1 Gm/24 hours for children *up to 6 years* of age and 2 Gm/24 hours for children *6 to 12 years* of age.

NURSING IMPLICATIONS

Carefully detailed history, complete physical, and laboratory examination including hemogram and urinalysis are advised before therapy is initiated.

White blood cell and differential counts should be repeated at frequent intervals during therapy.

Dipyrone should be discontinued if favorable response is not obtained within a few days. Fatal agranulocytosis has occurred even after short-term use.

Agranulocytosis onset is sudden and calls for prompt termination of dipyrone therapy to prevent fatality. Drug should be discontinued at first evidence of reduction in blood cell count or sign of agranulocytosis.

Instruct patient to report immediately any symptoms of impending infection (eg, sore throat, pain, swelling, tenderness, ulceration of mouth or throat), fever, skin rash, or other unexpected signs.

Monitor and report change in intake and output ratio and pattern. Report bloody or tarry stools.

Weight should be checked daily if possible. Report weight gain or edema to physician.

Aqueous solutions of dipyrone may acquire yellow discoloration, apparently without loss of pharmacologic activity.

DRUG INTERACTIONS: Possibility of severe hypothermia in patients receiving concomitant dipyrone and **phenothiazine** therapy. **Chlorpromazine** may increase antipyretic effect of dipyrone.

DISULFIRAM, N.F.
(ANTABUSE, RO-SULFIRAM)

Alcohol deterrent

ACTIONS AND USES

Antioxidant compound. Appears to act by inhibiting the hepatic aldehyde dehydrogenase necessary for oxidation of acetaldehyde to acetate during normal degradation of alcohol. When a small amount of alcohol is ingested, acetaldehyde concentration of blood rises to 5 to 10 times normal level, producing toxic systemic reaction (disulfiram-alcohol reaction or acetaldehyde syndrome), which serves as deterrent to further drinking. Possesses antithyroid and slight sedative actions, but usually these effects are not significant unless alcohol is ingested. Does not cause tolerance or dependence.

Used as adjunct in treatment of selected patients with chronic alcoholism who want to maintain a state of enforced sobriety.

ABSORPTION AND FATE

Rapidly but incompletely absorbed from GI tract. Full action may require 12 hours. Accumulates in fat depots. Greater part of drug is oxidized, probably largely by liver, and excreted slowly in urine. About 20% still remains in body between 1 and 2 weeks.

CONTRAINDICATIONS AND PRECAUTIONS

Hypersensitivity to disulfiram; severe myocardial disease; psychoses; pregnancy; patients receiving or patients who have recently received alcohol, metronidazole, paraldehyde. Use of disulfiram-alcohol test in patients over 50 years of age or patients who have cardiac or hepatic disease. Cautious use: diabetes mellitus, epilepsy, hypothyroidism, cerebral damage, chronic and acute nephritis, hepatic cirrhosis or insufficiency.

ADVERSE REACTIONS

Mild GI disturbances, headache, allergic dermatitis, urticaria, acneiform rash, aftertaste, drowsiness, fatigue, restlessness, tremor, impotence, psychotic reaction (usually with high doses), polyneuritis, peripheral neuritis, optic neuritis (rarely); possibly cholestatic hepatitis. Disulfiram-alcohol reaction: flushing, intense throbbing of head and neck, nausea, violent vomiting, thirst, sweating, marked uneasiness, confusion, weakness, vertigo, blurred vision, palpitation, chest pain, hypotension, arrhythmias, acute congestive failure, marked respiratory depression, unconsciousness, convulsions, sudden death.

ROUTE AND DOSAGE

Oral: initially a maximum of 500 mg daily in single dose for 1 to 2 weeks; maintenance: 250 mg daily (range 125 to 500 mg). Should not exceed 500 mg daily.

NURSING IMPLICATIONS

Patient should give permission for disulfiram therapy; patient and responsible family members must be fully informed of possible consequences of ingesting alcohol. Therapy is attempted only under careful medical and nursing supervision.

Disulfiram is used as an adjunct to supportive and psychiatric therapy and only in patients who are motivated and fully cooperative.

Therapy is not initiated until patient has abstained from alcohol and alcohol-containing preparations for at least 12 hours and preferably 48 hours.

Complete physical examination, especially of circulatory and nervous systems, and careful drug history are advised prior to therapy. Baseline and follow-up transaminase tests (in 10 to 14 days) are suggested to detect hepatic dysfunction. In addition, complete blood count and sequential multiple analysis 12 (SMA-12) test should be made every 6 months.

Daily dose should be taken in the morning, when the resolve not to drink should be strongest. May be prescribed at time of retiring for patients who experience sedative effect. To minimize sedative effect, dosage is adjusted downward. Tablets preferably are crushed and well mixed with liquid if compliance is a problem.

Caution patient to avoid alcohol in any form, including external applications. Inform patient of unusual sources of alcohol: liniments; shaving, face, or body lotions; backrub solutions; elixirs, fluid extracts, tinctures (eg, cough medicines, Geritol, paragoric); vinegars; among others.

Patient should be informed that prolonged administration of disulfiram does not produce tolerance; the longer one remains on therapy, the more sensitive one becomes to alcohol.

Disulfiram-alcohol reaction (see Adverse Reactions) occurs within 5 to 10 minutes following ingestion of alcohol and may last 30 to 60 minutes to several hours. After symptoms subside, patient usually enters sound sleep for several hours.

Intensity of reaction varies with each individual, but it is generally proportional to amount of alcohol ingested.

Warn patient that reaction to alcohol may occur as long as 2 weeks following a single dose of disulfiram.

Although psychotic reactions are usually associated with high dosages, disulfiram may unmask underlying psychosis in some patients stressed by alcohol withdrawal.

During first 2 weeks of therapy, patient may experience metallic or garliclike aftertaste and other mild side effects such as drowsiness, headache, fatigue, impotence, acneiform skin eruptions. These dose-related symptoms often disappear with continued therapy.

Advise patient to carry an identification card stating that he is on disulfiram therapy and describing the symptoms of disulfiram-alcohol reaction and the physician or institution to contact in emergency. Cards may be obtained from Ayerst Laboratories. Ask pharmacist for nearest address.

Supervised disulfiram-alcohol test reaction has now largely been abandoned in favor of detailed description of the reaction to the patient. It is sometimes performed in selected hospitalized patients as a guide to proper dosage level and to have the patient experience, under controlled conditions, what happens when alcohol is ingested. Usually done after 2 weeks of therapy; patient is asked to drink slowly 8 ml of alcohol U.S.P. (15 ml of 100-proof whiskey). Alcohol dose may be repeated only once.

Treatment of severe disulfiram-alcohol reaction: treatment for shock; oxygen or carbogen (95% O_2; 5% CO_2); large doses of intravenous vitamin C; ephedrine sulfate; antihistamines. Monitor potassium levels.

To be effective, disulfiram must be taken consistently for months or even years. Compliance should be determined periodically.

Behavior modification has been achieved for many patients through Alcoholics Anonymous, Al-Anon (for relatives and friends), and Alateen (for teenage children of alcoholic parents).

DRUG INTERACTIONS: Disulfiram may increase blood levels of **oral anticoagulants** (watch for altered anticoagulant effect when disulfiram is started or stopped), **barbiturates** and **phenytoin**. Patients on **isoniazid** therapy receiving disulfiram should be observed for coordination problems and marked changes in behavior. Disulfiram should be discontinued if these signs develop. Preliminary reports indicate that combined **metronidazole**-disulfiram therapy may result in psychotic episodes and confusional states. **Paraldehyde** is thought to be metabolized to acetaldehyde, and thus theoretically it could lead to a reaction like the disulfiram-alcohol reaction. Disulfiram may also decrease rates of metabolism of certain other drugs; therefore, be alert to the potential for toxicity of drugs given concurrently.

DOPAMINE HYDROCHLORIDE
(INTROPIN)

Adrenergic (sympathomimetic)

ACTIONS AND USES
Naturally occurring neurotransmitter and immediate precursor of norepinephrine. Major cardiovascular effects produced by direct action on α- and β-adrenergic receptors and on specific dopaminergic receptors in mesenteric and renal vascular beds. Positive inotropic effect on myocardium produces increased cardiac output with increase in systolic and pulse pressure and little or no effect on diastolic pressure. Improved circulation to renal vascular bed reflected in increased glomerular filtration rate and usually increased urinary output with sodium excretion. Blood flow to peripheral vascular bed may decrease while mesenteric flow increases. Less prone to cause substantial decrease in systemic vascular resistance (SVR), tachyarrhythmias, or increased myocardial oxygen consumption than are other catecholamines. More effective when therapy is started shortly after signs and symptoms of shock appear and before urine flow has decreased to approximately 0.3 ml/minute.
Used to correct hemodynamic imbalance in shock syndrome due to myocardial infarction, trauma, endotoxic septicemia, open heart surgery, and renal and congestive failure.

ABSORPTION AND FATE
Onset of action within 5 minutes; duration less than 10 minutes. Widely distributed in body, but does not cross blood–brain barrier. About 75% of dose is inactivated, chiefly by monoamine oxidase in liver, kidney, and plasma. Approximately 25% of dose is metabolized to norepinephrine within adrenergic nerve terminals. Excreted in urine primarily as metabolites; small portion excreted unchanged.

CONTRAINDICATIONS AND PRECAUTIONS
Pheochromocytoma; tachyarrhythmias or ventricular fibrillation. Safe use in pediatric patients not established. Cautious use: patients who have recently received MAO inhibitors; during pregnancy; patients with history of occlusive vascular disease (eg, Buerger's or Raynaud's disease), cold injury, diabetic endarteritis, arterial embolism.

ADVERSE REACTIONS
Most frequent: ectopic beats, nausea, vomiting, tachycardia, anginal pain, palpitation, dyspnea, headache, hypotension, vasoconstriction (indicated by disproportionate rise in diastolic pressure). Less frequent: piloerection, aberrant con-

duction, bradycardia, widening of QRS complex, azotemia, elevated blood pressure, necrosis and tissue sloughing with extravasation.

ROUTE AND DOSAGE

Intravenous infusion: initially 2 to 5 μg/kg/minute; may be increased gradually to 50 μg/kg/minute, if necessary. Contents of 5-ml ampul (containing 40 mg/ml) must be diluted with appropriate sterile solution recommended by manufacturer. See package insert.

NURSING IMPLICATIONS

Before initiation of dopamine therapy, hypovolemia should be corrected, if possible, with either whole blood or plasma.

Dilution should be made just prior to administration, although reportedly the solution may remain stable for 24 hours after dilution.

IV infusion rate and guidelines for adjusting rate of flow in relation to changes in blood pressure will be prescribed by physician. Microdrip or other reliable metering device should be used for accuracy of flow rate.

Monitor blood pressure, pulse, peripheral pulses, color and temperature of extremities (for peripheral ischemia), and urinary output at intervals prescribed by physician. Precise measurements are essential for accurate titration of dosage.

Indicators for decreasing or temporarily suspending dose: reduced urine flow rate in absence of hypotension, ascending tachycardia, dysarrhythmias, disproportionate rise in diastolic pressure (marked decrease in pulse pressure), change in skin color or temperature of extremities (due to compromised circulation).

Infusion rate must be continuously monitored for free flow, and care must be taken to avoid extravasation, which can result in tissue sloughing and necrosis. For this reason, infusions are made preferably into large veins of antecubital fossa.

Antidote for extravasation: infiltration should be made as soon as possible with 10 to 15 ml of normal saline containing 5 to 10 mg phentolamine, using syringe and fine needle.

Dopamine is a potent drug. Patient must be under constant observation.

In addition to improvement in vital signs and urine flow, other indices of adequate dosage and perfusion of vital organs include loss of pallor, increase in toe temperature, adequacy of nail bed capillary filling, and reversal of confusion or comatose state.

Signs and symptoms of overdosage generally respond to dosage reduction or temporary discontinuation of drug, since dopamine has short duration of action. However, have on hand an α-adrenergic blocking agent (eg, phentolamine) to antagonize peripheral vasoconstriction.

Protect dopamine from light. Discolored solutions should not be used.

DRUG INTERACTIONS: Pressor effects of dopamine are prolonged and intensified if **MAO inhibitors** have been administered within previous 2 or 3 weeks (initial dose of dopamine should be reduced by at least one-tenth the usual dose in these patients), a similar reaction may occur with concomitant use of **furazolidone** since it reportedly may cause dose-related inhibition of MAO. Possibility of enhanced response to dopamine in patients receiving or patients who have recently received **guanethidine.** Concurrent administration of dopamine and **diuretic agents** may produce additive or potentiating effect. **Cyclopropane** and related anesthetics may sensitize myocardium to action of dopamine. Dopamine should be used with extreme caution in these patients.

Central stimulant (respiratory), analeptic

ACTIONS AND USES*
Short-acting analeptic capable of stimulating all levels of cerebrospinal axis. Actions similar to those of nikethamide, but it is reported to have greater margin of safety because of minor effect on cortex. Respiratory stimulation by direct medullary action or possibly by indirect activation of peripheral chemoreceptors produces increased tidal volume and slight increase in respiratory rate. Decreases Pco_2 and increases Po_2 by increasing alveolar ventilation; may elevate blood pressure and pulse rate by stimulation of brain stem vasomotor areas. Also increases salivation, and release of gastric acids, and epinephrine.

Used as short-term adjunctive therapy to alleviate post anesthetic and drug-induced respiratory depression and to hasten arousal and return of pharyngeal and laryngeal reflexes. Also used as temporary measure (approximately 2 hours) in hospitalized patients with chronic pulmonary disease associated with acute respiratory insufficiency as an aid to prevent elevation of arterial CO_2 tension during administration of oxygen (not used in conjunction with mechanical ventilation).

ABSORPTION AND FATE
Onset of respiratory stimulation following a single IV injection occurs in 20 to 40 seconds and peaks in 1 or 2 minutes, with duration rarely more than 5 to 12 minutes. Rapidly metabolized. Believed to be excreted in urine as metabolites.

CONTRAINDICATIONS AND PRECAUTIONS
Known hypersensitivity to doxapram; epilepsy and other convulsive disorders; incompetence of ventilatory mechanism due to muscle paresis, pulmonary fibrosis, flail chest, pneumothorax, airway obstruction, extreme dyspnea, acute bronchial asthma; severe hypertension, coronary artery disease, uncompensated heart failure, cerebrovascular accident. Safe use during pregnancy and in patients 12 years of age or younger not established. Cautious use: cerebral edema, history of bronchial asthma, chronic obstructive pulmonary disease, cardiac disease, severe tachycardia, arrhythmias, hyperthyroidism, pheochromocytoma, hypertension, head injury, increased intracranial pressure, peptic ulcer, patients undergoing gastric surgery, acute agitation.

ADVERSE REACTIONS
Central and autonomic nervous systems: dizziness, sneezing, apprehension, confusion, involuntary movements, hyperactivity, paresthesia (feeling of warmth, burning, especially of genitalia, perineum), flushing, sweating, hyperpyrexia, headache, pilomotor erection, pruritus, muscle tremor, spasms, rigidity, convulsions (rarely), increased deep-tendon reflexes, bilateral Babinski sign, carpopedal spasm, pupillary dilation, mild delayed narcosis. **Respiratory:** dyspnea, tachypnea, cough, laryngospasm, bronchospasm, hiccups, rebound hypoventilation, hypocapnia with tetany. **Cardiovascular:** mild to moderate increase in blood pressure, phlebitis, sinus tachycardia, bradycardia, extrasystoles, lowered T waves, PVCs, chest pains, tightness in chest. **GI:** nausea, vomiting, diarrhea, salivation, sour taste. **Genitourinary:** retention, frequency, incontinence. Other (cause-and-effect relationship not established): decreased hemoglobin, hematocrit, and RBC count; elevated BUN; albuminuria.

ROUTE AND DOSAGE
Intravenous: 0.5 to 1 mg/kg body weight; single injection not to exceed 1.5 mg/kg body weight or 2 mg/kg when given as injections at 5-minute intervals. Intravenous infusion: recommended maximum dose is 4 mg/kg, not to exceed 3 Gm. Compatible with 5% or 10% dextrose in water or normal saline.

NURSING IMPLICATIONS

Adequacy of airway and oxygenation must be assured before initiation of doxapram therapy.

IV flow rate will be prescribed by physician. Infusion rate may start at 5 mg/minute until satisfactory respiratory response is observed. It should then be maintained at 1 to 3 mg/minute and be adjusted to maintain desired respiratory response.

Careful monitoring and accurate observations of blood pressure, pulse, deep-tendon reflexes, and airway are essential guides for determining minimum effective dosage and preventing overdosage.

Observe patient continuously during therapy and maintain vigilance (usually about 1 hour) until patient is fully alert and protective pharyngeal and laryngeal reflexes are completely restored.

Notify physician immediately of any side effects. Be alert for early signs of toxicity: tachycardia, muscle tremor, spasticity, hyperactive reflexes.

A mild to moderate increase in blood pressure commonly occurs; this is a matter of concern in patients with preexisting hypertension.

If sudden hypotension or dyspnea develops, doxapram should be discontinued.

Doxapram generally produces increased alertness in postoperative patients and earlier perception of pain than usual. However, since the action of doxapram is short, keep in mind that poststimulation narcosis may occur.

Oxygen, resuscitative equipment, and IV barbiturates should be readily available in the event of excessive CNS stimulation.

Determinations of blood gases, Po_2, Pco_2, and O_2 saturation are desirable to assess effectiveness of respiratory stimulation. In patients with chronic obstructive pulmonary disease, arterial blood gases should be drawn prior to initiation of doxapram infusion and oxygen administration and then at least every ½ hour during infusion.

Doxapram should be discontinued if arterial blood gases show evidence of deterioration and mechanical ventilation is initiated.

Extravasation or use of a single injection site for prolonged periods can cause thrombophlebitis.

Postoperative patients or patients in a state of narcosis with chronic pulmonary insufficiency should receive oxygen concomitantly. Respiratory stimulation produced by doxapram increases the work of breathing and thus increases oxygen consumption and CO_2 production.

DRUG INTERACTIONS: Synergistic pressor effects (increase in blood pressure arrhythmias) may occur in patients receiving **sympathomimetic agents** or **MAO inhibitors**. Initiation of doxapram should be delayed for at least 10 minutes following discontinuation of anesthetics that sensitize myocardium to catecholamines, such as halothane and related anesthetics.

DOXEPIN HYDROCHLORIDE
(ADAPIN, SINEQUAN)

Tricyclic antidepressant

ACTIONS AND USES

Pharmacologically related to imipramine (qv) and has similar actions, contraindications, precautions, and adverse reactions. In addition to antidepressant action, it also has mild tranquilizing properties and is reported to be well tolerated by elderly patients.

Used in treatment of anxiety and depression of psychoneurotic states, alcoholism, organic disease, psychotic depressive disorders including involutional depression, and manic–depressive reactions.

CONTRAINDICATIONS AND PRECAUTIONS

Hypersensitivity, glaucoma, tendency to urinary retention; pregnancy; use in children under 12 years of age; concomitant use of MAO inhibitors or within 2 weeks of their administration. See Imipramine.

ADVERSE REACTIONS

Drowsiness (common), dry mouth, blurred vision, constipation or diarrhea; urinary retention, anorexia, nausea, vomiting, taste disturbances, dizziness, tinnitus, weight gain. Infrequent: edema, alopecia, sweating, flushing, chills, hypotension, tachycardia, extrapyramidal symptoms, bone marrow depression. Also see Imipramine.

ROUTE AND DOSAGE

Oral: 10 to 50 mg 3 times daily. More severely ill patients may require gradual increase to 300 mg/day. Highly individualized.

NURSING IMPLICATIONS

Patients with suicidal tendencies should be watched closely during early stages of therapy.

Antianxiety effects may be apparent a few days after drug is initiated; however, optimal antidepressant effects may not be noted until after 2 or 3 weeks of drug therapy.

Drowsiness and anticholinergic effects (dry mouth, constipation, urinary retention, blurred vision) are usually mild and often subside with continued therapy. Reduction of dosage may be necessary if symptoms persist.

Caution patients about the incidence of drowsiness; patients should avoid driving a car or operating dangerous machinery while taking the drug.

Warn patient that doxepin may potentiate response to alcohol.

The oral concentrate should be diluted with approximately 120 ml of water or orange juice just prior to administration.

Protect drug from direct sunlight and strong artificial light.

See Imipramine Hydrochloride.

DRUG INTERACTIONS: Reportedly doxepin in doses less than 100 mg/day does not appear to be antagonistic to the effects of **guanethidine** and related compounds; however, at doxepin doses of 100 to 300 mg, significant antagonism of **guanethidine**'s antihypertensive effect does occur. Also see Imipramine.

DOXORUBICIN HYDROCHLORIDE
(ADRIAMYCIN)

Antineoplastic (antibiotic)

ACTIONS AND USES

Cytotoxic anthracycline glycoside antibiotic isolated from *Streptomyces peucetius,* with wide spectrum of antitumor activity and strong immunosuppressive properties. Intercalates with preformed DNA residues, blocking effective DNA and RNA transcription. Highly destructive to rapidly proliferating cells and slow-developing carcinomas; selectively toxic to cardiac tissue. No clinical cross-resistance to standard antineoplastics; therefore, it may be especially effective in patients with less advanced disease. Cytotoxicity precludes its use as antiinfective agent.

Used to produce regression in neoplastic conditions. Generally used in combined modalities with surgery, radiation, and immunotherapy. Also effective pretreatment to sensitize superficial tumors to local radiation therapy. One member of the ABVD, BACOP, CHOP combination chemotherapeutic regimen.

ABSORPTION AND FATE

Widely distributed in tissues, especially liver, lungs, heart, and kidneys. Absorbed by cells; binds to cellular components, particularly nucleic acids. Metabolized in liver and other tissues to active and inactive metabolites. Excreted predominantly in bile (about 50% as unchanged drug); 10% to 20% of single dose is excreted in feces in 24 hours, with 15% to 45% within 7 days. Less than 6% excreted in urine after 5 days, primarily as unchanged drug.

CONTRAINDICATIONS AND PRECAUTIONS

Myelosuppression, impaired cardiac function, obstructive jaundice, pregnancy. Safe use in patients of childbearing potential not established. Cautious use: impaired hepatic or renal function, patients having had radiotherapy to areas surrounding the heart.

ADVERSE REACTIONS

Cardiovascular: serious and irreversible myocardial toxicity with delayed congestive heart failure, acute left ventricular failure, and hypotension. **Hematopoietic:** high incidence of myelosuppression: leukopenia (principally granulocytes), thrombocytopenia, anemia. **GI:** stomatitis and esophagitis (common) with ulcerations, nausea, vomiting, inanition, diarrhea. **Dermatologic:** hyperpigmentation of nail beds and buccal mucosa (especially in blacks); hyperpigmentation of dermal creases (especially in children), facial flush, rash, complete alopecia, recall of skin reactions due to prior radiotherapy, hypersensitivity. Other: conjunctivitis (rare), lacrimation, drowsiness, fever. With extravasation: severe cellulitis, vesication, tissue necrosis, lymphangitis, thrombophlebitis.

ROUTE AND DOSAGE

Intravenous: 60 to 75 mg/m^2 administered at 21 day intervals. Alternatively 30 mg/m^2 for 3 successive days every 4 weeks. Total dosage should not to exceed 550 mg/m^2 body surface. Highly individualized; dosage based indirectly on weight. Reconstituted by adding 5 ml of 0.9% sodium chloride injection to the 10-mg vial, or 25 ml to the 50-mg vial. Shake vial and allow contents to dissolve.

NURSING IMPLICATIONS

Caution should be observed in preparing doxorubicin. If powder or solution contacts skin or mucosa, wash thoroughly with soap and water.

Administration directly into tubing of freely running infusion of normal saline or 5% dextrose in water is recommended to reduce the likelihood of extravasation. Do not mix this drug with other drugs.

Physician will order specific infusion rate. Transient flushing may occur if drug is administered too rapidly. Urticaria around injection site (due to histamine release) is usually self-limiting.

Care should be taken to avoid extravasation. Examine the injection site frequently during infusion. Provide meticulous site care to prevent infection. IV tubing should be dated and changed at least every 24 hours.

Give prompt attention to the patient's complaint of a stinging or burning sensation around injection site; stop infusion immediately, even though blood return can be demonstrated. Application of cold compresses may reduce severity of tissue damage.

Begin a flow chart to establish baseline data for future comparative purposes. Include temperature, pulse, respiration, blood pressure, body weight, laboratory values, and intake–output ratio and pattern.

Evaluation of hepatic, renal, hematopoietic, and cardiac functions should be performed prior to initiation of therapy, at regular intervals thereafter, and at end of therapy. Since cardiac failure may occur several weeks to months after cessation of therapy, ECG should also be performed at least monthly during this time.

Therapeutic response to doxorubicin is not likely to occur without some evidence of toxicity.

Myocardial toxicity (irreversible) becomes more of a threat as cumulative dose approaches 550 mg/m² body surface.

Be alert to early signs of cardiac toxicity (dyspnea, steady weight gain, hypotension, arrhythmias) to permit immediate medical treatment. Frequent pulse, blood pressure, and weight readings are important cumulative data for early detection of cardiopathy.

Objective signs of hepatic dysfunction (jaundice, dark urine, pruritus) or kidney dysfunction (changed intake–output ratio and pattern, local discomfort with voiding) demand prompt attention, since both conditions cause delayed drug elimination. Report to physician.

Stomatitis, generally maximal in second week of therapy, frequently begins with a burning sensation accompanied by erythema of oral mucosa that may progress to ulceration and dysphagia in 2 or 3 days. Fastidious oral hygiene is required, especially before and after meals. Patient should be referred to a dentist if dental caries or peridontal disease is present. See Mechlorethamine for mouth care.

Immunosuppressive properties of doxorubicin require careful screening of visitors and attending personnel to shield the patient from infection, especially during leukopenic periods.

The nadir of leukopenia (an expected 1000/mm³) typically occurs 10 to 14 days after single dose; prompt recovery within 5 to 7 days is usual.

Superinfections by microflora may result from antibiotic therapy during leukopenic period. Report black or furry tongue, diarrhea, and foul-smelling stools.

Complete alopecia (reversible) is an expected side effect. Regrowth of hair usually begins 2 to 3 months after drug is discontinued. Discuss this side effect with the patient in order to plan for cosmetic substitution, if desired. An awareness of the impact of the loss of scalp and body hair on one's concept of sexuality should guide this discussion.

Bloody diarrhea may result from an antiblastic effect on rapidly growing intestinal mucosal cells. The physician may prescribe an antidiarrheal medication. Avoid rectal medications and use of rectal thermometer in order to prevent trauma.

Advise patient that the drug imparts a red color to urine for 1 to 2 days after administration.

Increased lacrimation for 5 to 10 days after a single dose is a possibility. Caution patient to keep hands away from eyes to prevent conjunctivitis.

Consult the physician about his plan for disclosure of diagnosis, expected results of therapy, and prognosis to the patient and family in order to facilitate better communication with the patient.

Collaborate with dietitian and patient's family to help the patient maintain optimum nutritional status. Determine dietary preferences; try to support and augment rather than reform eating patterns during period of discomfort. Space pain medication so that peak effect is at mealtime; appropriately schedule fatiguing treatments to avoid presenting food to a tired patient.

Reconstituted solution is stable for 24 hours at room temperature and for 48 hours under refrigeration. Protect solution from sunlight; discard unused remainder.

(DOXY-II, DOXYCHEL, VIBRAMYCIN HYCLATE)
DOXYCYCLINE MONOHYDRATE
(DOXY-II, DOXYCHEL, VIBRAMYCIN MONOHYDRATE)

Antibacterial

ACTIONS AND USES

Tetracycline antibiotic synthetically derived from oxytetracycline. Similar to tetracycline (qv) in actions, uses, contraindications, precautions, and adverse reactions. More completely absorbed, effective blood levels maintained for longer periods, and excreted more slowly than most tetracyclines; thus, it requires smaller and less frequent doses. Reportedly, usual doses of doxycycline do not lead to excessive blood accumulation in patients with renal impairment.

ABSORPTION AND FATE

Almost completely absorbed following oral administration. Range of plasma protein binding reported: 25% to 90%. Half-life about 15 hours after single dose and up to 22 hours after repeated doses (essentially the same for patients with normal and impaired renal function). Metabolized in part by liver. Excreted primarily in bile and feces (up to 90%); also excreted slowly in urine.

CONTRAINDICATIONS AND PRECAUTIONS

Sensitivity to tetracyclines; use of IV doxycycline in children under 8 years of age. Also see Tetracycline.

ADVERSE REACTIONS

With oral drug: nausea, diarrhea, GI discomfort; renal impairment, hepatotoxicity with excessive dosage; increased intracranial pressure; discoloration of nails, onycholysis; permanent discoloration and inadequate calcification of deciduous and permanent teeth when used during period of tooth development (from fourth month of fetal development to 8 years of life); overgrowth of nonsusceptible organisms; photosensitivity. Also see Tetracycline.

ROUTE AND DOSAGE

Adults: Oral: 100 mg every 12 hours on first day, followed by maintenance dose of 100 mg/day as single dose or 50 mg every 12 hours (for severe infections 100 mg every 12 hours is recommended). Intravenous: 200 mg on first day administered in one or two infusions; subsequent daily dosage: 100 to 200 mg depending on severity of infection. **Children** (*weighing 100 lb or less*): Oral, intravenous: 2 mg/lb body weight on first day of treatment as single dose or divided into 2 doses; subsequent daily dosage: 1 or 2 mg/lb body weight as single dose or divided into 2 doses.

NURSING IMPLICATIONS

Check expiration date. Degradation products of tetracycline or its congeners are nephrotoxic and have caused Fanconilike syndrome.

Note that usual dosage and frequency of administration differ from those of other tetracyclines. Dosages in excess of those recommended may result in increased incidence of side effects.

Reportedly, absorption of oral drug is not markedly influenced by simultaneous ingestion of food or milk. However, iron preparations, sodium bicarbonate, and antacids containing aluminum, calcium, or magnesium may significantly interfere with absorption. Therefore, these medications should be spaced at least 3 hours after doxycycline.

Preparation and storage of solutions: all tetracycline solutions should be used before the manufacturer's stated expiration date. Reconstituted solutions may be stored up to 72 hours prior to start of infusion if refrigerated and protected from sun and artificial light.

For IV use, the reconstituted solution must be diluted further with NaCl, 5%

dextrose, or other diluents (named by manufacturer) before administration. Infusion must be completed within 12 hours of dilution. Date IV solution; bottle should be covered with foil or other light-resistant material during infusion.

When diluted with lactated Ringer's or dextrose 5% in lactated injection, infusion must be completed within 6 hours to ensure adequate stability.

IV infusion rate will be prescribed by physician. Duration of infusion will vary with dose, but it is usually 1 to 4 hours. Recommended minimum infusion time for 100 mg of 0.5-mg/ml solution is 1 hour.

Therapy should be continued at least 24 to 48 hours after symptoms have subsided.

Caution patient to avoid exposure to direct sunlight and ultraviolet light while taking doxycycline and for 4 or 5 days after therapy is terminated.

See Tetracycline Hydrochloride.

DOXYLAMINE SUCCINATE, N.F.
(DECAPRYN)

Antihistaminic

ACTIONS AND USES
Ethanolamine derivative with actions, uses, contraindications, precautions, and adverse reactions similar to those of diphenhydramine (qv).
ROUTE AND DOSAGE
Oral: **Adults and children** *12 years of age and over:* 12.5 to 25 mg every 4 to 6 hours, if necessary. **Children** *under 12 years:* 3.75 to 6.25 mg every 4 to 6 hours, if necessary.

NURSING IMPLICATIONS
High incidence of drowsiness.
See Diphenhydramine Hydrochloride.

DROMOSTANOLONE PROPIONATE, N.F.
(DROLBAN, MASTERONE)

Antineoplastic, androgen

ACTIONS AND USES
Synthetic steroid hormone chemically and pharmacologically related to testosterone (qv). Has lower incidence of androgenic side effects than parent compound. In advanced carcinoma, promotes weight gain and feeling of well-being, even though objective remission may not be obtained.
Used palliatively in advanced inoperable metastatic carcinoma of breast.
CONTRAINDICATIONS AND PRECAUTIONS
Carcinoma of male breast; premenopausal women. Cautious use: during pregnancy, liver disease, cardiac decompensation, nephritis, nephrosis, carcinoma of prostate. See Testosterone.
ADVERSE REACTIONS
Virilism; hypercalcemia; edema (occasionally); severe, reversible CNS side effects (rare); local reaction at injection site (rare). See Testosterone.
ROUTE AND DOSAGE
Intramuscular (in sesame oil): 100 mg 3 times weekly.

NURSING IMPLICATIONS

At least 8 to 12 weeks of therapy may be necessary to produce satisfactory results. If disease being treated progresses significantly during first 6 to 8 weeks of treatment, another form of therapy may be indicated.

Treatment may be continued as long as satisfactory results are obtained.

Patients with edema may require diuretic therapy before and during treatment with dromostanolone. Monitor weight and inspect dependent areas for signs of fluid retention. Report significant weight changes to physician.

Serum calcium and alkaline phosphatase levels should be determined before and periodically during therapy.

Advise patient to report symptoms of hypercalcemia, deep bone and flank pain, polyuria, muscle weakness, nausea, vomiting, anorexia, constipation.

Product should not be refrigerated.

See Testosterone.

DROPERIDOL, N.F.

(INAPSINE)

Neuroleptic, tranquilizer

ACTIONS AND USES

Butyrophenone derivative structurally and pharmacologically related to haloperidol and piperazine-type phenothiazines. Antagonizes emetic effects of morphinelike analgesics and other drugs that act on CTZ. Has slight α-adrenergic blocking activity and direct vasodilator effect that may cause hypotension. Potentiates other CNS depressants and reduces pressor effects of epinephrine. Has no apparent analgesic activity.

Used to produce tranquilizing effect and reduce nausea and vomiting during surgical and diagnostic procedures, for premedication, during induction, and as adjunct in maintenance of general or regional anesthesia. Principally used in combination with a potent narcotic analgesic such as fentanyl (eg, Innovar) to produce neuroleptanalgesia (quiescence and psychic indifference to environmental stimuli) to permit carrying out certain diagnostic and neurologic procedures.

ABSORPTION AND FATE

Onset of action within 3 to 10 minutes; peaks in about 30 minutes following single IM or IV dose. Duration of sedative and tranquilizing effects is generally 2 to 4 hours; however, tranquilization may persist 6 to 12 hours. Metabolized by liver and excreted in urine and feces. About 10% excreted in urine as unchanged drug. Reportedly crosses placenta.

CONTRAINDICATIONS AND PRECAUTIONS

Known intolerance to droperidol and other phenothiazines. Parkinsonism, hypotension. Safe use during pregnancy, women of childbearing potential, and in children younger than 2 years of age not established. Cautious use: elderly, debilitated, and other poor-risk patients; liver, kidney, or cardiac dysfunction.

ADVERSE REACTIONS

Most frequent: hypotension, tachycardia, drowsiness. Chills, shivering, dizziness, restlessness, anxiety, hallucinations, mental depression, laryngospasm, bronchospasm. Extrapyramidal symptoms: dystonia, akathisia, oculogyric crisis. See Haloperidol.

ROUTE AND DOSAGE

Adults: Intramuscular, intravenous (premedication): 2.5 to 10 mg 30 to 60 minutes before the procedure. **Children** *2 to 12 years of age:* 1 to 1.5 mg per each 20 to 25 lb body weight.

NURSING IMPLICATIONS

Monitor vital signs closely. Hypotension and tachycardia are common side effects of droperidol. Fluids and pressor agents, (other than epinephrine) eg, metaraminol, should be immediately available.

Because of possibility of orthostatic hypotension, exercise care in moving and positioning patients.

Patients who have received narcotic analgesic concurrently should be observed carefully for signs of impending respiratory depression (restlessness, apnea, rigidity). A narcotic antagonist and resuscitative equipment, including oropharyngeal airway or endotracheal tube, suction, and oxygen, should be readily available.

Elevated blood pressure has been reported following administration of droperidol with parenteral analgesics.

When patient is under the effect of another CNS depressant, the required dose of droperidol may be less than usual.

Postoperative narcotics or other CNS depressants are prescribed in reduced doses (as low as 25% or 30% of those usually recommended), since they have additive or potentiating effects with droperidol.

Extrapyramidal symptoms (see Haloperidol) may occur up to 24 hours postoperatively.

Droperidol may aggravate symptoms of acute depression.

Drug incompatibilities: do not mix with parenteral barbiturates, since a precipitate may occur.

Protect from light.

See Haloperidol.

DYDROGESTERONE, N.F., B.P.
(DUPHASTON, GYNOREST)

Progestin agent

ACTIONS AND USES

Synthetic progestational steroid. Promotes development of normal, full secretory endometrium in uterus previously sensitized by estrogen. Uniquely nonthermogenic; lacks estrogenic and androgenic activities of progesterone, but similarly may decrease glucose tolerance. Reduces uterine motility by unknown mechanism. Female masculinization has not been observed with use of this drug. Progestogen therapy may mask onset of climacteric.

Used to treat primary and secondary amenorrhea, dysmenorrhea, abnormal uterine bleeding due to hormone imbalance in absence of organic pathology, endometriosis.

ABSORPTION AND FATE

Absorption from GI tract is rapid (20 to 30 minutes) and almost complete. Plasma half-life about 5 minutes. Blood levels decline in 2 to 3 hours. Small amounts stored in body fat. Metabolized in liver. Some excretion in feces; most of dose excreted in urine within 24 hours. Crosses placenta and is detectable in breast milk.

CONTRAINDICATIONS AND PRECAUTIONS

Thrombophlebitis, thromboembolic disorders, pulmonary embolism, cerebral apoplexy, or patient with history of these conditions; marked liver disease or impairment; undiagnosed vaginal bleeding; known or suspected breast neoplasm; missed abortion; nursing mother. Cautious use: diabetes mellitus; history of psychosis, epilepsy, migraine, asthma; cardiac or renal dysfunction.

Some reactions are reportedly associated with use of estrogen-progestin combination drugs; whether they are specifically due to the progestin component has neither been confirmed nor disproved. **Cardiovascular**: thrombophlebitis, pulmonary embolism, cerebral thrombosis, hypertension. **GI**: changes in weight and appetite; diarrhea, nausea, vomiting; cholestatic jaundice. **Neurologic**: sudden partial or complete loss of vision, proptosis, diplopia, neuro-ocular lesions; mental depression, nervousness, dizziness, migraine, headache. **Genitourinary**: cystitislike syndrome, vaginal candidiasis, premenstruallike syndrome, breakthrough bleeding, spotting, change in menstrual flow, amenorrhea, cervical erosion and increased cervical secretions, changes in libido. **Other**: acne, rash with or without pruritus, erythema multiforme and nodosum; loss of scalp hair, hirsutism; backache, fatigue, breast changes (tenderness, enlargement, secretion); decreased glucose tolerance, mild leukocytosis.

ROUTE AND DOSAGE

Oral (*amenorrhea*): 10 to 20 mg daily in divided doses, day 15 through day 25 of cycle; (*oligomenorrhea*): 10 mg daily in divided doses for 5 days; this cycle is repeated for 3 to 6 months, then discontinued to determine if spontaneous menstrual pattern has been established; (*abnormal uterine bleeding*): initially 10 to 20 mg in divided doses for 5 to 10 days; thereafter, 10 mg daily in divided doses, day 21 through day 25 of cycle; (*endometriosis*): 20 mg in divided doses either daily or continuously without interruption, or from day 5 to day 25 of cycle.

NURSING IMPLICATIONS

Since dydrogesterone does not prevent ovulation, the usual cyclic changes can be expected, and conception can occur during treatment.

Accurate basal body temperatures to determine day of ovulation may be monitored, since drug does not alter basal body temperature.

Pretherapy and periodic physicals during dydrogesterone treatment should include examination of pelvic organs and breast, Papanicolaou smear, and glycosuria test.

Teach patient breast self-examination and emphasize importance of doing it on a regular monthly basis (after menstrual flow has stopped).

Warn patient to report promptly symptoms of jaundice (yellow skin, soft palate, and sclerae, dark urine, pruritus, clay-colored stools).

If liver or endocrine function tests are abnormal during dydrogesterone therapy, reevaluation following a 2- or 3-month interruption is recommended.

Patients with diabetes should be advised to report positive urine tests for sugar. Dosage of antidiabetic drug may require adjustment.

When history of psychic depression exists, a responsible member of patient's family should be advised to note and report evidence that might suggest recurrence.

Perineal itching and burning may signal onset of vaginal candidiasis (secondary to progestogen excess) or cystitislike syndrome. Urge patient to report promptly to physician for differential diagnosis and treatment.

Teach patient to differentiate between withdrawal and breakthrough bleeding: withdrawal bleeding follows discontinuation of drug within 3 or 4 days and is expected; breakthrough bleeding and spotting occur intermenstrually and should be reported. Dose adjustment or drug discontinuation may be indicated.

Teach patient how to elicit *Homan's sign:* pain in calf and popliteal region with forced dorsiflexion of foot (sign of thrombosis). Urge prompt reporting of pain, tenderness, and redness of extremity.

Monitor weight every other day; record for comparative purposes. Fluid retention has not been reported with dydrogesterone. However, counsel patient with history of conditions worsened by edema (eg, migraine, epilepsy) to report promptly signs of fluid retention (such as tight rings and shoes, increasing weight) to physician.

Visual changes are serious side effects. Advise patient to withhold medication and to report promptly their onset. If ophthalmic examination reveals papilledema or retinal-vascular lesion, medication will be withdrawn.

The pathologist should be notified of dydrogesterone therapy when relevant tissue specimens are submitted.

See Oral Contraceptives (general discussion).

DYPHYLLINE
(AIRET, CIRCAIR, DILIN, DYFLEX, DILOR, EMFABID, LUFYLLIN, NEOTHYLLINE)

Smooth-muscle relaxant

ACTIONS AND USES

Xanthine and derivative of theophylline (qv), with which it shares actions, uses, contraindications, precautions, and adverse reactions. Claimed to cause less gastric distress than theophylline because of its neutral pH and to be more uniformly and predictably absorbed, but blood levels and activity are lower. Used in treatment of acute bronchial asthma and for reversible bronchospasm associated with chronic bronchitis and emphysema. Available in several antiasthmatic preparations in combination with quaifenesin, eg, Dilor-G, Lufyllin-GG, Emfaseem, G-Bron.

CONTRAINDICATIONS AND PRECAUTIONS

Cautious use: in children; concomitant administration of other xanthine formulations or other CNS stimulating drugs. Also see Theophylline.

ROUTE AND DOSAGE

Adults: Oral: 200 mg 3 or 4 times daily. In acute asthma attack: 400 to 600 mg may be prescribed initially. Intramuscular: 250 to 500 mg. **Children:** Oral: 2 to 3 mg/lb in divided doses, not to exceed 6 mg/lb/day. All dosages titrated to individual patient requirements.

NURSING IMPLICATIONS

Administration of oral preparation after meals may prevent gastric discomfort.

For IM administration, aspirate carefully before injecting drug to avoid inadvertent intravascular injection. Inject drug slowly.

Discard ampul if a precipitate is present.

Report promptly early signs of overdosage: nausea, vomiting, headache, palpitation, CNS stimulation (irritability, restlessness).

Protect dyphylline from light.

See Theophylline.

DRUG INTERACTIONS: Concurrent administration of dyphylline (and other xanthines) with **ephedrine** or other **sympathomimetics** can cause excessive CNS stimulation. Also see Theophylline.

E

ECHOTHIOPHATE IODIDE, U.S.P.
(Phospholine Iodide)

Ophthalmic cholinergic (miotic)

ACTIONS AND USES

Extremely potent, long-acting, quaternary organophosphorus compound. Similar to demecarium in actions, uses, contraindications, precautions, and adverse effects. In contrast to the situation with demecarium, the cholinesterase inhibition produced by echothiophate is relatively irreversible, ie, cholinesterase activity returns only when new enzyme is formed.

Used particularly in treatment of open angle glaucoma and convergent strabismus. Use is usually reserved for patients not satisfactorily controlled by less potent miotics.

ABSORPTION AND FATE

Absorbed through conjunctival sac. Miotic action begins within 10 to 45 minutes following instillation and may persist 1 to 4 weeks.

CONTRAINDICATIONS AND PRECAUTIONS

Hypersensitivity to drug ingredients; acute-angle closure glaucoma, active uveal inflammation. Safe use during pregnancy not established. Cautious use: patients routinely exposed to organophosphate insecticides. Also see Demecarium Bromide.

ADVERSE REACTIONS

Brow ache, dimness or blurring of vision; reduced serum cholinesterases; decreased pseudocholinesterase activity; diarrhea, sweating, muscle weakness. See Demecarium Bromide.

ROUTE AND DOSAGE

Topical: 1 drop of 0.03% to 0.25% ophthalmic solution instilled into conjunctival sac once or twice daily (morning and evening). Not to exceed a twice-daily schedule. Highly individualized.

NURSING IMPLICATIONS

When possible, instillation of daily dose or one of the daily doses should be made at bedtime to minimize the disturbing effects of blurred vision produced by miosis.

Technique of administration: gentle finger pressure should be held against nasolacrimal sac for 1 or 2 minutes following instillation. This minimizes drainage into nose and throat and thus systemic absorption. Immediately remove excess solution around eye with tissue. Rinse hands thoroughly after handling drug.

If possible, tonometric measurements should be made each hour for 3 or 4 hours after initial instillation and periodically during therapy.

Brow ache or dimness or blurring of vision may occur at onset of therapy, but these usually disappear within 5 to 10 days. Patient may require an analgesic.

Physician may prescribe concomitant instillation of phenylephrine or epinephrine hydrochloride to improve visual acuity (dilates miotic treated eye without increasing intraocular pressure) and to reduce conjunctival redness.

All patients should remain under constant supervision while receiving echothiophate.

In most patients, serum pseudocholinesterase and erythrocyte cholinesterase levels will be depressed after a few weeks of eyedrop therapy, with resultant systemic effects.

Caution patient to report salivation, diarrhea, profuse sweating, urinary incontinence, or muscle weakness. These systemic effects indicate the need to terminate medication.

Warn patients of possible additive systemic effects from exposure to organophosphorus-type insecticides and pesticides, eg, parathion, malathion. If these are used, advise the patient to wear a respiratory mask, to wash frequently, and to change clothing.

Systemic effects occurring after topical application, skin contact, or accidental ingestion can be antagonized by parenteral atropine sulfate or pralidoxime.

Tolerance may develop after prolonged use, but the response is usually restored by a prescribed rest period from drug.

Aqueous solutions remain stable for 1 month at room temperature or for 12 months from date of reconstitution if refrigerated.

DRUG INTERACTIONS: Other **cholinesterase inhibitors** potentiate the action of echothiophate. With prolonged use of echothiophate, there is the possibility of severe reactions follow injections of **procaine** or administration of **succinylcholine.** Also see Demecarium Bromide.

EDETATE CALCIUM DISODIUM, U.S.P.
(Calcium Disodium Edathamil, CALCIUM DISODIUM VERSENATE, CaEDTA)
SODIUM CALCIUMEDETATE, B.P.

Metal complexing (chelating) agent

ACTIONS AND USES

Chelating agent that combines with divalent and trivalent metals to form stable, nonionizing, water-soluble complexes that can be readily excreted by kidneys. Action is dependent on ability of heavy metal to displace the less strongly bound calcium in the drug molecule.

Used principally as adjunct in treatment of acute and chronic lead poisoning (plumbism). May be used in combination with dimercaprol (BAL) in treatment of lead encephalopathy. Reported to be of some value in treatment of poisoning from other heavy metals such as chromium, manganese, nickel, zinc, and possibly vanadium, and also in removal of radioactive and nuclear fission products. Not effective in poisoning from arsenic, gold, or mercury. Also used to diagnose suspected lead poisoning.

ABSORPTION AND FATE

Approximately 5% to 10% of oral dose is absorbed; fecal excretion continues for about 2 or 3 days. Following IV administration, urinary excretion of chelated lead begins in about 1 hour. Peak excretion of chelates occurs within 24 to 48 hours.

CONTRAINDICATIONS AND PRECAUTIONS

Oral use in patients with severe renal disease or in acute lead poisoning, anuria, during pregnancy or in women of childbearing potential. Extreme caution in patients with renal dysfunction, active tuberculosis, or calcified tubercular lesions.

ADVERSE REACTIONS

Numbness, tingling sensations, headaches, muscle cramps, anorexia, nausea, vomiting, diarrhea, abdominal cramps, weakness, hypotension, burning sensation at injection site, thrombophlebitis, hypercalcemia, gout. With high doses or prolonged administration: proteinuria, hematuria, acute tubular necrosis, transient bone marrow depression, cheilosis and other mucocutaneous lesions. Febrile systemic reaction (malaise, fatigue, excessive thirst, fever, chills, severe myalgia, arthralgia, frontal headache, GI distress, urinary frequency and urgency), and accompanied by histaminelike reactions, sneezing, nasal congestion, lacrimation. Depletion of blood metals.

ROUTE AND DOSAGE

Oral (rarely) **Adults**: 4 Gm daily in divided doses. **Children**: 65 mg/kg/day in divided doses. Treatment may be continued for maximum of 2 weeks, followed by 2-week rest period prior to additional courses. Intravenous: 1 Gm in 250 to 500 ml 5% dextrose in water or isotonic sodium chloride injection twice daily (12-hour intervals) for 3 to 5 days. Therapy should then be interrupted for 2 days, followed by additional 5 days of treatment, if indicated. Intramuscular (preferred route for children): 50 mg/kg/day, in equally divided doses twice daily for 3 to 5 days. Second course may be given after rest period of 4 or more days. Procaine should be added to minimize pain at injection site (1 ml of procaine 1% to each ml of concentrated drug).

NURSING IMPLICATIONS

One gram edetate exchanges its calcium for 3 to 5 mg lead in the blood.

Adequacy of urinary output must be determined before therapy is initiated. Physician will prescribe specific IV infusion rate.

Rapid IV infusion can be lethal in patients with overt or incipient lead encephalopathy because of increase in intracranial pressure. Excess fluid intake should be avoided in these patients; consult physician regarding allowable intake.

Monitor vital signs. Report cardiac rhythm irregularities.

Be alert for occurrence of febrile systemic reaction that may occur 4 to 8 hours after drug infusion (see Adverse Reactions).

Monitor intake and output. Since drug is excreted almost exclusively via kidneys, toxicity may develop if output is inadequate. Therapy should be stopped if urine flow is markedly diminished or absent. Report any change in output or intake–output ratio to physician.

Home patients and responsible family members should be instructed to adhere to prescribed dosage regimen, to report adverse reactions immediately to physician, and to keep scheduled follow-up appointments.

Edetate calcium disodium can produce potentially fatal effects when higher than recommended doses are used or when it is continued after toxic effects appear.

Routine urinalysis including test for coproporphyrins, and BUN determination should be performed prior to therapy and daily during entire course of therapy. Presence of large renal epithelial cells or increasing hematuria and proteinuria are indications to terminate drug immediately.

Because edetate calcium disodium may chelate metals other than lead, patients on prolonged therapy should have periodic determinations of blood metals (eg, copper, zinc).

Lead poisoning is a persistent problem in certain occupations and in areas where older homes exist. Adequate measures should be instituted to eliminate sources of exposure to lead. In areas where lead poisoning is endemic, parents should be encouraged to take their children to lead-detection clinics.

Manifestations of lead poisoning include abdominal colic, pallor, anemia, blue-black pigmented line along gingival margins (in patients with poor oral hygiene), peripheral neuritis, encephalopathy (ataxia, vomiting, lethargy, stupor, followed by convulsions, mania, and coma). Normal whole blood lead level: 0 to 50 μg/dl. Clearcut symptoms of lead poisoning occur within a range of 80 to 100 μg/dl.

Antidote (curare principles), diagnostic aid (myasthenia gravis)

ACTIONS AND USES
Short-acting anticholinesterase quaternary ammonium compound similar to neostigmine in actions, contraindications, precautions, and adverse reactions. Acts as antidote to curariform drugs by displacing them from muscle cell receptor sites, thus permitting resumption of normal transmission of neuromuscular impulses. However, like neostigmine, it prolongs skeletal muscle relaxant action of succinylcholine chloride and decamethonium bromide.

Used for differential diagnosis and as adjunct in evaluation of treatment requirements of myasthenia gravis, for differentiating myasthenic from cholinergic crisis, and to reverse neuromuscular block produced by overdosage of curariform drugs. Not recommended for maintenance therapy for myasthenia gravis because of its short duration of action.

ABSORPTION AND FATE
Onset of effect within 30 to 60 seconds after injection; duration 5 to 10 minutes.

CONTRAINDICATIONS AND PRECAUTIONS
Hypersensitivity to anticholinesterase agents; intestinal and urinary obstruction. Safe use in women of childbearing potential and during pregnancy and lactation not established. Cautious use: bronchial asthma, cardiac arrhythmias. Also see Neostigmine.

ADVERSE REACTIONS
See Neostigmine.

ROUTE AND DOSAGE
Adults: *Edrophonium test for myasthenia gravis* (IV: dosage 10 mg in tuberculin syringe): initially 2 mg injected within 15 to 30 seconds; needle is left in situ; if there is no reaction after 45 seconds, the remaining 8 mg is injected; test may be repeated after 30 minutes. IM: 10 mg; if cholinergic reaction occurs, retest after 30 minutes with 2 mg to rule out false negative reaction. *Evaluation of myasthenic treatment:* 1 to 2 mg IV administered 1 hour after last oral dose of anticholinesterase medication used in treatment. *Myasthenic crisis evaluation* (2 mg in tuberculin syringe): initially 1 mg IV; if after an interval of 1 minute the patient's condition does not deteriorate, administer remaining 1 mg. *Curare antagonist:* 10 mg IV administered over 30 to 45 seconds; repeated as necessary; maximal dose 40 mg. **Children:** *Edrophonium test for myasthenia gravis: (Children weighing up to 75 lb):* 1 mg IV; if no response after 45 seconds, dose may be titrated up to 5 mg; alternatively, 2 mg IM. *(Children over 75 lb):* 2 mg IV; if no response after 45 seconds, dose may be titrated up to 10 mg; alternatively, 5 mg IM. *Infants:* recommended dose is 0.5 mg.

NURSING IMPLICATIONS
Edrophonium must be administered by a physician. Monitor vital signs. Observe for signs of respiratory distress. Patients over 50 years of age are particularly likely to develop bradycardia and hypotension.

Antidote (atropine sulfate) and facilities for endotracheal intubation, tracheostomy, suction, and assisted respiration should be immediately available for treatment of cholinergic reaction.

Edrophonium test for myasthenia gravis: Estimates of muscle strength should be made before and after administration of edrophonium, eg, width of palpebral fissure before and after 1 minute of sustained upward gaze, range of extraocular movements, grip strength, vital capacity, ability to elevate head and extremities, ability to cough, swallow, and talk.

Positive response to edrophonium test consists of brief improvement in muscle strength unaccompanied by lingual or skeletal muscle fasciculations. In nonmyasthenic patients, edrophonium produces a cholinergic reaction (muscarinic side effects): skeletal muscle fasciculations, muscle weakness.

Evaluation of myasthenic treatment: *Myasthenic response:* immediate subjective improvement with increased muscle strength (improvement of ptosis, respiration, ability to speak, swallow, and talk), absence of fasciculations; generally indicates that patient requires larger dose of anticholinesterase agent or longer-acting drug. *Cholinergic response* (muscarinic side effects): lacrimation, diaphoresis, salivation, abdominal cramps, diarrhea, nausea, vomiting; accompanied by decrease in muscle strength; fasciculations may be present or absent. Usually indicates overtreatment with anticholinergic drugs. *Adequate response:* no change in muscle strength; fasciculations may be present or absent; minimal cholinergic side effects (observed in patients at or near optimal dosage level).

Test to differentiate myasthenic crisis from cholinergic crisis (same principle as for evaluation of myasthenic treatment): respiratory exchange must be adequate before test is performed. **Myasthenic crisis** (may be secondary to sudden increase in severity of myasthenia gravis): edrophonium will cause improvement of respiration; indicates need for longer-acting anticholinesterase drug. **Cholinergic crisis** (caused by overstimulation by anticholinesterase drugs): edrophonium will produce increase in oropharyngeal secretions and further weakness of muscles of respiration; usually indicates need for discontinuing anticholinesterase drug.

When used as curare antagonist, the effect of each dose of edrophonium on respiration should be carefully observed before it is repeated, and assisted ventilation should always be employed.

EMETINE HYDROCHLORIDE, U.S.P., B.P.

Antiamebic

ACTIONS AND USES

Natural or synthetic alkaloid of ipecac with direct lethal action on *Entamoeba histolytica* in tissues. More effective against motile forms (trophozoites) than cysts. Causes degeneration of nucleus and cytoplasm of amebae and eradicates parasites, possibly by interfering with multiplication of trophozoites. Also has expectorant, diaphoretic, and emetic actions, but not used clinically for these effects.

Used in combination with other amebicides in management of acute fulminating amebic dysentery (intestinal amebiasis) or for acute exacerbations of chronic amebic dysentery. Highly effective in treatment of extraintestinal amebiasis (amebic abscess, amebic hepatitis). Also used in certain cases of balantidiasis, fascioliasis, and paragonimiasis.

ABSORPTION AND FATE

Readily absorbed and widely distributed in body. Highest concentration in liver; appreciable amounts also found in lung, kidney, and spleen. Appears in urine 20 to 40 minutes after injection; still present 40 to 60 days after being discontinued.

CONTRAINDICATIONS AND PRECAUTIONS

In patients who have received a course of emetine 6 weeks to 2 months previously; for treatment of mild symptoms or carriers of amebiasis; liver, heart, or kidney disease; pregnancy. Contraindicated in children except those with severe dysentery not controlled by other amebicides. Cautious use: debilitated or aged patients.

GI: nausea and vomiting associated with dizziness, faintness, and headache; diarrhea; abdominal cramps. **Neuromuscular:** skeletal muscle weakness, tenderness, stiffness, pain, tremors; loss of sense of taste. **Cardiovascular:** hypotension, tachycardia, precordial pain, dyspnea, ECG abnormalities, gallop rhythm, cardiac dilatation, congestive failure, death. **Local reactions at injection site:** (frequent) aching, tenderness, and local muscle weakness; eczematous, urticarial, or purpuric lesions. **Large doses:** acute lesions in heart, liver, kidney, intestinal tract, skeletal muscle.

ROUTE AND DOSAGE

Adults: Subcutaneous (deep), intramuscular: 65 mg daily or 32 mg twice daily (morning and evening). Some authorities recommend 1 mg/kg per day; dose should not exceed 65 mg/day. Never administered for more than 10 days, and a course should not be repeated in less than 6 weeks. **Children** *under 8 years of age:* no more than 10 mg daily; *over 8 years:* no more than 20 mg daily.

NURSING IMPLICATIONS

Emetine is a potent drug. Patients should be hospitalized and on absolute bed rest during therapy and for several days thereafter. Tachycardia may occur in patients permitted to ambulate. It is also advisable for patients to remain sedentary for several weeks after drug is terminated.

Isolation precautions are not required. However, use meticulous technique in disposal of feces and collection of stool specimens.

Emetine is administered by deep subcutaneous or IM injection. Aspirate carefully after needle is introduced.

IV injection is dangerous and is specifically contraindicated.

Make a record of injection sites and observe these sites daily. Muscle ache and tenderness at area of injection occur frequently.

Emetine is very irritating to tissues. Avoid contact of drug with eyes and mucous membranes. Wash hands thoroughly after handling drug.

Cumulative toxic action may occur. The patient should be closely observed and advised to report any unusual symptom, no matter how minor it may seem.

An ECG should be taken before emetine is inititated, as well as after the fifth dose, on completion of therapy, and 1 week later. ECG changes usually appear about 7 days after drug is administered; they are reversible.

ECG alterations may persist in some patients 2 months or more after discontinuation of drug. Some patients experience dyspnea until drug is stopped.

Pulse (rate and quality) and blood pressure should be recorded at least 3 times daily. Tachycardia frequently precedes appearance of ECG abnormalities.

Monitor neuromuscular function, especially of neck and extremities (most likely involved). Report immediately any signs of weakness and complaints of fatigability, listlessness, muscular stiffness, tenderness, or pain. These symptoms usually appear before more serious symptoms and thus may serve as guides to avoid overdosage.

Emetine should be discontinued on the appearance of tachycardia, a precipitous fall in blood pressure, marked weakness or other neuromuscular symptoms, and severe GI effects. These adverse reactions should be reported promptly.

Intake and output should be monitored. Report oliguria or change in intake–output ratio. Record number, unusual odor, and consistency of stools, as well as the presence of mucus, blood, or other foreign matter. Stool specimens should be delivered to the laboratory while they are still warm to facilitate identification of amebae.

Suspect emetine-induced reaction if stools increase in number following improvement of diarrhea.

Restoration of body fluids and nutrients is an important adjunct to drug therapy.

Emetine for treatment of acute fulminating amebic dysentery is administered only long enough to control symptoms (usually 3 to 5 days). For extraintestinal amebiasis (amebic hepatitis or abscess) it is generally given for 10 days; another amebicide should be given simultaneously or as an immediate follow-up to guarantee eradication of *E. histolytica* from primary lesions in intestines.

Patients to be discharged should be instructed about the amount of activity allowed and urged to remain under medical supervision until otherwise advised.

Repeated fecal examinations at intervals of up to 3 months are necessary to assure elimination of amebae. Patients with acute amebic dysentery often become asymptomatic carriers, depending on the adequacy of concomitant amebicide therapy to remove intestinal cysts.

Microscopic examination of the feces of household members and other suspected contacts should be supplemented by a search for direct contamination of water or other possible sources of infection.

A health teaching plan for patients and family members should include personal hygiene, particularly regarding sanitary disposal of feces, handwashing after defecation and before preparing or eating food, the risks of eating raw food, and control of fly contamination.

EPHEDRINE
(I-SEDRIN PLAIN)
EPHEDRINE SULFATE, U.S.P.
(BOFEDROL, ECTASULE MINUS, EPHEDSOL, NASDRO SLO-FEDRIN)

Adrenergic

ACTIONS AND USES

Indirect acting sympathomimetic amine.

Pharmacologically similar to epinephrine (qv), but less potent, with slower onset and more prolonged action; effective by oral route. Causes less elevation of blood sugar than epinephrine and has more pronounced central stimulatory actions. Thought to act indirectly by releasing tissue stores of norepinephrine and by direct stimulation of α and β adrenergic receptors. Cardiovascular effects persist 7 to 10 times as long as those of epinephrine; although bronchodilation is less prominent, it is more sustained. Like epinephrine, it contracts dilated arterioles of nasal mucosa, thus reducing engorgement and edema and facilitating ventilation and drainage. Local application to eye produces mydriasis without loss of light reflexes or accommodation or change in intraocular pressure. Its use in enuresis is based on its ability to contract urinary bladder sphincter and its central effects, which decrease depth of sleep. Potentiates action of acetylcholine at neuromuscular junctions; thus it may increase skeletal muscle tone in myasthenia gravis.

Used to relieve congestion of hay fever, allergic rhinitis, and sinusitis; and in treatment and prophylaxis of mild cases of acute asthma and in patients with chronic asthma requiring continuing treatment. Also has been used for its central actions: in treatment of narcolepsy, to improve respiration in narcotic and barbiturate poisoning, to combat hypotensive states, especially those associated with spinal anesthesia; in management of enuresis or impaired bladder control; as adjunct in treatment of myasthenia gravis; as mydriatic; to relieve dysmenorrhea; and for temporary support of ventricular rate in Adams-Stokes syndrome.

ABSORPTION AND FATE

Readily absorbed when given by oral and parenteral routes. Maximum bronchodilator effect occurs within 1 hour and persists approximately 3 hours. Widely distributed in body fluids; crosses blood–brain barrier. About 60% to 75% excreted unchanged in urine.

CONTRAINDICATIONS AND PRECAUTIONS

History of hypersensitivity to ephedrine; narrow-angle glaucoma; patients receiving MAO inhibitors, tricyclic antidepressants, digitalis, oxytocics. Safe use during pregnancy not established. Use with extreme caution in hypertension, arteriosclerosis, angina pectoris, chronic heart disease, diabetes mellitus, hyperthyroidism, prostatic hypertrophy, and in patients receiving cyclopropane or halogenated hydrocarbon anesthesics.

ADVERSE REACTIONS

Systemic (usually with large doses): headache, insomnia, nervousness, anxiety, tremulousness, giddiness; palpitation, tachycardia, precordial pain, cardiac arrhythmias; difficult or painful urination, acute urinary retention (especially older men with prostatism); vertigo, sweating, thirst, nausea, vomiting, anorexia, transient hypertension. **Topical use:** burning, stinging, dryness of nasal mucosa, sneezing. **Overdosage:** euphoria, confusion, delirium, hallucinations, CNS depression (somnolence, coma), hypertension, rebound hypotension, respiratory depression.

ROUTE AND DOSAGE

Adults: Oral, subcutaneous, intramuscular, intravenous (slowly): 15 to 50 mg every 3 to 4 hours as necessary (timed-action preparations usually administered every 8 to 12 hours). Maximum total 24-hour dose should not exceed 150 mg. Nasal solution (1% to 3%): 2 to 4 drops in each nostril no more than 4 times a day for 3 or 4 consecutive days (do not repeat before 2 hours). **Children:** Oral, subcutaneous, intravenous: 3 mg/kg/24 hours, divided into 4 to 6 doses (timed-action preparations administered every 12 hours).

NURSING IMPLICATIONS

Patients receiving ephedrine IV must be under constant supervision. Check blood pressure repeatedly during first 5 minutes then check every 3 to 5 minutes until stabilized.

Monitor intake–output ratio, especially in older male patients.

Ephedrine is a commonly abused drug. Patients should be advised of side effects and dangers and should be cautioned to take medication only as prescribed.

Insomnia is common, particularly with continued therapy. Timing of administration and size of dosage are important considerations.

Systemic effects can occur because of excessive dosage from rapid absorption of drug solution through nasal mucosa and from GI tract if swallowed. These are most likely to occur in the elderly.

Generally, nose drops are instilled with head in lateral, head-low position to avoid entry of drug into throat. Check with physician.

Instruct patient to rinse dropper or spray tip in hot water after each use in order to prevent contamination of nasal solution.

Tachyphylaxis (diminution of response) with rebound congestion may occur if drug is administered in rapidly repeated doses or over prolonged period of time. Prescribed withdrawal of drug over several days frequently enables the patient to attain former responsiveness.

In patients receiving ephedrine regularly for allergic conditions, the drug should be withdrawn at least 12 hours before sensitivity tests are made, in order to prevent false positive reactions.

Preserved in well-closed, light-resistant containers.

Also see Epinephrine.

DRUG INTERACTIONS: Severe hypertension may occur when ephedrine is used in conjunction with **furazolidone** and **MAO inhibitors.** Ephedrine may cause serious cardiac arrhythmias in combination with **halothane,** and related **anesthetics.** There is the possibility of increased insomnia, nervousness, and GI complaints in combination with **aminophylline.** Ephedrine may be less active in patients receiving **methyldopa,** and **reserpine.** Ephedrine may block antihypertensive effect of **guanethidine.**

EPINEPHRINE, U.S.P.

(ASMOLIN, ASTHMA METER, PRIMATENE MIST, SUS-PHRINE)

EPINEPHRINE BITARTRATE, U.S.P.

(ASMATANE MIST, E½, E$_1$, AND E$_2$ OPHTHALMIC SOLUTIONS, EPITRATE, MEDIHALER-EPI)

EPINEPHRINE BORATE (EPINEPHRYL BORATE)

(EPINAL, EPPY SOLUTIONS)

EPINEPHRINE HYDROCHLORIDE

(ADRENALIN CHLORIDE, EPIFRIN, GLAUCON, MISTURA E, VAPONEFRIN)

Adrenergic

ACTIONS AND USES

Naturally occurring catecholamine obtained from animal adrenal glands; also prepared synthetically. Acts directly on both alpha and beta receptors; the most potent activator of alpha receptors. Imitates all actions of sympathetic nervous system except those on facial artery and sweat gland effector cells. Strengthens myocardial contraction; increases blood pressure, cardiac rate, and cardiac output. Relaxes bronchial smooth muscle, constricts bronchial arterioles, and inhibits histamine release; thus reduces congestion and edema and increases tidal volume and vital capacity. Constricts arterioles, particularly in skin, mucous membranes, and kidneys, but dilates skeletal muscle blood vessels. Increases glycogenolysis, inhibits insulin release in pancreas, and stimulates metabolism. Relaxes uterine musculature and inhibits uterine contractions. CNS stimulation believed to result from peripheral effects. Also lowers intraocular pressure possibly by decreasing aqueous humor formation and by increasing facility of aqueous outflow; produces brief mydriasis, slight relaxation of ciliary muscle, and vasoconstriction. Has only slight effect on normal eye, and reportedly is more effective in light-colored eyes than in dark eyes.

Used for temporary relief of bronchospasm, acute asthmatic attack, mucosal congestion, hypersensitivity, and anaphylactic reactions, syncope due to heart block or carotid sinus hypersensitivity, and to restore cardiac rhythm in cardiac arrest; may be used with sodium bicarbonate to improve myocardial status and facilitate defibrillation. Effective in management of simple (open-angle) glaucoma, alone or in combination with a cholinergic agent, and effective as mydriatic and ophthalmic decongestant. Also used to relax myometrium and inhibit uterine contractions, to prolong action and delay systemic absorption of local and intraspinal anesthetics, and topically to control superficial bleeding.

Bronchodilation occurs within 3 to 5 minutes following subcutaneous injection of 1:1000 solution, with maximal effects in 20 minutes. Suspension forms provide both rapid and sustained action that may persist 8 to 10 hours or more. Bronchodilation occurs within 1 minute after oral inhalation. Topical application to conjunctiva reduces intraocular pressure within 1 hour; maximal effects in 4 to 8 hours; action may persist 12 to 24 hours or more. Mydriasis occurs within a few minutes and may last several hours. Pharmacologic actions terminated primarily by uptake and metabolism in sympathetic nerve endings. Circulating drug metabolized in liver and other tissues by MAO and catechol-o-methyl transferase. Inactive metabolites and small amount of unchanged drug excreted in urine. Crosses placenta, but not blood–brain barrier; enters breast milk.

CONTRAINDICATIONS AND PRECAUTIONS

Hypersensitivity to sympathomimetic amines; narrow-angle glaucoma; hemorrhagic, traumatic, or cardiogenic shock; cardiac dilatation, cerebral arteriosclerosis, coronary insufficiency, arrhythmias, organic heart or brain disease; during second stage of labor; for local anesthesia of fingers, toes, ears, nose, genitalia; during general anesthesia with cyclopropane or halogenated hydrocarbons; to treat overdosage of adrenergic blocking agents or phenothiazines. Cautious use: elderly or debilitated patients; prostatic hypertrophy; hypertension; diabetes mellitus; hyperthyroidism; Parkinson's disease; tuberculosis; psychoneurosis; during pregnancy; in patients with long-standing bronchial asthma and emphysema with degenerative heart disease; in children under 6 years of age.

ADVERSE REACTIONS

Systemic reactions: nervousness, restlessness, sleeplessness, fear, anxiety, tremors, severe headache, weakness, dizziness, syncope, pallor, nausea, vomiting, sweating, dyspnea, precordial pain, palpitation, hypertension, tachyarrhythmias including fatal fibrillation; bronchial and pulmonary edema, urinary retention, tissue necrosis, altered state of perception and thought, psychosis. **Altered laboratory values:** elevated serum cholesterol, blood glucose, serum lactate, and serum urate levels; increased urinary VMA excretion; lactic acidosis (with overdosage). **Ophthalmic use:** transient stinging or burning of eyes, lacrimation, brow ache, headache, rebound conjunctival hyperemia, allergy, iritis; with prolonged use: melaninlike deposits on lids, conjunctiva, and cornea; corneal edema; loss of lashes (reversible); maculopathy with central scotoma in aphakic patients (reversible). **Nasal use:** burning, stinging, dryness of nasal mucosa, sneezing, rebound congestion.

ROUTE AND DOSAGE

Adults: *Parenteral 1:1000* (0.1%) solution: Subcutaneous, intramuscular: 0.1 to 1 ml (0.1 to 1 mg) started with small dose and increased if required. *Parenteral suspension 1:400* (Asmolin): Subcutaneous, intramuscular: 0.2 to 0.6 ml (0.5 to 1.5 mg), not repeated within 4 hours. *Parenteral suspension 1:200* (Sus-Phrine): Subcutaneous only: 0.1 to 0.3 ml (0.5 to 1.5 mg), not repeated within 4 hours; initial test dose should not exceed 0.1 ml. *Cardiac resuscitation:* Intravenous, intracardiac: 1 mg (usually as 1 to 10 ml of a 1:10,000 solution). *Intraspinal use:* 0.2 to 0.4 ml of 1:1000 solution. *Use with local anesthetic:* 1:500,000 to 1:50,000. *Inhalation:* 1:100 (1%) solution administered by aerosol, nebulizer, or IPPB machine. *Nasal:* 1:1000 solution (drops or spray). *Ophthalmic:* 0.1% to 2% solution. *Topical hemostatic:* 1:50,000 to 1:1000 solution. **Children** *over 6 years: 1:1000 solution: Subcutaneous:* 0.01 ml/kg dose; maximum 0.5 ml. *Suspension 1:200:* 0.004 ml/kg/dose SC repeated every 8 to 12 hours. *Suspension 1:400:* 0.008 ml/kg/dose SC repeated every 8 to 12 hours.

NURSING IMPLICATIONS

Parenteral:

Medication errors associated with epinephrine have resulted in fatalities. For example, injection of the 1:100 solution intended for oral inhalation has caused death when mistaken for the 1:1000 solution designed for parenteral administration. Be certain to check type of solution prescribed, concentration, dosage, and route.

Since epinephrine is prescribed in very small doses, a tuberculin syringe is preferable for accuracy in measuring.

Epinephrine injection should be protected from exposure to light at all times. Do not remove ampul or vial from carton until ready to use.

Before withdrawing epinephrine suspension into syringe, shake vial or ampul thoroughly to disperse particles; then inject promptly.

Carefully aspirate before injecting epinephrine. Inadvertent IV injection of usual subcutaneous or IM doses can result in sudden hypertension and possibly cerebral hemorrhage.

Drug absorption (and action) can be hastened by massaging the injection site.

Repeated injections may cause tissue necrosis due to vascular constriction. Rotate injection sites and observe for signs of blanching.

In general, the IM route is not used because of the possibility of necrosis and gangrene. If prescribed, injection into buttocks should be avoided.

Monitor blood pressure and pulse and observe patient closely. Epinephrine may widen pulse pressure (elevate systolic with minimal rise or even decrease of diastolic).

When administered IV, blood pressure should be checked repeatedly during first 5 minutes, then checked every 3 to 5 minutes until stabilized.

When drug is given intracardially (by physician), it must be followed by external cardiac massage to permit drug to enter coronary circulation.

Oral inhalation:

Treatment should start with first symptoms. The least number of inhalations that provide relief should be used. To prevent excessive dosage, at least 1 or 2 minutes should elapse before taking additional inhalations of epinephrine. Dosage requirements vary with each patient. Caution patient that overuse or too frequent use can result in severe adverse effects.

Instruct the patient to rinse mouth and throat with water immediately after inhalation to avoid swallowing residual drug (causes epigastric pain and systemic effects) and to prevent dryness of oropharyngeal membranes.

If patient is also taking isoproterenol, it should not be used concurrently with epinephrine. An interval of 4 hours should elapse before changing from one drug to the other.

Patients should be advised to report to a physician if symptoms are not relieved in 20 minutes or if they become worse.

Advise patients to report bronchial irritation, nervousness, or sleeplessness. Dosage should be reduced.

Nasal:

Nose drops should be instilled with head in lateral, head-low position to prevent entry of drug into throat. Check with physician.

Forewarn patients that intranasal application may sting slightly.

Instruct patients to rinse nose dropper or spray tip with hot water after each use to prevent contamination of solution with nasal secretions.

Inform patients that intranasal applications frequently cause rebound congestion and that prolonged use may result in drug-induced rhinitis. Caution patients to use medication as prescribed and to inform a physician if drug is not effective.

Ophthalmic:

Ophthalmic preparation causes mydriasis with blurred vision and sensitivity to light in some patients being treated for glaucoma. Drug is usually administered at bedtime or following prescribed miotic to minimize these symptoms.

Repeated tonometer readings are advised during continuous therapy, especially in elderly patients.

When separate solutions of epinephrine and a topical miotic are used, the miotic should be instilled 2 to 10 minutes prior to epinephrine because of the limited capacity of the conjunctival sac. Consult physician.

Inform the patient that transitory stinging may follow initial administration and that headache and brow ache occur frequently at first, but usually subside with continued use. Advise the patient to report to a physician if symptoms persist. Local reactions are sometimes controlled by lower drug concentration.

Patients should be instructed to discontinue epinephrine and to consult a physician if signs of hypersensitivity develop (edema of lids, itching, discharge, crusting eyelids); if it is prescribed for irritation, patients should report if condition persists or becomes worse.

General:

Patients subject to acute asthmatic attacks and responsible family members should be taught how to administer epinephrine subcutaneously. Medication and equipment should be available for home emergency. Confer with physician.

Epinephrine reduces bronchial secretions and thus may make mucus plugs more difficult to dislodge. Physician may prescribe bronchial hygiene program, including postural drainage, breathing exercises, and adequate hydration (3000 to 4000 ml) to facilitate expectoration. Objective measures such as vital capacity and maximal expiratory flow rate may be used to assess response to therapy.

Tolerance ("epinephrine fastness") can occur with repeated or prolonged use (effectiveness often returns if drug is withheld 12 hours to several days). Caution the patient to report to a physician; continued use of epinephrine in the presence of tolerance can be dangerous.

Advise patient to report difficulty in voiding or urinary retention (especially male patients).

Epinephrine may increase blood glucose levels. Patients with diabetes should be observed closely for loss of diabetes control.

Instruct patients to take medication only as prescribed and to report the onset of systemic effects of epinephrine. A decrease in frequency of administration or concentration of drug or temporary discontinuation of therapy may be indicated.

Treatment of overdosage: The cardiac and bronchodilating effects of epinephrine are antagonized by β-adrenergic blocking agents such as propranolol; marked pressor effects are antagonized by α-adrenergic blocking agents such as phentolamine.

Oxidation of epinephrine imparts a color ranging from pink to brown. Discard discolored or precipitated solutions.

Preserved in tight, light-resistant containers. Commercial preparations vary in stability; therefore, follow manufacturer's directions with respect to expiration date and storage requirements for each product.

Epinephrine is readily destroyed by oxidizing agents, alkalies (including sodium bicarbonate), halogens, permanganates, chromates, nitrates, and salts of easily reducible metals such as iron, copper, and zinc.

LABORATORY TEST INTERFERENCES: False increases in bilirubin, SMA-12/60 method (in vitro).

DRUG INTERACTIONS: Effects of epinephrine may be potentiated by certain **antihistamines (diphenhydramine, tripelennamine, dexchlorpheniramine), thyroid hormones, tricyclic antidepressants,** and **sympathomimetic agents.**

Possibility of enhanced pharmacologic response to epinephrine in patients receiving or having received **guanethidine** (concurrent use not recommended). Epinephrine is administered with caution in patients already receiving **propranolol,** since bradycardia may result. IV administration of epinephrine during use of **halothane** and **related general anesthetics** may lead to serious ventricular arrhythmias (subcutaneous and IM administration is reported to be safe provided appropriate precautions are taken). Although epinephrine reportedly is not significantly affected by concurrent administration of **MAO inhibitors,** patients with cardiovascular disease receiving MAO inhibitors should be closely observed for possible increase in heart rate and blood pressure. Epinephrine-induced hyperglycemia may require increased dosage of **insulin** and **oral hypoglycemics.**

ERGONOVINE MALEATE, U.S.P., N.F.
(ERGOTRATE MALEATE)

Oxytocic

ACTIONS AND USES

Ergot alkaloid with slow but powerful oxytocic effect; less toxic and less prone to cause gangrene than other ergot derivatives. Exerts moderate cerebral vascular constriction, but is inferior to ergotamine (qv) as a migraine specific. Produces prolonged nonphasic uterine contractions. Like other oxytocics, may evoke severe hypertensive episodes in hypertensive or toxemic patients, or when regional anesthesia (caudal or spinal) containing vasoconstrictors has been used.

Used to prevent or reduce postpartum and postabortal hemorrhage due to uterine atony.

CONTRAINDICATIONS AND PRECAUTIONS

Use prior to delivery of placenta, threatened spontaneous abortion, prolonged use, hypersensitivity to ergot; uterine sepsis, hypertension, toxemia.

ADVERSE REACTIONS

Nausea, vomiting (especially with IV doses), severe hypertensive episodes, bradycardia, allergic phenomena ergotism. Also see Ergotamine.

ROUTE AND DOSAGE

Oral (*postpartum bleeding*): 0.2 to 0.4 mg every 6 to 12 hours until danger of atony passes (usually 48 hours). Intramuscular or (emergency) intravenous (*oxytocic*): 0.2 mg (1 ml) after delivery of placenta or anterior shoulder or during puerperium.

NURSING IMPLICATIONS

IM injection produces initial firm titanic contraction of the postpartum uterus; a succession of minor relaxations and contractions is superimposed over this, with relaxation increasing over next period of 1.5 hours. Vigorous rhythmic contractions continue for 3 hours or more after injection.

Desired oxytocic action of ergonovine may be antagonized by hypocalcemia. Treatment: cautious IV calcium gluconate (if patient is not also taking digitalis) before ergonovine administration.

Severe cramping following oral doses is evidence of effectiveness; however, it may also indicate need to reduce dose.

Monitor blood pressure, pulse, and uterine response following injection until postpartum condition is stabilized (about 1 or 2 hours).

Report sudden increase in blood pressure, pulse changes, and frequent periods of uterine relaxation. (Uterus may fail to respond in hypocalcemic patients.)

High incidence of nausea and danger of hypertensive and cerebrovascular accident have limited the use of IV route to emergency treatment.

Although it is possible that the hypersensitive person may develop ergotism (see Index), it is unreported thus far.

IV ergonovine given in second stage of labor as head is born induces contraction in 1 minute. IM injection as infant is being born produces, in 2 to 5 minutes, uterine contractions that separate placenta and prevent blood loss.

Oral tablets may also be administered on tongue (perlingually) or by rectum (suspended in water as retention enema).

Before labor is induced, consult with physician about route to be used for administration of ergonovine during delivery. Have drug prepared so that there is no delay.

Store drug in cool place (below 46 F). However, delivery room stocks may be kept at room temperature for up to 60 days.

Also see Ergotamine Tartrate.

ERGOTAMINE TARTRATE, U.S.P.
(ERGOMAR, ERGOSTAT, GYNERGEN, MEDIHALER ERGOTAMINE)

Analgesic (specific migraine)

ACTIONS AND USES
Natural amino acid alkaloid of ergot. Alpha adrenergic blocking agent with direct stimulating action on cranial and peripheral vascular smooth muscles and depressant effect on central vasomotor centers. In vascular headache, exerts vasoconstrictive action on previously dilated cerebral vessels, reduces amplitude of arterial pulsations, and antagonizes effects of serotonin (implicated in etiology of vascular headaches). Does not demonstrate intrinsic sedative or analgesic actions. By unknown mechanism, ergotamine activity can lead to damage of vascular endothelium, with subsequent occlusion, thrombosis, and gangrene. Large doses may induce slight elevation of blood pressure and diminish arterial blood flow sufficiently to cause tissue ischemia. Myometrium stimulation (oxytocic effect) becomes more prominent with dose increases and as uterine sensitivity to ergot develops during adolescence and pregnancy. Reportedly nonaddictive and does not promote development of tolerance.

Used as single agent or in combination with caffeine (Cafergot) to relieve pain of migraine, cluster headache (histamine cephalalgia), and other vascular headaches.

ABSORPTION AND FATE
Poorly and erratically absorbed from GI tract; effective oral dose must be 8 to 10 times that of an IM injection because response is delayed and unpredictable. Detoxification appears to be in liver; duration of action may be 24 hours. Data on excretion not available.

CONTRAINDICATIONS AND PRECAUTIONS
Hypersensitivity, pregnancy, use in children, sepsis, obliterative vascular disease, thromboembolic disease, prolonged use of excessive dosage, hepatic and renal disease, severe pruritus, marked arteriosclerosis, coronary heart disease, hypertension, infectious states, anemia, and malnutrition. Cautious use: during lactation, elderly patients.

ADVERSE REACTIONS
Acute ergotism (rare): vomiting, diarrhea, unquenchable thirst, paresthesias, convulsive seizures, rapid or weak pulse, confusion, itching and cold skin; (occasionally): gangrene of nose, digits, ears. **Chronic ergotism:** intermittent

claudication, muscle pains, numbness, coldness and cyanosis of digits (Raynaud's phenomenon). Also: complete absence of medium- and large-vessel pulsations in extremities; precordial distress and pain; transient bradycardia or tachycardia; elevated or lowered blood pressure; depression; drowsiness; mixed miosis (rare).

ROUTE AND DOSAGE

Oral, sublingual: initially 1 tablet (2 mg) at start of migraine repeated after 30 minutes if necessary. Dosage should not exceed 3 tablets (6 mg) in 24-hour period nor 5 (10 mg) tablets in any 1 week. Subcutaneous, intramuscular: initially 0.25 mg; repeated in 40 minutes if necessary. Total amount required to control headache is then used at prodrome of subsequent attacks. Maximum dose: 2 ml/week. Inhalation: each spray delivers 0.36 mg dose. Start with one inhalation; if not relieved in 5 minutes, use another. Space additional inhalations no less than 5 minutes apart; maximum dose, 6 inhalations in 24 hours.

NURSING IMPLICATIONS

Oral doses are less effective than parenteral, but they usually relieve mild or incipient attacks of migraine.

If an oral dose of 8 mg or more is required to give pain relief, it is better to resort to subcutaneous injection of 0.5 mg. Consult physician.

Sublingual tablet is preferred early in the attack because of its rapid absorption and effective lower dose.

Following parenteral administration, pain from migraine attack may disappear within 15 minutes to 2 hours or more; after an oral dose, relief may not come for 5 hours or longer, if at all.

Since degree of pain relief is proportional to rapidity of treatment, drug therapy should begin as soon after onset of attack as possible, preferably during prodrome (scintillating scotomas, visual field defects, paresthesias, usually on side opposite to that of the migraine).

Advise patient to lie down in a quiet, dark room for 2 to 3 hours after drug administration.

Acute ergot poisoning is rare; it frequently results from overdosing or attempts at abortion.

Instruct patient to report claudication and cold or numb digits. Dose adjustment is indicated. With avoidance of the drug for 1 to 3 days, vasoconstriction usually subsides. Carefully protect extremities from exposure to cold temperatures; provide warmth, but not heat, to ischemic areas.

Patients with migraine should be helped to identify underlying emotional and physical stresses that may precipitate attacks and should be assisted in learning how to deal with them. Adequate relaxation, recreation, and sleep may help to reduce severity and frequency of attacks.

Injection test (diagnostic): relief of throbbing recurrent headache after 1-ml IM injection of ergotamine is confirmation of vascular origin of headache.

Precordial pain in the susceptible individual may occur 5 to 10 minutes after IM injection of ergotamine and may last 30 to 45 minutes. Sublingual nitroglycerin (0.6 mg) usually relieves such chest pain in 5 minutes.

Warn the woman of childbearing age to avoid use of ergotamine if she suspects she is pregnant; this is because of its oxytocic effect.

Warn patients not to increase dosage without consulting physician; overdosage is the chief cause of untoward effects from the drug.

Preserved in light-resistant container away from excessive heat.

DRUG INTERACTIONS: **Propranolol** blocks natural pathway for vasodilation in patient receiving a vasoconstrictor; thus it may enhance vasoconstrictor activity of ergot alkaloids.

ERYTHRITYL TETRANITRATE, N.F.
(ANGINAR, CARDILATE, Erythrol Tetranitrate)

Vasodilator (coronary)

ACTIONS AND USES

Similar to nitroglycerin (qv), but has slower onset and longer duration of action. Used in prophylaxis and long-term treatment of angina pectoris, rather than in acute attacks, in patients with frequent and recurrent anginal pain and reduced exercise tolerance.

ABSORPTION AND FATE

Effects following administration of sublingual or chewable tablet occur after 5 to 10 minutes, with maximum action in 30 to 45 minutes. Following ingestion of oral tablet, effects appear in 30 minutes, with maximum effects in 60 to 90 minutes. Duration of action for all forms 2 to 4 hours.

ROUTE AND DOSAGE

Sublingual: initially 5 mg 3 times daily. Oral (tablet or chewable tablet): initially 10 mg 3 times daily. Dose may be increased in 2 or 3 days if needed. For the average patient, the following schedule of administration is suggested by manufacturer: 5 to 15 mg on arising, at lunch time, at 4 or 5 P.M., and at bedtime (p.r.n.).

NURSING IMPLICATIONS

Note that onset of action varies with preparation and route of administration.

Because of its more rapid onset of action, the physician may prescribe additional sublingual doses, as is done with nitroglycerin, prior to contemplated exertion or anticipated stress.

Combined rapid action and slower action may be obtained by allowing the tablet to dissolve partially under the tongue for 2 or 3 minutes, then swallowing remaining portion; consult physician about teaching the patient.

Sublingual administration may produce a tingling sensation at points of drug contact with mucous membranes. If the patient finds this objectionable, tablet may be placed in buccal pouch.

Mild GI disturbances and fall in blood pressure (lightheadedness) sometimes occur with large doses and may be controlled by dosage reduction.

Vascular headaches are common during first week of therapy because of disturbed cerebral hemodynamics. Advise patient to report to physician. Temporary reduction of dosage and administration of analgesics generally provide relief.

Oral tablet is reported less likely to produce headaches than other forms.

Since the patient may misinterpret freedom from anginal attacks as an indication to drop all restrictions, guidelines should be provided regarding allowable activities.

Tolerance to drug effect may develop with extended use.

Stored in cool place in airtight containers. Protect from light.

See Nitroglycerin.

(E-MYCIN, ERYTHROCIN, ILOTYCIN, KESSO-MYCIN, ROBIMYCIN, RP-MYCIN)

Antibacterial

ACTIONS AND USES
   Macrolide antibiotic produced by a strain of *Streptomyces erythreus*. Considered one of the safest antibiotics in use today. Bacteriostatic or bactericidal, depending on nature of organism and drug concentration used. Antibacterial spectrum is similar to that of penicillin; commonly used as penicillin substitute in hypersensitive patients for infections not requiring high antibiotic blood levels. More active against Gram-positive than Gram-negative bacteria. Acts by inhibiting protein synthesis of sensitive microorganisms. Resistant mutants are especially frequent among staphylococci.
   Used in treatment of pneumococcal and diplococcal pneumonia, *Mycoplasma pneumoniae* (primary atypical pneumonia), acute pelvic inflammatory disease caused by *Neisseria gonorrhoeae* in females sensitive to penicillin, infections caused by susceptible strains of staphylococci, streptococci, and certain strains of *Haemophilus influenzae*. Also used in intestinal amebiasis, in treatment of diphtheria as adjunct to antitoxin and for carrier state, and as alternate choice in treatment of primary syphilis in patients allergic to penicillins. Topical applications used in treatment of pyodermas and external ocular infections.
ABSORPTION AND FATE
   Peak plasma concentrations in about 4 hours following oral administration (absorption is delayed by presence of food in stomach). Adequate blood levels maintained by administration every 6 hours. Rectal administration produces demonstrable blood levels within 30 minutes that are maintained for 8 hours or longer. Diffuses readily into tissues and most body fluids, including pleural and peritoneal spaces and inflamed meninges. Concentrates in normal liver; excreted in active form primarily in bile and feces. About 2% to 5% of orally administered dose excreted in urine as active drug. Crosses placenta and is excreted in breast milk.
CONTRAINDICATIONS AND PRECAUTIONS
   Hypersensitivity to erythromycins. Safe use during pregnancy not established. Cautious use: impaired hepatic function.
ADVERSE REACTIONS
   Most frequent: abdominal cramping, discomfort, distention, diarrhea. Infrequent: nausea, vomiting, heartburn, anorexia, and hypersensitivity reactions: fever, eosinophilia, urticaria, skin eruptions, anaphylaxis (rare). Superinfections by nonsusceptible bacteria, yeasts, or fungi. Rectal suppository: anal or rectal irritation, pain, irregular bowel movements.
ROUTE AND DOSAGE
   Adults: Oral: 250 mg every 6 hours. For twice-a-day schedule, one-half total daily dose may be prescribed every 12 hours (usual dose range 1 to 4 Gm daily). Ophthalmic: ointment (5 mg/Gm): applied one or more times daily. Topical: ointment (1%): applied to affected skin areas 2 or 3 times daily. **Children:** Oral: 30 to 50 mg/kg/day in 4 equally divided doses; for more severe infections dose may be doubled. Rectal suppository *(children up to 20 lb):* 125 mg suppository every 8 hours; *(20 to 40 lb):* same dosage every 6 hours.

NURSING IMPLICATIONS
Culture and sensitivity testing should be done to determine organism susceptibility.
Activity of erythromycin may be decreased in acid medium and by the presence of food in the stomach. Therefore it is administered preferably

on an empty stomach 1 hour before or 3 hours after meals. Do not give with, or immediately before or after, fruit juices.

GI symptoms following oral administration are dose-related. Report their onset to physician. If symptoms persist following dosage reduction, physician may prescribe drug to be given with meals in spite of impaired absorption.

Before receiving erythromycin for gonorrhea, patients suspected of having syphilis should have microscopic examination for *Treponema pallidum* and monthly serologic tests for a minimum of 4 months.

In treatment of primary syphilis, spinal fluid examination should be done before treatment and as part of follow-up after therapy.

Observe for symptoms of overgrowth of nonsusceptible bacteria or fungi (fever, black furry tongue, sore mouth, enteritis, perianal irritation or itching, vaginal discharge). Emergence of resistant staphylococcal strains is highly predictable during prolonged therapy.

In treatment of streptococcal infections, erythromycin therapy should be continued for at least 10 days.

Hepatic function tests should be performed periodically during prolonged drug regimens.

Strict adherence of patient to prescribed dosage regimen should be stressed.

Insertion of suppository (suppository should be at room temperature): Following removal of foil wrapper, moisten suppository with water (lubricants interfere with absorption) and insert pointed end first past anal sphincter. If resistance to insertion is encountered, inserting blunt end first may be successful. Hold buttocks together for several minutes immediately after insertion.

If the patient has a bowel movement within 1 hour following insertion of suppository, repeat dosage should be given. Consult physician.

Information regarding use of rectal suppositories for longer than 5 days is not available; therefore, when practical, change to oral form should be made.

Mild transient discomfort sometimes occurs following suppository insertion. If significant local discomfort such as burning sensation or anal or rectal irritation or pain persists, rectal administration should be discontinued.

Suppositories should be stored in a cool place or refrigerated.

For topical applications to skin, consult physician about procedure to use for cleaning affected area prior to each application.

Ointment preparation for skin problems should not be used in eyes or in external ear if eardrum is perforated. Drug should be discontinued if signs of sensitivity or irritation appear.

For treatment of eye infections, use only preparations labeled for ophthalmic use.

LABORATORY TEST INTERFERENCES: False elevations of urinary catecholamines, urinary steroids, and transaminases (by colorimetric methods) have been reported.

DRUG INTERACTIONS: There is the possibility of cross-resistance between erythromycin and either **lincomycin** or **clindamycin;** concurrent use is not advised. Concurrent administration of erythromycin and **penicillin** may result in synergism of antibacterial activity. Routine concurrent use is not recommended, particularly for treatment of streptococcal infections.

Antibacterial

ACTIONS AND USES

Acid ester salt of erythromycin (qv). Reported to be acid-stable and thus less susceptible to action of gastric juices or food in stomach and to give higher, more predictable, and more prolonged antibiotic blood levels than other oral forms of erythromycin. Unlike other erythromycins it may produce hepatotoxicity.

ABSORPTION AND FATE

Peak blood levels in about 2 hours following oral administration. Serum half-life approximately 3 to 5 hours. About 0.8% of dose excreted in urine in 6 hours. Primarily excreted in bile. See Erythromycin.

CONTRAINDICATIONS AND PRECAUTIONS

Hypersensitivity to erythromycins; hepatic dysfunction; treatment of skin disorders such as acne or furunculosis or prophylaxis of rheumatic fever. Safe use during pregnancy not established. Also see Erythromycin.

ADVERSE REACTIONS

Cholestatic hepatitis syndrome (hypersensitivity reaction): malaise, nausea, vomiting, heartburn, abdominal cramps, right upper quadrant pain or tenderness, jaundice, fever, disturbance in color vision, headache, myalgia, abnormal liver function tests, eosinophilia, leukocytosis, slight increase in prothrombin time. Also see Erythromycin.

ROUTE AND DOSAGE

Oral: **Adults:** 250 mg every 6 hours; dosage may be increased up to 4 Gm or more per day according to severity of infection. **Children:** 30 to 50 mg/kg/day orally in divided doses; for more severe infections dosage may be doubled. For twice-a-day dosage, in both adults and children, one-half of total daily dose may be prescribed. Available forms: tablet, chewable tablet, capsule, suspension.

NURSING IMPLICATIONS

Culture and sensitivity testing should be done before initiation of treatment.

Cholestatic hepatitis syndrome appears most frequently after 1 to 2 weeks of continuous therapy or following several repeated courses of the drug, but it has also occurred after a few days of treatment; this condition is generally reversible within 3 to 5 days after cessation of therapy.

Premonitory symptoms of hepatitis may include abdominal cramps, nausea, and vomiting, followed by fever, leukocytosis, and eosinophilia. Advise patients to report immediately the onset of adverse reactions and to be on the alert for signs and symptoms associated with jaundice: dark urine, light-colored stools, pruritus, yellow skin, sclerae, and soft palate.

Hepatic function tests and blood cell counts should be conducted periodically if therapy is prolonged 10 days or more.

Serum levels are comparable whether taken after food or in the fasting state.

Chewable tablets should be chewed or crushed, not swallowed whole.

Therapeutic dosage should be continued for at least 10 days in treatment of group A β-hemolytic streptococcal infections.

After reconstitution, suspensions are stable for 14 days at room temperature, however palatability is retained if kept refrigerated.

See Erythromycin.

Antibacterial

ACTIONS AND USES

Acid-stable ester salt of erythromycin. Intramuscular preparation is used only when administration by other routes is not practical. See Erythromycin.

ABSORPTION AND FATE

Usually readily and reliably absorbed after oral ingestion; however, individual variability has been reported. Following IM administration of 100 mg in adults, peak serum levels are attained in 1 hour, gradually falling to 0.1 mg/ml in 6 to 8 hours. In children, peak levels are produced within 2 hours, gradually falling to low levels by 6 hours. Half-life 2 to 5 hours. Concentrates in liver; excreted primarily in bile. Also see Erythromycin.

CONTRAINDICATIONS AND PRECAUTIONS

Hypersensitivity to erythromycins or to butyl aminobenzoate (local anesthetic used in commercial IM preparation); IM use in small children or in serious infections when high dosage and/or frequent or prolonged administration is required. Safe use during pregnancy not established. Cautious use: impaired hepatic function.

ADVERSE REACTIONS

Pain on injection and possible sterile abscess and necrosis, abdominal cramps, diarrhea, anorexia, nausea, vomiting, skin eruptions, superinfections. See Erythromycin.

ROUTE AND DOSAGE

Adults: Oral: 400 mg every 6 hours; may be increased up to 4 Gm or more per day according to severity of infection. Intramuscular: 100 mg at 4- to 8-hour intervals (total daily dose 5 to 8 mg/kg). **Children:** Oral: 30 to 50 mg/kg/day in 4 equally divided doses; dosage may be doubled in more severe infections. Intramuscular (*children over 13.6 kg*); 50 mg repeated at 4- to 6-hour intervals (or approximately 12 mg/kg/day). For twice-a-day schedule in both adults and children, one-half the total daily dose may be prescribed every 12 hours. Available oral forms: tablet, chewable tablet, suspension.

NURSING IMPLICATIONS

Culture and sensitivity testing should be done.

Refrigeration of the parenteral preparation is not recommended, as the solution becomes thick and difficult to use. If drug has been refrigerated, manufacturer recommends warming solution slightly to make it less viscous.

Erythromycin ethylsuccinate IM is not miscible with water. Use only dry syringe and needle for administration. Needle should be no finer than 21 gauge.

The IM preparation is not intended for subcutaneous or IV use. Administer injections deep into large muscle mass; aspirate carefully before injecting drug. Rotate injection sites. Quantities larger than 100 mg may produce severe pain that persists for hours, despite the fact that it contains an anesthetic.

Small children do not have the large muscle mass required for IM injection; therefore, it is not recommended.

Observe injection sites daily. Sterile abscess formation and necrosis are possible.

Oral therapy should be instituted as soon as possible. Manufacturer cautions against repeated IM injections.

Commercially available chewable tablets should be chewed and not swallowed whole.

Oral formulations may be administered without regard to meals in patients 2 years of age or older. Drug should be administered on empty stomach in patients under 2 years of age pending results of bioavailability studies in this age group.

In treatment of group A β-hemolytic streptococcal infections, therapeutic oral dosage should be continued for at least 10 days.

Oral suspensions are stable for 10 days under refrigeration. Note expiration date.

See Erythromycin.

ERYTHROMYCIN GLUCEPTATE, U.S.P.
(ILOTYCIN GLUCEPTATE IV)

Antibacterial

ACTIONS AND USES

Soluble salt of erythromycin indicated for use when oral or rectal administration is not possible or the severity of infection requires immediate high serum levels. See Erythromycin.

ABSORPTION AND FATE

Peak serum level of 3 to 4 μg/ml achieved in 1 hour following administration of 200 mg IV; falls to 0.5 μg/ml at 6 hours. Principally eliminated via bile. Approximately 12% to 15% of dose is excreted in urine in active form. See Erythromycin.

CONTRAINDICATIONS AND PRECAUTIONS

Hypersensitivity to erythromycins. Safe use during pregnancy not established. Cautious use: impaired hepatic function.

ADVERSE REACTIONS

Pain and venous irritation following IV injection; allergic reactions, anaphylaxis (rare); superinfections and variations in liver function tests following prolonged or repeated therapy.

ROUTE AND DOSAGE

Adults and children: Intravenous: 15 to 20 mg/kg body weight daily. Higher doses may be given in very severe infections. Continuous infusion is preferable, but may also be administered in divided doses by intermittent infusion, over 20 to 60 minutes, and no less frequently than every 6 hours.

NURSING IMPLICATIONS

Culture and sensitivity testing should be done.

Initial solution is prepared by adding sterile water for injection *without preservatives* to the vial (see manufacturer's directions for dilution). Shake vial until drug is completely dissolved. Saline or other solutions may cause gel formation and therefore should not be used in this initial step. Stable up to 7 days if refrigerated.

Prior to administration, initial solution as prepared above may then be diluted with 0.9% sodium chloride injection or 5% dextrose in water, and buffered to neutrality (see manufacturer's directions). Stability of solution is dependent on pH and is optimal at 6 to 8.

Continuous infusion is administered slowly within 24 hours after dilution.

A physician will prescribe specific IV infusion rate. Rate should be sufficiently slow to avoid pain along course of vein.

IV infusion of large doses reported to be associated with thrombophlebitis.

Since hearing impairment has been associated with large IV doses of erythromycin lactobionate, it is possible that it may occur with large doses of erythromycin gluceptate (it has occurred as early as the second day and as late as the third week of therapy and has been completely reversible after discontinuation of drug).

Periodic hepatic function tests are advised in patients receiving daily high doses or prolonged therapy.

Oral therapy should replace IV administration as soon as possible.

See Erythromycin.

ERYTHROMYCIN LACTOBIONATE, U.S.P.
(ERYTHROCIN LACTOBIONATE-I.V.)

Antibacterial

ACTIONS AND USES
Lactobionate salt of erythromycin. Indicated for use when oral or rectal administration is not possible or severity of infection requires immediate high serum levels.

ABSORPTION AND FATE
Rapid IV infusion of 200 mg produces peak serum levels of 3 to 4 μg/ml almost immediately; levels gradually reduce to 0.5 μg/ml at 6 hours. Approximately 12% to 15% of dose is excreted in urine in active form. Primarily excreted in bile. See Erythromycin.

CONTRAINDICATIONS AND PRECAUTIONS
Hypersensitivity to erythromycins. Safe use during pregnancy not established. Cautious use: impaired hepatic function.

ADVERSE REACTIONS
Anorexia, abdominal discomfort, diarrhea, nausea, vomiting, allergic reactions, thrombophlebitis at injection site, impaired hearing associated with IV infusions of 4 Gm/day or more (reversible). Also see Erythromycin.

ROUTE AND DOSAGE
Adults and children: Intravenous: 15 to 20 mg/kg body weight daily. Higher doses may be given in very severe infections (up to 4 Gm/day). Continuous infusion is preferable, but may be administered in divided doses by intermittent infusion, over 20 to 60 minutes, at intervals not greater than every 6 hours.

NURSING IMPLICATIONS
Culture and sensitivity tests should be done.

Initial solution is prepared by adding sterile water for injection *without preservatives* to the vial (see manufacturer's directions for dilution). Shake vial until drug is completely dissolved. Saline or other solutions may cause precipitation and therefore should not be used in this initial step. Stable up to 2 weeks if refrigerated.

Prior to administration, initial solution as prepared above may then be diluted with 0.9% sodium chloride injection, lactated Ringer's, or other IV fluids recommended by manufacturer, and buffered to neutrality (see manufacturer's directions). The final diluted solution should be administered within 24 hours.

IV infusion rate will be prescribed by physician. Rate should be sufficiently slow to avoid pain along course of vein.

IV infusions of large doses reportedly are associated with thrombophlebitis at injection site and hearing difficulty. Hearing defects have appeared as early as the second day of therapy and as late as the third week; these are completely reversible after discontinuation of drug.

Periodic hepatic function tests are advised in patients receiving daily high
doses or prolonged therapy.
IV therapy should be replaced by oral dosage form as soon as possible.
See Erythromycin.

ERYTHROMYCIN STEARATE, U.S.P., B.P.
(BRISTAMYCIN, ERYPAR, ETHRIL, ERYTHROCIN STEARATE, PFIZER-E, SK-ERYTHROMYCIN, WINTROCIN)

Antibacterial

ACTIONS AND USES
Acid-labile stearic acid salt of erythromycin. Reportedly one of the most completely and reliabily absorbed forms of erythromycin.
ABSORPTION AND FATE
Readily absorbed, especially on empty stomach; but individual variations have
been observed. Oral dose of 250 mg produces average serum level of at least 0.6
μg/ml in 2 hours. Peak serum levels rise with repeated administration. Average
half-life is approximately 5.5 hours. Excreted primarily in bile. See Erythromy-
cin.
CONTRAINDICATIONS AND PRECAUTIONS
Hypersensitivity to erythromycins. Safe use during pregnancy not established.
Cautious use: impaired hepatic function.
ADVERSE REACTIONS
Abdominal cramps, diarrhea, nausea, vomiting, urticaria, skin eruptions, superinfections. See Erythromycin.
ROUTE AND DOSAGE
Adults: Oral: 250 mg every 6 hours; dosage may be increased up to 4 Gm/day
or more according to severity of infection. **Children:** 30 to 50 mg/kg/day orally
in 4 equally divided doses. For more severe infections, dosage may be doubled.
For twice-a-day schedule in both adults and children, one-half of total daily
dose may be prescribed every 12 hours.

NURSING IMPLICATIONS
Culture and sensitivity testing should be done.
Optimum blood levels are obtained when drug is given on empty stomach
(preferably 1 hour before or 3 hours after meals).
In treatment of group A β-hemolytic streptococcal infections, therapeutic
dosage should be administered for at least 10 days.
Protect tablets from light.
See Erythromycin.

ESTRADIOL, N.F.
(AQUADIOL, ESTRACE, PROGYNON)

Estrogen

ACTIONS AND USES
Natural or synthetic steroidal hormone produced by ovaries. Essential for normal maturation of the female and for maintenance of normal menstrual cycles
during reproductive years. Promotes endometrial lining development and increases volume, acidity, and glycogen content of vaginal secretions. Weakly
anabolic; large doses induce sodium and fluid retention. Decreases intestinal

motility but stimulates uterine motility. Decreases bone resorption rate; accelerates epiphyseal closure in long bones and is partially responsible for maintenance of blood vessel and skin structure in the female. Decreases platelet adhesiveness and increases serum levels of vitamin-K-dependent clotting factors. Increases serum triglycerides and α-lipoproteins, but reduces β-lipoproteins and plasma cholesterol. Prolonged therapy blocks anterior pituitary functions (inhibiting lactation, ovulation, androgenic secretion, and development of proliferative endometrium). Reportedly, estrogen therapy increases risk of thromboembolic disease (men and women), endometrial carcinoma, and gallbladder disease (in postmenopausal women). May mask onset of climacteric. Men receiving large doses of estrogen are more prone than nonusers to nonfatal myocardial infarction.

Used to treat natural or surgical menopausal symptoms, kraurosis vulvae, hypogonadism, acne, and postpartum lactation suppression. Also used as palliative for prostatic carcinoma and inoperable mammary cancer in women at least 5 years postmenopause. Has been used to prevent and treat postmenopausal osteoporosis.

ABSORPTION AND FATE

Readily absorbed through skin, mucous membranes, and GI tract. Absorption begins promptly following parenteral dose and continues for days. Half-life 50 minutes. Large amounts of free estrogen are excreted into bile, reabsorbed from GI tract, and recirculated through liver, which is the principle site of degradation. Excretion primarily in urine as sulfates and glucuronides; small amounts present in feces. Crosses placenta and appears in breast milk.

CONTRAINDICATIONS AND PRECAUTIONS

Estrogen hypersensitivity; known or suspected pregnancy, estrogenic-dependent neoplasms, breast cancer (except in selected patients being treated for metastatic disease); history of active thromboembolic disorders, arterial thrombosis, or thrombophlebitis; undiagnosed abnormal genital bleeding; adolescents with incomplete bone growth; hepatic disease; thyroid dysfunction; blood dyscrasias. Cautious use: endometriosis, lactation; conditions adversely affected by fluid retention; severe hypertension; diseases of calcium and phosphate metabolism; cerebrovascular or coronary artery disease; psychiatric disorders occurring during menopause; family history of breast or genital tract cancer or diabetes mellitus; gestational diabetes; gallbladder disease; preexisting fibromyomata; abnormal mammogram; history of idiopathic jaundice of pregnancy; varicosities.

ADVERSE REACTIONS

GI: nausea, vomiting, anorexia, diarrhea, abdominal cramps, bloating, cholestatic jaundice, thirst. **Dermatologic**: allergic rash, pruritus, acne, chloasma, melasma, loss of scalp hair, hirsutism, hyperpigmentation of areola. **CNS**: headaches, migraine, vertigo, mental depression, insomnia, paresthesias, nervousness, irritability, lassitude, anxiety, chorea, scotomata, intolerance to contact lenses. **Genitourinary**: mastodynia, breast secretion, breakthrough bleeding, spotting, changes in menstrual flow, vaginal candidiasis, reactivation of endometriosis, cystitislike syndrome, increased size of preexisting fibromyomata. In males: gynecomastia, testicular atrophy, feminization, impotence (reversible). **Other**: increased bromsulphalein retention and total thyroid circulation; increased serum renin substrate level; decreased response to metyrapone test; decreased glucose tolerance; hypercalcemia, hypertension, leg cramps, edema, weight gain or loss, aggravation of hepatic cutaneous porphyria, changes in libido, fatigue, backache.

ROUTE AND DOSAGE

Highly individualized. Oral: 1 to 2 mg daily (cyclic regimen). Intramuscular (aqueous or oil base): *Menopause*: 1 mg/week in divided doses for 2 to 3 weeks; thereafter, dosage gradually reduced to minimum requirements. *Kraurosis vulvae*: 1 to 1.5 mg one or more times per week. *Prostatic cancer*: 1.5 mg 3 times per week. Subcutaneous implantation: 25-mg pellet.

NURSING IMPLICATIONS

Roll vial of aqueous suspension vigorously between palms to assure uniform drug dispersion.

Implanted pellets (approximately 3.2 mm in diameter and 3.5 mm long) provide constant estrogen level for about 3 months.

To avoid continuous stimulation of reproductive tract tissues, estrogen administration is usually cyclic: 3 weeks on drug, followed by 1 week without (or first 25 days followed by rest period of remaining days of each month).

A complete history (including menstrual pattern) and physical examination with special reference to blood pressure, eyes, breasts, abdomen, and pelvic organs, and including Pap smear, should precede institution of estrogen therapy and be repeated periodically during treatment.

Urge patients to return at least annually for reassessment of continued need for estrogen therapy.

Estrogen-primed endometrium may bleed 48 to 72 hours after dose is discontinued. In cyclic therapy, estradiol is resumed on schedule before induced menstruation stops.

Withdrawal bleeding may occur even after oophorectomy and after menopause. Teach postmenopausal women that such bleeding is pseudomenstruation and does not indicate return of fertility.

If a patient has intermittent bleeding or begins to bleed without having previously done so, she should promptly report to her physician for an evaluation. Breakthrough bleeding may be stopped by increasing estrogen dose; however, if bleeding persists, the physician may recommend curettage.

If user becomes pregnant, she should be apprised of the potential risk of masculinization of female fetus.

Cyclic fluid retention should be reported. The physician may prescribe a low-salt diet and diuretic.

When estradiol is given for postpartum breast engorgement, fluids are usually restricted and a tight breast binder is worn for relief.

Nausea, frequently at breakfast time, seldom interferes with eating or causes weight loss and usually disappears after 1 or 2 weeks of drug use.

Be alert to the possibility of behavior changes or increasing mental depression, which are symptoms that may suggest recurrence of pretreatment psychic disorders. Report to physician; drug will usually be discontinued.

Teach patient to identify and promptly report signs of embolic disorders: sudden severe headache or chest pain, unexplained visual disturbances, tenderness, pain and swelling of legs, abdominal pain, edema.

Symptoms of vaginal candidiasis (thick, white, curdlike secretions and inflamed congested introitus) should be reported promptly to permit appropriate treatment.

Reassure male patients that estrogen-induced feminization and impotence are reversible with termination of therapy.

When estradiol is used for acne treatment, a period of worsened skin condition frequently precedes improvement.

History of jaundice in pregnancy increases the possibility of estrogen-induced jaundice. Instruct patients to report yellow skin and sclera, pruritus, dark urine, and light-colored stools. Estrogen is usually interrupted pending clinical investigation.

Advise patients to weigh themselves under standard conditions 1 or 2 times per week and to report sudden weight gain or signs of fluid retention.

Menopausal symptoms in well-controlled patients on estrogen therapy begin to return in full intensity by end of rest period without estrogen.

Advise diabetic users to report positive urine tests promptly. Dosage adjustment of the diabetic drug may be indicated. Emphasize necessity of periodic clinical evaluation for the potential diabetic (family history).

When hypercalcemia (normal Ca: 9 to 10.6 mg/dl) occurs in patients with breast cancer, it usually indicates progression of bone metastasis; estrogen treatment is usually terminated.

The pathologist should be advised of estrogen therapy when relevant specimens are submitted; the dentist also should be advised if extraction or periodontal surgery is anticipated.

If liver or endocrine function tests are abnormal, they should be repeated after estrogen has been withdrawn for two cycles.

DRUG INTERACTIONS: Estradiol effects are decreased by **barbiturates** (interfere with estrogen breakdown by liver). Estradiol decreases the activity of **oral anticoagulants** by increasing levels of prothrombin and other blood factors. **Anticonvulsant** dose may require adjustment (estradiol has fluid-retention properties and increases hepatic breakdown of anticonvulsant). Established dose requirements for **antidiabetic drug** may be increased because of lowered glucose tolerance. Estradiol potentiates antiinflammatory and glycosuric effects of **hydrocortisone** and increases action of **meperidine** by interfering with hepatic degradation. Estradiol may increase toxic reactions of **imipramine** and other **tricyclic antidepressants.**

ESTRADIOL BENZOATE, N.F., B.P.

Estrogen

ROUTE AND DOSAGE

Intramuscular (aqueous or sesame oil vehicle): *Menopause:* 1 mg/week, preferably in divided doses for 2 to 3 weeks; thereafter dosage is gradually reduced to minimal requirements. *Kraurosis vulvae:* 1 to 1.5 mg one or more times per week. *Prostatic cancer:* 1.5 mg 3 times per week.

NURSING IMPLICATIONS

When used for palliation of prostatic cancer, dosage is based on studies of efficacy rather than end organ response; therefore, thickening of the breast of the male is not used as a guideline for therapy.

In patients receiving treatment for kraurosis vulvae, continuous therapy with estradiol alone may induce functional bleeding. Advise patients to report any bleeding.

Protect solutions from light. Store at room temperature to prevent separation of crystals from oil solution.

See Estradiol.

ESTRADIOL CYPIONATE, U.S.P.
(DEPO-ESTRADIOL CYPIONATE, DURAESTRIN, ELONATE P.A., ESTRO-CYP, FEMOGEN CYP)

Estrogen

ACTIONS AND USES

See Estradiol for actions, absorption, fate, contraindications, and adverse reactions. Average duration of action is 3 to 8 weeks.

Intramuscular (cottonseed oil base): *Menopause:* 1 to 5 mg, repeated in 2 to 3 weeks. *Kraurosis vulvae:* 5 to 10 mg, repeated in 2 to 3 weeks. Highly individualized dosage and schedule.

NURSING IMPLICATIONS
Store at room temperature; protect from light.
See Estradiol.

ESTRADIOL VALERATE, U.S.P.
(DELESTROGEN, DURATRAD, ESTATE, ESTRAVAL-P.A., FEMOGEN LA, REP ESTRA)

Estrogen

ACTIONS AND USES
Provides 2 to 3 weeks of estrogen effects from single intramuscular injection. See Estradiol.

ROUTE AND DOSAGE
Intramuscular (in oil vehicle): *Castration, menopausal syndrome, senile vaginitis:* 10 to 20 mg any time; repeated 2 to 3 weeks after initial injection; stopped after second injection. *Prostatic carcinoma:* 30 mg or more every 1 or 2 weeks. *Postpartum breast engorgement:* 10 to 25 mg as single injection at end of first stage of labor.

NURSING IMPLICATIONS
Store at room temperature; protect from light.
See Estradiol.

ESTROGENS, CONJUGATED, U.S.P.
(CONEST, CO-ESTRO, ESTROPAN, FEMEST, FEM-H, MENOGEN, MENOTAB, PREMARIN, and others)

Estrogen, systemic hemostatic

ACTIONS AND USES
Short-acting estrogen preparation obtained from urine of pregnant mares. Contains mixture of conjugated estrogens, including sodium estrone sulfate (50% to 65%) and sodium equilin sulfate (20% to 35%). Topical preparations used for atrophic vaginitis and kraurosis vulvae and as adjunct in therapy for acne vulgaris. May be used parenterally to control or arrest uterine hemorrhage and for emergency treatment of spontaneous capillary bleeding. Other uses similar to those of estradiol (qv).

ROUTE AND DOSAGE
Oral: *Menopause:* 1.25 mg daily, adjusted up or down for maintenance at minimal level that provides effective control (usually 0.625 mg or less). *Female hypogonadism:* 2.5 to 7.5 mg daily in divided doses for 20 days followed by 10-day rest period; if there is no bleeding at end of this cycle, same dosage is repeated. *Senile vaginitis, kraurosis vulvae:* 1.25 to 3.75 mg daily. *Mammary cancer:* 30 mg daily in divided doses for at least 2 months for subjective response and 5 months for objective response. *Prostatic cancer:* 1.25 to 2.5 mg 3 times daily. Intravenous,

intramuscular: **Adults:** 25 mg. **Children:** 5 to 10 mg. Repeated in 6 to 12 hours if necessary. Topical (cream, 0.625 mg/Gm): 2 to 4 Gm/day; (lotion, 1 mg/ml in 30% isopropanol): 1 ml twice daily.

NURSING IMPLICATIONS

Store drug in refrigerator before reconstitution. To reconstitute add diluent to ampul and agitate *gently.*

If reconstituted solution is stored in refrigerator and protected from light, it will remain stable for 60 days. Discard precipitated or discolored solution.

Rapid IV injection may cause skin flushing.

Systemic hyperestrogenic effects (uterine bleeding, edema, mastalgia, reactivation of endometriosis) may result from overdosage of topical preparations, especially if skin surface is abraded or denuded. Caution patients to adhere to prescribed regimen and to report symptoms to a physician promptly.

Note that esterified estrogens (Amnestrogen, Femogen, Menest, SK-Estrogens) combine the same estrogenic substances but in different proportions.

See Estradiol.

ESTROGENS, ESTERIFIED, U.S.P.
(AMNESTROGEN, ESTRATAB, EVEX, FEMOGEN, GLYESTRIN, MENEST, SK-ESTROGENS, ZESTE)

Estrogen

ACTIONS AND USES

Estrogen preparations containing sodium estrone sulfate (75% to 85%) and sodium equilin sulfate (6.5% to 15%) calculated on basis of total esterified estrogen content. See Estradiol for uses, absorption and fate, contraindications, and adverse reactions.

ROUTE AND DOSAGE

Oral: *Menopause:* 1.25 mg daily; cyclic regimen recommended. Dosage adjusted up or down to minimal maintenance level effective for relief of symptoms. *Female hypogonadism:* 2.5 to 7.5 mg daily for 21 days, followed by 5 days of oral progestin therapy. If bleeding occurs before this regimen is concluded, therapy should be discontinued; otherwise, after 7 days without medication, therapy should be continued as before. *Prostatic carcinoma:* 3.75 mg or more per day for several weeks, then approximately half dosage for maintenance. Breast cancer: 30 mg daily for 2 months for subjective response, or total of 5 months for objective response. *Postpartum breast engorgement:* 5 mg daily for 2 days or more, started as soon as possible after delivery.

NURSING IMPLICATIONS

See Estradiol.

ESTRONE, N.F.
(ESTROVAG, ESTRUSOL, MENFORMON (A), THEELIN)
ESTRONE PIPERAZINE SULFATE, N.F.
(OGEN)

Estrogen

ACTIONS AND USES
Steroidal estrogen obtained from natural and synthetic sources. Conjugation with piperazine sulfate stabilizes estrone and renders it effective orally. See Estradiol.

ROUTE AND DOSAGE
Oral (estrone piperazine sulfate): *Menopause:* 2.5 mg daily. *Senile vaginitis and pruritus vulvae:* 0.625 to 2.5 mg daily. *Female hypogonadism:* 1.25 to 3.75 mg for first 3 weeks, followed by rest period of 8 to 10 days. *Postpartum breast engorgement:* 3.75 mg every 4 hours for 5 doses during first 20 hours after delivery. *Prostatic carcinoma:* 7.5 to 15 mg daily in 3 divided doses. Intramuscular (estrone): *Replacement therapy:* 0.1 to 1 mg weekly. Dosage adjusted to minimum required to gain symptomatic control. *Senile vaginitis:* 0.1 to 0.5 mg 2 to 3 times weekly. Suppository (0.2 mg): one at bedtime.

NURSING IMPLICATIONS

Estrone piperazine sulfate is given cyclically (eg, 3 weeks on, 1 week off) when used for menopause and for female hypogonadism symptoms.

Intramuscular preparations have either water or oil for the base. Oily preparation may become cloudy on chilling because of drug precipitation. Warm solution until it is clear before administration.

Oral estrone is given cyclically, with the exception of treatment modalities for cancer or for breast engorgement.

When estrone is used palliatively for cancer, response should be apparent within 3 months after start of therapy. If a response occurs, drug is continued until disease is again progressive.

See Estradiol.

ETHACRYNIC ACID, U.S.P., B.P.
(EDECRIN)
SODIUM ETHACRYNATE FOR INJECTION, U.S.P.
(SODIUM EDECRIN)

Diuretic

ACTIONS AND USES
Unsaturated ketone derivative of phenoxyacetic acid with rapid and potent diuretic action. Action mechanism is unclear, but it may involve blocking of sulfhydryl-catalyzed enzyme systems. Inhibits sodium reabsorption in proximal tubule and most segments of loop of Henle, induces potassium and hydrogen ion deficits, and decreases urinary ammonium ion concentration. Promotes calcium loss in hypercalcemia and nephrogenic diabetes insipidus. Paradoxic decrease in urine volume may follow drug-induced sodium loss. Fluid-electrolyte loss may exceed that produced by thiazides, but the effect on carbohydrate metabolism and blood glucose is less. Tends to promote urate excretion at high doses and retention at low doses; does not inhibit carbonic anhydrase. Action is independent of systemic acid–base balance. Appears to have little or no direct effect on renal blood flow or glomerular filtration rate. Aldosterone secretion

may be increased, thus contributing to hypokalemia. Hypotensive effect may be due to hypovolemia secondary to diuresis, and in part to decreased vascular resistance.

Used in treatment of severe edema associated with congestive heart failure, hepatic cirrhosis, renal disease, nephrotic syndrome, lymphedema. Also used in treatment of nephrogenic diabetes insipidus and hypercalcemia. Investigational use in treatment of mild to moderate hypertension and as adjunct to therapy of hypertensive crises complicated by pulmonary edema or renal failure.

ABSORPTION AND FATE

Diuretic effect occurs within 30 minutes following oral administration, peaks in 2 hours, and lasts 6 to 8 hours. Following IV injection, diuresis is apparent within 5 minutes; it reaches maximum within 15 to 30 minutes and persists approximately 2 hours. Half-life 30 to 70 minutes. Accumulates in liver. Metabolized to cysteine conjugate; approximately two-thirds of dose is excreted in urine; remainder is eliminated in bile. Rate of urinary excretion increases as pH increases. It is not known whether it crosses placenta or enters breast milk.

CONTRAINDICATIONS AND PRECAUTIONS

History of hypersensitivity to ethacrynic acid; anuria, hepatic coma, dehydration, electrolyte imbalance, hypotension, pregnancy, lactation, women of childbearing age, infants, parenteral use in pediatric patients. Cautious use: hepatic cirrhosis; elderly cardiac patients; diabetes mellitus; history of gout; concomitant administration with antihypertensive agents, other diuretics, aminoglycoside antibiotics, digitalis glycosides, corticosteroids.

ADVERSE REACTIONS

GI: anorexia, nausea, vomiting, dysphagia, abdominal discomfort or pain, malaise, diarrhea, GI bleeding (IV use), acute pancreatitis (increased serum amylase), abnormal liver function tests, jaundice, hepatic damage, hypoproteinemia. **Electrolyte imbalance:** hyponatremia, hypokalemia, hypochloremic alkalosis, hypomagnesemia, hypocalcemia, hypercalciuria, hypovolemia, hyperuricemia. **Dermatologic:** skin rash, pruritus. **Hematologic:** thrombocytopenia, agranulocytosis, severe neutropenia, Henoch's purpura (in patients with rheumatic fever). **Cardiovascular:** postural hypotension, thrombophlebitis, emboli. **Other:** tetany, acute gout, elevated BUN, hematuria, hyperglycemia, acute hypoglycemia (rare), gynecomastia, headache, fever, chills, blurred vision, fatigue, weakness, apprehension, confusion, local irritation of IV site, vertigo, tinnitus, sense of fullness in ears, temporary or permanent deafness.

ROUTE AND DOSAGE

Adults: Oral: initially 50 to 100 mg (single dose); maintenance (following diuresis) consists of minimal effective dose (50 to 100 mg once or twice daily after meals) administered on continuous or intermittent dosage schedule. Dosage adjustments are usually made in increments of 25 to 50 mg. Total daily dosage should not exceed 400 mg. **Children:** Oral: initial 25 mg followed by 25 mg increments to level of maintenance dose. **Adults only:** Intravenous (sodium ethacrynate): 0.5 to 1 mg/kg body weight. Single doses should not exceed 100 mg.

NURSING IMPLICATIONS

Follow manufacturer's directions for reconstitution of sodium ethacrynate. Solution should be used within 24 hours; discard solution if it becomes cloudy or opalescent.

Baseline and periodic determinations should be made of blood count, serum electrolytes, CO_2, BUN, creatinine, blood sugar, uric acid, and liver function. Frequent WBC determinations and liver function tests are advised during prolonged therapy.

Schedule doses to avoid nocturia and thus sleep interference.

Explain diuretic effect (increased volume and frequency of voiding) to the patient.

Diuretic effect tends to diminish with continuous therapy.

Administer oral drug after a meal or food to prevent gastric irritation.

Monitor blood pressure during initial therapy. Since orthostatic hypotension sometimes occurs, supervision of ambulation is advisable. Caution the patient to make position changes slowly, particularly from recumbent to upright position.

Patient should be observed closely when receiving the drug by IV infusion. Rapid, copious diuresis following IV administration can produce hypotension and peripheral vascular collapse. Check infusion site frequently. Extravasation causes local pain and tissue irritation.

Monitor intake–output ratio as an important measure of drug action. Drug should be discontinued if excessive diuresis, oliguria, hematuria, or sudden profuse diarrhea occurs. Report signs to physician.

Establish baseline weight prior to start of therapy; weigh patient under standard conditions. To initiate diuresis, the smallest dose required to produce weight loss of 1 to 2 lb per day is recommended. Report weight gain in excess of 2 pounds/day.

Once "dry weight" has been achieved, drug dosage and frequency of administration should be reduced.

Observe for and report warning signs and symptoms of electrolyte imbalance: anorexia, nausea, vomiting, thirst, dry mouth, polyuria, oliguria, weakness, fatigue, dizziness, headache, muscle cramps, paresthesias, drowsiness, mental confusion.

Fluid and electrolyte depletion is most apt to occur in patients on large doses or salt-intake restriction. Consult physician regarding allowable salt and fluid intake. Generally, salt intake is liberalized.

Elderly and debilitated patients require close observation. Excessive diuresis promotes dehydration and hypovolemia, both of which often precede circulatory collapse, cerebrovascular thrombosis, and pulmonary emboli, especially in these patients.

Report immediately possible signs of thromboembolic complications: pain in chest, back, pelvis, legs.

Monitor blood pressure and pulse of patients with impaired cardiac function. Diuretic-induced hypovolemia may reduce cardiac output, and electrolyte loss promotes cardiotoxicity in those receiving digitalis or other cardiac glycosides.

To reduce or prevent potassium depletion, the physician may prescribe daily ingestion of potassium-rich foods (banana, orange, peach, dried dates), potassium supplement, and intermittent dosage schedule.

GI side effects occur most frequently after 1 to 3 months of therapy or in patients on high dosage. Loose stools or other GI symptoms at any time during therapy should be reported in order to permit dosage adjustment or discontinuation of drug if indicated.

Report immediately any evidence of impaired hearing. Ototoxicity has been associated with renal insufficiency, concomitant administration of aminoglycoside antibiotics, and rapid IV administration. Hearing loss may be preceded by vertigo, tinnitus, or fullness in ears; it may be transient, lasting 1 to 24 hours, or it may be permanent.

In patients receiving aminoglycoside antibiotics concurrently with ethacrynic acid, renal status, audiograms, and vestibular function tests are advised before initiation of therapy and regularly throughout therapy.

Impaired glucose tolerance with hyperglycemia and glycosuria may occur in diabetic and diabetic-prone individuals and in patients with decompensated hepatic cirrhosis. Watch for signs of hypoglycemia when ethacrynic acid is withdrawn.

Acute hypoglycemia with convulsions reportedly has been associated with use of large doses in patients with uremia.

aminoglycoside antibiotics, potentiate the hypotensive effects of **antihypertensive drugs** (dosage of antihypertensive agent and possibly that of ethacrynic
acid should be reduced), and enhance the hypoprothrombinemic effects of **oral
anticoagulants.** A higher incidence of GI bleeding has been attributed to concurrent use of sodium ethacrynate (IV) and **heparin.** Ethacrynic-acid-induced
electrolyte imbalance may enhance the cardiotoxicity of **cardiac glycosides**
(primarily from loss of potassium and magnesium), and the neuromuscular
blockade produced by **tubocurarine** and other **neuromuscular blocking agents**
(from loss of potassium). Excessive potassium loss may result when given with
amphotericin B or **corticosteroids.** Ethacrynic acid may increase the possibility
of **lithium** toxicity (by promoting excretion of potassium and sodium). By
elevating serum urate levels, it may antagonize the actions of **uricosuric agents.**
Reportedly, ethacrynic acid may augment the effects of **alcohol** or produce
alcohol intolerance (caution patients of this possibility). There is the possibility
of nephrotoxicity if it is used with **cephaloridine** (concomitant administration
is generally avoided).

ETHCHLORVYNOL, N.F., B.P.
(PLACIDYL)

Sedative, hypnotic

ACTIONS AND USES
Tertiary acetylenic alcohol with CNS depressant effects similar to those of
chloral hydrate and barbiturates. Mechanism of action not known. Hypnotic
doses produce cerebral depression and quiet, deep sleep; sedative doses reduce
anxiety and apprehension. Also exhibits anticonvulsant and muscle relaxant
activity. Has no analgesic properties. Effect on REM sleep not known.
Used for short-term hypnotic therapy for simple insomnia and as daytime
sedative in mild anxiety or tension states.
ABSORPTION AND FATE
Rapidly absorbed from GI tract. Hypnotic dose induces sleep within 15 to 30
minutes. Maximal blood levels in 1 to 1.5 hours; duration of action about 5
hours. Localizes in adipose tissue, liver, kidney, spleen, brain, cerebrospinal
fluid, bile. Extensively metabolized, probably by liver. Approximately 10% of
dose is excreted unchanged in urine within 24 hours.
CONTRAINDICATIONS AND PRECAUTIONS
Known hypersensitivity to ethchlorvynol; porphyria; patients with uncontrolled pain; first and second trimesters of pregnancy. Safe use in children not
established. Cautious use: third trimester of pregnancy; patients with mental
depression or suicidal tendencies; addiction-prone individuals; impaired hepatic
or renal function; elderly or debilitated patients; patients receiving MAO inhibitors, including pargyline hydrochloride, and tricyclic antidepressants; patients
who respond unpredictably to alcohol or barbiturates.
ADVERSE REACTIONS
Hypotension, nausea, vomiting, aftertaste, blurred vision, dizziness, facial
numbness, urticaria, headache, mild hangover. In susceptible patients: giddiness, ataxia, prolonged hypnosis, profound muscular weakness, excitement,
hysteria, syncope. Rare: hypersensitivity reactions (urticaria, thrombocytopenia), cholestatic jaundice. Overdosage: stupor, coma, bradycardia, hypotension, respiratory failure. Chronic abuse: tremors, incoordination, slurred speech,
nystagmus, toxic amblyopia, permanent visual defects, peripheral neuropathy.

Oral: *sedative,* 100 to 200 mg 2 or 3 times a day; *hypnotic,* 500 mg to 1 Gm at bedtime.

NURSING IMPLICATIONS

Ethchlorvynol produces transient giddiness and ataxia in some patients who apparently absorb the drug very rapidly. Symptoms may be minimized by administering the drug with milk or other food.

Report the appearance of mental confusion, hallucinations, or drowsiness in patients receiving daytime sedation; dosage should be decreased, or drug should be discontinued.

The elderly may not tolerate average adult doses. Observe intensity and duration of drug action.

Report to physician if pain is present. Pain should be controlled before administration of ethchlorvynol.

Caution the patient to avoid driving a motor vehicle or engaging in other activities requiring mental alertness and physical coordination for at least 5 hours after he has taken the drug.

Psychologic and physical dependence is possible; therefore, prolonged administration is not recommended. Classified as schedule IV drug under federal Controlled Substances Act.

Severe withdrawal symptoms may occur if drug is discontinued abruptly in patients taking regular doses (unusual anxiety, tremors, ataxia, irritability, slurred speech, memory loss, hallucinations, delirium, convulsions).

Preserved in tight, light-resistant containers.

DRUG INTERACTIONS: Dosage of ethchlorvynol should be reduced in patients receiving **MAO inhibitors** or **tricyclic antidepressants.** Transient delirium has been reported when ethchlorvynol and **amitriptyline** have been used concurrently. Additive CNS depression may occur when ethchlorvynol is administered concomitantly with **alcohol, barbiturates,** or or other **CNS depressants;** caution the patient. Ethchlorvynol may decrease activity of **oral anticoagulants.**

ETHINAMATE, N.F.
(VALMID)

Sedative, hypnotic

ACTIONS AND USES

Carbamic acid derivative with central depressant effects similar to those produced by barbiturates, but with shorter duration of action. Also exhibits anticonvulsant activity.

Used chiefly as rapid-acting hypnotic in mild insomnia.

ABSORPTION AND FATE

Rapidly and almost completely absorbed from GI tract. Induces sleep in about 20 minutes; effects last 3 to 5 hours. Rapidly metabolized, primarily in liver; metabolites excreted in urine.

CONTRAINDICATIONS AND PRECAUTIONS

Known hypersensitivity to ethinamate; patients with uncontrolled pain. Safe use during pregnancy and lactation and in pediatric patients not established. Cautious use: elderly, debilitated patients; patients with mental depression or suicidal tendencies; addiction-prone individuals.

Infrequent: mild GI symptoms, skin rash, paradoxical excitement (especially in children), thrombocytopenic purpura and drug idiosyncrasy with fever (rare). Overdosage: hypotension, respiratory depression, coma.

ROUTE AND DOSAGE

Oral: 500 mg to 1 Gm 20 minutes before retiring.

NURSING IMPLICATIONS

Lower doses are generally prescribed for elderly and debilitated patients.

Psychic and physical dependence may occur with chronic use of large doses.

Gradual withdrawal in a controlled hospital setting and psychiatric follow-up are recommended after prolonged overdosage. Abrupt withdrawal can precipitate severe reactions (tremulousness, hyperactive reflexes, agitation, disorientation, severe insomnia, syncopal episodes, hallucinations, convulsions).

Caution the patient to avoid driving and other dangerous activities for at least 4 or 5 hours after taking ethinamate.

Patients should be informed that additive CNS effects may occur with concomitant administration of alcohol, barbiturates, or other CNS depressants.

Classified as schedule IV drug under federal Controlled Substances Act.

LABORATORY TEST INTERFERENCES: Falsely high urinary 17-ketosteroid levels (Holtorff-Koch modification of Zimmerman reaction) reported.

ETHINYL ESTRADIOL, U.S.P.
(ESTINYL, FEMINONE, LYNORAL, MENOLYN, OVOGYN)

Estrogen

ACTIONS AND USES

Active when taken by mouth, unlike estradiol; inactivation by liver or other tissues is slow. Combined with progestins in oral contraceptives to control ovulation.

ROUTE AND DOSAGE

Oral: *Menopause or postmenopause:* 0.02 to 0.05 mg daily; dosage adjusted to minimal effective level. *Postpartum breast engorgement:* 0.5 to 1 mg daily for 3 days, then gradually decreased to 0.1 mg after 7 days; therapy then discontinued. *Female hypogonadism:* 0.05 mg 1 to 3 times daily for 2 weeks, followed by 2 weeks of progesterone; regimen to be continued 3 to 6 months. *Breast cancer:* 1 mg 3 times daily. *Prostatic carcinoma:* 0.15 to 0.2 mg daily. *Contraception:* see Oral Contraceptives.

NURSING IMPLICATIONS

Given cyclically, except when used for treatment of postpartum breast engorgement and palliation of carcinoma.

See Estradiol.

(ZACTANE)

Analgesic

ACTIONS AND USES
Synthetic nonnarcotic analgesic structurally related to meperidine, but effective only for relief of mild to moderate pain. Produces analgesic effect by unknown action on CNS. Does not suppress cough reflex and has little or no antipyretic or antiinflammatory action. Reported to have low abuse potential.

Used in treatment of mild to moderate pain. Frequently used in combination with other agents such as aspirin, phenacetin, and meprobamate for relief of pain of arthritis and other musculoskeletal disorders.

ABSORPTION AND FATE
Readily absorbed from GI tract. Peak blood levels in 1 hour. Partially detoxified by liver. Excreted chiefly in urine within 48 hours as intact drug and metabolites.

CONTRAINDICATIONS AND PRECAUTIONS
History of hypersensitivity or intolerance to ethoheptazine citrate.

ADVERSE REACTIONS
Infrequent: nausea, vomiting, epigastric distress, dizziness, pruritus. Symptoms suggestive of cumulative toxicity: headache, visual disturbances, syncope, nervousness.

ROUTE AND DOSAGE
Oral: 75 to 150 mg 3 or 4 times daily, depending on severity of pain.

NURSING IMPLICATIONS
Warn patients that the drug may potentiate the depressant effects of alcohol, barbiturates, and other CNS depressants.

Zactirin, a commercially available compound, contains ethoheptazine citrate 75 mg with aspirin 325 mg. Equagesic contains ethoheptazine citrate 75 mg, aspirin 250 mg, meprobamate 150 mg.

When used with combination drugs, be alert to the possibility of toxic effects of other drugs.

Ethoheptazine citrate is not classified as a controlled substance.

ETHOSUXIMIDE, U.S.P., B.P.
(ZARONTIN)

Anticonvulsant

ACTIONS AND USES
Succinimide antiepilepsy agent. Reduces frequency of epileptiform attacks, apparently by depressing motor cortex and by elevating CNS threshold to stimuli. Usually ineffective in management of psychomotor or major motor seizures.

Used in management of petit mal epilepsy. May be administered in combination with other anticonvulsants when other forms of epilepsy coexist with petit mal.

ABSORPTION AND FATE
Essentially completely absorbed from GI tract. Peak plasma concentrations in 1 to 7 hours; however, 4 to 7 days are required for steady-state plasma concentrations. Plasma half-life 24 to 60 hours. No significant degree of plasma protein binding. Metabolized by liver. Excreted slowly in urine, about 50% as metabolites and 10% to 20% as unchanged drug. Small amounts excreted in bile and feces.

CONTRAINDICATIONS AND PRECAUTIONS
Hypersensitivity to succinimides; severe liver or renal disease; use alone in mixed types of epilepsy (may increase frequency of grand mal seizures). Safe use in women of childbearing potential or during pregnancy not established.

GI: nausea, vomiting, anorexia, weight loss, epigastric distress, abdominal pain, diarrhea, constipation. **Neurologic:** hiccups, ataxia, dizziness, drowsiness, headache, euphoria, restlessness, irritability, anxiety, hyperactivity, aggressiveness, depression, inability to concentrate, lethargy, confusion, sleep disturbances, night terrors, hypochondriacal behavior; rarely: psychosis, increased depression with overt suicidal intentions, auditory hallucinations. **Hematologic:** eosinophilia, leukopenia, thrombocytopenia, agranulocytosis, pancytopenia, aplastic anemia, positive direct Coombs' test. **Dermatologic:** Stevens-Johnson syndrome, pruritic erythematous skin eruptions, exfoliative dermatitis, systemic lupus erythematosus. **Ophthalmic:** blurred vision, myopia, photophobia, periorbital edema. **Genitourinary:** frequency, hematuria, albuminuria, renal damage. **Other:** increased libido, hirsutism, alopecia, vaginal bleeding, swelling of tongue, gum hypertrophy, muscle weakness.

ROUTE AND DOSAGE

Highly individualized. Oral: **Adults and children** *over 6 years:* 250 mg twice daily. **Children** *3 to 6 years:* 250 mg daily in divided doses. Dosage increases are made in small increments. One recommended method is to increase daily dose by 250 mg every 4 to 7 days until control is achieved with minimal side effects. A total daily dose exceeding 1.5 Gm should be administered only under strict medical supervision.

NURSING IMPLICATIONS

Baseline and periodic hematologic studies and tests of liver and renal function should be made.

Since ethosuximide may impair mental and physical abilities, caution the patient to avoid driving a motor vehicle and other hazardous activities.

GI symptoms, drowsiness, ataxia, dizziness, and other neurologic side effects occur frequently and indicate the need for dosage adjustment.

Close observation is required during the period of dosage adjustment and whenever other medications are added to or eliminated from the drug regimen.

Behavioral changes are most likely to occur in the patient with a prior history of psychiatric disturbances. Close supervision is indicated. Drug should be withdrawn slowly if these symptoms appear.

Abrupt withdrawal of ethosuximide (whether used alone or in combination therapy) may precipitate seizures or petit mal status.

Since long-term drug therapy is generally required, the occurrence of adverse drug effects is a possibility. Caution the patient and responsible family members to report any unusual sign or symptom to the physician. Stress the importance of follow-up visits.

Advise the patient to carry a wallet identification card or bracelet (eg, Medic Alert) indicating that he has epilepsy and is taking medication.

ETHOTOIN, B.P.

(Ethylphenyhydantoin, PEGANONE)

Anticonvulsant

ACTIONS AND USES

Hydantoin derivative structurally similar to phenytoin (qv). Reported to be less toxic but less effective than phenytoin and lacks its antiarrhythmic properties.

Used for control of grand mal and psychomotor seizures, usually as adjunct to other anticonvulsant medications.

ABSORPTION AND FATE

Probably metabolized by liver. Excreted in urine and bile as unchanged drug and metabolites; small quantities excreted in saliva.

CONTRAINDICATIONS AND PRECAUTIONS

Hypersensitivity to hydantoins; hepatic abnormalities; hematologic disorders. Risk potential during pregnancy and in women of childbearing age. Cautious use: elderly or gravely ill patients.

ADVERSE REACTIONS

Common: anorexia, nausea, vomiting, drowsiness, skin rash. Infrequent: lymphadenopathy, ataxia, gingival hyperplasia. Also see Phenytoin Sodium.

ROUTE AND DOSAGE

Adults: Oral: initially 1 Gm or less daily, in 4 to 6 divided doses. Subsequent dosage gradually increased over period of several days; maintenance: 2 to 3 Gm daily in 4 to 6 divided doses. **Children:** initial dose should not exceed 750 mg daily; maintenance: 500 mg to 1 Gm daily in divided doses. Optimum dosage determined on basis of individual response.

NURSING IMPLICATIONS

Doses should be spaced as evenly as practicable. Administer with or immediately after food to reduce incidence of gastric irritation.

Dosage reduction or substitution or discontinuation of other anticonvulsant medications should be accomplished gradually and with close observation of patient.

Blood counts and urinalyses are advised at start of therapy and at monthly intervals thereafter.

Patients with psychomotor epilepsy should be closely observed for symptoms of depression or other changes of behavior.

If drug is discontinued, withdrawal should be done slowly to prevent precipitating seizures or status epilepticus.

Ethotoin darkens on exposure to light and extreme heat.

See Phenytoin Sodium.

DRUG INTERACTIONS: Concurrent administration of ethotoin and **phenacemide** may cause paranoid symptoms. Also see Phenytoin Sodium.

ETHOXAZENE HYDROCHLORIDE
(SERENIUM)

Analgesic

ACTIONS AND USES

Azo dye structurally similar to phenazopyridine (qv). Chief value lies in its local anesthetic action on urinary tract mucosa. Imparts little or no antibacterial activity to urine.

Used to relieve pain associated with chronic infections of urinary tract such as cystitis, urethritis, pyelitis.

ABSORPTION AND FATE

Excreted in feces and urine.

CONTRAINDICATIONS AND PRECAUTIONS

Uremia, severe hepatitic disease, chronic glomerular nephritis, pyelonephritis of pregnancy with GI disturbances. Cautious use: GI conditions.

Adults: Oral: 100 mg 3 times daily before meals. **Children** *under 8 years:* 100 mg 2 times daily before meals.

NURSING IMPLICATIONS
Inform patient that the drug may impart an orange to orange red discoloration to urine.
See Phenazopyridine.

LABORATORY TEST INTERFERENCES: Ethoxazene reportedly may interfere with BSP and PSP excretion tests and urine bilirubin determinations (atypical color reactions with Bili-Labstix and Ictotest).

ETHOXZOLAMIDE, U.S.P.
(CARDRASE, ETHAMIDE)

Carbonic anhydrase inhibitor

ACTIONS AND USES
Nonbacteriostatic sulfonamide derivative similar to acetazolamide (qv) in actions, uses, contraindications, precautions, and adverse reactions. Used as adjunctive treatment for edema of congestive heart failure, and for chronic simple and secondary glaucoma.

ABSORPTION AND FATE
Onset of action in 2 hours; peak in 5 to 6 hours; duration 8 to 12 hours. Distributed in plasma, muscles, kidneys, liver, lungs, erythrocytes, aqueous humor, brain, and cerebrospinal fluid. Approximately 40% of dose is excreted unchanged in urine; fate of remainder not determined.

ROUTE AND DOSAGE
Oral: *Glaucoma:* 62.5 to 250 mg 2 to 4 times daily as indicated by tonometric measurements. *Edema of congestive heart failure:* 62.5 to 125 mg daily for 3 consecutive days of each week or on alternate days.

NURSING IMPLICATIONS
When given for edema of congestive heart failure, the drug is administered in the morning after breakfast.
With large dose, many patients exhibit drowsiness and paresthesias.
See Acetazolamide.

ETHYLESTRENOL
(MAXIBOLIN)

Anabolic

ACTIONS AND USES
Synthetic steroid hormone with relatively more anabolic than androgenic activity. Promotes body tissue-building and inhibits tissue-depleting processes; supports nitrogen, potassium, chloride, and phosphorus conservation. Enhances weight gain and combats depression and weakness in debilitating conditions. Stimulates bone growth, aids in bone matrix reconstitution, and may support calcification of metastatic lesions of breast cancer. Prevents or reverses profound nitrogen loss associated with corticosteroid therapy without compromising antiinflammatory activity. Mechanism of action in refractory anemias is unclear, but may be due to direct stimulation of bone marrow or protein anabolic activity, or to androgenic stimulation of erythropoiesis. Suppresses pituitary

gonadotropic functions, and may exert direct effect on testes. Potentially has all the side effects of testosterone.

Used to reverse catabolic effects of prolonged immobilization and debilitative states (severe burns, paraplegia, extensive surgery) and to control pain of metastasis in female breast cancer. Probably effective as adjunctive therapy for osteoporosis, pituitary dwarfism, and marked maturational delay and in selected types of refractory anemias and arthritis. Will not enhance athletic ability.

ABSORPTION AND FATE

Well absorbed from GI tract; metabolized in liver, and excreted in urine. Crosses placenta; appears in breast milk.

CONTRAINDICATIONS AND PRECAUTIONS

Hypersensitivity to drug; nephrosis; cardiac, hepatic, or renal decompensation; hypercalcemia; infancy. In males: known or suspected prostatic cancer, benign prostatic hypertrophy with obstruction, carcinoma of breast. In females: lactation, pregnancy, menstrual disorders. Cautious use: prepubertal males; patients easily stimulated sexually; concomitant ACTH, corticosteroid, or anticoagulant therapy; diabetes mellitus; history of coronary disease or myocardial infarction.

ADVERSE REACTIONS

Both sexes: nausea, vomiting, diarrhea, gastric irritation, burning of tongue, hypersensitivity, anaphylactoid reaction (rare), habituation, excitation, insomnia, increased or decreased libido, acne (especially females and prepubertal males), hypercalcemia, leukopenia, hepatocellular carcinoma (rare), chills, sodium and water retention, edema, jaundice. **Males** (*prepubertal*): premature epiphyseal closure, acne, priapism, growth of facial and body hair, phallic enlargement; (*postpubertal*): inhibition of testicular function, testicular atrophy, impotence, epididymitis, gynecomastia, bladder irritability. Females: virilization (hoarseness, acne, oily skin, hirsutism, enlarged clitoris, stimulation of libido, menstrual irregularities, male-pattern baldness). **Altered laboratory tests:** metyrapone; fasting blood sugar and glucose tolerance tests; thyroid function tests; blood coagulation tests (increased factors II, V, VII, X); decreased creatinine and creatinine excretion; increased 17-ketosteroid excretion; elevated BSP, transaminase, bilirubin, serum cholesterol.

ROUTE AND DOSAGE

Oral. **Adults:** 4 to 8 mg/day, reduced to minimum levels at first evidence of clinical response (daily dosage usually does not exceed 0.1 mg/kg body weight). **Children:** 1 to 3 mg/day; highly individualized. A single course of therapy for adults and children should not exceed 6 weeks. If necessary, treatment may be restarted after interval of 4 weeks.

NURSING IMPLICATIONS

Administer drug immediately before or with meals to diminish GI distress.

Reportedly, anabolic drugs are most effective when combined with a therapeutic dietary regimen (high in calories, protein, vitamins, and minerals), physical therapy, and optimum health-promoting habits. All these measures require the patient's understanding and cooperation.

Elicit support of responsible family member and nutritionist in development of dietary regimen that satisfies the anorexic, debilitated patient. Diet may be tolerated better if given in frequent small feedings.

Baseline and periodic determinations of liver function and serum electrolytes are indicated (drug may cause retention of sodium, chloride, water, potassium, and inorganic phosphates). Serial determinations of serum cholesterol are advised in patients with history of myocardial infarction or coronary artery disease. (Normal total cholesterol: 150 to 250 mg/dl.)

Reinforce adherence to scheduled appointments for physical therapy (if prescribed) and laboratory tests. Stress importance of good personal hygiene, including meticulous skin care (females and prepubertal males are especially likely to develop acne).

Teach patient to note and report symptoms of jaundice (dark urine, pruritus, yellow skin, or sclerae) to physician. Dose adjustment may reverse the condition; however, if liver function tests are abnormal, therapy will be discontinued.

Monitor intake–output ratio and pattern and weight, and check for edema; report significant changes. Edema is generally controllable with salt restriction and/or diuretic therapy.

Hypercalcemia symptoms (lassitude, anorexia, nausea, vomiting, constipation, dehydration, polyuria, polydipsia, asthenia, loss of muscle tone) may be difficult to distinguish from symptoms associated with condition being treated unless they are anticipated and thought of as a symptom cluster. Hypercalcemia is particularly likely to occur in patients with metastatic breast carcinoma and may indicate bone metastases. Anabolic therapy will be stopped if it develops; consult physician about hydration and activity of patient.

Be alert for voice changes in female patient. Onset of hoarseness or deepening of voice can easily be overlooked if its significance as an early sign of virilization is not appreciated. Virilization may be irreversible even after prompt discontinuation of therapy. Unless the benefits of the drug are considered to outweigh its distressing side effects, therapy will be discontinued.

Instruct female patient to report menstrual irregularities. Usually the physician will discontinue medication pending determination of etiology.

Record beneficial effects of anabolic therapy, such as stimulation of appetite, euphoria, and general feeling of renewed vigor and well-being.

When used in pediatrics, therapy is preceded by x-ray of wrist bones to establish level of bone maturation. During treatment, bone maturation may proceed more rapidly than linear growth; therefore intermittent dosage schedule and periodic x-rays are usual.

Since skeletal stimulation continues about 6 months after treatment has been stopped, x-rays are used as determinants of discontinuing therapy well before bone maturation reaches the norm for chronologic age. Teach parents the importance of keeping child's appointments for bone maturation studies.

Children under 7 years of age are particularly sensitive to androgenic effects and therefore should be closely observed for precocious development of male sexual characteristics or masculinization; they should be questioned about the presence of priapism (inappropriate and frequent erections). These symptoms may necessitate drug withdrawal.

Patient with congenital aplastic anemia usually requires continued maintenance doses and supplementary iron.

Anabolic treatment may cause reduction of blood glucose in some diabetic patients. Watch closely for symptoms of hypoglycemia and report to physician. Change in dosage of antidiabetic drug may be required.

Observe patient on concomitant anticoagulant therapy for ecchymotic areas, petechiae, or abnormal bleeding from any site. Close monitoring of prothrombin time is essential.

Since anabolic steroids may alter many laboratory tests, inform pathologist when tissues or body fluids are submitted for study. Several values remain altered for 2 to 3 weeks after discontinuation of drug.

DRUG INTERACTIONS: Anabolic steroids may potentiate **oral anticoagulants,** enhance hypoglycemic response to **antidiabetic drugs,** and increase **oxyphenbutazone,** and **phenylbutazone** plasma levels. **Barbiturates** decrease the effect of androgens by increasing their hepatic breakdown.

F

FENFLURAMINE HYDROCHLORIDE
(PONDIMIN)

Anorexiant

ACTIONS AND USES

Sympathomimetic amine related to amphetamine. Differs pharmacologically from amphetamine in that it generally produces CNS depression more often than stimulation. Exact mechanism of appetite-inhibiting action not clearly defined, but may be due to stimulation of hypothalamus. Believed to have intrinsic hypoglycemic activity; appears to increase glucose uptake by skeletal muscles, thus reducing glucose available for conversion to lipid.

Used as short-term (a few weeks) adjunct in treatment of exogenous obesity.

ABSORPTION AND FATE

Readily absorbed from GI tract. Onset of action 1 to 2 hours; duration of anorexigenic effect 4 to 6 hours. Widely distributed to most body tissues. Considerable individual variation in drug metabolism and elimination. Slowly excreted in urine, primarily as metabolites; small quantities excreted as unchanged drug. Rate of urinary excretion is increased in acid urine. Excreted in saliva and sweat in small amounts.

CONTRAINDICATIONS AND PRECAUTIONS

Hypersensitivity to sympathomimetic amines; hyperthyroidism; severe hypertension; glaucoma; symptomatic cardiovascular disease including arrhythmias; history of drug abuse; agitated states; during or within 14 days following administration of MAO inhibitors; concomitant use of CNS depressants or CNS stimulants. Safe use during pregnancy, in women of childbearing age, and in children under 12 years of age not established. Cautious use: mental depression, hypertension, diabetes mellitus.

ADVERSE REACTIONS

Common: drowsiness, diarrhea, dry mouth. **Less frequent:** GI: nausea, vomiting, unpleasant taste, abdominal pain, constipation. CNS: dizziness, confusion, incoordination, headache, elevated mood, dysphoria, mental depression, anxiety, nervousness, psychotic episodes, tremors, agitation, weakness, fatigue, dysarthria, insomnia, vivid dreams, nightmares. **Dermatologic:** skin rashes, urticaria, ecchymosis, erythema, burning sensation of skin. **Cardiovascular:** palpitation, tachycardia, chest pain, arrhythmias, hypotension, hypertension, fainting. **Miscellaneous:** sweating, fever, chills, blurred vision, mydriasis, eye irritation, myalgia, edema, dysuria, urinary frequency, bad taste, grinding teeth during sleep, eye irritation, increased or decreased libido, impotence, menstrual irregularities, hair loss. **Overdosage:** confusion, agitation, hyperventilation, exaggerated or depressed reflexes, convulsions, hyperpyrexia, dilated nonreactive pupils, rotatory nystagmus, coma, cardiac arrest.

ROUTE AND DOSAGE

Oral: initially 20 to 40 mg 3 times daily before meals. May be increased at weekly intervals by 20 mg daily to maximum of 40 mg 3 times daily. Timed-release tablet: 60 mg daily.

NURSING IMPLICATIONS

Dosage increases should be made gradually to minimize possibility of side effects.

Diarrhea may occur during first week of therapy; report it to physician; dose reduction or termination of therapy may be required.

Patients with diabetes maintained on insulin or other antidiabetic drugs should be observed for excessive hypoglycemic activity when fenfluramine is added to the therapeutic regimen.

If fenfluramine is prescribed for patients with hypertension, blood pressure should be monitored.

Mentally depressed patients may become more depressed during therapy and/or following withdrawal of fenfluramine.

Warn patient that fenfluramine may impair ability to perform hazardous tasks such as driving a motor vehicle.

If tolerance to anorexigenic effect develops, drug should be discontinued.

To achieve and maintain loss of weight, patient should be adequately instructed in dietary management.

Following excessive use, abrupt discontinuation of fenfluramine may be associated with irritability and mental depression.

Classified as schedule IV substance under federal Controlled Substances Act.

DRUG INTERACTIONS: Use of fenfluramine during or within 14 days following administration of **MAO inhibitors** may result in hypertensive crisis. Fenfluramine reportedly may alter the effects of **hypotensive drugs**, eg, **guanethidine, methyldopa, reserpine**. Effects of **CNS depressants** or **stimulants** may be additive (caution patient).

FENTANYL CITRATE
(SUBLIMAZE)

Narcotic analgesic

ACTIONS AND USES

Synthetic phenylpiperidine derivative. Pharmacologic actions qualitatively similar to those of morphine and meperidine, but action is more prompt and less prolonged, and fentanyl appears to have less emetic activity. On a weight basis, it is estimated to be about 80 times more potent than morphine. Histamine release occurs rarely.

Used for analgesic action of short duration preoperatively, during surgery, and in immediate postoperative period. Commercially available combination of fentanyl with neuroleptic drug droperidol (Innovar) is used to produce tranquilization and analgesia for surgical and diagnostic procedures.

ABSORPTION AND FATE

Onset of action is almost immediate following IV administration, with peak analgesic effect in 3 to 5 minutes; duration 30 to 60 minutes. Onset of action following IM injection occurs in 7 to 15 minutes; duration 1 to 2 hours. Metabolized primarily in liver. Excreted in urine chiefly as metabolites; about 10% excreted as unchanged drug.

CONTRAINDICATIONS AND PRECAUTIONS

Patients who have received MAO inhibitors within 14 days; myasthenia gravis. Safe use in women of childbearing potential, during pregnancy, and in children younger than 2 years of age not established. Cautious use: head injuries, increased intracranial pressure; elderly, debilitated, poor-risk patients; chronic obstructive pulmonary disease and other respiratory problems; liver and kidney dysfunction; bradyarrhythmias.

ADVERSE REACTIONS

Euphoria, miosis, blurred vision, nausea, vomiting, dizziness, diaphoresis, hypotension, muscle rigidity (especially muscles of respiration) following rapid IV infusion, laryngospasm, bronchoconstriction, respiratory depression, respiratory arrest, bradycardia, circulatory depression, cardiac arrest.

Adults: Intramuscular, intravenous (slow): 0.05 to 0.1 mg. **Children** *2 to 12 years of age:* 0.02 to 0.03 mg per 20 to 25 lb.

NURSING IMPLICATIONS

Monitor vital signs and observe patient for signs of skeletal and thoracic muscle (depressed respirations) rigidity.

Duration of respiratory depressant effect may be considerably longer than analgesic effect. Have immediately available: oxygen, resuscitative equipment, endotracheal tube, suction, narcotic antagonist such as naloxone, and skeletal muscle relaxant, eg, succinylcholine for muscular rigidity.

Physician will rely on accurate reporting of drug effect following initial dose to estimate effects of subsequent doses if needed.

Narcotics and other CNS depressants have additive or potentiating effects. If prescribed, initial dosage of narcotic analgesic should be reduced to one-fourth or one-third of those usually employed.

Fentanyl can produce dependence of the morphine type and therefore has abuse potential. Classified as schedule II drug under federal Controlled Substances Act.

Protect drug from light.

FERROCHOLINATE
(CHEL-IRON, FERROLIP, KELEX)

Hematinic

ACTIONS AND USES

Chelated iron compound not as well absorbed as ferrous sulfate, but reported to produce fewer adverse effects. Contains 12% elemental iron. See Ferrous Sulfate for actions, uses, contraindications, precautions, and adverse reactions.

ROUTE AND DOSAGE

Oral: **Adults and children** *over 6 years:* 330 mg (equivalent to 40 mg elemental iron) 3 times daily. **Infants and children** *under 6 years:* 104 mg (equivalent to 12.5 mg elemental iron) daily in divided doses. Dosage depends on severity of anemia. Available as tablets, liquid, drops, and syrup.

NURSING IMPLICATIONS
See Ferrous Sulfate.

FERROUS FUMARATE, U.S.P., B.P.
(ELDOFE, FEOSTAT, FERRANOL, FUMASORB, FUMERIN, IRCON, LAUD-IRON, PALMIRON, SPAN-FF, TOLERON)

Hematinic

ACTIONS AND USES

Comparable to ferrous sulfate in actions, uses, contraindications, and adverse reactions. Contains 33% elemental iron.

ROUTE AND DOSAGE

Oral: **Adults and children** *over 6 years:* 200 mg (equivalent to 66 mg elemental iron) 1 to 4 times daily. **Infants and children** *under 6 years:* 100 to 300 mg daily in 3 to 4 divided doses. Dosage depends on severity of anemia.

NURSING IMPLICATIONS
See Ferrous Sulfate.

FERROUS GLUCONATE, N.F., B.P.
(ENTRON, FERGON, FERRALET)

Hematinic

ACTIONS AND USES
   Claimed to cause less gastric irritation and to be better tolerated than ferrous
   sulfate. Has same actions, uses, contraindications, and adverse reactions as
   ferrous sulfate. Contains 11.6% ferrous iron.
ROUTE AND DOSAGE
   Oral: 200 to 600 mg daily (equivalent to 24 to 72 mg elemental iron). **Children**
   6 to 12 years: 100 to 300 mg 3 times daily. **Infants and children** *under 6 years:* 100
   to 300 mg/day in divided doses. Dosage depends on severity of anemia. Available as tablets, capsules, timed-release capsules, elixir.

NURSING IMPLICATIONS
See Ferrous Sulfate.

FERROUS SULFATE, U.S.P., B.P.
(FERO-GRADUMET, MOL-IRON)
FERROUS SULFATE, DRIED, U.S.P., B.P.
(FEOSOL TABLETS, FER-IN-SOL)

Hematinic

ACTIONS AND USES
   Standard iron preparation against which other oral preparations are usually
   measured. Corrects erythropoietic abnormalities and may reverse gastric, esophageal, and other tissue changes caused by lack of iron. Ferrous sulfate contains 20% ferrous iron; ferrous sulfate dried contains 29.7% ferrous iron.
   Used to correct simple iron deficiency and to treat iron-deficiency (microcytic,
   hypochromic) anemias. Also may be used prophylactically during periods of
   increased iron needs, as in infancy, childhood, and pregnancy.
ABSORPTION AND FATE
   Absorbed into small intestinal mucosal cells, where small fraction is changed to
   ferric iron and incorporated into apoferritin and ferritin; lost into feces when
   mucosal cells are shed at end of 5-day life cycle. When iron presented to gut
   is in excess of need, mucosal cell uptake is minimal ("mucosal block"). Larger
   fraction enters bloodstream and binds to transferrin. Distributed to functional
   and storage sites in bone marrow, spleen, liver, hemoglobin, myoglobin, metal-
   loenzymes. Plasma iron concentration and total iron-binding capacity vary with
   disease states and physiologic conditions (higher in men than in women and
   higher in morning than in evening); regulated principally by hemoglobin synthesis. Major excretion route in feces via shedding of mucosal cells; also lost in
   epithelial cells of skin, nails, hair, sweat, urine, and breast milk.

Peptic ulcer, regional enteritis, ulcerative colitis, hemolytic anemias (in absence of iron deficiency), hemochromatosis, hemosiderosis, patients receiving repeated blood transfusions.

ADVERSE REACTIONS

Generally minimal: nausea, anorexia, constipation, diarrhea, epigastric pain, abdominal distress, headache, iron-overload hemosiderosis (rare). Massive overdosage: lethargy, drowsiness, nausea, vomiting, abdominal pain, diarrhea, local corrosion of stomach and small intestines, acidosis, shock, cardiovascular collapse, convulsions, liver necrosis, coma, death. Large chronic doses in infants: rickets (due to interference with phosphorous absorption).

ROUTE AND DOSAGE

Adults: Oral: 300 mg to 1.2 Gm (the equivalent of 60 to 240 mg elemental iron) daily. Therapeutic dosages depend on severity of iron deficiency. Preferably given in divided doses rather than in single large daily doses. **Children** *6 to 12 years:* 120 to 600 mg daily in divided doses. **Children** *under 6 years:* 300 mg daily in divided doses.

NURSING IMPLICATIONS

Therapeutic dosages are prescribed only if indicated by appropriate diagnostic procedures. If hemoglobin and hematocrit determinations suggest anemia, a complete blood count, reticulocyte count, and serum bilirubin determination are usually obtained; bone marrow examination may also be done.

In addition to iron replacement, an important therapeutic goal is to determine the reason for iron loss to remedy or alleviate causative factors.

A searching health history should be recorded to determine, among other things, dietary iron intake, adequacy of diet in general, and possible drug-induced causes of anemia, such as aspirin in high dosages, sulfonamides, quinidine, antimalarial drugs, and phenylbutazone.

Since iron is potentially corrosive, tablets or capsules should not be taken within 1 hour of bedtime, and adequate liquid should accompany ingestion of medication to assure passage into stomach.

If the patient experiences difficulty in swallowing tablet or capsule, consult physician about prescribing a liquid formulation or a less corrosive form, such as ferrous gluconate. (Sustained contact of iron with esophageal mucosa can cause ulceration.)

Oral iron preparations are best absorbed when taken between meals. However, to minimize gastric distress it may be necessary to administer the drug with or immediately after meals; or the physician may prescribe smaller doses or a change to enteric-coated or extended-release dosage form.

Sustained-release preparations are generally not preferred over ferrous sulfate tablets because they tend to transport iron beyond sites of optimal absorption. Also, they are more expensive.

In general, liquid preparations should be well diluted and administered through a straw. Instruct the patient to rinse mouth with clear water immediately after ingestion to prevent temporary staining of teeth.

Feosol elixir may be mixed with water, but it is not compatible with milk, fruit juice, or wine vehicles. However, the preparation Fer-In-Sol drops may be given in water or in fruit or vegetable juice according to manufacturer.

Inform patients that iron preparations cause dark green or black stools. Advise patients to report constipation or diarrhea. These symptoms may be relieved by adjustments in dosage or diet or by change to another iron preparation.

Simple iron deficiency may be asymptomatic, but it is usually associated with ill-defined symptoms such as anorexia, easy fatigability, headache, dizziness, tinnitus, and sensitivity to cold. As iron depletion becomes more severe, signs and symptoms may include dyspnea on exertion, palpitation, menstrual disturbances, decreased libido, waxy pallor, paresthesias, epithelial changes including brittleness of hair and nails and flattening or concavity of nails, and Plummer-Vinson syndrome (severe anemia): dysphagia, stomatitis, atrophic glossitis.

Therapeutic response may be experienced within 48 hours as a sense of well-being, increased vigor, improved appetite, and decreased irritability (in children). Reticulocyte response may begin in 4 days; it usually peaks in 7 to 10 days (reticulocytosis) and returns to normal after 2 or 3 weeks. Hemoglobin generally increases by 2 Gm/dl and hematocrit by 6% in 3 weeks.

Hemoglobin and reticulocyte values should be monitored during therapy. In the absence of satisfactory response after 3 weeks of drug treatment, possible reasons for failure warrant investigation: eg, noncompliance, inadequate dosage, occult blood loss, malabsorption, infection, presence of other anemias.

RDA for iron in children 4 to 6 years is 10 mg; for adult males: 10 mg; adult females: 18 mg; pregnancy: 18 mg; lactation: 18 mg.

The average American diet provides approximately 6 mg of iron per 1000 calories. Foods high in iron content (> 5 mg/100 Gm): organ meats (liver, heart, kidney), brewer's yeast, wheat germ, egg yolk, dried beans, dried fruits, oysters. Other good sources (1 to 5 mg/100 Gm): most muscle meats, fish, fowl, most cereals and green vegetables, dark molasses.

Facilitate development of a dietary teaching plan for patient and family.

In patients with uncomplicated iron deficiency, there is little therapeutic indication for concurrent administration of ascorbic acid, since these patients are able to absorb oral iron adequately. However, ascorbic acid may be prescribed in patients who have difficulty in absorbing adequate quantities of iron, such as infants and young children with severe anemia.

At present there is no convincing evidence that iron utilization is influenced by concomitant administration of copper, molybdenum, magnesium, calcium, or chlorophyll.

Iron therapy is generally continued for 2 to 3 months after the hemoglobin level has returned to normal (roughly twice the period required to normalize hemoglobin concentration). Replenishment of iron stores is a slow process, because iron absorption decreases as hemoglobin approaches normal levels.

Ingested overdoses of iron preparations in children may be fatal. Caution patients to store these drugs out of reach of children (at least one death per month is reported).

Treatment of overdosage: Vomiting should be induced quickly, and eggs and milk should be fed to form iron complexes until gastric lavage can be done (within first hour of ingestion). Lavage solution: 1% sodium bicarbonate; iron chelating agent (eg, deferoxamine mesylate) should be administered. Measures to combat shock, dehydration, blood loss, and respiratory failure may be necessary. (Gastric lavage should not be performed after the first hour because of danger of perforation due to gastric necrosis. Dimercaprol should not be used because it may form toxic complexes.)

Preserved in well-closed containers.

LABORATORY TEST INTERFERENCES: Large iron doses may cause false positive tests for occult blood with *o*-toluidine (Hematest, Occultest, Labstix) and guaiac reagent); benzidine test is reportedly not affected.

DRUG INTERACTIONS: Absorption of oral iron is inhibited by **antacids, cholestyramine,** and **pancreatic extracts** (space doses as far apart as possible). There may be delayed or impaired hematologic response to iron therapy with **chloramphenicol** or **vitamin E** (in children). Simultaneous administration of oral iron interferes with absorption of **oral tetracyclines** and vice versa; if concurrent administration is necessary, patient should receive tetracycline 3 hours after or 2 hours before iron administration. Concurrent administration of **ascorbic acid** ($>$ 200 mg orally) increases GI absorption of elemental iron. Studies in humans do not support earlier animal studies indicating that **allopurinol** and iron interact adversely.

FIBRINOGEN, U.S.P.
(PARENOGEN)
HUMAN FIBRINOGEN, B.P.

Systemic hemostatic

ACTIONS AND USES
A sterile fraction prepared from normal human plasma. Fibrinogen is an essential factor in blood coagulation.
Used alone or as adjunct in treatment of congenital or acquired afibrinogenemia or hypofibrinogenemia.
ADVERSE REACTIONS
Serum hepatitis, intravascular thrombosis, visceral infarction. When administered rapidly: cyanosis, tachycardia, pulmonary edema. Rarely: generalized paresthesias, hemoglobinemia, hemoglobinuria, hypersensitivity reactions, increased rouleaux formation, positive Coombs' test.
ROUTE AND DOSAGE
Intravenous: 2 to 8 Gm. Subsequent doses based on results of plasma fibrinogen levels.

> **NURSING IMPLICATIONS**
> The solution should be used within 1 hour after reconstitution.
> Monitor vital signs and observe patient closely for adverse reactions.
> Except in extreme emergencies, use is determined by studies of blood coagulation, plasma fibrinogen, and fibrinolytic activity.
> Repeated determinations of plasma fibrinogen level should be obtained during therapy. Normal plasma fibrinogen level is 200 to 600 mg/dl, depending on the individual laboratory and methods used.
> Even though fibrinogen is irradiated and donors are tested for Australian antigen, the risk of viral hepatitis is present.
> Gamma globulin [immune serum globulin (human)] is sometimes used to reduce the possibility of serum hepatitis. It is administered IM (usually 10 ml) within 1 week after fibrinogen has been given, followed by a second injection 1 month later.
> Fibrinogen in dry form should be stored at temperatures between 2 and 8 C. It is inactivated by heat.

FLAVOXATE HYDROCHLORIDE
(URISPAS)

Urinary antispasmodic

ACTIONS AND USES
 Exerts spasmolytic (papaverinelike) action on smooth muscle. Reported to pro-
 duce an increase in urinary bladder capacity in patients with spastic bladder,
 possibly by direct action on detrusor muscle.
 Used for symptomatic relief of dysuria, frequency, urgency, nocturia, inconti-
 nence, and suprapubic pain associated with various urologic disorders.
ABSORPTION AND FATE
 Following oral administration of a single 100-mg dose, 10% to 30% is excreted
 in urine within 6 hours.
CONTRAINDICATIONS AND PRECAUTIONS
 Pyloric or duodenal obstruction, obstructive intestinal lesions, ileus, achalasia,
 GI hemorrhage, obstructive uropathies of lower urinary tract, use in children
 younger than 12 years of age, use during pregnancy and in women of childbear-
 ing potential. Cautious use: suspected glaucoma.
ADVERSE REACTIONS
 Nausea, vomiting, dry mouth and throat, nervousness, vertigo, headache,
 drowsiness, blurred vision, increased ocular tension, disturbances of eye accom-
 modation, urticaria, dermatoses, mental confusion (especially in the elderly),
 dysuria, tachycardia, palpitation, hyperpyrexia, eosinophilia, leukopenia, abdominal pain, difficulty with concentration, constipation (with high doses).
ROUTE AND DOSAGE
 Oral: 100 to 200 mg 3 to 4 times a day.

> **NURSING IMPLICATIONS**
> Because of the possibility of drowsiness, mental confusion, and blurred
> vision, advise patients to avoid driving and performing tasks that are
> hazardous or that require mental alertness and physical coordination.
> Advise patient to report to physician the lack of a favorable response. Also
> instruct patient to report adverse reactions.

FLORANTYRONE
(ZANCHOL)

Hydrocholeretic

ACTIONS AND USES
 Synthetic preparation with pharmacologic actions and clinical uses similar to
 those of dehydrocholic acid. Stimulates production of bile by liver and increases
 flow of low-viscosity, low-sediment bile.
 Used to facilitate bile flow in chronic gallbladder dysfunction, postcholecystec-
 tomy syndrome, and biliary dyskinesia and to prevent T-tube encrustation and
 plugging.
CONTRAINDICATIONS AND PRECAUTIONS
 Complete or threatened biliary tract obstruction, common duct obstruction,
 acute cholecystitis, cholangitis, cholestatic jaundice, use as laxative for simple
 constipation or belching or to improve hepatic function. Safe use during pregnancy or lactation not established. Cautious use: nonobstructive biliary calculi.

Increased number of stools, diarrhea, nausea, vomiting, abnormal liver function tests, allergic reactions: eosinophilia, pruritus.

ROUTE AND DOSAGE

Oral: 250 mg 3 or 4 times daily.

NURSING IMPLICATIONS

Florantyrone is administered with meals and at bedtime.

FLOXURIDINE, N.F.
(FUDR)

Antineoplastic (antimetabolite)

ACTIONS AND USES

Antimetabolite and pyrimidine antagonist. Catabolized to 5-fluorouracil in vivo. Highly toxic, with low therapeutic index. For absorption, fate, contraindications, precautions, see Fluorouracil.

Used effectively as palliative agent in treatment of selected patients considered incurable by surgery or other means. See Fluorouracil.

ADVERSE REACTIONS

Dermatologic: dermatitis, excoriation, maceration, pruritic ulcerations, rash. **GI:** stomatitis, cramps, enteritis, gastritis, duodenal ulcer. **Other:** ataxia, blurred vision, nystagmus, vertigo, convulsions, depression, dysuria, fever, hemiplegia, hiccups, hypoadrenalism, lethargy, hepatopathology, renal insufficiency, edema. **Altered laboratory values:** elevations of BSP, prothrombin, total proteins, sedimentation rate, alkaline phosphatase, serum transaminase, serum bilirubin, and lactic dehydrogenase. Also see Fluorouracil.

ROUTE AND DOSAGE

Intraarterial infusion (continuous): 0.1 to 0.6 mg/kg/day. Given with use of appropriate pump to overcome large artery pressure and to assure uniform rate of infusion. Higher dosages (0.4 to 0.6 mg/kg) required for hepatic artery infusion because of hepatic degradation of drug.

NURSING IMPLICATIONS

Floxuridine has a shelf life of 3 years in the dry state. Drug is reconstituted with sterile water. Can be refrigerated (36 F to 46 F) for not more than 2 weeks.

Patient should be hospitalized at least during the initial course of therapy.

Examine infusion site frequently for signs of blocked, leaking, or displaced catheter and for infections.

Therapeutic response will likely be accompanied by some evidence of toxicity; supervise patient carefully and be sure he is informed about expected toxic effects, particularly those in the mouth.

Usually 1 to 6 weeks of continuous therapy are required for adequate clinical response.

Therapy should be discontinued promptly with onset of any of the following: stomatitis, leukopenia, intractable vomiting, diarrhea, thrombocytopenia, abnormal bleeding from any site.

See Fluorouracil.

(ANCOBON, 5-FC, 5-Fluorocytosine)

Antifungal

ACTIONS AND USES
Fluorinated pyrimidine structurally related to fluorouracil, but lacks its antineo-plastic activity. Precise actions poorly understood, but may act as antimetabolite in fungal cells.
Used in treatment of serious systemic infections caused by susceptible strains of *Cryptococcus* and *Candida.*

ABSORPTION AND FATE
Well absorbed from GI tract and widely distributed in body tissues and fluid, including aqueous humor and cerebrospinal fluid. Peak serum levels in 2.5 to 6 hours. Half-life 3 to 4 hours (may be as long as 200 hours in renal failure). Slightly bound to plasma proteins. Minimally metabolized. Approximately 90% of dose is excreted unchanged in urine.

CONTRAINDICATIONS AND PRECAUTIONS
Safe use in women of childbearing potential and during pregnancy and lactation not established. Extreme caution in impaired renal function, bone marrow de-pression, hematologic disorders, patients being treated with or having received radiation or bone marrow depressant drugs.

ADVERSE REACTIONS
Hypoplasia of bone marrow: anemia, leukopenia, thrombocytopenia, agranulocytosis (rare); nausea, vomiting, diarrhea, abdominal bloating, bowel perforation (rare); rash; elevated levels of serum alkaline phosphatase, SGOT, SGPT, BUN, and serum creatinine. Less frequently: confusion, hallucinations, headache, sedation, vertigo, hepatomegaly, eosinophilia.

ROUTE AND DOSAGE
Oral: **Adults and children** *weighing more than 50 kg:* 50 to 150 mg/kg body weight at 6-hour intervals (dosage modified in patients with renal dysfunction); *weighing less than 50 kg:* 1.5 to 4.5 Gm/m² of body surface.

NURSING IMPLICATIONS
Incidence and severity of nausea and vomiting may be decreased by giving capsules a few at a time over a 15-minute period.
Culture and sensitivity tests should be performed before initiation of therapy and at weekly intervals during therapy. Organism resistance has been reported.
Hematologic, renal, and hepatic function tests should be performed on all patients prior to and at frequent intervals during therapy.
Especially in patients with impaired renal function, frequent assays of blood drug level are recommended to determine adequacy of drug excretion (therapeutic range reported to be 25 to 120 μg/ml).
Monitor intake and output. Report change in intake–output ratio.
Duration of therapy is generally 4 to 6 weeks, but it may continue for several months.
Flucytosine is preserved in light-resistant containers.

(FLORINEF)

Adrenocortical steroid (salt-regulating)

ACTIONS AND USES
Long-acting synthetic steroid with potent mineralocorticoid and glucocorticoid activity. Plasma half-life about 30 minutes. Small doses produce marked sodium retention, increased urinary potassium excretion, and elevated blood pressure, perhaps due to effects on electrolytes. If protein intake is inadequate, fludrocortisone induces negative nitrogen balance. Absorption, fate, contraindications, and adverse reactions are same as for hydrocortisone (qv).
Used as partial replacement therapy for primary and secondary adrenocortical insufficiency in Addison's disease; used for treatment of salt-losing adrenogenital syndrome.

ROUTE AND DOSAGE
Oral (*Addison's disease*): 0.1 mg daily (dosage may range from 0.1 mg 3 times a week to 0.2 mg daily); (*salt-losing adrenogenital syndrome*): 0.1 to 0.2 mg/day.

NURSING IMPLICATIONS
Concomitant oral cortisone or hydrocortisone therapy may be advisable to provide substitute therapy approximating normal adrenal activity.
Periodic checking of serum electrolyte levels is usual during prolonged therapy. Supplemental calcium and potassium chloride, as well as restricted salt intake, may be necessary during long-term therapy.
Monitor weight and intake-output ratio to observe onset of fluid accumulation, especially if patient is on unrestricted salt intake and without potassium supplement.
Instruct patient to report signs of potassium deficit (anorexia, paresthesias, drowsiness, muscle weakness, nausea, polyuria, postural hypotension, mental depression).
Advise patient on therapy for Addison's disease to eat foods with high potassium content (see Index).
Monitor and record blood pressure daily. If transient hypertension develops as a consequence of therapy, report to physician. Usually the dose will be reduced to 0.05 mg daily.
Store in airtight containers. Protect from light.
See Hydrocortisone.

FLUMETHASONE
(FLUCORT)
FLUMETHASONE PIVALATE, N.F.
(LOCORTEN)

Adrenocortical steroid (glucocorticoid)

ACTIONS AND USES
Synthetic steroid with antiinflammatory, antipruritic, and vasoconstrictive activity. Local antiinflammatory effect reportedly is more than 800 times that of hydrocortisone (qv). Systemic effects are virtually absent.
Used to treat a variety of dermatoses, such as sunburn, anogenital pruritus, atopic dermatitis, contact dermatitis, eczema, psoriasis, seborrhea dermatosis, insect bites, diaper rash.

CONTRAINDICATIONS AND PRECAUTIONS

Ophthalmic use, vaccinia, varicella, hypersensitivity to any ingredient. Also see Hydrocortisone.

ADVERSE REACTIONS

Local: burning sensation, pruritus, irritation, dryness, hypertrichosis, acneiform eruptions, hypopigmentation. With occlusive dressings: macerated skin, atrophy of skin, secondary infection, striae, miliaria.

ROUTE AND DOSAGE

Topical: gently apply thin layer of cream (0.03%) to affected areas until it disappears, 3 to 4 times daily until lesions have cleared. Occlusive dressings may be used to manage psoriasis or stubborn skin conditions such as neurodermatitis, lichen planus, or lichen simplex conditions.

NURSING IMPLICATIONS

See Hydrocortisone for nursing implications related to topical applications.

FLUOCINOLONE ACETONIDE, U.S.P., N.F., B.P.
(FLUONID, SYNALAR, SYNEMOL)

Adrenocortical steroid (glucocorticoid)

ACTIONS AND USES

Synthetic fluorinated corticosteroid with glucocorticoid action and strong antiinflammatory, antipruritic, and vasocontrictive actions, but negligible mineralocorticoid effects. More effective than hydrocortisone (qv).

Used to relieve inflammatory manifestations of corticosteroid-responsive dermatoses.

CONTRAINDICATIONS AND PRECAUTIONS

Infants under 2 years of age; ophthalmic use. Also see Hydrocortisone.

ADVERSE REACTIONS

See Hydrocortisone.

ROUTE AND DOSAGE

Topical: applied in thin layer over affected area 2 to 4 times daily. Supplied as cream, ointment, and solution in 0.025% and 0.01% strengths; 0.2% cream should be used only for restricted periods, and quantity used per day should not exceed 2 Gm.

NURSING IMPLICATIONS

Protect drug from light.

See Hydrocortisone for nursing implications related to topical application.

FLUOCINONIDE, U.S.P.
(LIDEX, TOPSYN)

Adrenocortical steroid (glucocorticoid)

ACTIONS AND USES

Synthetic fluorinated glucocorticoid used only topically for antiinflammatory effects in glucocorticoid-responsive dermatoses. For absorption, fate, contraindications, and adverse reactions see Hydrocortisone.

ROUTE AND DOSAGE

Topical: apply thin layer of ointment, cream, gel (0.05%) to affected area 3 or 4 times daily as needed.

FLUOROMETHOLONE, N.F.
(FML LIQUIFILM, OXYLONE)

Adrenocortical steroid (glucocorticoid)

ACTIONS AND USES
Glucocorticoid with actions, contraindications, and adverse reactions similar to those of hydrocortisone (qv).
Used topically in management of glucocorticoid-responsive dermatoses and ocular inflammations.

ROUTE AND DOSAGE
Topical (skin): 0.025% cream 1 or 2 times daily; (eye): 1 or 2 drops 0.1% ophthalmic suspension every hour the first 1 or 2 days, then 2 to 4 times daily.

FLUOROURACIL, U.S.P.
(FU, 5-FU, 5-Fluorouracil, EFUDEX, FLUOROPLEX)

Antineoplastic (pyrimidine antagonist)

ACTIONS AND USES
Antimetabolite and pyrimidine antagonist. Blocks action of enzymes essential to normal DNA and RNA synthesis, and may become incorporated in RNA to form a fraudulant molecule; unbalanced growth and death of cell follow. Highly toxic, especially to proliferative cells in neoplasms, bone marrow, and intestinal mucosa. Low therapeutic index with high potential for producing severe hematologic toxicity. One member of the CMFOP combination chemotherapeutic regimen.
Used for palliative treatment of inoperable neoplasms of breast, colon, urinary bladder, ovary, cervix, liver, pancreas. Also used topically for solar or actinic keratoses.

ABSORPTION AND FATE
No absorption from topically applied preparation (Efudex) if skin is intact. Unpredictable absorption from GI tract; therefore given intravenously. Following rapid infusion, intact drug leaves plasma in 3 hours; metabolized in liver; 15% of unchanged drug is excreted in urine in 6 hours, 60% to 80% as respiratory carbon dioxide in 8 to 12 hours. Crosses blood–brain barrier. Metabolic fate of topically applied drug unknown.

CONTRAINDICATIONS AND PRECAUTIONS
Poor nutritional status, pregnancy, myelosuppression, major surgery within previous month, serious infections. Cautious use: history of high-dose pelvic irradiation, metastatic cell infiltration of bone marrow, previous use of alkylating agents, men and women in childbearing ages, hepatic and renal impairment.

ADVERSE REACTIONS
GI: anorexia, nausea, vomiting, stomatitis, pharyngitis, diarrhea, paralytic ileus, GI bleeding. **Hematologic:** leukopenia, thrombocytopenia, anemia (common). **Topical use:** pain, pruritus, hyperpigmentation, burning at site of application. **Other:** alopecia, nail changes (including loss), pruritic maculopapular rash (ex-

tremities), photosensitivity, erythema, increased pigmentation, skin atrophy, epistaxis, photophobia, euphoria, acute cerebellar syndrome (dysmetria, nystagmus, ataxia); cardiotoxicity (rare).

ROUTE AND DOSAGE

Highly individualized. Intravenous: initially 12 mg/kg body weight daily for 4 successive days, followed by 7.5 mg/kg on alternate days if no toxicity develops. Discontinue at end of 12th day. Maximum daily dose 800 mg. Maintenance dosage individualized. Topical (1% to 5% cream or solution): apply twice daily (usually for 2 to 4 weeks).

NURSING IMPLICATIONS

Avoid skin exposure and inhalation of drug particles.

Fluorouracil solution may become discolored during storage without adverse effect. Store in controlled room temperature (59 F to 86 F) in tight, light-resistant container. Do not freeze. If solution precipitates, resolubilize by heating to 140 F. Shake ampul vigorously; cool to body temperature before administration.

Dose is determined by actual weight unless patient is obese, in which case ideal weight is used. Weigh patient under standard conditions and record weight every 3 or 4 days. Report unexplained gradual increase in weight.

Maintenance of adequate nutrition is imperative. Work with dietitian and family to provide adaptations in dietary habits and patterns called for by the mild but troublesome symptoms that must be tolerated (eg, anorexia, nausea, sore mouth).

Dysphagia and retrosternal burning, symptoms of enteric injury at different levels, should be reported. Any discomfort that may interfere with food intake deserves special attention.

A dose sufficient to create mild toxicity (anorexia, vomiting) may be necessary to produce antineoplastic effects.

Establish a reference data base for body weight, intake–output ratio and pattern, food preferences and dietary habits, bowel habit, and condition of mouth.

Monitor blood reports as indicators for design of patient care. During leukopenic period (nadir usually 9 to 14 days after first dose), restrict visitors and personnel with colds or infections.

Protect patient from trauma, unnecessary injections, and use of rectal thermometer or invasive tubing.

During thrombocytopenic period (7th to 17th day), watch for and report signs of abnormal bleeding from any source; inspect skin for ecchymotic and petechial areas.

Antiemetics may be ordered to alleviate nausea and vomiting. Monitor patient carefully if vomiting is intractable, and report to physician.

Indications for drug discontinuation: severe stomatitis, leukopenia (WBC below 3500/mm^3 or rapidly decreasing count), intractable vomiting, diarrhea, thrombocytopenia (below 100,000/mm^3), hemorrhage from any site.

Inform the patient of the importance of prompt reporting of the first signs of toxicity: anorexia, vomiting, nausea, stomatitis, diarrhea, GI bleeding.

Hospitalization and strict supervision during the first course of therapy with 5-FU is necessary.

Poor-risk patients and occasionally patients in fairly good condition may die from the severe toxicity characteristic of this drug.

Remissions are often short, lasting no longer than 5 to 6 months; some patients have received 9 to 45 courses of treatment over periods of time ranging from 12 to 60 months.

The maculopapular rash usually responds to symptomatic treatment and is reversible.

Stomatitis, a reliable early sign of toxicity, often precedes leukopenic period by days. Inspect patient's mouth daily. Promptly report cracked lips, dryness and erythema of buccal membranes, white patches. To help patient eat with comfort, ask physician for anesthetic solution to be applied before meals. See Index for nursing care of stomatitis.

Prepare patient for alopecia, an expected (reversible) toxic effect. Discuss plans for cosmetic substitution if patient desires, although new growth usually begins within several months.

Use of topical preparations: Advise patient to avoid prolonged exposure to sunlight. Avoid application of cream or solution near eyes, nose, and mouth.

Consult physician about pretreatment preparation of lesion, ie, should previous applications be removed? How?

Use a nonmetallic applicator or gloved fingers to apply medication. If unprotected fingers are used, immediately wash hands thoroughly.

Even if absorption is minimal, systemic toxicity may follow use on large ulcerated area (medicinal taste, lacrimation, photosensitivity, telangiectasia, insomnia) (also see Adverse Reactions).

If occlusive dressing is used, there may be inflammatory reaction of adjacent normal skin.

A skin lesion treated with topical fluorouracil heals without scarring in 1 to 2 months after cessation of therapy. Expected response of lesion to topical 5 FU: erythema followed by scaling, tenderness, vesiculation, ulceration, necrosis, reepithelialization. Applications are continued until ulcerative stage is reached (2 to 6 weeks after initial application) and then discontinued.

Remissions are usually marked by nearly complete relief from pain.

FLUOXYMESTERONE, U.S.P., B.P.
(HALOTESTIN, ORA-TESTRYL, ULTANDREN)

Androgen

ACTIONS AND USES

Short-acting orally effective halogenated derivative of testosterone (qv) with up to five times the androgenic/anabolic activity of methyltestosterone. Has hypercholesterolemic effect; causes minimum retention of sodium; thus hypertension and edema rarely complicate therapy. Reduces nitrogen, potassium, and calcium excretion and promotes recalcification of osseous metastases and regression of soft-tissue lesions.

Used in both sexes to treat debilitating conditions (such as those associated with burns, paraplegia, prolonged corticosterone therapy, chronic malnutrition). In males, used as replacement therapy in conditions associated with testicular hormone deficiency. In females, used to antagonize effects of estrogen in androgen-responsive inoperable breast cancer. Sometimes combined with estrogen to treat postmenopausal osteoporosis and to reduce side effects of long-term therapy. See Testosterone for absorption and fate.

CONTRAINDICATIONS AND PRECAUTIONS

Severe cardiorenal disease or liver damage; nephrosis or nephrotic phase of nephritis; history of myocardial infarct; athletes; infants; women with advanced inoperable mammary cancer less than 1 year or more than 5 years post menopause; pregnancy; lactation. Also see Testosterone.

Jaundice (reversible), hepatocellular carcinoma, peliosis hepatitis, nausea, vomiting, diarrhea, symptoms resembling peptic ulcer, anaphylactic reactions (rare). Altered laboratory values: metyrapone test; fasting blood sugar and glucose tolerance tests; increased BSP; increase or decrease in serum cholesterol; increased SGOT, serum bilirubin, and alkaline phosphatase; increased clotting factors II, V, VII, and X; increased creatine and creatinine excretion lasting up to 2 weeks after therapy is discontinued. Also see Testosterone.

ROUTE AND DOSAGE

Oral (male hypogonadism and climacteric): 2 to 10 mg daily (highly individualized); (metastatic carcinoma of female breast): 15 to 30 mg daily in divided doses; (postpartum breast engorgement): 2.5 mg when active labor has started, then 5 to 10 mg daily in divided doses for 4 to 6 days.

NURSING IMPLICATIONS

Administer drug with food to diminish GI distress.

Instruct patient to report priapism (symptom of overdosage) promptly; temporary interruption of regimen is indicated.

Explain to female patient on drug for palliation of mammary cancer that virilization usually occurs at dosage used. Give emotional support. Urge early reporting of voice change (hoarseness or deepening), increased libido (associated with clitoral enlargement), hirsutism. Usually, stopping therapy will end further development of symptoms but will not reverse hirsutism or voice change.

When used for palliation of mammary cancer, subjective effects of therapy may not be experienced for about 1 month; objective symptoms may be delayed for as long as 3 months.

Anabolic response may be evidenced by euphoria and gain in weight and appetite, especially in emaciated and debilitated patient.

Also see Testosterone.

FLUPHENAZINE DECANOATE
(PROLIXIN DECANOATE)
FLUPHENAZINE ENANTHATE, U.S.P.
(PROLIXIN ENANTHATE)
FLUPHENAZINE HYDROCHLORIDE, U.S.P., B.P.
(PERMITIL, PROLIXIN)

Antipsychotic agent (major tranquilizer)

ACTIONS AND USES

Potent phenothiazine of piperazine subgroup. Similar to aliphatic (eg, chlorpromazine) and piperidine (eg, thioridazine) phenothiazines, with the following exceptions: more potent on weight basis, higher incidence of extrapyramidal complications, lower frequency of sedative and hypotensive effects, longer duration of action. The hydrochloride has more rapid action and shorter duration of action and thus may be used initially to determine the patient's response or to establish appropriate dosage. Esterification of fluphenazine (decanoate and enanthate) slows rate of drug release from tissues, thereby prolonging duration of action; these forms are indicated primarily for maintenance therapy in patients who cannot be relied on to take oral antipsychotic drugs daily. See Chlorpromazine.

Used for manifestations of psychotic disorders.

Onset of action following subcutaneous or IM injection of fluphenazine decanoate or enanthate occurs in 24 to 72 hours; peak antipsychotic effect in 48 to 96 hours; duration of effect 4 weeks or longer for decanoate, 1 to 3 weeks for enanthate. Following oral or IM administration of fluphenazine hydrochloride, onset of action occurs within 1 hour; duration of action is 6 to 8 hours. See Chlorpromazine Hydrochloride.

CONTRAINDICATIONS AND PRECAUTIONS

Known hypersensitivity to phenothiazines; subcortical brain damage, comatose or severely depressed states, blood dyscrasias, renal or hepatic disease, patients receiving large doses of narcotics or other CNS depressants. Safe use in children, in women of childbearing potential, and during pregnancy or lactation not established. Cautious use: elderly patients; patients who have reacted adversely to other phenothiazines; cardiovascular diseases; pheochromocytoma; history of convulsive disorders; patients exposed to extreme heat or phosphorous insecticides; peptic ulcer; respiratory impairment. Also see Chlorpromazine.

ADVERSE REACTIONS

Nausea, headache, increased intraocular pressure, fecal impaction, peripheral edema, hypotension, drowsiness, dizziness, epigastric pain, blurred vision, dry mouth, urinary retention, polyuria, sweating, augmentation of epilepsy; mental depression, extrapyramidal symptoms. Rarely: transient leukopenia, abnormal liver function tests, cholestatic jaundice. Also see Chlorpromazine.

ROUTE AND DOSAGE

Fluphenazine decanoate, fluphenazine enanthate: Subcutaneous, intramuscular: 25 mg every 2 weeks (dosage may range from 12.5 to 100 mg at intervals from 1 to 3 weeks). Weekly dosage should not exceed 100 mg. Doses should be increased cautiously in increments of 12.5 mg in patients already receiving 50 mg or more. *Fluphenazine hydrochloride:* Oral: initially 2.5 to 10 mg daily, usually in divided doses at 6- to 8-hour intervals. (Sustained-release tablets also available.) Oral doses exceeding 20 mg should be used with caution. Maintenance: 1 to 5 mg daily. Intramuscular only: 2.5 to 10 mg in divided doses at 6- to 8-hour intervals (IM doses exceeding 10 mg should be used with caution.) Dosages for all forms are highly individualized to attain smallest effective drug level.

NURSING IMPLICATIONS

Dry syringe and needle (at least 21 gauge) should be used when administering fluphenazine decanoate or enanthate (both are in a sesame-oil vehicle). Moisture may cause solution to become cloudy.

Note that parenteral fluphenazine hydrochloride is given by IM route only. Fluphenazine decanoate and enanthate may be given subcutaneously or by IM route (as prescribed).

Mental depression and extrapyramidal symptoms occur with high frequency, particularly with long-acting forms (decanoate and enanthate). Be alert for the appearance of these side effects. See Chlorpromazine.

Since fluphenazine decanoate and enanthate have a long duration of action, early detection of adverse effects is critically important. Patient should be informed about adverse reactions and urged to report symptoms promptly to physician.

Renal function should be monitored in patients on long-term therapy. The drug should be discontinued if BUN becomes abnormal. (Normal BUN: 8 to 18 mg/dl).

Monitor blood pressure during period of dosage adjustment. Fluctuations in blood pressure occur in some patients.

Patients on large doses who undergo surgery should be observed closely for hypotensive reactions. Patients with cerebrovascular or renal insufficiency and those with severe cardiac reserve deficiency are also prone to hypotensive effects of fluphenazine.

Caution patient against driving motor vehicles or other hazardous activities until his reaction to the drug has been determned.

Gel-type antacids or those containing aluminum or magnesium should not be administered simultaneously with oral fluphenazine (since they may decrease its absorption); if prescribed administer 1 hour before or 2 hours after fluphenazine.

Warn patients that alcohol, barbituates, or other CNS depressants may potentiate drug effects.

Fluphenazine hydrochloride solutions should be protected from light. Solutions may safely vary in color from almost colorless to light amber; discard dark or otherwise discolored solutions.

See Chlorpromazine Hydrochloride.

FLUPREDNISOLONE, N.F.
(ALPHADROL)
FLUPREDISOLONE VALERATE

Adenocortical steroid (glucocorticoid)

ACTIONS AND USES
Synthetic adrenal glucocorticoid. On a dosage basis, 5 mg fluprednisolone are equivalent to 20 mg hydrocortisone. Has low sodium-retaining activity, and potassium depletion rarely occurs; cannot be used alone for treatment of Addison's disease. Shares actions, uses, and contraindications of hydrocortisone (qv).

ADVERSE REACTIONS
Negative nitrogen balance, weight gain, CNS hyperactivity. Also see Hydrocortisone.

ROUTE AND DOSAGE
Oral: Dosage range is wide and must be individualized according to patient's condition. Suppressive dose given 3 to 7 days. Dosage reduced gradually in decrements of 0.75 to 1.5 mg at intervals of 2 to 4 days until maintenance dose is established. Rheumatoid arthritis: **Adults**: initially: 2.25 to 6 mg daily; maintenance 0.75 to 4.5 mg daily. **Pediatric**: 2.25 to 4.5 mg daily; maintenance 0.75 to 3 mg daily.

NURSING IMPLICATIONS
Administer drug at meal times or with large glass of water to reduce gastric distress

If satisfactory response is not obtained in 7 days, reevaluation of diagnosis is in order.

Thiazide or mercurial diuretics may be given conjointly with fluprednisolone to induce diuresis in patient with resistant edema.

See Hydrocortisone.

Hypnotic

ACTIONS AND USES
Benzodiazepine derivative with hypnotic activity equal to or greater than that produced by barbiturates or chloral hydrate. Mode and site of action not known, but appears to act at limbic and subcortical levels of CNS to produce sedation, skeletal muscle relaxation, and anticonvulsant effects. Produces slight if any suppression of REM (dream sleep) time, but marked reduction of stage 4 sleep (deepest sleep stage). Significance of sleep alterations not understood. Appears to have little effect on respiratory or vasomotor centers.

Used as hypnotic in management of simple insomnia. Has been used investigationally as induction agent prior to general anesthesia.

ABSORPTION AND FATE
Rapidly absorbed from GI tract. Induces sleep within 15 to 30 minutes that lasts 7 to 8 hours. Widely distributed throughout body tissues. Rapidly metabolized, probably by liver. Excreted in urine as active and inactive metabolites. Small amount eliminated in feces.

CONTRAINDICATIONS AND PRECAUTIONS
Known hypersensitivity to flurazepam; prolonged administration; intermittent porphyria. Safe use in women of childbearing potential, in children under 15 years of age, and during pregnancy not established. Cautious use: impaired renal or hepatic function, mental depression, history of suicidal tendencies, addiction-prone individuals, elderly or debilitated patients.

ADVERSE REACTIONS
Residual sedation, drowsiness, lightheadedness, dizziness, staggering gait, ataxia; heartburn, nausea, vomiting, diarrhea, constipation, abdominal pain; headache, nervousness, apprehension, talkativeness, irritability; palpitation, chest pain; muscle and joint pain; genitourinary complaints. **Overdosage** or **intolerance**: severe sedation, disorientation, lethargy, coma. Rarely: leukopenia, granulocytopenia, sweating, flushing, blurred vision, burning eyes, shortness of breath, dry mouth, excessive salivation, bitter taste, swollen tongue, faintness, hypotension, allergic reactions (rash, pruritus); nightmares, euphoria, depression, hallucinations, confusion; paradoxic reactions (rarely): excitement, hyperactivity. Altered laboratory values: elevated SGOT and SGPT, elevated levels of total and direct bilirubins, elevated level of alkaline phosphatase.

ROUTE AND DOSAGE
Oral: 15 to 30 mg before retiring. Therapy is initiated with 15 mg for the elderly.

NURSING IMPLICATIONS
Effect may increase with repeated doses and continue 1 to 2 days after drug is stopped.

Excessive drowsiness, ataxia, vertigo, and falling occur more frequently in elderly or debilitated patients. Supervise ambulation. Bedsides may be advisable.

Warn patients that the drug may impair ability to perform hazardous activities such as driving a motor vehicle or operating machinery.

Advise patient to avoid alcohol. Concurrent ingestion with flurazepam causes an intensification of CNS depressant effects. Reportedly, symptoms may occur even when alcohol is ingested 10 hours after last flurazepam dose.

Caution patients about the possibility of additive depressant effects if combined with barbiturates, tranquilizers, or other CNS depressants.

With repeated use, blood counts and liver and kidney function tests are advised.

Prolonged use of large doses can result in psychic and physical dependence.

Subject to control under federal Controlled Substances Act. Classified as schedule IV drug.

Preserved in tight, light-resistant containers, protected from heat.

See Chlordiazepoxide.

FOLIC ACID, U.S.P., B.P.
(FOLVITE, Pteroylglutamic Acid)
FOLATE SODIUM
(FOLVITE SODIUM)

Vitamin (hematopoietic)

ACTIONS AND USES

Member of vitamin B complex group essential for nucleoprotein synthesis and maintenance of normal erythropoiesis. Folic acid is not metabolically active, but is reduced in body to the coenzyme tetrahydrofolic acid, which is involved in the 1-carbon transfer reactions in purine and thymidylate biosynthesis. In folic acid deficiency, impaired thymidylate synthesis results in the production of defective DNA that leads to megaloblast formation and arrest of bone marrow maturation.

Used in treatment of folate deficiency megaloblastic anemias associated with malabsorption syndromes, alcoholism, primary liver disease, inadequate dietary intake, certain drugs, pregnancy, infancy, and childhood.

ABSORPTION AND FATE

Readily absorbed from small intestine (primarily proximal portion). Peak folate activity in 30 to 60 minutes, following oral administration. Largely reduced and methylated in liver to metabolically active folate forms. Distributed to all body tissues, with high concentration in cerebrospinal fluid. Extensively bound to plasma proteins. Traces of unchanged drug excreted in urine with usual therapeutic doses, but large amounts eliminated following high doses. Excreted in breast milk.

CONTRAINDICATIONS AND PRECAUTIONS

Use of folic acid alone for treatment of pernicious anemia or other vitamin B_{12} deficiency states.

ADVERSE REACTIONS

Reportedly nontoxic. Rarely: allergic sensitization (rash, pruritus, general malaise, bronchospasm). Slight flushing and feeling of warmth following IV administration.

ROUTE AND DOSAGE

Oral, subcutaneous (deep), intramuscular, intravenous: therapeutic, 0.25 to 1 mg daily; maintenance, 0.1 to 0.4 mg daily; for pregnant and lactating women, 0.8 mg daily.

NURSING IMPLICATIONS

A careful dietary and drug history should be obtained. Drugs reported to cause folate deficiency include oral contraceptives, phenytoin, primidone, and barbiturates. Folate deficiency may also result from renal dialysis.

Folic acid may obscure diagnosis of pernicious anemia by alleviating hematologic manifestations of vitamin B_{12} deficiency while allowing irreparable neurologic damage to remain progressive.

Treatment of anemia with OTC vitamin preparations containing folic acid subject the patient with iron-deficiency anemia to needless expense and may delay early detection of pernicious anemia.

Normal serum folate levels have been reported to range from 0.005 to 0.025 μg/dl.

Folates are present in a wide variety of foods; high sources in folates include yeast, liver, fresh green vegetables, and fruits. Approximately 50% to 90% of folate content is destroyed by long cooking or by canning.

The recommended daily allowances of folic acid are as follows: infants 50 μg; children 100 to 300 μg; adults 400 μg; during pregnancy 800 μg; during lactation 600μg.

Therapeutic effects of folic acid therapy include a sense of well-being during first 24 hours of treatment, improvement in blood picture (reticulocytosis within 2 to 5 days, reversion to normoblastic hematopoiesis and eventually normal hemoglobin), gradual reversal of symptoms of folic acid deficiency (glossitis, diarrhea, weight loss, irritability, fatigue, insomnia, forgetfulness, pallor). Keep physician informed of patient's response.

Emphasize the need to remain under close medical supervision while receiving folic acid therapy. Adjustment of maintenance dose should be made if there is threat of relapse.

Folic acid injection should be protected from light.

LABORATORY TEST INTERFERENCES: Falsely low serum erythrocyte folate levels may occur with *L. cassei* assay method in patients receiving antibiotics such as tetracyclines.

DRUG INTERACTIONS: **Chloramphenicol** may antagonize response to folate therapy. Daily administration of 5 mg or more of folic acid may increase metabolism of **phenobarbitol** and also **phenytoin** and other **hydantoin** derivatives with resultant increased seizure frequency.

FURAZOLIDONE, N.F.
(FUROXONE)

Antiinfective, antiprotozoal

ACTIONS AND USES

Synthetic nitrofuran with antibacterial and antiprotozoal properties. Acts by interfering with several bacterial enzyme systems. Bactericidal against majority of GI pathogens, including species of *Aerobacter, Escherichia coli, Giardia lamblia, Proteus, Salmonella, Shigella, Staphylococcus,* and *Vibrio cholerae.* Also has MAO inhibitor action that is cumulative and dose-related (occurring after 4 or 5 days of therapy) and is thought to be due to a metabolite.

Used in treatment of bacterial or protozoal diarrhea and enteritis caused by susceptible organisms. Available in combination with nifuroxime (Tricofuron) for treatment of *Trichomonas vaginalis, Candida albicans,* and *Haemophilus vaginalis.*

ABSORPTION AND FATE

Poorly absorbed from GI tract. Catabolic end products excreted in urine.

CONTRAINDICATIONS AND PRECAUTIONS

Sensitivity to furazolidone, concurrent use of alcohol, other MAO inhibitors, tyramine-containing foods, indirect-acting sympathomimetic amines, infants under 1 month of age. Safe use in women of childbearing age and during pregnancy or lactation not established. Cautious use, if at all, in patients with glucose-6-phosphate dehydrogenase deficiency (G-6-PD).

Anorexia, nausea, vomiting, headache, malaise, hypoglycemia, hypersensitivity reactions (fever, arthralgia, hypotension, urticaria, vesicular or morbilliform rash), intravascular hemolysis in patients with G-6-PD deficiency (reversible), agranulocytosis (rare).

ROUTE AND DOSAGE

Oral: **Adults**: 400 mg daily in 4 equally divided doses up to maximum of 8.8 mg/kg/24 hours. **Pediatric** *over 1 month of age*: 5 mg/kg/day, in 4 equal doses.

NURSING IMPLICATIONS

Bed rest and fluid and electrolyte replacement (as indicated) are important adjuncts to drug therapy. Consult physician regarding dietary allowances.

Advise patient and family member to record number of stools passed, fluid intake, and daily weight (useful criteria for determining fluid loss).

Examine patient and keep physician informed of signs of dehydration and electrolyte imbalance: decreased skin turgor, sunken eyes; dry, furrowed tongue, low blood pressure, diminished or irregular pulse, muscle or abdominal cramps.

Caution patient not to exceed prescribed dosage and to contact physician if diarrhea persists or worsens or if adverse reactions develop. If satisfactory clinical response does not occur within 7 days, drug should be discontinued.

Faintness, weakness, and lightheadedness may be symptoms of hypersensitivity reaction or hypoglycemia and should be reported.

Foods high in tyramine may produce hypertensive reaction. Provide patient with list of high-tyramine foods (see Index). Hypertensive crisis is most likely to occur when drug is continued beyond 5 days or when large doses are given.

Warn patients not to drink alcohol during furazolidone therapy and for at least 4 days after drug is stopped. Ingestion of alcohol may cause disulfiramlike reaction: nausea, sweating, fever, flushing, pounding headache, palpitation, tachycardia, drop in blood pressure, dyspnea, sense of chest constriction; symptoms may last up to 24 hours. If treatment of hypotension is required, levarterenol or other direct-acting pressor agent is used; indirect-acting agents, eg, ephedrine, are contraindicated.

Drug history prior to therapy is advisable. Advise patient not to take over-the-counter medications unless approved by physician. Nasal sprays, cold and hay-fever remedies, and other medications containing indirect-acting amines expose patient to hazards of hypertensive reaction.

Patients with G-6-PD deficiency (eg, patients of Mediterranean or Near East origin and blacks) should be closely followed by blood and urine studies for intravascular hemolysis: hematuria (pink or red urine), hemoglobinuria, hemoglobinemia.

Inform patients that drug may impart a harmless brown color to urine.

Possible cause of diarrhea should be investigated, eg, contaminated foods or water, carriers, general sanitation. Fecal cultures of family members should be considered.

Preserved in tight, light-resistant containers.

LABORATORY TEST INTERFERENCES: Furazolidone metabolite reportedly may cause false positive reaction for urine glucose with Benedict's reagent.

DRUG INTERACTIONS: A disulfiram (Antabuse) type of reaction may occur with **alcohol.** Concomitant use of **antihistamines,** other **MAO inhibitors, narcotics, sedatives, indirect-acting sympathomimetic amines** (eg, **ephedrine,** phenylephrine), and **tyramine** predispose to hypertensive reactions. Concomitant use with **tricyclic antidepressants** may cause toxic psychosis.

FUROSEMIDE, U.S.P.
(LASIX)
FRUSEMIDE, B.P.

Diuretic

ACTIONS AND USES
Rapid-acting potent sulfonamide "loop" diuretic with pharmacologic effects and uses almost identical to those of ethacrynic acid (qv). Exact mode of action not clearly defined. As with ethacrynic acid, urinary pH falls after administration, but in some patients bicarbonate excretion may temporarily increase the pH. Renal vascular resistance decreases and renal blood flow may increase during drug administration. Enhances excretion of sodium, chloride, potassium, hydrogen, calcium, magnesium, ammonium, bicarbonate, and possibly phosphate. Reportedly may be less ototoxic than ethacrynic acid.
Used in treatment of edema associated with congestive heart failure, cirrhosis of liver, and renal disease, including nephrotic syndrome. May be used for treatment of hypertension, alone or in combination with other antihypertensive agents.

ABSORPTION AND FATE
Following oral administration, diuretic effect begins in 30 to 60 minutes, peaks in 1 to 2 hours, and persists 6 to 8 hours. Following IV injection, diuretic effect starts within 5 minutes (somewhat later after IM) and peaks in 20 to 60 minutes, with duration of 2 hours. Approximately 95% bound to plasma proteins. Small amount metabolized by liver. Rapidly excreted in urine, primarily as unchanged drug; approximately 50% of oral dose and 80% of IV dose are excreted within 24 hours. Small amounts excreted in feces. Crosses placenta.

CONTRAINDICATIONS AND PRECAUTIONS
History of sensitivity to furosemide or sulfonamides. Oliguria, anuria, fluid and electrolyte depletion states, hepatic coma; women of childbearing potential; pregnancy. Cautious use: elderly patients, hepatic cirrhosis, nephrotic syndrome, cardiogenic shock associated with acute myocardial infarction, history of gout, patients receiving digitalis glycosides or potassium-depleting steroids.

ADVERSE REACTIONS
Fluid and electrolyte imbalance: hypovolemia, dehydration, hyponatremia, hypokalemia, hypochloremia, metabolic alkalosis, hypomagnesemia, hyperuricemia (especially after large IV doses), hypercalciuria. **Cardiovascular**: postural hypotension with excessive diuresis, acute hypotensive episodes, circulatory collapse, thromboembolic episodes. **GI**: nausea, vomiting, diarrhea, mild to moderate abdominal and cramping pain (reported in children after IV administration). **Hematologic**: anemia, leukopenia, aplastic anemia, thrombocytopenic purpura, agranulocytosis (rare). **Dermatologic**: pruritus, urticaria, exfoliative dermatitis, erythema multiforme (rare). **Ototoxicity**: tinnitus, reversible or permanent hearing loss. **Genitourinary**: flank and loin pain, allergic interstitial nephritis, irreversible renal failure, bladder pressure or spasm, urinary frequency. **Other**: hyperglycemia, glycosuria; tetany (rare); increase in blood ammonia, elevated BUN, acute gout (rare); increased perspiration; paresthesias; photosensitivity, blurred vision. Also reported, but causal relationship not firmly established: sweet taste, oral and gastric burning, paradoxic swelling, headache, jaundice, acute pancreatitis with elevated serum amylase and lipase.

ROUTE AND DOSAGE
Adults: Oral (for diuresis): 20 to 80 mg, preferably in the morning, followed by second dose 6 to 8 hours later, if necessary; diuretic doses may be carefully

titrated up to 600 mg daily for severe edematous states; (for hypertension): 40 mg twice daily. Intramuscular, intravenous: (*for diuresis*): 20 to 40 mg (highly individualized). **Pediatric**: Oral: 2 mg/kg body weight as single dose; if necessary, may be increased by 1 or 2 mg/kg not sooner than 6 to 8 hours after previous dose; maintenance dosage adjusted to minimum effective level. Intramuscular, intravenous: initially 1 mg/kg body weight; if necessary, dosage may be increased by 1 mg/kg not sooner than 2 hours after previous dose; pediatric doses by any route greater than 6 mg/kg not recommended.

NURSING IMPLICATIONS

Hospitalization is recommended when therapy is initiated in patients with hepatic cirrhosis and ascites.

Frequent determinations should be made of blood count, serum electrolytes, CO_2, BUN, blood sugar, and uric acid during first few months of therapy and periodically thereafter.

Schedule doses to avoid nocturia and sleep disturbance (eg, a single dose is generally administered in the morning; twice-a-day doses may be prescribed for 8 A.M. and 2 P.M.).

Intermittent dosage schedule is frequently used to allow time for natural correction of electrolyte and acid–base imbalance; eg, drug may be given for 2 to 4 consecutive days each week.

Patients receiving the drug parenterally should be observed, and vital signs should be monitored. Sudden death from cardiac arrest has been reported. Parenteral administration should be replaced by oral administration when practical.

Infusion rate will be prescribed by physician and should be checked frequently (generally the rate should not exceed 4 mg/minute).

Close observation of the patient is essential during a period of diuresis. Sudden alteration in fluid and electrolyte balance may precipitate adverse reactions: weakness, fatigue, lightheadedness, dizziness, vomiting, perspiration, muscle cramps, bladder spasm, and urinary frequency. Report onset of these symptoms to physician.

Monitor intake–output ratio. Report decrease in output, excessive diuresis, or diarrhea.

Weigh patient daily under standard conditions. Rapid and excessive weight loss (from vigorous diuresis) can induce dehydration and acute hypotensive episodes.

Monitor blood pressure during periods of diuresis and through period of dosage adjustment.

Excessive dehydration is most likely to occur in the elderly, in those with chronic cardiac disease on prolonged salt restriction, or in those receiving sympatholytic agents. Resultant hypovolemia may lead to vascular thrombi and emboli (from hemoconcentration) or circulatory collapse.

Consult physician regarding allowable salt and fluid intake. To prevent hyponatruria and hypochloremia, salt intake is generally liberalized in most patients. However, patients with cirrhosis usually require at least moderate salt restriction.

Patients receiving antihypertensive drugs concurrently are subject to episodes of postural hypotension (dosage of other agents is generally reduced by at least 50% when furosemide is added to regimen). Caution patients to make position changes slowly, particularly from recumbent to upright position.

To reduce or prevent potassium depletion, the physician may prescribe daily ingestion of potassium-rich foods (eg, bananas, oranges, peaches, dried dates), potassium supplement, and intermittent administration of furosemide.

Be alert to signs of hearing loss, complaints of fullness in ears, or complaints of tinnitus. Hearing impairment is usually associated with renal insufficiency, uremia, rapid IV injection of large doses, or concomitant administration of other ototoxic drugs.

Furosemide may cause hyperglycemia. Diabetic and diabetic-prone individuals and patients with decompensated hepatic cirrhosis require careful monitoring of urine and blood glucose.

Acute gout can occur in susceptible patients. Advise the patient to report onset of joint redness, swelling, or pain.

Warning signs and symptoms of fluid and electrolyte imbalance are the following: anorexia, nausea, vomiting, thirst, dry mouth, weakness, fatigue, confusion, dizziness, leg cramps (see Index for symptoms of specific electrolyte depletion state).

Oral furosemide should be discontinued 1 week and parenteral furosemide 2 days before elective surgery.

Tablets and parenteral solutions are stored at room temperature protected from light and excessive heat. Slight discoloration of tablets reportedly does not alter potency; however, injection solutions having a yellow color should be discarded.

Store oral solution in refrigerator (avoid freezing).

DRUG INTERACTIONS: Furosemide potentiates ototoxicity of **aminoglycoside antibiotics** (and other drugs associated with ototoxicity); antagonizes hypoglycemic effect of **antidiabetic agents**; may potentiate hypotensive effect of **antihypertensive agents**; enhances nephrotoxicity of **cephalosporins**; may increase vasomotor instability with **chloral hydrate**; enhances K loss in patients receiving **corticosteroids**; increases possibility of toxicity of **digitalis glycosides** (by causing K, Ca, and Mg depletion); enhances the action of other **diuretic agents**; increases possibility of **lithium toxicity** (by promoting excretion of K and Na); may decrease arterial responsiveness to **pressor amines**; increases possibility of salicylate toxicity in patients receiving high doses of **salicylates**, may potentiate neuromuscular blocking effect of **skeletal muscle relaxants** such as **tubocurarine** (by causing hypokalemia); and may antagonize the action of **uricosuric agents** by causing hyperuricemia.

GALLAMINE TRIETHIODIDE, U.S.P., B.P.
(FLAXEDIL)

Skeletal muscle relaxant

ACTIONS AND USES
Synthetic, nondepolarizing neuromuscular blocking agent (curare substitute). Similar to tubocurarine (qv) in actions, uses, contraindications, precautions, and adverse reactions. About 20% as potent as tubocurarine; reported to produce less ganglionic blockade and to have no histamine-releasing properties except in very high doses. Has parasympatholytic effect on cardiac vagus, and may cause tachycardia and occasionally hypertension.

ABSORPTION AND FATE
Muscle relaxation peaks within 3 minutes, with duration of 15 to 20 minutes. Significantly bound to serum albumin. Excreted primarily unchanged in urine. Crosses placenta.

CONTRAINDICATIONS AND PRECAUTIONS
Hypersensitivity to gallamine or iodides; myasthenia gravis; impaired pulmonary or renal function; shock; patients weighing less than 5 kg, hyperthyroidism, hypertension, tachycardia, cardiac insufficiency, hypoalbuminemia. Also see Tubocurarine.

ROUTE AND DOSAGE
Intravenous: 1 mg/kg body weight. Single dose not to exceed 100 mg. Highly individualized.

NURSING IMPLICATIONS
Tachycardia occurs almost immediately after administration, reaches maximum within 3 minutes, and declines gradually to premedication level.
Patients with electrolyte imbalance, dehydration, or elevated temperature may be more sensitive to the effects of gallamine.
May be stored at room temperature, protected from light and excessive heat.
See Tubocurarine Chloride.

GAMMA BENZENE HEXACHLORIDE, U.S.P., B.P.
(GAMENE, KWELL)

Pediculicide, scabicide

ACTIONS AND USES
Used for eradication of itch mite of scabies *(Sarcoptes scabiei)* and for infestations of head lice *(Pediculus capitis)* and crab lice *(Phthirus pubis)* and their nits.

CONTRAINDICATIONS AND PRECAUTIONS
Hypersensitivity to any component of the drug; application to eyes, face, acutely inflamed skin areas; prolonged or repeated applications (can be absorbed through skin, especially in the young).

ADVERSE REACTIONS
Skin irritation, erythema, sensitization (eczematous eruptions). Highly toxic if absorbed through skin or ingested: vomiting; diarrhea; irritation of eyes, skin, and mucosa; paresthesias; CNS stimulation (tremors, convulsions); aplastic anemia; ventricular fibrillation; liver and kidney damage.

Topical: 1% cream, lotion, or shampoo.

NURSING IMPLICATIONS

Scabies: Take soapy bath or shower, rinse well, and dry thoroughly. Apply thin film of cream or lotion over entire body surface from neck down (avoid urethral meatus). Pay particular attention to intertriginous areas (finger webs and other body creases and folds), wrists, elbows, and belt line. After 24 hours, remove medication thoroughly by shower or tub bath. Put on clean clothing; change bed linen. A second application is usually not needed; but if necessary, treatment may be repeated after 1 week. Pediculosis: After a bath or shower, apply to hairy infested areas and adjacent areas. Leave on for 12 to 24 hours. Wash thoroughly and put on clean clothing; change bed linen. A second application is seldom needed; but if necessary, treatment may be repeated in 4 days.

Head and crab lice: Pour about 1 ounce (2 tablespoonsful) of shampoo onto affected area; rub vigorously, being sure to wet all hairy areas with shampoo. Add small amount of warm water and work into thick lather for at least 4 minutes. For head lice, pay particular attention to areas above and behind ears and back of head. Rinse completely; dry thoroughly with towel. Use fine-tooth comb to remove remaining nit shells. If necessary, treatment may be repeated in 24 hours, but not more than twice in 1 week. Inform patient that shampoo formulation is intended only for treatment of head and crab lice; it should not be used as a routine shampoo. Combs, brushes, and other washable items may be cleaned with the shampoo.

Advise patient to use medication only as directed by physician. Stress the importance of avoiding overdosage.

Shaving of hair is not necessary.

Instruct patients to discontinue medication and report to a physician if signs of irritation or sensitization occur.

Caution patients not to apply medication to face and to avoid contact with eyes. If accidental eye contact occurs, flush thoroughly with water.

Contaminated bed linen and clothing should be carefully washed (boiled if possible) or dry cleaned (if not washable) to prevent reinfestation. Particular attention should be paid to the seams of clothing. For dry cleaning, place clothing in a plastic bag, seal it carefully, and inform dry cleaner of contents.

Microscopic confirmation of scabies mites is recommended before treatment, if diagnosis is in doubt. Burrows occur in 15% to 18% of patients and can be seen by oblique light or hand lens.

Pruritic nodules sometimes develop after scabies infestation and may last for weeks, months, or years. Further scabicide treatment is not indicated; however, advise the patient to report to a physician. Intralesional steroids or surgical excision are sometimes required.

Patients with crab lice should be examined for venereal disease. In addition to close body contact, crab lice may also be transmitted by toilet seats, bedclothes, or clothing of infested persons.

Gamma benzene hexachloride is a highly toxic drug if taken internally. Caution patients to keep it out of reach of children. Accidental ingestion is treated by gastric lavage and saline cathartics. Oily liquids and epinephrine are contraindicated.

First infestations of scabies may exist 2 to 6 weeks before the patient becomes symptomatic. During this phase, scabies is highly contagious.

Scabies may be spread by contact with infested persons, clothing, and other fomites. A careful history should be taken to identify the source of infestation.

Case-finding efforts should include family members and other close-contact persons. Suspect scabies if a person complains of nocturnal itching (classic symptom).

Scabies is commonly called the 7-year itch, probably because reinfestations are common unless precautions are taken. Recurring, limited infestations of scabies may indicate a domestic animal source, especially dogs, cats, cattle, or poultry.

GENTAMICIN SULFATE, U.S.P., B.P. (GARAMYCIN)

Antibacterial

ACTIONS AND USES

Broad-spectrum aminoglycoside antibiotic derived from *Micromonospora purpurea,* an actinomyces. By acting directly on bacterial ribosome, inhibits protein bio-synthesis. Active against a wide variety of Gram-negative bacteria, including *Pseudomonas aeruginosa, Proteus* species (including indole-positive and -negative strains), *Escherichia coli,* and *Klebsiella, Enterobacter,* and *Serratia* species. Also effective against certain Gram-negative organisms, particularly penicillin-sensitive and some methicillin-resistant strains of *Staphylococcus aureus.* Cross-resistance and allergenicity with other members of aminoglycoside group thought to be possible. Has neuromuscular blocking action, in common with other amino-glycoside antibiotics.

Parenteral use restricted to treatment of serious infections of GI tract, respiratory tract, urinary tract, CNS, bone, skin, and soft tissue (including burns), when other less toxic antimicrobial agents are ineffective or are contraindicated. May be used in combination with other antibiotics. Also used topically for primary and secondary skin infections and for infections of external eye and its adnexa.

ABSORPTION AND FATE

Rapidly absorbed following IM injection. Peak serum concentrations in 30 to 90 minutes; effective serum levels persist 6 to 8 hours. Administration of IV infusion over 2-hour period produces similar concentrations. Serum levels higher and more prolonged in patients with impaired renal function. Widely distributed to extracellular fluids. Approximately 25% loosely bound to plasma proteins. Serum half-life about 1 to 2 hours. Excreted primarily in urine, largely as unchanged drug (excretion correlates with creatinine clearance). Slight absorption may occur following topical applications, especially with cream formulations. Crosses placenta.

CONTRAINDICATIONS AND PRECAUTIONS

Known hypersensitivity to gentamicin, concomitant use of other neurotoxic (ototoxic) and/or nephrotoxic drugs. Safe use during pregnancy not established. Cautious use: impaired renal function; topical applications to widespread areas; elderly, infants, and children.

ADVERSE REACTIONS

Neurotoxicity: ototoxicity (vestibular disturbances, impaired hearing), optic neuritis, peripheral neuritis, numbness, tingling of skin, muscle twitching, convulsions. **Nephrotoxicity:** rising levels of BUN, nonprotein nitrogen, serum creatinine; oliguria, renal damage. **Allergic reactions:** rash, pruritus, urticaria, eosinophilia, burning sensation of skin, fever, joint pains, laryngeal edema. **Hematologic:** granulocytopenia, agranulocytosis, thrombocytopenic purpura, anemia. **Other:** increased SGOT, SGPT, and serum bilirubin; decreased serum calcium; increased or decreased reticulocyte counts; transient hepatomegaly, splenomegaly; superinfections; anorexia, nausea, vomiting, weight loss, increased salivation; headache, drug fever, lethargy; loss of hair and eyebrows;

pulmonary fibrosis, hypotension or hypertension; local irritation and pain following IM use; neuromuscular blockade and respiratory paralysis (with high doses). Following topical use: photosensitivity, erythema, pruritus; burning, stinging, lacrimation with ophthalmic use.

ROUTE AND DOSAGE

Intramuscular, intravenous: **Adults:** 3 to 5 mg/kg/day in 3 equal doses every 8 hours. **Children:** 6 to 7.5 mg/kg/day in 3 equal doses every 8 hours. **Infants and neonates:** 7.5 mg/kg/day in 3 equal doses every 8 hours. **Premature or full-term neonates** *1 week of age or less:* 5 mg/kg/day in 2 equal doses every 12 hours. Dosages must be adjusted for patients with impaired renal function. Topical: 0.1% cream or ointment, applied gently to lesions 3 or 4 times daily. Ophthalmic solution (0.3%): 1 or 2 drops in affected eye every 4 hours. Ophthalmic ointment (0.3%): applied in small amount 2 or 3 times daily.

NURSING IMPLICATIONS

Culture and sensitivity tests should be performed initially and periodically during continued therapy. Drug is generally given for 7 to 10 days.

Renal function and vestibular and auditory function should be determined before initiation of therapy and at regular intervals during treatment, especially in patients with impaired renal function and in those receiving higher doses or longer treatment. Vestibular and auditory function should also be checked 3 to 4 weeks after drug is discontinued.

Ototoxic effect is greatest on vestibular branch of 8th cranial nerve (symptoms: headache, dizziness, nausea, and vomiting with motion, ataxia, nystagmus); however, auditory damage (tinnitus, roaring noises) may also occur. Hearing loss occurs particularly in high tone range; generally, conversational hearing range is not affected. Prompt reporting is critically essential to avoid permanent damage.

Drug plasma concentrations should be determined at frequent intervals for patients with impaired renal function (usually not allowed to exceed 10 μg/ml).

Physician may use creatinine clearance rate and serum creatinine concentration as guides to dosage scheduling when serum levels are not feasible (frequency of administration in hours is approximated by multiplying serum creatinine by 8).

Intake and output should be monitored. Consult physician about desirable intake; generally, patient is kept well hydrated during gentamicin therapy to prevent chemical irritation of renal tubules. Report oliguria and unusual change in intake–output ratio. A decrease in urinary output and increases in BUN, serum creatinine, and creatinine clearance are indications of nephrotoxicity.

Be alert for signs of bacterial overgrowth with nonsusceptible organisms (diarrhea, anogenital itching, vaginal discharge, stomatitis, glossitis).

In treatment of urinary tract infections, concomitant alkalinizing agent may be prescribed to raise urinary pH above 7, since gentamicin is less active in an acidic medium.

The usual duration of treatment for most patients is 7 to 10 days.

Topically treated lesions may be covered with gauze, if necessary.

Systemic absorption and toxicity are possible when topical applications, particularly cream preparations, are made to large denuded body surfaces.

In treatment of impetigo contagiosa, individual crusts should first be removed (gently) to allow topical medication to contact infected site. Removal may be facilitated by soaking crusts with warm soap and water or by application of wet compresses. Consult physician regarding specific procedure.

Caution patients using topical applications to avoid excessive exposure to sunlight because of danger of photosensitivity. Also advise patient to withhold medication and to notify physician if signs of irritation or sensitivity occur.

Gentamicin is incompatible in a syringe or in solution with any other drug.

DRUG INTERACTIONS: Possibility of additive nephrotoxic effects with combined use of gentamicin and **cephalosporins**. **Ethacrynic acid** and **furosemide** may enhance ototoxicity of gentamicin (and other aminoglycoside antibiotics); concurrent use is usually avoided. Combined or sequential use of **other aminoglycoside antibiotics** with gentamicin increases the probability of ototoxicity and nephrotoxicity. **Anti-motion-sickness drugs** may mask symptoms of ototoxicity. There is enhanced neuromuscular blockade with neuromuscular blocking drugs (eg, **decamethonium, ether, succinylcholine, tubocurarine,** and related anesthetics). Activity of gentamicin is diminished significantly by **carbenicillin**. If concurrent administration is prescribed, they should be given about 1 to 2 hours apart.

GITALIN, N.F.
(GITALIGIN)

Cardiotonic

ACTIONS AND USES
Mixture of amorphous glycosides obtained from *Digitalis purpurea*. Has same actions, uses, contraindications, and adverse reactions as other digitalis glycosides. Rate of elimination slower than that of digoxin, but faster than that of digitalis and digitoxin. See Digitalis.

ABSORPTION AND FATE
Following oral administration, action begins in 2 to 4 hours and peaks in 8 to 12 hours. Activity may persist 7 to 12 days. Rate of elimination closely correlated with duration of action.

ROUTE AND DOSAGE
Oral (rapid digitalization): 2.5 mg followed by 0.75 mg every 6 hours until desired therapeutic effect or mild toxicity occurs (usually after total dose of about 6 mg in 24 hours); (slow digitalization): 1.5 mg daily for 4 to 6 days; maintenance: 0.25 to 1.25 mg daily.

NURSING IMPLICATIONS
The maintenance dose is given preferably in the morning.
Preserved in tight, light-resistant containers.
See Digitalis.

GLUCAGON, U.S.P.

Antagonist, insulin

ACTIONS AND USES
Polypeptide hormone produced by alpha cells of islets of Langerhans. Actions appear to be related to increased synthesis of cyclic adenosine monophosphate (cAMP). Promptly elevates blood glucose concentration by increasing phosphorylase activity, thus stimulating breakdown of glycogen to glucose in liver. Intensity of hyperglycemia is dependent on hepatic glycogen reserve and presence of phosphorylase. Glucagon is of little value in starvation, adrenal insuffi-

ciency, or chronic hypoglycemia; juvenile or unstable diabetics do not respond satisfactorily. Exerts positive inotropic and chronotropic action on heart similar to that produced by catecholamines.

Used in emergency treatment of severe hypoglycemic reactions in patients on insulin therapy for diabetes and psychiatric patients receiving insulin-shock treatment, when dextrose is not available or its use is impractical. May be used together with dextrose for patients in very deep coma.

ABSORPTION AND FATE

Blood glucose level increases within 5 to 20 minutes after injection; falls to normal or hypoglycemic level within 1.5 hours. Metabolized primarily by liver.

CONTRAINDICATIONS AND PRECAUTIONS

Known hypersensitivity to protein compounds.

ADVERSE REACTIONS

Infrequent: nausea and vomiting, hypersensitivity reactions, anaphylaxis, hypotension (rare).

ROUTE AND DOSAGE

For hypoglycemia: subcutaneous, intramuscular, intravenous: 0.5 to 1 unit (dissolve lyophilized glucagon in accompanying solvent supplied by manufacturer). If no response occurs within 20 minutes, dose may be repeated once or twice depending on depth and duration of coma. Failure to respond may necessitate immediate administration of IV glucose. For insulin-shock therapy: subcutaneous, intramuscular, intravenous: after 1 hour of coma, 0.5 to 1 unit. If no response occurs in 10 to 25 minutes, dose may be repeated. In very deep state of coma, glucose may be given in addition to glucagon for more immediate response.

NURSING IMPLICATIONS

Hypoglycemic reactions require immediate treatment. Prolonged hypoglycemic coma can result in cortical damage.

Patient usually awakens from hypoglycemic coma 10 to 20 minutes following glucagon injection. As soon as possible after patient regains consciousness, oral carbohydrate should be given to restore liver glycogen and to prevent secondary hypoglycemic episode (physician may administer IV dextrose in cases of very deep coma or if patient fails to respond to glucagon).

Patients receiving glucagon following insulin-shock therapy should be fed orally as soon as possible after awakening, and the usual dietary regimen should be followed.

Vomiting sometimes occurs on awakening. Have emesis basin and suction equipment immediately available, and position patient to prevent aspiration.

Following recovery from hypoglycemic reaction, symptoms such as headache, nausea, and weakness may persist.

Physician may request that a responsible family member be taught how to administer glucagon subcutaneously or intramuscularly. Stress the importance of notifying the physician whenever a hypoglycemic reaction occurs so that the reason for the reaction can be ascertained to prevent further episodes.

A diabetic teaching plan should be reviewed for all patients and responsible family members. Commonly, hypoglycemic episodes follow delay of food intake or increased physical activity. Review the early symptoms of hypoglycemia (headache, weakness, hunger, tremor, irritability, lack of muscle coordination, apprehension, diaphoresis), and emphasize the importance of routinely carrying lump sugar, candy, or other readily available carbohydrate to take at first warning of oncoming reaction.

Because glucagon is a protein substance, the possibility of a hypersensitivity reaction should be borne in mind.

Glucagon solutions remain potent for 3 months if kept refrigerated (2 to 15 C). Lyophilized (dry powder) form is stable at room temperature. Glucagon should be considered incompatible in syringe with any other drug.

DRUG INTERACTIONS: Marked hypoprothrombinemic responses may occur when high doses of glucagon (25 mg for 2 days or more) are administered concomitantly with warfarin and possibly **oral anticoagulants.**

GLUTAMIC ACID HYDROCHLORIDE, N.F.
(ACIDULIN)

Acidifier, gastric

ACTIONS AND USES
Amino acid chemically combined with hydrochloric acid that is released on contact with water. May be prescribed instead of diluted hydrochloric acid for treatment of hypochlorhydria and achlorhydria because it is convenient to carry and does not injure dental enamel. Also available in OTC preparations in combination with pepsin to aid in digestion, eg, Muripsin, Glutasyn, Alidol-Pepsin, Normacid.
CONTRAINDICATIONS AND PRECAUTIONS
Gastric hyperacidity, peptic ulcer.
ADVERSE REACTIONS
Overdose: systemic acidosis.
ROUTE AND DOSAGE
Oral: 1 to 3 capsules or pulvules 3 times daily before each meal (each pulvule contains 340 mg of glutamic acid hydrochloride).

NURSING IMPLICATIONS
See Hydrochloric Acid, Diluted.

GLUTETHIMIDE, N.F., B.P.
(DORIDEN)

Sedative, hypnotic

ACTIONS AND USES
Piperidine derivative structurally related to methyprylon. Pharmacologic actions similar to those of barbiturates. Can induce hypnosis without producing reliable analgesic, antitussive, or anticonvulsant action. Produces less respiratory depression, but greater degree of hypotension, than barbiturates. Exhibits anticholinergic activity, especially mydriasis, and inhibits salivary secretions and intestinal motility. Significantly suppresses REM sleep (dreaming stage of sleep); but following drug withdrawal after chronic administration, REM rebound occurs, and patient may experience markedly increased dreaming, nightmares, and/or insomnia. Addiction liability similar to that of barbiturates. Stimulates hepatic microsomal enzymes and thus may alter metabolism of other drugs.
Used as short-term hypnotic in treatment of simple insomnia and for sedative effect preoperatively and during first stage of labor. Not indicated for routine sedation.

Erratic absorption from GI tract. Sleep is usually induced within 30 minutes following hypnotic dose, lasting 4 to 8 hours. Serum level decline is biphasic: first phase about 4 hours, second phase 10 to 12 hours. Widely distributed to body tissues; localizes particularly in adipose tissue, liver, kidney, brain, and bile. About 50% bound to plasma proteins. Almost completely metabolized in liver by hydroxylation; conjugates with glucuronic acid. Glucuronides are excreted slowly in urine; less than 2% of dose excreted unchanged. About 1% to 2% excreted in feces. Crosses placenta; small quantities may appear in breast milk.

CONTRAINDICATIONS AND PRECAUTIONS

Known hypersensitivity to glutethimide; uncontrolled pain; intermittent porphyria; severe hepatic and renal impairment; prolonged administration; children younger than 12 years of age. Safe use in women of childbearing potential and during pregnancy (except with caution during first stage of labor) not established. Cautious use: elderly or debilitated patients, prostatic hypertrophy, bladder neck obstruction, pyloroduodenal obstruction, stenosing peptic ulcer, narrow-angle glaucoma, hypotension, cardiac arrhythmias, mental depression (particularly in patients with suicidal tendencies), history of alcoholism or drug abuse.

ADVERSE REACTIONS

Generally infrequent: gastric irritation, nausea, hiccups, drug "hangover," dry mouth, blurred vision, generalized skin rash (occasionally, purpuric or urticarial), exfoliative dermatitis, paradoxic excitement, headache, vertigo, acute hypersensitivity reactions, porphyria, jaundice, blood dyscrasias (thrombocytopenic purpura, aplastic anemia, leukopenia), CNS depression in fetus. **Acute overdosage** (CNS depression): coma; depressed reflexes, including corneal reflex; dilated, fixed pupils; hypotension; hypothermia followed by hyperpyrexia; tachycardia; respiratory depression; cyanosis; sudden apnea; urinary bladder atony; decreased intestinal motility; adynamic ileus; facial twitching; intermittent spasticity; flaccid paralysis; pulmonary and cerebral edema; renal tubular necrosis; severe infections. **Chronic toxicity** (toxic psychosis): slurred speech, impaired memory, inability to concentrate, mydriasis, dry mouth, nystagmus, ataxia, hyporeflexia, tremors, peripheral neuropathy, osteomalacia (rare).

ROUTE AND DOSAGE

Oral: (for insomnia): 250 to 500 mg at bedtime, repeated if necessary, but not less than 4 hours before arising; (preoperatively): 500 mg the night before surgery and 500 mg to 1 Gm 1 hour before anesthesia; (first stage of labor): 500 mg at onset of labor, repeated once if necessary.

NURSING IMPLICATIONS

If administered for insomnia, glutethimide should be given 4 hours or more before the usual time of arising in order to avoid residual daytime effects.

Sedative-hypnotic effect of glutethimide is counteracted by pain. Consult physician about prescribing an analgesic for pain, if required.

Keep physician informed of patient's response to drug. Smallest effective dosage should be used for the shortest period of time compatible with patient's needs.

Advise patient to report onset of rash or any other unusual symptoms. Discontinuation of drug is indicated if a rash occurs.

Caution patient to avoid driving a motor vehicle or engaging in other activities requiring mental alertness for 7 to 8 hours following drug ingestion.

Warn patient about possible adverse reactions when glutethimide is combined with alcohol or other CNS depressants (see Drug Interactions).

Prolonged use of moderate to high doses of glutethimide can produce tolerance and psychologic and physical dependence.

Abrupt withdrawal following regular use may produce nausea, vomiting, nervousness, tremors, abdominal cramps, nightmares, insomnia, tachycardia, chills, fever, numbness of extremities, dysphagia, delirium, hallucinations, or convulsions. Withdrawal should be gradual, with stepwise dose reduction over a period of several days or weeks.

Overdosage of glutethimide is difficult to treat. Patients tend to go in and out of toxicity, possibly due to delayed absorption of the drug.

Treatment of acute overdosage: gastric lavage, regardless of time that has elapsed since drug ingestion. Some physicians lavage with a 1:1 mixture of castor oil and water (glutethimide is lipid-soluble). Supportive treatment is based on presenting signs and symptoms.

Classified as schedule III drug under federal Controlled Substances Act.

DRUG INTERACTIONS: Possibility of increased CNS depression with concomitant administration of **alcohol** (also enhances glutethimide absorption), **barbiturates,** and other **CNS depressants.** Additive anticholinergic effects may occur with **tricyclic antidepressants.** There is decreased anticoagulant response in patients receiving **oral anticoagulants.** Anticoagulant dosage may require adjustment during treatment and on cessation of glutethimide.

GLYCERIN, U.S.P., B.P.
(GLYCEROL, GLYROL, OSMOGLYN)
GLYCERIN ANHYDROUS
(OPHTHALGAN)

ACTIONS AND USES
Trihydric alcohol. When administered orally raises plasma osmotic pressure by withdrawing fluid from extravascular spaces; lowers ocular tension by decreasing volume of intraocular fluid. Also may decrease cerebrospinal fluid pressure and produce slight diuresis. Topical application to eye reduces edema by hygroscopic effect.

Used orally to reduce elevated intraocular pressure prior to or following surgery for glaucoma, retinal detachment, or cataract extraction and to reduce elevated CSF pressure. Sterile glycerin (anhydrous) is used topically to reduce superficial corneal edema resulting from trauma, surgery, or disease and to facilitate ophthalmoscopic examination.

ABSORPTION AND FATE
Rapidly absorbed from GI tract following oral administration and distributed through blood. Intraocular pressure begins to decline within 10 minutes; maximal effect occurs in 30 minutes to 2 hours and may persist 4 to 8 hours. Metabolized in liver to CO_2 and water, or utilized in glucose or glycogen synthesis. Approximately 7% to 14% excreted unchanged in urine.

CONTRAINDICATIONS AND PRECAUTIONS
Hypersensitivity to any of the ingredients. Cautious use: cardiac, renal, or hepatic disease; diabetes; dehydrated or elderly patients.

ADVERSE REACTIONS
Headache, dizziness, nausea, vomiting, thirst, diarrhea, hyperglycemia, glycosuria, dehydration, disorientation, convulsive seizures (rare).

ROUTE AND DOSAGE
Oral (50% to 75% glycerin): 1 to 1.5 Gm/kg body weight, repeated at approximately 5-hour intervals. Topical ophthalmic (sterile anhydrous glycerin): 1 or 2 drops instilled into eye every 3 to 4 hours for reduction of corneal edema.

NURSING IMPLICATIONS

Commercially available flavored solution may be poured over crushed ice and sipped through a straw. Lemon juice and 0.9% sodium chloride (if allowed) may be added to unflavored solution for palatability.

Headache (from cerebral dehydration) may be prevented or relieved by having patient lie down during and after administration of oral drug.

Consult physician regarding fluid intake in patients receiving drug for elevated intraocular pressure. Although hypotonic fluids will relieve thirst and headache caused by the dehydrating action of glycerin, these fluids may nullify its osmotic effect.

Slight hyperglycemia and glycosuria may occur with oral use. Patients with diabetes may require adjustment in insulin dosage.

Glycerin is also available in suppository form to promote defecation and it is used as a vehicle for many drugs applied to the skin. Undiluted glycerin (95% to 99%) adsorbs moisture and hence is somewhat dehydrating and irritating when applied to skin and mucous membranes. When diluted with water, it acts as an emollient and humectant. Dilution for mouth care: 2 parts glycerin to 1 part water; flavor with lemon juice.

GLYCOPYRROLATE, N.F.
(ROBINUL)

Anticholinergic

ACTIONS AND USES

Synthetic anticholinergic (antimuscarinic) quaternary ammonium compound with pharmacologic effects similar to those of atropine (qv). In contrast to atropine, glycopyrrolate is highly polar and therefore does not easily penetrate lipid membranes such as the blood–brain barrier. Has lower incidence of CNS-related side effects than atropine, and reportedly has longer vagal blocking and antisialogogue effects. Inhibits motility of GI tract and genitourinary tract and decreases volume of gastric and pancreatic secretions, saliva, and perspiration. Also antagonizes muscarinic symptoms (eg, excessive tracheal or bronchial secretions, bronchospasm, bradycardia, intestinal hypermotility) induced by cholinergic drugs, such as anticholinesterases, and anesthetic agents.

Used in adjunctive management of peptic ulcer and other GI disorders associated with hyperacidity, hypermotility, and spasm. Commercially available in combination with phenobarbital (eg, Robinul-PH). Also used parenterally as preanesthetic and intraoperative medication and to reverse neuromuscular blockade.

ABSORPTION AND FATE

Poorly and irregularly absorbed following oral administration; peak effects appear in about 1 hour and may persist 6 hours. Following subcutaneous or IM administration, peak effects occur in 30 to 45 minutes; vagal blocking effects may last 2 to 3 hours, and antisialogogue effects may persist up to 7 hours. Action following IV dose begins in 10 to 15 minutes; duration of action shorter than with other routes. Thought to be excreted primarily in urine and bile and as unchanged drug in feces.

CONTRAINDICATIONS AND PRECAUTIONS

Hypersensitivity to glycopyrrolate; glaucoma; asthma; prostatic hypertrophy; obstructive uropathy; obstructive lesions or atony of GI tract; severe ulcerative colitis; myasthenia gravis; tachycardia; during cyclopropane anesthesia; children under age 12 (except parenteral use in conjunction with anesthesia). Safe use during pregnancy or lactation not established. Also see Atropine.

Xerostomia, decreased sweating, urinary hesitancy or retention, blurred vision, mydriasis, constipation, palpitation, tachycardia, drowsiness, weakness, dizziness. Overdosage: Neuromuscular blockade (curarelike action) leading to muscular weakness and paralysis is theoretically possible. Also see Atropine.

ROUTE AND DOSAGE

Oral: **adults only:** initially 1 to 2 mg 3 times daily in morning, early afternoon, and evening. Dosage adjusted to needs of individual patient. Recommended maximum daily dosage is 8 mg. Maintenance: 1 mg 2 times daily. Subcutaneous, intramuscular, intravenous: 0.1 to 0.2 mg at 4-hour intervals 1 to 4 times a day; dilution not required.

NURSING IMPLICATIONS

Incidence and severity of side effects are generally dose-related.

Caution patient to avoid high environmental temperatures (heat prostration can occur due to decreased sweating).

Since glycopyrrolate may produce dizziness, drowsiness, and blurred vision, warn patient not to engage in activities requiring mental alertness, such as operating a motor vehicle or performing other hazardous tasks.

See Atropine Sulfate.

GOLD AU 198
(AURCOLOID-198, AUREOTOPE)

Antineoplastic, diagnostic aid

ACTIONS AND USES

Radiopharmaceutical with relatively short half-life (2.7 days). Prepared by neutron activation in a nuclear reactor: irradiated gold foil dissolved in aqua regia, then stabilized in colloid solution by gelatin. Mean effective life of emission (both beta and gamma rays) about 4 days. Administered into pleural and peritoneal cavities, gold becomes maximally concentrated at serosal and lymphatic metastatic deposits, permitting ionizing exposure to both fixed and free-floating tumor cells. Action mechanism not clear, but admixture and contact lead to decreased rate of fluid accumulation. Intracavitary radiation does not replace surgery or deep radiation treatment; it is costly and offers little therapeutic advantage over use of alkylating agents, talc, or quinacrine.

Used to treat recurrent malignant effusion of serous cavities, to control chronic intraarticular effusion, as palliative of inoperable prostatic carcinoma, and experimentally to irradiate lymphatic systems and to prevent spread of cancer. Also used diagnostically for imaging liver, bone marrow, lymph nodes, spleen.

ABSORPTION AND FATE

Reticuloendothelial cells and free macrophages phagocytize gold particles introduced into cavities. Injected radiogold rapidly cleared from blood, permitting imaging of liver within 5 minutes. Distribution largely to spleen, Kupffer cells, bone marrow, macrophages. Small amounts slowly excreted in urine (1%); most of the gold stays in tissue for long periods of time without extensive adhesion formation. The radionuclide decays in body.

CONTRAINDICATIONS AND PRECAUTIONS

Pregnancy; lactation; persons less than 18 years old, unless indications are compelling; after surgery, unless cavity wound healing is complete; exposed or ulcerated cavity surfaces; cavities with evidence of fluid loculation; dying patients.

Radiation sickness, myelodepression, chest pains, generalized skin rash, anorexia, nausea, vomiting; (intraperitoneal): diarrhea, abdominal pain, intestinal obstruction; myelosuppression, hypersensitivity (itching around injection site), skin rash, stomatitis, neuritis, nephritis.

ROUTE AND DOSAGE

Therapeutic (intrapleural): 25 to 100 mCi; (intraperitoneal): 35 to 125 mCi. Highly individualized. Diagnostic (intravenous): 150 to 500 mCi.

NURSING IMPLICATIONS

Administer only if solution is distinctly red in color.

IV diagnostic radiogold is administered with patient in supine position. Imaging may be performed 5 minutes to 48 hours after radiopharmaceutical administration.

Radiogold is carried from drug vial into the cavity by saline. Contaminated outlet tubing (vial to patient) and vial are set aside for radioactive decay and disposal.

Before intracavitary administration, most of fluid in the particular cavity is removed. Following administration, especially during first hour, the patient should change his position frequently to assure proper distribution of the drug.

In absence of peritoneal effusion, the cavity may be insufflated with air or nitrous oxide to prevent filtration or loculation when radiogold is introduced.

A polyethylene catheter may be used for intracavity injection to prevent infiltration.

Following administration of radiogold for therapy, the patient becomes a source of high-intensity gamma radiation and is thus a serious hazard to hospital personnel and other patients.

The patient is usually isolated in a single room during treatment period. The nurse can work within 2 feet of patient for a period of no more than 20 minutes daily and should wear a film badge or exposure meter.

Remove dressings by remote handling techniques; transport radioactive dressings, linen, and equipment to storage depot for the radiation decay period. Follow agency regulations.

Avoid contact of radiogold solution with aluminum; radionuclide will precipitate out of solution.

Hospitalization is usually required until body level of radioactivity is less than 30 mCi.

Favorable clinical response (3 to 4 weeks after treatment) is evidenced by posttherapeutic resorption of fluid or failure of fluid to reaccumulate after posttherapy paracentesis or thoracentesis.

Control of condition being treated may last from a few weeks to several months. If response is disappointing, treatment may be repeated after a period of 4 to 6 weeks.

Radiogold has an expiration date of 8 days after date of standardization.

Both solution and glass container may darken on standing as a result of radiation.

Solution may be refrigerated.

(MYOCHRYSINE)
SODIUM AUROTHIOMALATE, B.P.

Antirheumatic

ACTIONS AND USES
Similar to aurothioglucose (qv) in actions and uses. Contains approximately 50% gold.
Used in treatment of selected patients (adults and juveniles) with acute rheumatoid arthritis.

ABSORPTION AND FATE
Readily absorbed following IM injection. Peak plasma concentrations reached in 4 to 6 hours. Thought to be highly concentrated in kidney, liver, spleen, and synovial fluid. Bound to plasma protein. Half-life lengthens with successive injections. Excreted primarily in urine; appreciable amounts also eliminated in feces. After a course of treatment, traces may be found in urine for 6 months or more.

CONTRAINDICATIONS AND PRECAUTIONS
Severe toxicity from previous exposure to gold or other heavy metals, severe debilitation, systemic lupus erythematosus, Sjögren's syndrome in rheumatoid arthritis, renal disease, hepatic dysfunction, history of infectious hepatitis or hematologic disorders, uncontrolled diabetes or congestive heart failure. Safe use during pregnancy not established. Cautious use: history of drug allergies or hypersensitivity, hypertension.

ADVERSE REACTIONS
Skin and mucous membranes: transient pruritus, erythema, dermatitis (common), alopecia, shedding of nails, gray to blue pigmentation of skin (chrysiasis), stomatitis (common), glossitis, bronchitis, pharyngitis, gastritis, colitis, vaginitis, conjunctivitis (rare). **Renal**: nephrotic syndrome, glomerulitis with hematuria, proteinuria. **Hematologic** (rare): leukopenia, agranulocytosis, thrombocytopenia, hypoplastic and aplastic anemia, eosinophilia. **Allergic** (nitritoid-type reactions): flushing, fainting, dizziness, fall in blood pressure, sweating, nausea, vomiting, weakness. Less frequently: anaphylactic shock, bradycardia, edema of tongue, angioneurotic edema. **Other**: gold deposits in ocular tissues, hepatitis with jaundice, bilirubinemia, peripheral neuritis, encephalitis.

ROUTE AND DOSAGE
Highly individualized. **Adults:** intramuscular (weekly injections): 1st injection 10 mg, 2nd injection 25 mg, 3rd and subsequent injections to 16th or 20th injection 50 mg. If no improvement occurs after this amount, treatment is generally discontinued. If improvement occurs, patient is placed on maintenance schedule: 50 mg at 2-week intervals for 4 injections; 50 mg at 3-week intervals for 4 injections: 50 mg monthly until treatment is discontinued (length of treatment depends on patient response). **Pediatric:** Juvenile rheumatoid arthritis: dosage is proportional on weight basis to recommended adult dosage. No more than 25 mg in a single dose should be given to children under 12 years of age.

NURSING IMPLICATIONS
Agitate vial before withdrawing dose to assure uniform suspension
Baseline hemoglobin and erythrocyte determinations, WBC count, differential count, platelet count, and urinalysis should be obtained before initiation of therapy and at regular intervals thereafter.
Rapid reduction in hemoglobin level, WBC count below 4000/mm^3, eosinophil count above 5%, and platelet count below 100,000/mm^3 signify possible toxicity.

Prior to each injection, urine should be analyzed for protein, blood, and sediment. Drug should be discontinued promptly if proteinuria or hematuria develops.

Patient should be interviewed and examined before each injection to detect occurrence of transient pruritus or dermatitis (both are common early indications of toxicity), stomatitis (sore tongue, palate, or throat), metallic taste, indigestion, or other signs and symptoms of possible toxicity. Treatment should be interrupted immediately if any of these reactions occurs.

Drug is preferably administered intragluteally with patient lying down. Patient should remain recumbent for at least 30 minutes after injection because transient giddiness, vertigo, and facial flushing may occur. Observe for allergic reaction.

Allergic reaction may occur almost immediately after injection, 10 minutes after injection, or at any time during therapy; if it is observed, treatment should be discontinued. At time of injection have BAL on hand.

Patients who develop gold dermatitis should be warned that exposure to sunlight may aggravate the problem.

The appearance of purpura or ecchymoses is always an indication for a platelet count; report to physician.

Patients should be informed about possible adverse reactions and warned to report any symptom suggestive of toxicity as soon as it appears. Adverse reactions may occur at any time during drug therapy or even a few months after drug is discontinued; most reactions occur during second or third month of treatment (usually after the amount injected has reached about 250 to 500 mg).

Therapeutic effects may not appear until 6 to 8 weeks of therapy. Rapid improvement in joint swelling usually indicates that patient is closely approaching drug tolerance level; report to physician.

Preserved in tight, light-resistant containers. Drug should not be used if it is any darker than pale yellow.

GRISEOFULVIN, U.S.P., B.P.
(FULVICIN-U/F, GRIFULVIN V, GRISACTIN, GRISEOFULVIN MICROSIZE, GRISEOFULVIN ULTRAMICROSIZE, GRISOWEN, GRIS-PEG)

Antifungal agent

ACTIONS AND USES

Fungistatic antibiotic derived from species of *Penicillium.* Deposits in keratin precursor cells and has special affinity for diseased tissue. Tightly bound to new keratin of skin, hair, and nails, which becomes highly resistant to fungal invasion. Effective against various species of *Epidermophyton, Microsporum,* and *Trichophyton* (has no effect on other fungi, including candida, bacteria, and yeasts). Exerts fungistatic action primarily by arresting metaphase of cell division. Also has some direct vasodilatory activity. Efficacy of GI absorption of ultramicrosize formulation reported to be twice that of microsize griseofulvin.

Used in treatment of mycotic disease of skin, hair, and nails not amenable to conventional topical measures. Concomitant use of appropriate topical agent may be required, particularly for tinea pedis. Griseofulvin has been used investigationally in treatment of Raynaud's disease, angina pectoris, and gout.

ABSORPTION AND FATE

Absorbed primarily from duodenum (extent varies among individuals). Absorption of microsize griseofulvin is variable and unpredictable. Single 500-mg dose of microsize and 250-mg dose of ultramicrosize form produce roughly comparable peak plasma levels in about 4 hours. Concentrates in skin, hair, nails, liver, fat, and skeletal muscle. Can be detected in outer layers of stratum corneum soon after absorption. Metabolized in liver. Excreted in urine and feces chiefly as inactive metabolites and small amounts of unchanged drug. Also excreted in perspiration. Elimination half-life is 9 to 24 hours.

CONTRAINDICATIONS AND PRECAUTIONS

History of sensitivity to griseofulvin; porphyria; hepatic disease; systemic lupus erythematosus. Safe use during pregnancy or for prophylaxis against fungal infections not established. Cautious use: penicillin-sensitive patients (possibility of cross-sensitivity with penicillin exists; however, reportedly penicillin-sensitive patients have been treated without difficulty).

ADVERSE REACTIONS

Low incidence of side effects. **Neurologic**: headache, insomnia, peripheral neuritis, paresthesias, fatigue, mental confusion, impaired performance of routine functions, vertigo, blurred vision, diminished hearing (rare). **GI**: heartburn, nausea, vomiting, diarrhea, flatulence, dry mouth, thirst, decreased taste acuity, unpleasant taste, furred tongue, oral thrush. **Hematologic**: leukopenia, neutropenia, granulocytopenia, punctate basophilia, monocytosis. **Renal**: proteinuria, cylinduria. **Hypersensitivity**: urticaria, photosensitivity, lichen planus, skin rashes, serum sickness syndromes, severe angioedema. Other reported: hepatotoxicity, estrogenlike effects (in children), aggravation of systemic lupus erythematosus, overgrowth of nonsusceptible organisms, candidal intertrigo, elevated porphyrins in feces and erythrocytes.

ROUTE AND DOSAGE

Oral: **Adults:** 250 to 500 mg of ultramicrosize griseofulvin (Gris-PEG) or 500 mg to 1 Gm of microsize griseofulvin per day (best results reportedly obtained when calculated dose is divided into 4 equal parts and given at 6-hour intervals). **Children**: 5 mg ultramicrosize griseofulvin (Gris-PEG) or 10 mg microsize griseofulvin per kilogram body weight daily. All dosages highly individualized.

NURSING IMPLICATIONS

Note that griseofulvin ultramicrosize (Gris-PEG) is prescribed in lower doses (125 mg Gris-PEG is biologically equivalent to 250 mg griseofulvin microsize preparations, eg, Fulvicin-U/F, Grifulvin V, Grisactin).

Accurate laboratory identification of infecting organism is essential prior to initiation of treatment.

Giving the drug after meals may allay GI disturbances.

Serum levels may be increased by giving the microsize formulations with a high-fat-content meal (enhances drug absorption).

Headaches often occur during early therapy but frequently disappear with continued drug administration.

Blood studies should be performed at least once weekly during first month of therapy or longer. Periodic tests of renal and hepatic function are also advised.

Patient may experience symptomatic relief after 48 to 96 hours of therapy. Stress the importance of continuing treatment as prescribed to prevent relapse.

Treatment should be continued until there is clinical improvement, as well as negative potassium hydroxide mounts of lesion scrapings or cultures for 2 or 3 consecutive weeks.

Duration of treatment depends on time required for replacement of infected skin, hair, or nails and thus varies with site of infection. Average duration of treatment for tinea capitis (scalp ringworm) is 4 to 6 weeks; tinea corporis (body ringworm), 2 to 4 weeks; tinea pedis (athlete's foot), 4 to 8 weeks; tinea unguium (nail fungus), at least 4 months for fingernails, depending on rate of growth, and 6 months or more for toenails.

Caution patient to avoid exposure to intense natural or artificial sunlight, because photosensitivity-type reactions may occur.

Warn patient of possible reaction (tachycardia, flushing) on ingestion of alcohol during therapy.

Emphasize importance of cleanliness and keeping skin dry (moist skin favors growth of fungi). For athlete's foot, advise patient to wear well-ventilated shoes without rubber soles, to alternate shoes, and to change socks daily. Physician may prescribe a drying powder as necessary.

DRUG INTERACTIONS: Griseofulvin may potentiate the effects of **alcohol.** Activity of griseofulvin may be diminished by **barbiturates** (cause reduction of griseofulvin serum levels). In some patients, griseofulvin may decrease the hypoprothrombinemic effects of **warfarin** and possibly other **oral anticoagulants.** Close monitoring of prothrombin time is advised when griseofulvin is added to or withdrawn from anticoagulant drug regimen.

GUAIFENESIN, N.F., B.P.
(EXPECTRAN, Glyceryl Guaiacolate, GLYTUSS, G-200, GG-CEN, GLYCOTUSS, HYTUSS, MALOTUSS, ROBITUSSETS, ROBITUSSIN, 2/G)

Expectorant

ACTIONS AND USES

Enhances reflex outflow of respiratory tract fluids by irritation of gastric mucosa and thus aids in expectoration by reducing their adhesiveness and surface tension.

Used to combat dry, unproductive cough associated with colds and bronchitis. A common ingredient in cough mixtures. Reportedly may inhibit platelet function.

ADVERSE REACTIONS

Low incidence: GI upset, nausea, drowsiness.

ROUTE AND DOSAGE

Oral: **Adults:** 100 to 200 mg every 3 to 4 hours. **Children** *age 6 to 12:* 50 to 100 mg every 3 to 4 hours; *age 2 to 6:* 25 to 50 mg every 3 to 4 hours as required. Available forms: tablets, capsules, troches, liquid.

NURSING IMPLICATIONS

See Benzonate for patient teaching points.

LABORATORY TEST INTERFERENCES: Guaifenesin may produce color interferences with certain laboratory determinations of 5-hydroxyindoleacetic acid (5-HIAA) and vanillylmandelic acid (VMA).

DRUG INTERACTIONS: By inhibiting platelet function, guaifenesin may increase risk of hemorrhage in patients receiving **heparin** therapy.

Antihypertensive

ACTIONS AND USES

Potent, long-acting, postganglionic adrenergic blocking agent. Reduces responses to sympathetic nerve activation by depleting norepinephrine stores from adrenergic nerve endings. As a result, produces gradual prolonged fall in blood pressure that is usually associated with bradycardia and decreased pulse pressure. Chronic administration causes supersensitivity of effector cells to catecholamines. Antihypertensive effect results from venous dilatation with peripheral pooling, decreased venous return, and decreased cardiac output. Drug-induced sodium retention and edema may occur unless concomitant diuretic therapy is administered. Guanethidine also causes decreased plasma renin activity. It diminishes or eliminates cardiovascular reflexes and is therefore more effective in lowering orthostatic than supine blood pressure. Local instillation in eye causes miosis and reduces intraocular pressure in glaucomatous eyes. Marked increase in GI motility is the result of unopposed parasympathetic activity.

Major use: treatment of severe hypertension in conjunction with or following a course of treatment with a thiazide diuretic and/or hydralazine. Has been used investigationally to treat glaucoma and in the treatment of hyperthyroidism and thyroid crisis to reduce heart rate.

ABSORPTION AND FATE

Partially absorbed from GI tract (3% to 30% variability in absorption rate, but rate remains constant for each individual). Maximal antihypertensive effect in 3 days or more. Appears to be metabolized by hepatic microsomal enzymes. Highly concentrated in cells of kidney, liver, and lungs. Excreted in urine as active drug and less active metabolites; some excretion via feces. Small amounts may remain in body up to 14 days or longer. Appears in breast milk in negligible amounts.

CONTRAINDICATIONS AND PRECAUTIONS

Pheochromocytoma; frank congestive heart failure (not due to hypertension) within 1 week of administration of MAO inhibitors. Safe use during pregnancy not established. Cautious use: renal disease; nitrogen retention or rising BUN levels; limited cardiac reserve; coronary disease with insufficiency; recent myocardial infarction; cerebrovascular disease, especially with encephalopathy; febrile illnesses; history of peptic ulcer, colitis, or bronchial asthma.

ADVERSE REACTIONS

Common: severe diarrhea, marked orthostatic and exertional hypotension, dizziness, skeletal muscle weakness, lassitude, syncope, bradycardia, inhibition of ejaculation, psychologic impotence, edema, and weight gain with occasional development of dyspnea and congestive heart failure. **Less common:** fatigue, nausea, vomiting, nocturia, urinary retention or incontinence, constipation, rise in BUN, dermatitis, scalp hair loss, dry mouth, ptosis of eyelids, blurred vision, parotid tenderness, myalgia, muscle tremor, psychic depression, chest pains, paresthesias, nasal congestion, asthma (in susceptible individuals), complete A-V block, polyarteritis nodosa. Reported, but causal relationship not established: anemia, thrombocytopenia, leukopenia.

ROUTE AND DOSAGE

Oral: *Ambulatory patients:* initially 10 mg daily, depending on patient's response; incremental increases of 10 mg no more often than every 5 to 7 days; maintenance: 25 to 50 mg once daily. *Hospitalized patients:* 25 to 50 mg daily, increased by 25 or 50 mg daily or every other day as indicated. All dosages highly individualized.

NURSING IMPLICATIONS

During period of dosage adjustment, doses must be carefully titrated on the basis of orthostatic and supine blood pressures. The hypotensive effect of guanethidine is greater with patient in orthostatic position as opposed to supine position.

Physician generally prescribes taking blood pressure first in supine position and then again after patient has been standing for 10 minutes. Some physicians also request that it be taken immediately after mild exercise.

Since hospitalized patients are given higher initial doses than ambulatory patients, standing blood pressure determinations should be made regularly during the day, if possible. The full effect of guanethidine on standing blood pressure should be carefully evaluated before patient is discharged.

Caution patient not to get out of bed without assistance. Supervise ambulation.

Patients should be informed that orthostatic hypotension is most prominent shortly after arising from sleep and when too rapid changes are made to sitting or upright positions. Warn patients to move gradually to sitting position. Some physicians advise patient to slowly flex arms and legs prior to standing to augment venous return. These precautions should be observed throughout drug therapy and for several days after drug is withdrawn.

Patients should also be informed that orthostatic hypotension is intensified by prolonged standing, hot baths or showers, hot weather, alcohol ingestion, and physical exercise (particularly if followed by immobility).

Warn patients to lie down or sit down (in head-low position) immediately at the onset of dizziness, weakness, or faintness. Fainting or blackout occurs when such symptoms are ignored. To control these symptoms, the physician may reduce dosage of guanethidine and prescribe concomitant administration of a thiazide diuretic and another antihypertensive agent, eg, reserpine.

Intake and output should be monitored in patients with limited cardiac reserve or impaired renal function. Report changes in intake–output ratio.

Patients with limited cardiac reserve are particularly susceptible to guanethidine-induced sodium and water retention, with resulting edema, congestive failure, and drug resistance (a thiazide diuretic is generally prescribed to reduce the possibility of these effects).

Observe for evidence of edema, and weigh patients daily (or as prescribed) under standard conditions: same time (preferably in the morning before breakfast and after voiding), same clothing, same scale. Sudden weight gain of 2 lb or more should be reported to physician.

Consult physician regarding allowable salt intake. Generally, patients are advised to omit obviously salty foods and to avoid adding salt to served foods. Physician may prescribe greater restriction of sodium-containing foods for patients with limited cardiac reserve.

Because guanethidine has prolonged onset of action (3 days or more) and duration of effect (4 to 10 days), and since its effects are cumulative, dosage should be increased slowly in the ambulatory patient and only if there has been no decrease in standing blood pressure from previous levels. Blood pressure should be monitored during dosage adjustment.

A limited degree of tolerance may develop early in therapy. Dosage plateau is usually reached in 2 weeks.

Ideal dosage is that which reduces orthostatic blood pressure to within normal range without faintness, dizziness, weakness, or fatigue.

Advise the patient to report character and frequency of stools. Diarrhea due to accelerated GI motility may be manifested by increased frequency of bowel movements rather than loose stools and may be explosive and embarrassing to patient. Physician may prescribe an anticholinergic agent (eg, atropine) or paregoric; dosage adjustment or discontinuation of drug may be required. State of hydration and electrolyte levels should be checked in patients with severe and persistent diarrhea.

Dosage requirements may be reduced in presence of febrile illnesses. Advise patient to report fever to physician.

Guanethidine may sensitize the patient to some sympathomimetic agents found in OTC cold remedies and cause hypertensive crisis. Caution patient to consult physician before taking any OTC drug.

Guanethidine is reported to have antidiabetic activity (mechanism unknown). Patients on antidiabetic therapy should be observed closely for signs of hypoglycemia.

Candidates for home blood pressure measurements are selected on the basis of ability to follow directions, emotional stability, cooperation, and normal hearing.

Assist the patient to develop a record system for sitting and standing blood pressures (as prescribed) to provide physician with information on degree of control achieved.

To reinforce patient compliance in taking drug regularly, suggest that it be taken to coincide with some routine activity, such as brushing teeth in the morning.

A patient teaching plan should include the following: knowledge of the medical problem; drug action (reason for taking drug); dosage regimen; follow-up plans; symptoms to be reported; diet restrictions, if prescribed (eg, salt regulation); weight control plans; instruction in the importance of avoiding alcohol, tobacco, and excessive caffeine (coffee, tea, and colas), as well as emotionally charged situations and self-medication; instruction in the importance of hobbies and regular vacations. The need for long-term therapy should be reinforced continually.

Periodic blood counts and liver and kidney function tests are advised during prolonged therapy.

In patients undergoing elective surgery, guanethidine is generally discontinued or dosage is lowered 2 weeks prior to surgery to reduce the possibility of vascular collapse and cardiac arrest during anesthesia. If emergency surgery is indicated, preanesthetic and anesthetic agents should be administered cautiously in reduced dosages.

DRUG INTERACTIONS: Drugs reported to antagonize the antihypertensive effects of guanethidine include **amphetamines, butyrophenones** (eg, **haloperidol**), **cocaine, diethylpropion, ephedrine, MAO inhibitors, methylphenidate, oral contraceptives, phenothiazines, thioxanthenes** (eg, **thiothixene**), and **tricyclic antidepressants.** Drugs reported to enhance the hypotensive effects of guanethidine include **alcohol, levodopa, methotrimeprazine, rauwolfia derivatives,** and **thiazides** and **related diuretics.** Guanethidine may augment the response to predominantly direct-acting α-adrenergic sympathomimetic amines, eg, **dopamine, epinephrine, levarterenol, metaraminol, methoxamine,** and **phenylephrine.** Additive bradycardic effect may be produced by concomitant administration with **cardiac glycosides.**

H

HALOPERIDOL, U.S.P.
(HALDOL)

Antipsychotic (major tranquilizer)

ACTIONS AND USES

Potent, long-acting butyrophenone derivative with many pharmacologic actions similar to those of piperazine-type phenothiazines, although there is little structural resemblance. Like phenothiazines, it causes a higher incidence of extrapyramidal effects and less sedation and hypotension than other major tranquilizers. Precise mechanism of action not known. Appears to depress CNS at subcortical level, midbrain, and brain-stem reticular formation. Has strong antiemetic effect acting directly on CTZ; inhibits action of catecholamines, including dopamine and norepinephrine. Also has weak central anticholinergic properties, and produces peripheral α-adrenergic blockade.

Used in treatment of agitated states associated with acute and chronic psychoses, including schizophrenia, manic phase of manic–depressive psychosis, psychotic reactions in adults with organic brain syndrome or mental retardation; used in management of tics and vocal utterances of Gilles de la Tourette's disease.

ABSORPTION AND FATE

Well absorbed from GI tract. Plasma levels peak within 2 to 6 hours following oral administration and within 10 minutes following IM administration (peak effect occurs in 30 to 45 minutes). Blood levels may plateau for as long as 72 hours, with detectable blood levels persisting for weeks. Concentrates in liver; about 15% excreted in bile. Approximately 40% of single dose is excreted in urine during first 5 days; small amounts continue to be excreted for about 28 days. Appears in breast milk.

CONTRAINDICATIONS AND PRECAUTIONS

Hypersensitivity to haloperidol; Parkinson's disease; severe mental depression; CNS depression. Safe use during pregnancy and in women of childbearing potential, in nursing mothers, and in pediatric age group not established. Cautious use: history of drug allergies, elderly or debilitated patients, severe cardiovascular disorders, patients receiving anticonvulsant therapy.

ADVERSE REACTIONS

CNS effects (high incidence of extrapyramidal reactions): parkinsonlike symptoms, motor restlessness, dystonia, akathisia, hyperreflexia, torticollis, opisthotonos, oculogyric crisis, persistent tardive dyskinesia (rarely). Other CNS effects: insomnia, restlessness, anxiety, euphoria, agitation, drowsiness, mental depression, lethargy, headache, confusion, vertigo, grand mal seizures, exacerbation of psychotic symptoms. **Autonomic:** dry mouth (or hypersalivation), constipation (or diarrhea), urinary retention, diaphoresis, blurred vision. **Cardiovascular:** tachycardia, hypotension, hypertension (with overdosage). **Hematologic:** mild and usually transient leukopenia, leukocytosis, anemia, tendency toward lymphomonocytosis, agranulocytosis (rarely). **Respiratory:** laryngospasm, bronchospasm, increased depth of respiration, bronchopneumonia, respiratory depression. **Endocrine:** menstrual irregularities, breast pain, lactation, gynecomastia, impotence, increased libido, hyperglycemia, hypoglycemia. **Dermatologic:** maculopapular and acneiform rash and (rarely) photosensitivity and loss of hair. **Other:** anorexia, nausea, vomiting, jaundice (occasionally), variations in liver function tests, possibility of ocular and cutaneous changes, decreased serum cholesterol.

Oral: initially 0.5 to 5 mg 2 or 3 times daily (daily dosages up to 100 mg may be necessary to achieve optimal response in some patients). Following satisfactory response, dosage is gradually decreased to lowest effective maintenance level. Intramuscular: 2 to 5 mg; may be repeated every hour or every 4 to 8 hours as necessary.

NURSING IMPLICATIONS

Although orthostatic hypotension is not common, take necessary safety precautions. Have patient recumbent at time of parenteral administration and for about 1 hour following injection (levarterenol or phenylephrine is prescribed when a vasopressor is indicated; epinephrine is contraindicated).

Extrapyramidal reactions occur frequently during first few days of treatment. Symptoms are usually dose-related and are controlled by dosage reduction or concomitant administration of antiparkinson drugs. Discontinuation of therapy may be necessary. Reactions appear to be more prominent in younger patients. (See Chlorpromazine for description of extrapyramidal effects.)

Be alert for behavioral changes in patients also receiving antiparkinson drugs (eg, benztropine, trihexyphenidyl).

Patients receiving antiparkinson drugs with haloperidol may require their continuation beyond termination of haloperidol therapy to avoid extrapyramidal symptoms (they have different excretion rates).

Haloperidol is administered cautiously to patients receiving anticonvulsant medication because it may lower the convulsant threshold.

When haloperidol is used to control mania or cyclic disorders, the patient should be closely observed for rapid mood shift to depression. Depression may represent a drug side effect or a reversion from a manic state.

Differential diagnosis between extrapyramidal side effects and psychotic reaction requires sensitive observation and prompt reporting.

Fatal bronchospasm associated with use of major tranquilizers has been postulated to result from drug-induced lethargy, reduced sensation of thirst, dehydration, hemoconcentration, and reduced ventilation. Adequate fluid intake and regularly scheduled breathing exercises may help to prevent its occurrence.

Ambulatory patients and responsible family members should be completely informed about drug regimen, symptoms to be reported, and the importance of compliance and follow-up.

Caution the patient to avoid driving a motor vehicle and engaging in other dangerous activities requiring mental alertness and physical coordination.

Periodic blood studies and liver function tests are advised in patients on prolonged therapy.

Preserved in tight, light-resistant containers.

DRUG INTERACTIONS: Haloperidol is additive to or may potentiate the action of other **CNS depressants** (such as **alcohol, barbiturates,** and other **sedatives**), **narcotics** and other **analgesics,** and **tranquilizers.** Haloperidol antagonizes the stimulant effect of **amphetamines**; antagonizes the pressor effects of **epinephrine** (causes paradoxic lowering of blood pressure) and may antagonize the antihypertensive effect of **guanethidine.** Haloperidol may reduce the prothrombin time of **anticoagulants** (close monitoring of prothrombin time is required during concurrent therapy and when haloperidol is discontinued). There is the possibility of increased intraocular pressure when **anticholinergic drugs,** including **antiparkinson agents,** are administered concomitantly.

(DEPO-HEPARIN, HEPATHROM, HEPRINAR, LIPO-HEPIN,
LIQUAEMIN SODIUM, PANHEPRIN)

Anticoagulant

ACTIONS AND USES

Mucopolysaccharide with rapid anticoagulant effect prepared from bovine lung or porcine intestinal mucosa. Believed to exert direct effect on blood coagulation by enhancing action of heparin cofactor (an inhibitor of thrombin), blocking conversion of prothrombin to thrombin and fibrinogen to fibrin. No evidence of fibrinolytic activity and does not block hepatic prothrombin synthesis. Prolongs clotting time but bleeding time usually unaffected. Also reported to exhibit antilipemic, antiinflammatory, and diuretic effects.

Used in prophylaxis and treatment of thromboses and emboli and to prevent thromboembolic complications arising from arterial and cardiac surgery. Also used as anticoagulant in blood transfusions, extracorporeal circulation, dialysis procedures, and blood samples for laboratory purposes. Value in treatment of hyperlipemia and as prophylaxis in myocardial infarction and angina pectoris not definitely established.

ABSORPTION AND FATE

Almost immediate action following IV administration. Peak effect in 5 to 10 minutes; clotting time returns to normal within 2 to 6 hours. Onset of action following SC administration occurs in about one hour; effects may persist 12 to 16 hours. Extensively bound to plasma proteins. Some uptake with storage in mast cells. Inactivated in liver and excreted slowly in urine as partially degraded heparin; 20% to 25% of single dose excreted in active form. Does not cross placenta or appear in breast milk.

CONTRAINDICATIONS AND PRECAUTIONS

Contraindications: hypersensitivity to heparin, uncontrollable bleeding, bleeding tendencies, (hemophilia, purpura, jaundice, thrombocytopenia), ulcerative lesions, open wounds, ascorbic acid deficiency; severe liver or kidney disease, subacute bacterial endocarditis, continuous tube drainage of stomach or small intestines, threatened abortion; during or following surgery of brain, spinal cord, or eye; shock. Safe use during pregnancy and in persons of childbearing potential not established. Cautious use: hypertension, mesenteric thrombosis, biliary tract surgery, mild liver or kidney disease, alcoholism, history of allergy or asthma; during menstruation, immediate postpartum period, patients with indwelling catheters; when administering ACD-converted blood (may contain heparin); patients in hazardous occupations.

ADVERSE REACTIONS

Spontaneous bleeding, injection site reactions, diarrhea, transient alopecia, paresthesias; acute reversible thrombocytopenia, hypofibrinogenemia (usually following IV). Rarely priapism; hypersensitivity reactions: fever, chills, urticaria, pruritus, burning sensations, rhinitis, lacrimation, anaphylactoid reactions. Large doses for prolonged periods: osteoporosis with spontaneous fractures, hypoaldosteronism, suppressed renal function. Rebound hyperlipemia (after discontinuation of heparin).

ROUTE AND DOSAGE

(Dose determination depends upon patient's partial thromboplastin time). Deep subcutaneous (intrafat), intramuscular (rarely used): initial, 10,000 to 20,000 units, then 8,000 to 10,000 units every 8 hours or 12,000 to 20,000 units every 12 hours. Intravenous (continuous infusion): 10,000 to 40,000 units added to 1000 ml of infusion solution (utilizing IV infusion pump and a volumetric administration set if available). Intravenous (intermittent injection): 5,000 to 10,000 units every 4 to 6 hours (undiluted or diluted with 50 to 100 ml Isotonic Sodium Chloride Injection). Total body perfusion (open heart surgery): 150 to 400 units/kg IV. Hyperlipemia: 20,000 to 40,000 units deep SC, 2 or 3 times

arterial blood line prior to dialysis; usual sustaining dose: 1,000 to 2,500 units/
hour throughout dialysis. Follow equipment manufacturer's directions.

NURSING IMPLICATIONS

Read label carefully. Heparin comes in various strengths and in regular as
well as repository forms.

Patient should be hospitalized during heparin therapy.

Before administering heparin, coagulation (clotting) time results must be
checked by physician and dose order obtained. Follow agency policy.

Coagulation assays, HCT, leukocyte, and platelet counts should be made
before therapy is initiated to establish baseline measurements.

Commonly used test to monitor heparin therapy is the activated partial
thromboplastin time (APTT). In general, dosage is adjusted to keep APTT
between 1½ and 2½ times control level.

Accurate observations of clinical response and careful titration of doses
based on blood coagulation tests are critically important. Patients vary
widely in their response to heparin.

Since thrombocytopenia has recently been observed in a significant number
of patients during heparin treatment, careful monitoring of platelet count
advised. Reduction in platelet count reported to occur 2 to 10 days after
initiation of heparin; returns to normal levels 3 to 5 days following discontinuation of therapy.

For SC (intrafat) and IM administration, clotting time is usually determined
before each injection.

Deep SC heparin injection is made preferably into fatty layer of abdomen or above iliac crest. Do not use areas within 2 inches of um-
bilicus or any scar. Discard needle used to withdraw medication from
container. For accuracy, use a tuberculin syringe and a 25 or 26 gauge,
½ to ⅝ inch needle. Sponge selected area with alcohol and allow to
dry (rubbing may traumatize tissue). Suggested technic for intrafat injection: gently bunch up a defined roll of fat tissue without pinching,
and insert needle at 90° angle to skin surface. Do not withdraw plunger to check entry into blood vessel. Still maintaining hold of tissue
roll and keeping needle steady, slowly inject drug. Withdraw needle in
same direction as introduced while simultaneously releasing tissue.
Apply gentle pressure to puncture site for 5 to 10 seconds but do not
massage. Rotate injection sites.

During dosage adjustment period, coagulation tests are performed before
each SC or IM injection. After dosage is established, tests may be done
once daily (4 hours after last IV injection or 1 hour before next SC dose).

The "Z track" technic may also be used: skin layer of a fat roll is grasped and
lifted upward. Needle is inserted at approximately 45° angle to skin surface. Following drug injection, remove needle rapidly while simultaneously releasing tissue. Do not aspirate to see if blood vessel has been
entered and do not massage following injection.

IM route is generally not ordered because of risk of hemorrhage and
hematoma.

If other drugs are ordered IM, their administration should be timed when
patient has minimal prolongation of coagulation time. This also pertains
to invasive procedures, eg, catheterizations, enemas.

Construct a flow sheet indicating date, coagulation time determinations,
heparin doses, and location of injection sites.

When intermittent IV doses are given, clotting times should be determined
prior to each injection.

Prescribed flow rate for continuous IV infusions must be closely monitored
to assure accuracy in dosage. Clotting times should be determined at

4-hour intervals and dosage adjusted accordingly. Check at least hourly for signs of infiltration. In the event of infiltration or phlebitis, site should be changed. Follow hospital policy for daily care of IV infusion site.

When a roller pump is used, care should be taken to avoid negative pressure at infusion site which may increase rate of heparin administered into system. Check level in drip chamber at least every 2 hours to evaluate actual dosage being infused and to make sure pump is working properly. Pump should be out of reach of patient; check frequently for kinks or leaks.

Absorption of repository preparation is irregular in rate and quantitatively unpredictable; therefore, risk of unexpected bleeding is greater than with rapid-acting forms. Observe patient closely.

Inform patient that heparin may have a diuretic effect beginning 36 to 48 hours after initial dose and continuing 36 to 48 hours after termination of therapy.

Examine urine and stools for evidence of bleeding; instruct ambulatory patient to report dark colored or black stools or unusual color of urine.

Some physicians prescribe serial hematocrit, urine and stool studies to detect occult bleeding.

Monitor vital signs. Report fever, drop in blood pressure, rapid pulse, or other signs of bleeding.

Have on hand protamine sulfate (neutralizes effect of heparin). In some cases whole blood or plasma transfusion may be necessary.

Most common bleeding sites: GI and GU tracts, wounds, nose. Examine body daily, especially hands, lower legs, feet, sacrum for evidence of bruises, petechiae, or purpura. Petechiae of soft palate, conjunctiva, and retina are characteristic signs of thrombocytopenia. Low back pain may be indicative of abdominal bleeding.

Preliminary reports indicate that risk of hemorrhage is greatest in women over 60 years of age. Regardless of sex and age, hemorrhagic complications occur with high frequency when drug is given prophylactically following surgery, and when administered intermittently by IV injection (in contrast to continuous IV infusion).

Menstruation may be increased and prolonged. Usually this is not a contraindication to continued therapy if bleeding is not excessive and patient has no underlying pathology.

In the absence of a low platelet count, patient may carry out normal activities such as shaving with a safety razor. (Usually heparin does not affect bleeding time.)

Transient alopecia sometimes occurs several months after heparin therapy. Reassure patient that condition is temporary.

Smoking and alcohol consumption may cause altered responses to heparin and therefore are not advised. Caution patient not to take aspirin, cough preparations containing glyceryl guaiacolate or any other OTC medications without physician's approval.

Abrupt withdrawal of heparin may precipitate increased coagulability. Generally, full dose heparin is followed by oral anticoagulant prophylactic therapy.

Administration of an oral anticoagulant usually overlaps that of heparin for 3 to 5 days while heparin is being tapered off. To obtain valid prothrombin time, a period of 4 to 5 hours after last IV dose, and 12 to 24 hours after last SC dose of heparin should elapse before blood is drawn.

Heparin should be protected from freezing.

LABORATORY TEST INTERFERENCES: False elevations of: plasma corticosteroids (heparin containing benzyl alcohol), and sulfobromophthalein test (BSP).

DRUG INTERACTIONS: Drugs that may increase risk of bleeding; **oral anticoagulants, aspirin, cancer chemotherapeutic agents, dextran, dipyridamole, ethacrynic acid (IV), glyceryl guaiacolate, phenylbutazone, probenecid, quinine.** Drugs that may partially counteract anticoagulant action of heparin: **antihistamines, digitalis, nicotine, protamine** (may be used clinically as antagonist) **tetracyclines.** Many drugs are incompatible with parenteral heparin; therefore, avoid mixing with any drug unless specifically prescribed by physician or clinical pharmacist.

HETACILLIN POTASSIUM
(VERSAPEN, VERSAPEN-K)

Antibacterial

ACTIONS AND USES
Semisynthetic penicillin prepared by reaction of ampicillin with acetone. Rapidly converted to ampicillin in body. Actions, uses, contraindications, precautions, and adverse reactions essentially identical to those of ampicillin (qv).

ABSORPTION AND FATE
Well absorbed from GI tract. Peak serum levels in 2 to 3 hours. Blood levels decrease slowly; low concentrations still present in serum 8 hours after administration. About 20% bound to plasma proteins. Penetrates cerebrospinal fluid only when meninges are inflamed. Partially metabolized in liver. Excreted largely unchanged in urine and bile. Crosses placenta and appears in breast milk.

ROUTE AND DOSAGE
Oral: *Patients weighing 40 kg or more:* 225 to 450 mg 4 times daily. *Patients weighing less than 40 kg:* 22.5 to 45 mg/kg/day. All dosages individualized according to severity of infection.

NURSING IMPLICATIONS
Food retards drug's absorption; administer in fasting state (eg, at least 1 hour before or 2 hours after meals). Absorption is enhanced by giving drug with a full glass of water.
Infections due to group A β-hemolytic streptococci should be treated for a minimum of 10 days.
Patients with urinary or GI tract infections may require therapy for several weeks and bacteriologic and/or clinical follow-up for several months after drug is discontinued.
Reconstituted oral liquid formulations are stable 14 days under refrigeration. See Ampicillin.

HEXACHLOROPHENE, U.S.P.
(GAMOPHEN, PHISOHEX, SOY-DOME CLEANSER, WESCOHEX)
HEXACHLOROPHANE, B.P.

Topical antiinfective, detergent

ACTIONS AND USES
Polychlorinated phenol derivative. Bacteriostatic against Gram-positive bacteria, especially strains of staphylococci. Less active against Gram-negative organisms; has little effect on spores. Effectiveness depends on adsorption of antibacterial residue on skin that resists removal by water, soaps, and detergents for several days. Cumulative antibacterial action develops with repeated use. The Food and Drug Administration now disapproves of incorporating hexachlorophene in cosmetics and OTC deodorant soaps and powders because of potential systemic absorption.

Used for surgical scrub and as bacteriostatic skin cleanser. May also be used, only as long as necessary, to control an outbreak of Gram-positive infection when other procedures have been unsuccessful.

CONTRAINDICATIONS AND PRECAUTIONS

Sensitivity to any of its components; primary light sensitivity to halogenated phenol derivatives; use with premature infants; use on burned or denuded skin; use as occlusive dressing, wet pack, or lotion; use for vaginal pack or tampon; application to any mucous membranes, to large surface areas, or for prophylactic total body bathing.

ADVERSE REACTIONS

Sensitization (photosensitivity, dermatitis, erythema, scaling). **Systemic toxicity** (from absorption or accidental ingestion): CNS irritation manifested by dizziness, headache, confusion, diplopia, miosis, twitching, irritability, convulsions, respiratory arrest; diarrhea; abdominal distention and pain; anorexia; nausea; vomiting; hypotension; shock.

ROUTE AND DOSAGE

Topical: 3% emulsion, liquid soap.

NURSING IMPLICATIONS

A single application has little more effect than nonmedicated soaps. Regular and repeated applications are required to build up antibacterial residue (maximal concentration reached in 2 to 4 days).

Presence of organic matter (eg, pus, serum) reduces activity of hexachlorophene, but activity is retained in the presence of soaps, oils, and vehicles for topical application.

Infants, especially premature infants or those with dermatoses, are particularly susceptible to hexachlorophene absorption.

Hexachlorophene should be rinsed thoroughly with clear water, especially from sensitive areas such as scrotum, to prevent possibility of systemic absorption. Do not use alcohol or alcohol-containing products, since they remove the antibacterial residue.

Hexachlorophene may produce erythema, dryness, and scaling in patients with sensitive skin, especially when combined with excessive rubbing or exposure to heat or cold.

Discontinue immediately if signs of cerebral irritability or other adverse reactions (suggestive of absorption) occur.

If drug contacts eyes, rinse out promptly and thoroughly with water.

Accidental ingestion: If patient is seen early, stomach is evacuated by emesis or gastric lavage. Olive oil or vegetable oil (60 ml) may then be given to delay drug absorption, followed by a saline cathartic to hasten removal. IV fluids, electrolyte replacement, and vasopressor therapy may then be required.

Do not pour hexachlorophene into a medicine cup, medicine bottle, or similar container, since it may be mistaken for baby formula or other medication.

Preserved in tightly covered, light-resistant containers.

HEXOCYCLIUM METHYLSULFATE
(TRAL)

Anticholinergic

ACTIONS AND USES

Synthetic quaternary ammonium compound with antisecretory and antispasmodic effects qualitatively similar to those of atropine. Contraindications,

precautions, and adverse effects essentially as for atropine (qv).
Used in adjunctive management of peptic ulcer and other GI disorders associated with hyperacidity, hypermotility, and spasm.

ABSORPTION AND FATE
Degree of absorption varies among individuals. Effects persist 3 to 4 hours (approximately 10 hours with sustained-release tablet). Metabolic fate and route of excretion not known.

CONTRAINDICATIONS AND PRECAUTIONS
Safe use during pregnancy or lactation and in children not established. Also see Atropine.

ADVERSE REACTIONS
Blurred vision, dry mouth, urinary hesitancy or retention, drowsiness, palpitation, tachycardia, mental confusion and/or excitement, especially in the elderly. Also see Atropine.

ROUTE AND DOSAGE
Oral: 25 mg 4 times daily, before meals and at bedtime. Sustained-release tablet: 50 mg 2 times daily, before lunch and at bedtime or before breakfast and before evening meal. Highly individualized.

NURSING IMPLICATIONS
Because of the possibility of drowsiness and blurred vision, caution the patient to avoid hazardous work and activities requiring mental alertness, such as operating a motor vehicle or dangerous machinery, while taking the drug. Also advise elderly patients to be careful when climbing or descending stairs and when getting out of bed.

First signs of overdosage may be flushing of skin and increased intensity of mouth dryness.

Sustained-release tablet should not be chewed.

Caution patients to avoid high environmental temperature; heat prostration can occur due to decreased sweating.

See Atropine Sulfate.

HOMATROPINE HYDROBROMIDE, U.S.P., B.P.
(HOMATROCEL, ISOPTO HOMATROPINE)

Anticholinergic (ophthalmic)

ACTIONS AND USES
Synthetic alkaloid with actions, contraindications, precautions, and adverse reactions similar to those of atropine (qv). Preferred to atropine for certain ophthalmologic purposes because its mydriatic and cycloplegic actions occur more rapidly and are less prolonged. Cycloplegia is usually incomplete unless applications are made repeatedly.
Used as mydriatic for ocular examination and as cycloplegic to measure errors of refraction. Also used in treatment of iritis, iridocyclitis, and ciliary spasm and as cycloplegic and mydriatic in preoperative and postoperative conditions.

ABSORPTION AND FATE
Following instillation, maximal paralysis of accommodation and mydriatic effects occur in 30 to 60 minutes, with recovery in 1 to 3 days.

CONTRAINDICATIONS AND PRECAUTIONS
Hypersensitivity; glaucoma; children under 6 years of age. Cautious use: patients with narrow anterior chamber angle; children; the elderly; hypertension; hyperthyroidism; diabetes. Also see Atropine.

Increased intraocular pressure. With prolonged use: local irritation, congestion, and edema; eczema; follicular conjunctivitis. Excessive dosage: symptoms of atropine poisoning. See Atropine.

ROUTE AND DOSAGE

Topical: 1 or 2 drops of 1% to 5% solution instilled in eye 1 to 3 times a day. For refraction: 1 or 2 drops of 2% solution every 10 to 15 minutes for 5 doses; or 1 or 2 drops of 5% solution, repeated in 15 minutes.

NURSING IMPLICATIONS

Determinations of intraocular pressure and width of anterior chamber angle (gonioscopy) are advised before and during drug use, particularly if therapy is intensive or prolonged. Drug may increase intraocular pressure even in the normal eye.

Systemic absorption may be minimized by applying pressure against inner canthus of eye (lacrimal duct) for 1 or 2 minutes after each instillation. This is particularly advisable when stronger solutions are used. See Demecarium Bromide for instillation technique.

Recommended dosage should not be exceeded.

Frequent and continued use or overdosage may produce symptoms of atropine poisoning.

Advise the patient to report immediately the onset of eye pain, changes in visual acuity, rapid pulse, or dizziness. Drug should be discontinued if these symptoms occur.

Advise the patient to report dryness of mouth. This symptom may be relieved by reduction in dosage.

Photophobia associated with mydriasis may require patient to wear dark glasses.

Since the drug produces blurred vision, advise the patient against driving and other hazardous activities until effect disappears.

See Atropine Sulfate.

HOMATROPINE METHYLBROMIDE, N.F.
(HOMAPIN, MALCOTRAN, NOVATRIN)

Anticholinergic, antispasmodic

ACTIONS AND USES

Semisynthetic quaternary ammonium derivative of belladonna alkaloids. Actions, contraindications, precautions, and adverse reactions as for atropine (qv). Has less antimuscarinic activity than atropine, but is reported to be 4 times more potent as a ganglionic blocking agent, and has no CNS action.

Used in treatment of peptic and duodenal ulcer, pylorospasm, functional diarrhea, hypermotility states, spasticity of colon and biliary tract. Also used in dysmenorrhea to relieve uterine hypertonicity. Commercially available in combination with phenobarbital, eg, Homapin PB, Spasticol S.A.

ROUTE AND DOSAGE

Oral: 2.5 to 10 mg 4 times a day, before meals.

NURSING IMPLICATIONS

Since the drug may produce dizziness and blurred vision, advise the patient against driving and other hazardous activities until his reaction to the drug has been determined.

Preserved in tight, light-resistant containers.

See Atropine Sulfate.

(ALIDASE, WYDASE)

Spreading agent

ACTIONS AND USES
   Mucolytic enzyme prepared from purified bovine testicular hyaluronidase. Hydrolyzes hyaluronic acid, which normally obstructs intercellular diffusion of invasive substances. Promotes diffusion and consequently absorption of transudates, exudates, and injected fluids.
   Used to enhance dispersion and absorption of other injected drugs; used for hypodermoclysis, and as adjunct in subcutaneous urography for improving resorption of radiopaque agents.

CONTRAINDICATIONS AND PRECAUTIONS
   Injection into or around inflamed, infected, or cancerous areas; congestive heart failure; hypoproteinemia.

ADVERSE REACTIONS
   Infrequent: sensitivity, spread of infectious processes, overhydration.

ROUTE AND DOSAGE
   For absorption and dispersion of injected drugs: 150 N.F. units. *Hypodermoclysis:* 150 N.F. units added to clysis (injected into rubber tubing, close to needle) or injected subcutaneously prior to clysis (150 N.F. units will facilitate absorption of 1000 ml or more of solution). *Subcutaneous urography:* 75 N.F. units.

NURSING IMPLICATIONS

Preliminary skin test for sensitivity is advised. Approximately 0.02 ml is injected intradermally by physician; positive reaction consists of wheal with pseudopods and localized itching within 5 minutes, persisting 20 to 30 minutes. Erythema alone is not a positive reaction.

Addition of hyaluronidase to hypodermoclyses may promote overhydration because it speeds water absorption. Infusion flow rate should be prescribed by physician.

When it is used to increase diffusion of a drug, bear in mind that absorption will be enhanced. Therefore, watch for adverse reactions and expect a shorter duration of action.

Lyophilized form is reconstituted with sodium chloride injection just before use (usually in the proportion of 1 ml per 150 N.F. units of hyaluronidase).

Store in cool, dry place.

HYDRALAZINE HYDROCHLORIDE, N.F.

(APRESOLINE, LOPRESS)

HYDRALLAZINE HYDROCHLORIDE, B.P.

Antihypertensive

ACTIONS AND USES
   The only phthalazine used clinically in North America. Reduces blood pressure by direct relaxation of vascular smooth muscles, with greater effect on arterioles than on veins. Diastolic response is often greater than systolic. Resulting vasodilation reduces peripheral vascular resistance and increases renal and cerebral blood flow. Has little effect on capacitance blood vessels. Antihypertensive effect may be limited by sympathetic reflexes, which cause increased heart rate, stroke volume, and cardiac output. Postural hypotensive effect is reportedly less than that produced by ganglionic blocking agents. Usually increases plasma renin activity.

Used alone, but most commonly as adjunct with other drugs, for management of essential hypertension. May be used in early malignant hypertension and in hypertension that persists after sympathectomy.

ABSORPTION AND FATE

Following oral administration, peak plasma concentrations reached in 3 to 4 hours; small amounts detectable for as long as 24 hours. Antihypertensive effect occurs gradually over 15 minutes following IM injection and lasts 3 to 4 hours. Blood pressure begins to fall within a few minutes following IV injection; maximal effect in 10 to 80 minutes. Metabolized in liver. Less than 5% excreted unchanged in urine together with approximately same amount of metabolites. Excretion rate greatest between 2 and 10 hours after dose.

CONTRAINDICATIONS AND PRECAUTIONS

Hypersensitivity to hydralazine, coronary artery disease, mitral valvular rheumatic heart disease, myocardial infarction, tachycardia, lupus erythematosus (LE). Safe use during pregnancy not established. Cautious use: cerebrovascular accident; advanced renal impairment; use with MAO inhibitors.

ADVERSE REACTIONS

Common: headache, palpitation, angina pectoris, anorexia, tachycardia, nausea, vomiting, diarrhea, sweating. **Less frequent:** nasal congestion, flushing, lacrimation, hypotension, paradoxic pressor response, conjunctivitis, peripheral neuritis, vertigo, dyspnea on exertion, tremors, muscle cramps, psychotic reactions (depression, anxiety, disorientation), hypersensitivity (rash, urticaria, pruritus, fever, chills, hepatitis [rare]), dysuria, difficult micturition, paralytic ileus, constipation, rheumatoid or LE-like syndrome (fever, arthralgia, malaise, splenomegaly, lymphadenopathy, edema, dermatitis, positive direct Coombs' test, presence of LE cells in peripheral blood), blood dyscrasias (reduced hemoglobin and red cell count, leukopenia, agranulocytosis, purpura). **Overdosage:** headache, generalized skin flushing, myocardial ischemia, arrhythmias, profound shock.

ROUTE AND DOSAGE

Oral: initially 10 mg 4 times daily for 2 to 4 days, increased to 25 mg 4 times daily for balance of first week; for second and subsequent weeks 50 mg 4 times daily. For maintenance, dosage is adjusted to lowest effective level. Highly individualized. Intramuscular, intravenous: 10 to 40 mg repeated every 6 hours, if necessary.

NURSING IMPLICATIONS

Complete blood count, LE cell preparation, and antinuclear antibody titer determinations are advised before initiation of therapy and periodically during prolonged therapy.

Observe mental status; note anxiety, depression, obtundation (signs of cerebral ischemia from too rapid reduction in blood pressure).

Blood pressure should be closely monitored in patients receiving parenteral hydralazine. Check every 5 minutes until stabilized at desired level, then every 15 minutes thereafter throughout hypertensive crisis.

A marked fall in blood pressure may further compromise renal blood flow in patients with renal damage and result in reduced urinary output.

Intake and output should be monitored when drug is given parenterally and in those with renal dysfunction. Output may be increased in some patients because of improved renal blood flow.

Instruct patient to monitor weight and to check for edema. Advise patient to report sudden gain or apparent slow increase in weight, and the onset of edema.

Most patients receiving parenteral hydralazine are transferred to oral form within 24 to 48 hours.

It may help home patients to remember to take oral medication if it is scheduled after meals and at bedtime (when ordered 4 times daily).

Some patients experience headache and palpitation within 2 to 4 hours after first oral dose. Symptoms usually subside spontaneously. Advise patients to inform physician of adverse reactions; most can be controlled by dose reduction.

Physician may prescribe pyridoxine (vitamin B_6) for patients who develop symptoms of peripheral neuritis (paresthesias, numbness). This complication is believed to result from antipyridoxine effect of hydralazine.

Because of the possibility of postural hypotension, caution patients to make position changes slowly, particularly from lying to sitting position and from sitting to standing, and to avoid standing still, taking hot baths and showers, strenuous exercise, and excessive alcohol intake.

Caution patient to lie down or sit down (in head-low position) if he feels faint or dizzy. Patients who engage in potentially hazardous activities such as driving or operating machinery should be advised of the possibility of these symptoms.

In patients with marked blood pressure reduction, withdrawal of hydralazine is accomplished gradually to avoid sudden rise in pressure.

An LE cell preparation is indicated if patient manifests arthralgia, fever, chest pain, malaise, or other unexplained signs and symptoms.

LE manifestations usually regress after drug is withdrawn; however, some residual effects may continue 7 to 8 years.

Stress the importance of follow-up care. Some patients develop tolerance during chronic drug administration requiring higher dosages or a change in drug regimen.

DRUG INTERACTIONS: Intensification of vasodilatory effects (reduced pressor response) may occur when hydralazine is used concomitantly with **epinephrine.** An additive hypotensive effect is possible with concomitant administration of hydralazine and other **antihypertensive agents, diuretics, MAO inhibitors, procainamide** and **quinidine.**

HYDROCHLORIC ACID, DILUTED, U.S.P., B.P.

Acidifier (gastric)

ACTIONS AND USES
Gastric hydrochloric acid is essential for conversion of pepsinogen to active pepsin (important for protein digestion), activation of pancreatic and hepatic secretions, stimulation of secretin, and neutralization of bicarbonates of intestinal secretions, thus helping to maintain electrolyte balance. It also has germicidal effects on numerous bacteria.

Used in hydrochloric acid deficiency states, as in pernicious anemia, gastric carcinoma, chronic gastritis, and idiopathic achlorhydria.

CONTRAINDICATIONS AND PRECAUTIONS
Hyperacidity, peptic ulcer.

ADVERSE REACTIONS
Prolonged use of high doses; depletion of bicarbonate and rise of serum chloride; metabolic acidosis.

ROUTE AND DOSAGE
Oral: 2 to 8 ml (10% solution) 3 times daily.

NURSING IMPLICATIONS
Administer well diluted (at least 150 to 250 ml of water) through glass drinking tube in order to prevent damage to tooth enamel. Tell the patient

that the taste is sour, and instruct him to place tube well back into mouth and to sip slowly.

Medication may be prescribed to be taken during meals or immediately after meals. If taken after meals, follow immediately with alkaline mouthwash.

Observe and record therapeutic effects. Symptoms of achlorhydria are poorly defined, but may consist of vague epigastric distress after meals, belching, abdominal distension, coated tongue, nausea, vomiting, and morning diarrhea.

Physician may prescribe high-alkaline diet consisting of citrus fruits and green vegetables or alkalinizing salts to help maintain acid–base balance.

With large doses, acid–base status should be checked every few days after start of therapy and periodically during therapy.

HYDROCHLOROTHIAZIDE, U.S.P., B.P.
(DIUCEN-H, ESIDRIX, HydroDIURIL, HYDROMAL, HYDRO-Z-50, LEXOR, ORETIC, RO-HYDRAZIDE, THIURETIC, X-AQUA)

Diuretic (thiazide), antihypertensive

ACTIONS AND USES

Benzothiadiazine (thiazide) derivative. Similar to chlorothiazide (qv) in actions, uses, contraindications, precautions, and adverse reactions. Causes less carbonic anhydrase inhibition and (on weight basis) is reported to have 5 to 10 times more natriuretic activity than chlorothiazide. Available in combination with several antihypertensive agents.

ABSORPTION AND FATE

Onset of diuretic effect in 2 hours; peaks in 4 to 6 hours; duration 6 to 12 hours. Excreted unchanged by kidneys within 24 hours. Also see Chlorothiazide.

CONTRAINDICATIONS AND PRECAUTIONS

Hypersensitivity to thiazides or sulfonamides; anuria; nursing mothers. Cautious use: bronchial asthma, allergy, hepatic cirrhosis.

ADVERSE REACTIONS

Nausea, vomiting, vertigo, pulmonary edema (rarely), allergic pneumonitis, activation of gout, lupus erythematosus, hyperglycemia. Also see Chlorothiazide.

ROUTE AND DOSAGE

Oral: **Adults:** *Edema:* initially 25 to 200 mg daily for several days or until nonedematous weight is attained; maintenance: 25 to 100 mg daily or intermittently; some patients may require up to 200 mg daily. *Hypertension:* initially 75 mg daily; may be given as single dose every morning; maintenance: after 1 week, dosage adjusted downward to as little as 25 mg/day or upward to as much as 100 mg daily (dosage determined by patient's blood pressure response). Some patients may require up to 200 mg daily. **Pediatric:** usual dosage based on 1 mg/lb body weight. Infants under 6 months of age may require up to 1.5 mg/lb daily in 2 doses.

NURSING IMPLICATIONS

See Chlorothiazide.

HYDROCODONE BITARTRATE, N.F.
(DICODID, Dihydrocodeinone Bitartrate)

Antitussive (narcotic)

ACTIONS AND USES
Morphine derivative similar to codeine, but more addicting and with slightly greater antitussive activity. See Morphine.
Used for symptomatic relief of hyperactive or nonproductive cough. A common ingredient in a variety of proprietary mixtures.

ROUTE AND DOSAGE
Adults: Oral: 5 to 10 mg 3 or 4 times a day, if necessary. **Children:** 0.6 mg/kg daily in divided doses.

NURSING IMPLICATIONS
Administer the syrup undiluted for optimum effect.
Antitussive action may last 4 to 6 hours.
Caution patients not to take larger doses than prescribed. Psychic and physical dependence and tolerance may develop with repeated administration.
Classified as schedule II drug under federal Controlled Substances Act of 1970.
Preserved in tight, light-resistant containers.
See Morphine Sulfate.

HYDROCORTISONE, U.S.P., B.P.
(CORT-DOME, CORTEF, DERMACORT, HYDROCORTONE, ROCORT and others)
HYDROCORTISONE ACETATE, U.S.P., B.P.
(CORTEF ACETATE, CORTIFOAM, HYDROCORT, and others)
HYDROCORTISONE CYPIONATE, N.F.
HYDROCORTISONE SODIUM PHOSPHATE, U.S.P.
HYDROCORTISONE SODIUM SUCCINATE, U.S.P., B.P.
(SOLU-CORTEF)

Adrenocortical steroid (glucocorticoid, mineralocorticoid)

ACTIONS AND USES
Short-acting synthetic steroid with strong glucocorticoid actions and, in high doses, mineralocorticoid properties. Promotes synthesis of glucose in liver, but decreases glucose utilization by all but hepatic cells, thus predisposing patient on high doses to diabetes mellitus. Stimulates synthesis of enzyme protein in liver, but inhibits peripheral protein synthesis, leading to severe protein wasting. Interrupts normal linear growth in children. Required for mobilization of fatty acids, but inhibits their production. Displays anti-vitamin-D activity (leading to interference with calcium absorption from GI tract), and produces tendency toward gastroduodenal ulceration; supports peripheral vascular responsiveness to catecholamine. Antiinflammatory effects: prevents or suppresses clinical phenomena of inflammation and interferes with tissue granulation and repair. Immunosuppressive effects: decreased number of circulating eosinophils and lymphocytes, reduction in antibody titers, and suppressed cell-mediated hypersensitivity reactions. Does not prevent antigen–antibody union; may block induction of immune response. Mineralocorticoid effects result in

sodium retention and potassium excretion, preservation of normal water distribution, and ability to excrete water load normally. High doses may cause cerebral dysfunction leading to depression, disorientation, and euphoria. Suppresses ACTH and melanocyte-stimulating hormone elaboration. Used as replacement therapy in adrenocortical insufficiency, to suppress undesirable inflammatory or immune responses, to produce temporary remission in nonadrenal disease, and to block ACTH production in diagnostic tests. Specific indications include: connective-tissue diseases, pemphigus, alopecia areata, shock unresponsive to conventional therapy, ocular inflammatory conditions, neoplastic disease of lymphatic system, metastatic mammary carcinoma, allergic states, chronic ulcerative colitis, nephrotic syndrome.

ABSORPTION AND FATE

Absorbed from skin and synovial membranes. Complete and rapid absorption from GI tract; absorption following IM injection is slow, continuing 24 to 48 hours. Enters circulation, where it is irreversibly bound to transcortin. Biotransformation in liver; plasma half-life 60 to 90 minutes, with maximum effects 2 to 8 hours after oral dose. Excreted in urine principally as 17-hydroxycorticosteroids and 17-ketogenic steroids. Crosses placenta.

CONTRAINDICATIONS AND PRECAUTIONS

Active or latent peptic ulcer, psychoses, acute glomerulonephritis, systemic fungal disease, viral diseases of skin, active or arrested tuberculosis, Cushing's syndrome, infections not controlled by antibiotics, ocular herpes simplex, myasthenia gravis. Safe use in women of childbearing potential and during pregnancy and lactation not established. Topical steroids are contraindicated in presence of varicella, vaccinia, and markedly impaired circulation. Cautious use: in children, diabetes mellitus, hepatitis, cardiovascular and renal disease, glaucoma, osteoporosis, convulsive disorders, hypothyroidism, infectious diseases, diverticulitis, nonspecific ulcerative colitis.

ADVERSE REACTIONS

Fluid and electrolyte disturbances (such as calcium and potassium loss, sodium retention). **Cardiovascular:** hypertension, hypotension, thrombophlebitis, necrotizing angiitis. **Musculoskeletal:** muscle wasting, osteoporosis, pathologic fractures. **GI:** nausea, vomiting, peptic ulcer, pancreatitis, abdominal distension, ulcerative esophagitis. **Dermatologic:** hyperhydrosis, purpura, striae, thin or fragile skin, acneiform eruptions, hypopigmentation, hirsutism. **Neurologic:** convulsions, increased intracranial pressure with papilledema, syncope, headache, insomnia, mood swings, personality changes, aggravation of preexisting psychiatric disorders. **Endocrine:** iatrogenic hyperadrenocorticism, menstrual irregularities, sterility, virilization, suppressed linear growth in children, steroid diabetes (reversible), activation of latent diabetes mellitus. **Ophthalmic:** posterior subcapsular cataracts (usually irreversible), increased intraocular pressure, glaucoma, exophthalmos. Other: impaired healing, masked infections, negative nitrogen balance, hypersensitivity, anaphylactic reactions, renal calculi, obesity. **Altered laboratory test values:** elevated serum cholesterol and triglycerides, moderate elevation of serum uric acid, decreased ^{131}I uptake, retarded erythrocyte sedimentation rate.

ROUTE AND DOSAGE

Oral initial dose large enough to suppress symptoms of condition under treatment, then reduced to lowest effective level; daily schedule, usually 4 times per day; (replacement): 10 to 25 mg daily; (antiinflammatory): 40 to 80 mg daily. Intravenous (emergency, surgery, trauma): 100 mg infused slowly over period of 2 to 10 hours depending on severity of condition. Intramuscular: 50 to 300 mg. Intraarticular (acetate): 5 to 50 mg. Topical: creams, ointments, lotions, solutions 0.125% to 2.5%. **Children:** approximately 80% of cortisone dose.

NURSING IMPLICATIONS

Carefully check label for recommended route of administration.

Before corticosteroid therapy is started, a skin test for tuberculosis may be done.

Inject IM preparation deep into upper outer quadrant of buttock. Avoid inadvertent subcutaneous injection, which may produce "pseudoatrophy" with persistent depression of overlying dermis, lasting several weeks or months.

Cortisol concentrations in human plasma are maximal between 2 A.M. and 8 A.M. and minimal between 4 P.M. and 12 midnight. Exogenous corticosteroids suppress adrenal cortex activity less when given in the morning, the time of maximum activity; to minimize, suppression replacement steroid may be given in divided doses: two-thirds in morning, one-third in evening.

Establish baseline and continuing data regarding blood pressure, intake-output ratio and pattern, weight, and sleep pattern. Start flow chart as reference for planning individualized patient care indicated by drug response.

Two-hour postprandial blood glucose, serum potassium, chest x-ray, and routine laboratory studies are performed at regular intervals during long-term steroid therapy. If patient has a history of diabetes mellitus, urine should be tested for glucosuria daily.

Opthalmoscopic examinations including tonometer tests are recommended every 2 to 3 months, especially if patient is receiving topical steroid treatment.

Monitor patient's weight under standard conditions. Inform the patient that a slight weight gain with improved appetite is expected, but after dosage stablization has been achieved, a sudden or slow but steady weight increase (5 lb/week) should be reported.

Check and record blood pressure during dose stabilization period at least two times daily. Report an ascending pattern.

Facilitate a conference between dietician and patient if therapeutic diet is ordered. Teach food sources of potassium (leafy vegetables, avocado, wheat, citrus fruit, bananas, whole grains), as well as foods to avoid in order to decrease sodium intake (snack foods, prepared luncheon meats, bouillon, sauces, processed cheese, and salt added to diet).

Because of decreased capacity to fight infection and the possibility of masked infection, warn patient to report incidence of slow healing or persistent inflammation in an abrasion, wound, or joint, or any vague feeling of being sick without clear etiologic definition. Urge patient to be fastidious about personal hygiene and to give special attention to foot care.

To continue beneficial effect of intraarticular injection, teach the patient proper joint alignment, appropriate posttreatment exercises, when to begin the exercises, and how long to avoid weight-bearing activities.

Exaggerated sense of well-being and analgesic effects may encourage patient to increase physical activity. However, since corticosteroids fail to check underlying disease processes, amount and degree of activity should be prescribed to prevent additional deterioration of painless joints. Discuss with physician, and work with family and patient, to plan reasonable and safe range of activities of daily living.

Compression and spontaneous fractures present hazards, particularly in rheumatoid arthritis, diabetes, immobilized patients and the elderly. Report persistent backache or chest pain (possible symptoms of rib or vertebral fracture). Patient's mattress should be firm or supported by a bedboard.

Be aware of previous history of psychotic tendencies. Drug-induced cerebral dysfunction tends to copy previous state. Changes in behavior, emotional stability, sleep pattern, or psychomotor activity may signal the onset of recurrence and should be reported to physician.

Dyspepsia with hyperacidity should not be ignored. Encourage patient to report symptoms to physician.

"Steroid" ulcers with long-term therapy are frequently treated with antacid regimen (1 hour after meals and at bedtime). Encourage patient to avoid alcohol (increases acid output) and caffeine (secretagogue).

When given for rheumatoid arthritis, complete relief is not sought, because of the hazards of continuous treatment. A regimen of rest, physical therapy, and salicylates continues during steroid therapy.

Ordinarily, long-term corticosteroid therapy is not interrupted when patient undergoes major surgery, but dosage may be increased.

To prevent withdrawal symptoms and permit adrenals to recover from drug-induced partial atrophy following therapy, doses are reduced over time by scheduled decrements. Instruct patient not to change dosage schedule.

Abrupt withdrawal of glucocorticosteroids promotes exacerbation of inflammatory processes and development of adrenal insufficiency.

Patient is supervised about 1 year beyond termination of long-term corticosteroid therapy because asymptomatic adrenal insufficiency can persist. Severe stress (eg, trauma, surgery) within that time may require a rapid-acting steroid to prevent precipitation of a crisis.

To minimize corticosteroid withdrawal symptoms, patient may be placed on alternate-day steroid therapy, a dosing regimen in which twice the usual daily dose is administered every other morning, as a method of maintaining patient on long-term steroid therapy. Regimen also minimizes pituitary-adrenal suppression, cushingoid state, and growth suppression in children.

Single doses, or use for a short period (less than 1 week), do not produce serious side effects when discontinued, even with moderately large doses.

Protect drug from light.

Patient and family should be advised to tell a new physician or surgeon about recently prolonged corticosteroid treatment.

Advise patient receiving adrenocorticosteroid to carry an identification card or jewelry with recorded diagnosis, drug therapy, and name of physician.

Urge patient to adhere to scheduled appointments with physician for regimen reevaluation.

Topical applications: Cleansing and application of prescribed ointments or creams should be done with extreme gentleness because of easy bruisability and poor healing; patient with moon facies is especially vulnerable. Inspect skin daily; purpura, petechiae, ecchymoses, and abrasions should be reported. Advise patient to avoid injury and exposure to temperature extremes.

Ointment, cream, or lotion should be massaged into affected area gently and thoroughly until it disappears. If occlusive dressing is used, sparingly apply medication, rub until it disappears, and then reapply, leaving a thin coat over lesion. Completely cover area with pliable nonporous film or corticoid tape. Consult physician.

If lesion is essentially dry, make dressing as airtight and watertight as possible. Prevent evaporation by sealing occlusive dressing to adjacent normal skin. If lesion is essentially moist, incomplete sealing of film edges or punctures in film will allow excess moisture to escape.

An occlusive dressing over corticosteroid-treated skin increases percutaneous penetration as much as 10%. Discomfort and warmth may be troublesome. Inspect skin carefully between applications for maceration, secondary infection, skin atrophy, striae, or miliaria; if they are present, stop medication and notify physician.

Rates of penetration of topical corticosteroid differ in various anatomic sites;

thus comparatively small doses are used on face, scalp, scrotum, axilla, and groin; usually, occlusive dressings are not applied to these areas. Caution should be used when plastic-film occlusive dressing is used on children to avoid possibility of accidental suffocation.

Instruct ambulatory patient receiving topical corticosteroid to report promptly if initial therapeutic response is followed by relapses. Contact sensitivity or sensitivity to corticosteroid impurities may be presenting. The medication will be changed either in kind or in dose.

Although adrenal suppression from topical therapy occurs infrequently, whole-body applications of potent corticosteroid, and stress such as surgery may present hazards. Replacement therapy before surgery may be given to prevent adrenal crisis.

LABORATORY TEST INTERFERENCES: Corticosteroids may produce glucosuria and may produce or exacerbate proteinuria. Topical application has been shown to decrease excretion of 17-ketogenic steroids and 17-hydroxycorticosteroids.

DRUG INTERACTIONS: Hyperglycemic action of corticosteroids may decrease hypoglycemic effects of **chlorpropamide, acetohexamide, tolazamide,** or **tolbutamide.** Corticosteroids may increase renal excretion of **aspirin,** thereby lowering salicylate levels during concurrent therapy. **Phenobarbital** and other **barbiturates, phenytoin,** and possibly other **hydantoins** reduce the effectiveness of corticosteroids by increasing their metabolism by hepatic microsomal drug-metabolizing activity. Topical **vitamin A** reverses corticosteroid-induced impairment of wound healing. **Oral contraceptives** augment antiinflammatory and mineralocorticoid actions of corticosteroids. **Amphotericin B, thiazide diuretics, furosemide,** and **ethacrynic acid** augment potassium depletion effects of adrenocorticosteroid therapy. **Indomethacin** and **salicylates** may enhance ulcerogenic effect. Prolonged concurrent **antibiotic** and corticosteroid treatment can result in severe superinfection.

HYDROFLUMETHIAZIDE, N.F.
(DIUCARDIN, SALURON)

Diuretic (thiazide), antihypertensive

ACTIONS AND USES
Benzothiadiazine (thiazide) derivative. Similar to chlorothiazide in actions, uses, contraindications, precautions, and adverse reactions. Reported to have approximately 5 to 10 times the diuretic potency of chlorothiazide on a weight basis.

ABSORPTION AND FATE
Onset of diuretic effect in 1 to 2 hours; duration 18 to 24 hours. Presumed to be distributed and excreted similarly to other thiazides. See Chlorothiazide.

ROUTE AND DOSAGE
Oral: **Adults:** *diuretic:* 25 to 200 mg daily; *antihypertensive:* 50 to 100 mg daily. Highly individualized according to patient's requirements and response. Single doses should not exceed 100 mg. **Children:** 1 mg/kg once daily.

NURSING IMPLICATIONS
See Chlorothiazide.

HYDROMORPHONE HYDROCHLORIDE, N.F.
(DILAUDID, Dihydromorphinone Hydrochloride)

Analgesic (narcotic)

ACTIONS AND USES
Semisynthetic phenanthrene derivative structurally similar to morphine (qv), but with more potent analgesic effect. Has more rapid onset and shorter duration of action than morphine, and reported to have less hypnotic action and less tendency to produce nausea and vomiting.
Used for relief of moderate to severe pain. Available in syrup form (in combination with guaifenesin) as antitussive.

ABSORPTION AND FATE
Onset of analgesic effect in 15 to 30 minutes; peaks in 30 to 90 minutes, and lasts 4 to 5 hours. Metabolized primarily in liver. Excreted chiefly in urine as glucuronide conjugate.

ROUTE AND DOSAGE
Oral, subcutaneous, intramuscular, intravenous (slowly): 2 mg every 4 to 6 hours. For severe pain, parenteral dose may be increased to 3 to 4 mg every 4 to 6 hours. Rectal suppository: 3 mg.

> **NURSING IMPLICATIONS**
> When sleep follows administration of hydromorphone, it is usually due to relief of pain rather than hypnosis.
> Produces physical dependence after prolonged administration.
> Classified as schedule II drug under federal Controlled Substances Act.
> Produces physical dependence after prolonged administration.
> High drug abuse potential. Very high "street demand."
> Withdrawal symptoms are similar to those of morphine dependence but occur sooner.
> Preserved in tight, light-resistant containers.
> See Morphine Sulfate.

HYDROXOCOBALAMIN, N.F.

(ALPHA-REDISOL, ALPHA-RUVITE, COBALPHAMEAD, COBAVITE LA, CODROXOMIN, CRYSTI-12 GEL, DROXOVITE, HYCOBAL-12, NEO-BETALIN 12, RUBESOL-LA 1000, SYTOBEX-H)

Hematopoietic vitamin

ACTIONS AND USES
Cobalamin derivative similar to cyanocobalamin (vitamin B_{12}) in actions, uses, contraindications, precautions, and adverse reactions. More slowly absorbed from injection site than cyanocobalamin, and may be taken up by liver in larger quantities. Results in higher and more sustained serum cobalamin levels and significantly less urinary excretion of cobalamin than produced by similar doses of cyanocobalamin; however, some patients reportedly develop antibody to plasma B_{12}-binding protein.

ROUTE AND DOSAGE
Intramuscular: **Adults:** doses as low as 30 μg daily for 5 to 10 days, followed by 100 μg once monthly, and doses as high as 1000 μg on alternate days until remission, then 1000 μg monthly. **Children:** 100 μg over 2 or more weeks to total dosage of 1 to 5 mg. Maintenance: 60 μg/month.

HYDROXYAMPHETAMINE HYDROBROMIDE, U.S.P. (PAREDRINE)

Adrenergic

ACTIONS AND USES
Sympathomimetic amine similar to ephedrine in many actions, but almost lacking in CNS stimulant activity. Indirectly stimulates α- and β-adrenergic receptors by releasing catecholamine stores. Pressor effects probably due more to direct cardiac stimulation than to enhanced peripheral resistance. Topical application to eye produces mydriasis without cycloplegia, thus sparing patient of long-lasting residual blurred vision.
Used topically to produce mydriasis and vasoconstriction for diagnostic eye examinations; used during surgery, and used to prevent synechiae in uveitis. Oral drug is used for selected patients with heart block and for temporary relief of postural hypotension.

ABSORPTION AND FATE
Produces mydriasis in 45 to 60 minutes, with recovery in about 6 hours following topical application to eye. Duration of action following oral administration is about 90 to 120 minutes.

CONTRAINDICATIONS AND PRECAUTIONS
Hypersensitivity or idiosyncrasy to sympathomimetic amines, severe hypertension, heart disease, thyrotoxicosis, narrow-angle glaucoma, agitated states, patients receiving tricyclic antidepressants, use with anesthetics that sensitize heart to catecholamines (eg, halothane, cyclopropane), use within 2 weeks of MAO inhibitors, use in children under 12 years of age. Safe use during pregnancy and in women of childbearing potential not established. Cautious use: advanced arteriosclerosis, coronary artery disease, diabetes, impaired renal function, hyperthyroidism, the elderly.

ADVERSE REACTIONS
Cardiovascular: marked elevation of blood pressure, palpitation, precordial pain, ventricular arrhythmias. **CNS:** restlessness, dizziness, weakness, tremors, headache. **GI:** dry mouth, unpleasant taste, diarrhea, nausea, vomiting. **Allergic:** urticaria. **Other:** prolonged mydriasis.

ROUTE AND DOSAGE
Oral: 20 to 60 mg 3 or 4 times a day. Dosage varies with condition and response of patient. Topical: 1% ophthalmic solution: 1 or 2 drop into the conjunctival sac.

DRUG INTERACTIONS: Hydroxyamphetamine may antagonize the effects of concurrently administered **guanethidine** or **reserpine.** In common with other vasopressors, hydroxyamphetamine may cause serious cardiac arrhythmias with **halothane** and related **anesthetics,** and pressor effects may be potentiated by **MAO inhibitors, oxytocics,** and **tricyclic antidepressants.**

HYDROXYCHLOROQUINE SULFATE, U.S.P., B.P.
(PLAQUENIL SULFATE)

Antimalarial, suppresant (lupus erythematosus)

ACTIONS AND USES

A 4-aminoquinoline derivative closely related to chloroquine and with similar actions, uses, contraindications, precautions, and adverse reactions.

CONTRAINDICATIONS AND PRECAUTIONS

Known hypersensitivity to 4-aminoquinoline compounds; psoriasis, porphyria, long-term therapy in children, pregnancy. Safe use in juvenile arthritis not established. Cautious use: hepatic disease, alcoholism with hepatotoxic drugs, impaired renal function, metabolic acidosis, patients with tendency toward dermatitis. Also see Chloroquine.

ADVERSE REACTIONS

GI distress, retinopathy, muscle weakness, vertigo, tinnitus, nerve deafness, dermatologic and hematologic reactions. With overdosage: respiratory depression, cardiovascular collapse, shock. Also see Chloroquine.

ROUTE AND DOSAGE

Oral: *Acute malaria:* **Adults:** initially 800 mg, followed by 400 mg after 6 to 8 hours, then 400 mg on each of next 2 days to total of 2 Gm. **Children** *11 to 15 years:* 600 mg, then 2 doses of 200 mg after 8 and 24 hours; *6 to 10 years:* 400 mg, then 2 doses of 200 mg at 8-hour intervals; *2 to 5 years:* 400 mg, then 200 mg 8 hours later; *1 year and under:* 100 mg, then 3 doses of 100 mg every 6 to 8 hours. *Malaria suppression:* **Adults:** 400 mg once weekly on same day of each week. If possible, suppressive therapy should begin 2 weeks prior to exposure and be continued for 8 weeks after leaving endemic area; failing this, an initial double (loading) dose of 800 mg in adults or 10 mg base/kg in children administered in 2 divided doses 6 hours apart. *Lupus erythematosus:* **Adults:** 400 mg once or twice daily for several weeks or months, depending on patient response; maintenance 200 to 400 mg daily. *Antirheumatic:* **Adults:** initially 400 to 600 mg daily; dosage increased gradually to optimum response level, then reduced slowly to maintenance level; maintenance 200 to 400 mg daily.

NURSING IMPLICATIONS

Administration of drug with food or milk may reduce incidence of GI distress.

All patients on long-term therapy should have baseline and periodic (every 3 months) ophthalmoscopic examinations (including visual acuity, slit lamp, fundoscopy, and visual fields) and blood cell counts.

Hydroxychloroquine has cumulative actions. In patients requiring long-term therapy, therapeutic effect may not appear until after several weeks, and maximal benefit may not occur for 6 months.

Patients receiving prolonged therapy should be informed about adverse symptoms and advised to report their onset immediately. Patients should be questioned about possible symptoms and examined periodically (include tests for muscle weakness, knee and ankle reflexes, and opthalmoscopic examinations). Drug should be discontinued if weakness, visual symptoms, or skin eruptions occur.

Caution patients to keep drug out of reach of children. Children are especially sensitive to 4-aminoquinoline compounds. A number of fatalities have been reported.

Preserved in tightly closed, light-resistant containers.

See Chloroquine Hydrochloride.

HYDROXYPROGESTERONE CAPROATE (IN OIL), U.S.P.
(CORLUTIN L.A., DELALUTIN, DURALUTIN, ESTRALUTIN, GESTEROL L.A., HYDROXON, HYLUTIN, HYPROVAL-P.A., LUTATE, PRO-DEPO, RELUTIN)

Progestin

ACTIONS AND USES

Long-acting (9 to 17 days), synthetic progestational hormone. Has slower onset and longer action than dydrogesterone (qv). Does not prevent conception. Lacks estrogenic and androgenic activity.

Used to treat irregular estrus cycle, amenorrhea, advanced uterine cancer, and postpartum pains. Has been used as test for endogenous estrogen production.

ADVERSE REACTIONS

Coughing, dyspnea, chest constriction, allergylike reactions (especially at high doses). Also see Dydrogesterone.

ROUTE AND DOSAGE

Intramuscular (in sesame oil or castor oil vehicle): *Menstrual disorders:* 125 to 250 mg per cycle. *Uterine adenocarcinoma:* 1000 mg or more at once; repeated one or more times weekly. Stop at time of relapse and after 12 weeks if no objective response. *Test for endogenous estrogen production:* 250 mg started any time. Repeated for confirmation 4 weeks after first injection; stopped after second injection.

NURSING IMPLICATIONS

Test for endogenous estrogen production: If patient is not pregnant and has a responsive endometrium (producing estrogen), bleeding (progesterone withdrawal sign) occurs 7 to 14 days after injection, indicating endogenous estrogen.

Protect from light. Stored at room temperature.

See Dydrogesterone.

HYDROXYUREA, U.S.P.
(HYDREA)

Antineoplastic

ACTIONS AND USES

Synthetic analogue of urea with antimetabolite activity. Blocks incorporation of thymidine into DNA and may damage already formed DNA molecules; does not affect synthesis of RNA or protein. Cytotoxic effect limited to tissues with high rates of cell proliferation. May reduce iron utilization by erythrocytes; reportedly does not alter erythrocyte survival time. No cross-resistance with other antineoplastics has been demonstrated.

Used in palliative treatment of metastatic melanoma, chronic myelocytic leukemia, and recurrent metastatic or inoperable ovarian cancer. Also used as adjunct to x-ray therapy for treatment of advanced epidermoid carcinoma of head and neck, including lip. Used investigationally in treatment of psoriasis.

ABSORPTION AND FATE

Readily absorbed from GI tract; peak serum concentrations in 2 hours. Undetectable in blood after 24 hours. Degraded in liver. Over 80% recovered as respiratory CO_2 and as urea in urine within 12 hours; remainder excreted unchanged. No cumulative effect. Passes blood–brain barrier.

CONTRAINDICATIONS AND PRECAUTIONS

Pregnancy; men and women of childbearing age; children; severe anemia or myelosuppression. Cautious use: following recent use of other cytotoxic drugs or irradiation; renal dysfunction; elderly patients.

ADVERSE REACTIONS

Hematologic (bone marrow suppression): leukopenia, thrombocytopenia, megaloblastic erythropoiesis, anemia. **GI** (occasional): stomatitis, anorexia, nausea, vomiting, diarrhea, constipation. **Dermatologic:** maculopapular rash, facial erythema, postirradiation erythema, alopecia (rare). **Neurologic** (rare): headache, dizziness, drowsiness, hallucinations, disorientation, convulsions. **Renal:** dysuria (rare), elevated BUN, serum uric acid, and creatinine levels.

ROUTE AND DOSAGE

Oral: Dosage individualized on basis of patient's actual or ideal weight, whichever is less. *Intermittent therapy:* 80 mg/kg body weight as single dose every third day. *Continuous therapy:* 20 to 30 mg/kg body weight daily.

NURSING IMPLICATIONS

Incidence of toxicity is as high as 66% with doses of 40 mg/kg body weight. Inform patient of potential side effects and of importance of reporting symptoms promptly.

Status of kidney, liver, and bone marrow function and blood status should be determined prior to and periodically during therapy. Hemoglobin, WBC, and platelet counts are monitored weekly throughout therapy.

If WBC count decreases to 2500/mm³ and platelet count decreases to 100,000/mm³, therapy will be interrupted. Drug-induced anemia is usually treated by whole blood replacement without interrupting drug therapy.

Monitor body weight and report either a steady, slow change or a precipitous change to physician.

If patient cannot swallow capsule, contents may be emptied into glass of water and taken immediately. Small amounts of inert material used as drug vehicle may not dissolve, but can be ingested.

Patients with marked renal dysfunction may rapidly develop visual and auditory hallucinations and hematologic toxicity. Changes in intake–output ratio or pattern may be significant indicators of impending nephrotoxicity and should be reported.

An adequate trial period for antineoplastic efficacy (tumor shrinking or growth arrest) is reported to be 6 weeks.

In patients receiving concomitant irradiation therapy, hydroxyurea is generally initiated 7 days before start of irradiation treatment and is continued during and for an indefinite period after radiotherapy.

See Fluorouracil for additional nursing implications.

Antianxiety agent (minor tranquilizer), antiemetic

ACTIONS AND USES
Piperazine derivative of diphenylmethane, structurally and pharmacologically related to other cyclizine compounds, eg, buclizine, chlorcyclizine. In common with such agents, it causes CNS depression and has anticholinergic, antispasmodic, antiemetic, local anesthetic, and antihistaminic activity. Its ataractic effect is produced primarily by depression of hypothalamus and brain-stem reticular formation, rather than cortical areas. Also reported to have skeletal muscle relaxant effect and antisecretory, analgesic, and mild antiarrhythmic activity.

Used for treatment of emotional or psychoneurotic states characterized by anxiety, tension, or psychomotor agitation; to relieve anxiety, control emesis, and reduce narcotic requirements prior to or following surgery or delivery; used as adjunctive therapy in allergic conditions, chronic urticaria, pruritus, and alcoholism; and to control nausea and vomiting due to various disease processes.

ABSORPTION AND FATE
Onset of effects within 15 to 30 minutes following oral administration; duration of action 4 to 6 hours. Metabolic fate not known.

CONTRAINDICATIONS AND PRECAUTIONS
Known hypersensitivity to hydroxyzine; use as sole treatment in psychoses or depression. Safe use during early pregnancy not established.

ADVERSE REACTIONS
Drowsiness, dry mouth, headache. Rarely: involuntary motor activity, tremor, convulsions, dizziness, urticaria, erythematous macular eruptions, erythema multiforme. Following inadvertent intraarterial, intravenous, or subcutaneous injection: pain and induration at injection site, endarteritis, thrombosis, digital gangrene.

ROUTE AND DOSAGE
Oral (hydroxyzine hydrochloride or pamoate): **Adults:** 25 mg to 100 mg 3 or 4 times daily. **Children** *under 6 years:* 50 mg daily in divided doses; *over 6 years:* 50 to 100 mg daily in divided doses. Intramuscular (hydroxyzine hydrochloride): **Adults:** 25 to 100 mg; dose repeated in 4 to 6 hours, as needed. **Children:** 0.5 mg/lb body weight.

NURSING IMPLICATIONS
IM administration should be made deep into body of a relatively large muscle. In adults, the preferred site is the upper outer quadrant of buttock or the midlateral thigh. In children, the recommended site is the midlateral muscle of thigh.

Carefully aspirate to avoid inadvertent injection into blood vessel. Hydroxyzine must not be administered by subcutaneous, intraarterial, or IV injection. See Adverse Reactions.

Rotate injection sites and observe daily.

Drowsiness may occur, but it usually disappears with continued therapy or following reduction of dosage.

Forewarn the patient about the possibility of drowsiness and dizziness, and caution against driving a car or performing hazardous tasks requiring mental alertness and physical coordination while taking hydroxyzine.

Patients should know the possible additive effects of hydroxyzine with

alcohol, and other drugs. See Drug Interactions. When prescribed concomitantly, dosage of CNS depressant is reduced up to 50%.
Protect hydroxyzine from light.

LABORATORY TEST INTERFERENCES: Possibility of false positive urinary
17-hydroxycorticosteroid determinations (modified Glenn-Nelson technique).

DRUG INTERACTIONS: Hydroxizine is additive with or may potentiate other
CNS depressants such as **alcohol, analgesics, anesthetics, barbiturates,** and
other **sedatives, narcotics,** and **tranquilizers.**

IBUPROFEN
(MOTRIN)

Antiinflammatory

ACTIONS AND USES
  Phenylpropionic acid derivative with nonsteroid antiinflammatory activity and significant antipyretic and analgesic properties. Compared to aspirin, higher doses are required for antiinflammatory effect than for analgesia; also reported to cause fewer GI symptoms than aspirin in equieffective doses. Although ibuprofen may enhance platelet aggregation, it reportedly causes less GI occult bleeding than aspirin. Antiinflammatory action postulated to be due to inhibition of prostaglandin synthesis and/or release. Antipyretic effect is thought to result from action on hypothalamus; heat dissipation accompanies vasodilation and peripheral blood flow. Cross-sensitivity with aspirin has been reported. Used in chronic, symptomatic treatment of active rheumatoid arthritis and osteoarthritis.

ABSORPTION AND FATE
  Rapidly absorbed. Peak plasma levels occur in 1 to 2 hours and decline to about one-half peak level in 4 hours. Approximately 90% to 99% bound to plasma proteins; plasma half-life reported to be 2 to 4 hours. Metabolized by oxidation to inactive metabolites. Excretion almost completed within 24 hours after last dose. About 50% to 60% excreted in urine as inactive metabolites and less than 10% as unchanged drug. Some biliary excretion occurs.

CONTRAINDICATIONS AND PRECAUTIONS
  History of hypersensitivity to ibuprofen; patients with nasal polyps, angioedema, and history of aspirin-induced bronchospasm (allergy); active peptic ulcer; children 14 years of age or younger; pregnancy. Cautious use: history of GI ulceration, impaired hepatic or renal function, cardiac decompensation.

ADVERSE REACTIONS
  GI (most common): heartburn, nausea, vomiting, anorexia, diarrhea, constipation, bloating, flatulence, stomatitis, epigastric or abdominal pain, GI ulceration, bleeding. **CNS:** headache, dizziness, lightheadedness, tinnitus, deafness (rare), fatigue, malaise, drowsiness, anxiety, confusion, depression. **Ophthalmic:** toxic amblyopia (rare), blurred vision, visual-field defects. **Dermatologic:** maculopapular and vesicobullous skin eruptions, erythema multiforme, pruritus, rectal itching, acne. **Hematologic:** leukopenia; decreased hemoglobin and hematocrit; transitory rise in SGOT, SGPT, serum alkaline phosphatase; rise in Ivy bleeding time. **Other:** sore throat, epistaxis, flushing, fluid retention with edema.

ROUTE AND DOSAGE
  Oral: 300 or 400 mg 3 or 4 times a day; total daily dosage not to exceed 2400 mg. Highly individualized.

NURSING IMPLICATIONS
Absorption rate is slower and drug plasma level is reduced when ibuprofen is administered with food; therefore it is usually given on an empty stomach, eg, 1 hour before or 2 hours after meals.
If GI intolerance occurs, physician may prescribe administration of drug with food or milk or may decrease dosage.
Patients with history of cardiac decompensation should be observed closely for evidence of fluid retention and edema.

Patients who experience any visual disturbances should have ophthalmo-scopic evaluation, including examination of central visual fields.

Side effects appear to be dose-related. Physician will rely on accurate obser-vation and reporting to estimate lowest effective dosage level.

Inform patients about possible CNS effects (lightheadedness, dizziness, drowsiness), and caution them to avoid dangerous activities until their reactions to the drug have been determined.

Patients should be advised to report immediately to physician the onset of GI disturbances, skin rash, blurred vision, or other eye symptoms.

Optimum therapeutic response generally occurs within 2 weeks (eg, relief of pain, stiffness, or swelling or improved joint flexion and strength). When satisfactory response occurs, dosage should be reviewed by physician and adjusted as required.

DRUG INTERACTIONS: Ulcerogenic effect may be potentiated by concomitant administration of ibuprofen and **indomethacin, phenylbutazone,** or **salicy-lates.** There is also the possibility (based on animal studies) that **aspirin** may cause lower blood levels and decrease the antiinflammatory activity of ibu-profen. Although ibuprofen has not been shown to enhance the hypoprothrom-binemic effects of **oral anticoagulants,** cautious use is advised if they are given concurrently, since ibuprofen enhances platelet aggregation.

IDOXURIDINE, U.S.P., B.P.
(DENDRID, HERPLEX, IDU, STOXIL)

Antiviral (ophthalmic)

ACTIONS AND USES

Topical antiviral agent structurally similar to thymidine, a metabolite essential for synthesis of DNA. Complexes with viral DNA and inhibits DNA replica-tion, thereby blocking cell reproduction of herpes simplex virus. Epithelial infections, especially initial attacks, characterized by dendritic figures respond better than stromal infections. Has no effect on scarring, vascularization, or resultant loss of vision. Some resistant strains of herpes simplex have been reported.

Used in treatment of dendritic (herpetic, herpes simplex) keratitis.

CONTRAINDICATIONS AND PRECAUTIONS

Hypersensitivity to any of its components. Cautious use: women of childbearing potential; during pregnancy; corticosteroids used with extreme caution if at all.

ADVERSE REACTIONS

Occasionally, local irritation, pain, pruritus, inflammation, or edema of eyes, lids, and surrounding face; photophobia; local allergic reaction (rare); corneal clouding, stippling, and small punctate defects; corneal ulceration.

ROUTE AND DOSAGE

Topical: Ophthalmic solution 0.1%: initially 1 drop instilled in conjunctival sac of each infected eye every hour during the day and every 2 hours at night until improvement occurs. Dosage may then be reduced to 1 drop every 2 hours during the day and every 4 hours at night. Ophthalmic ointment 0.5%: 5 instillations daily into conjunctival sac of infected eye; given approximately every 4 hours, with last dose at bedtime.

NURSING IMPLICATIONS

Boric acid should not be used during therapy with idoxuridine, since irrita-tion may occur.

Idoxuridine should not be mixed with other medications.

The recommended frequency and duration of therapy must not be exceeded.

Patients should be closely supervised by ophthalmologist.

To prevent recurrence, applications are usually continued for at least 3 to 5 days after corneal healing appears complete, as demonstrated by loss of staining with fluorescein.

Epithelial infections usually improve within 7 or 8 days. If patient continues to improve, therapy is generally continued up to 21 days. If no improvement is noted after 7 or 8 days, physician may institute another form of therapy.

Preserved in tightly covered, light-resistant containers.

IMIPRAMINE HYDROCHLORIDE, U.S.P., B.P.
(ANTIPRESS, IMAVATE, JANIMINE, PRESAMINE, SK-PRAMINE, TOFRANIL)
IMIPRAMINE PAMOATE
(TOFRANIL-PM)

Tricyclic antidepressant

ACTIONS AND USES

Dibenzazepine-derivative tricyclic antidepressant. Action mechanism unknown; appears to inhibit reuptake of serotonin and norepinephrine by nearby cells, thus restoring neurotransmitter concentration within synaptic gap. Has anticholinergic, antihistaminic, hypotensive, mild peripheral vasodilator, and prominent sedative effects; may exhibit quinidinelike action on heart. Action in treatment of enuresis reportedly involves anticholinergic effect and/or CNS stimulation resulting in earlier arousal to sensation of full bladder.

Used in endogenous depression; occasionally used for reactive depression. Less effective in presence of organic brain damage or schizophrenia. Sometimes used concomitantly with electroconvulsive therapy and antipsychotic drugs. Imipramine is the only tricyclic used for temporary adjuvant therapy in symptomatic treatment of enuresis in children 6 years of age and older.

ABSORPTION AND FATE

Readily absorbed from GI tract. Peak plasma levels within 1 to 2 hours after oral administration and 30 minutes after IM injection. Wide distribution, with high concentrations in heart, brain, liver, lungs; binds to plasma and tissue proteins. Plasma half-life 8 to 16 hours. Metabolized primarily in liver; may enter enterohepatic circulation. Evidence suggests genetic basis for variations in protein binding and ability to metabolize tricyclics. Approximately 40% of dose is excreted in urine within 24 hours (inactive metabolites); 70% excreted within 72 hours. About 22% eliminated in feces via bile. Believed to cross placenta.

CONTRAINDICATIONS AND PRECAUTIONS

Sensitivity to tricyclic compounds; use during acute recovery period following myocardial infarction; severe renal or hepatic impairment; use of the hydrochloride in pediatric conditions other than enuresis in children at least 6 years of age; use of the pamoate in children of any age; concomitant use or use within 2 weeks of MAO inhibitors. Safe use during pregnancy and lactation and in women of childbearing potential not established. Cautious use: children, adolescents, and elderly patients, especially with history of cardiovascular disease; increased intraocular pressure; narrow-angle glaucoma; urinary retention; seizure disorders; those with suicidal tendencies; prostatic hypertrophy; hiatal hernia; pyloric stenosis; hyperthyroidism; patients on thyroid medication; concomitant use of electroconvulsive therapy.

Anticholinergic (atropinelike) effects: dry mouth and rarely associated sublingual adenitis, blurred vision, disturbances of accommodation, mydriasis, constipation, paralytic ileus, urinary retention, delayed micturition, dilatation of urinary tract (rare). **Cardiovascular:** hypotension, hypertension, palpitation, tachycardia, arrhythmias, myocardial infarction, congestive heart failure, heart block, thrombophlebitis, shock. **Psychiatric:** disturbed concentration, confusion, disorientation, hallucinations, delusions, involuntary staring, anxiety, restlessness, irritability, agitation, insomnia, nightmares, hypomania, mania, exacerbation of psychoses. **Neurologic:** drowsiness, fatigue, weakness, headache, dizziness, tinnitus, paresthesias, peripheral neuritis, extrapyramidal symptoms (rigidity, tremors, twitching, ataxia, incoordination, hyperreflexia), seizures. **GI:** nausea, vomiting, diarrhea, epigastric pain, delayed gastric emptying, esophageal reflux, anorexia, stomatitis, parotid swelling, black tongue, peculiar taste. **Endocrinologic:** testicular swelling, gynecomastia (males), galactorrhea and breast enlargement (females), increased or decreased libido, ejaculatory or other potency disturbances, elevation or depression of blood sugar levels. **Allergic:** skin rashes, petechiae, urticaria, pruritus, photosensitization, edema (face, tongue, or generalized), drug fever. **Hematologic:** (believed to be due to hypersensitivity): bone marrow depression: agranulocytosis, eosinophilia, purpura, thrombocytopenia, leukopenia. **Other:** jaundice, altered liver function tests, weight gain or loss, nasal congestion, excessive perspiration, flushing, paradoxic urinary frequency, nocturia.

ROUTE AND DOSAGE

For depression: Oral, intramuscular: (Hospitalized patients): 50 mg 2 times a day, gradually increased up to 200 mg daily, as required; if no response after 2 weeks, increased to 250 to 300 mg/day. (Outpatients): initially 75 mg/day, gradually increased to 150 mg/day, as required; maximum dosage 200 mg/day. Adolescents and geriatric patients: initially 30 to 40 mg/day; rarely exceeds 100 mg/day. Maintenance: 50 to 150 mg/day. *For childhood enuresis* (imipramine hydrochloride only): Oral: initially 25 mg/day 1 hour before bedtime. If response is not satisfactory within 1 week, dose may be increased to 50 mg nightly in children under 12 years of age; children 12 years of age and older may receive up to 75 mg nightly.

NURSING IMPLICATIONS
General:
Complete health and drug history and baseline determinations of standing and recumbent blood pressures are recommended before initiation of tricyclic therapy.
Preliminary and periodic leukocyte and differential counts, liver function tests, and determinations of cardiac status are advised in patients with preexisting cardiovascular disease and those receiving high doses or prolonged therapy.
The user of tricyclics is frequently advised to avoid alcohol or OTC drugs during and for 2 weeks following termination of therapy (many OTC preparations contain alcohol and sympathomimetic amines; conjoint administration with imipramine might precipitate potentially lethal reactions).
Warn patients that the drug may impair mental and physical abilities to perform hazardous tasks such as driving a motor vehicle or operating machinery, particularly during early therapy.
Caution patients to avoid exposure to strong sunlight (photosensitivity reactions can occur). Suggest use of sun screening agent during summer months for sun-sensitive patients.
Leukocyte and differential counts are indicated if patient develops fever, malaise, or sore throat or mouth (early signs of agranulocytosis). With-

hold drug and institute protective isolation pending evaluation of hematologic status.

Tricyclic therapy should be discontinued several days prior to elective surgery.

Onset of toxic effects is sudden with overdosage. Treatment (for oral ingestion): emesis or lavage, preferably followed by instillation of activated charcoal slurry. Physostigmine, pyridostigmine, neostigmine, propranolol, anticonvulsants (diazepam, short-acting barbiturate), paraldehyde, methocarbamol, and equipment for respiratory support should be available. Constant ECG monitoring and close observation for at least 4 to 5 days are recommended because relapses reportedly occur after apparent recovery.

Crystals may form in some ampuls of injectable imipramine. To dissolve, immerse intact ampul in hot water for about 1 minute.

Preserved in tightly covered, light-resistant containers.

Antidepressant therapy:

Preparation and education of patient and significant family members, in collaboration with physician, from start of therapy may help to promote patient compliance. Summary of pertinent teaching points: (1) Stress biochemical nature of endogenous depression, and stress that the tricyclic compound is given to correct this condition, much as insulin is given to a diabetic. (2) Permanent remission occurs in most cases (75% to 80%). (3) Expect a therapeutic lag of 2 to 3 weeks before onset of symptom relief. (4) Side effects may occur, but these indicate that drug is "working." Tolerance to these effects often develops after the first few days or weeks of treatment. Keep physician informed, as dosage adjustment may be necessary. (5) Drug must be taken exactly as prescribed, not on an "as needed" basis. (6) Keep follow-up appointments. (7) Advise significant family members to encourage physical and diversional activities (do not allow patient to vegetate). (8) See the general statements and other statements in this section for additional teaching points.

Side effects are most likely to occur in elderly patients and those receiving more than 200 mg/day. Supervised ambulation and bedsides may be indicated, particularly during early therapy.

Tricyclic antidepressants may cause grand mal seizures in certain susceptible patients, eg, those with seizure disorders or family history of epilepsy, organic brain disease, cerebral arteriosclerosis, alcoholism, or barbiturate withdrawal, as well as those having had previous electroconvulsive therapy and those receiving high doses of imipramine.

Accurate observation and early reporting of patient's response to drug therapy are essential in preventing serious adverse effects and in designing an individualized therapeutic regimen.

Since imipramine is long-acting, physician may prescribe administration of entire daily dose at bedtime to reduce daytime sedation, or in the morning for patients who experience insomnia and stimulation.

Risk of suicide and need for psychologic support are particularly great when the patient begins to recover. Supervise drug ingestion to make certain that the patient does not "cheek" the pill, and observe necessary environmental precautions.

Monitor vital signs during early phase of therapy, particularly in patients receiving high doses, those with pretreatment hypotension or hypertension, and the elderly. Measurements should be made during peak drug effect period. Note that wide interpatient variations may exist.

Orthostatic hypotension tends to be mild in normotensive individuals, but it may be marked in patients with pretreatment hypertension.

Instruct patient to make position changes slowly, especially from recumbent to upright posture, and to dangle legs over bed for a few minutes before ambulating. Caution against standing still for prolonged periods and taking hot showers and baths (vasodilation caused by heat may potentiate drug hypotensive effect). Instruct the patient to lie down or sit down (in head-low position) immediately if lightheadedness or faintness occurs.

If orthostatic hypotension is a problem, elastic stockings (if prescribed) and elevation of legs while sitting may help.

Extrapyramidal symptoms may occur in patients receiving large doses (especially the elderly), indicating need for dosage reduction, dosage change, or discontinuation of drug.

Report promptly the appearance of psychogenic reactions (eg, transition from depression to hypomania or mania, hallucinations, delusions), which are especially apt to occur in patients with organic brain damage or history of psychosis. Tricyclic therapy will be discontinued.

Monitor intake and output, at least until maintenance dosage is stabilized, to detect urinary retention or frequency, constipation, or paralytic ileus. Palpate for bladder distention, and auscultate for peristalsis as indicated. Note depressed patient's interest in food and fluids. Some patients may require increases in bulk foods or fluids and a laxative to overcome drug-induced constipation.

Mouth dryness may be relieved by rinsing with clear water and by increasing fluid intake (if allowed).

Meticulous mouth care may help prevent drug-induced stomatitis, sublingual adenitis, and parotitis. Since depressed patients tend to neglect personal hygiene, also supervise general care (excessive perspiration is a drug side effect).

Weigh patients under standard conditions at least biweekly. Edema and weight gain sometimes occur during early therapy.

Be alert to signs of cholestatic jaundice: flulike symptoms (general malaise, nausea, vomiting, fever, upper abdominal pain), yellow skin or sclerae, dark urine, light-colored stools.

Hyperglycemia or hypoglycemia may occur in some patients. Diabetics should be monitored, particularly during early therapy.

Therapeutic effectiveness of tricyclic antidepressant therapy may be evidenced by renewed interest in surroundings and personal appearance, elevation of mood, increased physical activity, improved appetite and sleep patterns, and reduction in morbid preoccupations.

Onset of therapeutic effectiveness may not be apparent before 2 to 3 weeks of therapy. If no improvement occurs after a 4- to 8-week trial, drug is usually discontinued. With satisfactory response, maintenance dosage can be instituted.

Maintenance therapy is usually continued 3 to 6 months after a 2-month period of apparent remission.

Some patients experience complete recovery within 4 to 6 weeks; others may require drug therapy for several years.

Drug withdrawal should be gradual. Abrupt termination of therapy, especially in patients receiving high doses for 2 months or more, may result in nausea, headache, malaise, muscle aches, irritability, coryza, and insomnia.

Enuresis:

Note that imipramine pamoate is not intended for children of any age because of its high unit potency.

For early evening bedwetters, imipramine may be more effective if one-half the daily dose is prescribed for midafternoon and the second half at bedtime.

With adequate dosage, positive results generally occur in 1 to 2 weeks. Some physicians recommend maintenance dosage until the child is dry every night for 3 months. Children who relapse when drug is withheld do not always respond to restart of therapy.

Imipramine should be withdrawn as soon as satisfactory results are achieved. Long-term effects of drug in children is not known.

When imipramine is to be withdrawn, dosage is tapered off gradually to reduce the possibility of relapse. In some patients, effectiveness decreases with continued drug administration. Counsel parent to inform physician if this occurs.

Most frequent side effects in children are headache, dizziness, irritability, insomnia, and GI complaints. Advise parent to report symptoms to physician. Dosage reduction or termination of therapy may be indicated.

Enuresis is generally associated with an emotional component, such as guilt feelings and anxiety, even when it is not primarily psychogenic in origin; ample time should be given to parent and child to discuss problems of management.

Counsel parent in the proper use and care of imipramine. Lethal poisoning in children has been reported.

DRUG INTERACTIONS: Potentiated effects may occur with concurrent administration of tricyclic antidepressants and **acetazolamide** (may increase renal tubular absorption of tricyclic agent), **alcohol** (additive sedation and psychomotor impairment), and **amphetamines** (may increase tricyclic serum levels). There may be additive anticholinergic activity with **anticholinergics,** including **antihistamines** (may increase tricyclic serum levels) and **antiparkinson agents, barbiturates** (may potentiate toxic doses of tricyclic agents), **chlordiazepoxide** (impaired motor function and additive anticholinergic effects), **estrogenic substances** (may increase tricyclic toxic reactions), **epinephrine** and other **sympathomimetics** (increased pressor response and arrhythmias), **ethchlorvynol** (transient delirium), **haloperidol** (increases tricyclic blood levels), **MAO inhibitors** (hyperpyrexia, fluctuations in blood pressure, muscle rigidity, coma), **meperidine** and possibly other **narcotics** and **sedatives** (enhanced respiratory depression and additive anticholinergic effects), **meprobamate** (enhanced sedation and dizziness), **methylphenidate** (increased tricyclic serum levels), **phenothiazines** (mutually potentiating effects), **reserpine** and related alkaloids (possibility of excessive CNS stimulation), **thyroid compounds** (possibility of mutually potentiating effects), and **thioxanthene tranquilizers** (mutually potentiating effects).

Clinical effects of tricyclics may be decreased by **ammonium chloride, ascorbic acid** in large doses (decrease renal tubular absorption), or **barbiturates** (possibility of decreased tricyclic serum levels; however, may potentiate adverse effects of toxic doses of tricyclic agent).

Tricyclics may decrease **phenylbutazone** effect (possibly by inhibiting GI absorption of phenylbutazone).

Tricyclics may antagonize the antihypertensive effects of **bethanidine, debrisoquine, guanethidine** (with exception of **doxepin**) and other related agents, and **methyldopa.**

Close monitoring of **anticoagulant** response is advised when a tricyclic is added to or withdrawn from regimen.

Antiinflammatory agent, analgesic, antipyretic

ACTIONS AND USES

Potent nonsteroid arylacetic acid compound with antiinflammatory, analgesic, and antipyretic effects similar to those of aspirin. Antipyretic and antiinflammatory actions may be related to ability to block prostaglandin biosynthesis. Appears to inhibit motility of polymorphonuclear leukocytes, development of cellular exudates, and vascular permeability in injured tissue. Apparently has no antihistaminic, antiserotonin, or uricosuric action.

Used for palliative treatment in active stages of moderate to severe rheumatoid arthritis, rheumatoid spondylitis, acute gouty arthritis, and osteoarthritis of hip in patients intolerant to or unresponsive to adequate trials with salicylates and other therapy.

ABSORPTION AND FATE

Promptly and almost completely absorbed from GI tract. Onset of action in 1 to 2 hours. Peak plasma levels within 3 hours following single oral dose; duration of action 4 to 6 hours. Approximately 90% bound to plasma protein, and also extensively bound in tissues; low concentrations in cerebrospinal fluid. Largely metabolized in liver and kidneys. Excreted primarily in urine, mainly as glucuronide and about 10% to 20% as unchanged drug. Some elimination in bile and feces. Appears in breast milk.

CONTRAINDICATIONS AND PRECAUTIONS

Allergy to indomethacin or aspirin, history of GI lesions; pregnancy, nursing mothers, children 14 years of age or younger. Cautious use: history of psychiatric illness, epilepsy, or parkinsonism; impaired renal or hepatic function, in patients with infection, elderly patients, persons in hazardous occupations.

ADVERSE REACTIONS

CNS: headache (common), dizziness, vertigo, lightheadedness, syncope, ataxia, insomnia, nightmares, drowsiness, narcolepsy, confusion, coma, convulsions, peripheral neuropathy, psychic disturbances (hallucinations, depersonalization, depression), aggravation of epilepsy, parkinsonism. **GI** (common): nausea, vomiting, diarrhea, ulcerative stomatitis, GI ulceration, hemorrhage, perforation. **Hematologic:** hemolytic anemia, aplastic anemia (sometimes fatal), agranulocytosis, leukopenia, thrombocytopenic purpura. **Eye and ear:** blurred vision, lacrimation, eye pain, visual field changes, corneal deposits, retinal disturbances including macula, tinnitus, hearing disturbances, deafness (rarely). **Hypersensitivity:** rash, purpura, pruritus, urticaria, angioedema, angiitis, rapid fall in blood pressure, dyspnea, asthma syndrome (in aspirin-sensitive patients). **Other:** epistaxis, hair loss, erythema nodosum, vaginal bleeding, hyperglycemia and glycosuria (rare), toxic hepatitis, pancreatitis, edema, elevated blood pressure, hematuria. **Altered laboratory findings:** increased BUN, SGOT, SGPT, serum alkaline phosphatase, cephalin flocculation, thymol turbidity, and serum amylase; positive direct Coombs' test.

ROUTE AND DOSAGE

Oral: *Rheumatoid arthritis:* 25 mg 2 or 3 times daily; if tolerated, may be increased by 25 mg at weekly intervals until satisfactory response is obtained or total daily dosage of 150 to 200 mg is reached. *Acute gouty arthritis:* 50 mg 3 times daily until pain is tolerable; then dose is rapidly reduced to complete termination of drug therapy.

NURSING IMPLICATIONS

Indomethacin is contraindicated in patients allergic to aspirin. Question patient carefully regarding aspirin sensitivity prior to initiation of therapy.

Administer immediately after meals, or with food or antacid (if prescribed).

Incidence of adverse reactions is high (especially in elderly patients) and is dose-related in most patients. Physician will rely on accurate and prompt reporting of patient's response and tolerance to establish lowest possible effective dosage.

Indomethacin can cause severe GI complications (reported to be the most common side effect). Be alert to suspicious signs and symptoms and report immediately.

Patient should be carefully observed and should be instructed to report adverse reactions in order to prevent serious and sometimes irreversible or fatal effects.

Frontal headache is the most frequent CNS side effect; it should be reported. If it persists, dosage reduction or cessation of drug may be indicated. Usually it is more severe in the morning, but it may occur within 1 hour after drug ingestion. A dose scheduled at bedtime, with milk, may reduce the incidence of morning headache.

Complete blood counts, renal and hepatic function tests, ophthalmoscopic examinations, and hearing tests should be performed periodically during prolonged therapy.

Following control of acute flairs of chronic rheumatoid arthritis, physician may make repeated attempts to reduce daily doses until drug is finally discontinued.

Expected therapeutic effects in rheumatoid arthritis are reduced fever, increased strength, and relief of pain, swelling, and tenderness. If improvement is not noted in 2 to 3 weeks, alternate therapy is generally prescribed.

Therapeutic effect in acute gouty attack (relief of joint tenderness and pain) is usually apparent in 24 to 36 hours; swelling generally disappears in 3 to 5 days. Keep physician informed; dosage should be reduced once pain is tolerable.

Bear in mind that indomethacin may mask signs and symptoms of latent infections.

Because of the possibility of dizziness and lightheadedness, caution the patient to avoid activities requiring mental alertness and motor coordination.

Advise the patient not to take aspirin, because it may potentiate the ulcerogenic effects of indomethacin. Also see Drug Interactions.

Green coloration of urine has been reported in patients who develop indomethacin-induced hepatitis.

Preserved in tight, light-resistant containers.

DRUG INTERACTIONS: Ulcerogenic effects of indomethacin may be potentiated by concomitant administration of **corticosteroids, phenylbutazone,** or **salicylates.** Concurrently administered **aspirin** may delay or decrease indomethacin absorption and thus may interfere with its therapeutic effectiveness. Recent reports indicate that indomethacin does not enhance the hypoprothrombinemic effects of **oral anticoagulants;** however, since indomethacin inhibits platelet aggregation and may cause GI ulceration and bleeding, cautious use is advised. **Probenecid** may increase indomethacin serum levels; patients receiving these drugs concurrently should be observed closely for indomethacin toxicity. Indomethacin may predispose patients to severe reactions from **smallpox vaccine.**

Antidiabetic

ACTIONS AND USES

Fast-acting, clear, colorless solution of antidiabetic principle secreted by beta cells in beef or pork pancreas (or both, as indicated on label). Enhances transmembrane passage of glucose into most body cells; by unknown mechanism, may itself enter the cell to actuate selected intermediary metabolic processes. Promotes conversion of glucose to glycogen, inhibits fatty acid mobilization from fat depots, promotes triglyceride synthesis, stimulates protein production, and induces net potassium movement into liver and adipose and muscle tissues. In the diabetic, insulin temporarily restores efficient sugar and fat utilization, maintains blood sugar within normal parameters, and prevents glucosuria, diabetic acidosis, and coma. The only form of insulin that can be given IV.

Used to supplement or replace endogenous insulin in treatment of juvenile-onset (brittle) diabetes mellitus and complicated maturity-onset diabetes. Also used to improve appetite and increase weight in selected cases of nondiabetic malnutrition; used therapeutically in selected cases of schizophrenia by inducing hypoglycemic shock. IV insulin therapy is used for emergency treatment of diabetic ketoacidosis.

ABSORPTION AND FATE

Following administration, circulates widely in extracellular fluid as free hormone. Action begins in 30 to 60 minutes, peaks in 2 or 3 hours, and lasts 5 to 8 hours. Plasma half-life following IV injection less than 9 minutes. Metabolized primarily by liver; less than 10% of dose eliminated in urine.

CONTRAINDICATIONS AND PRECAUTIONS

Hypersensitivity to insulin animal protein.

ADVERSE REACTIONS

Hypoglycemia (hyperinsulinism): profuse sweating, hunger, nausea, tremulousness, palpitation, tachycardia, weakness, paresthesias, circumoral pallor, numb mouth and tongue, visual disturbances (diplopia, blurred vision, mydriasis), apprehension, irritability, inability to concentrate, fatigue, delirium, convulsions, Babinski reflex, negative ketone and sugar urine tests, coma. **Diabetic ketoacidosis:** poor skin turgor, soft eyeballs, dry tongue, flushed and dry skin, polydipsia, polyuria, anorexia, weakness, hyperventilation; nausea, vomiting, diarrhea, abdominal pain, fruity-smelling breath, drowsiness, inattentiveness, Kussmaul breathing, acetonuria, glucosuria. **Other:** posthypoglycemic hyperglycemia (Somogyi effect); injection site atrophy and scar tissue, insulin resistance.

ROUTE AND DOSAGE

Supplement or replacement (subcutaneous): maintenance dosage highly individualized according to blood and urine glucose determinations. Available concentrations: U 40, U 80, U 100, U 500 (indicating number of U.S.P. units of insulin protein in 1 ml of solution). *Ketoacidosis* (subcutaneous, intravenous):**Adults**: 50 to 150 units; additional doses may be given hourly until patient is out of acidosis, then maintenance subcutaneous doses every 6 hours. **Children:** initially 1 to 4 U/kg body weight (according to presence of glycosuria, acetonuria, or acidosis and level of consciousness). Subsequent dosage highly individualized. IV route used during emergency period only.

NURSING IMPLICATIONS

Insulin injection (variously called "regular," "neutral," "plain," "ordinary," "unmodified," or just "insulin") should not be confused with modified insulins.

In general, dosage is adjusted to maintain postprandial blood glucose below 160 mg/dl. Normal fasting blood sugar is 60 to 100 mg/dl; normal 2-hour postprandial blood sugar is 70 to 130 mg/dl.

During early period of dosage regulation, some patients experience visual difficulties. Advise patients to postpone changing prescription lenses until vision stabilizes (usually 3 to 6 weeks).

In the event of unavoidable insulin shortage, advise patients to reduce dosage temporarily, decrease food intake by one-third of usual quantity, and drink generous amounts of liquids with little or no caloric value (water, coffee, tea, clear soup, broth).

Storage, preparation, and administration:

Advise patient to keep extra vial of insulin, syringe, and needle on hand.

Insulin in use is stable at room temperature up to 1 month. Avoid exposure to temperature extremes or to direct sunlight. Refrigerate stock supply.

Avoid injection of cold insulin; it can lead to lipodystrophy, reduced rate of absorption, and local reactions.

VNA nurses often prepare a week's supply of daily insulin doses for selected patients. Syringes are refrigerated until ready for use. Patient should be instructed to remove syringe from refrigerator about 1 hour before administration time.

Do not administer discolored or turbid solution.

Check expiration date on label. Discard outdated vials and partially used vials that have not been in use for several weeks.

Insulin injection is compatible with all modified insulin preparations. When mixing insulins, they should have the same concentration.

Always use a syringe that coordinates with strength of insulin to be administered. Standardized color code for cap and syringe markings: red indicates U 40, green indicates U 80, orange indicates U 100.

If possible, select a strength of insulin that can be given within the range of 0.25 to 0.75 ml.

Insulin should be administered 15 to 30 minutes before a meal so that peak action will coincide with postprandial hyperglycemia.

Eliminate air bubble within syringe and hub of needle (dead space) for accurate dosage. In syringes with detachable needles, dead space may be equivalent to 0.1 cc. Some disposable syringes with permanently attached needles have no dead space and thus provide more accurate measurement.

Prepare skin with alcohol, allow skin to dry (alcohol precipitates insulin), and inject insulin into area that has a substantial layer of fat and is free of large blood vessels and nerves. Commonly used injection sites: upper arms, thighs, abdomen (avoid area over urinary bladder and 2 inches around navel), buttocks, and upper back (if fat is loose enough to pick up).

Traditional method of injecting insulin: use 25-gauge ½-inch needle, and insert at right angle to skin. Another method (reportedly reduces lipodystrophy): lift skin and fat away from muscle, insert ⅝- to ⅞-inch needle at 20- to 45-degree angle into base of fold, and inject into pocket between fat and muscle layer.

Avoid IM injection (which is irritating and is followed by erratic absorption rate) and superficial subcutaneous injection (may cause local allergic reaction or irritation).

Aspirate needle carefully; intravascular injection can cause immediate hypoglycemic response. Following removal of needle, apply pressure (without massage) to puncture site for 2 or 3 seconds.

If patient is engaged in active sports it has been suggested that injection of insulin be made into the abdomen rather than into a muscle that will be heavily taxed since this may increase insulin absorption too quickly.

Available injection sites are lost when lipodystrophy (dimpling) (seen predominantly in women and children) or hypertrophy (thickening) de-

velops. To prevent this, avoid reuse of a site for 6 to 8 weeks if possible.
Maintain an injection record to assure systematic site rotation. Allow approximately 1 inch between injection sites, and use all designated sites in one body part before proceeding to next body area.

Care of reusable equipment:

Reusable syringe and needle may be sterilized by boiling (in a strainer) for 10 minutes. Avoid heavily chlorinated water. Soft tap water, distilled water, or clean rainwater is ideal.

Long-acting insulins may form a precipitate in the syringe; to remove crust use vinegar-soaked cotton swab, and rinse thoroughly before sterilization.

Use dry syringe and needle; each time after administration of insulin, rinse syringe thoroughly with water, and clean needle with wire.

Adverse reactions:

Local allergic reaction at injection site sometimes develops 1 to 3 weeks after therapy starts and usually appears 1 to 12 hours after an injection. Symptoms may last several hours to days, but they usually disappear with continued use. Advise patient to report symptoms; physician may prescribe an antihistamine. Injection technique should be checked.

Generalized allergic reaction (sensitivity to animal source of insulin) is treated by antihistaminic, by substituted insulin from another source, or by an oral hypoglycemic drug.

Patients highly sensitive to insulin who cannot be maintained on oral hypoglycemics may be rapidly desensitized with subcutaneous administration of small and frequent doses of insulin. Observe patient closely for anaphylaxis and onset of hypoglycemia during desensitization period. Monitor vital signs.

Hypoglycemic reaction may occur from excess insulin, insufficient food intake (eg, skipped or delayed meals), unaccustomed exercise (burns up sugar and thus adds to insulin effect of lowering blood sugar), or nervous or emotional tension.

Symptomatic hypoglycemia occurs when blood sugar becomes lowered to 50 mg/dl or when fall in blood sugar is sudden and rapid. Onset generally corresponds to peak action of insulin.

Restlessness and diaphoresis occurring during sleep are suggestive of hypoglycemia in the diabetic.

Instruct patient and responsible family members to respond promptly to beginning symptoms of hypoglycemia (often vague): profuse sweating, hunger, fatigue, inability to concentrate, headache, drowsiness, anxiety.

Hypoglycemic reaction is an emergency situation, since prolonged hypoglycemia can cause irreversible brain damage. Advise patient to take 10 Gm of fast-acting carbohydrate: 4 ounces of orange juice (1.5 to 3 ounces for child). If orange juice is not available, any one of the following may be taken: 4 ounces of apple juice or ginger ale, 3 ounces of 7-Up, 2.5 teaspoons of sugar, 2 teaspoons of honey or corn syrup, 5 Life-Savers.

Failure to show signs of recovery within 30 minutes indicates necessity for emergency treatment.

Patients with severe hypoglycemia may receive glucagon, epinephrine, or IV glucose 10% to 50%. As soon as patient is fully conscious, oral carbohydrate should be given to prevent secondary hypoglycemia.

Since severe hypoglycemia develops suddenly in some patients, physician may advise patient to keep a supply of glucagon on hand for emergency use; a responsible family member may be taught how to administer it.

Glutol, Glutorea, and Instant Glucose are commercial glucose products for emergency use by family when patient in hypoglycemia is unconscious. Prescribed amount squeezed into buccal cavity adheres to mucous membrane and is absorbed or swallowed by reflex action.

Advise patient to carry Life-Savers or other candy or lump of sugar at all times.

Diabetic ketoacidosis as a sequel to insulin deficiency or resistance is a medical emergency that appears over a period of weeks in controlled diabetics or in a few hours in noncontrolled patients. Precipitating factors: rapid growth in juveniles, infection, illness, emotional stress, surgery, pregnancy. Patient/family education is critically important.

Severe ketoacidosis is treated with insulin injection IV. To prevent hypoglycemia during treatment, 1 Gm dextrose is usually administered concomitantly for each unit of insulin being given. Blood sugar is monitored hourly at bedside until values improve, then every 2 to 4 hours, as prescribed.

During treatment for ketoacidosis with IV insulin, check blood pressure, intake–output ratio, and urinary levels of sugar and acetone every hour. Observe level of consciousness; be alert for signs of hypoglycemia (patient may pass from hyperglycemia into insulin shock without regaining consciousness). Also observe for signs of hyperkalemia (see Index).

The juvenile diabetic generally is more prone to hypoglycemia and ketoacidosis than the mature diabetic. Both child and parent must know signs of impending complications (see Adverse Reactions).

Activity and insulin requirement vary inversely; thus insulin requirements of the normally active diabetic child tend to decrease in the summer (when activity increases) and increase in the fall. The abnormally active child with diabetes requires added food before and during anticipated activity.

The vascular complications seen in adults do not present a problem during childhood. Foot care, cuts, broken bones, bruises, and related conditions are of no more significance to the diabetic child than to the nondiabetic child; however, prevention of infection is important in all age groups.

In the event of an illness, advise patient to continue taking insulin, go to bed, and drink liberally (every hour if possible) of noncaloric liquids. Do not force liquids if nauseated or vomiting. If unable to eat prescribed diet, replace with liquid or semiliquid carbohydrate according to food exchange list. Test urine for sugar and acetone four times a day, before meals and at bedtime. Consult physician for insulin regulation if unable to eat prescribed diet, or if 4 meals of liquid or semiliquid carbohydrates have been taken or if urine tests are unusual (eg, high sugar, sugar with acetone).

Urine testing:

For reliability of results, advise patient to use only the prescribed type of urine test. Review the instructions on the package insert with the patient.

Test of first voiding reflects a summation of blood sugars; test of second voiding (preferred and usually prescribed) reflects an instantaneous measurement of sugar in the blood.

Check with physician about frequency of urine testing (dependent on extent of glycosuria and insulin type). In the labile diabetic, urine may be tested four times daily, before meals and at bedtime. Occasionally, tests are done at times of peak and minimum insulin effects.

In general, glycosuria indicates unsuitable insulin dosage or dietary imbalance or indiscretion and a renal threshold exceeding 180 mg/dl (some physicians prefer to have their patients show an occasional trace or positive reading).

Usually urine test for ketones is not done routinely in stabilized diabetics. It is checked routinely in new, unstable, and juvenile diabetics, and if patient has lost weight, exercises vigorously, or has an illness.

Presence of acetone without sugar usually signifies insufficent carbohydrate intake. Acetone with sugar may indicate onset of ketoacidosis. Notify physician promptly.

Since women in third trimester of pregnancy and nursing mothers have lactose in urine, cupric sulfate reagents such as Benedict's test or Clinitest should not be used. Glucose oxidase reagents, eg, Tes-Tape or Clinistix may be used.

Caution patients to avoid over-the-counter medications (may have high sugar content) unless approved by physician. Aspirin or ascorbic acid in large doses may cause positive urine glucose test.

Other:

Emphasize need for maintaining optimum skin care and foot care to prevent vascular-related complications and infection.

Hypoglycemic reaction is sometimes the first indication of pregnancy in the diabetic woman. Patient should report promptly to physician.

Insulin requirements during first trimester of pregnancy frequently decrease by one-third (utilization of glucose by fetus). During second and third trimesters, hormonal changes induced by pregnancy and action of placental insulinase may necessitate increased dosage (decreased insulin requirement during this period suggests a failing placenta). On day of delivery, physician may omit insulin dose and administer IV glucose.

After delivery, maternal insulin requirements usually are less than prepregnant dosage. Patient should be observed closely for hypoglycemia. Insulin requirement gradually returns to prepregnancy level within 1 to 6 weeks.

During lactation, frequent blood sugar determinations are advised. Both Benedict's test and Clinitest give positive readings for lactose; therefore they should not be used during this period. Greater reliance will be placed on blood sugar analyses.

When the patient plans to travel, advise him to carry ample insulin (in event of delay in flight), at least 2 or 3 syringes, and an adequate supply of emergency carbohydrate in hand luggage or handbag (travel kits are available).

Insulin dosage adjustment when traveling requires preplanning with physician, particularly when changes in time zones are involved.

If foreign languages are spoken in countries to be visited, advise the patient to learn emergency vocabulary: "Sugar." "May I have orange juice?" "I am a diabetic." "I need a doctor."

For information about diabetic care in foreign countries, patients may write to International Diabetes Foundation, 3–6 Alfred Place, London WC1, England.

Advise patient that at all times he should wear medical identification bracelet, necklace, or card (available in local pharmacies), with patient's and physician's names, addresses, and telephone numbers, as well as diagnosis, dosage, and type of antidiabetic agent being taken.

Avoid alcohol, since it may reduce gluconeogenesis and thus precipitate hypoglycemic crisis.

Be familiar with the information on insulin package insert, which is also available to the patient, and consult with physician for directions the patient is to follow. Prepare a teaching plan in collaboration with physician, dietitian, patient, and responsible family members.

Summary of patient/family teaching plan:

Nature of diabetes mellitus.

Insulin: action, administration, storage, syringe-insulin coordination.

What to do in the event of unavoidable insulin shortage.

Adjustments of insulin dosage (as prescribed) in relation to urine tests, illness, changes in activity, diet, travel, pregnancy.

Urine testing and recording.

Cause, symptoms, prevention, and treatment of hypoglycemia and ketoacidosis.

Importance of adhering to prescribed diet and optimal body weight.

Exercise schedule (approved by physician).

Personal hygiene: foot care, skin and dental care, prevention of infection.

Over-the-counter medications and alcohol.

Referral to VNA to assure continued health supervision.

Importance of regular follow-up visits for check of blood sugar and adjustment of insulin dosage and diet, if necessary.

DRUG INTERACTIONS: Additive hypoglycemic effects may occur with **alcohol, anabolic steroids, fenfluramine, guanethidine, MAO inhibitors, oxytetracyclines,** and **phenylbutazone.** Additive hyperglycemic effects (through varied mechanisms of action) may occur with concomitant use of **corticosteroids, diazoxide, dextrothyroxine, epinephrine, estrogens, ethacrynic acid, furosemide, lithium, oral contraceptives, phenothiazines, thiazides, thyroid preparations,** and **triamterene. Propranolol** blocks warning symptoms of hypoglycemia and may produce hypoglycemia and possibly hyperglycemia by interfering with carbohydrate metabolism. **Glucagon** and **chlorthalidone** antagonize hypoglycemic effects of insulin. **Cyclophosphamide** inhibits insulin antibody formation, thus increasing the hypoglycemic action of insulin.

INSULIN INJECTION, CONCENTRATED
(REGULAR [CONCENTRATED] ILETIN)

Antidiabetic

ACTIONS AND USES

Concentrated insulin from pork pancreas unmodified by any agent that might prolong its action. For contraindications, precautions, and adverse reactions, see Insulin Injection.

Used for the occasional patient who develops insulin resistance and requires daily doses greater than 200 U (even as high as several thousand units).

ABSORPTION AND FATE

May show activity over 24-hour period. See Insulin Injection.

ROUTE AND DOSAGE

Subcutaneous, intramuscular: 1 to 3 times daily. Highly individualized dosage.

NURSING IMPLICATIONS

Label on U 500 insulin is brown-and-white striped.

Do not administer this preparation IV.

Discard solution that is not clear and colorless.

Measure accurately; slight variation can mean a large overdose or underdose.

There seems to be no condition of absolute resistance. All insulin-resistant patients will respond if dose is large enough.

Patients receiving concentrated insulin are kept under medical surveillance until dosage is established.

Deep secondary hypoglycemia reactions may develop 18 to 24 hours after administration of drug.

Frequently responsiveness to insulin effect is regained after a short period of concentrated insulin therapy.

See Insulin Injection.

Antidiabetic

ACTIONS AND USES
Clear, yellowish insulin solution modified by addition of zinc chloride and nonallergenic globin derived from blood of cattle. For actions, contraindications, precautions, and adverse reactions, see Insulin Injection.
Used to treat patients who are sensitive to protamine zinc insulin or who cannot be controlled with other forms of insulin.

ABSORPTION AND FATE
Intermediate-acting insulin preparation. Action begins in 2 hours, peaks in 8 to 16 hours, and lasts for about 24 hours. See Insulin Injection.

ROUTE AND DOSAGE
Subcutaneous (individualized): concentrations available are U 40, U 80, and U 100 (per milliliter).

NURSING IMPLICATIONS
Do not administer drug intravenously.
Preparation is not suitable for emergency use.
Administer by deep subcutaneous injection 30 to 60 minutes before break-fast.
Initial dosage is usually two-thirds to three-fourths of total daily dose of insulin injection.
Effective diabetic control is usually provided by one injection per 24 hours with dietary regulation.
Globin zinc is not a suspension; therefore it does not require shaking. Discard cloudy and outdated solutions.
Hypoglycemia is most apt to occur in the late afternoon. Notify the physician promptly if symptoms present; treatment is ingestion of soluble carbohydrate (hard candy, sugar, orange juice, honey).
See Insulin Injection.

INSULIN, ISOPHANE, SUSPENSION, U.S.P.
(ISOPHANE INSULIN, NPH ILETIN, NPH INSULIN)

Antidiabetic

ACTIONS AND USES
Suspension of crystals of protamine zinc insulin in neutral buffer with sufficient protamine to bind the insulin with pH 7.1 to 7.4. Combines some of the advantages and eliminates some of the disadvantages of both very short-acting and very long-acting preparations. Therapeutic effect is prompt enough to control postprandial hyperglycemia, which formerly called for supplemental doses of insulin injection. For actions, contraindications, and adverse reactions, see Insulin Injection.

ABSORPTION AND FATE
Intermediate-acting insulin preparation. Action begins within 60 to 90 minutes, peaks in 8 to 12 hours, and usually lasts for as long as 24 hours. See Insulin Injection.

ROUTE AND DOSAGE
Subcutaneous (individualized): concentrations available are U 40, U 80, and U 100 (per milliliter).

NURSING IMPLICATIONS

Gently rotate vial between palms and invert end to end several times. If suspension or vial walls display granules or clumps, discard vial.

Do not give this preparation IV.

Administer drug 30 to 90 minutes before first meal of the day.

Isophane insulin may be mixed with insulin injection without altering either solution.

If dosage is very high, may be given in divided doses: two-thirds in morning and one-third in late afternoon.

Mixing solutions: When preparing a mixture of insulins, make sure that both solutions are of the same concentration. Use same procedure every day to assure accuracy and safety: To give 5 U insulin injection and 10 U isophane insulin, use aseptic technique and inject 10 U air into isophane insulin bottle. Withdraw needle. Inject 5 U air into insulin injection bottle. Withdraw 5 U insulin. Eliminate all air bubbles from hub of needle and syringe barrel. Insert needle into bottle of isophane injection (make sure needle tip is below level of liquid). Withdraw 10 U isophane insulin. The physician may order the reverse of this sequence (ie, withdraw isophane insulin first); the important point is to follow the same order or sequence with the same stock bottle every day.

A hypoglycemic episode is most apt to occur between midafternoon and dinnertime, when insulin effect is peaking. Patient should be told to eat a snack in midafternoon and to carry candy to treat a reaction. A snack at bedtime will prevent insulin reaction during the night.

The patient should always consult his physician before making changes in dosage to accommodate anticipated stress or exercise. Also see Insulin Injection.

INSULIN, PROTAMINE ZINC SUSPENSION, U.S.P.

(PROTAMINE, ZINC and ILETIN; PROTAMINE, ZINC INSULIN, PZI)

Antidiabetic

ACTIONS AND USES

Cloudy suspension of insulin modified by addition of zinc (approximately 0.2 mg zinc per 100 U insulin and 1.25 mg protamine sulfate). See Insulin Injection for actions, contraindications, precautions, and adverse reactions.

Used to treat diabetes mellitus in patients who are inadequately controlled by unmodified insulin.

ABSORPTION AND FATE

Long-acting insulin preparation. Effects become evident in 4 to 8 hours; peak effect in 14 to 20 hours; duration of action in excess of 36 hours. See Insulin Injection.

ROUTE AND DOSAGE

Subcutaneous (individualized): concentrations available are U 40, U 80, and U 100 (per milliliter).

NURSING IMPLICATIONS

Gently rotate vial between palms and invert end to end several times. If suspension or vial walls display granules or clumps, discard vial.

Not to be administered IV.

Administer 30 to 60 minutes before breakfast.

Teach patient that prolonged insulin effect requires careful distribution of carbohydrates in a balanced diet. Patient should not redistribute food or alter dose or time of taking insulin.

If one dose of insulin has controlled diabetes for some time, the patient may test his urine once a day or two or three times weekly. In the event of infection, emotional stress, or change in activity, he should increase number of tests per day.

When mixing insulin injection with PZI, prepare solution immediately before administration. Withdraw insulin injection into syringe before PZI so that vial of insulin injection will not be contaminated with excess protamine. See Isophane Insulin for guidelines for mixing insulins.

The usual proportion of PZI to insulin injection is 1:2 or 1:3, in order to provide a preparation with both rapid onset and prolonged duration of action.

Blood sugar levels fall slowly after injection of PZI; thus, marked hypoglycemia may develop without producing apparent (clustered) symptoms. Teach patient and responsible other to be alert to the significance of sweating or fatigue unwarranted by patient's activities, as well as other vague symptoms such as lassitude, drowsiness, tremulousness. The physician should be notified immediately; without prompt and adequate treatment, patient may become unconscious.

Treatment of PZI-induced hypoglycemia requires both soluble and slowly digestible carbohydrate: eg, corn syrup or honey with bread, followed in 1 or 2 hours by additional carbohydrate, such as milk and crackers. Emergency treatment: 10 to 20 Gm D-glucose IV followed later by food.

During early period of adjustment to PZI, hypoglycemia may be prevented by eating small amount of food (2 or 3 crackers) between daytime meals and having a bedtime snack of milk and a small sandwich or some crackers.

Full therapeutic effect of PZI may be delayed several days following institution of treatment; during this interval, small supplemental doses of insulin injection are often necessary.

Also see Insulin Injection.

INSULIN ZINC SUSPENSION, U.S.P., B.P.
(LENTE ILETIN, LENTE INSULIN)

Antidiabetic

ACTIONS AND USES

Cloudy insulin suspension modified by addition of zinc chloride (approximately 0.2 mg zinc per 100 U insulin), so that solid phase of suspension consists of a mixture of amorphous and crystalline insulin in a 3:7 ratio. Because this form has no foreign protein (protamine or globin), allergic reactions are rare. Time action is intermediate between those of prompt and extended insulins and is so close to that of NPH insulin that the two forms may be used interchangeably. For contraindications, precautions, and adverse reactions, see Insulin Injection. Used for treatment of diabetes in patients allergic to other preparations of insulin. Also used for patients with evidence pointing toward thrombotic phenomena in which protamine may be a factor. See Insulin Injection.

ABSORPTION AND FATE

Intermediate-acting, with effect beginning within 60 to 90 minutes; peak action reached in 8 to 12 hours; duration 24 hours. See Insulin Injection.

ROUTE AND DOSAGE

Subcutaneous (individualized): concentrations available are U 40, U 80, and U 100 (per milliliter).

NURSING IMPLICATIONS

Administer 30 to 60 minutes before breakfast.

Do not administer IV.

This preparation is not suitable for emergency treatment.

Zinc insulin preparations (Ultralente, Lente, Semilente) can be mixed with one another, but they must not be mixed with other modified insulin.

Active principle is in the milky white precipitate. To assure complete dispersion, mix thoroughly by gently rotating the vial between the palm and by inverting it end to end several times. If the suspension or vial walls display clumps of precipitate after mixing, discard vial.

Symptoms of hypoglycemia are most apt to occur between midafternoon and dinnertime (an early symptom may be a sense of extreme fatigue). Notify the physician promptly and give patient emergency soluble carbohydrate. If the period of time between the midday meal and evening meal is prolonged, an afternoon snack may be ordered.

The possibility of nocturnal hypoglycemia should not be overlooked, especially during dose adjustment of Lente Iletin. Watch the sleeping patient carefully for signs of restlessness or profuse sweating.

Since time action of insulin zinc suspension (Lente) approximates that of isophane insulin suspension, the patient can usually be transferred directly to the latter on a unit-for-unit basis. Duration of action with Lente may be longer than with isophane insulin.

Also see Insulin Injection.

INSULIN ZINC SUSPENSION, EXTENDED, U.S.P.
(ULTRALENTE ILETIN, ULTRALENTE INSULIN)

Antidiabetic

ACTIONS AND USES

Cloudy suspension of insulin modified by addition of zinc chloride (approximately 0.2 mg zinc per 100 U insulin). Large particle size and high zinc content delay absorption and prolong action. No modifying protein (protamine or globin) is added; therefore, incidence of allergic reactions is low. See Insulin Injection for actions, uses, contraindications, and adverse reactions.

ABSORPTION AND FATE

Long-acting insulin preparation. Action begins within 4 to 8 hours, peaks in 16 to 18 hours, and continues for more than 36 hours. See Insulin Injection.

ROUTE AND DOSAGE

Subcutaneous (individualized): concentrations available are U 40, U 80, and U 100 (per milliliter).

NURSING IMPLICATIONS

This drug is not to be used IV.

Administered 30 to 90 minutes before breakfast by deep subcutaneous injection.

Active principle is in the milky white precipitate. To assure complete dispersion, mix thoroughly by gently rotating vial between palms and by inverting it end to end several times. If suspension on vial walls display clumps of precipitate after mixing, discard vial.

May be mixed with Lente and Semilente, but must not be mixed with other modified insulin preparations.

Hypoglycemia is most apt to occur during the night or early morning. Notify physician promptly if it occurs (watch sleeping patient carefully for signs of restlessness or profuse sweating). Hypoglycemia is treated by administering soluble carbohydrate (orange juice, sugar, honey) plus a slowly digestible carbohydrate (bread, crackers). Supplemental feedings may be prescribed.

Also see Insulin Injection.

INSULIN ZINC SUSPENSION, PROMPT, U.S.P.
(SEMILENTE ILETIN, SEMILENTE INSULIN)

Antidiabetic

ACTIONS AND USES

Cloudy suspension of insulin modified by addition of zinc chloride (approximately 0.2 mg zinc per 100 U insulin) so that solid phase of suspension is amorphous. No modifying protein (protamine or globin) is added; therefore, incidence of allergic reactions is low. See Insulin Injection for actions, contraindications, precautions, and adverse reactions.

Used for routine management of diabetes, especially for patients allergic to other types of insulin. Also used for patients with evidence pointing toward thrombotic phenomena in which protamine may be a factor.

ABSORPTION AND FATE

Rapid-acting insulin preparation. Action begins within ½ to 1 hour, peaks in 5 to 7 hours and lasts 12 to 16 hours. See Insulin Injection.

ROUTE AND DOSAGE

Subcutaneous (individualized): concentrations available are U 40, U 80, and U 100 (per milliliter).

NURSING IMPLICATIONS

Never administer this preparation IV.

Preparation not suitable for emergency use.

Administered 30 minutes before breakfast.

Active principle is in the milky white precipitate. To assure complete dispersion, mix thoroughly by gently rotating vial between palms and by inverting it end to end several times. If the suspension on vial walls displays clumps of crystalline precipitate after mixing, discard vial.

Symptoms of hypoglycemia are most apt to appear before lunch; glucosuria is most apt to appear during the night.

A mixture of prompt insulin zinc suspension (Semilente) and insulin zinc suspension (Lente) may be indicated when glucosuria after meals cannot be controlled by Lente insulin alone.

The zinc insulin preparations (Ultralente, Lente, Semilente) can be mixed with one another, but they must not be mixed with other modified insulin.

This preparation should not be substituted for another insulin preparation without direction by a physician.

Also see Insulin Injection.

IODINATED GLYCEROL
(ORGANIDIN)

Expectorant

ACTIONS AND USES

Stable complex of iodine and glycerol. Liquefies thick, tenacious respiratory tract fluid and facilitates expectoration. Contains approximately 50% organically bound iodine, little or no inorganic iodine, and no free iodine.

Used as adjunctive treatment in bronchial asthma, bronchitis, emphysema, and other respiratory disorders and after surgery to help prevent atelectasis.

CONTRAINDICATIONS AND PRECAUTIONS

History of marked sensitivity to inorganic iodides; hypersensitivity to iodinated glycerol (or any of its ingredients) and related compounds.

ADVERSE REACTIONS

Rarely: GI irritation, rash, hypersensitivity, iodism (dose-related and reversible).

ROUTE AND DOSAGE

Oral: **Adults:** 60 mg 4 times a day. **Children:** up to one-half the adult dosage, based on child's weight. Available as tablets (30 mg each), 5% solution (50 mg/ml), and elixir (60 mg/5 ml).

NURSING IMPLICATIONS

All preparations should be administered with liquid.

Drug should be discontinued if skin rash or other evidence of hypersensitivity occurs.

IODOCHLORHYDROXYQUIN, N.F.
(MYCOQUIN, QUINOFORM, TOROFOR, VIOFORM)
CLIOQUINOL, B.P.

Local antiinfective

ACTIONS AND USES

Halogenated hydroxyquinoline with antifungal, antibacterial, and antiamebicidal actions. Oral and vaginal suppository forms have been temporarily withdrawn from U.S. market pending further study of toxicity.

Used topically for treatment of inflamed skin conditions such as eczema, athlete's foot, and other fungal conditions and for simple wounds, ulcers, and burns.

ABSORPTION AND FATE

May be absorbed through skin. Some is excreted rapidly in urine in conjugated form; remainder is excreted slowly, persisting in body for 1 month or more.

CONTRAINDICATIONS AND PRECAUTIONS

Hypersensitivity to iodine; tuberculosis; vaccinia, varicella, or other viral skin conditions; severe renal disease; hepatic damage; thyroid disorder.

ADVERSE REACTIONS

Infrequent: local burning, irritation, pruritus ani, staining of hair. Systemic reactions (not reported with topical applications but possible): iodism (furunculosis, dermatitis, chills, fever, sore throat, brassy taste, stomatitis, coryza, swelling of salivary glands), diarrhea, constipation, abdominal discomfort, slight enlargement of thyroid gland, hair loss, agranulocytosis, subacute myelooptic neuropathy.

ROUTE AND DOSAGE

Topical (3% cream, lotion, or ointment; powder): applied to affected areas 2 to 4 times daily.

NURSING IMPLICATIONS

Systemic absorption is enhanced by application to widespread areas and use of occlusive dressings.

Inform patients that the drug may stain fabric or hair yellow on contact.

Warn patients to avoid contact of drug with eyes.

Drug should be discontinued if skin irritation, persistent diarrhea, rash, or other signs of sensitivity develop.

Caution patients to apply the drug as directed and only for the period of time prescribed.

Preserved in tightly covered, light-resistant containers.

LABORATORY TEST INTERFERENCES: Possibility of elevated PBI and decreased ^{131}I thyroidal uptake. May yield a false positive ferric chloride test for phenylketonuria if iodochlorhydroxyquin is present on diaper or in urine.

IPECAC SYRUP, U.S.P.
IPECACUANHA, B.P.

Emetic

ACTIONS AND USES

Derived from dried rhizomes and roots of *Cephaelis ipecacuanha;* contains several alkaloids, of which emetine comprises over 50%. Acts locally on gastric mucosa and centrally on chemoreceptor trigger zone to induce vomiting. Also has expectorant action that is thought to result from increased bronchial secretions caused by reflex stimulation of gastric mucosa and lowered sputum viscosity.

Used as emergency emetic to remove ingested poisons. An ingredient in many OTC expectorant mixtures.

CONTRAINDICATIONS AND PRECAUTIONS

Comatose, semicomatose, inebriated, or deeply sedated patients; patients in shock; when danger of convulsions is present; impaired cardiac function; arteriosclerosis; for treatment of ingested strong alkalis, acids, strychnine, petroleum distillates, volatile oils.

ADVERSE REACTIONS

If drug is not vomited but absorbed, or for overdosage: persistent vomiting, bloody diarrhea, shock, cardiac arrhythmias, cardiotoxicity, convulsions, coma.

ROUTE AND DOSAGE

Oral: **Adults and children** *over 1 year of age:* 15 ml (3 teaspoonsful). Dose may be repeated once in 20 minutes, if vomiting has not occurred. **Children** *less than 1 year of age:* 5 to 10 ml (1 to 2 teaspoonsful).

NURSING IMPLICATIONS

Not to be confused with ipecac fluidextract, which is 14 times stronger and has caused deaths when mistakenly given at the same dosage as ipecac syrup.

Action of ipecac is facilitated by following the dose with 200 to 300 ml of milk (preferably evaporated milk); smaller volumes for small children. (Reportedly absorption of toxic substances may be increased by large volumes of water.) Emetic effect occurs in 15 to 30 minutes.

Activated charcoal should not be given simultaneously because charcoal adsorbs ipecac and renders it completely ineffective.

In small children, emetic effect may be enhanced by gently bouncing the child.

Available without prescription in quantity of 30 ml for emergency use as emetic. Food and Drug Administration requires labeling to include the following cautions before use: call a physician, a poison control center, or a hospital emergency room immediately for advice; keep the drug out of reach of children.

If vomiting does not occur within 30 minutes after the repeat administration, dosage should be recovered by gastric lavage and activated charcoal. Stored in tight containers, preferably at temperature not exceeding 25 C (77 F).

IRON DEXTRAN, U.S.P., B.P.
(FERRODEX, HEMATRAN, IMFERON, K-FeRON)

Hematinic

ACTIONS AND USES
Complex of ferric hydroxide with dextran in 0.9% sodium chloride solution for injection. Reticuloendothelial cells of liver, spleen, and bone marrow separate iron from iron dextran complex; ferric iron is gradually released into plasma, combines with transferrin, and is transported to bone marrow, where it is incorporated into hemoglobin.
Used in treatment of microcytic, hypochromic anemia due to iron deficiency when oral administration is not feasible or is ineffective.

ABSORPTION AND FATE
Following IM administration, most of drug is absorbed from injection site through lymphatic system. Approximately 60% absorbed after 3 days, and up to 90% after 1 to 3 weeks. The remainder is gradually absorbed over several months or longer. Slowly cleared from plasma by reticuloendothelial system. Small amounts of iron dextran cross the placenta. Traces are excreted in breast milk, urine, bile, and feces.

CONTRAINDICATIONS AND PRECAUTIONS
Hypersensitivity to the product; all anemias except iron-deficiency anemia. Safe use during pregnancy and childbearing period not established. Cautious use: rheumatoid arthritis, ankylosing spondylitis, impaired hepatic function, history of allergies.

ADVERSE REACTIONS
Headache, arthralgia, myalgia, transient paresthesias, nausea, vomiting, faintness, syncope, dizziness, tinnitus, hypotension, tachycardia, precordial pressure sensation, sweating, fever, chills, transient loss of taste, metallic taste, peripheral vascular flushing (rapid IV), local phlebitis (IV), soreness and inflammation of IM injection site, brown discoloration of skin (IM injection site), regional lymphadenopathy, abdominal pain, rash, urticaria, pruritus, convulsions, circulatory collapse, hemosiderosis (following unwarranted therapy), anaphylactic reactions (particularly with rapid IV): nausea, dizziness, fall in blood pressure, chest pain, fatal cardiac arrhythmias. Risk of carcinogenesis reportedly appears to be extremely small.

ROUTE AND DOSAGE
Total dosage may be calculated by formula: Wt in lbs $\times$ (100 $-$ % Hgb) $\times$ 0.3 = mg of iron. Requirements of individuals weighing 30 lb or less should be reduced to 80% of the amount calculated by this formula. Each milliliter of iron dextran contains 50 mg of elemental iron. A test dose of 25 mg IM or IV is administered on first day; if no adverse reactions are apparent, subsequent doses are given as follows until the calculated amount has been given (doses indicated should not be exceeded): Intramuscular: **Infants** *under 10 lb:* up to 25 mg/day. **Children** *10 to 20 lb:* up to 50 mg/day. *Patients 20 to 110 lb:* up to 100 mg/day. *Patients over 110 lb:* up to 250 mg/day. Intravenous: Within 2 or 3 days after test dose, dosage may be raised to 2 ml/day until calculated dose has been administered.

NURSING IMPLICATIONS

Diagnosis of iron-deficiency anemia should be corroborated by appropriate laboratory investigations, with the cause being determined and if possible corrected, before therapy is initiated.

Regardless of route used, initial test doses are advised to observe patient's response to the drug. Fatal anaphylactic reactions have occurred.

IM injections should be given only into upper outer quadrant of buttock, using a 2- or 3-inch, 19- or 20-gauge needle. The Z-track technique is recommended in order to avoid the possibility of drug leakage along the needle track and brown staining of subcutaneous tissue. Staining of skin may also be minimized by using one needle to withdraw drug from container and another needle for injection. Brown staining of skin may persist 1 to 2 years, since drug is absorbed slowly from subcutaneous tissue.

Z-track technique: Firmly displace skin laterally prior to injection. After needle is inserted, withdraw plunger carefully to check that there is no entry into a blood vessel. Inject slowly. Rotate injection sites. No more than 5 ml should be injected into a single IM site.

The multiple-dose vial is used only for IM injections. Since it contains a preservative (phenol), it is not suitable for IV use.

The IV route is preferred and recommended for patients with insufficient muscle mass, those with impaired absorption (as in edema), when uncontrolled bleeding is a possibility, or when massive and prolonged parenteral therapy is indicated.

Following IV administration, the patient should remain in bed for at least 30 minutes to prevent orthostatic hypotension.

IV administration may exacerbate or reactivate joint pain in patients with rheumatoid arthritis or ankylosing spondylitis. For this reason, the IM route is generally preferred in these patients.

When given by IV infusion, flow rate should be prescribed by physician. If a reaction occurs, stop IV immediately and report to physician. (The use of 5% dextrose injection instead of 0.9% sodium chloride injection is reportedly associated with a high incidence of local pain and phlebitis.)

Bear in mind that systemic reactions may occur over a 24-hour period after parenteral iron has been administered. Instruct patient to report any unusual symptoms.

Periodic determinations of hemoglobin, hematocrit, and reticulocyte count should be made as a guide to therapy. Oral iron therapy should replace parenteral therapy as soon as feasible.

Anticipated response to parenteral iron therapy is an average weekly hemoglobin rise of about 1 Gm/dl. As with oral therapy, peak levels are generally reached in about 4 to 8 weeks.

Blood typing and cross matching are reportedly not affected by iron dextran.

Mixing any other drug in syringe or solution with iron dextran is not advised.

LABORATORY TEST INTERFERENCES: There is the possibility of falsely elevated serum bilirubin and falsely decreased serum calcium values. Large doses of iron dextran may color the serum brown.

Hematinic

ACTIONS AND USES
    Chemical complex of iron, sorbitol, and citric acid. Similar to iron dextran (qv), and reported to produce comparable therapeutic response. Contains the equivalent of 50 mg elemental iron per milliliter.
    Used in iron-deficiency anemia not amenable to oral iron therapy.

ABSORPTION AND FATE
    Rapidly absorbed from injection site directly into bloodstream; minimal portions absorbed via lymphatic system. Maximal serum levels obtained within 2 hours; bone marrow uptake occurs within 24 to 72 hours. Iron sorbitex not utilized for hemoglobin synthesis is stored chiefly in liver. Approximately one-third of a single dose is excreted in urine within 24 hours. Small amounts excreted in saliva and feces. Crosses placenta.

CONTRAINDICATIONS AND PRECAUTIONS
    Known hypersensitivity to parenteral iron; all anemias other than iron-deficiency anemia; folic acid deficiency; concomitant use of oral iron; kidney disease; active urinary tract infections; severe liver damage; pediatric use, IV use.

ADVERSE REACTIONS
    Nausea, vomiting, transient alterations in taste perception, flushing, dizziness, headache, urinary frequency, hematuria, albuminuria, blurred vision, faulty hearing, transient pain and staining at IM site, hemosiderosis, anaphylactic-type reaction: nausea, chest pain, dizziness, fall in blood pressure, cardiac arrhythmias.

ROUTE AND DOSAGE
    Intramuscular: 1.5 mg/kg body weight daily. Total dosage to be given is based on formula (see Iron Dextran).

NURSING IMPLICATIONS
Diagnosis of iron-deficiency anemia should be corroborated by appropriate laboratory investigations before therapy is initiated.
Administer by deep IM injection into upper outer quadrant of buttock. The Z-track technique (see Iron Dextran) is advised to minimize the possibility of skin staining (unlike the situation with iron dextran, staining usually persists for only a few weeks). Rotate injection sites.
IV injection is specifically contraindicated. After needle is inserted into muscle, carefully withdraw plunger to check that there is no entry into a blood vessel.
Incidence and severity of systemic side effects increase in patients receiving doses of 200 mg or more.
Monitor vital signs and observe patient closely for at least 2 hours after injection. Observe for and report the occurrence of fever, sweating, myalgia, palpitation, precordial pain, or fall in blood pressure. These symptoms may occur 30 minutes to 2 hours after drug administration and usually subside within with a few hours.
Some patients experience altered taste perception within 30 minutes after drug administration; it may persist for 10 to 12 hours.
Inform patients that urine may turn dark brown or black on standing and that this is no cause for alarm.

(MARPLAN)

Antidepressant

ACTIONS AND USES
  MAO inhibitor of the hydrazide group. Similar in actions, uses, contraindica-
  tions, precautions, and adverse reactions to phenelzine (qv).
  Recommended only for treatment of depressed patients refractory to or intoler-
  ant to tricyclic antidepressants or to electroconvulsive therapy.
ROUTE AND DOSAGE
  Oral: initially 30 mg daily in single or divided doses; maintenance 10 to 20 mg
  (or less) daily. Doses larger than 30 mg daily not recommended.

NURSING IMPLICATIONS
A complete review of prior drug therapy is advised before initiation of
  isocarboxazid.
Most adverse reactions occur because of failure to recognize cumulative
  effects of isocarboxazid (see Phenelzine Sulfate).
Therapeutic effects may be apparent within a week or less, but in some
  patients there may be time lag of 3 to 4 weeks before improvement occurs.
Dosage is individually adjusted on basis of careful observations of patient.
Physician will reduce dosage to maintenance level as soon as improvement
  is observed, because drug has a cumulative effect.
Although therapeutic effect is delayed, toxic symptoms from overdosage or
  from ingestion of contraindicated substances (eg, foods high in tyramine)
  may occur within hours.
See Phenelzine Sulfate.

ISOFLUROPHATE, U.S.P.
(DFP, Diisopropyl Fluorophosphate, FLOROPRYL)

Anticholinesterase (ophthalmic), miotic

ACTIONS AND USES
  Potent, long-acting organophosphorous cholinesterase inhibitor. Actions similar to those of demecarium; however, unlike demecarium, it produces virtually
  irreversible inactivation of cholinesterase. Topical application to eye results in
  intense and prolonged miosis and ciliary muscle contraction due to inhibition
  of cholinesterase.
  Used in treatment of primary open-angle glaucoma in patients resistant to
  short-acting miotics; used as diagnostic aid and in management of accommodative (nonparalytic) convergent strabismus (esotropia) in patients with essen-
  tially equal visual acuity.
ABSORPTION AND FATE
  Rapidly absorbed from mucous membranes and skin following contact. Miosis
  is produced within 20 minutes, with maximal effect in about 4 hours; effect may
  last 2 weeks or more.
CONTRAINDICATIONS AND PRECAUTIONS
  Sensitivity to organophosphorous compounds. See Demecarium Bromide.
ADVERSE REACTIONS
  Ocular pain, headache, lenticular opacities (long-term use). Also see
  Demecarium Bromide.
ROUTE AND DOSAGE
  Topical (0.025% ophthalmic ointment): *Glaucoma:* initially one quarter inch strip
  in conjunctival sac every 8 to 72 hours. *Strabismus:* not more than one quarter

inch strip administered every night for 2 weeks. If eye becomes straighter, an accommodative factor is demonstrated. *Esotropia:* not more than one quarter inch strip at a time, every night for 2 weeks; dosage is then reduced to one quarter inch strip every other day or one quarter inch strip once a week for 2 months, after which patient's status is reevaluated.

NURSING IMPLICATIONS

May be prescribed at night before retiring to reduce discomfort of blurred vision and ciliary spasm.

During initial therapy for glaucoma, tonometric measurements every 3 or 4 hours are advised to detect any immediate rise in intraocular pressure.

Isoflurophate is rapidly absorbed from skin and can cause contact dermatitis. After administration, immediately blot excess medication from eyelid with tissue and wash hands thoroughly.

Isoflurophate is unstable in the presence of water. Containers should be tightly closed to prevent absorption of moisture. Do not wash tip of tube or allow it to touch eyelid or any other moist surface.

Patients receiving isoflurophate should remain under medical supervision.

Warn patient of possible additive effects from exposure to carbamate or organophosphate insecticides and pesticides, eg, parathion, malathion.

See Demecarium Bromide.

ISONIAZID, U.S.P., B.P.
(INH, Isonicotinic Acid Hydrazide, HYZYD, LANIAZID, NICONYL, NYDRAZID, ROLAZID TEEBACONIN)

Antibacterial (tuberculostatic)

ACTIONS AND USES

Hydrazide of isonicotinic acid with highly specific action against *Mycobacterium tuberculosis.* Exerts bacteriostatic action against actively growing tubercle bacilli; may be bactericidal in higher concentrations. Postulated to act by interfering with metabolism of bacterial proteins, nucleic acid, carbohydrates, and lipids. Reported to have some MAO-inhibiting properties and to act as a competitive antagonist of pyridoxine (vitamin B_6).

Used in treatment of all forms of active tuberculosis caused by susceptible organisms and as preventive in high-risk persons. May be used alone or with other tuberculostatic agents.

ABSORPTION AND FATE

Peak blood levels in 1 to 2 hours following oral administration and sooner following IM injection. Levels decline to 50% or less within 6 hours. Diffuses readily into body tissues, organs, and fluids, notably saliva, bronchial secretions, and pleural, ascitic, and cerebrospinal fluids. Metabolized in liver primarily by acetylation and dehydrazination (rate of acetylation is genetically determined). Half-life 2 to 4 hours (prolonged in hepatic insufficiency and in "slow" inactivators). About 75% to 95% of dose is excreted in urine within 24 hours as metabolites; small amounts excreted in saliva and feces. Crosses placenta and passes into breast milk.

CONTRAINDICATIONS AND PRECAUTIONS

History of isoniazid-associated hypersensitivity reactions, including hepatic injury; acute liver damage of any etiology; pregnancy (unless risk is warranted). Cautious use: chronic liver disease, renal dysfunction, history of convulsive disorders.

Usually dose-related. **Neurologic:** paresthesias, peripheral neuritis, visual disturbances, optic neuritis and atrophy, tinnitus, vertigo, ataxia, somnolence, excessive dreaming, insomnia, amnesia, euphoria, toxic psychosis, changes in affect and behavior, depression, impaired memory, hyperreflexia, muscle twitching, convulsions. **Hypersensitivity:** fever, chills, skin eruptions (morbilliform, maculopapular, purpuric, urticarial), lymphadenitis, vasculitis, keratitis. **Hepatotoxicity:** elevated SGOT and SGPT, bilirubinemia, jaundice, fatal hepatitis. **Metabolic and endocrine:** pyridoxine (vitamin B_6) deficiency, pellagra, gynecomastia, hyperglycemia, glycosuria, acetonuria, metabolic acidosis, proteinuria. **Hematologic:** agranulocytosis, hemolytic or aplastic anemia, thrombocytopenia, eosinophilia, methemoglobinemia. **GI:** nausea, vomiting, epigastric distress, constipation. **Other reported:** headache, tachycardia, dyspnea, dry mouth, urinary retention (males), postural hypotension, rheumatic and lupus-erythematosus-like syndromes.

ROUTE AND DOSAGE

Oral and IM dosages are identical. Administered in single or divided doses. *Treatment:* **Adults:** 5 mg/kg body weight (up to 300 mg) daily. **Infants and children:** 10 to 30 mg/kg (up to 300 to 500 mg) daily. *Preventive therapy:* **Adults:** 300 mg daily. **Infants and children:** 10 mg/kg (up to 300 mg) daily.

NURSING IMPLICATIONS

Appropriate mycobacteriologic studies and susceptibility tests should be performed before initiation of therapy and periodically thereafter to detect possible bacterial resistance.

Vision testing and ophthalmoscopic examinations are recommended initially and periodically during drug therapy, as well as whenever visual symptoms appear. Early cessation of therapy usually results in resolution of ocular reactions.

In patients with GI reactions, drug may be prescribed in smaller divided doses or administered simultaneously with food.

Isoniazid in solution tends to crystallize at low temperatures; if this occurs, solution should be allowed to warm to room temperature to redissolve crystals prior to use.

Local transient pain may follow IM injections. Massage injection site following drug administration. Rotate injection sites.

Adverse reactions occur most frequently in malnourished patients, the elderly, and in "slow" isoniazid inactivators (approximately 50% of blacks and Caucasians are "slow" inactivators; the majority of Eskimos and Orientals are "rapid" inactivators).

Pyridoxine (vitamin B_6) may be prescribed concomitantly to prevent neurotoxic effects of isoniazid. Peripheral neuritis, the most common reaction, is usually preceded by paresthesias of feet and hands (numbness, tingling, burning). Patients particularly susceptible include malnourished patients, diabetics, adolescents, and "slow" inactivators.

Monitor tuberculin precipitation reaction and blood pressure during period of dosage adjustment. Some patients experience orthostatic hypotension; therefore, caution against rapid positional changes. Supervision of ambulation may be indicated, particularly in the elderly.

Diabetic patients should be observed for loss of diabetes control. Both true glycosuria and false positive Benedict's tests have been reported. See Laboratory Test Interferences.

Isoniazid hepatitis (sometimes fatal) usually develops during the first 4 to 6 months of treatment, but it may occur at any time during drug therapy; it is most common in patients 50 years of age and older and in those who ingest alcohol daily.

Patients should be carefully interviewed and examined at regular intervals for early detection of signs and symptoms of hepatotoxicity (loss of appetite, fatigue, malaise, dark urine, jaundice or scleral icterus). Instruct patient to withhold medication and report promptly to physician if any of these effects occur. Some physicians order monthly liver function tests.

Hypersensitivity reactions should be reported immediately and all drugs withheld. Generally, they occur within 3 to 7 weeks following initiation of therapy.

Therapeutic effects of isoniazid usually become evident within the first 2 to 3 weeks of therapy and may include reduction of fever and night sweats, diminished cough and sputum, increased appetite and weight gain, reduction of fatigue, and sense of well-being. Over 90% of patients receiving optimal therapy have negative sputum by the 6th month.

Check weight at least twice weekly under standard conditions.

Isoniazid may produce a sense of euphoria, which tempts the patient to do more than he should. Stress the importance of planned rest periods.

Antituberculous agents permit therapy to continue on an outpatient basis after initial hospitalization. Patients and responsible family members must understand the importance of continuous medical supervision and uninterrupted drug therapy to prevent relapse and spread of infection to others.

In general, isoniazid therapy is continued for a minimum of 18 months to 2 years for original treatment of active tuberculosis. When used for preventive therapy, isoniazid is usually continued for 12 months.

Preserved in tightly closed, light-resistant containers.

LABORATORY TEST INTERFERENCES: There is the possibility of false positive results with Benedict's solution, but usually not with Clinitest or glucose oxidase methods (eg, Clinistix, Dextrostix, Tes-Tape).

DRUG INTERACTIONS: Daily ingestion of **alcohol** may increase risk of isoniazid-induced hepatotoxicity. Simultaneous administration of large doses of **aluminum hydroxide** and other aluminum-containing antacids may delay or decrease absorption of isoniazid; to minimize risk of interaction, schedule isoniazid at least 1 hour prior to antacid administration. Concurrent administration of isoniazid and **phenytoin** (diphenylhydantoin) and possibly other hydantoin derivatives may result in a significant rise in serum phenytoin levels and toxicity (ataxia, drowsiness, nystagmus); reduced phenytoin dosage is recommended, in "slow" inactivators particularly, when isoniazid is added to the therapeutic regimen.

ISOPROPAMIDE IODIDE N.F.
(DARBID)

Anticholinergic

ACTIONS AND USES
Synthetic quaternary ammonium compound; long acting anticholinergic with actions similar to those of atropine (qv).
Used primarily for adjunctive treatment of peptic ulcer. See Atropine.

CONTRAINDICATIONS AND PRECAUTIONS
Hypersensitivity to iodine; tachycardia. Cautious use: elderly patients, autonomic neuropathy, hepatic and renal disease, ulcerative colitis, hyperthyroidism, coronary disease, hypertension, cardiac arrhythmias, children under 12 years of age. Also see Atropine.

ADVERSE REACTIONS
Iodine rash (rare): acneiform eruptions, exfoliative dermatitis. **Overdosage:** depression, circulatory collapse, curarelike action: weakness in short muscles (ie, eye, eyelids, fingers and toes) and in muscles of jaw, neck, leg; hypotension. Also see Atropine.

ROUTE AND DOSAGE
Oral: **Adults and children** *over 12:* 5 to 10 mg every 12 hours.

NURSING IMPLICATIONS

Isopropamide may alter PBI level and suppress ^{131}I uptake; therefore usually drug is discontinued one week before these tests are made. Patient should inform a new physician that he is taking this drug.

If patient is on continuous therapy, teach him to check his pulse periodically. Advise him to consult his physician if pulse rate increases above 96 beats/minute.

Patient should understand importance of prompt reporting of the following symptoms: hazy vision, drooping of eyelids, weakness in hand muscles. While curarelike symptoms seldom occur, their appearance necessitates discontinuation of the drug.

Preserve drug in well closed, light-resistant container.

Also see Atropine Sulfate.

ISOPROTERENOL HYDROCHLORIDE, U.S.P.
(IPRENOL, ISUPREL HYDROCHLORIDE, NORISODRINE AEROTROL, PROTERNOL, VAPO-N-ISO)
ISOPROTERENOL SULFATE, N.F.
(ISO-AUTOHALER, LUF-ISO, MEDIHALER-ISO, NORISODRINE SULFATE)

Adrenegic, bronchodilator

ACTIONS AND USES
Synthetic sympathomimetic amine chemically and pharmacologically similar to epinephrine, but acts almost exclusively on β-adrenergic receptors. Primary therapeutic effects include cardiac stimulation (positive inotropic and chronotropic actions), relaxation of bronchial tree, and peripheral vasodilation. Usually increases cardiac output and work, but may diminish efficiency. Lowers peripheral vascular resistance, and increases venous return to heart. Decreases both diastolic and mean pressures, but maintains or slightly increases systolic pressure, especially when patient is in shock. Large doses cause substantial drop in blood pressure, and repeated large doses may result in cardiac enlargement and focal myocarditis. Relaxes GI and uterine smooth muscles; inhibits histamine release. Increases hepatic glycogenolysis; but, unlike epinephrine, stimulates insulin secretion and thus rarely produces hyperglycemia. Can also cause central excitation.

Used as bronchodilator in acute and chronic asthma and other respiratory disorders and in bronchospasm induced by anesthesia. Also effective as cardiac stimulant in cardiac arrest, carotid sinus hypersensitivity, cardiogenic and bacteremic shock, Stokes-Adams syndrome, or ventricular arrhythmias due to A-V block.

ABSORPTION AND FATE
Readily absorbed following parenteral injection and oral inhalation. Absorption following oral, sublingual, and rectal routes reportedly not as predictable. Bronchodilation occurs promptly and persists 1 to 2 hours following inhalation and

sublingual tablet (variable), up to 2 hours following subcutaneous injection, and 2 to 4 hours following rectal administration. Action begins about 30 minutes following timed-release tablet and lasts 6 to 8 hours. Pharmacologic action appears to terminate primarily by tissue uptake. Metabolized by conjugation in GI tract, liver, lungs, and other tissues. Metabolism in children may be more rapid and extensive. Secreted in urine within 24 to 48 hours. Small quantities of inactive metabolites excreted in feces.

CONTRAINDICATIONS AND PRECAUTIONS

Preexisting cardiac arrhythmias associated with tachycardia; use of extended-release form in patients with coronary sclerosis; central hyperexcitability; simultaneous use with epinephrine. Safe use in women of childbearing potential and during pregnancy and lactation not established. Cautious use: sensitivity to sympathomimetic amines; elderly and debilitated patients; hypertension; coronary insufficiency and other cardiovascular disease; renal dysfunction; hyperthyroidism; diabetes; prostatic hypertrophy; glaucoma; tuberculosis.

ADVERSE REACTIONS

Facial flushing, sweating, mild tremors, nervousness, anxiety, headache, palpitation, tachycardia, lightheadedness, vertigo, insomnia, excitement, weakness, fatigue, precordial pain or distress, severe prolonged asthma attack, bad taste, buccal ulcerations (sublingual administration), bronchial irritation and edema (particularly with inhalations of powder), swelling of parotid glands (prolonged use), paradoxic Stokes-Adams seizure (rare). **Overdosage:** nausea, vomiting, cardiac excitability, extrasystoles, arrhythmias, elevation followed by fall in blood pressure, severe bronchoconstriction, cardiac arrest, sudden death (especially following excessive use of aerosols).

ROUTE AND DOSAGE

Isoproterenol hydrochloride: Inhalation: *Metered-dose nebulizer* (120 to 250 μg): Start with 1 inhalation; if no relief after 2 to 5 minutes, inhalation may be repeated. Maintenance: 1 or 2 inhalations 4 to 6 times daily at not less than 3- to 4-hour intervals. No more than 2 inhalations at any one time. *Hand-bulb nebulizer* (1:200 solution): 5 to 15 deep inhalations; (1:100 solution): 3 to 7 deep inhalations. If necessary, repeated once after 5 to 10 minutes. Treatment intervals not less than 3 to 4 hours up to 5 times daily. *Nebulization by oxygen, compressed air, or IPPB apparatus:* 0.5 ml of 1:200 solution diluted to 2 to 2.5 ml with water or isotonic saline. Flow rate regulated to administer over 10 to 20 minutes; may be repeated up to 5 times daily, if necessary. Oral: *Sustained-action tablet:* 30 to 180 mg daily. Sublingual, rectal **(adults):** 10 to 20 mg 3 or 4 times daily; maximum 60 mg/day; **(children):** 5 to 10 mg 3 or 4 times daily; maximum 30 mg/day. Subcutaneous: 0.15 to 0.2 mg. Intramuscular: 0.02 to 1 mg. Intravenous infusion: 5 μg/minute, 1:250,000 solution. Intravenous (direct): 0.01 to 0.2 mg (0.5 to 10 ml) of 1:50,000 solution. Intracardiac: 0.02 mg.

Isoproterenol sulfate: *Metered powder inhaler* (10%, 25%): 1 or 2 inhalations of normal depth; if necessary, second dose repeated in 5 minutes and third dose 10 minutes after second dose; not to exceed 3 doses for each attack. *Metered aerosol nebulizer* (75 to 150 μg): start with 1 inhalation; if necessary, repeat after 2 to 5 minutes; maintenance, 1 or 2 inhalations 4 to 6 times daily, not to exceed 2 inhalations at any one time or more than 6 inhalations in an hour.

NURSING IMPLICATIONS

IV administration is regulated by continuous ECG monitoring.

Patient must be observed constantly, and response to therapy must be carefully monitored by frequent determinations of heart rate, ECG pattern, blood pressure, and central venous pressure, as well as (for patients with shock) urine volume, blood pH, and Pco$_2$ levels.

IV infusion rate should be prescribed by physician, with specific guidelines for regulating flow or terminating infusion in relation to heart rate, premature beats, ECG changes, precordial distress, BP, and urine flow.

Constant-infusion pump apparatus is recommended to prevent sudden influx of large amounts of drug.

Facilities for administration of oxygen mixtures and respiratory assistance should be immediately available.

High frequency of arrhythmias reported, particularly when administered IV to patients with cardiogenic shock or ischemic heart disease, digitalized patients, and those with electrolyte imbalance.

Intracardiac injection for cardiac standstill must be accompanied by cardiac massage to perfuse drug to myocardium.

Solutions intended for oral inhalation must not be injected.

Sublingual or oral tablet: Patient taking either form should be forewarned of potential transient facial flushing, palpitation, and precordial discomfort. (Systemic effects reported to occur more frequently by these routes than by inhalation.)

Sublingual tablet administration: Instruct patient to allow tablet to dissolve under tongue, without sucking, and not to swallow saliva (may cause epigastric pain) until drug has been completely absorbed.

Sublingual tablet may be administered rectally, if prescribed.

Prolonged use of sublingual tablets reportedly can damage teeth, possibly because of drug acidity. Patient should be advised to rinse mouth with water between doses.

Sustained-release tablet should be swallowed whole and not broken or chewed.

Oral inhalations: Note that dosage and recommended method of inhaling may vary with type of nebulizer and formulation used. Patient should be carefully instructed in use of nebulizer and cautioned to take the lowest effective dose necessary to obtain relief.

Patient instructions for administration by metered-dose nebulizers: Place mouthpiece well into mouth, aimed at back of throat. Close lips and teeth around mouthpiece. Exhale through nose as completely as possible, then inhale through mouth slowly and deeply while actuating the nebulizer to release dose. Hold breath several seconds, remove mouthpiece, and then exhale slowly.

Instructions for metered powder inhaler: Caution patient *not* to take forced deep breathing, but to breathe with normal force and depth. Observe patient closely for exaggerated systemic drug action.

Patients requiring more than 3 aerosol treatments within 24 hours should be under close medical supervision.

Inhalation via oxygen aerosolization: Administered over 15- to 20-minute period, generally, with oxygen flow rate adjusted to 4 liters/minute. Turn on oxygen supply before patient places nebulizer in mouth. Lips need not be closed tightly around nebulizer opening. Placement of Y tube in rubber tubing permits patient to control administration.

Advise patient to rinse mouth immediately after inhalation therapy to help prevent dryness and throat irritation.

Rinse mouthpieces thoroughly with warm water at least once daily to prevent clogging.

Volume of solution placed in nebulizer should be sufficient for not more than 1 day's supply. Change solution daily.

Inform patient that saliva and sputum may appear pink following inhalation treatment.

Tolerance to bronchodilating effect and cardiac stimulant effect may develop with prolonged or too frequent use, and rebound bronchospasm may occur when effects of drug end.

Caution patient to take medication as prescribed, and advise patient to report to physician if usual dosage does not produce expected relief. Once tolerance has developed, continued use can result in serious adverse effects.

Parotid swelling following prolonged use has been reported. Drug should be discontinued if this occurs.

Inform patient taking repeated doses, as well as responsible family members, about adverse reactions, and advise them to report onset of such reactions to physician.

Preserved in tight, light-resistant containers. Solutions gradually become pink to brownish pink from exposure to air, light, or heat or contact with metal or alkali. Do not use if precipitate or discoloration is present.

DRUG INTERACTIONS: Effects of isoproterenol are antagonized by **pro-pranolol** (β-adrenergic blocking agent). Possibility of additive effects and increased cardiotoxicity when administered concomitantly with **epinephrine** or most other sympathomimetic bronchodilators (may be alternated if given at least 4 hours apart). Administration of isoproterenol in patients receiving **cyclo-propane** or **halogenated hydrocarbon general anesthetics** may result in arrhythmias.

ISOXSUPRINE HYDROCHLORIDE, N.F.
(ISOLAIT, ROLISOX, VASODILAN, VASOPRINE)

Vasodilator

ACTIONS AND USES

Sympathomimetic agent with β-adrenergic stimulant activity and with slight effect on α-receptors. Produces direct relaxation of vascular and uterine smooth musculature. Vasodilating action on arteries supplying skeletal muscles is greater than on cutaneous vessels. Also exhibits bronchodilatory effect and mild inhibition of GI motility.

Used for relief of symptoms associated with cerebral vascular insufficiency and peripheral vascular disease, such as arteriosclerosis obliterans, thromboangiitis obliterans (Buerger's disease), and Raynaud's disease. Also has been used in treatment of dysmenorrhea, premature labor, and threatened abortion.

ABSORPTION AND FATE

Therapeutic blood levels are achieved within 1 hour and persist for almost 3 hours. Partly conjugated in blood; excreted primarily in urine.

CONTRAINDICATIONS AND PRECAUTIONS

Contraindicated immediately post partum; in presence of arterial bleeding; parenteral use in presence of hypotension, tachycardia.

ADVERSE REACTIONS

Infrequent and mild: nausea, vomiting, severe rash, postural hypotension, fainting, dizziness, lightheadedness, palpitation, muscular weakness, nervousness. With large doses or parenteral administration: hypotension, tachycardia.

ROUTE AND DOSAGE

Oral: 10 to 20 mg 3 or 4 times daily. Intramuscular: 5 to 10 mg 2 or 3 times a day. Single IM doses exceeding 10 mg not recommended.

NURSING IMPLICATIONS

Advise patient to report adverse reactions; they are usually effectively controlled by dosage reduction.

Parenteral administration may cause hypotension and tachycardia. Monitor blood pressure and pulse. Supervise ambulation.

Therapeutic response to isoxsuprine in treatment of peripheral vascular disorders is manifested by relief of intermittent claudication, rest pain, and the sensations of numbness, coldness, and burning in extremities.

Patients should be completely informed about skin care of legs and feet and care of toenails. Properly fitted shoes and stockings and the importance of avoiding mechanical, chemical, and thermal trauma should be emphasized. Cessation of smoking and control of weight are crucial adjuncts to pharmacotherapeutic regimen.

Discuss with physician the rehabilitative management of the patient with peripheral vascular disease. Prescribed adjuncts to drug therapy may include the following: elevation of head of bed with 4- to 6-inch blocks to relieve rest pain (by enhancing blood flow to extremities); Buerger-Allen exercises; graduated exercise program to develop collateral blood supply.

For treatment of menstrual cramps, isoxsuprine is usually started 1 to 3 days before onset of menstruation and continued until pain is relieved or menstrual flow stops.

KANAMYCIN, U.S.P.
(KANTREX)

Antibacterial (aminoglycoside)

ACTIONS AND USES

Aminoglycoside antibiotic derived from *Streptomyces kanamyceticus* and similar to neomycin in chemical structure and antibacterial properties. Active against many Gram-negative microorganisms, especially *Klebsiella pneumoniae, Enterobacter aerogenes, Proteus* species, *E. coli, Serratia marcescens,* and Mima-Herellea. Also effective against many strains of *Staphylococcus aureus,* but it is not the drug of choice. Cross-resistance between kanamycin and neomycin is complete. Like other aminoglycosides, exerts curarelike effect on neuromuscular junction. Oral kanamycin reportedly decreases serum cholesterol.

Used orally to reduce ammonia-producing bacteria in intestinal tract as adjunctive treatment of hepatic coma; used for preoperative bowel antisepsis and for treatment of intestinal infections. Parenteral drug is used in short-term treatment of serious infections. Also used intraperitoneally following fecal spill during surgery; used as irrigation solution and as aerosol treatment.

ABSORPTION AND FATE

Poorly absorbed from GI tract. Excreted in feces as unchanged drug; absorbed portion, if any, excreted unchanged in urine. Completely absorbed following IM injection in about 1.5 hours. Peak serum concentrations reached in about 1 hour, declining to very low levels by 12 hours. Serum half-life 2 to 4 hours. Diffuses to most body fluids, including cerebrospinal fluid, but only if meninges are inflamed. Also readily absorbed from peritoneal cavity. Excreted by kidneys (mostly by glomerular filtration); 81% excreted in urine as unchanged drug. Approximately one-half of IM dose eliminated in 4 hours; excretion complete within 24 to 48 hours (prolonged in patients with renal impairment). Crosses placenta and appears in breast milk.

CONTRAINDICATIONS AND PRECAUTIONS

History of hypersensitivity to kanamycin or other aminoglycosides; history of drug-induced ototoxicity; long-term therapy; concurrent or sequential administration with other ototoxic, nephrotoxic, and/or neurotoxic agents; potent diuretics; oral use in intestinal obstruction; intraperitoneally to patients under effects of anesthetics or muscle relaxants; IV administration to patients with renal impairment; nursing mothers. Safe use in pregnancy not established. Cautious use: impaired renal function, myasthenia gravis.

ADVERSE REACTIONS

GI: nausea, vomiting, diarrhea, appetite changes, abdominal discomfort, stomatitis, malabsorption syndrome (with prolonged oral administration). **Nephrotoxicity:** hematuria, proteinuria, cylinduria, elevated serum creatinine and BUN, acute tubular necrosis (rare). **Ototoxicity:** deafness (may be irreversible), vertigo, tinnitus. **Neurotoxicity:** circumoral and other paresthesias, optic neuritis, peripheral neuritis, headache, restlessness, acute brain syndrome, bulging fontanelles, arachnoiditis, convulsions; rarely: neuromuscular paralysis, repiratory depression, sensory involvement of glossopharyngeal (IX) cranial nerve. **Hypersensitivity:** eosinophilia, maculopapular rashes, pruritus, anaphylaxis. **Hematologic:** anemia, increased or decreased reticulocytes, decreased plasma fibrinogen, granulocytopenia, agranulocytosis, thrombocytopenia, purpura. **Other:** superinfections; laryngeal edema; blurred vision; fever; joint pain; pulmonary fibrosis; hypotension; hypertension; tachycardia; increased salivation; weight loss; decreased serum calcium; increased SGOT, SGPT, and serum bilirubin; transient hepatomegaly; splenomegaly; local pain; nodular formation at injection site.

ROUTE AND DOSAGE

Oral: *Preoperative intestinal antisepsis:* 1 Gm every hour for 4 doses, then 1 Gm every 6 hours for 36 to 72 hours. *Intestinal infections:* **Adults:** 3 to 4 Gm/day in divided doses. **Children:** 50 mg/kg daily in 4 to 6 equally divided doses, usually continued 5 to 7 days. *Hepatic coma:* 8 to 12 Gm/day in divided doses. Intramuscular: **Adults and children:** 7.5 mg/kg in 2 to 4 equally divided and spaced doses. Maximum daily dose is 1.5 Gm regardless of body weight. Intravenous: not to exceed 15 mg/kg body weight daily in 2 or 3 equal doses. Intraperitoneal: **Adults only:** 0.05 Gm diluted in 20 ml sterile distilled water, instilled through wound catheter. Inhalation (aerosol): **Adults and children:** 250 mg 2 to 4 times a day. Irrigation solution: (0.25%).

NURSING IMPLICATIONS

Culture and sensitivity studies should be performed at initiation of therapy and periodically thereafter (therapy may be started prior to return of results).

Urinalysis and kidney function tests should be assessed before and at regular intervals during therapy.

Risk of ototoxicity is high in patients with impaired renal function, the elderly, poorly hydrated patients, and patients in whom therapy is expected to last 5 days or more. Close monitoring of kidney function and pretreatment and repeat audiograms are advised in these patients.

Administer IM injection deep into upper outer quadrant of buttock (often associated with pain). Observe sites daily for signs of irritation; rotate injection sites.

Monitor intake and output. Report decrease in urine output or change in intake–output ratio.

Check reports of urinalysis and kidney function test and notify physician immediately of signs of renal irritation: albuminuria, casts, red and white cells in urine, increasing NPN, BUN, and serum creatinine, and edema. Audiogram should be obtained if any of these signs are present. Physcian may terminate kanamycin therapy.

Since parenteral kanamycin is highly concentrated in the urinary system, patient should be well hydrated to prevent chemical irritation of renal tubules. Fluid intake should be sufficient to produce output of at least 1500 ml/day. Consult physician.

Lower than usual dosages are prescribed for patients with renal dysfunction. One suggested method of estimating dosage interval is to multiply serum creatinine value by 9 and to use resulting figure as interval in hours between doses: eg, if creatinine level is 2 mg/dl ($2 \times 9 = 18$), dose should be administered every 18 hours.

Monitoring of antibiotic blood levels is advised in patients with impaired renal function (generally maintained around 25 μg/ml).

Drug should be stopped if patient complains of tinnitus, dizziness or vertigo, sense of fullness in ears, or subjective hearing loss or if follow-up audiograms show loss of high-frequency perception. High-frequency deafness usually occurs first, but it can be detected only by audiometry (auditory toxicity occurs more commonly than vestibular toxicity).

In patients with impaired renal function, deafness has occurred 2 to 7 days after termination of therapy.

If no objective clinical response occurs within 3 to 5 days of parenteral therapy, sensitivity tests should be rechecked and therapy terminated.

Patients receiving kanamycin in the postoperative period should be closely monitored for neuromuscular and respiratory depression. Have on hand parenteral neostigmine, calcium gluconate, and sodium bicarbonate.

Some vials may darken with time, but this does not indicate loss of potency.
Kanamycin should not be mixed in the same syringe with other drugs.
Discard partially used vials within 48 hours.
Advise home patients to discard remaining drug after therapy is completed.

DRUG INTERACTIONS: There is the possibility of additive nephrotoxic effects
with **cephalosporins.** Combined or sequential use of kanamycin with other
aminoglycoside antibiotics increases the possibility of nephrotoxicity and ototoxicity. Concurrent use with potent diuretics (eg, **ethacrynic acid, furosemide**)
potentiates ototoxicity.
Enhanced neuromuscular blockade and respiratory depression may occur with
ether, related **inhalation anesthetic agents,** and **skeletal muscle relaxants**
(surgical), eg, **succinylcholine, tubocurarine.**

LANATOSIDE C, N.F.
(CEDILANID)

Cardiotonic

ACTIONS AND USES
Rapid-acting cardiac glycoside obtained from leaves of *Digitalis lanata*. Shares actions, uses, contraindications, and adverse reactions of digitalis.

ABSORPTION AND FATE
Poorly and irregularly absorbed from GI tract. Cardiac effects begin within 1 to 2 hours and peak within 4 to 6 hours. Effects may persist 1 to 3 days. About 20% excreted in urine daily.

ROUTE AND DOSAGE
Oral: *Digitalization:* total digitalizing dose 8 to 10 mg. Highly individualized. Recommended schedule: first day 3.5 mg; second day 2.5 mg; third day 2 mg; thereafter 1.5 mg daily until full digitalization achieved. *Maintenance:* 0.5 to 1.5 mg daily.

NURSING IMPLICATIONS
During digitalization period, before administering lanatoside C, check laboratory reports if available (know what the physician regards as acceptable parameters for serum levels of potassium, magnesium, and calcium), take apical pulse for 1 full minute, noting rate, rhythm, and quality; check for signs and symptoms of lanatoside C toxicity (see Digitalis).
Preserved in tightly covered, light-resistant containers.
See Digitalis.

LEUCOVORIN CALCIUM, U.S.P.
(CALCIUM FOLINATE, Citrovorum Factor, Folinic Acid)

Antianemic, antidote (to folic acid antagonists)

ACTIONS AND USES
Tetrahydrofolic acid derivative and active form of folic acid, an essential compound required for nucleoprotein synthesis and maintenance of normal erythropoiesis.
Used for treatment of folate deficient megaloblastic anemias due to sprue, pregnancy, and nutritional deficiency when oral therapy is not feasible. Also used to diminish toxicity of inadvertent overdosage of folic acid antagonists, particularly methotrexate.

CONTRAINDICATIONS AND PRECAUTIONS
Undiagnoised anemia.

ADVERSE REACTIONS
Allergic sensitization. See Folic Acid.

ROUTE AND DOSAGE
Intramuscular (megaloblastic anemias): no more than 1 mg daily; (overdosage of folic acid antagonists): amount equal to weight of antagonist given.

NURSING IMPLICATIONS
Solution should be used as soon as possible following reconstitution since a precipitate may form with prolonged standing.

Duration of treatment depends on hematologic response to leucovorin.
To be effective as antidote for overdosage of folic acid antagonist, leukovorin should be administered within 1 hour if possible; ineffective after a delay of 4 hours.
See Folic Acid.

LEVALLORPHAN TARTRATE, N.F., B.P.
(LORFAN)

Narcotic antagonist

ACTIONS AND USES
N-allyl analogue of levorphanol. Similar to nalorphine in having both narcotic antagonist and agonist (morphinelike) effects. Antagonizes severe narcotic-induced respiratory depression, but exerts little action against mild respiratory depression and may even increase it. Largely replaced by naloxone, which has little or no agonistic activity.
Used in treatment of significant narcotic-induced respiratory depression.

ABSORPTION AND FATE
Acts within 1 to 2 minutes; effects last about 2 to 5 hours. Readily crosses placenta.

CONTRAINDICATIONS AND PRECAUTIONS
Mild narcotic-induced respiratory depression; respiratory depression due to barbiturates or other sedatives and hypnotics, anesthetics, other nonnarcotic CNS depressants, or pathologic causes; narcotic addiction (may precipitate severe and possibly fatal withdrawal symptoms).

ADVERSE REACTIONS
Dysphoria, miosis, pseudoptosis, sweating, pallor, lethargy, drowsiness, dizziness, nausea, sense of heaviness in limbs, respiratory depression. High doses: weird dreams, visual hallucinations, disorientation, feelings of unreality. Neonates: irritability, increased crying.

ROUTE AND DOSAGE
Intravenous: **Adults:** 1 mg; if required, this may be followed by 1 or 2 additional doses of 0.5 mg at 10- to 15-minute intervals. Total dose not to exceed 3 mg. **Neonates** (approximately one-tenth adult dose): 0.05 to 0.1 mg diluted to 2 ml with 0.9% sodium chloride injection and injected into umbilical cord vein immediately after delivery. If vein cannot be used, injection may be given subcutaneously or intramuscularly.

NURSING IMPLICATIONS
Not to be confused with levorphanol tartrate, a narcotic analgesic.
Artificial respiration with oxygen and other resuscitative measures may accompany drug administration.
Monitor vital signs. Since duration of narcotic action is often longer than that of levallorphan, observe patient closely for return of respiratory depression. Additional dose of levallorphan may be necessary.
Patient should be closely observed for a day or more, even if he shows signs of apparent improvement.

(LEVOPHED, Norepinephrine Bitartrate)
NORADRENALINE ACID TARTRATE, B.P.

Adrenergic (vasoconstrictor)

ACTIONS AND USES

Identical to body catecholamine norepinephrine. Acts directly and predominantly on α-adrenergic receptors; little action on β-receptors except in heart (β_1 receptors). Main therapeutic effects are vasoconstriction and cardiac stimulation. Has powerful constrictor action on resistance and capacitance blood vessels. Reduces blood flow to kidney, other vital organs, skin, and skeletal muscle. Peripheral vasoconstriction (α-adrenergic action) and moderate inotropic stimulation of heart (β-adrenergic action) result in increased systolic and diastolic blood pressure, myocardial oxygenation, coronary artery blood flow, and work of heart. Cardiac output varies reflexly with systemic blood pressure. Reflex increase of vagal activity in response to pronounced effect on arterial blood pressure may cause bradycardia. Causes less CNS stimulation and has less effect on metabolism than does epinephrine; however, in large doses it can increase glycogenolysis and inhibit pancreatic insulin release, with resulting hyperglycemia. May cause contraction of pregnant uterus.

Used to restore blood pressure in certain acute hypotensive states such as sympathectomy, pheochromocytomectomy, spinal anesthesia, poliomyelitis, myocardial infarction, septicemia, blood transfusion, and drug reactions. Also used as adjunct in treatment of cardiac arrest.

ABSORPTION AND FATE

Pressor activity occurs rapidly and lasts 1 to 2 minutes following termination of IV infusion. Pronounced localization in sympathetic nerve endings. Inactivated in liver and other tissues, primarily by catechol-*o*-methyl transferase and to smaller extent by monamine oxidase. Excreted in urine mainly as inactive metabolites; 4% to 16% of dose is excreted unchanged. Crosses placenta.

CONTRAINDICATIONS AND PRECAUTIONS

Use as sole therapy in hypovolemic states, except as temporary emergency measure; mesenteric or peripheral vascular thrombosis; profound hypoxia or hypercarbia; pregnancy; use during cyclopropane or halothane anesthesia. Cautious use: hypertension, hyperthyroidism, severe heart disease, elderly patients, patients receiving MAO inhibitors or tricyclic antidepressants.

ADVERSE REACTIONS

Headache, palpitation, hypertension, reflex bradycardia, fatal arrhythmias (large doses), respiratory difficulty, restlessness, anxiety, tremors, dizziness, weakness, insomnia, pallor, tissue necrosis at injection site (with extravasation), swelling of thyroid gland (rare). **Overdosage or individual sensitivity:** blurred vision, photophobia, hyperglycemia, retrosternal and pharyngeal pain, profuse sweating, vomiting, severe hypertension, violent headache, cerebral hemorrhage, convulsions. **With prolonged administration:** plasma volume depletion, edema, hemorrhage, intestinal, hepatic, and renal necrosis.

ROUTE AND DOSAGE

Highly individualized according to response of patient. Intravenous infusion: suggested initial infusion rate: 2 to 3 ml per minute. Average maintenance dose: 0.5 to 1 ml/minute of a 0.004 mg/ml solution.

NURSING IMPLICATIONS

IV infusion of levarterenol in saline alone is not recommended. Dextrose (in distilled water or saline solution) is used to prevent oxidation and thus loss of potency.

Risk of extravasation is reportedly reduced if infusion is administered through a plastic catheter inserted deep into vein (preferably antecubital).

Catheter tie-in technique is not recommended, as it promotes stasis.

A double-bottle setup is advisable (1 bottle without levarterenol) so that IV can be kept running in the event that levarterenol must be stopped.

In patients with severe hypotension after myocardial infarction, the physician may prescribe addition of heparin to levarterenol infusion to prevent thrombosis of infused vein and perivenous reaction.

An infusion pump or apparatus to control levarterenol flow rate is generally used. Regulation of flow rate is determined by blood pressure response. Consult physician for specific guidelines.

Blood volume depletion must be continuously corrected by appropriate fluid and electrolyte replacement therapy to maintain tissue perfusion and to avoid recurrence of hypotension when levarterenol is stopped.

Whole blood or plasma are incompatible with levarternol and therefore should be administered separately.

Patient should be attended constantly while receiving levarterenol. Take baseline blood pressure and pulse before start of therapy, then every 2 minutes from initiation of drug until stabilization occurs at desired level, then every 5 minutes during drug administration.

In normotensive patients it is recommended that flow rate be adjusted to maintain blood pressure at low normal (usually 80 to 100 mm Hg systolic). In previously hypertensive patients, systolic is generally maintained no higher than 40 mm Hg *below* preexisting systolic level.

In addition to vital signs, carefully observe and record mentation (index of cerebral circulation), skin temperature of extremities, and color (especially of earlobes, lips, nail beds).

Flow rate must be constantly monitored. Check infusion site frequently for free flow (adhesive tape should not obscure injection site). Report immediately any evidence of extravasation: blanching along course of infused vein (may occur without obvious extravasation), cold, hard swelling around injection site.

Antidote for extravasation ischemia: Phentolamine, 5 to 10 mg in 10 to 15 ml normal saline injection, is infiltrated throughout affected area (using syringe with fine hypodermic needle) as soon as possible. Some physicians prefer to add phentolamine (5 to 10 mg) to each liter of infusion solution as a preventive against sloughing should extravasation occur.

Monitor intake and output. Urinary retention and renal shutdown are possibilities, especially in hypovolemic patients. Urinary output is a sensitive indicator of the degree of renal perfusion. Report decrease in urinary output or change in intake–output ratio.

Headache, vomiting, palpitation, arrhythmias, chest pain, photophobia, and blurred vision are possible symptoms of overdosage. Reflex bradycardia may occur as a result of rise in blood pressure.

Emergency drugs should be immediately available in the event of cardiac irregularities. Atropine is an antidote for bradycardia; cardiac arrhythmias may be treated with propranolol.

If therapy is to be prolonged, it may be advisable to change infusion sites at intervals to allow effect of local vasoconstriction to subside.

When therapy is to be discontinued, infusion rate is slowed gradually. Abrupt withdrawal should be avoided. Continue to monitor vital signs and observe patient closely after cessation of therapy for clinical sign of circulatory inadequacy.

Do not use solution if discoloration or precipitate is present.

Preserved in tightly closed, light-resistant containers.

DRUG INTERACTIONS: Levarterenol should be used cautiously and in small doses in patients receiving drugs that may potentiate its pressor effects: some

390

antihistamines (especially **dexchlorpheniramine, diphenhydramine, tripelennamine), parenteral ergot alkaloids, guanethidine, methyldopa,** and **tricyclic antidepressants.** Levarterenol should be administered with extreme caution in patients receiving **MAO inhibitors** (possibility of severe and prolonged hypertension in some patients). Concurrent administration of levarterenol with **cyclopropane** or **halothane** and related general anesthetics may lead to ventricular arrhythmias. Administration of levarterenol to patients already receiving **propranolol** may result in high elevations of blood pressure.

LEVODOPA, U.S.P.
(BENDOPA, BIO/DOPA, DOPAR, LARODOPA, LEVOPA, L-DOPA, PARDA, RIO-DOPA)

Antiparkinsonian

ACTIONS AND USES

Metabolic precursor of dopamine, a catecholamine neurotransmitter. Unlike dopamine, levodopa readily crosses the blood–brain barrier. Precise mechanism of action unknown. It is hypothesized that levodopa is rapidly decarboxylated to dopamine and thus restores dopamine levels in extrapyramidal centers (believed to be depleted in parkinsonism). Cardiac stimulation may be produced by action of dopamine on β-adrenergic receptors. Also may augment secretion of growth hormone, which in turn is postulated to affect glucose utilization. Used in treatment of idiopathic Parkinson's disease, postencephalitic and arteriosclerotic parkinsonism, and parkinsonian symptoms associated with manganese and carbon monoxide poisoning. Also commercially available in combination with carbidopa (eg, as Sinemet), a decarboxylase inhibitor, to permit lower dosage range of levodopa and thus reduce incidence of adverse reactions.

ABSORPTION AND FATE

Rapidly and completely absorbed from GI tract. Peak plasma concentrations within 1 to 3 hours. Converted to dopamine by decarboxylation in GI tract and liver; small amount of levodopa reaches CNS, where it is metabolized to dopamine by dopa decarboxylase. Major metabolite is homovanillic acid; minute amounts of dopamine are converted to norepinephrine. About 80% of dose is excreted in urine within 24 hours; negligible amounts are eliminated in feces.

CONTRAINDICATIONS AND PRECAUTIONS

Known hypersensitivity to levodopa, narrow-angle glaucoma patients with suspicious pigmented lesion or history of melanoma, acute psychoses, severe psychoneurosis, within 2 weeks of MAO inhibitors. Safe use in women of childbearing potential, during pregnancy and lactation, and in children under 12 years of age not established. Cautious use: cardiovascular, renal, hepatic, or endocrine disease, history of myocardial infarction with residual arrhythmias, peptic ulcer, convulsions, psychiatric disorders, chronic wide-angle glaucoma, diabetes, pulmonary diseases, bronchial asthma, patients receiving antihypertensive drugs.

ADVERSE REACTIONS

GI (common): anorexia, nausea, vomiting, abdominal distress, flatulence, dry mouth, dysphagia, sialorrhea; (less frequent): burning sensation of tongue, bitter taste, diarrhea or constipation; (rarely): duodenal ulcer, GI bleeding. **Cardiovascular** (common): orthostatic hypotension; (less frequent): palpitation, tachycardia, hypertension, phlebitis. **Neuropsychiatric** (frequent): choreiform and involuntary movements, increased hand tremor, bradykinetic episodes (on–off phenomena), trismus, grinding of teeth (bruxism), ataxia, muscle twitching, numbness, weakness, fatigue, headache, opisthotonos, confusion, agitation, anxiety, euphoria, insomnia, nightmares; (less frequent): psychotic episodes with paranoid delusions or hallucinations, severe depression, hypomania; (rare): convulsions. **Ophthalmic:** blepharospasm, diplopia, blurred vision, dilated pupils, widening of palpebral fissures, oculogyric crises (rare). **Hematologic:** hemolytic anemia, agranulocytosis, reduced hemoglobin and hematocrit, leukopenia. **Altered laboratory values:** elevated BUN, SGOT, SGPT, alkaline phosphatase, LDH, bilirubin, protein-bound iodine, serum level of growth hormone; decreased glucose tolerance. Other: rhinorrhea, flushing, skin rashes, increased sweating, bizarre breathing patterns, urinary retention or incontinence, increased sexual drive, priapism, weight gain or loss, edema; (rarely): hiccups, loss of hair, activation of Horner's syndrome and malignant melanoma.

ROUTE AND DOSAGE

Oral: initially 0.5 to 1 Gm daily divided into two or more equal doses with food; daily dosage increased gradually in increments of not more than 0.75 Gm every 3 to 7 days, as tolerated. Total daily dosage not to exceed 8 Gm. Highly individualized.

NURSING IMPLICATIONS

The incidence of GI side effects is lessened by administering drug with food.

If patient is unable to swallow capsule or tablet form, consult pharmacist about preparing a liquid formulation.

Rate of dosage increase is determined primarily by patient's tolerance and response to levodopa. Make accurate observations and report promptly adverse reactions (generally dose-related and reversible) and therapeutic effects.

Monitor vital signs, particularly during period of dosage adjustment. Report alterations in blood pressure, pulse, and respiratory rate and rhythm.

Orthostatic hypotension is usually asymptomatic, but some patients experience dizziness and syncope. Caution patient to make positional changes slowly, particularly from recumbent to upright position, and to dangle legs a few minutes before standing. Supervision of ambulation is indicated. Tolerance to this effect usually develops within a few months of therapy. Elastic stockings may help some patients; consult physician.

Muscle twitching and spasmodic winking (blepharospasm) are early signs of overdosage; report them promptly.

All patients should be closely monitored for behavior changes. Patients in depression should be closely observed for suicidal tendencies.

Elevation of mood and sense of well-being may precede objective improvement. Stress the importance of resuming activities gradually and observing safety precautions in order to avoid injury. The patient with a history of cardiac problems should be cautioned against overactivity.

Patients with chronic wide-angle glaucoma should be monitored during therapy for changes in intraocular pressure.

Patients with diabetes should be observed carefully for alterations in diabetes control. Frequent monitoring of blood sugar is advised.

All patients on extended therapy should be checked periodically for symptoms of diabetes and acromegaly and for functioning of hematopoietic, hepatic, and renal systems.

About 80% of patients on full therapeutic doses for 1 year or longer develop abnormal involuntary movements such as facial grimacing, exaggerated chewing, protrusion of tongue, rhythmic opening and closing of mouth, bobbing of head, jerky arm and leg movements, and exaggerated respiration. Symptoms tend to increase if dosage is not reduced.

Patients receiving large doses may show cyclic exacerbation of parkinsonism, with profound weakness. Attacks develop within minutes, last 1 to 3 hours, and usually appear at same time each day; this on–off phenomenon probably is due to excessive levodopa level.

Therapeutic effects: significant improvement usually appears during second or third week of therapy, but it may not occur for 3 to 4 months or more in some patients.

Inform patients that a metabolite of levodopa may cause urine to darken on standing and may also cause sweat to be dark-colored.

Caution patients not to take over-the-counter preparations or fortified cereals unless approved by physician. Multivitamins, antinauseants, and fortified cereals usually contain pyridoxine (vitamin B_6); 5 mg or more of pyridoxine daily may reverse the effects of levodopa.

In the event a patient requires general anesthesia, levodopa therapy is continued as long as patient is able to take fluids and medication by mouth (generally discontinued 6 to 24 hours prior to anesthesia). Therapy usually is resumed as soon as patient is able to take oral medication.

Patient and responsible family members require guidance and supervision of drug regimen.

Physical therapy is an important adjunct to drug therapy.

LABORATORY TEST INTERFERENCES: There is the possibility of false negative glucose oxidase tests (eg, Clinistix, Tes-Tape) and false positive results with the copper reduction method (Clinitest), especially in patients receiving large doses. It is reported that Clinistix and Tes-Tape may be used if reading is taken at margin of wet and dry tape. There is the possibility of false positive tests for urinary ketones by dip-stick tests, eg, Acetest (equivocal), Ketostix, Labstix, false elevations of serum and urinary uric acid levels by colorimetric methods, but not uricase, false increases in urinary protein by Lowry method, false decreases in urinary vanillylmandelic acid by Pisano method.

DRUG INTERACTIONS: Drugs that may inhibit or decrease therapeutic effects of levodopa include **anticholinergics, diazepam** and possibly other **phenothiazines** (mutually antagonistic), **phenylbutazone, pyridoxine,** (vitamin B_6 in doses of 5 mg or more), and **reserpine.** Levodopa may enhance the hypotensive effects of **guanethidine** and **methyldopa;** methyldopa may enhance antiparkinsonian effects of levodopa (used therapeutically). Concomitant use of **MAO inhibitors** may produce hypertension (levodopa contraindicated with MAOIs, but may be used concurrently in carbidopa-levodopa combination product). **Propranolol** may enhance the therapeutic effect of levodopa and may also enhance levodopa-induced stimulation of growth hormone secretion.

LEVOPROPOXYPHENE NAPSYLATE, N.F.
(NOVRAD)

Antitussive

ACTIONS AND USES

Levo isomer of propoxyphene with centrally acting antitussive action and local anesthetic properties. Unlike the dextro isomer of propoxyphene (Darvon), it has little or no analgesic activity.

Used as adjunct in symptomatic relief of nonproductive cough.

CONTRAINDICATIONS AND PRECAUTIONS

When it is inadvisable to decrease frequency and intensity of cough; known sensitivity to drug.

ADVERSE REACTIONS

Usually minor: headache, drowsiness, dizziness, nervousness, diarrhea, epigastric burning, urinary frequency or urgency, dry mouth, visual disturbances, skin rash, urticaria. Overdosage: vomiting, muscle tremors, agitation.

Oral: **Adults:** 50 to 100 mg every 4 hours; maximum recommended daily dosage 600 mg. **Pediatric:** (*children weighing 23 to 45 kg*): 50 mg every 4 hours; **infants and children** *up to 23 kg:* 25 mg every 4 hours, as required.

NURSING IMPLICATIONS

Antitussive action usually lasts about 4 hours.

Caution patients that mental and physical abilities for performance of hazardous tasks such as driving a car or operating machinery may be impaired.

Advise patients to report symptoms of CNS stimulation (tremors, nervousness, agitation, vomiting) or CNS depression (drowsiness); dosage should be reduced or drug discontinued.

Recommended treatment of overdosage is gastric lavage along with supportive and symptomatic therapy. No specific antagonist for levopropoxyphene is known.

See Benzonatate for nursing measures to relieve nonproductive cough.

LEVORPHANOL TARTRATE, N.F., B.P.
(LEVO-DROMORAN)

Analgesic (narcotic)

ACTIONS AND USES

Synthetic morphinan derivative with actions, uses, contraindications, precautions, and adverse reactions similar to those of morphine (qv). More potent as an analgesic and has somewhat longer duration of action than morphine. Reported to cause less nausea, vomiting, and constipation than equivalent doses of morphine, but may produce more sedation, smooth-muscle stimulation, and respiratory depression. Unlike morphine, can be given by mouth.

ABSORPTION AND FATE

Peak analgesia within 60 to 90 minutes following subcutaneous injection; duration of action 6 to 8 hours. Metabolized primarily in liver. Excreted in urine mainly as glucuronide conjugate.

ROUTE AND DOSAGE

Oral, subcutaneous: 2 to 3 mg. Dosage is reduced in poor-risk patients, very young or very old patients, and patients receiving other CNS depressants.

NURSING IMPLICATIONS

Not to be confused with levallorphan tartrate, a narcotic antagonist, and sometimes used as an antidote for levorphanol.

Levorphanol should be given in the smallest effective dose and as infrequently as possible to minimize the possibility of tolerance and physical dependence.

Classified as schedule II drug under federal Controlled Substances Act.

See Morphine Sulfate.

(CYTOLEN, LETTER, LEVOID, NOROXINE, RO-THYROXINE,
ROXSTAN, SYNTHROID, T_4)

Hormone, thyroid

ACTIONS AND USES

Synthetically prepared monosodium salt levo isomer of thyroxine, with similar
actions and uses; 0.1 mg is equivalent to 65 mg desiccated thyroid and is about
600 times more potent. For contraindications, precautions, and adverse reactions, see Thyroid.

Used as specific replacement therapy for diminished or absent thyroid function
resulting from primary or secondary atrophy of gland, surgery, excessive radiation or antithyroid drugs, congenital defect. Administered orally for hypothyroid state; administered IV for myxedematous coma or other thyroid dysfunc-
tions demanding rapid replacement, as well as in failure to respond to oral
therapy.

ABSORPTION AND FATE

Following absorption, binds to plasma protein. Circulation half-life 6 or 7 days.
Distributed widely; gradually released into tissue cells, where it causes increased
metabolic rate, usually after 12 to 48 hours. One milligram of levothyroxine
increases heat production about 1000 calories.

ROUTE AND DOSAGE

All doses individualized and initiated cautiously according to age, physical
condition, severity, and duration of hypothyroidism. Oral (thyroid replacement): **Adults:** 0.1 mg daily, with gradual increments of 0.05 to 0.1 mg every
1 to 3 weeks until desired response is attained; maintenance 0.1 to 0.2 mg daily.
Children: initially no more than 0.05 mg daily, with increments of 0.025 to 0.05
mg daily until desired response is attained; maintenance 0.3 to 0.4 mg daily.
Intravenous (myxedematous coma or stupor): 0.2 to 0.4 mg first day; 0.1 to 0.2
mg or more on second day if there is no evidence of progressive improvement;
daily doses of lesser amounts are continued until patient can accept daily dose.
Intramuscular: may be used when oral route is not feasible and rapid onset is
not desired.

NURSING IMPLICATIONS

Administered as single dose, preferably before breakfast.

Parenteral preparation should be reconstituted with NaCl injection USP
immediately before administration. Shake vial until solution is clear. Discard unused portion. (Do not use bacteriostatic sodium chloride).

Transfer from levothyroxine to liothyronine: discontinue levothyroxine before starting small dose of liothyronine. Transfer from liothyronine to
levothyroxine: start levothyroxine; then, after several days, discontinue
liothyronine.

Levothyroxine may aggravate severity of previously obscured symptoms of
diabetes mellitus, Addison's disease, or diabetes insipidus. Therapeutic
measures directed at these disorders may require adjustment.

There is great urgency in achieving full thyroid replacement in infants or
children because of the critical importance of the hormone in sustaining
growth and development.

Therapy with levothyroxine results in euthyroidism, with expected protein-
bound iodine levels of 4 to 9 μg/dl or more. Other laboratory determinations usually fall within normal range.

Also see Thyroid.

LIDOCAINE HYDROCHLORIDE, U.S.P.
(ANESTACON SOLUTION, LIDA-MANTLE CREME, XYLOCAINE HYDROCHLORIDE)
LIGNOCAINE HYDROCHLORIDE, B.P.

Antiarrhythmic, local anesthetic

ACTIONS AND USES

Aminoacyl amide with anesthetic and antiarrhythmic properties. Cardiac actions similar to those of procainamide and quinidine, but has little effect on myocardial contractility, A-V and intraventricular conduction, cardiac output, and systolic arterial pressure in equivalent doses. Exerts antiarrhythmic action by suppressing automaticity in His-Purkinje system and by elevating electrical stimulation threshold of ventricle during diastole. Progressive depression of CNS occurs with increasing blood concentrations. Action as local anesthetic is more prompt, more intense, and longer lasting than that of procaine.

Used for rapid control of ventricular arrhythmias occurring during acute myocardial infarction, cardiac surgery, and cardiac catheterization and those caused by digitalis intoxication. Preparations also available for surface and infiltration anesthesia and for nerve block, and caudal anesthesia. Topical preparations are used to relieve local discomfort of skin and mucous membranes.

ABSORPTION AND FATE

Following IV bolus dose, action begins within 10 to 90 seconds and lasts up to 20 minutes. Following IM injection, effective antiarrhythmic blood levels occur within 5 to 15 minutes and persist 60 to 90 minutes. Rapidly distributed to most body tissues. Plasma half-life is about 2 hours (longer in patients with renal or hepatic disease). About 50% to 75% bound to plasma proteins. Approximately 90% metabolized by liver and excreted in urine as metabolites; 10% excreted as unchanged drug. Average duration of anesthetic action is 90 to 120 minutes. Crosses placenta.

CONTRAINDICATIONS AND PRECAUTIONS

History of hypersensitivity to amide-type local anesthetics; application or injection of lidocaine anesthetic in presence of severe trauma or sepsis; supraventricular arrhythmias; Stokes-Adams syndrome; untreated sinus bradycardia; severe degrees of sinoatrial, atrioventricular, and intraventricular heart block. Safe use in children not established. Cautious use: liver or renal disease, congestive heart failure, marked hypoxia, respiratory depression, hypovolemia, shock, myasthenia gravis.

ADVERSE REACTIONS

CNS: drowsiness, dizziness, lightheadedness, restlessness, confusion, disorientation, irritability, apprehension, euphoria, wild excitement, tinnitus, decreased hearing, blurred or double vision, impaired color perception, numbness of lips or tongue and other paresthesias including sensations of heat and cold, chest heaviness, difficulty in speaking, difficulty in breathing or swallowing, muscular twitching, tremors, psychosis. With high doses: convulsions, respiratory depression and arrest. **Cardiovascular** (with high doses): hypotension, bradycardia, conduction disorders including heart block, cardiovascular collapse, cardiac arrest. **Other reported:** anorexia, nausea, vomiting, excessive perspiration, soreness at IM site, local thrombophlebitis (with prolonged IV infusion), hypersensitivity reactions (urticaria, rash, edema, anaphylactoid reactions).

ROUTE AND DOSAGE

Intravenous (direct): 50 to 100 mg, administered at rate of 25 to 50 mg/minute; if indicated, may be repeated after 5 minutes. No more than 200 to 300 mg in a 1-hour period are advised. Intravenous infusion: 20 to 50 μg/kg/minute for average 70-kg man (1 to 4 mg/minute). Intramuscular: approximately 4.3 mg/kg body weight; if necessary, may be repeated once after interval of 60 to 90 minutes. Topical (jelly, ointment, cream, solution): 2.5% to 5%.

NURSING IMPLICATIONS

Only lidocaine hydrochloride injection without preservatives or epinephrine that is specifically labeled for IV use should be used for IV injection or infusion.

For IV infusion, use fluid administration set calibrated to provide 60 micro-drops/ml. Physician will prescribe specific rate of flow. Flow rate must be closely monitored.

Lidocaine should not be added to transfusion assemblies.

Constant ECG monitoring and frequent determinations of blood pressure are essential to avoid potential overdosage and toxicity.

Auscultate lungs for basilar rales, especially in patients who tend to metabolize the drug slowly (eg, congestive heart failure, cardiogenic shock, hepatic dysfunction).

In patients with sinus bradycardia, administration of IV lidocaine to eliminate ventricular ectopic beats is usually preceded by prior acceleration of heart (eg, by isoproterenol or electric pacing) to avoid provoking more frequent and serious ventricular arrhythmias.

Watch for neurotoxic effects, particularly in patients receiving IV infusions of lidocaine or those with high lidocaine blood levels (drowsiness, confusion, paresthesias, visual disturbances, excitement, behavioral changes).

IV infusion should be terminated as soon as patient's basic cardiac rhythm stabilizes or at earliest signs and symptoms of toxicity (infusions are rarely continued beyond 24 hours). An oral antiarrhythmic is used for maintenance therapy.

If ECG signs of excessive cardiac depression such as prolongation of P-R interval and QRS complex or the appearance or aggravation of arrhythmias occur, infusion should be stopped immediately.

Reports of convulsions are common. Resuscitative equipment and emergency drugs should be immediately available for management of convulsions and respiratory depression.

Deltoid muscle is recommended as the preferred IM site, since faster and higher peak blood levels are produced than by injection into gluteus or lateral thigh.

IM injection should be made with frequent aspirations to avoid inadvertent intravascular administration.

Lidocaine blood levels of approximately 2 to 5 μg/ml are reported to provide "usually effective" antiarrhythmic activity. Blood levels greater than 5 μg/ml are potentially toxic.

Anesthetic use: Lidocaine solutions containing preservatives should not be used for spinal or epidural (including caudal) block.

Oral topical anesthetics may interfere with swallowing. Food should not be ingested within 60 minutes following drug application, especially in pediatric, elderly, or debilitated patients.

Partially used solutions of lidocaine without preservatives should be discarded after initial use.

LABORATORY TEST INTERFERENCES: Increases in creatine phosphokinase level may occur for 48 hours following IM use and may interfere with test for presence of myocardial infarction.

DRUG INTERACTIONS: Additive cardiac depressant effects may occur when lidocaine is used concurrently with **phenytoin (diphenylhydantoin)**, **procainamide** (also additive neurologic effects), **propranolol**, and **quinidine**. Lidocaine (in high doses) may enhance muscle relaxant effects of **succinylcholine** and other **neuromuscular blocking agents.**

Antibacterial

ACTIONS AND USES

Derived from *Streptomyces lincolnensis*. Principally bacteriostatic, it acts by binding exclusively to 50S subunits of bacterial ribosomes, thus suppressing protein synthesis. Similar to erythromycin in antibacterial activity, and demonstrates some cross-resistance with it. Effective against most of the common Gram-positive pathogens, particularly streptococci, pneumococci, and staphylococci. Also effective against *Bacteroides* and other anaerobes; however, little activity against most Gram-negative organisms, and ineffective against viruses, yeasts, or fungi. Resistance by *Staphylococcus* is acquired in stepwise manner. Lincomycin is reported to have neuromuscular blocking properties.

Use reserved for treatment of serious infections caused by susceptible bacteria in penicillin-allergic patients or patients for whom penicillin is inappropriate.

ABSORPTION AND FATE

Rapidly but only partially (20% to 35%) absorbed from GI tract. Peak plasma concentrations in 2 to 4 hours after oral dose; levels maintained above minimal inhibitory concentration for 6 to 8 hours. IM injection produces maximal plasma concentrations within 30 minutes; effective levels persist 12 to 14 hours. IV infusion of 600 mg over a 2-hour period produces therapeutic levels that persist for 14 hours. Following subconjunctival injection, ocular fluid drug levels last 5 hours. Distributed to most body tissues and fluids. Significant concentrations in bone, aqueous humor, and cerebrospinal fluid (particularly when meninges are inflamed). Half-life about 5 hours. Excreted in urine, bile, and feces as bioactive metabolite and active drug. Crosses placenta and may appear in breast milk.

CONTRAINDICATIONS AND PRECAUTIONS

Previous hypersensitivity to lincomycin and clindamycin; liver disease; known monilial infections (unless treated concurrently); use in treatment of nursing mothers; use in newborns. Safe use in pregnancy not established. Cautious use: impaired renal function; history of GI disease, particularly colitis; history of liver, endocrine, or metabolic diseases; history of asthma or allergies.

ADVERSE REACTIONS

GI: glossitis, stomatitis, nausea, vomiting, anorexia, decreased taste acuity, unpleasant or altered taste, abdominal cramps, diarrhea, acute enterocolitis, pseudomembranous colitis (potentially fatal). **Hematopoietic:** neutropenia, leukopenia, agranulocytosis, thrombocytopenic purpura, and aplastic anemia and pancytopenia (rare). **Hypersensitivity:** pruritus, urticaria, skin rashes, exfoliative and vesiculobullous dermatitis, erythema multiforme resembling Stevens-Johnson syndrome (rare), angioedema, photosensitivity, serum sickness, anaphylaxis. **Cardiovascular:** hypotension, cardiopulmonary arrest (particularly after rapid IV). **Other:** superinfections, vaginitis, tinnitus, vertigo, dizziness, headache, generalized myalgia, thrombophlebitis (following IV use), pain at IM injection site (infrequent), jaundice and abnormal liver function tests (direct relationship to lincomycin not established).

ROUTE AND DOSAGE

Oral: **Adults:** 500 mg every 6 to 8 hours. **Children** *over 1 month of age:* 30 to 60 mg/kg divided into 3 or 4 equal doses. Intramuscular: **Adults:** 600 mg every 12 to 24 hours. **Children** *over 1 month of age:* 10 mg/kg every 12 to 24 hours. Intravenous: **Adults:** 600 mg to 1 Gm every 8 to 12 hours. Maximum recommended dose 8 Gm (1 Gm of lincomycin is diluted in not less than 100 ml of 5% dextrose in water or saline or other appropriate solution recommended by manufacturer and infused over period of not less than 1 hour). **Children** *over 1 month of age:* 10 to 20 mg/kg/day divided equally and infused every 8 to 12 hours. Subconjunctival injection: 75 mg.

NURSING IMPLICATIONS

A careful history should be taken of previous sensitivities to drugs or other allergens.

Culture and sensitivity tests should be performed initially and during therapy to determine continued microbial susceptibility.

Absorption is delayed by the presence of food in stomach or intestines. Administer oral drug at least 1 to 2 hours before meals or 2 to 3 hours after meals. Administer with water, and advise the patient to take nothing by mouth except water for 1 to 2 hours after oral administration.

Administer IM injection deep into large muscle mass; inject slowly to minimize pain. Rotate injection sites.

Monitor blood pressure and pulse in patients receiving parenteral drug. Have patient remain recumbent following drug administration until blood pressure stability is assured.

Relatively high incidence of diarrhea (20%) is associated with use of lincomycin. Monitor patients closely and report changes in bowel frequency. If significant diarrhea occurs, drug should be discontinued; large bowel endoscopy has been recommended.

Antiperistaltic agents such as opiates or diphenoxylate with atropine (Lomotil) may prolong and worsen diarrhea. Medical management consists of fluid, electrolyte, and protein supplements, as indicated, and possibly corticosteroids.

Diarrhea, acute colitis, or pseudomembranous colitis (suspect this if patient develops high temperature, diarrhea, or ileus) may occur up to several weeks following cessation of therapy. Advise patients to report promptly the onset of perianal irritation, diarrhea, or blood and mucus in stools.

Advise patients to report immediately symptoms of hypersensitivity. Drug should be discontinued.

Serum drug levels should be monitored closely in patients with severe impairment of renal function (levels tend to be higher). Recommended dosage for these patients is 25% to 30% that for patients with normal renal function.

Periodic hepatic and renal function studies and blood cell counts are indicated during prolonged drug therapy.

Superinfections by nonsusceptible organisms are most likely to occur when duration of therapy exceeds 10 days.

Drug therapy should continue at least 10 days in patients with β-hemolytic streptococcal infections to reduce the possibility of rheumatic fever or glomerulonephritis.

Lincomycin is incompatible with Novobiocin and Kanamycin.

DRUG INTERACTIONS: Activity of lincomycin (and clindamycin) theoretically can be antagonized by **erythromycin.** Concurrent use not recommended. **Kaolin-pectin antidiarrheal compounds** (eg, Kaopectate) and **sodium or calcium cyclamate** interfere with intestinal absorption of oral lincomycin. If used, space at least 2 hours before lincomycin (or clindamycin). Concurrent administration of lincomycin (or clindamycin) with **neuromuscular blocking agents** may cause neuromuscular weakness.

Hormone, thyroid

ACTIONS AND USES

Synthetic form of natural thyroid hormone. Shares actions and uses of thyroid (qv), but has more rapid action and more rapid disappearance of effect, permitting quick dosage adjustment if necessary; 25 μg are equivalent to approximately 65 mg of thyroid or thyroglobulin. May be used in T_3 suppression test to differentiate suspected hyperthyroidism from euthyroidism. See Thyroid for absorption, fate, contraindications, precautions, and adverse reactions.

ROUTE AND DOSAGE

All doses gradually increased from initial to maintenance levels with 12.5- to 25-μg increments at 1- or 2-week intervals. Oral: **Adults** (*hypothyroidism*): initially 25 μg daily; maintenance 25 to 100 μg daily; (*myxedema*): initially 5 μg daily; maintenance 50 to 100 μg daily; (*male infertility due to hypothyroidism*): initially 5 μg; maintenance 25 to 50 μg daily; (*goiter*): initially 5 μg daily; maintenance 75 μg daily. **Children:** (*cretinism*): initially 5 μg daily, with a 5-μg increment every 3 to 4 days until desired response is attained; at 1 year of age, 50 μg daily; more than 3 years, full adult dosage.

NURSING IMPLICATIONS

Since this drug is bound less firmly to serum protein than thyroxine, PBI (normal: 4 to 8 μg/dl) may remain at hypothyroid level, even though patient is euthyroid.

Metabolic effects persist a few days after drug withdrawal.

Infants with thyroid dysfunction (mother provides little or no thyroid hormone to fetus) are started on replacement therapy as soon as possible to prevent permanent mental and physical changes.

When changing to liothyronine from thyroid, levothyroxine, or thyroglobulin, discontinue other medication, initiate liothyronine at low dosage, with gradual increases according to patient's response.

Residual actions of other thyroid preparations may persist for weeks; therefore, during early period of liothyronine substitution for another preparation, watch for possible additive effects, particularly if the patient is elderly, has cardiovascular disease, or is a child.

With onset of overdosage symptoms, drug is withheld for 1 or 2 days; usually therapy can be resumed with small dosage.

T_3 suppression test: when thyroid uptake of ¹³¹I (radioactive iodine, RAI) is in borderline high range, give 75 to 100 μg liothyronine daily for 7 days, then repeat RAI uptake test. In hyperthyroidism, 24-hour RAI uptake will not be significantly affected; in euthyroid patient, 24-hour RAI uptake will decrease to less than 20%.

Depresses RAI uptake, especially when dose is above 75 μg daily. This effect disappears in 2 weeks after drug withdrawal.

Also see Thyroid.

(EUTHROID, THYROLAR)

Hormone, thyroid

ACTIONS AND USES
Synthetic levothyroxine (T_4) and liothyronine (T_3) combined in a constant 4:1 ratio by weight; actions and uses like those of thyroid (qv). Products by different manufacturers differ in total amounts of each drug included in the formulation. See Thyroid for uses, fate, and adverse reactions.

CONTRAINDICATIONS AND PRECAUTIONS
Morphologic hypogonadism, nephrosis, adrenal deficiency due to hypopituitarism. Cautious use: concomitant anticoagulant therapy; myxedema, diabetes mellitus. See Thyroid.

ROUTE AND DOSAGE
Dosage individualized to approximate thyroid replacement need. Oral: **Adults and children:** initially 0.25 to 0.5 grain daily, with gradual increases every 1 or 2 weeks for adults, every 2 weeks for children. Eventual maintenance dosage in growing child may be higher than in adult.

NURSING IMPLICATIONS
Usually administered as a single daily dose, preferably before breakfast.
Therapy results in euthyroidism, with PBI levels that fall within the normal range (4 to 8 μg/dl).
Available liotrix preparations contain variable amounts of T_3 and T_4; eg, preparations said to be equivalent to desiccated thyroid may contain 60 μg T_4 and 15 μg T_3 (Euthroid) or 50 μg T_4 and 12.5 μg T_3 (Thyrolar). Instruct patients to have their prescriptions filled with the same brand currently being taken.
Changeover from another thyroid preparation can be made by direct substitution of liotrix for current dose of the other product, with gradual dose increase every 1 or 2 weeks.
Liotrix tablets have an expiration period of 2 years.
Store in heat-, light-, and moisture-proof container.
Also see Thyroid.

LITHIUM CARBONATE, U.S.P., B.P.
(ESKALITH, LITHANE, LITHONATE, LITHOTABS, PFI-LITHIUM)

Antidepressant

ACTIONS AND USES
Alkali metal salt which behaves in body much like sodium ion.
Accumulates within neurons since Na pump is less efficient in transporting it out than Na, and thus alters electrophysiological characteristics of neurons. Introduction of lithium (Li) in body is followed by cation balance between Na, K, and Li.
Subsequent lithium-induced increase in Na and K excretion places particular importance on Na and fluid balance. Enhances reuptake (thus inactivation) of biogenic amines, 5-HT and norepinephrine at nerve terminals, but apparently does not affect dopaminergic systems in brain. Specific relationship of these actions in treatment of mania not known. May induce several endocrinologic effects. Decreases amount of circulating thyroid hormones, but normal functioning usually returns through pituitary feedback. Other possible effects: blocking of renal response to ADH, elevation of serum growth hormone levels (clinical significance not determined); and decrease in glucose tolerance.
Used for control and prophylaxis of manic episodes in manic-depressive psy-

chosis. May be given simultaneously with an antipsychotic agent during acute manic episode until clinical response to Li occurs. Effect in prevention of depression not established.

ABSORPTION AND FATE

Rapidly but sometimes variably absorbed from GI tract. Peak serum levels in 2 to 4 hours. Decreases in plasma concentrations are biphasic: steep drop after 5 to 6 hours, followed by slower elimination over next 24 or more hours. Widely distributed in body water; later drug shifts intracellularly. High concentrations in kidneys, saliva; moderate amounts in muscle, bone, liver. No evidence of protein binding. Crosses blood-brain barrier slowly with appreciable amounts in cerebrospinal fluid, once steady state established.

Half-life about 24 hours, after chronic treatment (longer in elderly patients). Following glomerular filtration about 80% reabsorbed. Approximately 50% to 75% of single dose excreted in urine within 24 hours, followed by slower excretion over several days.

Alkalinization of urine increases excretion. Less than 1% eliminated in feces and sweat. Crosses placenta; enters breast milk.

CONTRAINDICATIONS AND PRECAUTIONS

Significant cardiovascular or renal disease, brain damage, schizophrenia, organic brain syndrome, severe debilitation, dehydration or Na depletion; patients on low salt diet or receiving diuretics; pregnancy (especially first trimester), nursing mothers. Safe use in children under age 12 not established. Cautious use: elderly patients, thyroid disease, epilepsy.

ADVERSE REACTIONS

CNS: dizziness, headache, lethargy, drowsiness, fatigue, slurred speech, psychomotor retardation, giddiness, tinnitus, incontinence, restlessness, seizures, confusion, blackout spells, disorientation, recent memory loss, stupor, coma. **Neuromuscular:** fine hand tremors (common), coarse tremors, choreoathetotic movements; fasciculations, clonic movements, incoordination including ataxia, muscle weakness, hyperreflexia, extrapyramidal symptoms (parkinsonism, dyskinesias). **GI:** nausea, vomiting, anorexia, abdominal pain, diarrhea, dry mouth, metallic taste. **Cardiovascular:** arrhythmias, hypotension, peripheral circulatory collapse, ECT changes. **Hormonal:** diffuse thyroid enlargement, elevated ^{131}I uptake, lowered T_3, T_4 and PBI; hypothyroidism; diabetes insipidus-like syndrome, transient hyperglycemia, glycosuria. **Dermatologic** (most believed to be signs of toxicity rather than allergy): pruritus, maculopapular rash, hyperkeratosis, chronic folliculitis, transient acneiform papules (face, neck intertriginous areas), anesthesia of skin, cutaneous ulcers, drying and thinning of hair, allergic vasculitis. **Other:** elevated WBC count (especially neutrophils and lymphocytes); albuminuria, oliguria, increased uric acid excretion; transient scotomata, blurred vision, edema, weight gain (common) or loss, exacerbation of psoriasis, flu-like symptoms, EEG changes.

ROUTE AND DOSAGE

Oral: (Acute mania): 600 mg 3 times daily. Highly individualized according to serum Li levels and clinical response. Maintenance: 300 mg 3 or 4 times daily.

NURSING IMPLICATIONS

During acute treatment period, check Li blood level report before administering morning dose. If level exceeds 1.5 mEq/liter (or other value indicated by physician) consult physician before giving drug. Physician may withhold drug and resume treatment at lower dosage after 24 hours.

GI symptoms may be minimized by taking drug with meals. Transient nausea and general discomfort appear to coincide with peak rise in serum Li levels. Report persistent symptoms; physician may reduce and divide total daily dose or order sustained release form (provides consistent serum levels without high peaks).

Keep physician informed of patient's progress. Observe for normalization of the following common symptoms of mania: aggressiveness, grandiose or flight of ideas, distractability, inappropriate mood elevation, irritability, poor judgment, hyperactivity, talkativeness, disturbed sleep pattern.

Patient's tolerance for Li is greatest during acute manic phase and decreases as manic symptoms subside. Physician will reduce dosage rapidly when therapeutic effect is achieved, to prevent toxicity.

Peak therapeutic effects usually occur 7 to 10 days after initiation of therapy; some evidence of control may be apparent within a few days. If no therapeutic effect within 2 weeks, drug is usually discontinued.

Weigh patient daily; check ankles, tibiae, and wrists for edema. Report changes in intake-output ratio, sudden weight gain, or edema.

Normal excretion of Li depends upon normal kidney function and adequate salt and fluid intake. Fluid intake of 2500 to 3000 ml/day (at least during initial stabilization period) and well balanced diet with adequate salt intake are advised. Marked reduction in Na and/or fluid intake can accelerate Li retention with subsequent toxicity. Conversely, marked increase in Na intake can increase Li excretion and reduce drug effect.

Instruct patient/family to report to physician significant events that affect salt and water balance: e.g., vomiting, diarrhea, diuresis, infection, fever, excessive perspiration. Supplemental salt and fluids may be prescribed. If symptoms are severe, temporary reduction or cessation of the drug may be required to avoid toxicity.

Lithium may be given to selected patients during pregnancy with close surveillance of Na balance and weekly Li levels. Observe patient closely for signs of Li toxicity. Although serum Li excretion may increase markedly during pregnancy, often necessitating increase in dosage, excretion tends to stop abruptly at delivery. Physician may prescribe half-dose during week prior to expected delivery; after delivery, prepregnancy Li dosage is usually reinstated.

Polydipsia and polyuria, apparently not dose related, are common side effects particularly in the elderly. Symptoms appear during early therapy, then lessen but may reappear after several months or years in patients on maintenance therapy. Some patients develop a diabetes insipidus syndrome (inability to concentrate urine). Test urine periodically for specific gravity and report lower than normal value (1.015 to 1.025). Discontinuation of Li may be necessary.

Fine hand tremor may occur during early treatment and in some patients may persist throughout therapy. Discontinuation of Li may be necessary if tremor interferes with normal function.

Blood samples for Li determinations should be drawn 8 to 12 hours after last dose (usually before morning dose) and at the same time for each individual patient so that consistant data are obtained.

Since toxicity can occur even at therapeutic levels, discontinuation of medication and prompt reporting of changes in behavior and mood and appearance of adverse reactions are critically important. Dizziness, headache, feeling of dullness occur frequently and may worsen with impending toxicity. Physical status of patient and serum Li levels should be evaluated promptly.

Initially, serum Li levels should be determined every other day until desired level reached and clinical condition is stabilized; during maintenance therapy determinations are made at monthly intervals. Urge patient to keep follow-up appointments.

Therapeutic serum Li levels: 1 to 1.5 mEq/liter (not to exceed 2 mEq/liter during acute treatment phase); maintenance levels: 0.6 to 1.2 mEq/liter (not to exceed 1.5 mEq/liter). Therapeutic and maintenance levels are usually lower for elderly patients, who may exhibit toxicity at levels normally tolerated by younger patients. In these patients, physician may also use urinary creatinine clearance as an index of patient's ability to process Li. Lithium clearance is about one-fifth that of creatinine (approximately 15 to 30 mg/min).

Caution patient not to engage in activities requiring alertness and coordination such as driving a car or operating machinery until physician has determined his reaction to drug.

Diffuse thyroid enlargement, generally without change in thyroid function, may occur in some patients (mostly women) after 5 months to 2 years of Li therapy. Palpate thyroid periodically and report size increase.

Be alert to and report symptoms of hypothyroidism (an occasional side effect): lethargy, puffed face, cold intolerance, fatigue, headache, weight gain. Symptoms are reversible with discontinuation of lithium.

Treatment of overdosage: induced vomiting, or gastric lavage if patient is conscious. Have available acetazolamide, aminophylline, mannitol, sodium bicarbonate, urea (to increase lithium excretion), and supportive measures for maintenance of airway and respiratory function, and correction of fluid and electrolyte imbalance. Dialysis may be required for severe intoxication. Supportive therapy should continue for several days since brain tissue releases lithium slowly.

DRUG INTERACTIONS: The following drugs decrease lithium effect by increasing its renal excretion: **acetazolamide, aminophylline, sodium bicarbonate, sodium chloride** (in excessive amounts). Concurrent use of **haloperidol** with lithium may produce additive meurological toxicity. Addition of **methyldopa** to lithium therapy may result in lithium toxicity (by unknown mechanism). **KI** and other **iodine-containing compounds,** and **tricyclic antidepressants** may enhance hypothyroid effect of lithium. Additive hyperglycemic effects may occur with concurrent use of **chlorpromazine** and other **phenothiazines.** **Thiazides** and other potassium losing **diuretics** may potentiate neurotoxic and cardiotoxic effects of lithium (enhanced Na and K excretion decreases Li excretion). Lithium may inhibit effects of **amphetamines.**

LOMUSTINE
(CeeNU, CCNU)

Antineoplastic (alkylating agent)

ACTIONS AND USES
Lipid-soluble alkylating nitrosurea with actions like those of carmustine (qv). Used as palliative therapy in addition to other modalities or with other chemotherapeutic agents in primary and metastatic brain tumors and as secondary therapy in Hodgkin's disease.

ABSORPTION AND FATE
Rapidly absorbed from GI tract. Serum half-life of drug and/or metabolites ranges from 16 to 48 hours. 50% of dose is excreted in urine within 24 hours; 75% within 4 days. Because of high lipid solubility and relatively no ionization at physiologic pH, crosses blood–brain barrier readily. CSF levels are 50% greater than concurrent plasma levels.

CONTRAINDICATIONS AND PRECAUTIONS
History of hypersensitivity to lomustine. Safe use in pregnancy not established. Reported to be carcinogenic in laboratory animals. Cautious use: patients with decreased circulating platelets, leukocytes, or erythrocytes.

Delayed (cumulative) myelosuppression, stomatitis, alopecia, anemia, hepato-toxicity, nausea, vomiting. Neurologic reactions (relationship to drug unclear): lethargy, ataxia, dysarthria.

ROUTE AND DOSAGE

Oral: **Adults and children:** 130 mg/m² as single dose, repeated in 6 weeks. Subsequent doses adjusted to patient's hematologic response.

NURSING IMPLICATIONS

Blood counts should be monitored weekly for at least 6 weeks after last dose. Liver function tests should be performed periodically.

Since hematologic toxicity is delayed and cumulative, a repeat course is not given before 6 weeks and not until platelets have returned to above 100,000 mm³ and leukocytes to above 4000 mm³.

Nausea and vomiting may occur 3 to 6 hours after drug administration, usually lasting less than 24 hours. Symptoms may be controlled by administering drug to fasting patient, or physician may prescribe an antiemetic prior to dosage.

Thrombocytopenia occurs about 4 weeks and leukopenia about 6 weeks after a dose, persisting 1 to 2 weeks.

Store capsules away from excessive heat (over 40 C).

See Carmustine.

LYPRESSIN
(DIAPID)

Hormone, antidiuretic, vasoconstrictor

ACTIONS AND USES

Lysine vasopressin; synthetic polypeptide with pharmacologic action similar to that of vasopressin (qv). Possesses antidiuretic activity, with very little oxytoxic and minimal cardiovascular pressor activity in therapeutic doses.

Used to control or prevent complications of diabetes insipidus due to deficiency of endogenous posterior pituitary antidiuretic hormone. Particularly useful in patients who are nonresponsive to other forms of therapy and who experience allergic or other undesirable effects from vasopressin of animal origin.

ABSORPTION AND FATE

Following intranasal application of 1 or 2 sprays (approximately 7 μg/spray), onset of action in about 1 hour; antidiuretic effect lasts 3 to 8 hours. Plasma half-life about 15 minutes. Metabolized in kidney and liver and excreted in urine.

CONTRAINDICATIONS AND PRECAUTIONS

Pregnant women or women of childbearing potential. Cautious use: patients for whom pressor effects would be undesirable, coronary artery disease, known sensitivity to antidiuretic hormone. Also see Vasopressin.

ADVERSE REACTIONS

Infrequent and mild: hypersensitivity, rhinorrhea, nasal congestion and irritation, pruritus and ulceration of nasal passages, headache, conjunctivitis, heartburn secondary to excessive nasal administration with postnasal drip, abdominal cramps, increased bowel movements. With inadvertent inhalation: substernal tightness, coughing, and transient dyspnea. Overdosage: marked but transient fluid retention. Also see Vasopressin.

ROUTE AND DOSAGE

Topical (intranasal): **Adults and children:** 1 or 2 sprays in each nostril 4 times daily. One spray provides approximately 2 U.S.P. Posterior Pituitary (Pressor) Units.

NURSING IMPLICATIONS

Lypressin solution has expiration period of 1 year following date of manufacture.

Warn patient not to inhale the spray.

Instruct patient to clear nasal passages well before administering the spray.

Hold bottle upright and insert nozzle into nostril with patient's head in a vertical position.

If more than 2 sprays for each nostril are needed every 4 to 6 hours to give relief, the frequency of administration rather than number of sprays per dose should be increased. Large doses (excess) will drain posteriorly into digestive tract, where drug will be inactivated. Warn patients not to increase dosage without physician's order.

If nocturia is a problem, physician may prescribe an additional dose at bedtime.

If the patient develops a cold or allergy, absorption of lypressin will be diminished. Advise the patient to report to physician; adjustment of therapy may be required.

Lyopressin dosage is individualized to control symptoms of diabetes insipidus: frequent urination and excessive thirst.

Also see Vasopressin.

MAFENIDE ACETATE CREAM
(SULFAMYLON CREAM)

Antibacterial, topical

ACTIONS AND USES
Synthetic topical sulfonamide. Bacteriostatic against many Gram-positive and Gram-negative organisms, including *Pseudomonas aeruginosa*, and certain strains of anaerobes. Topical applications produce marked reduction of bacterial growth in avascular tissue. Active in presence of pus and serum, and not affected by changes in pH of tissue environment. Major metabolite of mafenide inhibits carbonic anhydrase, which may result in alkaline urine and metabolic acidosis when large amounts of drug are absorbed from application sites. Cross-sensitivity with other sulfonamides not established.

Used as adjunctive therapy in second- and third-degree burns to prevent sepsis.

ABSORPTION AND FATE
Rapidly absorbed from burn surface. Peak plasma concentrations in 2 to 4 hours following systemic absorption; rapidly eliminated through kidneys.

CONTRAINDICATIONS AND PRECAUTIONS
History of hypersensitivity to mafenide, respiratory (inhalation) injury, pulmonary infection, women of childbearing potential. Safe use during pregnancy not established. Cautious use: impaired renal or pulmonary function.

ADVERSE REACTIONS
Intense pain, burning, or stinging at application sites (common); bleeding of skin; excessive body water loss; delayed eschar separation; excoriation of new skin; superinfections (fungal colonization in and below burn eschar); allergic manifestations (pruritus, rash, urticaria, blisters, facial edema, eosinophilia); metabolic acidosis; fatal hemolytic anemia (rare); bone marrow suppression (rare).

ROUTE AND DOSAGE
Topical (cream contains equivalent of 85 mg of mafenide base per gram): applied to burn areas to thickness of approximately 1/16 inch once or twice daily.

NURSING IMPLICATIONS

It is frequently difficult to distinguish between adverse reactions to mafenide and the effects of severe burns. Accurate observations are critical.

Wound cleaning and removal of debris should be carried out before each reapplication of mafenide cream.

Mafenide cream is applied aseptically to cleansed, debrided burn areas with sterile gloved hand.

To aid in debridement, patient should be bathed daily by whirlpool bath (preferable) or shower or in bed.

Dressings are not usually required, but if they are necessary, only a thin layer should be used. Some physicians prescribe dressings when eschar begins to separate (about 16 to 20 days) to expedite its removal.

Burn areas must be covered with cream at all times. When necessary, reapplications should be made to areas from which cream has been removed (eg, by patient's activity).

Intensity of local pain caused by mafenide may require administration of analgesic. Report to physician.

Monitor vital signs. Report immediately changes in blood pressure, pulse, and respiratory rate and volume.

Monitor intake and output. Report oliguria or changes in intake–output ratio. Physician may request urinary pH determinations (excessive renal alkaline loss can result in metabolic acidosis).

Acid–base balance should be monitored in patients with extensive burns and in those with pulmonary or renal dysfunction. Be alert to signs and symptoms of metabolic acidosis: dull headache, weakness, abdominal pain, nausea, vomiting, diarrhea, stupor, disorientation, Kussmaul respirations, reduced Pco_2 and blood pH.

In patients with extensive burns, it is advisable to maintain a flow chart to monitor mental status, vital signs, intake and output, weight, burn wound care, medications, and laboratory data.

Allergic reactions have reportedly occurred 10 to 14 days following initiation of mafenide therapy. Temporary discontinuation of drug may be necessary.

Mafenide therapy is usually continued until healing is progressing well (usually up to 60 days) or site is ready for grafting (after about 35 to 40 days). It is not withdrawn while there is a possibility of infection, unless adverse reactions intervene.

MAGALDRATE, U.S.P.
(RIOPAN)

Antacid

ACTIONS AND USES

Chemical combination of aluminum and magnesium hydroxides. Nonsystemic antacid with true buffering action and high acid-consuming capacity. Reportedly does not produce alkalosis or acid rebound. Low sodium content (not more than 0.7 mg of sodium per 400 mg of drug).

Used for symptomatic relief of hyperacidity associated with peptic ulcer, gastritis, peptic esophagitis, and hiatal hernia.

ABSORPTION AND FATE

Minimal absorption from GI tract. Buffering action may persist for about 60 minutes.

CONTRAINDICATIONS AND PRECAUTIONS

Sensitivity to components. Cautious use: impaired renal function.

ADVERSE REACTIONS

Infrequent: constipation (with prolonged use), hypermagnesemia (in patients with impaired renal function).

ROUTE AND DOSAGE

Oral: 400 to 800 mg 4 times daily. Physician may prescribe hourly administration initially to control severe symptoms. Available as suspension, chew tablets, and swallow tablets.

NURSING IMPLICATIONS

Preferably administered between meals and at bedtime.

Suspension should be taken with sufficient water to ensure passage of drug into stomach.

Chewable tablet should be completely chewed before swallowing. Swallow tablet should be taken with enough water to ensure prompt swallowing.

DRUG INTERACTIONS: Based on limited clinical data, there is a possibility that simultaneous administration of aluminum- and/or magnesium-containing antacids may delay absorption of **chlorpromazine** and other **phenothiazines, isoniazid, quinidine, warfarin,** and **dicumarol.** It may be advisable to space antacid so that it is not taken within 1 to 2 hours of these drugs. Antacids may significantly decrease intestinal absorption of **tetracyclines** (antacid should not be taken for at least 3 hours after tetracycline administration).

MAGNESIUM SULFATE, U.S.P., B.P.
(EPSOM SALTS, MgSO$_4 \cdot$7H$_2$O)

Anticonvulsant, saline cathartic, electrolyte replenisher

ACTIONS AND USES

When taken orally, acts as cathartic by osmotic retention of fluid, which distends colon, increases water content of feces, and causes mechanical stimulation of bowel activity. When given parenterally, acts as CNS depressant and also depressant of smooth, skeletal, and cardiac muscle. Anticonvulsant properties believed to be produced by CNS depression, principally by decreasing the amount of acetylcholine liberated from motor nerve terminals, thus producing peripheral neuromuscular blockade. Believed to act on myocardium by slowing rate of S-A node impulse formation and prolonging conduction time. In excessive doses, produces vasodilation by ganglionic blockade and direct action on blood vessels.

Used orally to relieve acute constipation and to evacuate bowel in preparation for x-ray of intestines. Used parenterally to control convulsions in toxemia of pregnancy, epilepsy, acute nephritis, and hypothyroidism, as well as to counteract muscle stimulating effects of barium poisoning; as replacement therapy in acute magnesium deficiency, and as adjunct in hyperalimentation. Also has been used to control hypertension, cerebral edema, uterine tetany, and paroxysmal atrial tachycardia. Used topically to reduce edema, inflammation, and itching.

ABSORPTION AND FATE

Following oral administration, cathartic action within 1 to 2 hours; excreted primarily in feces. Absorbed magnesium (20%) is rapidly eliminated by kidney. Immediate action following IV injection; duration about 30 minutes. Following IM administration, acts in approximately 1 hour and lasts 3 to 4 hours.

CONTRAINDICATIONS AND PRECAUTIONS

Myocardial damage; heart block; IV administration during the 2 hours preceding delivery; oral use in patients with abdominal pain, nausea, vomiting, fecal impaction, or intestinal irritation, obstruction, or perforation. Cautious use: impaired renal function, digitalized patients, concomitant use of other CNS depressants or neuromuscular blocking agents.

ADVERSE REACTIONS

Hypermagnesemia: flushing, sweating, extreme thirst, hypotension, sedation, confusion, depressed reflexes or no reflexes, muscle weakness, flaccid paralysis, hypothermia, depressed cardiac function, complete heart block, circulatory collapse, respiratory paralysis. **Repeated cathartic use:** dehydration, electrolyte imbalance.

ROUTE AND DOSAGE

Oral: 5 to 15 Gm. Intramuscular: 1 to 2 Gm in a 25% to 50% solution. Intravenous: 1 to 2 Gm in a 10% or 20% solution; rate of administration should not exceed 1.5 ml/minute of 10% solution or its equivalent for other concentrations. Parenteral doses highly individualized. Topical (hot or cold compresses): 25% to 50% solution; antipruritic: 2% to 4% solution.

NURSING IMPLICATIONS

For cathartic action, magnesium sulfate is best administered in the morning or midafternoon in a glass of water. Bitter, salty taste may be disguised by chilling medication or adding ice chips. It may be flavored with lemon or orange juice.

Sufficient water should be taken during the day when drug is administered orally to prevent net loss of body water.

When magnesium sulfate is given intravenously, patient requires constant observation. Check blood pressure and pulse every 10 to 15 minutes or more often if indicated.

Early indicators of magnesium toxicity include profound thirst, feeling of warmth, sedation, confusion, depressed deep tendon reflexes, and muscle weakness.

Before each repeated parenteral dose, knee jerks (patellar reflex) should be tested. Depressed reflexes or absence of patellar reflexes is a useful, objective index of early magnesium intoxication. Also check respiratory rate and character and urinary output, especially in patients with impaired renal function. Therapy is generally not continued if urinary output is less than 100 ml during the 4 hours preceding each dose.

Monitor intake and output (in patients receiving drug parenterally). Report oliguria and changes in intake–output ratio.

Resuscitation equipment and facilities for maintaining artificial respiration must be immediately available, as well as specific antidote: calcium gluconate or calcium gluceptate.

Newborns of mothers who have received parenteral magnesium sulfate within a few hours of delivery should be observed for signs of magnesium toxicity.

Monitoring of plasma magnesium levels is advised in patients receiving drugs parenterally (normal: 1.8 to 3.0 mg/dl). Plasma levels in excess of 4 mEq/liter are reflected in depressed deep tendon reflexes.

Patients receiving the drug for treatment of hypomagnesemia should be observed for improvement in these signs of deficiency: irritability, choreiform movements, tremors, tetany, twitching, muscle cramps, tachycardia, hypertension, psychotic behavior (hypomagnesemia is usually associated with other electrolyte deficiencies, especially calcium and potassium deficiencies).

Recommended daily allowances of magnesium (350 mg/day for men; 300 mg/day for women; 450 mg/day during pregnancy and lactation) are obtained in a normal diet. Rich sources are found in whole-grain cereals, legumes, most green leafy vegetables, and bananas.

DRUG INTERACTIONS: Additive CNS depression may occur when magnesium sulfate is administered with CNS depressants, eg, **barbiturates, narcotics, general anesthetics** (dosage of these agents should be adjusted). Excessive neuromuscular blockade has occurred in patients receiving magnesium sulfate and another **neuromuscular blocking agent** concomitantly.

MAGNESIUM TRISILICATE, U.S.P., B.P.
(TRISOMIN)

Antacid

ACTIONS AND USES

Nonsystemic antacid. Forms magnesium chloride and hydrated silicon dioxide by reaction with gastric juices. Onset of antacid action is slow but prolonged.

Gelatinous consistency of silicon dioxide provides adsorptive and protective properties. Magnesium chloride reacts with intestinal carbonate to form magnesium carbonate, a mild laxative. Commonly combined with aluminum hydroxide gel to overcome its constipating effects and to prolong antacid action (eg, A-M-T, Gelusil, Malcogel, Trisogel).

Used for relief of gastric hyperacidity and as adjunct in treatment of peptic ulcer.

ABSORPTION AND FATE

About 5% magnesium and 1% silica absorbed. Excreted in feces.

CONTRAINDICATIONS AND PRECAUTIONS

Concomitant administration of tetracyclines. Cautious use: renal insufficiency.

ADVERSE REACTIONS

Diarrhea, abdominal pain, nausea, hypermagnesemia in patients with renal insufficiency (flushed skin, thirst, hypotension, depressed reflexes, muscle weakness), silica kidney stones, intestinal impaction from magnesium trisilicate concretions (chronic use).

ROUTE AND DOSAGE

Oral: 1 to 4 Gm 4 times a day, between meals and at bedtime.

NURSING IMPLICATIONS

For maximum effectiveness, tablets should be thoroughly chewed (or dissolved) and taken with half a glass of water.

See Aluminum Hydroxide Gel.

MANNITOL, U.S.P.
(D-MANNITOL, OSMITROL, RESECTISOL)

Osmotic diuretic, diagnostic aid (renal function determination)

ACTIONS AND USES

Hexahydric alcohol prepared commercially by reduction of dextrose. Induces diuresis by raising osmotic pressure of glomerular filtrate, thereby inhibiting tubular reabsorption of water and solutes. In large doses, may increase rate of electrolyte excretion, particularly sodium, chloride, and potassium. Reduces elevated intraocular and cerebrospinal pressures by increasing plasma osmolality, thus inducing diffusion of water from these fluids back into plasma and extravascular space.

Used to promote diuresis in prevention and treatment of oliguric phase of acute renal failure following cardiovascular surgery, severe traumatic injury, surgery in presence of severe jaundice, hemolytic transfusion reaction. Also used to reduce elevated intraocular and intracranial pressures, to measure glomerular filtration rate (GFR), to promote excretion of toxic substances, and as irrigating solution in transurethral prostatic reaction to minimize hemolytic effects of water.

ABSORPTION AND FATE

Diuresis occurs within 1 to 3 hours. Elevated intraocular pressure is lowered within 30 to 60 minutes for period of 4 to 6 hours; elevated cerebrospinal fluid pressure may be reduced within 15 minutes, with effect lasting 3 to 8 hours. Confined to extracellular space; does not cross blood–brain barrier, except with very high plasma concentrations or in the presence of acidosis. Half-life is about 100 minutes. Small quantity metabolized to glycogen in liver. Rapidly excreted by kidney. Approximately 80% of 100 Gm dose appears in urine within 3 hours.

CONTRAINDICATIONS AND PRECAUTIONS

Anuria, marked pulmonary edema or congestive heart failure, metabolic edema, organic CNS disease, intracranial bleeding, shock, severe dehydration, history

ADVERSE REACTIONS

Dry mouth, thirst, blurred vision, marked diuresis, urinary retention, edema, headache, circulatory overload with pulmonary congestion, congestive heart failure, fluid and electrolyte imbalance, acidosis, nausea, vomiting, rhinitis, arm pain, anginalike pains, tachycardia, backache, transient muscle rigidity, tremors, convulsions, chills, fever, dizziness, hypotention, hypertension, allergic reactions, nephrosis, uricosuria, thrombophlebitis; with extravasation: local edema, skin necrosis.

ROUTE AND DOSAGE

Intravenous infusion: 50 to 200 Gm in 24-hour period. *Test dose:* 0.2 Gm/kg body weight infused over 3 to 5 minutes. If response is not adequate, dose may be repeated. *Measurement of GFR:* 100 ml of 20% solution (20 Gm) diluted with 180 ml sodium chloride injection; infusion rate 20 ml/minute. All dosages highly individualized. *Urogenital irrigation:* 2.5% to 5% solution.

NURSING IMPLICATIONS

IV infusion flow rate (prescribed by physician) is generally adjusted to maintain urine flow of at least 30 to 50 ml/hour.

A test dose is given to patients with marked oliguria. Response is considered adequate if urine flow of at least 30 to 50 ml/hour is produced over 2 to 3 hours after drug administration.

Serum and urine electrolytes (particularly sodium, potassium, and chloride), central venous pressure, and renal function should be closely monitored during therapy.

Intake and output must be accurately measured and recorded to achieve proper fluid balance. Increasing oliguria is an indication to terminate therapy; report immediately (if urinary output is not adequate, mannitol may accumulate and cause circulatory overload, with resulting pulmonary edema, water intoxication, and congestive heart failure).

Consult physician regarding allowable oral fluid intake volume. In general, volume of total fluid intake (all sources) should be no more than 1 liter in excess of urinary output.

Monitor vital signs, and be alert for indications of fluid and electrolyte imbalance (eg, thirst, muscle cramps or weakness, paresthesias, distended neck veins, dyspnea, chest rales, tachycardia, blood pressure changes).

Accurate daily weight under standard conditions provides another reliable index of fluid balance.

Care should be taken to avoid extravasation. Observe injection site for signs of inflammation or edema.

To measure GFR, urine is collected by catheter for a specific time period and analyzed for amount of mannitol excreted (mg/minute). Blood samples are drawn at start and end of time period, and plasma concentrations of mannitol are determined (mg/ml). Normal rate for men is 125 ml/minute; for women, 116 ml/minute.

Parenteral mannitol may crystalize when exposed to low temperatures. If crystallization occurs, place bottle in hot water bath (approximately 50 C) and periodically shake vigorously. Cool to body temperature before administration. Do not use solution if crystals cannot be completely dissolved.

Concentrations higher than 15% have a greater tendency to crystallize. Administration set with filter should be used when infusing 20% mannitol.

If blood is to be given simultaneously, at least 20 mEq of sodium chloride should be added to each liter of mannitol solution to avoid pseudoagglutination.

Patients receiving urologic irrigations of mannitol should be observed closely for systemic reactions.

Vasodilator (coronary)

ACTIONS AND USES
Long-acting organic nitrate with actions, contraindications, precautions, and adverse reactions similar to those of nitroglycerin.
Used in prophylactic management of angina pectoris (not intended for acute anginal attacks because action is too slow).

ABSORPTION AND FATE
Action begins within 15 to 30 minutes and persists 4 to 6 hours.

ADVERSE REACTIONS
Headache, rises in intraocular tension and intracranial pressure, methemoglobinemia, cardiovascular collapse. Also see Nitroglycerin.

ROUTE AND DOSAGE
Oral: 32 to 64 mg every 4 to 6 hours.

NURSING IMPLICATIONS
Tolerance to therapeutic effects develops rather quickly. Abstention for a few days (as prescribed by physician) may restore responsiveness.
See Nitroglycerin.

MAZINDOL
(SANOREX)

Anorexiant

ACTIONS AND USES
Imidazoisoindole derivative with pharmacologic properties similar to those of amphetamines. Produces CNS and cardiac stimulation and has amphetamine-like actions. Appears to exert primary effects on limbic system; also appears to alter norepinephrine metabolism by inhibiting normal neuronal uptake mechanism.
Used in short-term management of exogenous obesity.

ABSORPTION AND FATE
Readily absorbed from GI tract. Onset of action in 30 to 60 minutes; duration 8 to 15 hours. Excreted primarily in urine as unchanged drug and conjugated metabolites.

CONTRAINDICATIONS AND PRECAUTIONS
Glaucoma; hypersensitivity to the drug; severe hypertension; symptomatic cardiovascular disease, including arrhythmias; agitated states; history of drug abuse; during or within 14 days following administration of MAO inhibitors; children under age 12. Safe use in women of childbearing potential or during pregnancy not established.

ADVERSE REACTIONS
GI: dry mouth, unpleasant taste, diarrhea, constipation, nausea, vomiting. **CNS:** restlessness, dizziness, insomnia, dysphoria, depression, tremor, headache, drowsiness, weakness. **Cardiovascular:** palpitation, tachycardia. **Skin:** rash, excessive sweating, clamminess. **Endocrine:** impotence, changes in libido (rare).

ROUTE AND DOSAGE
Oral: 1 mg 3 times daily 1 hour before meals or 2 mg once daily 1 hour before lunch.

NURSING IMPLICATIONS

Drug may be taken with meals if GI discomfort occurs.

Possibility of abuse potential should be kept in mind.

Rate of weight loss is greatest during first few weeks of therapy and tends to decrease thereafter.

Tolerance may develop within a few weeks. When it occurs, drug should be discontinued.

Insulin requirements of patients with diabetes may be decreased in association with use of mazindol and concomitant caloric restriction and weight loss.

Caution patients that mazindol may impair ability to perform hazardous activities such as driving a car or operating machinery.

Classified as schedule III drug under federal Controlled Substances Act.

DRUG INTERACTIONS: Mazindol may decrease the hypotensive effects of **guanethidine** and potentiate pressor amines, eg, **levarterenol, isoproterenol** (patient should be closely monitored if given concomitantly). Administration of mazindol with or within 14 days of **MAO inhibitors** can produce hypertensive crisis.

MECAMYLAMINE HYDROCHLORIDE, N.F., B.P. (INVERSINE)

Antihypertensive

ACTIONS AND USES

Potent, long-acting secondary amine ganglionic blocking agent. Reduces blood pressure in both normotensive and hypertensive individuals. Generally produces greater change in standing blood pressure than in supine or sitting blood pressures. Tolerance rarely develops; CNS effects may be produced by large doses.

Used in treatment of moderately severe to severe hypertension and in uncomplicated malignant hypertension.

ABSORPTION AND FATE

Almost completely absorbed from GI tract. Effects appear in 30 minutes to 2 hours and last 6 to 12 hours or longer. Absorbed into extracellular spaces, and crosses blood–brain barrier; high concentrations accumulate in liver and kidney. Excreted slowly by kidney in unchanged form. Rate of renal elimination is markedly influenced by urinary pH (excretion promoted by acid urine and diminished in alkaline urine). Crosses placenta.

CONTRAINDICATIONS AND PRECAUTIONS

Coronary insufficiency, pyloric stenosis, glaucoma, uremia, recent MI; unreliable uncooperative patients. Cautious use: rising or elevated BUN; concomitant use with antibiotics or sulfonamides; renal, cerebral, or coronary vascular pathology; chronic pyelonephritis, recent CVA; prostatic hypertrophy, bladder neck obstruction, urethral stricture.

ADVERSE REACTIONS

GI: anorexia, glossitis, xerostomia, nausea, vomiting, constipation, diarrhea, ileus, abdominal distention. **CNS:** weakness, fatigue, sedation, orthostatic hypotension, dizziness, syncope, paresthesias, mydriasis, blurred vision, choreiform movements, tremor, confusion, seizures, mania, or depression. **Other:** decreased libido, hyperuricemia, interstitial pulmonary edema and fibrosis.

ROUTE AND DOSAGE

Oral: initially 2.5 mg 2 times daily, after meals; increased by increments of 2.5 mg at intervals of not less than 2 days until desired blood pressure response is

414 attained. Average total daily dosage: 25 mg, usually in 3 divided doses. Highly individualized.

NURSING IMPLICATIONS

Initial regulation of dosage should be dictated by blood pressure readings in standing position at time of maximal drug effect, as well as symptoms of orthostatic hypotension (faintness, dizziness, lightheadedness).

Because of diurnal variations in blood pressure, physician may prescribe relatively small dose in the morning (or omission of morning dose) and larger doses for afternoon or evening administration.

Administration of drug after meals may result in more gradual absorption and smoother control of blood pressure. Timing of doses in relation to meals should be consistent.

Adverse reactions should be reported immediately, since drug effects may last for hours to days after drug is discontinued.

Constipation, abdominal distension, or decreased bowel sounds may be the first signs of paralytic ileus and should be reported promptly.

Constipation is sometimes preceded by small, frequent stools. Physician may prescribe a laxative such as milk of magnesia if constipation is a problem. Bulk laxatives are not recommended.

Patients should be informed of factors that may potentiate the action of mecamylamine: excessive heat, fever, infection, alcohol, vigorous exercise, salt depletion (vomiting, diarrhea, excessive sweating).

Sodium intake is generally not restricted. Consult physician.

Seasonal variations may alter the hypotensive effect, eg, usually smaller doses are required in summer than in winter.

Partial tolerance may develop in some patients, necessitating dosage adjustment.

Mecamylamine withdrawal should be accomplished slowly. Sudden discontinuation of drug can result in severe hypertensive rebound. Usually, other antihypertensive therapy must be substituted; this must be done gradually, and patient must be supervised daily during period of dosage adjustment.

See Pentolinium Tartrate.

DRUG INTERACTIONS: Mecamylamine may potentiate **sympathomimetics** (use reduced dose). There may be potentiated hypotensive effects with **alcohol,** other **antihypertensive agents, bethanechol,** and **thiazide diuretics** (used therapeutically). Mecamylamine toxicity may result with agents that increase urine pH such as **acetazolamide** and **sodium bicarbonate.**

MECHLORETHAMINE HYDROCHLORIDE, U.S.P., B.P.
(MUSTARGEN, NITROGEN MUSTARD)

Antineoplastic

ACTIONS AND USES

Analogue of mustard gas and standard of reference for nitrogen mustards. Forms highly reactive carbonium ion, which alkylates groups such as guanine of DNA, thereby interfering with DNA replication and RNA and protein synthesis. Actions simulate those of x-ray therapy, but nitrogen mustards produce more acute tissue damage and more rapid recovery. Highly toxic to rapidly proliferating cells at any time during cell cycle. Has vesicant, myelosuppressive, and powerful CNS stimulant properties. One member of the MOPP combination chemotherapeutic regimen.

Use generally confined to nonterminal stages of neoplastic disease. Employed as single agent or in combination with other agents in palliative treatment of malignant lymphomas including Hodgkin's disease, lymphosarcomas, mycosis fungoides. Produces brief remissions in bronchogenic carcinoma and chronic lymphocytic leukemia. Sometimes preceded by or alternated with x-ray treatment.

ABSORPTION AND FATE

Rapid intramolecular transformation after administration; less than 0.01% of unchanged drug excreted in urine. Interruption of blood supply to given tissue a few minutes during and immediately after drug injection protects area from drug effects.

CONTRAINDICATIONS AND PRECAUTIONS

Pregnancy, at least until third trimester; myelosuppression produced by x-ray therapy, other antineoplastics, or infiltration of malignant cells; foci of acute or chronic suppurative inflammation; infectious granuloma. Cautious use: patients with lymphosarcoma or chronic leukemia, men or women in childbearing age.

ADVERSE REACTIONS

Dermatologic: maculopapular skin eruptions (rare); herpes zoster; severe induration, sloughing, thrombophlebitis at injection site; alopecia. **Reproductive:** amenorrhea, impaired spermatogenesis. **CNS:** temporary aphasia and paresis (rare), convulsions, progressive muscular paralysis. **GI:** stomatitis, anorexia, nausea, vomiting, diarrhea, peptic ulcer, jaundice. **Hematopoietic:** leukopenia, thrombocytopenia, lymphocytopenia, agranulocytosis, anemia, hyperheparinemia (rare). **Other:** hyperuricemia, metallic taste immediately after dose, weakness, fever, drowsiness, tinnitus, deafness, headache.

ROUTE AND DOSAGE

Intravenous: 0.4 mg/kg body weight given either in 2 to 4 daily consecutive injections or in a single dose. Intraarterial and intracavitary routes and dosages highly individualized. Another course of therapy may be repeated after recovery of bone marrow function.

NURSING IMPLICATIONS

Solution should be prepared and administered while wearing surgical gloves for protection of skin. Avoid inhalation of vapors and contact of drug with eyes. Irrigate immediately any contaminated area with copious amounts of water for 15 minutes, followed by 2% sodium thiosulfate solution. Irritation may appear after a latent period.

Solution is administered as soon as reconstituted; unused portion should be discarded. Solution is injected into tubing of a flowing IV infusion to dilute concentration of vesicant.

Give preferably late in the day to prevent interference with sleep by side effects.

If drug extravasates, prompt subcutaneous or intradermal injection with isotonic sodium thiosulfate solution (1/6 molar) and application of cold compresses intermittently for 6 to 12 hours may reduce local tissue damage and discomfort. Tissue induration and tenderness may persist a long time, and tissue may slough.

Begin flow chart with established baseline data relative to body weight, intake–output ratio and pattern, and blood picture as reference for design of drug and nursing care regimens.

Mechlorethamine dosage is determined on basis of actual body weight unaugmented by edema or ascites. Record daily weight. Alert physician to sudden weight gain or slow but steady weight gain.

Immediately after intracavitary administration, patient should be positioned (prone, supine, right side, left side, knee-chest) every 60 seconds for 5 minutes to assure full contact of drug with all parts of the cavity. Paracentesis may be done 24 to 36 hours later to remove any remaining fluid.

Avoid suggesting to the patient who is receiving the drug for first time that nausea may develop. A strong positive approach with this symptom is often better than an anticipatory one.

Nausea and vomiting may occur 1 to 3 hours after drug injection; vomiting usually subsides within 8 hours, but nausea may persist. Chlorpromazine alone or with barbiturate may be prescribed before or at time of injection to help control nausea and vomiting.

Anorexia and nausea (of central origin) often persist more than 24 hours. Attempt to schedule treatments, other drugs, and meals so as to avoid peak times of nausea.

Prolonged vomiting and diarrhea can produce blood volume depletion (physical signs: decreased skin turgor, shrunken and dry tongue, postural hypotension, weakness, confusion). Carefully monitor and record patient's fluid losses. Discuss with physician the supportive measures that will restore and maintain fluid balance.

Myelosuppressive symptoms appear by the fourth day after treatment begins and are maximal by 10th day. Lymphocytopenia usually occurs within 24 hours, with maximum in 6 to 8 days. Leukopenia appears a few days after therapy begins and persists 10 to 21 days.

Courses of treatment are usually spaced at least 6 weeks apart because of delayed myelosuppression. At end of treatment period, mild anemia appears in 2 to 3 weeks; hematopoietic depression may last 7 weeks or more.

Thrombocytopenia usually manifests 2 to 3 weeks after a course of treatment. Explain its significance to patient. Petechiae, ecchymoses, or abnormal bleeding from intestinal and buccal membranes should be reported immediately. Warn patient to prevent bruising or falls. During period of thrombocytopenia, injections should be kept at a minimum.

Be alert for symptoms of agranulocytosis, and report them immediately (profound weakness, high fever, chills, rapid and weak pulse, sore throat, dysphagia, pharyngeal, buccal, and rectal ulcerations).

Stomatitis demands continuous fastidious measures to prevent superimposed oral infection and to relieve discomfort: Keep oral membranes well hydrated by frequent rinses with warm water or with 1:1 hydrogen peroxide (H_2O_2) solution (1 tablespoon H_2O_2 mixed with 1 tablespoon water immediately before use). Note: H_2O_2 must be stored in light- and air-resistant container. Avoid the use of commercial mouth rinses; they may have an alcohol (irritating) base. Avoid the use of a dry or hard-bristled toothbrush. If gums are painful, cleanse teeth with gauze-covered finger or with rubber tip on toothbrush. Cleansing before and after meals is important. Encourage patient to floss teeth gently with unwaxed floss at least once a day; do it for him if necessary. Apply petroleum jelly to cracked dry lips. If marked discomfort is associated with eating, consult physician for anesthetizing spray or solution to be applied before meals. In presence of ulcerations or dysphagia, avoid hot or cold foods and drinks; avoid spicy, sour, dry, rough, or chunky foods, as well as smoking and alcoholic beverages. Tea at room temperature seems to be especially soothing.

Work with dietitian and patient's family to help patient maintain optimum nutritional status. Anorexia should not be ignored. Determine dietary preferences; support and augment (rather than attempt to reform) eating patterns during periods of discomfort and leukopenia.

Prolonged immunosuppression may encourage overgrowth of opportunistic organisms on mucous membranes. Report signs: furry or black tongue, diarrhea, foul-smelling stools. Drug will probably be discontinued.

Constipation will add irritation to already ulcerated anal membranes. Gentle laxative may be required. Encourage patient to maintain adequate fluid intake. Avoid use of rectal thermometer or rectal tube.

Inspect skin (eg, over chest, antecubital surfaces) for petechiae, and dependent areas for ecchymoses. Report if present.

Rapid neoplastic cell and leukocyte destruction releases large amounts of purines, which are subsequently converted to uric acid. Allopurinol (qv) may be prescribed to prevent this conversion, thereby reducing the chance of urate deposition or renal calculi.

Discuss the problem of alopecia (reversible) with the patient. If desired, facilitate cosmetic substitution. Keep in mind the psychologic importance of hair to one's self-image and concept of sexuality.

Maculopapular skin eruptions usually do not necessitate stopping drug.

Herpes zoster may be precipitated by mechlorethamine treatment; it usually necessitates interrupting therapy.

Amenorrhea after a course of therapy is usually temporary, but it may persist for several months.

High doses of mechlorethamine may cause tinnitus and deafness. Alert patient to report symptoms promptly.

Consult physician about plans for disclosure of diagnosis, prognosis, and particulars about treatment so that discussions with patient and family will be supportive and nonconflicting.

MECLIZINE HYDROCHLORIDE, U.S.P.
(ANTIVERT, BONINE)
MECLOZINE HYDROCHLORIDE, B.P.

Antiemetic, antihistamine

ACTIONS AND USES

Long-acting piperazine derivative of diphenylmethane structurally and pharmacologically related to cyclizine compounds. Has marked effect in blocking histamine-induced vasopressive response, but only slight anticholinergic action. In common with similar agents, also exhibits CNS depression, antispasmodic, antiemetic, and local anesthetic activity. Has marked depressant action on labyrinthine excitability and on conduction in vestibular-cerebellar pathways.

Used in management of nausea, vomiting, and dizziness associated with motion sickness and in vertigo associated with diseases affecting vestibular system.

ABSORPTION AND FATE

Slow onset of action; duration of action 8 to 24 hours. Metabolic fate unknown.

CONTRAINDICATIONS AND PRECAUTIONS

Hypersensitivity to meclizine; use during pregnancy and in women of childbearing potential; use in pediatric age group. See Diphenhydramine.

ADVERSE REACTIONS

Drowsiness, dry mouth, blurred vision.

ROUTE AND DOSAGE

Oral: Motion sickness: 25 to 50 mg once a day. Vertigo: 25 to 100 mg daily in divided doses, depending on clinical response.

NURSING IMPLICATIONS

Forewarn patients about side effects such as drowsiness, and advise patients not to drive a car or engage in other hazardous activities until their reactions to the drug are known.

Caution patients that the sedative action may be additive to that of alcohol, barbiturates, narcotic analgesics, or other CNS depressants.

Recommended dosage when used to prevent motion sickness: 25 to 50 mg

1 hour before anticipated departure. Thereafter, dose may be repeated every 24 hours for duration of journey.

Also see Diphenhydramine.

MEDROXYPROGESTERONE ACETATE, U.S.P.
(AMEN, DEPO-PROVERA, PROVERA)

Progestin

ACTIONS AND USES

Synthetic progestational hormone effective on estrogen-primed endometrium, with actions, uses, absorption, fate, contraindications, and adverse reactions similar to those of dydrogesterone (qv).

ROUTE AND DOSAGE

Oral: *Amenorrhea and functional bleeding:* 5 to 10 mg daily for 5 to 10 days beginning on the assumed 16th to 21st day of menstrual cycle. Intramuscular: *Endometrial carcinoma:* 400 mg to 1 Gm weekly.

NURSING IMPLICATIONS

See Dydrogesterone.

MEFENAMIC ACID, B.P.
(PONSTEL)

Analgesic

ACTIONS AND USES

Anthranilic acid derivative with analgesic, antiinflammatory, and antipyretic actions. Analgesic effect similar to that of aspirin, but indicated for short-term therapy only because it can cause serious toxicity.

Used for short-term relief of mild to moderate pain, such as musculoskeletal and post-dental-extraction pain.

ABSORPTION AND FATE

Absorbed slowly from GI tract. Peak analgesic effect in 2 to 4 hours, may persist up to 6 hours. Firmly bound to plasma proteins. Partly detoxified in liver. Excreted in urine and feces as free drug and conjugated metabolites. Approximately 50% of dose is excreted in urine within 48 hours.

CONTRAINDICATIONS AND PRECAUTIONS

Hypersensitivity to drug, GI inflammation or ulceration. Safe use in women of childbearing potential, in children under age 14 and during pregnancy or lactation not established. Cautious use: history of renal or hepatic disease, history of blood dyscrasias, asthma, diabetes mellitus.

ADVERSE REACTIONS

GI: diarrhea (common), may be associated with GI ulceration and bleeding; nausea; vomiting; cramps; flatus; constipation. **Hematopoietic:** severe autoimmune hemolytic anemia (prolonged use), leukopenia, eosinophilia, agranulocytosis, thrombocytopenic purpura, megaloblastic anemia, pancytopenia, bone marrow hypoplasia. **Renal:** mild renal toxicity, dysuria, albuminuria, hematuria, elevation of BUN. **CNS:** drowsiness, insomnia, dizziness, vertigo, unsteady gait, nervousness, confusion, headache. **Dermatologic:** urticaria, rash, facial edema. **Other reported:** eye irritation, loss of color vision (reversible), blurred vision, ear pain, perspiration, increased need for insulin in diabetic patients, mild hepatic toxicity, palpitation, dyspnea (rare).

Oral: initially 500 mg, followed by 250 mg every 6 hours, as needed.

NURSING IMPLICATIONS
Drug should be administered with food to minimize GI adverse effects.
Administration of the drug for a period exceeding 1 week is not recommended.
Mefenamic acid should be discontinued promptly if diarrhea, dark stools, hematemesis, ecchymoses, epistaxis, or rash occur and should not be used thereafter. Advise patients to report these signs of hypoprothrombinemia.
Since the drug may cause dizziness and drowsiness, caution patients to avoid driving a car and other hazardous activities.

LABORATORY TEST INTERFERENCES: There may be false positive reactions for urinary bilirubin (using diazo tablet test).

DRUG INTERACTIONS: Mefenamic acid may prolong prothrombin time in patients receiving **anticoagulants** (displaces anticoagulant from protein-binding sites) and may enhance ulcerogenic effects of **corticosteroids, indomethacin, phenylbutazone,** and **salicylates.**

MELPHALAN, U.S.P., B.P.
(ALKERAN, L-PAM, L-PHENYLALANINE MUSTARD, PAM)

Antineoplastic (alkylating agent)

ACTIONS AND USES
Nitrogen mustard compound chemically and pharmacologically related to mechlorethamine (qv). Has strong immunosuppressive and myelosuppressive effects, but unlike mechlorethamine, lacks vesicant properties.
Used chiefly for treatment of multiple myelomas. Investigational use in treatment of many other neoplasms, including Hodgkin's disease and carcinomas of breast, bronchus, and ovary. Regional perfusion alone or with other antineoplastics is investigational.
ABSORPTION AND FATE
Well absorbed from GI tract. Half-life in infusion solution at 20 C is 13 hours; in circulation it is reported to be 2 to 6 hours. Widely distributed to all tissues; metabolism and excretion data not known.
CONTRAINDICATIONS AND PRECAUTIONS
Recent treatment with other chemotherapeutic agent; concurrent administration with radiation therapy; severe anemia, neutrophilia, or thrombocytopenia. Cautious use during pregnancy or in men and women of childbearing age should be preceded by complete understanding of possible hazards.
ADVERSE REACTIONS
Hematologic: leukopenia, agranulocytosis, thrombocytopenia, anemia. Other: mild thrombophlebitis at site of infusion, uremia, angioneurotic peripheral edema, minor neurologic toxicity (rare). See Mechlorethamine.
ROUTE AND DOSAGE
Oral: 6 mg daily for 2 to 3 weeks; drug is then withdrawn for up to 4 weeks. When WBC and platelet counts start to rise, maintenance dose is instituted: 2 mg/day. See package insert for other dosage regimens.

NURSING IMPLICATIONS

Stored in light-resistant airtight containers at room temperature.

Administer oral drug with meals to reduce nausea and vomiting. An antiemetic may be ordered if dose is high and side effects are increased.

Leukocyte and platelet counts are done 2 to 3 times each week during dosage adjustment period; WBC is usually determined each 6 to 8 weeks during maintenance therapy.

Nadirs of platelets and leukocytes occur within a few weeks after therapy begins; recovery is rapid.

Dosage adjustment is primarily based on blood counts. Usually, drug is discontinued after 2 to 3 weeks treatment for about 4 weeks. When WBC and platelet counts begin to rise, maintenance dose of 2 mg daily is instituted.

Monitor laboratory reports to anticipate leukopenic and thrombocytopenic periods in order to adapt nursing care accordingly.

A degree of myelosuppression is maintained during therapy so as to keep leukocyte count in range of 3000 to 3500/mm^3.

The combination of reduced capacity for normal antibody production (characteristic of multiple myeloma) and melphalan-induced toxic hematopoietic depression makes the patient particularly susceptible to infections and prolonged responses to trauma. Be alert to onset of fever, profound weakness, chills, tachycardia, cough, sore throat, changes in kidney function, or prolonged infections, and report them to physician.

A favorable response to oral melphalan in patients with multiple myeloma may be very gradual over many months. Encourage patient not to abandon treatment too soon to receive maximum benefit.

See Mechlorethamine.

MENADIOL SODIUM DIPHOSPHATE, N.F., U.S.P.
(KAPPADIONE, SYNKAYVITE)

Prothrombogenic vitamin, vitamin K supplement

ACTIONS AND USES

Synthetic, water-soluble vitamin K analogue, derived from menadione (qv). Has same actions, uses, contraindications, and precautions as menadione, but is reported to be about one-half as potent. Its use as liver function test has generally been replaced by newer methods. It has been suggested that when used in combination with radiotherapy it may selectively increase radiosensitivity of tumor cells through an unknown action. Also reported to reduce adenosine triphosphate level in tumor cells.

ABSORPTION AND FATE

Absorbed directly into bloodstream after oral administration, even in the absence of bile. Following subcutaneous or IM administration, bleeding may be controlled within 1 to 2 hours; prothrombin time usually returns to normal in 8 to 24 hours. Response after IV administration is more prompt, but action is less sustained.

ROUTE AND DOSAGE

Oral, subcutaneous, intramuscular, intravenous: 5 to 15 mg once or twice daily. Liver function test: 75 mg IV. **Children:** 5 to 10 mg 1 or 2 times daily.

NURSING IMPLICATIONS

Dosage and duration of treatment are determined by prothrombin times and clinical response.

Concomitant administration of bile salts is not required for intestinal absorption, but their use is recommended by some physicians for patients with obstructive jaundice or biliary fistula.

Stored in tight, light-resistant containers at room temperature.

Parenteral drug is incompatible with protein hydrolysate.

See Menadione.

MENADIONE, N.F.
(VITAMIN K_3)
MENAPHTHONE, B.P.

Prothrombogenic vitamin, vitamin K supplement

ACTIONS AND USES

Synthetic, fat-soluble vitamin K analogue. Similar in activity to naturally occurring vitamin K in hepatic biosynthesis of blood clotting factors II, VII, IX, X. Mechanism by which liver synthesis of clotting factors is promoted is unknown. Used in treatment of hypoprothrombinemia caused by vitamin K deficiency secondary to oral antibacterial therapy and salicylate. Also effective in prevention and treatment of hypothrombinemia resulting from inadequate absorption and synthesis of vitamin K, as in obstructive jaundice, biliary fistula, ulcerative colitis, celiac disease, intestinal resection, regional enteritis, cystic fibrosis of pancreas. Has been used as liver function test. Largely replaced by phytonadione (vitamin K_1) as an antidote for oral anticoagulant overdosage and in prophylaxis and treatment of hemorrhagic disease of newborns because of its greater margin of safety.

ABSORPTION AND FATE

Absorbed directly into bloodstream after oral administration (requires bile for absorption), with effects occurring in 6 to 10 hours; effects appear 1 to 2 hours after parenteral injection. Hemorrhage usually controlled within 3 to 6 hours. Normal prothrombin time may be obtained in 12 to 14 hours. Limited storage in fat tissue for short time. Completely metabolized. Crosses placenta.

CONTRAINDICATIONS AND PRECAUTIONS

Hypersensitivity to menadione or its derivatives; administration to mothers during last few weeks of pregnancy as prophylaxis against hemorrhagic disease of newborn; neonates. Effect on human fertility and teratogenic potential not known. Cautious use: depressed liver function.

ADVERSE REACTIONS

Gastric upset, headache (after oral dose), allergic reactions (skin rash, urticaria), erythrocyte hemolysis (persons with glucose-6-phosphate dehydrogenase deficiency and newborns). With large doses: BSP retention, prolonged prothrombin time, further depression of liver function (patients with hepatic disease). In infants (particularly prematures, or when administered to mother prior to delivery): hyperbilirubinemia, kernicterus, brain damage, death.

ROUTE AND DOSAGE

Oral, intramuscular: 2 to 10 mg daily.

NURSING IMPLICATIONS

Dosage and duration of treatment are determined by prothrombin times and clinical response.

Patients with bile deficiency receiving oral menadione will require concomitant administration of bile salts for adequate absorption.

Drugs that inhibit or interfere with vitamin K activity, such as oral antibiotics, sulfonamides, quinidine, quinine, and salicylates, may be discontinued or given in reduced dosages.

Therapeutic response to menadione is indicated by shortening of prothrombin, bleeding, and clotting times and by a decrease in hemorrhagic tendencies.

Advise the patient stabilized on menadione to maintain a well-balanced diet and to avoid significant increases in daily intake of vitamin K-rich foods (eg, green leafy vegetables, egg yolks, liver, cheese).

Use of menadione to correct anticoagulant-induced prothrombin deficiency may promote the same clotting hazards that existed prior to anticoagulant therapy.

Normal prothrombin time: 12 to 14 seconds; bleeding times (Ivy): 1 to 6 minutes; clotting time (3 tubes): 5 to 15 minutes.

Patients receiving large doses of menadione may develop temporary resistance to coumarin or indandione-type anticoagulants. When anticoagulant therapy is reinstituted, larger doses of anticoagulant may be needed until prothrombin reaches a satisfactory level. Some patients may require a change to heparin, which acts on a different principle.

Alcoholic solution of menadione is a vesicant, and the noncommercial powder is irritating to skin and respiratory tract.

Stored in tight, light-resistant containers.

LABORATORY TEST INTERFERENCES: Falsely elevated urine steroid determinations (by modifications of Reddy, Jenkins, Thorn procedure) may be found.

DRUG INTERACTIONS: Menadione and its derivatives antagonize the effects of **warfarin** and other **oral anticoagulants.** Concurrent administration of **mineral oil** may interfere with absorption of oral menadione.

MENOTROPINS
(PERGONAL, HUMEGON, PREGOVA)

Gonad-stimulating principle

ACTIONS AND USES

Purified preparation of gonadotropins, extracted from postmenopausal urine and standardized biologically for follicle-stimulating hormone (FSH) and luteinizing hormone (LH) gonadotropic activities. Promotes growth of graafian follicles in women who do not have primary anovulation. Treatment usually results only in ovarian follicular growth and maturation. With clinical proof of follicular maturation, ovulation is induced by sequential administration of human chorionic gonadotropin (HCG).

Used to treat infertility in selected women with primary amenorrhea, secondary amenorrhea with or without galactorrhea, irregular menses, anovulatory cycles, and polycystic ovary syndrome.

ABSORPTION AND FATE

Disposition factors following parenteral administration not known. Approximately 8% of dose is excreted unchanged in urine. Urinary estrogen excretion during treatment reflects level of follicular enlargement.

CONTRAINDICATIONS AND PRECAUTIONS

Pregnancy, primary anovulation, thyroid and adrenal dysfunction, organic intracranial lesion, infertility caused by factors other than anovulation, abnormal bleeding of unknown origin, ovarian cysts or enlargement not due to polycystic ovary syndrome.

Dose-related: mild to moderate ovarian enlargement, abdominal distention and pain, ovarian hyperstimulation syndrome (sudden ovarian enlargement accompanied by ascites with or without pain and/or pleural effusion); hemoperitoneum, fever, nausea, vomiting, diarrhea, arterial thromboembolism (rare), hypovolemia, multiple ovulations, follicular cysts, birth defects.

ROUTE AND DOSAGE

Intramuscular (individualized): initially 75 IU each of FSH and LH (1 ampul) daily for 9 to 12 days followed by HCG (10,000 IU) one day after last dose of menotropins. Menotropins should not be given beyond 12 days. If ovulation occurs without pregnancy, regimen may be repeated at least twice at same dosage before increasing dosage to 150 IU each of FSH and LH daily for 9 to 12 days. As before, HCG (10,000 IU) is given 1 day after last dose of menotropins. If ovulation occurs without pregnancy, treatment may be repeated at monthly intervals for two more courses.

NURSING IMPLICATIONS

Treatment with menotropins is preceded by a thorough gynecologic and endocrinologic examination to rule out early pregnancy, primary ovarian failure, neoplastic lesion; husband's fertility is also evaluated.

Drug is prepared immediately before administration by dissolving ampul contents in 1 to 2 ml of sterile NaCl injection. Unused portion should be discarded.

Most reliable index of follicular maturation is the rate of urinary estrogen excretion. Other indirect estimates include serial examination of vaginal smears and cervical mucus specimens (Spinnbarkeit, ferning) and changes in appearance and volume of cervical mucus.

Teach patient to recognize indirect indices of progesterone production: rise in basal body temperature, menstruation following shift in basal temperature, increased volume of thin and watery vaginal secretion. Urinary pregnanediol levels are usually determined.

The couple should be encouraged to have intercourse daily beginning on day prior to administration of HCG until ovulation becomes apparent from indices of progestational activity. Care must be taken to insure insemination.

When total estrogen excretion level is more than 100 μg/24 hours, HCG is not administered because hyperstimulation syndrome is more likely to occur.

Patient should be examined at least every other day and for 2 weeks following HCG injection to detect excessive ovarian stimulation. Examiner should proceed with caution in performing pelvic examination to avoid rupture of possible ovarian cysts and consequent hemoperitoneum.

If significant ovarian enlargement occurs after ovulation, patient should refrain from intercourse.

Warn patient to report immediately if symptoms of hyperstimulation syndrome occur: abdominal distention and pain, dyspnea, vaginal bleeding. Discontinuation of intercourse, as well as hospitalization, may be necessary.

Advise patient to weigh herself every other day to detect sudden weight gain (hyperstimulation syndrome develops rapidly over a 3- to 4-day period and usually occurs within 2 weeks following therapy). Patient should understand the range of weight gain that is unacceptable and that should be reported to physician.

Mild ovarian enlargement (with or without abdominal distention and pain) usually regresses without treatment in 2 to 3 weeks.

Patient should be aware of statistics related to pregnancy after menotropins/HCG treatment. Reportedly, there is a 20% frequency of multiple births, 15% of which may be twins; 5% of total pregnancies result in 3 or more fetuses, of which 20% are viable.

Generally, pregnancy occurs within four to six courses of therapy.

MEPENZOLATE BROMIDE, N.F.
(CANTIL)

Anticholinergic

ACTIONS AND USES

Synthetic anticholinergic quaternary ammonium compound. Qualitatively similar to atropine in actions, contraindications, precautions, and adverse reactions. Acts predominantly on GI tract. Reduces motility of stomach, small intestine, and particularly colon. Large oral doses can reduce gastric secretion of hydrochloric acid. Also relaxes sphincter of Oddi. As with other quaternary anticholinergic agents, high doses may block ganglionic and skeletal neuromuscular transmission.

Used in adjunctive treatment of peptic ulcer, irritable bowel syndrome, neurogenic bowel disturbances, diverticulitis, and diarrhea. Commercially available in combination with phenobarbital.

ABSORPTION AND FATE

Irregular GI absorption. Onset of action in about 1 hour, lasting 3 to 4 hours. Excreted primarily in urine and bile and as unchanged drug in feces.

ROUTE AND DOSAGE

Oral: 25 to 50 mg 3 times a day and at bedtime. Low doses are used initially and are increased gradually until desired effects are obtained or side effects intervene.

NURSING IMPLICATIONS

Administered preferably before or with meals.

Caution patients not to engage in activities requiring mental alertness, such as driving a car, if drowsiness or blurred vision occurs.

See Atropine Sulfate.

MEPERIDINE HYDROCHLORIDE, U.S.P.
(DEMEROL HYDROCHLORIDE)
PETHIDINE HYDROCHLORIDE, B.P.

Narcotic analgesic

ACTIONS AND USES

Synthetic morphinelike compound (phenylpiperidine derivative). Chemically dissimilar to morphine, but in equianalgesic doses it is qualitatively comparable in regard to analgesic effects, sedation, euphoria, pupillary constriction, and respiratory depression. Reported to differ from morphine in having a somewhat more rapid onset and shorter duration of action and in producing less depression of cough reflex, constipation, urinary retention, and smooth muscle spasm. Usual doses produce either no pupillary change or slight miosis, but overdosage results in marked miosis or mydriasis. Also, unlike morphine, has little or no antidiarrheic or antitussive action and produces CNS stimulation in toxic doses. In common with morphine, it causes sensitization of labyrinthine apparatus, stimulation of chemoreceptor trigger zone, and depression of medullary vasomotor center; it also has vagolytic and anticholinergic actions and may inhibit release of ACTH and gonadotropic hormones. Promote release of histamine and antidiuretic hormone, and elevation of blood sugar.

Used for relief of moderate to severe pain, for preoperative medication, for support of anesthesia, and for obstetric analgesia.

ABSORPTION AND FATE

Well absorbed from GI tract; analgesic effect begins in 15 minutes, peaks in about 1 hour and subsides over 2 to 4 hours. Onset of action following subcutaneous or IM administration occurs within 10 minutes; action peaks within 60 minutes, duration of action for both routes 2 to 4 hours. Onset of action following IV administration in about 5 minutes; duration approximately 2 hours. About 40% bound to plasma proteins. Metabolized chiefly in liver to active and inactive metabolites. Excreted in urine, mostly as metabolites and about 5% unchanged drug. Excretion of unchanged drug is enhanced by acidification of urine. Crosses placenta and appears in breast milk.

CONTRAINDICATIONS AND PRECAUTIONS

Hypersensitivity to meperidine, convulsive disorders, acute abdominal conditions prior to diagnosis, use of MAO inhibitors within 14 days, pregnancy (prior to labor), nursing mothers. Cautious use: head injuries, increased intracranial pressure, asthma and other respiratory conditions, supraventricular tachycardias, prostatic hypertrophy, urethral stricture, glaucoma, elderly or debilitated patients, impaired renal or hepatic function, hypothyroidism, Addison's disease.

ADVERSE REACTIONS

CNS: dizziness, weakness, euphoria, dysphoria, sedation, headache, uncoordinated muscle movements, disorientation, decreased cough reflex, miosis, corneal anesthesia, respiratory depression. Toxic doses: muscle twitching, tremors, hyperactive reflexes, excitement, hypersensitivity to external stimuli, agitation, confusion, hallucinations, dilated pupils, convulsions. **Cardiovascular:** facial flushing, lightheadedness, hypotension, syncope, palpitation, bradycardia, tachycardia, cardiovascular collapse, cardiac arrest (toxic doses). **GI:** dry mouth, nausea, vomiting, constipation, biliary tract spasm. **Allergic:** pruritus, urticaria, skin rashes, wheal and flare over IV site. **Other reported:** oliguria; urinary retention; profuse perspiration; respiratory depression in newborn; bronchoconstriction (large doses); phlebitis (following IV use); pain, tissue irritation and induration, particularly following subcutaneous injection; increased levels of serum amylase, BSP retention, bilirubin, SGOT, SGPT.

ROUTE AND DOSAGE

Oral, subcutaneous, intramuscular, intravenous (given slowly IV and as diluted solution): **Adults:** 50 to 150 mg every 3 or 4 hours as necessary; *preoperative:* 50 to 100 mg IM or subcutaneously 30 to 90 minutes before anesthesia; *obstetric analgesia:* 50 to 100 mg IM or subcutaneously when pains become regular; may be repeated at 1- to 3-hour intervals. **Children:** 1 mg/kg IM, subcutaneously, or orally up to 100 mg, every 4 hours as necessary.

NURSING IMPLICATIONS

Narcotic analgesics should be given in the smallest effective dose and for the least period of time compatible with patient's needs.

Evaluate the patient's need for p.r.n. medication; check time of last dose and validity of physician's order. Follow health facility policy regarding time limit on narcotic orders. Record time of onset, duration, and quality of pain, preferably in patient's words.

In patients receiving repeated doses, note respiratory rate, depth, and rhythm and size of pupils. If respirations are 12 per minute or below and pupils are constricted or dilated (see Actions and Uses) or breathing is shallow, or if signs of CNS hyperactivity are present, consult physician before administering drug.

Carefully aspirate before giving IM injection in order to avoid inadvertent

IV administration. IV injection of undiluted drug can cause a marked increase in heart rate and syncope.

Although the subcutaneous route is sometimes prescribed, it is painful and can cause local irritation. The IM route is generally preferred when repeated doses are required.

A high incidence of severe untoward effects is associated with IV use. Facilities for administration of oxygen and control of respiration should be immediately available, as well as a narcotic antagonist (eg, naloxone, nalorphine).

Vital signs should be monitored closely. Heart rate may increase markedly, and hypotension may occur.

The syrup formulation should be taken in half a glass of water. Undiluted syrup may cause topical anesthesia of mucous membranes.

Before administering meperidine, provide maximum comfort measures and reduce environmental stimuli. Caution patients not to smoke and not to ambulate without assistance after receiving the drug. Bedsides may be advisable for some patients.

Use of comfort measures, as well as displays of thoughtfulness and interest by those attending the patient, is as important as medication in control of pain.

Monitor vital signs, particularly in patients receiving repeated doses. Meperidine may cause severe hypotension in postoperative patients and those with depleted blood volume.

Deep breathing, coughing (unless contraindicated), and changes in position at scheduled intervals may help to overcome the respiratory depressant effects of meperidine.

Parenteral administration has caused corneal anesthesia and thus abolishment of corneal reflex in some patients. Be alert for this possibility.

Ambulatory patients are more likely than supine patients to manifest nausea, vomiting, dizziness, and faintness associated with fall in blood pressure (these symptoms may also occur in patients without pain who are given meperidine); symptoms are lessened by the recumbent position and aggravated by the head-up position. Report to physician; dosage reduction or drug discontinuation may be indicated.

Caution ambulatory patients to avoid driving a car or engaging in other hazardous activities until any drowsiness and dizziness have passed.

Chart the patient's response to meperidine and evaluate continued need for the drug. Suggest to physician a change to a milder analgesic when in your judgment it is indicated.

Repeated use of meperidine can lead to tolerance and psychic and physical dependence of the morphine type. High abuse potential has been reported among nurses and physicians.

Abrupt discontinuation of meperidine following repeated use results in withdrawal symptoms resembling those caused by morphine, but symptoms develop more rapidly (within 3 hours, peaking in 8 to 12 hours) and are of shorter duration. Nausea, vomiting, diarrhea, and pupillary dilatation are less prominent, but muscle twitching, restlessness, and nervousness are greater than with morphine.

Classified as schedule II drug under federal Controlled Substances Act.

Preserved in tightly closed, light-resistant containers.

DRUG INTERACTIONS: CNS stimulation or depression induced by meperidine and its congeners may be enchanced by **amphetamines, MAO inhibitors, phenothiazines, tricyclic antidepressants,** and **other CNS depressants,** including **alcohol.**

Adrenergic (vasoconstrictor)

ACTIONS AND USES

Synthetic noncatecholamine with α- and predominant β-adrenergic activity. Acts both directly and indirectly (by releasing norepinephrine from tissue storage sites). Elevation of blood pressure probably results primarily from positive inotropic action and increased cardiac output, and to lesser extent to increase in peripheral resistance caused by peripheral vasoconstriction. Heart rate may be reflexly slowed. Antiarrhythmic action results from decrease in A-V conduction time, atrial refractory period, and conduction time in ventricular muscle. CNS effects are usually not prominent except with large doses.

Used mainly as pressor agent in treatment of hypotension secondary to ganglionic blockade or spinal anesthesia. Also has been used as an emergency measure in therapy of shock secondary to hemorrhage until whole blood replacement is available; as adjunct in treatment of cardiogenic shock, and to abolish certain cardiac arrhythmias.

ABSORPTION AND FATE

Onset of pressor effect following IM injection in 5 to 15 minutes; duration 1 to 2 hours. Following IV administration, pressor response begins almost immediately and lasts 30 to 45 minutes. Rapidly metabolized. Excreted in urine. Alkaline urine favors drug retention and tends to produce higher plasma levels.

CONTRAINDICATIONS AND PRECAUTIONS

History of sensitivity to mephentermine; patients receiving cyclopropane or halothane; in combination with or within 2 weeks of MAO inhibitors; shock secondary to hemorrhage (except in emergency). Safe use in women of childbearing age and during pregnancy or lactation not established. Cautious use: arteriosclerosis, cardiovascular disease, hypertension, hyperthyroidism, patients with known hypersensitivities, chronically ill patients.

ADVERSE REACTIONS

Infrequent: euphoria, anorexia, weeping, nervousness, anxiety, tremor. With large doses: cardiac arrhythmias, marked elevation of blood pressure, incoherence, drowsiness, convulsions.

ROUTE AND DOSAGE

Intramuscular, intravenous: 15 to 45 mg. Intravenous infusion: 0.1% solution (prepared by adding two 10-ml vials of the 30-mg/ml concentration to 500 ml of 5% dextrose in water).

NURSING IMPLICATIONS

Close observation of patient and monitoring of blood pressure, heart rate, ECG, and central venous pressure (CVP) are essential.

During IV administration, check blood pressure and pulse every 2 minutes until stabilized at prescribed level, then every 5 minutes thereafter during therapy. Continue monitoring vital signs for at least the duration of drug action (see Absorption and Fate) and longer if indicated.

IV flow rate should be prescribed by physician. Infusion rate is more easily regulated with a microdrip.

Tolerance may occur after repeated injections.

Preserved in tightly closed, light-resistant containers.

Mephentermine is incompatible with epinephrine hydrochloride and hydralazine hydrochloride.

DRUG INTERACTIONS: Mephentermine may be ineffective in patients receiving **reserpine** or **guanethidine** (these drugs reduce quantity of available norepinephrine in sympathetic nerve endings). Pressor response may be potentiated by **sympathomimetic amines, MAO inhibitors, and tricyclic antidepressants.** Administration of mephentermine during **cyclopropane** or **halothane** anesthesia may result in serious arrhythmias.

MEPHENYTOIN, N.F.
(MESANTOIN)
METHOIN, B.P.

Anticonvulsant

ACTIONS AND USES

Hydantoin derivative, with actions, contraindications, precautions, and adverse reactions similar to those of phenytoin. Reported to have lower incidence of ataxia, gingival hyperplasia, gastric distress, and hirsutism, but produces more sedative and hypnotic action than phenytoin and causes serious toxic reactions, including fatal blood dyscrasias, more frequently. Relatively ineffective for petit mal seizures.

Used for control of grand mal, focal, jacksonian, and psychomotor seizures in patients refractory to less toxic anticonvulsants. Usually used concomitantly with other antiepilepsy agents.

ABSORPTION AND FATE

Rapidly absorbed following oral administration. Onset of action in 30 minutes; duration 24 to 48 hours. Demethylated in liver to phethenylate (Nirvanol), an active metabolite believed to have both therapeutic and toxic properties. Excreted in urine.

CONTRAINDICATIONS AND PRECAUTIONS

History of hypersensitivity to mephenytoin; use in conjunction with oxazolidinedione antiepilepsy agents, eg, paramethadione, trimethadione (toxic synergism). Safe use during pregnancy not established. Cautious use: history of drug hypersensitivities. Also see Phenytoin.

ADVERSE REACTIONS

Drowsiness, dizziness, skin and mucous membrane manifestations (exfoliative dermatitis, erythema multiforme, toxic epidermal necrolysis, other skin rashes), blood dyscrasias (leukopenia, neutropenia, agranulocytosis, thrombocytopenia, aplastic anemia), hepatic damage, periarteritis nodosa, systemic lupus erythematosus syndrome. Also see Phenytoin.

ROUTE AND DOSAGE

Oral: **Adults and children:** initially 50 to 100 mg daily during first week; increased weekly by same amount until maintenance level. Maintenance: **Adults:** 200 to 600 mg daily administered in 3 equally divided doses (some patients require 800 mg daily). **Children:** 3 to 15 mg/kg/day administered in 3 equally divided doses.

NURSING IMPLICATIONS

Patients should be kept under close supervision at all times, since drug is associated with severe adverse effects. Serious blood dyscrasias have occurred 2 weeks to 30 months after initiation of therapy.

Screening tests of liver function, total white cell count, and differential count should precede initiation of therapy.

Blood studies should be performed every 2 weeks and should be continued until patient is on maintenance dosage for 2 weeks; then they should be repeated monthly for 1 year, and thereafter every 3 months (unless neutrophil count drops to 2500/mm^3 or 1600/mm^3, then performed every 2 weeks).

Medication should be discontinued if neutrophil count falls to 1600/mm³.
The most frequent side effect of mephenytoin therapy is drowsiness, which
may usually be diminished by reduction of dosage. Caution patients to
avoid hazardous activities until their reactions to the drug have been
determined. Supervision of ambulation and bedsides may be indicated for
some patients during early therapy.

Advise patients to report immediately the onset of drowsiness, ataxia, skin
rash, sore throat, fever, mucous membrane bleeding, or glandular swelling. All are indications of developing toxic reaction.

When mephenytoin replaces another antiepilepsy agent, the dosage of mephenytoin should be gradually increased while the drug being discontinued is gradually decreased over period of 3 to 6 weeks.

Discontinuation of mephenytoin should be accomplished gradually to minimize the risk of precipitating seizures or status epilepticus.

See Phenytoin (Diphenylhydantoin).

MEPHOBARBITAL, N.F.

(MEBARAL, MENTA-BAL, MEPHORAL, Methylphenobarbital)

Anticonvulsant, sedative

ACTIONS AND USES

Long-acting barbiturate with pharmacologic properties similar to those of
phenobarbital (qv); however, larger doses are required to produce comparable
anticonvulsant effects. Exerts strong sedative action, but relatively mild hypnotic effect. Clinical uses, contraindications, precautions, and adverse reaction
are as for phenobarbital.

Used to control grand mal and petit mal epilepsy, alone or in combination with
other antiepilepsy agents, and for sedative effect in management of delirium
tremens and other acute agitation and anxiety states.

ABSORPTION AND FATE

Approximately 50% absorbed following oral ingestion. Onset of action in 20 to
60 minutes; duration 6 to 8 hours. About 75% metabolized in liver to phenobarbital in 24 hours. Excreted in urine both unchanged and as metabolites. Alkalinization of urine or increase of urinary flow significantly hastens rate of phenobarbital excretion.

CONTRAINDICATIONS AND PRECAUTIONS

Hypersensitivity to barbiturates. Safe use during pregnancy not established.
Also see Phenobarbital.

ROUTE AND DOSAGE

Oral: (Anticonvulsant): **Adults:** 400 to 600 mg daily. **Children** *under 5 years:* 16
to 32 mg 3 or 4 times daily; *over 5 years:* 32 to 64 mg 3 or 4 times daily. (Sedative):
Adults: 32 to 100 mg 3 or 4 times daily; for delirium tremens 200 mg 3 times
daily. **Children:** 16 to 32 mg 3 or 4 times daily.

NURSING IMPLICATIONS

Change from other antiepilepsy agents to mephobarbital should be accomplished by gradually tapering off the former as mephobarbital doses are
increased to maintain seizure control.

When mephobarbital is prescribed concurrently with phenobarbital, the
dose should be about one-half the amount of each used alone. When
prescribed concurrently with phenytoin (diphenylhydantoin), the dose of
phenytoin is usually reduced.

Mephobarbital may be prescribed as a single dose at bedtime (if seizures generally occur at night) or during the day (if attacks are diurnal).

When mephobarbital antiepilepsy therapy is to be discontinued, dosage should be reduced gradually over 4 or 5 days to avoid precipitating seizures or status epilepticus.

Abrupt cessation after prolonged mephobarbital therapy may result in withdrawal symptoms (tremulousness, weakness, insomnia, delirium, convulsions).

Since mephobarbital may cause drowsiness and dizziness, caution patients to avoid hazardous activities such as driving a car.

Classified as schedule IV drug under federal Controlled Substances Act. See Phenobarbital.

MEPROBAMATE, U.S.P., B.P.

(AMOSENE, EQUANIL, KESSO-BAMATE, MEPRIAM, MEPROSPAN, MEPROTABS, MILTOWN, QIDbamate, SARONIL, SEDABAMATE, SK-BAMATE, TRANMEP)

Antianxiety agent (minor tranquilizer), skeletal muscle relaxant

ACTIONS AND USES

Propanediol carbamate derivative structurally and pharmacologically related to carisoprodol. CNS depressant actions similar to those of barbiturates. Acts on multiple sites in CNS and appears to block cortical-thalamic impulses. Has no effect on medulla, reticular activating system, or autonomic nervous system. Skeletal muscle relaxant effect is probably related to sedative rather than to direct action. Hypnotic doses suppress REM sleep.

Used to relieve anxiety and tension of psychoneurotic states and as adjunct in disease states associated with anxiety and tension. Also used to promote sleep in anxious, tense patients, and used to control spasms of tetanus elicited by somatic stimuli.

ABSORPTION AND FATE

Onset of sedative action within 1 hour following oral administration and within 10 to 15 minutes after IM injection. Plasma half-life ranges 6 to 16 hours. Uniformly distributed throughout body. Rapidly metabolized in liver. About 90% of dose is excreted in urine and 10% in feces, mainly as inactive metabolites, within 24 hours. Can induce hepatic microsomal enzymes. Crosses placenta and enters breast milk in high concentrations.

CONTRAINDICATIONS AND PRECAUTIONS

History of hypersensitivity to meprobamate or related compounds such as carisoprodol, carbromal, mebutamate, and tybamate; history of porphyria; IM injection in patients with renal insufficiency. Safe use during pregnancy and in women of childbearing potential or children under 6 years of age not established. Cautious use: impaired renal or hepatic function, convulsive disorders, history of alcoholism or drug abuse, patients with suicidal tendencies.

ADVERSE REACTIONS

CNS: drowsiness and ataxia (most frequent), dizziness, vertigo, slurred speech, headache, weakness, paresthesias, impaired visual accommodation, euphoria, paradoxic excitement, rapid EEG activity. **Allergy or idiosyncrasy:** itchy, urticarial, or erythematous maculapapular rash; exfoliative dermatitis; petechiae; purpura; ecchymoses; eosinophilia; peripheral edema; angioneurotic edema; adenopathy; fever; chills; proctitis; stomatitis; bronchospasm; oliguria; anuria; Stevens-Johnson syndrome; anaphylaxis. **Hematologic** (rare): leukopenia, agranulocytosis, aplastic anemia, thrombocytopenic purpura, erythroid hypoplasia, pancytopenia. **Cardiovascular:** hypotension, syncope, palpitation,

tachycardia, arrhythmias, transient ECG changes. **Other reported:** nausea, **431**
vomiting, diarrhea, exacerbation of porphyria, grand mal attack (patients with
epilepsy), respiratory depression and circulatory collapse (toxic doses), pain and
irritation at injection site, decreased radioactive iodine uptake.

ROUTE AND DOSAGE
Adults: Oral: 400 mg 3 or 4 times daily. Doses greater than 2400 mg/day not
recommended. Intramuscular: 400 mg every 3 or 4 hours (for tetanus). **Children**
6 to 12 years: Oral: 25 mg/kg daily divided into 2 or 3 doses. Intramuscular: 50
to 70 mg/kg/day in 6 to 8 divided doses (for tetanus).

NURSING IMPLICATIONS
Carefully aspirate before injecting IM; solution contains propylene glycol,
which if injected IV may cause thrombosis and hemolysis. Rotate injection sites.
Elderly patients are prone to drowsiness and hypotensive effects of meprobamate, particularly during early therapy. Generally, lower doses are prescribed and dosage increases are made gradually.
Caution patients to make position changes slowly, especially from recumbent to upright, and to dangle legs for a few minutes before standing.
Supervise ambulation, during early therapy particularly.
Hypnotic doses may cause increased motor activity during sleep. Bedsides
are advisable.
Drug therapy for relief of anxiety and neurosis is not a substitute for sympathetic understanding and investment of time exploring the patient's concerns and problems.
Warn patients that tolerance to alcohol will be lowered. Since meprobamate
may impair mental and physical abilities, caution patients to avoid driving
a car or engaging in other hazardous activities until their reactions have
been determined.
Periodic blood cell counts and liver function tests are advised in patients
receiving high doses.
Patients should be instructed to report immediately the onset of sore throat,
fever, early bruising, bleeding. All are possible indicators of hemolytic
toxicity.
Tolerance and psychologic and physical dependence may occur with long-
term use of high doses. Dosage of drug prescribed should be carefully
supervised, and prolonged use should be avoided.
Sudden withdrawal in physically dependent patients may precipitate preexisting anxiety and neuroses and withdrawal symptoms within 12 to 48
hours: vomiting, ataxia, muscle twitching, confusion, hallucinations, delirium, coma, convulsions (symptoms usually subside within 12 to 48
hours).
Treatment of meprobamate physical dependence consists of gradual drug
withdrawal over 1 to 2 weeks.
Treatment of overdosage: removal of drug from stomach (emesis or lavage),
administration of activated charcoal, general supportive measures, careful
monitoring of urinary output and fluid intake.
Classified as schedule IV drug under federal Controlled Substances Act.

LABORATORY TEST INTERFERENCES: There is the possibility that meprobamate may cause falsely high urinary steroid determinations.

DRUG INTERACTIONS: Possibility of additive CNS depressant effects with
concurrent use of meprobamate and **alcohol** and other **CNS depressants** and
imipramine and other **psychotropic drugs.**

Diuretic (mercurial)

ACTIONS AND USES

Organic mercurial complexed with thioglycolate, which improves absorption from injection site and slows release of mercuric ions, thereby helping to reduce risk of nephrotoxicity and cardiotoxicity. Each milliliter contains approximately 40 mg mercury and 0.1 mg edetate disodium. In therapeutic doses, liberated mercury ions depress tubular reabsorption of sodium and chloride and secondarily increase excretion of water devoid of bicarbonate. Excretion of chloride in excess of sodium may produce hypochloremic alkalosis, rendering mercurials ineffective. To provide the required acid pH at the tubular site of action, an acidifier salt such as ammonium chloride is often administered a few days prior to or concomitantly with the mercurial agent. May increase excretion of potassium, but to a lesser degree than that produced by thiazides.

Usually reserved for use in patients resistant to other diuretics for treatment of edema secondary to congestive heart failure, nephrotic syndrome, nephrotic stage of glomerulonephritis, and hepatic cirrhosis or portal obstruction.

ABSORPTION AND FATE

Rapidly and completely absorbed following parenteral injection. Diuretic response usually occurs in 1 to 3 hours, peaks in 5 to 9 hours, and lasts 12 to 24 hours. Extensively bound to plasma proteins. Localizes primarily in renal cortex; also distributed to tissue cells and liver. Metabolized mainly by kidneys. Rapidly excreted, primarily in urine (95%); small quantities (up to 5%) excreted in feces.

CONTRAINDICATIONS AND PRECAUTIONS

Hypersensitivity to mercury or other ingredients, severe renal insufficiency, acute and subacute nephritis, ulcerative colitis, dehydration, malignant hypertension. Safe use in women of childbearing potential and during pregnancy or lactation not established. Cautious use: BUN above 60 mg/dl, myocardial infarction, cardiac arrhythmias, hepatic insufficiency, gout, patients receiving digitalis glycosides, and elderly patients.

ADVERSE REACTIONS

Fluid and electrolyte imbalance: hyponatremia, hypochloremic alkalosis, hypokalemia, hypomagnesemia, hypovolemia, dehydration. **Hypersensitivity:** flushing, pruritus, cutaneous lesions (may become exfoliative), nausea, vomiting, fever, chills, vertigo, anaphylactic reactions (respiratory distress, cardiac irregularities, sudden hypotension). **Hematologic:** thrombocytopenia, neutropenia, leukopenia, agranulocytosis. **Mercurialism:** stomatitis, sore gums, excessive salivation, metallic taste, foul breath, gastritis, vomiting, diarrhea, colitis, diuresis, shock, renal damage. **Other:** hyperuricemia; headache; acute urinary retention; local pain and tenderness at IM site; pain, ecchymoses, nodule formation, and (rarely) sloughing at subcutaneous site. Inadvertent IV or intraarterial injection: severe cardiac irregularities, sudden death.

ROUTE AND DOSAGE

Subcutaneous, intramuscular: 0.2 to 2 ml (25 to 250 mg) daily, or once or twice weekly administered at intervals that best maintain "dry" (normal) weight. Test dose: 0.5 ml (62.5 mg) injected 24 hours before initiation of therapy.

NURSING IMPLICATIONS

Explain to the patient that the drug will increase voiding amounts. Have urinal or bedpan and call light readily available.

Since hypersensitivity reactions commonly occur with mercurial diuretics, a test dose is recommended.

If possible, administer drug early in the morning so that sleep will not be interrupted by diuresis.

Generally well tolerated by subcutaneous route when properly administered. Avoid edematous areas, adipose tissue, and areas of poor circulation. Rotate injection sites, and observe daily.

The IM route may be better tolerated by obese patients, emaciated patients, and those with skin susceptible to trauma.

Preferred IM site for mercurials is upper outer quadrant of gluteus maximus. Insert needle deep into muscle mass. Draw back plunger to make sure needle is not in blood vessel (see Adverse Reactions). Follow administration by gentle massage of injection site.

Monitor intake and output. Report lack of diuretic response, excessive diuresis, and oliguria. In some patients a urine output of 8 to 9 liters may be produced following initial effective dose.

Weigh patients daily under standard conditions. Loss of 2.5% body weight (approximately 2 to 4 lb) is an average diuretic response.

Monitor vital signs. Too rapid or prolonged diuresis may induce dehydration. Resultant hypovolemia can lead to hypotensive episodes, vascular thromboses, and emboli; these are most likely to occur in the elderly, in patients with chronic cardiac disease on prolonged salt restriction, and in patients receiving sympatholytic (adrenergic blocking) agents.

Measurements of abdominal girth, if ordered, should be taken at the same time each morning with the patient in the same position.

In patients with congestive heart failure, note and record the effect of therapy on dyspnea, orthopnea, moist rales in lung bases, and edema.

Serum electrolyte levels (sodium, potassium, chloride, magnesium), CO_2, and BUN determinations, and urine examinations for albumin, casts, blood, and specific gravity should be monitored in patients receiving repeated doses.

Observe for and instruct the patient to report signs and symptoms of electrolyte imbalance: weakness, fatigue, lassitude, faintness, confusion, muscle cramps, hyporeflexia, headache, paresthesias, thirst, anorexia, nausea, vomiting, abdominal discomfort.

Dietary sodium intake should be reduced, but not severely restricted; consult physician. Excessively low salt intake (especially in hot weather) may produce hypochloremic alkalosis with resultant drug refractoriness.

Daily ingestion of potassium-rich foods (citrus fruit, banana, dried dates, peaches) may reduce or prevent potassium depletion.

Diabetic patients receiving insulin or oral hypoglycemics should be observed for possible loss of diabetes control (see Drug Interactions; also note Laboratory Test Interferences).

Dimercaprol is used to reverse the early toxic effects of mercurial diuretics.

Mercaptomerin should be refrigerated and protected from light. Avoid freezing. Examine solution before use; do not use if discolored or precipitated.

LABORATORY TEST INTERFERENCES: Possibility of falsely decreased PBI (with acid distillation and chloric acid methods) and false negative results for urinary glucose by glucose oxidase methods (ie, Clinistix, Tes-Tape).

DRUG INTERACTIONS: There is risk of fatal ventricular fibrillation if **epinephrine** is given to patients receiving high doses of mercurial diuretics. Concomitant administration of mercaptomerin with **chlorothiazide** or **ethacrynic acid** may result in additive diuretic effect. Diuretic-induced hypokalemia (also loss of magnesium and calcium) potentiates the cardiotoxicity of **digitalis glycosides;** hypokalemia interferes with the hypoglycemic effect of **insulin** and **oral hypoglycemics;** loss of sodium and potassium may increase the possibility of **lithium** toxicity. Uricosuria produced by mercaptomerin (rare) may interfere with the effects of **probenecid** or **sulfinpyrazone.**

MERCAPTOPURINE, U.S.P., B.P.
(6-MP, 6-MERCAPTOPURINE, PURINETHOL)

Antineoplastic (purine antagonist)

ACTIONS AND USES

Antimetabolite and purine analogue. Antagonizes purine metabolism by unclear mechanism. Blocks conversion of inosinic acid to adenine and xanthine ribotides within sensitive tumor cells. Also inhibits adenine-containing coenzymes, suggesting an influence over multiple cellular reactions. Has delayed immunosuppressive properties. One member of the POMP combination therapeutic regimen.

Used primarily for treatment of acute leukemia. Response in adults is less than in children, but mercaptopurine is initial drug of choice. In chronic granulocytic leukemia, produces temporary remission.

ABSORPTION AND FATE

Oral preparations readily absorbed without damage to intestinal mucosa. Half-life following IV route, 90 minutes. Rapid distribution to sensitive tumor cells; crosses blood–brain barrier. Partial degradation in liver with rapid excretion in urine as metabolites, including 6-thiouric acid and inorganic sulfates. Small proportion excreted for as long as 17 days.

CONTRAINDICATIONS AND PRECAUTIONS

First trimester of pregnancy, infections. Cautious use: impaired renal or hepatic function, concomitant use with allopurinol.

ADVERSE REACTIONS

Hematologic: leukopenia, anemia, eosinophilia, pancytopenia, thrombocytopenia, abnormal bleeding, bone marrow hypoplasia. **GI:** stomatitis, esophagitis, anorexia, nausea, vomiting, diarrhea, steatorrhea (rare), intestinal ulcerations. **Other:** impaired liver function, hyperuricemia, skin rash, oliguria, renal impairment, drug fever.

ROUTE AND DOSAGE

Highly individualized. Oral: **Adults and children** *5 years of age and over:* 2.5 mg/kg/day in single or divided doses. If no clinical improvement in 4 weeks, dose is increased to 5 mg/kg/day, if tolerated. Maintenence: 2.5 to 5 mg/kg/day; usually continued during remission.

NURSING IMPLICATIONS

Start flow chart at beginning of therapy to record baseline data related to intake–output ratio and pattern and body weight. Dosage determination and clues to onset of renal dysfunction depend on accurate comparative data.

Monitor daily laboratory reports for suggested adaptations in nursing management. Blood picture may change dramatically in a short period, and counts may continue to decrease several days after drug is withdrawn.

During periods of leukopenia, protect patient from exposure to trauma, infections, or other stresses (restrict visitors and personnel who have colds).

Check vital signs daily.

Oral ulcerations are rare; those that occur resemble lesions of thrush (creamy white exudative patches on inflamed painful mucosa). Inspect buccal membranes if patient complains of discomfort. Amphotericin B or nystatin may be ordered for relief. See Index for nursing care of stomatitis.

Nausea, vomiting, and diarrhea are uncommon during drug administration, but they may signal excessive dosage, especially in adults.

In acute leukemia, mercaptopurine may be continued in spite of thrombocytopenia and bleeding. Often, bleeding stops and platelet count rises during treatment.

If thrombocytopenia develops, watch for signs of abnormal bleeding (ecchymoses, petechiae, melena, bleeding gums); report them immediately.

Jaundice signals onset of hepatic toxicity and may necessitate terminating use. Report other signs such as clay-colored stools or frothy dark urine. In some instances, jaundice appears and subsequently disappears during mercaptopurine therapy; it may persist days after drug is discontinued.

Weigh patient under standard conditions once weekly and record weight.

When allopurinol is ordered to reduce or prevent hyperuricemia (due to increased nucleoprotein breakdown), mercaptopurine dosage will be decreased by one-third or one-fourth of usual dosage.

Hyperuricemia therapy includes adequate fluid intake. Consult physician about desirable volume, particularly if patient is receiving IV infusions. Report sudden change in intake–output ratio that could suggest renal insufficiency.

Consult physician about plans for disclosure of diagnosis, prognosis, and particulars about treatment so that discussions with family and patient will be supportive and nonconflicting.

Store tablets in light- and air-resistant container.

DRUG INTERACTIONS: **Allopurinol** retards metabolism of mercaptopurine and therefore enhances antineoplastic activity and toxicity.

MESTRANOL, U.S.P., B.P.

Estrogen

ACTIONS AND USES

A 3-methoxy analogue of estrone with actions similar to those of estradiol (qv). Principal use is in combination with a progestin for contraceptive purposes. Not marketed as a single entity.

METAPROTERENOL SULFATE
(ALUPENT, METAPREL)
ORCIPRENALINE SULFATE, B.P.

Bronchodilator

ACTIONS AND USES

Potent synthetic sympathomimetic amine similar to isoproterenol in chemical structure and pharmacologic actions. Acts selectively on β_2-adrenergic receptors to relax smooth muscle of bronchi, uterus, and blood vessels supplying skeletal muscles. Reportedly has less stimulant action on β_1 receptors of heart than does isoproterenol.

Used as bronchodilator in symptomatic relief of asthma and reversible bronchospasm associated with bronchitis and emphysema. Has been used investigationally in treatment and prophylaxis of heart block and to avert progress of premature labor.

ABSORPTION AND FATE

Only 40% reaches general circulation after oral administration, due to metabolism in liver. Onset of action within 15 minutes after oral ingestion and within 1 minute following inhalation. Peak effects within 1 hour by either route; effects may persist 4 hours or more after single oral dose and 1 to 5 hours after inhalation. Excreted primarily as glucuronic acid and conjugates.

Sensitivity to other sympathomimetic agents, cardiac arrhythmias associated with tachycardia. Safe use during pregnancy and in women of childbearing potential, inhaler use in children under 12 not established. See Isoproterenol.

ADVERSE REACTIONS

Nervousness, weakness, drowsiness, tremor (particularly after oral administration), tachycardia, hypertension, palpitation, nausea, vomiting, bad taste; occasional difficulty in micturition and muscle cramps; cardiac arrest (excessive use). See Isoproterenol.

ROUTE AND DOSAGE

Oral: 20 mg 3 or 4 times daily. Inhalation (metered aerosol): 2 or 3 inhalations; usually not repeated more often than every 3 to 4 hours. Total daily dosage should not exceed 12 inhalations (each metered dose from inhaler delivers 0.65 mg of metaproterenol).

NURSING IMPLICATIONS

To administer metered aerosol dose: Instruct patient to shake container, exhale through nose as completely as possible, administer aerosol while inhaling deeply through mouth, and hold breath a few seconds before exhaling slowly. At least 2 minutes should elapse between inhalations.

Drug may have shorter duration of action after long-term use. Instruct patients to report failure to respond to usual dose.

Warn patients not to increase dose or frequency unless ordered by physician; there is the possibility of serious adverse effects.

Protect from light.

See Isoproterenol Hydrochloride.

METARAMINOL BITARTRATE, U.S.P.
(ARAMINE, PRESSONEX, PRESSOROL)
METARAMINOL TARTRATE, B.P.

Adrenergic

ACTIONS AND USES

Potent synthetic sympathomimetic amine. Overall effects similar to those of levarternol; but metaraminol is not as potent, has more gradual onset and longer duration of action, and usually lacks CNS stimulant effects. Acts directly on α-adrenergic receptors (vasoconstriction) and β_1 receptors of heart (positive inotropic effect); indirectly causes release of norepinephrine from storage sites. Tachyphylaxis may occur with prolonged use by depletion of epinephrine stores in nerve endings; in addition, metaraminol may function as weak or false neurotransmitter by replacing norepinephrine in sympathetic nerve endings, with resultant worsening of shock state. Vasoconstrictor action increases pulmonary arterial pressure, produces sustained rise in systolic and diastolic pressures, and reduces blood flow to kidneys and other vital organs and probably skin and skeletal muscles.

Used for prevention and treatment of acute hypotensive states occurring with spinal anesthesia, and as adjunct in treatment of hypotension due to hemorrhage, reaction to medication, surgical complications, brain damage, cardiogenic shock, and septicemia.

ABSORPTION AND FATE

Onset of pressor effect occurs within 1 to 2 minutes after start of IV infusion, within 10 minutes after IM injection, and in 5 to 20 minutes after subcutaneous administration. Effects last 20 to 90 minutes, depending on route of administration. Drug effects appear to be terminated primarily by uptake into tissues and urinary excretion.

Use with cyclopropane, halothane, MAO inhibitors; peripheral or mesenteric thrombosis; pulmonary edema, cardiac arrest; untreated hypoxia, hypercapnia, and acidosis; as sole therapy in hypovolemia. Safe use during pregnancy not established. Cautious use: digitalized patients, hypertension, thyroid disease, diabetes mellitus, cirrhosis of liver, history of malaria (may produce relapse).

ADVERSE REACTIONS

Apprehension, restlessness, headache, tremor, nausea, vomiting, weakness, flushing, pallor, sweating, precordial pain, palpitation, tachycardia, bradycardia, decreased urinary output, metabolic acidosis (hypovolemic patients), hyperglycemia. **Excessive dosage:** severe hypertension, headache, convulsions, acute pulmonary edema, arrhythmias, cardiac arrest. Injection site reactions (especially following subcutaneous): abscess formation, tissue necrosis, sloughing. **Prolonged use:** plasma volume depletion with recurrence of shock state.

ROUTE AND DOSAGE

Adults: Subcutaneous, intramuscular: 2 to 10 mg. At least 10 minutes should elapse before additional dose is given, to prevent cumulative effect. Intravenous (direct): *for grave emergency:* 0.5 to 5 mg. Intravenous infusion: 15 to 100 mg in 500 ml of 5% dextrose injection or sodium chloride injection. **Children:** Subcutaneous, intramuscular: 0.1 mg/kg. Intravenous (direct): 0.01 mg/kg. Intravenous infusion: 0.4 mg/kg (each 1 mg diluted in 25 ml of 5% dextrose or sodium chloride injection).

NURSING IMPLICATIONS

Except in emergency situations, blood volume should be corrected as fully as possible before therapy is initiated.

Subcutaneous injection is especially likely to cause tissue necrosis and sloughing; therefore, it is generally not prescribed.

Patients receiving drug IV must be constantly attended, with infusion flow rate being closely monitored. Changes in flow rate must be made cautiously, since the drug has cumulative effect and prolonged action.

Intravenous flow rate will be prescribed by physician (usually, systolic blood pressure is maintained at 80 to 100 mm Hg for previously normotensive patients; for previously hypertensive patients, it is maintained at 30 to 40 mm Hg below the usual pressure).

During IV infusion, check blood pressure every 5 minutes until it is stabilized at prescribed level, then every 15 minutes thereafter throughout therapy. Also note pulse rate and quality. Continue monitoring at regular intervals for several hours after infusion is complete.

When infusion is to be discontinued, flow rate should be reduced gradually, and abrupt withdrawal avoided. Equipment for reinstituting therapy should be immediately available.

Care should be taken to avoid extravasation during IV infusion. Injury to local tissue and necrosis may result.

Have on hand phentolamine (may be used to decrease pressor effects), propranolol (to treat cardiac arrhythmias), atropine (for bradycardia).

Observe intake–output ratio and pattern. Keep physician informed of renal response. Urinary output may decrease initially, then increase as blood pressure approaches normal levels. With excessive dosage, output may again decrease.

Metaraminol may cause diuresis in patients with cirrhosis of liver. Patients should be carefully monitored for excessive losses of water, sodium, and potassium.

Patients with diabetes should be closely monitored for loss of diabetes control.

Avoid exposure of drug to excessive heat, and protect it from light.

DRUG INTERACTIONS: There may be an enhanced pressor response to metaraminol in patients receiving (parenteral) **ergot alkaloids, furazolidone, guanethidine, MAO inhibitors,** or **tricyclic antidepressants.** There is the possibility that **digitalis** and **mercurial diuretics** may sensitize myocardium to the effects of metaraminol. Response to metaraminol may be altered by **reserpine** (based on limited studies). IV administration of metaraminol during use of **cyclopropane** or **halothane** or related general anesthetics may lead to serious ventricular arrhythmias.

METHACYCLINE HYDROCHLORIDE, N.F., B.P.
(RONDOMYCIN)

Antibacterial (tetracycline)

ACTIONS AND USES
    Synthetic broad-spectrum antibiotic derived from oxytetracycline. Similar to tetracycline (qv) in actions, uses, contraindications, precautions, and adverse reactions.
ABSORPTION AND FATE
    Readily but incompletely absorbed; 80% bound to plasma proteins. Half-life 16 hours. About 50% excreted unchanged in urine and about 5% in feces over 72 hours.
ROUTE AND DOSAGE
    Oral: **Adults:** 150 mg every 6 hours or 300 mg every 12 hours. **Children:** 6 to 12 mg/kg daily in 2 to 4 equally divided doses.

NURSING IMPLICATIONS
Check expiration date before administration. Outdated tetracyclines can
    cause serious reactions.
Food interferes with absorption. Administer at least 1 hour before or 2 hours
    following meals. Do not give with milk or with antacids containing aluminum, calcium, or magnesium.
Therapy should be continued for at least 24 to 48 hours after symptoms and
    fever have subsided.
Preserved in tight, light-resistant containers.
See Tetracycline Hydrochloride.

METHADONE HYDROCHLORIDE, U.S.P., B.P.
(DOLOPHINE, WESTADONE)

Narcotic analgesic

ACTIONS AND USES
    Synthetic diphenylheptane derivative with pharmacologic properties qualitatively similar to those of morphine (qv), but is orally effective and has longer duration of action. A single oral dose produces less sedation and euphoria than does morphine, but repeated doses produce marked sedation (cumulative action). Causes less constipation than morphine, but respiratory depressant effect (principal danger of overdosage) and antitussive actions are comparable. Highly addictive, with abuse potential that matches that of morphine; abstinence syndrome develops more slowly; withdrawal symptoms are less intense, but more prolonged.
    Used to relieve severe pain; used for detoxification and temporary maintenance treatment in hospital. Also used in federally controlled maintenance programs for ambulatory patients with opiate dependence.

Well absorbed from GI tract. Following single oral dose, analgesic effect occurs in 30 to 60 minutes, with duration of 6 to 8 hours; with repeated doses, effects may last 36 to 48 hours (cumulative effect). Widely distributed to tissues; about 85% firmly bound to plasma proteins. Metabolized chiefly in liver. Metabolites excreted in urine and in feces via bile; less than 10% excreted unchanged in urine. Crosses placenta and enters breast milk.

CONTRAINDICATIONS AND PRECAUTIONS

Obstetric analgesia. Safe use during pregnancy and for treatment of narcotic addiction in adolescent patients not established.

ADVERSE REACTIONS

Drowsiness, nausea, vomiting, dry mouth, constipation, lightheadedness, dizziness, transient fall in blood pressure, bone and muscle pain, hallucinations, impotence. Also see Morphine.

ROUTE AND DOSAGE

Oral, subcutaneous, intramuscular: *Relief of pain:* **Adults:** 2.5 to 10 mg; repeated, if necessary, every 3 to 4 hours. Parenteral doses larger than 10 mg not recommended. **Children:** 0.7 mg/kg/24 hours divided into 4 to 6 doses. *Detoxification treatment:* **Adults:** 15 to 40 mg; highly individualized and adjusted to keep withdrawal symptoms at a tolerable level. *Maintenance treatment:* 20 to 120 mg daily; highly individualized. Special state and federal approval required for doses in excess of 120 mg daily.

NURSING IMPLICATIONS

For analgesic effect, methadone should be administered in the smallest effective dose to minimize the possibility of tolerance and physical and psychic dependence.

IM route is preferred when repeated parenteral administration is required (subcutaneous injections may cause local irritation and induration). Aspirate carefully before injecting drug to avoid inadvertent IV administration. Rotate injection sites.

Evaluate the patient's continued need of methadone for pain. With repeated use (and because of cumulative effects), adjustment of dosage and lengthening of between-dose intervals may be possible.

Orthostatic hypotension, sweating, constipation, drowsiness, GI symptoms, and other transient side effects of therapeutic doses appear to be more prominent in ambulatory patients. Most side effects disappear over a period of several weeks.

Instruct patients to make position changes slowly, particularly from recumbent to upright position, and to sit or lie down if they feel dizzy or faint.

Patients should be informed that methadone may impair mental and physical abilities required for performance of potentially hazardous activities, such as driving a car or operating machinery.

Principal danger of overdosage, as with morphine, is extreme respiratory depression.

Due to the cumulative effects of methadone, abstinence symptoms may not appear for 36 to 72 hours after last dose and may last 10 to 14 days. Symptoms are usually of mild intensity (anorexia, insomnia, anxiety, abdominal discomfort, weakness, headache, sweating, hot and cold flashes). Purposive behavior is prominent by the sixth day.

In detoxification treatment, methadone is administered in decreasing doses, over a period not exceeding 21 days, to suppress abstinence symptoms during narcotic withdrawal. If more than 21 days of treatment are required, patient is said to be on maintenance.

Narcotic antagonists such as naloxone (preferred), nalorphine, and levallorphan terminate methadone intoxication by competing for narcotic binding sites. Since antagonist action is shorter (1 to 3 hours) than that of methadone (36 to 48 hours or more), repeated doses for 8 to 24 hours may be required. Patient should be watched closely for recurrence of respiratory depression.

Methadone maintenance consists of substituting stable doses of oral methadone to eliminate compulsive craving and euphoric effects of parenterally administered narcotics.

Maintenance treatment frequently begins with daily doses at an ambulatory clinic. Later, large take-home doses of methadone are dispensed as oral liquid (dissolved in juice to discourage parenteral injection).

Since opiate dependence is symptomatic of a wide variety of individual and social problems, methadone maintenance programs usually include coordinated psychiatric, social, and vocational rehabilitation services.

Methadone is classified as a schedule II drug under federal Controlled Substances Act. Also subject to strict regulations by Food and Drug Administration and state authorities; use for treatment of narcotic addiction is restricted to approved formal programs.

Preserved in tight, light-resistant containers.

See Morphine Sulfate.

DRUG INTERACTIONS: Methadone is used with caution and in reduced dosage in patients concurrently receiving other **CNS depressants** (including **alcohol**). Patients addicted to heroin or those who are on methadone maintenance may experience withdrawal symptoms when given **pentazocine** or **rifampin.**

METHALLENESTRIL
(VALLESTRIL)

Estrogen

ACTIONS AND USES
Synthetic estrogen with uses, actions, contraindications, and adverse reactions like those of estradiol (qv).

ROUTE AND DOSAGE
Oral: Menopause: 6 mg/day for 3 weeks, then 3 mg/day. Postpartum breast engorgement: 40 mg/day for 5 days. Postmenopausal vaginitis: 6 mg/day for 4 weeks. Prostatic carcinoma: 20 mg/day.

NURSING IMPLICATIONS
See Estradiol.

METHAMPHETAMINE HYDROCHLORIDE, U.S.P.

(Desoxyephedrine Hydrochloride, DESOXYN, FETAMIN, METHAMPEX, OBEDRIN-LA, STIMDEX)
METHYAMPHETAMINE HYDROCHLORIDE, B.P.

CNS stimulant, anorexiant

ACTIONS AND USES
Sympathomimetic amine chemically related to amphetamine and ephedrine. CNS stimulant actions (mood elevation, depression of appetite, decreased fa-

tigue) approximately equal to those of amphetamine, but accompanied by less peripheral activity. However, larger doses produce increased cardiac output, possibly reflex slowing of heart rate, and sustained increase in blood pressure, chiefly by cardiac stimulation. Excessive doses depress myocardium. Also see Amphetamine Sulfate.

Used as short-term adjunct in management of exogenous obesity, as adjunctive therapy in minimal brain dysfunction, narcolepsy, epilepsy, and postencephalitic parkinsonism, and in treatment of certain depressive reactions, especially when characterized by apathy and psychomotor retardation.

ABSORPTION AND FATE

Readily absorbed from GI tract; duration of effects 6 to 12 hours, but may continue up to 24 hours after large oral doses. From 55% to 70% of dose excreted unchanged in urine; 6% to 7% eliminated as amphetamine. Excretion is markedly increased in acid urine.

CONTRAINDICATIONS AND PRECAUTIONS

During pregnancy, especially first trimester; use as anorexiant in children under age 12; patients receiving MAO inhibitors; arteriosclerotic parkinsonism. Cautious use: even in mild hypertension; psychopathic personalities; hyperexcitability states; history of suicide; elderly or debilitated patients. Also see Amphetamine Sulfate.

ADVERSE REACTIONS

CNS (stimulation): restlessness, tremor, hyperreflexia, insomnia, headache, nervousness, anxiety, dizziness, euphoria or dysphoria. **Cardiovascular:** palpitation, arrhythmias, hypertension, hypotension, circulatory collapse. **GI:** dry mouth, unpleasant taste, nausea, vomiting, diarrhea, constipation. **Other:** psychotic episodes (rare), depression. Also see Amphetamine Sulfate.

ROUTE AND DOSAGE

Oral: **Adults:** 2.5 to 5 mg 1 to 3 times daily. Long-acting form: 10 to 15 mg once a day in the morning. Usual dose range: 2.5 to 30 mg daily. **Children:** (*minimal brain dysfunction*): initially 2.5 to 5 mg once or twice daily; may be increased by 5 mg increments until optimum response achieved. Usual effective dose: 20 to 25 mg daily.

NURSING IMPLICATIONS

If possible, medication should be taken early in the day to avoid insomnia.

When used for treatment of obesity, drug is administered 30 minutes before each meal. If insomnia results, advise patient to inform physician.

Duration of methamphetamine use in treatment of obesity should not exceed a few weeks.

Paradoxic increase in depression or agitation sometimes occurs in depressed patients. Report immediately; drug should be withdrawn.

Tolerance develops readily, and prolonged use may lead to drug dependence. High abuse potential. Commonly known as "speed" or "crystal" among drug abusers.

Withdrawal after prolonged use is frequently followed by lethargy that may persist several weeks.

Classified as schedule II drug under federal Controlled Substances Act.

Preserved in tight, light-resistant containers.

See Amphetamine Sulfate.

METHANDROSTENOLONE, N.F.
(DIANABOL)

Anabolic agent

ACTIONS AND USES
Androgenic steroid with relatively strong anabolic and weak androgenic and estrogenic activity. Actions, uses, and limitations similar to those of ethylestrenol (qv). Probably effective in osteoporosis and pituitary dwarfism. In prepubertal children, use is restricted to selected cases of severe maturational delay when growth hormone is unavailable.

ROUTE AND DOSAGE
Oral: **Adults:** initially 2.5 to 5 mg daily; in severe debilitated states 10 mg/day for up to 3 weeks; maintenance 2.5 to 5 mg daily. **Children:** up to 0.05 mg/kg body weight daily.

NURSING IMPLICATIONS
Intermittent therapy is advised. Drug is administered for no longer than 6 weeks, followed by an interval of 2 to 4 weeks before schedule is resumed.
Reportedly, methandrostenolone may lower fasting blood sugar in both diabetic and nondiabetic patients.
See Ethylestrenol.

METHANTHELINE BROMIDE, N.F.
(BANTHINE)

Anticholinergic

ACTIONS AND USES
Synthetic quaternary ammonium compound chemically related to propantheline. Peripheral effects, contraindications, precautions, and adverse reactions similar to those of atropine (qv). Differs from atropine in having a greater ratio of ganglionic blocking activity to antimuscarinic activity.
Used as adjunct in management of peptic ulcer, pylorospasm, spastic colon, pancreatitis, ureteral and bladder spasms.

ABSORPTION AND FATE
Onset of effects in 30 to 45 minutes, persisting 4 to 6 hours after oral administration. Duration of effects following IM about 2 to 4 hours. Excreted through all body fluids, but chiefly through urine and bile.

CONTRAINDICATIONS AND PRECAUTIONS
Hypersensitivity to methantheline or propantheline. See Atropine.

ADVERSE REACTIONS
Urinary retention, anhidrosis, dry mouth, constipation, mydriasis, blurred vision, dizziness, drowsiness, impotence, flushing, postural hypotension, tachycardia, palpitation, respiratory paralysis (large doses). Also see Atropine.

ROUTE AND DOSAGE
Adults: Intramuscular, intravenous: initially 50 to 100 mg 4 times daily at 6-hour intervals; maintenance generally one-half initial dose. **Children:** Oral: 6 mg/kg daily in 4 doses; (intramuscular): 3 mg/kg in 4 doses.

NURSING IMPLICATIONS
Generally administered about 10 minutes before meals or with meals and at bedtime. Advise patient not to chew oral preparation, as it is extremely bitter.

Urinary retention may be avoided by having patient void just prior to each dose.

Patients receiving parenteral therapy should be observed closely for curare-like effect on skeletal muscles, particularly respiratory depression or paralysis. Equipment for artificial respiration should be readily available.

Restlessness, euphoria, fatigue, and occasionally acute psychotic episodes occur in some patients.

Advise patient to report appearance of skin rash to physician.

Increase in fluid intake (if allowed) may help to prevent constipation.

Sugarless hard candy or gum, rinsing mouth with cool tap water, and mouth care after meals may relieve mouth dryness.

See Atropine Sulfate.

METHAPYRILENE HYDROCHLORIDE, N.F.
(DORMIN, HISTADYL, LULLAMIN, SEMIKON, SOMNI-CAPS)

Antihistaminic

ACTIONS AND USES
Ethylenediamine-type antihistamine. Analog of tripelennamine; reportedly not as potent, and produces somewhat less sedative effect. Similar to tripelennamine in actions, uses, contraindications, precautions, and adverse reactions.

ROUTE AND DOSAGE
Oral: **Adults:** 25 to 50 mg 4 or 5 times daily; estimated maximum dose 100 mg every 4 hours. **Children:** 0.88 to 1.32 mg/kg, repeated every 4 to 6 hours if needed. Subcutaneous, intramuscular: **Adults:** 20 to 40 mg repeated every 4 to 6 hours. **Children:** 0.3 to 0.6 mg/kg repeated every 4 to 6 hours. Intravenous: **Adults:** 10 to 20 mg injected slowly over 1 minute; subsequent doses may be increased to 40 mg if necessary, depending on patient's tolerance. Dose may be added to 250 mg of sterile normal saline and administered by IV drip over 30-minute interval. All dosages are highly individualized.

NURSING IMPLICATIONS
Methapyrilene may exert a relatively strong sedative effect in some individuals. Caution patients to avoid potentially hazardous activities such as driving a car or operating machinery.

In very small children methapyrilene may produce strong paradoxical excitation.

Included in several OTC preparations for insomnia in combination with scopolamine or other ingredients (eg, Compoz, Devarex, Nite Rest, Nytol, San-Man, Sominex).

Stress the importance of storing drug out of reach of children.

Preserved in tight, light-resistant containers.

See Tripelennamine Hydrochloride.

(QUAALUDE, SOPOR)
METHAQUALONE HYDROCHLORIDE, N.F.
(PAREST, SOMNAFAC)

Sedative, hypnotic

ACTIONS AND USES

Mechanism of action not known. Produces sedation and hypnosis without analgesia. CNS depressant effects similar to those of barbiturates and glutethimide; in common with these drugs, it may induce liver microsomal enzymes (although to a lesser extent) and thus may alter metabolism of other drugs. In 300-mg doses, it suppresses REM (dreaming) stage of sleep. On basis of molecular weights, 87 mg of methaqualone is approximately equivalent to 100 mg of the hydrochloride.

Used for simple insomnia and for daytime sedation.

ABSORPTION AND FATE

Almost entirely absorbed from GI tract in 2 hours (absorption of the hydrochloride is reported to be somewhat faster). Hypnotic effect in 10 to 20 minutes, persisting 6 to 8 hours. Extensive tissue localization, particularly in adipose tissue. Metabolized in liver and excreted in urine, bile, and feces. About 2% excreted unchanged in urine.

CONTRAINDICATIONS AND PRECAUTIONS

Known hypersensitivity to methaqualone; use during pregnancy, in women of childbearing potential, and in children. Cautious use: impaired hepatic function, history of porphyria, mental depression, suicidal tendencies, drug abuse, or drug experimentation.

ADVERSE REACTIONS

Neuropsychiatric: headache, fatigue, dizziness, torpor, transient paresthesias, restlessness, anxiety, hangover. **GI:** dry mouth, cheilosis, nausea, vomiting, epigastric discomfort, diarrhea, anorexia. **Dermatologic:** diaphoresis, foul-smelling perspiration (bromhidrosis), urticaria, skin eruptions. **Other:** necrotizing cystitis, aplastic anemia (rare), sensory and motor neuropathy of hands and feet (rare). **Acute toxicity:** delirium, tachycardia, pupillary dilation, pyramidal signs (hypertonia, hyperreflexia, myoclonus, convulsions), nasal and gastric bleeding, spontaneous vomiting with aspiration, pulmonary and cutaneous edema, shock, respiratory depression, coma, hepatic damage, renal insufficiency.

ROUTE AND DOSAGE

Oral: (*sedative*): 75 mg 3 or 4 times a day; (*hypnotic*): 150 to 300 mg at bedtime.

NURSING IMPLICATIONS

Prepare the patient for sleep before administering hypnotic dose. Drowsiness usually occurs in 10 to 20 minutes. In some patients, anxiety and restlessness occur instead of sedation or sleep. Bedsides may be advisable.

Explain to patients that tingling and numbness of extremities may be experienced prior to onset of hypnotic effect.

Smallest effective dosage should be given. Keep physician informed of patient's response to the drug and continued need of drug.

Because the potential for tolerance and both physical and psychologic dependence is high, it is recommended that methaqualone not be taken for periods longer than 3 months.

Pattern of insomnia and possible reasons why patient cannot sleep should be explored and ways suggested to promote relaxation, eg, warm bath; control of room temperature, humidity, and ventilation; soft music.

Patients who are changed from barbiturates or other sedative hypnotics may not experience a satisfactory hypnotic effect before 5 to 7 consecutive nights of methaqualone administration.

Sudden discontinuation of methaqualone in physically dependent patients may produce severe withdrawal symptoms: nausea, vomiting, abdominal cramps, anorexia, tremulousness, anxiety, headache, insomnia, confusion, weakness, diaphoresis, hallucinations, convulsions.

To treat physical dependence, a stabilizing dose of methaqualone is established; drug dosage is then gradually reduced over period of days or weeks. Patients require close monitoring, preferably in hospital.

REM rebound (marked increase in dreaming and nightmares) and insomnia may occur following drug withdrawal.

Since even sedative doses may produce drowsiness, excessive sedation, and dizziness, warn patients to avoid driving a car or engaging in other potentially hazardous activities.

Caution patient that alcohol, barbiturates, or other CNS depressants have additive effects and therefore should not be taken without the consent of the physician.

Stress the importance of keeping the drug out of reach of children.

Treatment of overdosage: evacuation of gastric contents, maintenance of blood pressure and respiration, and other supportive measures. Analeptics are contraindicated. Prolonged convulsions may require administration of succinylcholine or tubocurarine. Dialysis may be helpful.

Classified as schedule II drug under federal Controlled Substances Act.

Protect drug from light.

METHARBITAL, N.F.
(GEMONIL, METHARBITONE)

Anticonvulsant

ACTIONS AND USES
Long-acting barbiturate derivative with greater sedative effect and less antiepileptic activity than phenobarbital. Actions, contraindications, precautions, and uses as for phenobarbital (qv).

Used alone or in combination with other antiepileptic drugs for control of grand mal, petit mal, myoclonic, and mixed-type seizures.

ABSORPTION AND FATE
Onset of action in 2 to 4 hours; duration 6 to 12 hours. Demethylated in liver to barbital, which is then excreted in urine; less than 2% of dose is excreted unchanged.

ADVERSE REACTIONS
Usually infrequent and mild: drowsiness, dizziness, increased irritability, skin rash, gastric distress. See Phenobarbital.

ROUTE AND DOSAGE
Oral: **Adults:** initially 100 mg 1 to 3 times daily; gradually increased to level required to control seizures; usual dose range 100 to 800 mg daily. **Children:** 5 to 15 mg/kg/day.

NURSING IMPLICATIONS
Not to be confused with mephobarbital.

Abrupt discontinuation of drug in patients taking regular daily doses may precipitate status epilepticus.

Classified as schedule II drug under federal Controlled Substances Act.

See Phenobarbital.

(NEPTAZANE)

Carbonic anhydrase inhibitor

ACTIONS AND USES
Nonbactericidal sulfonamide derivative similar to acetazolamide, but with slower onset and longer duration of action. Appears to cause more drowsiness and fatigue than does acetazolamide, and has less diuretic activity. Actions, contraindications, precautions, and adverse reactions as for acetazolamide (qv). Used as adjunctive treatment in chronic simple (open-angle) glaucoma and secondary glaucoma and preoperatively in acute-angle-closure glaucoma when delay of surgery is desired in order to lower intraocular pressure. May be used concomitantly with miotic and osmotic agents.

ABSORPTION AND FATE
Intraocular pressure begins to fall within 2 to 4 hours; duration of action 6 to 12 hours or more. Distributed in plasma, erythrocytes, aqueous humor, extracellular and cerebrospinal fluids, and bile. Partially metabolized in liver. About 20% to 30% of dose is excreted in urine as active substance; fate of remainder not known. Crosses placenta.

CONTRAINDICATIONS AND PRECAUTIONS
Glaucoma due to severe peripheral anterior synechiae, severe or absolute glaucoma, hemorrhagic glaucoma. Also see Acetazolamide.

ADVERSE REACTIONS
Malaise, drowsiness, fatigue, mild GI disturbance, headache, vertigo, paresthesias, mental confusion, depression. Also see Acetazolamide.

ROUTE AND DOSAGE
Oral: 50 to 100 mg 2 or 3 times daily.

NURSING IMPLICATIONS
See Acetazolamide.

METHENAMINE HIPPURATE
(HIPREX, UREX)

Urinary antibacterial

ACTIONS AND USES
Chemical combination of methenamine (44%) and hippuric acid (56%). Antibacterial action depends on formaldehyde, which is liberated from methenamine in acidic urine; hippuric acid contributes to urinary acidification and also provides weak antibacterial action. See Methenamine Mandelate for actions, uses, contraindications, precautions.

ABSORPTION AND FATE
Over 90% of single dose is excreted in urine within 24 hours. See Methenamine Mandelate.

ROUTE AND DOSAGE
Oral: **Adults and children** *over 12 years:* 1 Gm twice daily (morning and night). **Children** *age 6 to 12 years:* 0.5 to 1 Gm twice daily (morning and night).

NURSING IMPLICATIONS
Elevated serum transaminase levels have been reported; therefore periodic liver function studies are recommended.
See Methenamine Mandelate.

(MANDELETS, MANDALAY, MANDELAMINE, METHAVIN,
PROV-U-SEP, RENELATE, THENDELATE)

Urinary antibacterial

ACTIONS AND USES

Chemical combination of methenamine (48%) and mandelic acid (52%). Antibacterial action depends on liberation of formaldehyde from methenamine in acidic (pH 5.5 or less) urine. Mandelic acid contributes to urine acidification and also provides weak antibacterial action. Active against a variety of Gram-negative and Gram-positive organisms, including *Escherichia coli, Staphylococcus aureus, S. albus,* and certain streptococci. Drug activity diminishes in infections caused by urea-splitting organisms such as *Pseudomonas* and *Proteus,* since they raise urinary pH.

Used for prophylactic or suppressive treatment of bacteriuria associated with chronic urinary tract infections. Sometimes used prophylactically prior to urinary tract instrumentation and catheterization.

ABSORPTION AND FATE

Readily absorbed from GI tract. Half-life approximately 4 hours. Rapidly excreted in urine by glomerular filtration and tubular secretion. In acidic urine, methenamine is hydrolyzed to ammonia and formaldehyde.

CONTRAINDICATIONS AND PRECAUTIONS

Impaired renal function, hepatic disease (because ammonia is produced), severe dehydration, combined therapy with sulfonamides. Safe use during pregnancy not established.

ADVERSE REACTIONS

Gastric upset, abdominal discomfort, dysuria, hypersensitivity (skin rash, urticaria, pruritus), tinnitus, muscle cramps. Large doses: bladder irritation, frequent and painful urination, albuminuria, hematuria, crystalluria.

ROUTE AND DOSAGE

Oral: **Adults and children** *over 12 years:* 1 Gm 4 times daily, after meals and at bedtime. **Children** *6 to 12 years:* 0.5 Gm 4 times daily; *under 6 years:* 50 mg/kg body weight divided into 3 doses.

NURSING IMPLICATIONS

Periodic urine culture and sensitivity tests should be performed.

Administration of drug after meals may minimize gastric distress.

Methenamine oral suspension (eg, Mandelamine) contains a vegetable oil base and therefore should be administered with caution to elderly or debilitated patients because of the possibility of lipid (aspiration) pneumonia.

Monitor intake and output. Methenamine is reportedly most effective when fluid intake is maintained at 1500 to 2000 ml/day and urinary pH is kept at 5.5 or below; consult physician. Increased urine volume (through increased fluid intake or diuretics) and a urinary pH over 5.5 significantly decrease the formaldehyde concentration in urine that is essential for antibacterial action.

Urinary pH should be monitored during methenamine therapy. Supplementary urinary acidification, if required, may be achieved by limiting intake of alkaline-producing foods such as vegetables, milk, peanuts, and fruits and fruit juices (except cranberry, plum, and prune, which are acid-forming) and by concomitant administration of acidifying drugs, eg, ascorbic acid, ammonium chloride.

Patients should be taught to check urine pH with Nitrazine paper to ensure consistent acidification. Some physicians instruct patients to adjust urine acidity by use of prescribed acidifying salt or diet when necessary.

LABORATORY TEST INTERFERENCES: Methenamine may produce falsely elevated values for urinary catecholamines and urinary steroids (17-hydroxycorticosteroids) (by Reddy method). Possibility of false urine glucose determinations with Benedict's test. Methenamine interferes with urine bilinogen and possibly urinary VMA determinations.

DRUG INTERACTIONS: Drugs that alkalinize urine decrease methenamine effectiveness, eg, **acetazolamide, sodium bicarbonate, thiazide diuretics.** Formaldehyde liberated from methenamine reacts with **sulfonamides** to form insoluble precipitates in urine (crystalluria).

METHENAMINE SULFOSALICYLATE
(HEXALET)

Urinary antibacterial

ACTIONS AND USES
Chemical combination of methenamine (39%) and sulfosalicylic acid (61%). Antibacterial action depends on formaldehyde, which is liberated from methenamine in acidic urine; sulfosalicylic acid contributes to urinary acidification and also provides weak antibacterial action. See Methenamine Mandelate.
CONTRAINDICATIONS AND PRECAUTIONS
Sensitivity to salicylates. Also see Methenamine Mandelate.
ROUTE AND DOSAGE
Oral: **Adults** and **children** *over 12 years:* 1 Gm with half a glass of water 4 times daily. **Children** *6 to 12 years:* one-half the adult dose.

NURSING IMPLICATIONS
Preferably administered after meals and at bedtime to minimize gastric irritation. Advise patients to report skin rash; drug should be discontinued. See Methenamine Mandelate.

METHICILLIN SODIUM, U.S.P., B.P.
(AZAPEN, CELBENIN, STAPHCILLIN)

Antibacterial

ACTIONS AND USES
Semisynthetic salt of penicillin with antimicrobial spectrum similar to that of penicillin G; differs from the latter in its high resistance to penicillinase-producing strains of staphylococci. Not as effective as penicillin G against non-penicillinase-producing staphylococci, streptococci, or pneumococci. A growing number of methicillin-resistant strains are reported to be developing.
Used primarily in infections caused by penicillinase-producing staphylococci. May be used to initiate therapy in suspected staphylococcal infections pending results of culture and sensitivity tests.
ABSORPTION AND FATE
Peak plasma concentrations within 30 minutes to 1 hour following IM injection and within 15 minutes after IV injection; serum levels decline within 4 hours after IM and within 2 hours after IV administration. Well distributed in various body tissues and fluids. Little diffusion to cerebrospinal fluid unless meninges are inflamed. About 40% bound to plasma proteins. Approximately two-thirds of 1-Gm dose is eliminated unchanged in urine in 4 hours; 20% or more excreted

in feces via bile (rate of elimination is extremely slow in infants). Crosses placenta.

CONTRAINDICATIONS AND PRECAUTIONS

Hypersensitivity to penicillins or cephalosporins; IV use in infants and children. Safe use during pregnancy not established. Cautious use: history of allergy, asthma, impaired renal function. See Penicillin G Potassium.

ADVERSE REACTIONS

Hypersensitivity reactions: skin rash, pruritus, urticaria, eosinophilia, serum sickness, anaphylactic reaction, interstitial nephritis. Also reported: bone marrow depression (anemia, neutropenia, granulocytopenia, agranulocytosis), neuropathy, irritation at IM site, thrombophlebitis (following IV administration), oral and rectal monilial superinfections. See Penicillin G Potassium.

ROUTE AND DOSAGE

Intramuscular: **Adults:** 1 Gm every 4 to 6 hours. **Children:** 25 mg/kg every 6 hours. Intravenous: **Adults** only: 1 Gm every 6 hours.

NURSING IMPLICATIONS

Culture and sensitivity tests should be performed initially and periodically during therapy.

A careful history must be obtained concerning previous hypersensitivity reactions to penicillins, cephalosporins, or any other allergens.

Reportedly well tolerated by deep intragluteal injection, although it may be painful. Rotate injection sites.

Periodic assessments of renal, hematopoietic, and hepatic function are advised during prolonged therapy.

Observe all injection sites for evidence of irritation or inflammation.

Frequent blood level measurements are advised in infants, since urinary excretion of drug is slower in this age group.

Febrile reactions are reported to occur in some patients 1 to 2 hours following IV administration.

Monitor patients for signs and symptoms of interstitial nephritis a hypersensitivity reaction that occurs 2 to 4 weeks following initiation of therapy: spiking fever, anorexia, skin rash, oliguria, hematuria, cloudy urine (pyuria, albuminuria), eosinophilia. Usually reversible following prompt termination of drug.

Drug therapy is generally continued at least 48 hours, or in the case of serious systemic infections, for at least 1 to 2 weeks after patient has become afebrile and asymptomatic and cultures are negative. Treatment of osteomyelitis may require several weeks of intensive therapy.

Methicillin is reconstituted with sterile water for injection or sodium chloride injection. Shake vial vigorously before withdrawing contents.

Reconstituted methicillin solutions are stable for 24 hours at room temperature and for 4 days under refrigeration. Most solutions for IV use are stable for 8 hours at room temperature (see manufacturer's literature).

Methicillin is reported to be incompatible with many drugs; therefore, do not mix it with other drugs, including other antibiotics. Use only solutions recommended by manufacturer.

(TAPAZOLE)

Thyroid inhibitor

ACTIONS AND USES

Thioamide with actions and uses similar to those of propylthiouracil, but 10 times as potent. Actions are less consistent, but effects appear more promptly than those of propylthiouracil. For absorption, fate, contraindications, and adverse reactions, see Propylthiouracil.

Used frequently to treat hyperthyroidism in pregnancy adjunctively with thyroid to prevent hypothyroidism in fetus and mother.

ROUTE AND DOSAGE

Oral: **Adults:** initially 15 to 60 mg daily every 8 hours; maintenance 5 to 15 mg daily. **Children:** initially 0.4 mg/kg body weight daily divided into 3 doses and given at 8 hour intervals; maintenance approximately half initial dose.

NURSING IMPLICATIONS

Dosage may be suspended about 2 weeks before anticipated delivery and restored in postpartum period if required.

Skin rash, a frequent adverse reaction, indicates need to discontinue drug and change to another antithyroid agent.

Stored in light-resistant containers.

Also see Propylthiouracil.

METHOCARBAMOL, N.F.
(ROBAXIN, ROMETHOCARB, METHO-500)

Skeletal muscle relaxant

ACTIONS AND USES

Propanediol-derivative monocarbamate with actions similar to those of carisoprodol, but it produces higher plasma levels more rapidly and for longer periods. Exerts skeletal muscle relaxant action by depressing multisynaptic pathways in spinal cord and possibly by sedative effect. Has no direct action on skeletal muscles.

Used as adjunct to physical therapy and other measures in management of discomfort associated with acute musculoskeletal disorders. Also used intravenously as adjunct in management of neuromuscular manifestations of tetanus.

ABSORPTION AND FATE

Rapidly absorbed following oral administration, with peak plasma concentrations after about 1 hour, duration of action about 24 hours. Muscle relaxant effects usually apparent within 10 minutes after IV injection. Metabolized in liver. Excreted in urine.

CONTRAINDICATIONS AND PRECAUTIONS

Hypersensitivity to any of the ingredients; acidosis; renal dysfunction (injectable methocarbamol contains polyethylene glycol 300 in vehicle, which may aggravate acidotic renal problems). Safe use during pregnancy and lactation and in women of childbearing potential and children under age 12 (except for tetanus) not established. Cautious use: epilepsy.

ADVERSE REACTIONS

Oral use: drowsiness, dizziness, lightheadedness, syncope (rare), headache, nausea. **Allergic manifestations** (parenteral or oral use): urticaria, pruritus, rash, conjunctivitis, nasal congestion, headache, blurred vision, fever, anaphylactic reaction. **Parenteral use:** thrombophlebitis, pain, sloughing (with ex-

travasation), flushing, metallic taste, nausea, nystagmus, diplopia, muscle **451**
spasms, muscle incoordination, vertigo, weakness, syncope, hypotension,
bradycardia, convulsions. **Other:** slight reduction of white cell count with prolonged therapy.

ROUTE AND DOSAGE

Adults: Oral: initially 1.5 Gm 4 times daily; maintenance 1 Gm 4 times daily,
or 750 mg every 4 hours, or 1.5 Gm 3 times daily. Intramuscular: 0.5 to 1 Gm
(5 to 10 ml) repeated at 8-hour intervals, if necessary. Intravenous: 1 to 3 Gm.
Maximum rate (direct) IV is 300 mg (3 ml) per minute. Intravenous infusion:
1 Gm diluted to not more than 250 ml with sodium chloride injection or 5%
dextrose injection. Parenteral doses not to exceed 3 Gm/day or to be given for
more than 3 consecutive days, except in treatment of tetanus. *Tetanus:* **Adults:**
initially 1 to 2 Gm (10 to 20 ml) administered directly into tubing of previously
inserted indwelling needle; up to 3 Gm may be given. May be repeated every
6 hours until nasogastric tube insertion is possible. Via nasogastric tube: total
daily dose up to 24 Gm (tablets should be crushed and suspended in water or
saline). **Children:** initially 15 mg/kg repeated every 6 hours as indicated.

NURSING IMPLICATIONS

Patient should be recumbent during and for at least 15 minutes following IV
injection in order to reduce the possibility of orthostatic hypotension and
other adverse reactions. Monitor vital signs and IV flow rate.

Supervise ambulation following parenteral administration. Advise patient to
make position changes slowly, particularly from recumbent to upright
position, and to dangle legs before standing.

Care should be taken to avoid extravasation of IV solution, which may result
in thrombophlebitis and sloughing.

IM dose should not exceed 5 ml (0.5 Gm) into each gluteal region. Insert
needle deep, and carefully withdraw plunger to make sure needle is not
in blood vessel. Inject drug slowly. Rotate injection sites, and observe
daily for evidence of irritation.

Oral administration should replace parenteral use as soon as feasible. Keep
physician informed of patient's response to therapy.

Adverse reactions following oral administration are usually mild and transient and subside with dosage reduction. Caution patients regarding
drowsiness and dizziness. Advise against activities requiring mental alertness and physical coordination until response to drug action is known.

Periodic WBC counts are advised during prolonged therapy.

Urine may darken to brown, black, or green on standing.

LABORATORY TEST INTERFERENCES: Methocarbamol may cause false increases in urinary 5-HIAA (with nitrosonaphthol reagent) and VMA (Gitlow
method).

DRUG INTERACTIONS: Inform patients that concurrent ingestion of methocarbamol and **alcohol** produces enhanced CNS depression (drowsiness and impaired judgment and coordination).

(BREVITAL SODIUM)
METHOHEXITONE INJECTION, B.P.

Anesthetic (intravenous)

ACTIONS AND USES

Rapid, ultra-short-acting barbiturate anesthetic agent. More potent than thiopental (qv), but has less cumulative effect and shorter duration of action, and recovery is more rapid. Abnormal muscle movements, coughing, sneezing, and laryngospasm reportedly occur more frequently than with thiopental.

Used for induction of anesthesia, as supplement for other anesthetics, and as general anesthetic for brief operative procedures.

ROUTE AND DOSAGE

Intravenous (induction): 5 to 12 ml of a 1% solution (50 to 120 mg) at rate of 1 ml every 5 seconds; (maintenance): 2 to 4 ml (20 to 40 mg) every 4 to 7 minutes as required. Continuous drip (0.2% solution): flow rate 1 drop per second.

NURSING IMPLICATIONS

Fall in blood pressure may occur in susceptible patients receiving drug in upright position.

Hiccups are not uncommon, particularly with rapid injection; they sometimes persist after anesthesia.

Facilities for assisting respiration and administration of oxygen should be readily available.

Stable in sterile water for injection at room temperature for at least 6 weeks. Solutions prepared with isotonic sodium chloride injection or 5% dextrose injection are stable for about 24 hours. Only clear, colorless solutions should be used.

See Thiopental Sodium.

METHOTREXATE, U.S.P., B.P.
(Amethopterin, MTX)
METHOTREXATE SODIUM

Antineoplastic, folic acid antagonist

ACTIONS AND USES

Antimetabolite and folic acid antagonist. Blocks folinic acid (active principle of folic acid) participation in nucleic acid synthesis, thereby interfering with mitotic process. Highly toxic to rapidly proliferating cells; some evidence of toxicity usually accompanies therapeutic response. Induces remission slowly; use often preceded by other antineoplastic therapies.

Used principally in combination regimens to maintain induced remissions. One member of the CMFOP, COMA, POMP combination chemotherapeutic regimens. Effective in treatment of gestational choriocarcinoma and hydatidiform mole and as immunosuppressant in kidney transplantation, for acute and subacute leukemias and leukemic meningitis, especially in children. Also used in lymphosarcoma, in certain inoperable tumors of head, neck, and pelvis, and in mycosis fungoides. Investigational use in therapy of severe psoriasis nonresponsive to other forms of therapy, SLE, and rheumatoid arthritis.

ABSORPTION AND FATE

Rapidly absorbed from GI tract; peak serum levels 1 to 4 hours after oral administration and one-half to 2 hours after parenteral administration. Serum half-life 2 to 4 hours after IM and oral administration; approximately one-half of drug is bound to serum proteins. Wide distribution, with highest concentrations in kidneys, gallbladder, spleen, liver, skin. Unchanged drug is retained several weeks in impaired kidneys, several months in the liver, and about 6 days in cerebrospinal fluid following intrathecal injection. Up to 90% of drug is cleared by kidneys; small amounts also excreted in stools through enterohepatic route. Crosses placenta; minimal passage across blood–brain barrier.

CONTRAINDICATIONS AND PRECAUTIONS

Pregnancy, hepatic and renal insufficiency, men and women in childbearing age, concomitant administration of hepatotoxic drugs and hematopoietic depressants, alcohol; preexisting blood dyscrasias. Cautious use: infections, peptic ulcer, ulcerative colitis, very young or old patients, cancer patients with preexisting bone marrow impairment, poor nutritional status.

ADVERSE REACTIONS

Dose-related and reversible. **GI:** hepatotoxicity, GI ulcerations and hemorrhage, ulcerative stomatitis, glossitis, gingivitis, pharyngitis, nausea, vomiting, diarrhea. **Hematologic:** marked myelosuppression, aplastic bone marrow, telangiectasis, thrombophlebitis at intraarterial catheter site, hyperuricemia. **Dermatologic:** erythematous rashes, pruritus, urticaria, folliculitis, vasculitis, photosensitivity, depigmentation, hyperpigmentation, alopecia. **Urogenital:** defective oogenesis or spermatogenesis, nephropathy. **Neurologic:** headache, drowsiness, blurred vision, dizziness, aphasia, hemiparesis, convulsions (after intrathecal administration), mental confusion, tremors, ataxia, coma. **Other:** malaise, undue fatigue, systemic toxicity (after intrathecal and intraarterial administration), chills, fever, decreased resistance to infection, septicemia, osteoporosis, metabolic changes precipitating diabetes and sudden death, pneumonitis.

ROUTE AND DOSAGE

Oral, intramuscular, intravenous, intraarterial, intrathecal: dosage individualized according to disease being treated, concurrent drug therapy, response, and tolerance of patient.

NURSING IMPLICATIONS

Avoid skin exposure and inhalation of drug particles.

Oral preparations should be given 1 to 2 hours before or 2 to 3 hours after meals.

Preserve drug in tight, light-resistant container.

Hepatic and renal function tests, blood tests (including blood type and group, bleeding time, coagulation time) and chest x-rays should be part of the health data base in case of emergency surgery or need for transfusion during therapy. Tests are repeated at weekly intervals during methotrexate therapy.

Hepatic function tests may be abnormal 1 to 3 days after methotrexate administration, and GI symptoms may be absent.

Monitor all laboratory reports daily as indicators for adaptations in nursing and drug regimens.

Patient should be fully informed of dangers of this drug and warned to report promptly any abnormal symptoms.

Alcohol ingestion increases the incidence and severity of methotrexate hepatotoxicity.

Leucovorin calcium (citrovorin factor) given a few hours after methotrexate protects normal tissues from lethal effects of the drug (leucovorin "rescue").

If an overdosage of methotrexate is given, leucovorin may be employed as antidote (must be given within 4 hours of overdosage).

Prolonged treatment with small frequent doses may lead to hepatotoxicity, which is best diagnosed by liver biopsy.

Ulcerative stomatitis with glossitis and gingivitis, often the first signs of toxicity, necessitate interruption of therapy or dosage adjustment. Inspect mouth daily; report patchy necrotic areas, bleeding and discomfort, or overgrowth (black, furry tongue).

Fastidious mouth care prevents infection, provides comfort, and is essential to maintenance of adequate nutritional status. See Index for nursing care of stomatitis.

In presence of hyperuricemia, patient may be kept well hydrated (urinary output about 2000 ml/24 hours) to dilute hyperuric fluids and given allopurinol to prevent urate deposition.

Monitor intake–output ratio and pattern. Severe nephrotoxicity (hematuria, dysuria, azotemia, oliguria) fosters drug accumulation and renal damage and requires dosage adjustment or discontinuation.

During leukopenic periods, prevent patient exposure to personnel and visitors with infections or colds. Be alert to onset of agranulocytosis (cough, extreme fatigue, sore throat, chills, fever), and report symptoms promptly. Methotrexate therapy will be interrupted and appropriate antibiotic drugs prescribed.

Be alert for and report symptoms of thrombocytopenia: ecchymoses, petechiae, epistaxis, melena, hematuria, vaginal bleeding, slow and protracted oozing following trauma.

Alopecia is reversible; hair regrowth begins after drug discontinuation, but it may require several months.

Methotrexate may precipitate gouty arthritis. Instruct the patient to report joint pains to physician.

Bloody diarrhea necessitates interruption of therapy to prevent perforation or hemorrhagic enteritis. Report to physician.

Warn patient not to self-medicate with vitamins. Some over-the-counter compounds may include folic acid (or its derivatives), which alters methotrexate response.

Diabetes may be precipitated; therefore, tests for glucosuria should be performed periodically, and significant symptoms such as polydipsia and polyuria should be reported.

Burning and erythema may occur in psoriatic areas after each dose of methotrexate.

Concomitant exposure to ultraviolet light may aggravate psoriatic lesions in patients on methotrexate therapy.

Deaths have been reported with use of this agent in the treatment of psoriasis.

Consult physician about plans for disclosure of diagnosis, prognosis, and treatment so that discussions with patient and family will be supportive and nonconflicting.

DRUG INTERACTIONS: **Salicylates, sulfonamides, phenytoin (diphenyl-hydantoin), tetracycline, chloramphenicol,** and **PABA** displace methotrexate from plasma protein binding, causing increased toxicity. Animal studies suggest that **probenecid** increases methotrexate plasma levels, with resultant increase in its toxicity. **Vitamin preparations** containing **folic acid** and derivatives may alter response to methotrexate. Hepatotoxicity caused by **alcohol** is increased by concomitant administration of methotrexate. Hypoprothrombinemia produced by **anticoagulants** is enhanced by this antineoplastic.

Analgesic

ACTIONS AND USES

Propylamino phenothiazine derivative with actions similar to those of chlor-promazine (qv). Extrapyramidal symptoms and dry mouth reportedly occur less commonly than with chlorpromazine, but orthostatic hypotension and sedation are more prominent. Raises pain threshold and may also produce amnesia. Analgesic effect comparable to that of morphine. Unlike morphine-type analgesics, psychic and physical dependence not reported with methotrimepra-zine, and it has no antitussive activity; it rarely produces respiratory depression. Used to relieve moderate to severe pain in nonambulatory patients; used for obstetric analgesia and sedation when respiratory depression is to be avoided, and as preanesthetic medication.

ABSORPTION AND FATE

Maximum analgesic effects within 20 to 40 minutes; duration about 4 hours. Enters cerebrospinal fluid. Probably metabolized in liver. Metabolites exhibit some activity, but less than parent drug. Excreted slowly in urine and feces, primarily as metabolites and about 1% as unchanged drug. Elimination in urine may continue 1 week after a single dose. Crosses placenta; small amounts may enter breast milk.

CONTRAINDICATIONS AND PRECAUTIONS

Hypersensitivity to phenothiazines; severe cardiac, renal, or hepatic disease; significant hypotension; comatose states; premature labor; children under 12 years of age; concomitant use with antihypertensive agents, including MAO inhibitors. Cautious use: elderly and debilitated patients with heart disease; history of convulsive disorders; women of childbearing potential; use during early pregnancy.

ADVERSE REACTIONS

Profound orthostatic hypotension with faintness or syncope, weakness, dizzi-ness; excessive sedation, amnesia, disorientation, euphoria, headache, slurred speech; blurred vision; nausea, vomiting, abdominal discomfort; dry mouth, nasal congestion, dysuria, tachycardia, bradycardia, palpitation; chills, hypo-tonic uterine inertia (rare); injection site reactions; elevated serum bilirubin (rare); respiratory depression (infrequent). With prolonged high dosage: in-creased weight, jaundice, severe blood dyscrasias including agranulocytosis and pancytopenia. Also see Chlorpromazine.

ROUTE AND DOSAGE

Intramuscular: 10 to 20 mg every 4 to 6 hours, if necessary. Doses may range from 5 to 40 mg at 1- to 24-hour intervals. *Elderly patients:* initially 5 to 10 mg; subsequent doses increased slowly according to patient's response.

NURSING IMPLICATIONS

Administer IM injection deep into large muscle mass (subcutaneous injection causes severe local irritation). Carefully withdraw plunger to avoid inad-vertent injection into blood vessel.

Pain at injection site and local inflammatory reaction occur commonly. Ro-tate injection sites and observe daily.

Drop in blood pressure (orthostatic hypotension), faintness, weakness, and dizziness may occur within 10 to 20 minutes after drug administration and may last 4 to 6 hours and occasionally up to 12 hours. Ambulation should be avoided or at least carefully supervised for at least 6 hours, but prefera-bly 12 hours.

Excessive sedation and amnesia also occur frequently during early drug therapy.

Tolerance to orthostatic hypotension, drowsiness, and other minor side effects usually occurs with successive doses and is generally maintained unless several days elapse between subsequent doses.

Blood pressure and pulse should be checked frequently until dosage regulation and response are stabilized. Elderly and debilitated patients require close monitoring.

Severe hypotensive effects have been treated with phenylephrine or methoxamine; levarterenol is reserved for hypotension not reversed by other vasopressors. Epinephrine is specifically contraindicated (may cause paradoxic decrease in blood pressure).

Methotrimeprazine is rarely administered beyond 30 days, except when narcotic drugs are contraindicated or in terminal illness.

When drug is used for prolonged periods, periodic blood studies and liver function tests are recommended.

Although it is not subject to narcotic controls, drug abuse is a possibility.

The manufacturer states that methotrimeprazine may be given in the same syringe with either atropine sulfate or scopolamine hydrochloride, but it should not be mixed with other drugs (dosage of atropine or scopolamine is reduced).

Protect drug from light.

DRUG INTERACTIONS: Methotrimeprazine is additive with and may potentiate **CNS depressants** (including **alcohol, general anesthetics, barbiturates, narcotics**), **anticholinergic agents** (eg, **atropine, scopolamine**), **aspirin, meprobamate** and other **tranquilizers,** other **phenothiazines,** and **skeletal muscle relaxants** (such as **succinylcholine** and **tubocurarine**). It has additive hypotensive effects with **antihypertensive agents,** including **MAO inhibitors** (concomitant use contraindicated). Methotrimeprazine reverses the vasopressor effects of **epinephrine** (concurrent use contraindicated).

METHOXAMINE HYDROCHLORIDE, U.S.P. (VASOXYL)

Adrenergic (vasopressor), antiarrhythmic

ACTIONS AND USES

Direct-acting sympathomimetic amine pharmacologically related to phenylephrine. Acts almost exclusively on α-adrenergic receptors. Pressor action is due primarily to direct peripheral vasoconstriction, which in turn causes rise in arterial blood pressure. Has no direct effect on heart, but tends to slow ventricular rate by vagal stimulation in response to elevated blood pressure. Large doses may produce bradycardia. Markedly reduces renal blood flow. Free of CNS stimulating action. True tachyphylaxis not reported.

Used for supporting, restoring, or maintaining blood pressure during anesthesia and to terminate some episodes of paroxysmal supraventricular tachycardia.

ABSORPTION AND FATE

Acts within 15 minutes following IM injection; effects may persist 1.5 hours. Acts almost immediately after IV injection and lasts about 1 hour. Widely distributed in body fluids. Excreted in urine.

CONTRAINDICATIONS AND PRECAUTIONS

Severe coronary or cardiovascular disease; in combination with local anesthetics for tissue infiltration; within 2 weeks of MAO inhibitors. Cautious use: history of hypertension or hyperthyroidism; following use of ergot alkaloids.

Paresthesias, feeling of coldness (particularly with high dosage), high blood pressure with projectile vomiting, severe headache, pilomotor erection (gooseflesh), urinary urgency, bradycardia.

ROUTE AND DOSAGE

Adults: Intramuscular: 10 to 15 mg, repeated if necessary, but not before about 15 minutes. Intravenous (emergencies): 3 to 5 mg injected slowly. **Pediatric:** Intramuscular: 0.25 mg/kg. Intravenous: one-third of IM dose (slowly).

NURSING IMPLICATIONS

Patients should be under close supervision.

Monitor vital signs. Report any increase in blood pressure above level prescribed by physician; report slowing of heart rate.

Have atropine on hand for excessive bradycardia.

Be alert for sudden changes in blood pressure and pulse after drug has been discontinued.

Monitor intake and output. Urinary frequency with retention is a possibility. Report oliguria or change in intake–output ratio.

Protect drug from light.

DRUG INTERACTIONS: There is the possibility of enhanced pharmacologic response to methoxamine in patients receiving or having recently received **guanethidine.**

METHOXYPHENAMINE HYDROCHLORIDE, N.F. (ORTHOXINE)

Adrenergic

ACTIONS AND USES

Direct-acting synthetic amine structurally and pharmacologically related to ephedrine (qv). Main sympathomimetic action is on β receptors of bronchial smooth muscles. Causes fewer cardiovascular effects than does ephedrine and has less pressor activity, but bronchodilator effect is greater and more prolonged. Has minimal CNS stimulant action and α receptor activity, and exhibits weak antihistaminic properties.

Used in treatment of bronchial asthma, acute urticaria, allergic rhinitis, GI allergy, and allergic headaches.

ABSORPTION AND FATE

Readily absorbed from GI tract. Effects appear within 30 minutes and may persist 3 to 4 hours.

CONTRAINDICATIONS AND PRECAUTIONS

History of previous adverse reactions to the drug; use within 2 weeks of MAO inhibitors. Cautious use: hypertension, hyperthyroidism, acute coronary disease, cardiac decompensation, diabetes mellitus. See Ephedrine.

ADVERSE REACTIONS

Nausea, dizziness, drowsiness, faintness, dry mouth. With high doses: palpitation, psychomotor stimulation, anxiety, wakefulness.

ROUTE AND DOSAGE

Oral: **Adults:** 50 to 100 mg every 3 to 4 hours, if necessary. **Children:** 25 to 50 mg every 4 to 6 hours, if necessary.

NURSING IMPLICATIONS
See Ephedrine Sulfate.

METHSCOPOLAMINE BROMIDE, N.F.
(Hyoscine Methylbromide, PAMINE BROMIDE, SCOLINE, Scopolamine Methylbromide)
METHSCOPOLAMINE NITRATE
(PARASPAN)

Anticholinergic

ACTIONS AND USES
Quaternary ammonium derivative of scopolamine, but lacks scopolamine's CNS actions. Its spasmolytic and antisecretory actions are quantitatively similar to those of atropine, but they last longer. Has greater selectivity in blocking vagal impulses from GI tract than either scopolamine or atropine (qv).
Used as adjunct in treatment of peptic ulcer, irritable bowel syndrome, and a variety of other GI conditions. Also may be used to control excessive sweating and salivation, migraine headaches, and premenstrual cramps.

ABSORPTION AND FATE
Erratic absorption following oral administration; effects appear in about 1 hour and persist 4 to 6 hours. Excreted primarily in urine and bile; some unchanged drug excreted in feces.

CONTRAINDICATIONS AND PRECAUTIONS
Hypersensitivity to any of the drug's constituents, prostatic hypertrophy, pyloric obstruction, tachycardia, cardiac disease. Safe use during pregnancy not established. Also see Atropine.

ADVERSE REACTIONS
Dry mouth, blurred vision, dizziness, drowsiness, constipation, flushing of skin, urinary hesitancy or retention. See Atropine.

ROUTE AND DOSAGE
Adults: Oral: 2.5 to 5 mg 3 or 4 times daily. Sustained-release form: 5 mg every 8 to 12 hours. Subcutaneous, intramuscular: 0.25 to 1 mg at 6- to 8-hour intervals. **Pediatric:** Oral: 0.2 mg/kg/24 hours, divided into 4 doses.

NURSING IMPLICATIONS
Oral preparation is usually administered 30 minutes before meals and at bedtime.
Incidence and severity of side effects are generally dose-related and therefore may be controlled by dosage reduction. Dosage is usually maintained at a level that produces slight dryness of mouth.
Patients receiving drug parenterally should be transferred to oral therapy once acute symptoms have subsided (about 24 to 48 hours).
Since methscopolamine may cause dizziness and drowsiness, warn patients not to engage in activities requiring mental alertness, such as driving a car.
Dryness of mouth may be relieved by sugarless chewing gum or candy or by rinsing mouth with water.
Preserved in tight, light-resistant containers.
See Atropine Sulfate.

DRUG INTERACTIONS: There is the theoretical possibility that concurrent use of methscopolamine and the slow-dissolving brand of **digoxin** may cause increased serum digoxin levels (decreased GI motility enhances digoxin absorption). Interaction is not likely to occur with liquid digoxin formulation or with fast-dissolving brand of digoxin.

METHSUXIMIDE, N.F.
(CELONTIN)

Anticonvulsant

ACTIONS AND USES
Succinimide derivative with actions, contraindications, precautions, and adverse reactions similar to those of ethosuximide (qv). Associated with high incidence of adverse effects.
Used for control of petit mal, psychomotor, and minor motor seizures refractory to other anticonvulsants. May be used in combination with other anticonvulsants in mixed types of epilepsy.

ABSORPTION AND FATE
Rapidly absorbed and metabolized. Peak plasma levels in 1 to 3 hours. Plasma half-life 2 to 4 hours. Not significantly bound to plasma proteins. Metabolized in liver to an active metabolite tentatively believed to be responsible for anticonvulsant action. Excreted in urine as active and inactive metabolites; less than 1% excreted unchanged.

CONTRAINDICATIONS AND PRECAUTIONS
Hypersensitivity to succinimides; drug allergies; hepatic or renal disease; blood dyscrasias. Also see Ethosuximide.

ADVERSE REACTIONS
CNS (most frequent): drowsiness, dizziness, ataxia; also headache, insomnia, diplopia, photophobia, severe mental depression, behavioral changes. **GI** (frequent): nausea, vomiting, anorexia, diarrhea, constipation, epigastric or abdominal pain, weight loss. **Hypersensitivity:** skin eruptions, fever, hiccups, periorbital edema and hyperemia, blood dyscrasias including aplastic anemia, systemic lupus erythematosus. **Other:** renal and hepatic damage. Also see Ethosuximide.

ROUTE AND DOSAGE
Oral: **Adults and children:** initially 300 mg daily for first week. If required, dosage may be increased by 300 mg at weekly intervals to maximum daily dosage of 1.2 Gm administered in divided doses. Highly individualized.

NURSING IMPLICATIONS
Drug tolerance varies among patients. Patient must be closely observed when dosage is increased or decreased, or when adding or eliminating other medication.
Advise patient to report immediately the onset of adverse effects (often controlled by dosage reduction). Development of a rash may herald more serious reactions.
Observe patient closely for behavioral changes. Drug should be withdrawn (slowly) at first appearance of depression, aggression, or other unusual behavioral manifestations in order to prevent progression to acute psychosis.
Abrupt drug withdrawal may precipitate petit mal status.
Periodic blood cell counts, tests of liver function, and urinalyses should be performed during therapy.
Since drug may cause drowsiness, dizziness, and visual disturbances, caution patients to avoid potentially hazardous activities such as driving a car.

Advise patient to carry a wallet identification card or jewelery indicating that he has epilepsy and is taking medication.

Store capsules away from heat.

METHYCLOTHIAZIDE, N.F.
(AQUATENSEN, ENDURON)

Diuretic (thiazide), antihypertensive

ACTIONS AND USES

Benzothiadiazine (thiazide) derivative. Similar to chlorothiazide in actions, uses, contraindications, precautions, and adverse reactions. Has natriuretic activity approximately 100 times that of chlorothiazide on a weight basis.

ABSORPTION AND FATE

Onset of diuretic effect occurs within 2 hours; effect peaks in about 6 hours; duration 24 hours. Excreted unchanged by kidneys. See Chlorothiazide.

ROUTE AND DOSAGE

Oral: **Adults:** 2.5 to 5 mg once daily; maximum effective single dose is 10 mg. **Children:** 0.05 to 0.2 mg/kg daily.

NURSING IMPLICATIONS

See Chlorothiazide.

METHYLCELLULOSE, U.S.P.
(CELLOTHYL, COLOGEL, HYDROLOSE, METHULOSE, VISCULOSE)

Cathartic (bulk-forming), ophthalmic lubricant

ACTIONS AND USES

Hydrophilic semisynthetic cellulose derivative. Oral preparation swells on contact with water to form a demulcent nonabsorbable gel that facilitates passage of stool and reflexly stimulates peristalsis.

Used orally as adjunct in treatment of chronic constipation. Also used in ophthalmic preparations for relief of dry eyes and eye irritation associated with deficient tear production, for corneal exposure from half-open eye during coma, and used as ocular lubricant for artificial eyes and contact lenses.

CONTRAINDICATIONS AND PRECAUTIONS

Nausea, vomiting, abdominal pain, intestinal obstruction, ulceration or stenosis, diarrhea.

ADVERSE REACTIONS

Oral form: diarrhea, nausea, vomiting, fecal impaction, esophageal obstruction.

ROUTE AND DOSAGE

Oral: 1 to 1.5 Gm 2 to 4 times a day. Ophthalmic (0.25% to 1%): 1 or 2 drops in eye 3 or 4 times daily or as needed.

NURSING IMPLICATIONS

Each oral dose should be taken with 1 or more glasses of water; additional fluids should be taken during the day. Fecal impaction can occur if fluid intake by mouth is insufficient.

Caution the patient not to chew the tablet form because it may start to swell in the esophagus and cause obstruction.

Effect generally occurs in 12 to 24 hours; however, some patients may require 2 or 3 days of medication.

Review proper bowel hygiene: adequacy of fluid and dietary intake, exercise, habit time.

Ophthalmic preparation (artificial tears) is a sterile, viscous, water-soluable, nongreasy lubricant.

Advise patient to discontinue use of ophthalmic preparation if eye discomfort or irritation occurs and to report to physician.

METHYLDOPA, U.S.P., B.P.
(α-METHYLDOPA, ALDOMET)
METHYLDOPATE HYDROCHLORIDE, U.S.P.
(ALDOMET ESTER HYDROCHLORIDE)

Antihypertensive

ACTIONS AND USES

Structurally related to catecholamines and their precursors. Exact mechanism of action unknown; metabolic product of the drug appears to act on both CNS and peripheral vasculature by displacing norepinephrine from its storage sites. Has weak neurotransmitter properties; inhibits decarboxylation of dopa, thereby reducing concentration of dopamine, a precursor of norepinephrine; also inhibits precursor of serotonin. Lowers standing and supine blood pressures, and unlike adrenergic blockers, it is not so prone to produce orthostatic hypotension, diurnal blood pressure variations, or exercise hypertension. Reduces renal vascular resistance; maintains cardiac output without acceleration, but may slow heart rate; tends to support sodium and water retention. Although it has sedative effect, it also increases REM sleep.

Used in treatment of sustained moderate to severe hypertension, particularly in patients with renal dysfunction. Also used in selected patients with carcinoid disease. Parenteral form may be used for treatment of hypertensive crises. Methyldopa is commercially available in combination with chlorothiazide (Aldoclor) and hydrochlorothiazide (Aldoril).

ABSORPTION AND FATE

About 50% of oral dose is absorbed from GI tract. Maximal antihypertensive effect in 4 to 6 hours; action may persist 24 hours after single dose. Following IV injection, decline in blood pressure may begin in 4 to 6 hours; duration 10 to 16 hours. Appears to be weakly bound to plasma proteins. Metabolized in GI tract and liver. About 85% excreted in urine within 24 hours; some unabsorbed oral drug excreted in feces.

CONTRAINDICATIONS AND PRECAUTIONS

Hypersensitivity to methyldopa, active hepatic disease, pheochromocytoma, blood dyscrasias, mild or labile hypertension amenable to treatment with mild sedation or thiazide diuretics. Safe use in women of childbearing potential and during pregnancy not established. Cautious use: history of impaired liver function or disease; angina pectoris.

ADVERSE REACTIONS

Neuropsychiatric: sedation, headache, weakness, fatigue, dizziness, paresthesias, Bell's palsy, decrease in mental acuity, involuntary choreoathetotic movements, parkinsonism, mild psychoses, depression, nightmares. **Cardiovascular:** orthostatic hypotension, aggravation of angina pectoris, bradycardia, myocarditis, edema, weight gain, paradoxic hypertensive reaction (especially with IV administration). **Hematologic:** positive direct Coombs test (common), myelosuppression. **GI:** distension, constipation, diarrhea, nausea, vomiting, dry mouth, sore or black tongue, sialadenitis. **Allergic:** fever, skin eruptions, ulcerations of soles of feet, eosinophilia. **Hepatotoxicity** (believed to be allergic reaction): abnormal liver function tests, jaundice, hepatitis. Other: nasal stuffiness (common), gynecomastia, lactation, decreased libido, impotence, hypothermia (large doses). Altered laboratory values: positive tests for lupus and rheumatoid factor, rise in BUN, increased serum amylase levels, pancreatitis, decreased urinary excretion of 5-hydroxyindoleacetic acid.

ROUTE AND DOSAGE

Adults: Oral: 250 mg 2 or 3 times a day for first 48 hours; daily dosage may then be increased or decreased, preferably at intervals of not less than 2 days, until adequate response is achieved. Maintenance 500 mg to 2 Gm in 2 to 4 divided doses daily. Maximum recommended daily dosage 3 Gm. Intravenous (methyldopate hydrochloride): 250 to 500 mg at 6-hour intervals, as required. Maximum recommended dose 1 Gm every 6 hours. Desired dose usually added to 100 ml of 5% dextrose injection and given slowly over 30 to 60 minutes. **Children:** Oral: 10 to 65 mg/kg/24 hours given in 2 to 4 divided doses. Intravenous: 20 to 65 mg/kg/24 hours in 4 equally divided doses at 6-hour intervals.

NURSING IMPLICATIONS

During period of dosage adjustment, physician may request blood pressures to be taken in lying, sitting, and standing positions.

During IV infusion of methyldopate, check blood pressure and pulse at least every 30 minutes until stabilized, and observe for adequacy of urinary output.

Transient sedation and drowsiness, sometimes associated with mental depression, weakness, and headache, commonly occur during first 24 to 72 hours of therapy or whenever dosage is increased. Symptoms tend to disappear with continuation of therapy or with dosage reduction. Advise patient to report extreme weakness and fatigue; drug discontinuation may be indicated.

To minimize daytime sedation, physician may prescribe dosage increases to be made in the evening.

Advise patient to report fever. Drug-induced fever, usually associated with myalgia, nausea, vomiting, and diarrhea, and less commonly with allergic manifestations, may occur between the 9th and 19th day of therapy.

Orthostatic hypotension with dizziness and lightheadedness may occur during period of dosage adjustment; this indicates need for dosage reduction. Elderly patients and patients with impaired renal function are particularly likely to manifest this drug effect. Supervision of ambulation may be advisable.

Caution patient that hot baths and showers may enhance orthostatic hypotension. Instruct patient to make position changes slowly, particularly from recumbent to upright, and to dangle legs a few minutes before standing.

Monitor intake and output. Report oliguria and changes in intake–output ration.

Weigh patient daily under standard conditions, and check for edema. Concomitant administration of a diuretic may be prescribed, if necessary.

Methyldopa hepatotoxicity (reversible) resembles viral hepatitis and commonly develops in 8 to 10 weeks, but it may occur from 1 week to 1 year after start of therapy; it is manifested by chills, fever, headache, pruritus, and anorexia and is sometimes associated with rash, arthralgia, enlarged liver, and positive Coombs test. Report to physician; drug should be discontinued.

Regularly scheduled blood counts and liver function tests are advised during first 6 to 12 weeks of therapy or if patient develops unexplained fever.

Positive Coombs test may or may not indicate hemolytic anemia; it usually develops between 6 and 12 months of therapy and may remain positive for several months after drug is discontinued. If for any reason the need for transfusion arises, both direct and indirect Coombs tests should be performed. Positive tests may interfere with accurate cross-matching of blood.

Caution the patient that methyldopa may affect the ability to perform activities requiring concentrated mental effort; therefore the patient should avoid potentially hazardous tasks such as driving a car or operating machinery.

Inform the patient that urine may darken on standing (thought to be due to breakdown product of drug or its metabolite) and that urine contaminated with a hypochlorite toilet bleaching agent may first turn red, then brown and black.

Compliance tends to be poor in patients receiving antihypertensive agents, for a variety of reasons. Urge the patient to keep follow-up visits. Some patients acquire tolerance about the second or third month of therapy, necessitating dosage increases, and rebound hypertension has been reported as a result of acute methyldopa withdrawal.

LABORATORY TEST INTERFERENCES: Methyldopa may interfere with creatinine measurements using alkaline picrate method, SGOT by colorimetric methods, and uric acid measurements by phosphotungstate method (in patients with high methyldopa blood levels); it may produce false elevations of urinary catecholamines.

DRUG INTERACTIONS: Hypotensive effect of methyldopa may be decreased by **amphetamines; tricyclic antidepressants** may block hypotensive response to methyldopa. Methyldopa partially inhibits the effects of systemically administered **ephedrine;** it increases the degree and duration of pressor response to **levarterenol.** Methyldopa produces additive hypotensive effects with **levodopa** (and possibly toxic CNS effects) and **methotrimeprazine;** there is the possibility of excitatory CNS effects with **MAO inhibitors.** Concomitant administration with **phenothiazines** or **propranolol** may result in paradoxic hypertensive response.

METHYLENE BLUE, U.S.P., B.P.
(M-B TABS, MG-BLUE, UROLENE BLUE)

Antimethemoglobinemic, antidote to cyanide poisoning

ACTIONS AND USES

Mildly antiseptic dye with oxidation–reduction action and tissue-staining property. In relatively high concentrations, it oxidizes ferrous iron of reduced hemoglobin to the ferric form, thus producing methemoglobin (methemoglobin so formed complexes with cyanide). In contrast, low concentrations act as catalytic intermediary electron acceptor in conversion of methemoglobin to hemoglobin. Prolonged administration accelerates destruction of erythrocytes.

Used for idiopathic and drug-induced methemoglobinemia and as antidote for cyanide poisoning; used as diagnostic agent and indicator dye. Its use in management of oxalate and phosphate urinary tract calculi is under clinical investigation. Formerly used as urinary antiseptic.

ABSORPTION AND FATE

Poorly absorbed from GI tract. Rapidly reduced in tissues to leuko form, which is excreted slowly in urine together with some unchanged drug. Also excreted in bile and feces.

History of allergy to methylene blue, renal insufficiency. Methylene blue is ineffective in patients with glucose-6-phosphate dehydrogenase deficiency.

ADVERSE REACTIONS

Bladder irritation, nausea, vomiting, diarrhea. Large doses: fever, methemoglobinemia, cardiovascular abnormalities. With continued administration: marked anemia.

ROUTE AND DOSAGE

Oral: 65 to 130 mg 2 or 3 times daily.

NURSING IMPLICATIONS

Should be administered after meals with full glass of water.

Inform patients that drug may impart blue-green color to urine and feces.

Since continued administration may cause marked anemia, frequent hemoglobin determinations are advised.

Methylene blue stain may be removed with a hypochlorite solution. Consult pharmacist.

METHYLERGONOVINE MALEATE, N.F. (METHERGINE)

Oxytocic

ACTIONS AND USES

Ergot alkaloid and congener of LSD. Induces rapid, sustained titanic uterine contraction that shortens third stage of labor and reduces blood loss. Has minimal vasoconstrictive activity. For absorption, fate, contraindications, and adverse reactions, see Ergotamine (ergot prototype).

Used for routine management after delivery of placenta and for postpartum atony, subinvolution, and hemorrhage. With full obstetric supervision, may be used during second stage of labor.

ROUTE AND DOSAGE

Oral: 0.2 mg 3 to 4 times daily in puerperium for maximum of 1 week. Intramuscular: 1 ml (0.2 mg) every 2 to 4 hours as necessary after delivery of placenta, after delivery of anterior shoulder, or during puerperium. Intravenous (emergency use only): 1 ml (0.2 mg), given slowly over 60-second period.

NURSING IMPLICATIONS

Ampuls with discolored solution should not be used. Store in cold place; protect from light.

Onset of action after oral administration, 5 to 10 minutes; after IV, immediate; after IM injection, 2 to 5 minutes.

Monitor vital signs (particularly blood pressure) and uterine response during and following parenteral administration of methylergonovine until partum period is stabilized (about 1 or 2 hours).

Notify physician if blood pressure suddenly increases or if there are frequent periods of uterine relaxation.

Also see Ergotamine Tartrate (ergot prototype).

(RITALIN HYDROCHLORIDE)

CNS stimulant

ACTIONS AND USES
   Piperidine derivative with pharmacologic actions and abuse potential qualitatively similar to those of amphetamine. Acts mainly on cerebral cortex. Exerts
   mild CNS and respiratory stimulation, with potency intermediate between
   those of amphetamine and caffeine. Effects more prominent on mental than on
   motor activities. Also believed to have an anorexigenic effect.
   Used as adjunctive therapy in minimal brain dysfunction in children (hyperkinetic behavior disorders), narcolepsy, mild depression, and apathetic or withdrawn senile behavior.
ABSORPTION AND FATE
   Well absorbed from GI tract. Effects may persist 3 to 6 hours. Widely distributed
   in body fluids; crosses blood–brain barrier. Excreted in urine as metabolites.
CONTRAINDICATIONS AND PRECAUTIONS
   Known hypersensitivity to the drug, marked anxiety, tension, agitation, severe
   depression, glaucoma, treatment of normal fatigue states, seizure disorders, EEG
   abnormalities. Safe use during pregnancy and in women of childbearing potential and children under age 6 not established. Cautious use: history of convulsive
   disorders, hypertension, patients receiving pressor agents or MAO inhibitors,
   emotionally unstable patients (eg, history of drug dependence, alcoholism).
ADVERSE REACTIONS
   Anorexia, dizziness, drowsiness, headache, insomnia, nervousness, blood pressure and pulse changes, palpitation, angina, tachycardia, arrhythmias, hypersensitivity reactions, visual disturbances, dyskinesia, seizures, abdominal pain,
   weight loss (especially in children). Also reported: leukopenia, anemia, scalp
   hair loss. Overdosage: hypertension, arrhythmias, vomiting, agitation, toxic
   psychosis, dry mucous membranes, mydriasis, hyperpyrexia, hyperreflexia,
   convulsions.
ROUTE AND DOSAGE
   Oral: **Adults:** 10 mg 2 or 3 times a day; usual dose range 20 to 60 mg daily.
   Highly individualized. **Children:** initially 5 mg before breakfast and lunch, with
   gradual increments of 5 to 10 mg weekly. Daily dosage above 60 mg not recommended.

NURSING IMPLICATIONS
Administer 30 to 45 minutes before meals. To avoid insomnia, last dose
   should be taken before 6 P.M.
Nervousness and insomnia (most common side effects) may require reduction of dosage or omission of afternoon or evening dose; however, they
   may diminish with time. Advise patients to report these and other adverse
   effects or paradoxic aggravation of symptoms.
Blood pressure and pulse should be monitored at appropriate intervals.
Advise patients to check weight at least 2 or 3 times weekly and to report
   weight loss. Height and weight should be checked in children, and failure
   to gain in either should be reported.
Periodic CBC and differential and platelet counts are advised during prolonged therapy.
Drug therapy in children should not be indefinite. If improvement is not
   observed after 1 month, drug should be discontinued. During prolonged
   therapy, periodic drug-free periods are recommended to assess the child's
   condition.
Chronic abusive use can lead to tolerance, psychic dependence, and psychoses.

Careful supervision is required for drug withdrawal following prolonged use. Abrupt withdrawal may result in severe depression and psychotic behavior.

Classified as schedule II drug under federal Controlled Substances Act.

DRUG INTERACTIONS: Methylphenidate may inhibit metabolism and thus potentiate the actions of **anticonvulsants, coumarin anticoagulants, phenylbutazone, tricyclic antidepressants,** and **vasopressors** (reduced dosage of these drugs may be required when given concomitantly with methylphenidate). Methylphenidate may decrease the hypotensive effect of **guanethidine.** There is possibility of hypertensive crisis with **furazolidone** and **MAO inhibitors.** Methylphenidate may be antagonized by **phenothiazine derivatives** and **propoxyphene.**

METHYLPREDNISOLONE, N.F., B.P.
(MEDROL)
METHYLPREDNISOLONE ACETATE, U.S.P., N.F.
(DEPO-MEDROL, MEDROL ACETATE)
METHYLPREDNISOLONE SODIUM SUCCINATE, U.S.P., N.F.
(SOLU-MEDROL)

Adrenocortical steroid (glucocorticoid)

ACTIONS AND USES

Synthetic adrenal steroid with similar glucocorticoid activity as hydrocortisone, but considerably less sodium and water retention effects than hydrocortisone (qv). Plasma half-life 3 to 4 hours. On weight basis, 4 mg methylprednisolone are equivalent to 20 mg hydrocortisone. Acetate has longer duration of action and more rapid onset of activity than parent compound. Sodium succinate is characterized by rapid onset of action; used for emergency therapy of short duration.

Used as potent antiinflammatory agent in management of ulcerative colitis, rheumatic fever, allergic and dermatologic disorders.

ROUTE AND DOSAGE

Adults: Oral: methylprednisolone 4 to 48 mg. Intraarticular (acetate): 4 to 80 mg. Intracutaneous, intralesional (acetate): 20 to 60 mg. Intramuscular (acetate): 40 to 120 mg daily or weekly; (succinate): 10 to 40 mg every 6 to 24 hours. Intravenous (succinate): 10 to 500 mg, depending on condition and response (large dose for septicemia). Topical (acetate): retention enema 4 to 120 mg every other day for 2 weeks or more. Ointment (acetate): 0.25% to 1%.

NURSING IMPLICATIONS

Alternate-day regimen (see Hydrocortisone) may be employed when methylprednisolone is given over long period of time.

Methylprednisolone sodium succinate solution should be used within 48 hours after preparation.

Protect from light.

Also see Hydrocortisone.

(ANDROID, METANDREN, NEO-HOMBREOL-M, ORAVIRON,
ORETON METHYL, SYNADROTABS, TESTRED)

Androgen

ACTIONS AND USES
Orally effective, short-acting steroid with androgen/anabolic activity ratio (1:1) similar to that of testosterone (qv), but less effective than its esters. Fails to produce full sexual maturation when administered to prepubertal male with complete testicular failure unless preceded by testosterone therapy.

Used as treatment for hypogonadism that starts in adult life after puberty; also used alone or combined with estrogen to treat menopausal symptoms and functional menstrual disorders. See Testosterone.

ABSORPTION AND FATE
Absorbed from oral mucosa and GI tract. All metabolites excreted in urine.

CONTRAINDICATIONS AND PRECAUTIONS
Hepatic dysfunction. Also see Testosterone.

ADVERSE REACTIONS
Cholestatic hepatitis with jaundice. Also see Testosterone.

ROUTE AND DOSAGE
Oral (replacement): 10 to 50 mg/day in divided doses, given after full androgenic effects are established by IM testosterone; (postpartum breast engorgement): 40 to 80 mg/day; (inoperable breast cancer in female): 200 mg/day for duration of therapeutic response or for no longer than 3 months if no remission. Buccal (linguet): one-half oral dose.

NURSING IMPLICATIONS
Buccal tablet should be placed in upper or lower buccal pouch between cheek and gum. Instruct patient not to chew or swallow tablet and to avoid eating, drinking, or smoking until absorption is complete. Tablet requires 30 to 60 minutes to dissolve. Change location of absorption site with each dose.

Good oral hygiene should be stressed as a means to decrease infection of cheek membranes irritated by buccal formulation.

Instruct patient to report inflamed or painful oral membranes. In addition to physical discomfort, absorption rate is changed by altered mucosal surface.

Creatinuria is a frequent finding with use of this drug, but its significance is unclear. Normal urinary creatine: Males: 0 to 40, females; 0 to 100 mg/24 hours.

Treatment of breast cancer is usually restricted to women who are more than 1 year but less than 5 years post menopause. If androgen treatment is going to be effective, it will be apparent within 3 months after therapy is instituted. When the disease again becomes progressive, therapy is stopped.

Since dosage sufficient to produce remission in breast cancer is quantitatively similar to that used for androgen replacement in the male, the female patient should be prepared for distressing and undesirable side effects of virilization (see index).

Advise female patient to report promptly if signs of virilization appear. Voice change and hirsutism may be irreversible, even after drug is withdrawn.

Instruct the male patient to report priapism or other signs of excess sexual stimulation. The physician will terminate methyltestosterone therapy.

Jaundice with or without pruritus appears to be dose-related. Instruct patient to report symptoms to physician. If liver function tests are altered at the same time, this drug will be withdrawn.

Also see Testosterone.

(NOLUDAR)

Hypnotic

ACTIONS AND USES

Piperidine derivative structurally related to glutethimide. Produces CNS depressant effects similar to those of short-acting barbiturates. Hypnotic doses suppress REM sleep.

Used as hypnotic for relief of simple insomnia. Sometimes used as sedative, but value for this purpose not established.

ABSORPTION AND FATE

Hypnotic dose induces sleep within 45 minutes; duration 5 to 8 hours. Plasma half-life 3 to 6 hours. Conjugated in liver; metabolites are secreted in bile and reabsorbed. Most of dose is excreted in urine as metabolites and their glucuronide conjugates; approximately 3% excreted unchanged.

CONTRAINDICATIONS AND PRECAUTIONS

Porphyria, known hypersensitivity to methyprylon. Safe use during pregnancy and in women of childbearing potential, nursing mothers, and children under 3 months of age not established. Cautious use: hepatic or renal impairment, addiction-prone individuals, mental depression, history of suicidal tendencies.

ADVERSE REACTIONS

Infrequent: morning drowsiness, dizziness, nausea, vomiting, diarrhea, esophagitis, headache, paradoxic excitation, skin rash, exacerbation of intermittent porphyria. Reported, but causal relationship not established: neutropenia, thrombocytopenia. **Acute toxicity:** somnolence, confusion, constricted pupils, hyperpyrexia, hypothermia, shock, pulmonary edema, respiratory depression; occasionally during recovery: excitation, convulsions, delirium, hallucinations.

ROUTE AND DOSAGE

Oral: **Adults:** 200 to 400 mg before retiring; total daily intake should not exceed 400 mg. **Pediatric** *over 3 months:* initially 50 mg at bedtime, increased up to 200 mg if required.

NURSING IMPLICATIONS

Hypnotic dose is administered 15 minutes before retiring. Prepare patient for sleep before administering drug.

In some patients, suppression of REM sleep may cause irritability, tension, confusion, and tremors.

Although tolerance develops to suppression of REM sleep, during chronic administration REM rebound may occur when drug is withdrawn: increased dreaming, nightmares, insomnia.

Tolerance may develop to hypnotic and sedative effects, but not to toxic effects.

Psychologic and physical dependence may occur, especially after prolonged use of large doses. Patient's continued need for methyprylon should be evaluated regularly.

Periodic blood counts are advised if drug is used repeatedly or over prolonged periods.

Warn patient about possible additive effects with alcohol and other CNS depressants.

Caution patient to avoid driving a car or engaging in other activities requiring mental alertness.

Gradual drug withdrawal is advised after prolonged use. Sudden discontinuation of drug may result in withdrawal symptoms similar to those following barbiturate dependence: confusion, marked nervousness, insomnia, sweating, polyuria, hyperreflexia, delirium, miosis, hallucinations, convulsion, death.

Treatment of overdosage: gastric lavage, general supportive measures (airway maintenance, assisted respiration, oxygen, IV fluids), pressor agent (levarterenol, metaraminol), short-acting barbiturate for convulsions and excitation, close monitoring of vital signs and urinary output.

Classified as schedule III drug under federal Controlled Substances Act.

Preserved in tightly closed, light-resistant containers.

METHYSERGIDE, N.F.
(SANSERT)

Specific: migraine

ACTIONS AND USES

Ergot derivative and congener of LSD. Unlike ergotamine (qv), has weak vasoconstrictor and oxytoxic actions, but exerts potent inhibition or blockade of serotonin (5-hydroxytryptamine), which may be implicated in mechanism of vascular headaches. Mode of action in prevention of migraine not clear; ineffective in treatment of acute attacks. Prolonged use has been known to promote fibrotic processes.

Used in prophylactic management of severe recurrent migraine, cluster, and other vascular headaches unresponsive to other antimigraine drugs. Also has been used to combat diarrhea and malabsorption associated with GI hypermotility in carcinoid disease, as well as for postgastrectomy dumping syndrome.

ABSORPTION AND FATE

Metabolic fate unknown, but thought to be well absorbed. Widely distributed to all tissues, and metabolized in liver.

CONTRAINDICATIONS AND PRECAUTIONS

Fibrotic processes, pulmonary or collagen diseases, edema, serious infections, debilitated states. Also see Ergotamine Tartrate.

ADVERSE REACTIONS

GI: nausea, vomiting, heartburn, abdominal pain, diarrhea, constipation. **CNS:** insomnia, drowsiness, vertigo, mild euphoria, confusion, excitement, feelings of unreality or depersonalization, distortions of body image, depression, anxiety, hallucinations, nightmares, ataxia, hyperesthesia, paresthesias. **Cardiovascular:** peripheral edema, thrombophlebitis, claudication, impaired circulation, angina of effort, ECG changes, postural hypotension, tachycardia. **Dermatologic:** facial flushing, telangiectasia, rash, excessive hair loss. **Fibrotic complications:** retroperitoneal (fatigue, malaise, fever, urinary obstruction with girdle or flank pain, dysuria, oliguria, polyuria, increased BUN and sedimentation rate), pleuropulmonary (dyspnea, chest pain and tightness, pleural friction rubs and effusion), cardiac (fibrotic thickening of valves with murmurs). **Other:** neutropenia, eosinophilia, weakness, arthralgia, myalgia, weight gain, scotoma, nasal stuffiness, positive direct Coombs' test.

ROUTE AND DOSAGE

Oral: 4 to 8 mg daily in divided doses.

NURSING IMPLICATIONS

GI side effects can frequently be prevented by gradual introduction of medication and by administering drug with meals.

Therapeutic trial period of 3 weeks is advised to determine patient's response to methysergide. If no response occurs in this time, it is unlikely that longer administration will be of benefit.

Pretreatment and periodic assessments of cardiac status, renal function, blood count, and sedimentation rate are advised.

Since incidence of side effects is relatively high (usually reversible with discontinuation of drug), patient should be examined regularly for development of fibrotic and vascular complications (auscultate heart and lungs; check peripheral pulses, and auscultate major vessels for bruits; observe for signs of phlebitis or venous obstruction). Also, observe and question patient concerning presence of CNS symptoms and other possible adverse effects (see Adverse Reactions).

Instruct patient to report the following immediately: onset of abdominal, back, or chest pain; dyspnea; leg pains while walking; cold, numb, or painful extremities; fever; dysuria or other urinary problems; edema; weight gain; other unusual signs and symptoms.

Counsel patient to weigh self daily, and teach patient how to check extremities for edema.

Caloric restriction and reduction of salt intake may be prescribed. Consult physician and instruct patient accordingly.

Since postural hypotension is a possible side effect, advise patient to make position changes slowly, particularly from recumbent to upright posture, and to dangle legs a few minutes before standing. Also instruct patient to lie down if faintness occurs.

Continuous administration of methysergide should not exceed 6 months without a medication-free interval of 3 to 4 weeks. Drug may be readministered after drug-free interval, if necessary.

To avoid "headache rebound," drug should be withdrawn gradually over 2- or 3-week period preceding discontinuation. Caution patient not to stop medication abruptly because of this possibility.

Patients with migraine should be helped to identify underlying emotional and physical stresses that may precipitate attacks and should learn how to deal with them. Adequate relaxation, recreation, and sleep may help to reduce severity and frequency of attacks.

Preserved in tight, light-resistant containers.

METRONIDAZOLE, U.S.P., B.P.
(FLAGYL)

Antiprotozoal

ACTIONS AND USES

Nitroimidazole compound with systemic antiprotozoal actions. Especially effective against *Trichomonas vaginalis* and *Entamoeba histolytica.* In amebiasis, effective at all sites of infection. Ineffective against *Candida albicans* or other fungi.

Used in treatment of trichomoniasis in both men and women; used in acute intestinal amebiasis and amebic liver abscess. Other clinical uses are investigational.

ABSORPTION AND FATE

Rapidly absorbed from GI tract. Maximum serum concentrations in about 1 hour; effective levels maintained at least 12 hours. Widely distributed; metabolized in liver. Metabolites excreted through enterohepatic and renal routes; traces also excreted in saliva, semen, vaginal secretions. Approximately 60% to 70% of dose is excreted in urine as unchanged drug. Crosses placenta and appears in breast milk.

CONTRAINDICATIONS AND PRECAUTIONS

History of hypersensitivity to metronidazole; blood dyscrasias; active CNS disease; pregnancy, especially first trimester; nursing mothers. Cautious use: coexistent candidiasis.

GI: nausea, vomiting, anorexia, epigastric distress, abdominal cramps, diarrhea, constipation, dry mouth, metallic or bitter taste. **CNS:** vertigo, headache, ataxia, incoordination (rare), confusion, irritability, depression, restlessness, weakness, fatigue, drowsiness, insomnia, sensory neuropathy, paresthesias. **Allergic:** rash, urticaria, pruritus, flushing. **Genitourinary:** polyuria, dysuria, pyuria, incontinence, cystitis, decreased libido, dyspareunia, dryness of vagina and vulva, sense of pelvic pressure. **Other:** moderate neutropenia, leukopenia, nasal congestion, fever, fleeting joint pains, ECG changes (flattening of T wave), fungal overgrowth.

ROUTE AND DOSAGE

Oral: *Trichomoniasis:* Women: 250 mg 3 times daily for 7 days. If further treatment is required, an interval of 4 to 6 weeks should elapse between courses. Men: 250 mg 3 times daily for 7 days. *Amebiasis:* **Adults:** 750 mg 3 times daily for 5 to 10 days. **Children:** 35 to 50 mg/kg/24 hours in 3 equal doses for 10 days.

NURSING IMPLICATIONS

Presence of trichomonads should be confirmed by wet smear and/or by culture prior to start of therapy for trichomoniasis.

Administer oral preparation immediately before, with, or immediately after meals or with food or milk to reduce GI distress.

Sexual partners should receive concurrent treatment. Asymptomatic trichomoniasis in the male is a frequent source of reinfection of the female.

Total and differential leukocyte counts are recommended before, during, and after therapy, especially if a second course is necessary.

Therapy should be discontinued immediately if symptoms of CNS toxicity develop, eg, ataxia, tremor, incoordination, paresthesias, numbness, impairment of pain or touch sensation.

Warn patients that ingestion of alcohol during metronidazole therapy may produce disulfiram-type reactions (sweating, diarrhea, nausea, vomiting, headache, flushing, modification of alcohol taste, thirst), hypotension, vertigo, blurred vision.

Inform patients that urine may appear dark or reddish brown (especially likely to occur with higher than recommended doses). This is thought to be caused by the metabolite and is reported to be of no clinical significance.

Women with trichomoniasis should be advised not to wear pantyhose or tight underwear and to avoid bubble baths. Also review perineal hygiene technique.

Metronidazole may encourage sudden candidal overgrowth. Advise patients to report symptoms: furry tongue, color changes of tongue, glossitis, stomatitis, vaginitis, curdlike milky vaginal discharge, proctitis. Treatment with a candicidal agent may be indicated.

Methods of controlling and preventing amebiasis include health education in personal hygiene, particularly hand washing after defecation and before preparing or eating food, sanitary disposal of feces, sanitary water supply, and fly control.

Repeated feces examinations, usually up to 3 months, are necessary to assure that amebae have been eliminated.

Preserved in tightly closed, light-resistant containers.

DRUG INTERACTIONS: There have been preliminary reports of psychotic episodes and confusional states associated with combined use of metronidazole and **disulfiram.** Concurrent ingestion of metronidazole and **alcohol** may produce a mild disulfiramlike effect in some patients.

(MAGNESIA MAGMA, MAGNESIUM HYDROXIDE)

Antacid, cathartic

ACTIONS AND USES

Aqueous suspension of magnesium hydroxide (approximately 8%) with rapid and long-acting neutralizing action. Although classified as nonsystemic antacid, 5% to 10% of the magnesium may be absorbed and also may cause slight acid rebound. Acts as antacid in low doses and as mild saline cathartic in higher doses. Reacts with hydrochloric acid in stomach to form magnesium chloride, which has neutralizing as well as cathartic action. Each milliliter reportedly is capable of neutralizing approximately 2.7 mEq of gastric acid.

Used for short-term treatment of occasional constipation, for relief of GI symptoms associated with hyperacidity, and as adjunct in treatment of peptic ulcer. Also has been used in treatment of poisoning by mineral acids and arsenic and as mouthwash to neutralize acidity.

ABSORPTION AND FATE

Absorbed magnesium ions are usually excreted rapidly by kidney. Cathartic action occurs in about 4 to 8 hours, depending on dosage.

CONTRAINDICATIONS AND PRECAUTIONS

Abdominal pain, nausea, vomiting, diarrhea, renal dysfunction, fecal impaction, intestinal obstruction or perforation.

ADVERSE REACTIONS

Excessive dosage: nausea, vomiting, diarrhea, alkalinization of urine, hypermagnesemia (patients with impaired renal function). **Prolonged use:** rectal stones (rare), electrolyte imbalance.

ROUTE AND DOSAGE

Oral: Antacid: **Adults:** 5 ml 4 times a day. Cathartic: **Adults:** 15 to 30 ml. **Children:** 2.5 to 5 ml.

NURSING IMPLICATIONS

Shake bottle well before pouring to assure administration of suspension and not supernatant liquid.

For antacid action, usually given 20 minutes to 1 hour before meals and at bedtime. Mix with about 30 ml of water to assure that it reaches the stomach.

When intended for antacid use, the cathartic effect of milk of magnesia can be minimized by coadministering or alternating with calcium carbonate or aluminum hydroxide gel, each of which has constipating effects. Consult physician. Commercially available in combination with aluminum hydroxide (Aludrox, Alurex, Maalox, and others).

For cathartic effect, follow the drug with a glass of water to enhance drug action. Administered in the morning or at bedtime. Commercially available in emulsion containing mineral oil (Haley's M-O). Evaluate the patient's continued need for drug.

Prolonged and frequent use in cathartic doses may lead to dependence.

See Bisacodyl for patient teaching points.

Stored at room temperature in tightly covered container. Slowly absorbs carbon dioxide on exposure to air. Avoid freezing.

DRUG INTERACTIONS: Alkalinization of urine caused by repeated use of milk of magnesia may decrease urinary excretion of weakly basic drugs (eg, **quinidine**). Simultaneous administration may increase serum **dicumarol** levels by enhancing its absorption. Milk of magnesia should not be taken within 1 to 2

hours of dicumarol. Simultaneous administration with **phenothiazines** may
produce lower phenothiazine serum levels due to decreased GI absorption.
Administer milk of magnesia at least 1 hour before or 2 hours after a phenothiazine. Milk of magnesia may complex with **tetracyclines** if administered simultaneously, resulting in significant reduction in serum antibiotic level. If prescribed, administer milk of magnesia at least 3 hours after tetracycline
derivative. There is the theoretical possibility of additive muscular relaxation
with **neuromuscular blocking agents** (eg, **succinylcholine, tubocurarine**).

MINERAL OIL, U.S.P.
(CLYSEROL OIL RETENTION, FLEET MINERAL OIL ENEMA, HEAVY
LIQUID PETROLATUM, KONDREMUL, NUJOL, PETROGALAR PLAIN,
WHITE MINERAL OIL)
LIQUID PARAFFIN, B.P.

Lubricant cathartic, emollient

ACTIONS AND USES
  Mixture of hydrocarbons obtained from petroleum. Lubricates and softens
  feces, retards water absorption from fecal content, and eases passage of stool.
  Used for temporary relief of constipation, and when straining at stool is contraindicated (eg, hypertension, certain cardiac disorders, following anorectal
  surgery). Given by retention enema to relieve fecal impaction and to avoid
  possible adverse effects of oral administration. Also used as pharmaceutical
  solvent and vehicle.
ABSORPTION AND FATE
  Limited absorption from intestinal tract with distribution to mesenteric lymph
  nodes, intestinal mucosa, liver, spleen. Eliminated in stool in 6 to 8 hours.
CONTRAINDICATIONS AND PRECAUTIONS
  Nausea, vomiting, abdominal pain, intestinal obstruction, oral administration to
  dysphagic patients. Cautious use: oral use in elderly or debilitated patients,
  during pregnancy.
ADVERSE REACTIONS
  Occasionally: pruritus ani; interference with postoperative anorectal wound
  healing; lipid pneumonitis. Prolonged use: anorexia, nausea, vomiting, nutritional deficiencies, hypoprothrombinemia.
ROUTE AND DOSAGE
  Oral: 15 to 45 ml. Rectal (retention enema) **Adults:** 90 to 120 ml; **Children** *2
  years or older:* one-fourth to one-half the adult dose, depending on age.

NURSING IMPLICATIONS
Usually administered in the evening. Digestion and passage of food from
  stomach may be delayed if taken within 2 hours of mealtime.
Potentiality of lipid pneumonia from aspiration of orally administered mineral oil is especially high in the elderly and debilitated patient. Administer
  with patient in upright position, and avoid giving just before patient
  retires.
Mineral oil is tasteless and odorless when cold (stored in refrigerator).
Although tasteless, consistency may be objectionable. Many patients prefer
  to drink orange juice or suck on slice of orange after taking oil; others
  prefer to mix it in orange juice.
Emulsified preparations are reportedly more palatable; however, this form
  may enhance absorption of oil through intestinal mucosa.
Prolonged use (more than 2 weeks) can reduce absorption of fat-soluble
  vitamins A, D, E, and K, carotene, calcium, and phosphates. For these

reasons, mineral oil base for low-calorie salad dressing is not advised.

Repeated oral use or rectal administration may result in oil seepage from rectum with soiling of clothing or bedding. Forewarn patient to be prepared for this possibility to avoid embarrassment.

Administration of retention enema is generally followed by a cleansing enema in 30 minutes to 1 hour. Consult physician.

Application of mineral oil to nasal passages to relieve dryness should be avoided because of danger of migration of droplets from pharynx into lungs, with resulting lipid pneumonia. Aqueous vehicles are safer.

Frequent or prolonged use of mineral oil may result in dependence. See Bisacodyl for patient teaching points concerning management of chronic constipation.

DRUG INTERACTIONS: By reducing absorption of vitamin K, mineral oil may potentiate effect of oral anticoagulants; on the other hand, ingestion of large amounts of mineral oil may decrease effectiveness of **oral anticoagulants** by impairing absorption (opposing mechanisms). Mineral oil may interfere with action of **nonabsorbable sulfonamides.**

MINOCYCLINE HYDROCHLORIDE
(MINOCIN, VECTRIN)

Antibacterial

ACTIONS AND USES

Semisynthetic tetracycline derivative with actions, uses, contraindications, precautions, and adverse reactions as for tetracycline (qv). Appears to be active against strains of staphylococci resistant to other tetracyclines, and photosensitivity occurs only rarely. Reported to be more completely absorbed than other tetracyclines because it is more lipid-soluble.

ABSORPTION AND FATE

Well absorbed by oral route. About 70% to 75% bound to plasma proteins. Serum half-life following single 200-mg dose approximately 11 to 17 hours. Slow renal clearance. About 12% of dose excreted in urine; remainder persists in body in fatty tissues. Crosses placenta, and appears in breast milk.

CONTRAINDICATIONS AND PRECAUTIONS

Hypersensitivity to tetracyclines, oral administration in meningococcal infections. Safe use during pregnancy not established. Cautious use: renal impairment. See Tetracycline.

ADVERSE REACTIONS

Most frequent: CNS side effects (weakness, lightheadedness, ataxia, dizziness or vertigo), nausea, cramps, diarrhea, flatulence. Also see Tetracycline.

ROUTE AND DOSAGE

Adults: Oral: 200 mg followed by 100 mg every 12 hours; alternatively, 100 or 200 mg initially, followed by 50 mg 4 times daily. Intravenous: 200 mg followed by 100 mg every 12 hours. Not to exceed 400 mg/24 hours. **Children:** 4 mg/kg initially, followed by 2 mg/kg every 12 hours (orally or IV). See manufacturers directions for preparation of parenteral solution.

NURSING IMPLICATIONS

Check expiration date. Outdated tetracyclines can cause severe adverse reactions.

Studies to date indicate that minocycline is not significantly influenced by food and dairy products, in contrast to other tetracyclines.

Since lightheadedness, dizziness, or vertigo occur frequently, caution patient to avoid driving vehicles and other hazardous activities while on minocycline. (Lightheadedness is usually transient and often disappears during therapy.)

Advise patient to report vestibular side effects (CNS symptoms). They usually occur within first week of therapy and are reversible when drug is stopped.

Serum drug level determinations are advised in patients receiving prolonged therapy.

Reconstituted solution is stable for 24 hours at room temperature, but final dilution for administration should be used immediately.

See Tetracycline Hydrochloride.

MITHRAMYCIN, U.S.P.
(MITHRACIN)

Antineoplastic

ACTIONS AND USES

Cytotoxic antibiotic produced by *Streptomyces plicatus,* with minimal immunosuppressive activity. Complexes with DNA, thus inhibiting DNA-directed RNA systhesis. May lower serum calcium levels by unclear mechanism. Appears to block hypercalcemic action of vitamin D, and may inhibit parathyroid hormone effect on osteoclasts. Interferes with synthesis of various clotting factors. High toxicity with low therapeutic index limits clinical use; little or no immunosuppressive properties.

Used to treat hospitalized patients with hypercalcemia or hypercalciuria associated with advanced neoplasms. Has been used to treat testicular malignancy and investigationally in Paget's disease and glioblastomas.

ABSORPTION AND FATE

Information on absorption, fate, and excretion is limited. Crosses blood–brain barrier, and appears to localize in areas of active bone resorption; excreted in urine. Has cumulative and irreversible toxicity.

CONTRAINDICATIONS AND PRECAUTIONS

Bleeding and coagulation disorders, myelosuppression, electrolyte imbalance (especially hypocalcemia, hypokalemia, hypophosphatemia), pregnancy, women of childbearing age. Cautious use: patients with prior abdominal or mediastinal radiology; liver or renal impairment.

ADVERSE REACTIONS

Hematologic: thrombocytopenia, bleeding and coagulation disorders (dose-related), leukopenia (mild). **GI:** stomatitis, anorexia, nausea, vomiting, diarrhea, widespread intestinal hemorrhage. **Other:** fever, drowsiness, irritability, dizziness, weakness, headache, mental depression, marked facial flushing, hemoptysis, nonspecific or acneiform skin rash, phlebitis, hypophosphatemia, hypokalemia, hypocalciuria, abnormal liver and renal function (reflected in laboratory values).

ROUTE AND DOSAGE

Intravenous: dosage and duration of therapy highly individualized on basis of hematologic and clinical responses.

NURSING IMPLICATIONS

Reconstituted with sterile water for injection. See manufacturer's directions for dilution. Reconstitute immediately before injection; discard unused portion. Vials should be kept refrigerated (2 to 8 C).

When edema, ascites, or hydrothorax is present, drug dose is based on ideal body weight.

A single intravenous dose may be sufficient to reduce elevated serum calcium to normal level within 24 to 48 hours for 3 to 15 days.

Watch IV flow rate (established by physician); GI side effects increase when rate is too fast.

Terminate infusion if extravasation occurs. Apply moderate heat to disperse the drug and to minimize tissue irritation. Infusion should be restarted in another vein.

Tumor response to therapy is usually observed within 3 to 4 weeks.

Electrolyte imbalance will be corrected prior to instituting or restarting mithramycin therapy; thereafter, weigh patient daily under standard conditions.

Establish flow chart at beginning of therapy, permitting continuous record of weight, intake–output ratio and pattern, and bowel pattern for comparative data on which to base patient care plan.

Frequent assessments of liver, hematologic (platelet count, bleeding and prothrombin times), and renal function are performed throughout therapy and for several days after last dose.

An antiemetic drug given before and concomitantly with drug administration may prevent nausea and vomiting.

Therapy is interrupted if leukocyte count is below 4000/mm^3, if platelet count is below 150,000/mm^3, or if prothrombin time is more than 4 seconds higher than control. (Normal: 12 to 14 seconds).

Thrombocytopenia, frequently evidenced by a single or persistent episode of epistaxis or hematemesis, may be rapid in onset during or after a course of treatment. Report marked facial flushing, which is often an early symptom.

Inspect skin daily for signs of purpura. Hemoptysis may occur because of bleeding into metastasis; report this immediately.

Rebound hypercalcemia (normal value 9 to 10.6 mg/dl) following mithramycin-induced hypocalcemia may persist 2 to 4 days. Hypercalcemia symptoms: nausea, vomiting, GI atony, polyuria, nocturia, thirst, dehydration, skeletal muscle weakness, confusion, drowsiness, shortened Q-T interval, bradycardia.

The hypercalcemic patient may be dehydrated. Monitor intake–output ratio to assure adequate fluid intake.

Signs of antiblastic action on GI mucosal cells (hematemesis, melena) necessitate stopping drug use.

Check patient's bowel function daily to prevent high fecal impaction due to diminished action of intestinal musculature.

Consult physician about dietary calcium intake, and coordinate dietary planning with dietitian, patient, and family.

DRUG INTERACTIONS: Concomitant administration of **vitamin D** may enhance hypercalcemia.

(MITOMYCIN C, MUTAMYCIN)

Antineoplastic

ACTION AND USES
Potent antineoplastic compound produced by *Streptomyces caespitosus* with wide range of antibacterial activity and described extensively in the literature as Mitomycin C. Effective in certain tumors nonresponsive to surgery, radiation or other chemotheraputic agents.

Action mechanism not clear but reportedly combines with DNA (attachment site unknown), thereby interfering with cellular and enzymatic RNA and protein synthesis. Mitomycin has been shown to be carcinogenic in mice and rats; thus selected patients must be aware of the inherent risk in spite of possible therapeutic benefits.

Used in combination with other chemotherapeutic agents in palliative, adjunctive treatment of disseminated adenocarcinoma of breast, pancreas or stomach squamous cell carcinoma of head, neck, lung and cervix. Not recommended to replace surgery and/or radiotherapy, nor as a single primary therapeutic agent.

ABSORPTION AND FATE
Following IV injection in dogs, 18 to 29% of drug is recovered within one hour; in children, 5 to 20% is recovered in one hour and all in two hours.

CONTRAINDICATIONS AND PRECAUTIONS
Hypersensitivity or idiosyncracy reaction; thrombocytopenia; coagulation disorders or bleeding tendencies; pregnancy. Cautions use: renal impairment, myelosuppression.

ADVERSE REACTIONS
Bone marrow toxicity (thrombocytopenia, leukopenia occurring 4 to 8 weeks after treatment onset); fever, anorexia, stomatitis, nausea, vomiting, alopecia; desquamation, induration, pruritus, pain, bleeding, paresthesias, necrosis, sloughing at injection site; hemoptysis, dyspnea, coughing, pneumonia, elevated BUN. Following symptoms may or not be drug induced: headache, blurred vision, drowsiness, fatigue, edema, syncope, confusion, thrombophlebitis, anemia, hematemesis, diarrhea, pain.

ROUTE AND DOSAGE
Intravenous: 2 mg/m^2/day for 5 days; after drug-free interval of 2 days, 2 mg/m^2/day for 5 days; thereafter dosage and schedule highly individualized.

NURSING IMPLICATIONS

Patient receiving mitomycin should be hospitalized so that emergency treatment and laboratory facilities will be available.

Avoid extravasation when drug is administered, to prevent extreme tissue reaction (cellulitis) to the toxic drug.

Because of cumulative myelosuppression, laboratory studies of platelet counts, prothrombin and bleeding times, differential and hemoglobin studies, serum creatinine are performed frequently during treatment and for at least 7 weeks after treatment is terminated.

Usually drug is not administered if serum creatinine is greater than 1.7 mg%.

If platelet count falls below 75,000 and WBC down to 3000 or prothrombin or bleeding times are prolonged, treatment is suspended or modified.

Monitor intake-output ratios. Any sign of impaired kidney function should be reported: change in ratio, dysuria, hematuria, oliguria, frequency, urgency. Keep patient hydrated (at least 2,000 to 2,500 ml orally daily if tolerated). Drug is nephrotoxic.

Observe closely for signs of infection. Monitor body temperature frequently.

Instruct patient to report immediately if signs of common cold present. See Mechlorethamine for Nursing Implications related to mouth care (for stomatitis).

MORPHINE SULFATE, U.S.P., B.P.

Narcotic analgesic (opium derivative)

ACTIONS AND USES
Suggested mechanisms of analgesic action include elevation of pain threshold, interference with pain conduction or CNS response to pain, or altered pain perception. Relieves pain without obtunding other sensory modalites, and may produce euphoria; drowsiness occurs commonly, and higher doses promote deep sleep. Also depresses respiratory center and cough reflex and may induce nausea and vomiting by increasing vestibular sensitivity and by CTZ stimulation (initial doses stimulate and subsequent doses depress vomiting center). Causes constriction of pupils, even in total darkness, and greatly enhances pupillary response to light (tolerance to miotic effect is rare). Generally, has no major effect on blood pressure or heart rate or rhythm when patient is supine; however, orthostatic hypotension may occur in head-up position, possibly by dilatation of peripheral vessels (histamine release) or by depression of medullary vasomotor center. Delays digestion by decreasing stomach motility and hydrochloric acid, biliary and pancreatic secretions. Decreases intensity and frequency of propulsive peristalsis, and enhances amplitude of nonpropulsive contractions, thus causing desiccation of feces and resultant constipation. Increases tone of smooth muscles and sphincters in GI, biliary, and genitourinary systems. Reduction of urinary outflow may be mediated by antidiuretic hormone release or by decreased renal blood flow. Release of ACTH, FSH, LH, and TSH may be suppressed.
Used for symptomatic relief of severe pain after nonnarcotic analgesics have failed and as preanesthetic medication; also used to relieve dyspnea of acute left ventricular failure and pulmonary edema and pain of myocardial infarction.

ABSORPTION AND FATE
Absorption from GI tract is complete, but variable in rate. Well absorbed following parenteral injection. Peak analgesia within 50 to 90 minutes following subcutaneous administration and 20 minutes after IV injection. Analgesia may be maintained up to 7 hours. Wide distribution, with concentration mainly in kidney, liver, lung, spleen; lower concentrations in brain and muscle. Metabolized chiefly in liver. About 90% of dose is excreted in urine within 24 hours, largely in conjugated form, with small amounts as unchanged drug; 7% to 10% excreted via bile through feces. Crosses placenta; small amounts appears in breast milk.

CONTRAINDICATIONS AND PRECAUTIONS
Hypersensitivity to opiates, increased intracranial pressure, convulsive disorders, acute alcoholism, acute bronchial asthma, chronic pulmonary diseases, severe respiratory depression, chemical-irritant-induced pulmonary edema, prostatic hypertrophy, undiagnosed acute abdominal conditions, pancreatitis, acute ulcerative colitis, severe liver or renal insufficiency, Addison's disease, hypothyroidism. Safe use during pregnancy not established. Cautious use: toxic psychosis, cardiac arrhythmias, cardiovascular disease, emphysema, kyphoscoliosis, cor pulmonale, severe obesity, reduced blood volume; very old, very young or debilitated patients; use during labor.

ADVERSE REACTIONS
CNS: respiratory depression, decreased cough reflex, euphoria, dysphoria, paradoxic CNS stimulation (restlessness, tremor, delirium, insomnia), drowsiness,

dizziness, weakness, headache, miosis, hypothermia. **GI:** nausea, vomiting, anorexia, constipation, dry mouth, biliary colic. **Cardiovascular:** bradycardia, orthostatic hypotension, syncope, flushing of face, neck, and upper thorax. **Genitourinary:** urinary retention or urgency, dysuria, reduced libido and/or potency (prolonged use). **Allergic:** pruritus, skin rashes, contact dermatitis, urticaria, hemorrhagic urticaria (rare), sneezing, wheal and flare and pain over injection site, edema, anaphylactoid reaction (rare). **Other:** sweating, prolonged labor and respiratory depression of newborn, decreased urinary VMA excretion, elevated transaminase levels, precipitation of porphyria. **Acute intoxication:** deep sleep, coma, marked miosis, severe respiratory depression (as low as 2 to 4/minute) or arrest, pulmonary edema, hypothermia, skeletal muscle flaccidity, oliguria, hypotension, bradycardia, convulsions (infants and children), cardiac arrest.

ROUTE AND DOSAGE

Oral (generally not recommended): 5 to 15 mg every 4 hours. Subcutaneous: **Adults:** 5 to 15 mg every 4 hours, if necessary. **Children:** 0.1 to 0.2 mg/kg per dose (single dose not to exceed 15 mg). Intravenous (rarely used): **Adults:** 2.5 to 15 mg in 4 to 5 ml water for injection, administered slowly over a 4- to 5-minute period.

NURSING IMPLICATIONS

Narcotic analgesics should be given in smallest effective dose and for the shortest time compatible with patient's needs.

Evaluate the patient's need for p.r.n. medication, and check time of last dose and validity of physician's order. Follow health facility policy regarding time limit on narcotic orders. Record time of onset, duration, and quality of pain (preferably in patient's own words).

Fullest analgesic effect is achieved if drug is administered before the patient experiences intense pain (morphine relieves continuous dull pain more effectively than sharp intermittent pain, which generally requires higher doses).

Note that the patient's cultural background may influence response to pain. Some patients tend to be stoic, but others may overtly show that they feel pain.

Elevated pulse or respiratory rate, restlessness, anorexia, or drawn facial expression may indicate need for analgesia.

Differentiate among restlessness as a sign of pain and the need for medication, restlessness associated with hypoxia, and restlessness caused by morphine-induced CNS stimulation (a paradoxic reaction that is particularly common in women and elderly patients).

Provide maximum comfort measures, and reduce environmental stimuli before preparing medication.

Before administering the drug, note respiratory rate, depth, and rhythm and size of pupils. Respirations of 12/minute or below and miosis are signs of toxicity (miosis is replaced by pupillary dilatation in asphyxia). Withhold drug and report these signs to physician.

Pupillary size is best judged in good room light (with patient facing away from window light) rather than by flashlight, which causes immediate miosis.

Caution patients not to smoke or ambulate without assistance after receiving the drug. Bedsides may be advisable.

Monitor vital signs at regular intervals. Morphine-induced respiratory depression may occur even with small doses, and it increases progressively with higher doses (generally reaching maximum within 90 minutes following subcutaneous and 7 minutes after IV administration). However, respiratory minute volume may remain below normal 4 to 5 hours following therapeutic doses.

Narcotic analgesics also depress cough and sigh reflexes and thus may induce atelectasis, especially in postoperative patients. Purposefully encourage changes in position, deep breathing, and coughing (unless contraindicated) at regularly scheduled intervals.

Narcotic antagonists (eg, naloxone) and facilities for oxygen and support of respiration should be available.

Nausea and orthostatic hypotension (with lightheadedness and dizziness) most often occur in ambulatory patients or when a supine patient assumes the head-up position or in patients not experiencing severe pain. (Morphine decreases the ability of the cardiovascular system to respond to gravitational shifts.)

Transient fall in blood pressure (even in the supine position) is apt to occur in patients with acute myocardial infarction.

Monitor intake–output ratio and pattern. Report oliguria or urinary retention. Morphine may dull perception of bladder stimuli; therefore, encourage the patient to void at least every 4 hours. Palpate lower abdomen to detect bladder distension.

Monitor bowel pattern. Inattention to the defecation reflex and desiccation of feces contribute to the constipating effects of morphine. Check for abdominal distension and intestinal peristaltic sounds during postoperative period.

Record relief of pain and duration of analgesia. Evaluate the patient's continued need for morphine. If indicated, suggest that the physician prescribe a less potent analgesic.

Tolerance as well as physiologic and psychologic dependence may develop with repeated use. There is high abuse liability.

Be alert to purposive behavior (manipulations) to get more drug; this usually begins shortly before next scheduled dose. Such behavior may signal the onset of tolerance and addiction.

Abrupt cessation of drug use in the presence of physiologic dependence initiates the abstinence syndrome, usually within 24 to 48 hours after last dose. Without treatment, withdrawal symptoms ("cold turkey") develop, with increasing intensity and a common sequence: drug craving and anxiety (within 6 hours of last dose); irritability, perspiration, yawning, rhinorrhea, itchy nose, sneezing, lacrimation (within 14 hours); pupil dilation, piloerection ("gooseflesh"), tremulousness, muscle jerks, bone and muscle aches, nausea, hot and cold flashes, tossing, restless sleep ("yen"), elevated systolic blood pressure, dilated pupils, elevated temperature, pulse, and respiration rates (within 24 to 36 hours); curled-up position, vomiting, diarrhea, weight loss, hemoconcentration, increased blood sugar, spontaneous ejaculation or orgasm (within 36 to 48 hours).

Severity and character of withdrawal symptoms depend on the interval between doses, duration of drug use, total daily dose, and health and personality of the addicted individual.

Classified as schedule II drug under federal Controlled Substances Act.

Morphine is reported to be physically and chemically incompatible with many solutions. Do not mix with other drugs without the advice of a pharmacist.

Preserved in tight, light-resistant containers.

LABORATORY TEST INTERFERENCES: There is the possibility of false positive urine glucose determinations using Benedict's solution. Plasma amylase and lipase determinations may be falsely positive for 24 hours after use of morphine.

DRUG INTERACTIONS: CNS depressant effects of morphine and other narcotic analgesics may be exaggerated and prolonged by concurrent administration of

alcohol, general **anesthetics, antianxiety drugs, phenothiazines,** tricyclic an-
tidepressants, barbiturates, other **sedatives, hypnotics,** and **MAO inhibitors.**
Narcotic analgesics may enhance the neuromuscular blocking action of **skeletal**
muscle relaxants.

NAFCILLIN SODIUM U.S.P.
(NAFCIL, UNIPEN)

Antibacterial, antibiotic

ACTIONS AND USES

Semisynthetic penicillin resistant to penicillinase and acids. Effective against penicillin-sensitive and penicillin-resistant strains of *Staphylococcus aureus*. Also active against pneumococci and group A β-hemolytic streptococci.

Used primarily in treatment of infections caused by penicillinase-producing staphylococci. May also be used to initiate treatment when staphylococcal infection is suspected.

ABSORPTION AND FATE

Incompletely and irregularly absorbed after oral administration. Peak serum levels within 30 to 60 minutes following oral and IM administration; duration 4 hours following oral and 4 to 6 hours following IM injection. Penetrates pleural, pericardial, and synovial fluids, with predominant concentration in liver. About 90% bound to plasma proteins. Enters enterohepatic circulation. Primarily eliminated in bile; 10% to 30% of dose is excreted unchanged in urine.

CONTRAINDICATIONS AND PRECAUTIONS

Hypersensitivity to penicillins, cephalosporins, and other allergens; use of oral route in patients with severe infections or patients who have gastric dilatation, cardiospasm, or intestinal hypermotility; IV use in neonates and infants. Safe use during pregnancy not established. Also see Penicillin G.

ADVERSE REACTIONS

Nausea, vomiting, diarrhea. Allergic reactions: urticaria, pruritus, rash, fever, anaphylaxis (particularly following IV), allergic interstitial nephritis, thrombophlebitis (following IV administration), pain, irritation, increase in serum transaminase activity (following IM administration). Also see Penicillin G.

ROUTE AND DOSAGE

Oral: **Adults:** 250 mg to 1 Gm every 4 to 6 hours; **infants and children:** 25 to 50 mg/kg/day in 4 divided doses; **neonates:** 10 mg/kg 3 or 4 times daily. Intramuscular: **Adults:** 500 mg every 4 to 6 hours; **infants and children:** 25 mg/kg twice daily; **neonates:** 10 mg/kg twice daily. Intravenous: **Adults:** 500 mg to 1 Gm every 4 hours.

NURSING IMPLICATIONS

Culture and sensitivity tests should be performed prior to and periodically during therapy.

A careful history should be obtained before therapy to determine any prior allergies.

Oral dose is best taken on an empty stomach at least 1 hour before or 2 hours after meals (although nafcillin is acid-stable, food interferes with absorption, and GI absorption of nafcillin is erratic).

Oral solution should be dated after reconstitution and refrigerated. Discard unused portions after 1 week.

IM injection in adults: administered by deep intragluteal injection. Make certain solution is clear. Select site carefully. Injection into or near major peripheral nerves or local vessels can result in neurovascular damage. Aspirate before injecting drug to avoid intraarterial administration. Rotate injection sites.

IM injection in children: intragluteal injection is contraindicated in young children because gluteal muscles are underdeveloped. In general, the per-ferred IM site in children under 3 years of age is the midlateral or an-terolateral thigh. Follow agency policy.

Reconstitution for IM injection should be with sterile water for injection. Follow manufacturer's direction for making 250 mg/ml concentration. Date vial after reconstitution. Keep under refrigeration; storage time var-ies with manufacturer.

For IV injection, required dose should be diluted in 15 to 30 ml of sterile water for injection or isotonic sodium chloride and administered over 5- to 10-minute period, either directly or through tubing of running IV

For continuous IV infusion, concentration of drug should be within range of 2 to 30 mg/ml. Compatible IV infusion solutions are isotonic sodium chloride, 5% dextrose in water, or 0.4% sodium chloride, Ringer's, or sodium lactate (30 mg/ml concentration only). Discard unused portions 24 hours after reconstitution.

Observe for signs of thrombophlebitis following IV administration, particu-larly in the elderly. IV therapy is usually not given for more than 24 to 48 hours.

Allergic reactions, principally rash, occur most commonly. Nausea, vomiting, and diarrhea may occur with oral therapy. Advise patient to report these symptoms promptly.

Periodic assessments of hepatic, renal, and hematopoietic functions are ad-vised during prolonged therapy.

Infections caused by β-hemolytic streptococci should be treated for at least 10 days to prevent possible development of acute rheumatic fever or glomerulonephritis.

Be alert for signs of bacterial or fungal superinfections in patient on pro-longed therapy.

See Penicillin G Potassium.

NALIDIXIC ACID, N.F.
(NegGram)

Antibacterial

ACTIONS AND USES
Synthetic naphthyridine derivative with marked bactericidal activity against Gram-negative organisms, including majority of *Proteus* strains, *Klebsiella,* En-terobacter *(Aerobacter),* and *Escherichia coli.* Ineffective against *Pseudomonas* species. Gram-positive bacteria are relatively resistant. Appears to act by inhibiting DNA synthesis of bacteria. Bacterial resistance has occurred.

Used in treatment of urinary tract infections caused by susceptible Gram-negative organisms.

ABSORPTION AND FATE
Rapidly and almost completely absorbed from GI tract. Peak serum levels may occur in 1 to 2 hours, but unpredictably because of high plasma protein binding (93% to 97%). Mostly metabolized in liver. Approximately 80% of single dose is excreted in urine within 24 hours as intact drug and conjugates. Small amounts are excreted in feces. Crosses placenta; negligible excretion in breast milk.

CONTRAINDICATIONS AND PRECAUTIONS
Known hypersensitivity to nalidixic acid, history of convulsive disorders, first trimester of pregnancy, infants younger than 3 months of age. Cautious use: second and third trimesters of pregnancy, renal or hepatic disease, epilepsy, severe cerebral arteriosclerosis.

GI (common): nausea, vomiting, abdominal pain, diarrhea; (occasionally): bleeding. **CNS:** drowsiness, dizziness, vertigo, muscle weakness, myalgia, visual disturbances; (with overdosage): headache, intracranial hypertension, convulsions, toxic psychosis (rare), 6th cranial nerve palsy (lateral rectus muscle of eye). **Allergic:** photosensitivity, angioedema, pruritus, urticaria, rash, fever, arthralgia (with joint swelling), eosinophilia, anaphylactoid reaction (rare). **Other reported:** cholestasis; metabolic acidosis (with overdosage); paresthesias; thrombocytopenia, leukopenia, hemolytic anemia (especially in glucose-6-phosphate dehydrogenase deficiency); increased BUN and SGOT; glycosuria and hyperglycemia (overdosage).

ROUTE AND DOSAGE

Oral: **Adults:** initially 1 Gm 4 times a day for 1 or 2 weeks; reduced to 500 mg 4 times a day for prolonged therapy. **Children** *over 3 months to age 12:* initially 55 mg/kg/day in 4 equally divided doses; for prolonged therapy, may be reduced to 33 mg/kg/day.

NURSING IMPLICATIONS

Culture and sensitivity tests are advised prior to initiation of treatment and periodically during therapy. Bacterial resistance sometimes develops within 48 hours after start of therapy. Follow-up cultures are also advised to determine if infection is eliminated.

Reportedly, blood levels are higher when drug is administered on empty stomach than when taken with food, but how this affects outcome of urinary level is unknown (because of high plasma protein binding). May be administered with food or milk if patient complains of GI distress.

CNS reactions tend to occur 30 minutes after initiation of treatment or after second or third dose. Infants, children, and geriatric patients are especially susceptible. Observe for and report immediately the onset of marked irritability, vomiting, bulging of anterior fontanelle (infants), headache, excitement or drowsiness, papilledema, vertigo.

Subjective visual distrubances may occur during first few days of therapy. Report to physician. Symptoms usually disappear promptly with reduction of dosage or discontinuation of therapy.

Blood counts and renal and hepatic function tests are recommended if therapy is continued longer than 2 weeks.

Caution patient to avoid exposure to direct sunlight or ultraviolet light while receiving drug. Therapy should be discontinued if photosensitivity occurs (erythema or bullae on exposed skin surfaces). Susceptible patients may continue to be photosensitive up to 3 months after termination of drug.

LABORATORY TEST INTERFERENCES: False positive urine tests for glucose with copper reduction methods (eg, Benedict's, Clinitest, Fehling's), but not with glucose oxidase methods (eg, Clinistix, Tes-Tape). May cause elevation of urinary 17-ketosteroids (Zimmerman method).

DRUG INTERACTIONS: Absorption of nalidixic acid may be decreased by **antacids;** however, **sodium bicarbonate** may increase absorption (clinical significance not determined). **Nitrofurantoin** may antagonize effect of nalidixic acid. Nalidixic acid may enhance effects of **oral anticoagulants** (by displacing them from protein binding sites).

(NALLINE HYDROCHLORIDE)

Narcotic antagonist

ACTIONS AND USES

N-allyl analog of morphine with narcotic antagonist and agonist (morphinelike) properties. In presence of narcotic depression, acts as antagonist; in absence of narcotic effects, exhibits morphinelike properties. Almost as effective as morphine in relief of pain, but dysphoria precludes its use as an analgesic, and psychotomimetic effects discourage its misuse and abuse. Ineffective against mild opioid-induced respiratory depression and that produced by nonnarcotic CNS depressants or pathologic causes, and may increase it. Believed to act in part by competing with morphinelike drugs for stereospecific opioid receptor sites.

Used in treatment of significant respiratory depression induced by natural and synthetic narcotics; used in asphyxia neonatorum from maternal narcotization, and for diagnosis of possible narcotic dependence.

ABSORPTION AND FATE

Acts within minutes following IV injection and within 5 to 20 minutes following subcutaneous administration. Duration of action 2 to 4 hours. High concentrations in brain. Largely metabolized in liver, and excreted as conjugates within 4 hours. Crosses placenta.

CONTRAINDICATIONS AND PRECAUTIONS

Hypersensitivity to nalorphine, narcotic addiction (except as diagnostic agent), respiratory depression induced by nonnarcotic CNS depressants, mild respiratory depression.

ADVERSE REACTIONS

Drowsiness, lethargy, dysphoria, pallor, miosis, pseudoptosis, sweating, hypotension, dizziness, nausea, vomiting, headache, salivation, ataxia, sensation of limb heaviness, slurred speech, hot and cold flashes, respiratory depression. **High doses:** euphoria, psychotomimetic effects (anxiety, hallucinations, disturbed sleep, weird dreams and daydreams, disorientation, panic, feelings of unreality).

ROUTE AND DOSAGE

Adults: Intravenous: 2 to 10 mg at 10- to 15-minute intervals, if necessary; not to exceed 3 doses. Initial dose should not exceed 5 mg if respiratory depression is caused by unknown agents. Subcutaneous (diagnosis of narcotic addiction): 1 to 3 mg; if withdrawal symptoms have not appeared within 20 to 30 minutes, second dose (5 mg) and third dose (8 mg) given 20 to 30 minutes apart, if necessary. **Pediatric:** Intravenous, intramuscular: 0.1 mg/kg/dose; maximum 3 doses. Asphyxia neonatorum: initially 0.2 mg into umbilical vein; if necessary, repeated at close intervals to maximum of 0.5 mg. If umbilical vein cannot be used, may be given IM or subcutaneously: use neonatal concentration (0.2 mg/ml).

NURSING IMPLICATIONS

Monitor respiratory rate and volume and other vital signs.

In treatment of respiratory depression, nalorphine is administered in conjunction with oxygen, artificial respiration, airway maintenance, and other resuscitative measures.

Nalorphine does not affect morphine-induced drowsiness. Anticipate that patient will remain sedated and drowsy for hours.

Since antagonistic effects of nalorphine are generally shorter than action of narcotic, respiratory depression may return as effects of nalorphine disappear. Patient should be closely observed for at least a day or more regardless of apparent improvement.

Diagnostic test for detection of narcotic addiction is administered only by physician in presence of reliable witness. Before test is started, physician will inform patient of risks involved and possible reactions if narcotics have been used. Physical examination and thorough medical and drug history should be completed before test.

Negative test results: abstinence symptoms not produced; only direct effects of nalorphine may be observed: yawning, miosis (mydriasis or no pupil change if administered within 24 hours after 1 or 2 therapeutic doses of morphine), lacrimation, respiratory depression (see Adverse Reactions).

Positive test results: appearance of withdrawal symptoms within 20 minutes indicates narcotic dependence: mydriasis, profuse sweating, yawning, rhinorrhea, lacrimation, hyperpnea, gooseflesh, fainting, sensation of heat, sensations of electric shocks in head, abdominal cramps, nausea, vomiting, defecation. Symptoms begin to wane in about 1 hour and usually disappear by 3 hours.

Withdrawal symptoms may be precipitated in patients who have received several doses of a narcotic for therapeutic analgesia. Produces symptoms in meperidine addicts only if taking 1.6 Gm or more daily. Symptoms will be particularly severe in methadone addicts.

Following completion of diagnostic test, continue to observe patient closely until effects of nalorphine disappear (for at least 4 hours, or longer if indicated).

Nalorphine should not be mixed with solutions of meperidine, as precipitation may occur.

Classified as schedule III drug under federal Controlled Substances Act. Protect drug from light.

NALOXONE HYDROCHLORIDE, U.S.P.
(NARCAN)

Narcotic antagonist

ACTIONS AND USES

N-allyl analog of oxymorphone. A "pure" narcotic antagonist, essentially free of agonistic (morphinelike) properties. Thus, unlike other narcotic antagonists (nalorphine and levallorphan), produces no significant analgesia, respiratory depression, psychotomimetic effects, or miosis when administered in the absence of narcotics, and possesses more potent narcotic antagonist action. In common with other narcotic antagonists, is not effective against non-opioid-induced respiratory depression. Tolerance and psychic or physical dependence not reported.

Used in treatment of narcotic overdosage and to reverse respiratory depression induced by natural and synthetic narcotics, and by pentazocine, and propoxyphene. Drug of choice when nature of depressant drug is not known, and for diagnosis of suspected acute narcotic overdosage.

ABSORPTION AND FATE

Onset of action following IV injection occurs within 2 minutes and within 2 to 5 minutes after subcutaneous or IM administration. Duration of action 3 to 5 hours, depending on dosage and route. Plasma half-life 60 to 90 minutes. Rapidly metabolized in liver, primarily by conjugation with glucuronic acid. Based on limited studies, 25% to 40% of IV dose is excreted in urine as metabolites in 6 hours and 60% to 70% in 72 hours. Readily crosses placenta.

CONTRAINDICATIONS AND PRECAUTIONS

Known hypersensitivity to naloxone; respiratory depression due to non-opioid drugs. Safe use during pregnancy (other than labor) not established. Cautious use: in neonates and children; known or suspected narcotic dependence; cardiac irritability.

ADVERSE REACTIONS

Excessive dosage in narcotic depression: reversal of analgesia, increased blood pressure, tremors, hyperventilation, slight drowsiness, elevated partial thromboplastin time. Too rapid reversal: nausea, vomiting, sweating, tachycardia.

ROUTE AND DOSAGE

Subcutaneous, intramuscular, intravenous: **Adults:** 0.4 mg; may be repeated IV at 2- to 3-minute intervals, if necessary, for 2 or 3 doses; **Pediatric:** 0.01 mg/kg; may be repeated as for adult administration.

NURSING IMPLICATIONS

Resuscitative measures such as maintaining airway, artificial ventilation, cardiac massage, and vasopressor agents may be required.

Monitor respirations and other vital signs. In some patients, respirations may "overshoot" to higher level than that prior to respiratory depression.

Duration of action of some narcotics may exceed that of naloxone; therefore, patient must be closely observed. Keep physician informed; repeat naloxone dose may be necessary.

Narcotic abstinence symptoms induced by naloxone generally start to diminish 20 to 40 minutes after administration and usually disappear within 90 minutes.

Surgical and obstetric patients should be closely monitored for bleeding. Naloxone has been associated with abnormal coagulation test results. Also observe for reversal of analgesia, which may be manifested by nausea, vomiting, sweating, tachycardia.

Not listed in controlled substance inventory list (1977 revision).

Protect drug from excessive light.

NANDROLONE DECANOATE, N.F.
(DECA-DURABOLIN)
NANDROLONE PHENPROPIONATE, N.F.
(DURABOLIN)

Anabolic agent

ACTIONS AND USES

Synthetic steroid with high ratio of anabolic activity to androgenic activity. Both esters have same actions and uses, but differ in action duration: decanoate action lasts 3 to 4 weeks; phenpropionate ester continues to exert anabolic effect for 1 to 3 weeks. See Ethylestrenol for actions, uses, and limitations.

ROUTE AND DOSAGE

Intramuscular: **Adults:** 50 to 100 mg *decanoate* every 3 to 4 weeks (100 to 200 mg weekly may be required for severe disease states); 25 to 50 mg *phenpropionate* weekly; 50 to 100 mg weekly may be required for severe disease states; **Children** *2 to 13 years:* 25 to 50 mg *decanoate* every 3 to 4 weeks; 12.5 to 25 mg *phenpropionate* every 2 to 4 weeks.

NURSING IMPLICATIONS

Inject drug deep IM, preferably into gluteal muscle in adult; follow agency policy regarding IM site in small child.

Intermittent therapy is usually recommended.(4 months course of treatment followed by 6 to 8 weeks rest period).
Also see Ethylestrenol.

NAPHAZOLINE HYDROCHLORIDE, U.S.P.
(CLEAR EYES, PRIVINE, VASOCON)

Adrenergic (vasoconstrictor)

ACTIONS AND USES

Direct-acting imidazoline derivative with marked α-adrenergic activity. Produces rapid and prolonged vasoconstriction of arterioles, thereby decreasing fluid exudation and mucosal engorgement. Differs from other sympathomimetic amines in that systemic absorption may cause CNS depression rather than stimulation.

Used topically as nasal decongestant and as topical ocular vasoconstrictor.

CONTRAINDICATIONS AND PRECAUTIONS

Hypersensitivity to any ingredients of preparation; narrow-angle glaucoma; concomitant use with MAO inhibitors or tricyclic antidepressants. Safe use during pregnancy or in infants or children not established. Cautious use: hypertension, cardiac irregularities, advanced arteriosclerosis, diabetes, hyperthyroidism, elderly patients.

ADVERSE REACTIONS

Nasal use: transient stinging or burning, dryness of nasal mucosa, hypersensitivity reactions. **Ophthalmic use:** pupillary dilation, increased intraocular pressure. **Overdosage** (systemic absorption): headache, lightheadedness, hypertension, palpitation, tachycardia, arrhythmias, hyperglycemia, marked sedation (accidental swallowing in children), hypothermia, cardiovascular collapse, respiratory depression.

ROUTE AND DOSAGE

Topical (nasal solution 0.05%): 2 drops in each nostril, no more frequently than every 3 hours; (nasal spray 0.05%): 2 sprays in each nostril every 4 to 6 hours; (ophthalmic solution 0.012% to 0.1%): 1 or 2 drops into conjunctival sac of affected eye every 3 or 4 hours (frequency depends on response).

NURSING IMPLICATIONS

Note that some commercial nasal solution preparations are designed to instill 2 drops with a single compression of dropper bulb (maximum dose is 2 drops).

Insomnia has not been reported; therefore, one dose may be scheduled at bedtime.

Instill nasal spray with patient in upright position. If administered in reclining position, a stream rather than a spray may be ejected, with possibility of systemic reaction.

Naphazoline is incompatible with aluminum. Do not use atomizers made of aluminum or that have moving aluminum parts.

When instilling nose drops, the amount of drug swallowed can be minimized by taking care not to direct the flow toward nasopharynx and by proper positioning of patient. Position used depends on condition being treated. Consult physician. Parkinson position: patient supine, head over edge of bed and turned to affected side (used for treating nasal passages and frontal and maxillary sinuses). Proetz position: patient supine, with head hanging straight back over edge of bed (used to treat ethmoid and sphenoid sinuses). Both positions can also be accomplished be placing pillow under patient's shoulders.

Following nasal instillation or spray, rinse dropper or spray top in hot water to prevent contamination of solution.

Rebound congestion and chemical rhinitis can occur with frequent and continued use.

Advise patient not to exceed prescribed regimen. Explain that systemic effects can result from swallowing excessive medication.

If nasal congestion is not relieved after 5 days, advise patient to discontinue medication and to contact physician.

To prevent contamination of eye solution, care should be taken not to touch eyelid or surrounding area with dropper tip.

Warn patient to keep drug out of reach of children.

Preserved in tight, light-resistant containers.

DRUG INTERACTIONS: Possibility of enhanced pressor effect when administered concomitantly with or within 2 weeks of **MAO inhibitors** or with **tricyclic antidepressants.**

NEOMYCIN SULFATE, U.S.P., B.P.
(MYCIFRADIN SULFATE, MYCIGUENT, NEOBIOTIC)

Antibacterial (aminoglycoside)

ACTIONS AND USES

Aminoglycoside antibiotic obtained from *Streptomyces fradiae;* reported to be the most potent in neuromuscular blocking action and the most nephrotoxic of this group. Broad spectrum of antibacterial activity, and actions similar to those of kanamycin (qv).

Used in treatment of severe diarrhea caused by enteropathogenic *Escherichia coli;* and for preoperative intestinal antisepsis; used to inhibit nitrogen-forming bacteria of GI tract in patients with cirrhosis or heptic coma and for treatment of urinary tract infections caused by susceptible organisms. Also used topically for short-term treatment of eye, ear, and skin infections. Available in a variety of creams, ointments, and sprays in combination with other antibacterials and corticosteroids.

ABSORPTION AND FATE

About 3% absorbed from GI tract following oral administration (neonates and prematures may absorb up to 10%). Peak plasma levels in 1 to 4 hours; still present in low levels at 8 hours. Half-life in adults about 2 hours (longer in patients with renal impairment and premature infants). About 90% bound to serum proteins. May be absorbed through ear, eye, denuded or inflamed skin, and body cavities following topical applications. Wide distribution in body tissues and fluids following IM administration; 30% to 50% of dose is excreted unchanged in urine, and about 97% of oral dose is excreted unchanged in feces.

CONTRAINDICATIONS AND PRECAUTIONS

History of sensitivity to topical or systemic neomycin or to any ingredient in formulations; use of oral drug in patients with intestinal obstruction; ulcerative bowel lesions; topical applications over large skin areas; parenteral use in patients with renal disease or impaired hearing; myasthenia gravis. Safe use during pregnancy not established. Cautious use: topical otic applications to patients with perforated eardrum. Also see Kanamycin.

ADVERSE REACTIONS

Oral use: mild laxative effect, diarrhea, nausea, vomiting; prolonged therapy: malabsorptionlike syndrome including cyanocobalamin (vitamin B_{12}) deficiency, low serum cholesterol. **Topical use:** redness, scaling, pruritus, dermatitis. **Systemic absorption:** nephrotoxicity, ototoxicity, neuromuscular blockade with muscular and respiratory paralysis, hypersensitivity reactions. See Kanamycin.

ROUTE AND DOSAGE

> **Adults:** Oral: (intestinal antisepsis): 1 Gm every hour for 4 doses, then 1 Gm every 4 hours for balance of 24 hours; alternatively 88 to 100 mg/kg daily in 6 divided doses for not more than 3 days; Coma: 4 to 12.5 Gm daily in 4 divided doses for 5 or 6 days. Retention enema: 1% or 2% solution; Diarrhea: 50 mg/kg in 4 divided doses for 2 or 3 days (average 3 Gm/day in divided doses). Intramuscular: 15 mg/kg in divided doses every 6 hours (infrequently used). Topical (5 mg/Gm): ointment, cream. **Pediatric:** Oral: 10 to 50 mg/kg daily divided into 4 to 6 doses; **Older infants and children:** 50 to 100 mg/kg daily divided into 4 to 6 doses.

NURSING IMPLICATIONS

Patients with renal or hepatic dysfunction receiving IM or extended oral neomycin therapy should have audiometric studies twice weekly, daily urinalysis for albumin, casts, and cells, and BUN every other day. Baseline determinations should be done before initiation of therapy. Serum drug levels also advised (toxic levels reportedly range from 8 to 30 μg/ml, although individual variations exist).

Neomycin can cause irreversible damage to auditory branch of 8th cranial nerve (occurs more frequently than vestibular damage). At first, loss of hearing most often involves high-frequency sounds, then may progress to include normal hearing frequencies. In general, severity and persistence of ototoxic symptoms depend on dosage and duration of drug therapy; these have occurred in patients on prolonged therapy even when serum drug levels have been low. Early reporting is essential.

Advise patient to report any unusual symptom related to ears or hearing: eg, tinnitus, roaring sounds, loss of hearing acuity, dizziness.

For treatment of diarrhea: Neomycin is used as adjunct to fluid and electrolyte replacement and bed rest.

Patients with hepatic coma: When neomycin therapy is initiated, protein is usually restricted from diet, and carbohydrate intake is increased. Diuretics are generally withheld. As symptoms subside and cerebral functions clear (eg, handwriting improves), protein intake is gradually increased.

Neomycin retention enema is sometimes prescribed for patients with hepatic coma. Recommended dilution for adults: 200 ml to 1 liter of 1% solution or 100 ml of 2% solution, to be retained for 20 minutes to more than 1 hour, as prescribed.

Monitor intake and output in patients receiving oral or parenteral therapy. Report oliguria or changes in intake–output ratio. Inadequate neomycin excretion results in high serum drug levels and risk of nephrotoxicity and ototoxicity.

Preoperative bowel preparation: Low-residue diet should be prescribed. Saline cathartic is generally given immediately before neomycin therapy is initiated. Daily enemas may also be ordered.

Topical use: The possibility of systemic absorption and sensitization should be considered. High incidence of allergic dermatitis is associated with topical neomycin. Sensitivity may be manifested as persistent dermatitis. Caution patient to stop treatment and report to physician if irritation occurs.

Patients who develop sensitivity should be informed that they will probably continue to be sensitive to neomycin and to other aminoglycoside antibiotics (gentamycin, kanamycin, neomycin, streptomycin).

For applications to skin: Consult physician about what to use for cleansing the part to be treated before each neomycin application.

Topical therapy of external ear is most effective if canal is clean and dry prior to instillation of neomycin. Consult physician. Duration of treatment should be limited to 7 to 10 days.

Caution patient not to exceed prescribed dosage or duration of therapy.

Parenteral solutions should be stored in refrigerator (2 C to 15 C) to minimize possibility of contamination and discoloration and should be used as soon as possible, preferably within 1 week after reconstitution.

DRUG INTERACTIONS: Neomycin may reduce **cyanocobalamin** (vitamin B_{12}) absorption. Also see Kanamycin.

NEOSTIGMINE BROMIDE, U.S.P., B.P.
(PROSTIGMIN BROMIDE)
NEOSTIGMINE METHYLSULFATE, U.S.P., B.P.
(PROSTIGMIN METHYLSULFATE)

Cholinergic (cholinesterase inhibitor)

ACTIONS AND USES

Synthetic quaternary ammonium analog of physostigmine, but less likely to cause disturbing side effects. Produces reversible cholinesterase inhibition or inactivation, and thus allows intensified and prolonged effect of acetylcholine at cholinergic synapses (basis for use in myasthenia gravis). Also produces generalized cholinergic response, including miosis, increased tonus of intestinal and skeletal muscles, constriction of bronchi and ureters, slower pulse rate, and stimulation of salivary and sweat glands. Has direct stimulant action on voluntary muscle fibers and possibly on autonomic ganglia and CNS neurons. Use in amenorrhea or as pregnancy test is based on premise that delayed menstruation may be due to diminished vascular responsiveness to acetylcholine.

Used to prevent and treat postoperative abdominal distension and urinary retention; for symptomatic control of and sometimes for differential diagnosis of myasthenia gravis; and to reverse the effects of nondepolarizing muscle relaxants, eg, tubocurarine. Also has been used for treatment of delayed menstruation and as screening test for early pregnancy. Used investigationally in treatment of supraventricular tachycardia resulting from overdosage of tricyclic antidepressants.

ABSORPTION AND FATE

Poorly and irregularly absorbed from GI tract. Onset of action occurs in 2 to 4 hours following oral administration and in 10 to 30 minutes following parenteral injection; duration of effect is 2.5 to 4 hours. Does not cross blood–brain barrier, except at extremely high doses. Metabolized in liver by microsomal enzymes. Excreted in urine.

CONTRAINDICATIONS AND PRECAUTIONS

Known hypersensitivity to neostigmine or bromide (oral formulation); mechanical, intestinal, or urinary obstruction; megacolon; peritonitis; acute peptic ulcer; urinary tract infection; hyperthyroidism. Safe use during pregnancy not established. Cautious use: bronchial asthma, bradycardia, cardiac arrhythmias, hypotension, recent coronary occlusion, epilepsy, vagotonia, patients receiving other anticholinergic drugs.

ADVERSE REACTIONS

Muscarinic effects: nausea, vomiting, eructation, epigastric discomfort, abdominal cramps, diarrhea, involuntary or difficult defecation or micturition, increased salivation (common) and bronchial secretions, tightness in chest, sneezing, cough, dyspnea, diaphoresis, lacrimation, miosis, blurred vision, bradycardia, hypotension. **Nicotinic effects:** muscle cramps, fasciculations (common), twitching, pallor, elevated blood pressure, fatigability, generalized weakness, respiratory depression and paralysis. **Cholinergic crisis (overdosage):** any or all of the above; with extremely high doses, also CNS stimulation, fear, agitation, restlessness.

ROUTE AND DOSAGE

Neostigmine bromide: Oral (myasthenia gravis): initially 15 to 30 mg 3 or 4 times daily, increased gradually until maximum benefit obtained. Maintenance dose range 15 to 375 mg daily, depending on patient's needs and tolerance. Neostigmine methylsulfate: Subcutaneous, intramuscular: (myasthenia gravis): 0.5 mg; subsequent doses based on individual response; (myasthenia gravis diagnosis): 0.022 mg/kg IM; to prevent postoperative distension and urinary retention: 0.25 mg subcutaneously or IM every 4 to 6 hours for 2 or 3 days; (for treatment): 0.5 to 1 mg subcutaneous or IM (for urinary retention, dose may be repeated every 3 hours for 5 doses after bladder has been emptied); (screening test for pregnancy): 1 mg IM daily for 3 successive days; (antidote for tubocurarine): 0.5 to 2 mg IV administered slowly, repeated as required.

NURSING IMPLICATIONS

Note that size of oral dose is considerably larger than that of parenteral dose because drug is poorly absorbed when taken orally (15 mg of oral drug is approximately equivalent to 0.5 mg of parenteral form).

Check pulse before giving drug to bradycardic patients. If below 80/minute, consult physician. Atropine will be ordered to restore heart rate.

For treatment of myasthenia gravis: monitor pulse, respiration, and blood pressure during period of dosage adjustment.

If patient has difficulty chewing, physician may prescribe oral neostigmine 30 to 45 minutes before meals. If patient has difficulty swallowing, the parenteral form may be necessary. Some patients require a nasogastric tube.

GI (muscarinic) side effects occur especially during early therapy and may be reduced by taking drug with milk or food. Physician may prescribe atropine or other anticholinergic agent with each dose or every other dose to suppress side effects (note: these drugs may mask toxic symptoms of neostigmine).

Regulation of dosage interval is extremely difficult; dosage must be adjusted for each patient to deal with unpredictable exacerbations and remissions.

Report promptly and record accurately the onset of myasthenic symptoms and drug side effects in relation to last dose in order to assist physician in determining lowest effective dosage schedule.

Encourage patient to keep a diary of "peaks and valleys" of muscle strength.

Frequently, drug therapy is required both day and night, with larger portions of total dose being given at times of greater fatigue, as in the late afternoon and at mealtimes.

All activities should be appropriately spaced to avoid undue fatigue.

Deep breathing, coughing, and range-of-motion exercises should be regularly scheduled. Consult physician.

Respiratory depression may appear abruptly in myasthenic patients. Report unusual apprehension (a frequent manifestation of inadequate ventilation), and be alert for tachypnea, tachycardia, restlessness, rising blood pressure.

Have the following immediately available: atropine, facilities for endotracheal intubation, tracheostomy, suction, oxygen, assisted respiration.

In myasthenic patients, the time that muscular weakness appears may indicate whether patient is in cholinergic or myasthenic crisis. Weakness that appears approximately 1 hour after drug administration suggests *cholinergic crisis (overdosage)* and is treated by prompt withdrawal of neostigmine and immediate administration of atropine. Weakness that occurs 3 hours or more after drug administration is more likely to be due to *myasthenic crisis (underdosage or drug resistance)* and is treated by more intensive anticholinesterase therapy.

Manifestations of neostigmine overdosage often appear first in muscles of neck and those involved in chewing and swallowing, with muscles of shoulder girdle and upper extremities affected next.

Signs and symptoms of myasthenia gravis that may be relieved by neostigmine: lid ptosis; diplopia; drooping facies; difficulty in chewing, swallowing, breathing, or coughing; weakness of neck, limbs, and trunk muscles. Record drug effect and duration of action.

Lid ptosis, especially in the elderly, may continue despite drug therapy. Often, patients are helped by means of an adhesive lid crutch attached to rim of eyeglasses.

Some patients become refractory to neostigmine after prolonged use and require change in dosage or medication.

Drug therapy for myasthenia gravis is lifesaving and must be continued throughout patient's life. Patient may require help to overcome psychologic problems associated with prolonged disability.

Patient and responsible family members should be taught to keep an accurate record for physician of patient's response to drug, as well as how to recognize side effects, how to modify dosage regimen according to patient's changing needs, or how to administer atropine if necessary. They should be aware that certain factors may require an increase in size or frequency of dose (eg, physical or emotional stress, infection, menstruation, surgery), whereas remission requires a decrease in dosage.

Advise patient to wear identification bracelet (such as Medic Alert) indicating the presence of myasthenia gravis. Also inform patient and family of educational resources provided by Myasthenia Gravis Foundation, Inc., New York Academy of Medicine Building, 2 East 103rd Street, New York, N.Y. 10029.

Neostigmine test for myasthenia gravis: The neostigmine test has been largely replaced by the edrophonium (Tensilon) test. All anticholinesterase medications should be discontinued at least 8 hours before test. Accurate recordings are made of grip strength, vital capacity, range of extraocular movements, ptosis, etc, before test (usually, atropine sulfate 0.6 mg IM is given prior to or concomitantly with neostigmine methylsulfate to prevent muscarinic effects). After neostigmine is given, muscle strength is retested at 15-minute intervals for 1 hour. Objective and subjective improvement in strength and movement indicates positive test. Nonmyasthenic patient may experience weakness, abdominal cramps, diarrhea, diaphoresis, dysuria.

When neostigmine is used as antidote for tubocurarine (or other nondepolarizing neuromuscular blocking agents), monitor respiration, maintain airway or assisted ventilation, and give oxygen as indicated. Respiratory assistance is continued until recovery of respiration and neuromuscular transmission is assured.

For relief of postoperative abdominal distension: Rectal tube (prescribed by physician) is inserted following drug administration to facilitate expulsion of gas. Lubricated tube is inserted just past rectal sphincter and kept in place for about 1 hour. In some cases, a small low enema may be prescribed. Record results: passage of flatus, decrease in abdominal distension, pain, rigidity.

For relief of urinary retention: Report to physician if patient does not urinate within 1 hour after first dose. Generally, catheterization will be prescribed if patient fails to void.

Screening test for early pregnancy and treatment of delayed menstruation: Patient is assumed to be pregnant if bleeding does not occur within 72 hours after third consecutive daily dose, providing other causes are ruled out. Positive diagnosis of pregnancy is not made until results are checked by biologic tests.

DRUG INTERACTIONS: Parenteral neostigmine antagonizes the effects of **nondepolarizing neuromuscular blocking agents,** eg, **gallamine, metocurine, pancuronium, tubocurarine** (interaction used therapeutically). Upward adjustment of neostigmine dosage may be required in myasthenic patients receiving drugs that interfere with neuromuscular transmission, eg, **aminoglycoside antibiotics (gentamicin, kanamycin, neomycin, streptomycin),** local anesthetics and some **general anesthetics,** and **antiarrhythmic agents,** eg, **procainamide, quinidine** (all used with extreme caution, if at all). Neostigmine may prolong the action of depolarizing muscle relaxants, eg, **decamethonium, succinylcholine.** Muscarinic effects of neostigmine are antagonized by **atropine** (interaction used therapeutically).

NIACIN, N.F.

(DIACIN, NIAC, NIACELS, NICAMIN, NICOBID, NICO-400, NICOCAP, NICOLAR, NICO-SPAN, NICOTINEX, Nicotonic Acid, TEGA-SPAN, TINIC, VASOTHERM, WAMPOCAP)

Vitamin (enzyme cofactor), antipellagra vitamin

ACTIONS AND USES

Water-soluble, heat-stable B-complex vitamin vaguely related chemically to nicotine, but possesses none of its pharmacologic properties. Functions with riboflavin as a control agent in coenzyme system that converts protein, carbohydrate, and fat to energy through oxidation–reduction. In large doses, capable of lowering serum cholesterol, triglyceride, and free fatty acid levels by an unknown mechanism. Also produces vasodilation (primarily of cutaneous vessels) by direct action on vascular smooth muscles, and is capable of causing histamine release. Niacin and its precursor tryptophan are essential for prevention of pellagra.

Used in prophylactic treatment of pellagra, usually in combination with other B-complex vitamins, and in deficiency states accompanying carcinoid syndrome, isoniazid therapy, and Hartnup's disease. Has been used as adjunctive treatment in hyperlipidemia (no clear evidence that it is beneficial or detrimental) and as vasodilator in peripheral vascular disorders, Meniere's disease, and labyrinthine syndrome, as well as to counteract LSD toxicity and to distinguish between psychoses of dietary and nondietary origin.

ABSORPTION AND FATE

Readily absorbed following oral or parenteral administration; however, individual variations may exist. Widely distributed to all body tissues, with minimal storage. Metabolized in liver. Small doses excreted in urine, chiefly as metabolites; large doses excreted primarily as unchanged vitamin.

CONTRAINDICATIONS AND PRECAUTIONS

Hypersensitivity to niacin or niacinamide; hepatic dysfunction, active peptic ulcer, gastritis, hemorrhage, severe hypotension. Safe use during pregnancy and lactation and in women of childbearing age and children not established. Cautious use: glaucoma, gout, diabetes, angina, gallbladder disease, allergies, history of peptic ulcer, jaundice, or liver disease.

Flushing of face and neck, pruritus, burning, tingling, dryness of skin, increased sebaceous gland activity, headache, dizziness, faintness, mild hypotension, increased GI motility, flatulence, diarrhea, anorexia, heartburn, nausea, vomiting (all the preceding are usually transient). Keratosis nigricans, toxic amblyopia, activation of peptic ulcer, impaired liver function (reversible), jaundice, hyperglycemia, glycosuria, hyperuricemia, gout, allergic reactions, fall in blood pressure, anaphylaxis (following IV).

ROUTE AND DOSAGE

Oral: *Antipellagra:* 25 to 50 mg 1 to 10 times daily; timed-release form: 125 or 250 mg morning and evening. Subcutaneous, intramuscular, intravenous: 25 to 50 mg 2 or more times daily; *Antihyperlipidemia:* initially ½ to 3 Gm daily; if no response dosage is increased to 4.5 Gm/day and then after several weeks to maximum of 6 Gm/day. *Vasodilation:* 50 mg 3 times daily.

NURSING IMPLICATIONS

With exception of timed-release forms, oral niacin should be administered with or shortly after meals to reduce incidence of GI side effects. If necessary to facilitate swallowing, take with cold water (avoid hot beverages).

Blood glucose and liver function tests are recommended during early drug therapy.

Diabetics and potential diabetics will require close monitoring. Hyperglycemia, glycosuria, ketonuria, and increased insulin requirements have been reported in high-dosage regimens.

Inform patient that vasodilation effects occur within minutes after oral ingestion (and immediately after parenteral administration) and may last a few minutes to 1 hour.

Caution patient to sit or lie down if weakness or dizziness is experienced and to report these symptoms and persistent flushing to physician. Relief may be obtained by reduction of dosage, by increasing subsequent doses in small increments, or by changing to sustained-action form. If drug is being used solely for niacin deficiency, physician may prescribe niacinamide, which is devoid of vasodilatory effects.

In treatment of hyperlipidemia, dosage is individualized according to effect on serum lipid levels. Patients who do not exhibit anticipated fall in serum lipid values may respond if tablets are chewed and followed with adequate amounts of water.

For treatment of niacin deficiency, small doses given frequently during the day are reported to be more effective than single large daily doses, since a considerable amount of the latter is excreted in urine.

Therapeutic response usually begins within 24 hours. Note and record effect of therapy on clinical manifestations of deficiency.

Caution patient with skin manifestations to avoid exposure to direct sunlight until lesions have entirely cleared.

Subclinical niacin deficiency is often associated with poverty, chronic alcoholism, dietary fads, pregnancy, cachexia of malignancy, isoniazid therapy, and chronic GI disease.

Recommended dietary allowance expressed in niacin equivalents is 6.6 mg/1000 kcal.

Rich niacin food sources: liver, kidney, lean meats, poultry, fish, brewer's yeast, wheat germ, and peanuts and other legumes. Milk and eggs contain small amounts, and they are excellent sources of tryptophan, a precursor of niacin (1 mg of niacin is derived from each 60 mg of dietary tryptophan).

Collaborate with physician, dietitian, patient, and a responsible family member in development of a teaching plan that includes total nutritional needs. Niacin deficiency is invariably accompanied by deficiencies in other B-complex vitamins.

LABORATORY TEST INTERFERENCES: False elevations with certain fluorometric methods of determining urinary catecholamines.

DRUG INTERACTIONS: Niacin may potentiate vasodilating and postural hypotension effects of **antihypertensives** (ganglionic blocking type).

NIACINAMIDE, U.S.P.
(NICOTINAMIDE)

Vitamin (enzyme cofactor)

ACTIONS AND USES
Amide of niacin used as alternative in prevention and treatment of pellagra. Has same actions as those of niacin (qv). Preferred to niacin in treatment of deficiency because it lacks unpleasant vasodilatory action and the hypolipemic, hepatic, and GI effects of niacin.

ROUTE AND DOSAGE
Oral (antipellagra): 25 to 50 mg 1 to 10 times daily. Subcutaneous, intramuscular, intravenous: 25 to 50 mg 2 times or more daily. Highly individualized.

NURSING IMPLICATIONS
See Niacin.

NICOTINYL ALCOHOL
(RONIACOL)
NICOTINYL TARTRATE
(RONIACOL TARTRATE)

Vasodilator (peripheral)

ACTIONS AND USES
Almost identical to niacin (nicotinic acid) in pharmacologic properties, but reportedly has more prolonged action. Converted to nicotinic acid in body. Produces peripheral vasodilation by direct action on vascular smooth muscle. Also reported to have antilipemic activity in higher doses, but may intensify carbohydrate intolerance. See Niacin.

Used in conditions associated with deficient circulation, as in peripheral vascular disease, vascular spasm, varicose ulcers, decubital ulcers, chilblains, Meniere's syndrome, and vertigo.

CONTRAINDICATIONS AND PRECAUTIONS
Cautious use: during pregnancy.

ADVERSE REACTIONS
Flushing of face and neck, nausea, paresthesias (especially in high doses), minor skin rashes, allergies (urticaria, localized angioedema), dizziness (occasionally). Also see Niacin.

ROUTE AND DOSAGE
Oral: 50 to 100 mg 3 times daily. Timed-release form (nicotinyl tartrate): 150 or 300 mg twice daily, morning and night.

NURSING IMPLICATIONS

Administered before meals.

Inform patient to expect blushing and sensation of warmth.

Caution patient that alcohol and large doses of niacin (in vitamin preparations) used simultaneously may produce additive vasodilation and dizziness.

Tolerance may develop with prolonged use.

See Isoxsuprine Hydrochloride for patient teaching points.

NIKETHAMIDE, N.F., B.P.
(CORAMINE)

Central and respiratory stimulant (analeptic)

ACTIONS AND USES

Diethyl derivative of nicotinamide, the pellagra-preventive vitamin. Similar to doxapram in actions and toxic effects (qv), but generally regarded to be less effective and to have less margin of safety.

Used to overcome CNS depression, respiratory depression, and circulatory failure, particularly when due to CNS depressant drugs. May be combined with electroshock therapy to restore respiration more quickly and to reduce number of required treatments.

ABSORPTION AND FATE

Readily absorbed following oral or IM administration; maximum effect in 10 to 30 minutes; duration about 1 hour. Duration of action following IV is 5 to 10 minutes, but may increase with succeeding doses. Converted in part to nicotinamide in body.

ADVERSE REACTIONS

Burning or itching, especially at back of nose, is the most common side effect. Also see Doxapram.

ROUTE AND DOSAGE

Adults: Intravenous, intramuscular: 1 to 15 ml of 25% solution (250 mg/ml). Oral (maintenance): 3 to 5 ml of 25% oral solution every 4 to 6 hours. **Pediatric:** 25 mg/kg, IV or IM, well diluted.

NURSING IMPLICATIONS

Difference between clinically effective dose and that producing side effects is often small. Therefore, any side effects should be construed to be the result of overdosage.

Widespread CNS stimulation may occur with repeated doses. Observe for and report increases in vital signs, coughing, sneezing, flushing, itching, nausea, vomiting, tremors, muscle rigidity.

See Doxapram Hydrochloride.

(CYANTIN, FURACHEL, FURADANTIN, FURALAN, FURALOID, J-DANTIN, MACRODANTIN, NITREX, NITRODAN, NITROFOR, PARFURAN, SARODANT, TRANTOIN, UROTOIN)
NITROFURANTOIN SODIUM
(FURADANTIN SODIUM)

Antibacterial (urinary)

ACTIONS AND USES

Synthetic nitrofuran derivative related to nitrofurazone. Active against wide variety of Gram-negative and Gram-positive microorganisms, including strains of *Escherichia coli, Staphylococcus aureus, Streptococcus faecalis,* enterococci, and *Klebsiella-Aerobacter. Pseudomonas aeruginosa* and many strains of *Proteus* are resistant. Presumed to act by interfering with several bacterial enzyme systems. Highly soluble in urine and reportedly most active in acid urine. Antimicrobial concentrations in urine exceed those in blood.

Used in treatment of pyelonephritis, pyelitis, and cystitis caused by susceptible organisms.

ABSORPTION AND FATE

Rapidly and almost completely absorbed from GI tract (macrocrystalline form appears to be absorbed more slowly than conventional tablets, but urinary concentrations are not significantly reduced). Half-life 18 minutes to 1 hour. Crosses blood–brain barrier. Degraded by all body tissues (except blood) to inactive metabolites. Excreted rapidly in urine, about 40% of dose as unchanged drug; small amounts may be eliminated in feces. Crosses placenta; enters breast milk.

CONTRAINDICATIONS AND PRECAUTIONS

Known hypersensitivity to nitrofuran derivatives, anuria, oliguria, significant impairment of renal function (creatinine clearance under 40 ml/minute), patients with glucose-6-phosphate dehydrogenase deficiency, infants under 1 month of age, parenteral use in children under 12 years of age. Safe use in women of childbearing potential, during pregnancy, pregnancy at term, and in nursing mothers not established. Cautious use: history of asthma, anemia, diabetes, vitamin B deficiency, electrolyte imbalance, debilitating disease.

ADVERSE REACTIONS

GI (most frequent): anorexia, nausea, vomiting, abdominal pain, diarrhea. **Hypersensitivity:** allergic pneumonitis, eosinophilia, skin eruptions, pruritus, urticaria, angioedema, anaphylaxis, asthmatic attack (patients with history of asthma), drug fever, arthralgia, cholestatic jaundice. **Hematologic** (rare): hemolytic or megaloblastic anemia (especially in patients with glucose-6-phosphate dehydrogenase deficiency), granulocytosis. **Neurologic:** peripheral neuropathy, headache, nystagmus, drowsiness, vertigo. **Others:** transient alopecia, genitourinary superinfections (especially with *Pseudomonas*), tooth straining from direct contact with oral suspension and crushed tablets (infants), and crystalluria (elderly patients); causal relationship not established: interstitial pneumonitis and/or fibrosis.

ROUTE AND DOSAGE

Adults: Oral: 50 to 100 mg 4 times daily. Intramuscular, intravenous (over 120 lb): 180 mg 2 times daily; (under 120 lb): 6.5 mg/kg daily divided into 2 equal doses. **Children** *over 1 month:* Oral: up to 5 to 7 mg/kg/24 hours divided into 4 equal doses.

NURSING IMPLICATIONS

Drug must be given at equally spaced intervals to maintain therapeutic urinary drug levels.

Administer oral drug with meals or milk to minimize gastric irritation.

Nausea occurs fairly frequently and may be relieved by using macrocrystalline preparation (Macrodantin) or by reduction in dosage. Consult physician.

Possibility of tooth staining (reportedly associated with direct contact of oral suspension or crushed tablets with teeth) remains equivocal. As precautionary measure, avoid crushing tablets and dilute oral suspension in milk, infant formula, water, or fruit juice.

Administration by IM route should not exceed 5 days. If therapy is still needed, oral or IV route is used.

Forewarn patient that IM injection of nitrofurantoin may be painful (pain may be severe enough to warrant discontinuation of drug by this route).

Inform patient that nitrofurantoin may impart a harmless brown color to urine (due to drug metabolite).

Monitor intake and output. Report oliguria and any change in intake–output ratio. Drug should be discontinued if oliguria or anuria develops or creatinine clearance falls below 40 ml/minute. (Normal: 115+20 ml/minute).

Consult physician regarding fluid intake. Generally, fluids are not forced, since drug is highly soluble; however, intake should be adequate.

Culture and sensitivity tests are performed prior to therapy and are recommended in patients with recurrent infections.

Be alert to signs of urinary tract superinfections: milky urine, foul-smelling urine, perineal irritation, dysuria.

Acute pulmonary sensitivity reaction usually occurs within first week of therapy and appears to be more common in the elderly. May be manifested by mild to severe flulike syndrome: fever, dyspnea, cough, chest pains, chills, decreased breath sounds, rhonchi and crepitant rates on auscultation. Eosinophilia generally develops in a few days. Recovery usually occurs rapidly after drug is discontinued.

Subacute or chronic pulmonary sensitivity reaction is associated with prolonged therapy. Commonly manifested by insidious onset of malaise, cough, dyspnea on exertion, altered pulmonary function (x-ray findings: interstitial pneumonitis and/or fibrosis).

Peripheral neuropathy can be severe and irreversible. Be alert for and advise the patient to report onset of muscle weakness, tingling, numbness, or other sensations. Reportedly, these are most likely to occur in patients with renal impairment, anemia, diabetes, electrolyte imbalance, vitamin B deficiency, or debilitating disease. Drug should be discontinued immediately.

Treatment is continued for at least 3 days after sterile urines are obtained. Course of treatment for acute infections rarely exceeds 14 days.

Nitrofurantoin sodium should be reconstituted with sterile water *without preservatives* (these cause drug precipitation). See manufacturer's directions.

Dispensed in amber-colored containers; strong light darkens drug. Nitrofurantoin decomposes on contact with metals other than stainless steel or aluminum.

LABORATORY TEST INTERFERENCES: Nitrofurantoin metabolite may produce false positive results with Benedict's reagent.

DRUG INTERACTIONS: Drugs that tend to alkalinize urine (eg, **acetazolamide, thiazides**) may decrease the effect of nitrofurantoin. There is the possibility that **antacids** may delay absorption of nitrofurantoin. Nitrofurantoin may antagonize the effects of **nalidixic acid.** Concomitant administration with **probenecid** (particularly in high doses) and possibly **sulfinpyrazone** may increase nitrofurantoin in serum to toxic levels by decreasing renal clearance (also decreasing effectiveness in urinary tract infections).

NITROFURAZONE, N.F.
(FURACIN, NISEPT, NITRAZONE, NITROFURASTAN, NITROZONE)

Antiinfective (topical)

ACTIONS AND USES

Synthetic nitrofuran related to nitrofurantoin. Bactericidal against most microorganisms causing surface infections, including many that have developed antibiotic resistance. Activity against *Pseudomonas aeruginosa* and certain strains of *Proteus* is limited; has no activity against fungi or viruses. Acts by inhibiting aerobic and anaerobic cycles in bacterial carbohydrate metabolism.

Used topically as adjunctive therapy to combat bacterial infection in second- and third-degree burns; used to prevent infection of skin grafts and/or donor sites. Has been used orally in other countries for treatment of late stage of African trypanosomiasis. Available in combination with other drugs for treatment of bacterial urethritis.

CONTRAINDICATIONS AND PRECAUTIONS

History of sensitization to nitrofuran derivatives. Safe use in women of childbearing potential and during pregnancy not established.

ADVERSE REACTIONS

Allergic contact dermatitis (most frequently reported), irritation, sensitization, superinfections.

ROUTE AND DOSAGE

Topical (available as 0.2% soluble dressing, solution, cream, ointment, powder). Soluble dressing: applied directly to lesions or placed on gauze; reapplied once daily or weekly. Solution: sprayed on painful lesions or burns; 1:1 dilution used for saturating dressing for skin grafts. Powder: applied directly to lesion (with shaker). Cream: applied directly to lesion or placed on gauze; reapplied once daily or every few days.

NURSING IMPLICATIONS

Solutions for wet dressings are prepared by diluting nitrofurazone solution with equal volume of sterile distilled water (preferred to saline). Solution should be used within 24 hours after preparation. Discard if cloudy.

Dressing removal may be facilitated by soaking with nitrofurazone solution (as described in preceding statement) or by flushing with sterile isotonic saline solution.

Confine applications of nitrofurazone to the part being treated. When wet dressings are used, normal skin surrounding the wound should be protected with an agent such as sterile petrolatum, petrolatum gauze, or zinc oxide. Consult physician.

Consult physician regarding procedure for cleaning wound following each dressing removal.

Drug should be discontinued if symptoms of sensitization or allergy occur: redness, itching, burning, swelling, rash, failure to heal.

Preserved in tight, light-resistant containers, away from heat. Drug darkens slowly on exposure to light, but reportedly this does not appreciably affect potency. Discoloration and deterioration may occur with repeated autoclaving.

(CARDABID, GLY-TRATE, NIGLYCON, NITORA, NITRINE-TDC,
NITRO-BID, NITROBON, NITRODYL, NITROGLYN, NITROL,
NITRO-LOR, NITRONG, NITROPRN, NITRO-SA, NITROSPAN,
NITRO-T.D., NITROSTAT, NITROTEST, NITROVAS, NTG, TRATES,
VASOGLYN)

Vasodilator (coronary)

ACTIONS AND USES
Organic nitrate produced from volatile liquid with explosive potential, rendered nonexplosive by addition of carbohydrates. Relaxes all smooth muscle by direct action, with most prominent effect on vascular smooth muscle. Resulting vasodilation produces lowered peripheral resistance, fall in blood pressure, and decreased cardiac output due to reduced venous return to heart. Precise action mechanism in treatment of angina pectoris not established, but appears to be due to reduction in myocardial oxygen consumption. Cross tolerance with other nitrites and nitrates may occur.
Used in prevention and treatment of acute anginal episodes. Sustained release tablets available for longer prophylaxis. Topical application used particularly for patients who fear nocturnal anginal attack. Has been used for temporary pain relief of biliary colic and to relieve paroxysmal nocturnal dyspnea.

ABSORPTION AND FATE
Sublingual tablet acts in 1 to 3 minutes; duration up to 30 minutes. Sustained release tablet acts in about 1 hour; action peaks in 3 to 4 hours and persists 8 to 12 hours. Topical ointment acts in 30 to 60 minutes with duration of 3 or more hours.

CONTRAINDICATIONS AND PRECAUTIONS
Sensitivity or tolerance to nitrites; early myocardial infarction; severe anemia, hypotension, increased intracranial pressure, glaucoma (sustained release forms).

ADVERSE REACTIONS
Transient headache, dizziness, flushing, postural hypotension, palpitation, increased heart rate, nausea, vomiting. Allergic reactions (skin rash, exfoliative dermatitis). **Hypersensitivity:** blurred vision, dry mouth, weakness, restlessness, pallor, perspiration, collapse. **Overdosage:** violent headache, syncope, tachycardia, paradoxical angina, circulatory collapse, coma, respiratory failure; methemoglobinia (toxic doses).

ROUTE AND DOSAGE
Sublingual: 0.4 to 0.6 mg (1/150 gr to 1/100 gr). Individualized dosage. Sustained release form: 1 capsule or tablet every 8 to 12 hours (usually before breakfast and at bedtime). Topical (2% ointment): 1 to 2 inches, as squeezed from tube, every 3 to 4 hours as necessary; some patients may require 4 or 5 inches.

NURSING IMPLICATIONS
Sublingual tablet (discuss following points with physician). Instruct patient to sit or lie down upon first indication of oncoming anginal pain, and place tablet under tongue or in buccal pouch (hypotensive effect of drug is intensified in the upright position). Advise patient to allow tablet to dissolve naturally and not to swallow until drug is entirely dissolved.
As soon as pain is completely relieved, any remaining tablet may be expelled from mouth, especially if patient is experiencing any unpleasant side effects such as headache.
Advise patient to relax 15 to 20 minutes after taking tablet to prevent dizziness or faintness.

If pain not relieved after one tablet, additional tablets may be taken at 5 minute intervals, but no more than 3 tablets per attack. Taking more tablets than necessary can further decrease coronary blood flow by producing systemic hypotension.

Pain not relieved after 15 minutes may indicate acute myocardial infarction or severe coronary insufficiency. Advise patient to contact physician immediately or have someone take him directly to emergency room.

For hospitalized patient, tablets should be kept at bedside. Allocate a specific number (usually 10 tablets) in an appropriate container, label, and make sure patient knows location and use. Request patient to report all attacks. Count tablets at 7 A.M. and 7 P.M.

Transient headache a frequent side effect, usually lasts about 5 minutes after sublingual administration and seldom longer than 20 minutes. Report to physician if persistent or severe. (Patients who do not have coronary disease may experience severe disabling headaches.)

Sublingual tablets may be taken prophylactically 3 to 5 minutes prior to exercise or other stimulus known to trigger anginal pain (drug effect will last up to 30 minutes).

Instruct patient to keep record for physician of number of anginal attacks, number of tablets required for relief of each attack, and possible precipitating factors.

Patient instruction for care of sublingual tablets: Write purchase date on new bottle.

Once bottle is opened, remove cotton filler. Keep bottle tightly capped. Store stock supply in cool, dry place or at controlled room temperature not exceeding 86 F (30 C). Inactivation of nitroglycerin is increased by time, heat, air, moisture.

Inform family members of location of stock supply.

Open stock bottle once weekly to remove week's supply of tablets. Carry these on person at all times, away from body heat (eg, in jacket pocket, handbag).

An empty nitroglycerin bottle is an ideal container for carrying week's supply (amber colored bottle with metal cap). Tablets lose considerable potency in containers made of metal, plastic, or cardboard and when mixed with other capsules or tablets.

After one week, discard unused tablets and replenish supply from stock bottle.

References vary with respect to how long stock supply retains potency: some report 1 month, others 3 months. Positive indication of potency is ability of drug to produce burning or stinging sensation under tongue. (Nitrostat is more stable than other sublingual tablets; it is dispensed in small bottle holding 25 tablets.

Sustained release tablet or capsule should be swallowed whole.

Nitroglycerin ointment (discuss following points with physician).

Before initiation of treatment take baseline blood pressure and heart rate, with patient in sitting position. (Have patient rest approximately 10 minutes before taking measurements.)

One hour after medication has been applied, check blood pressure and pulse again with patient in sitting position. Report measurements to physician. (Appropriate dosage is that which produces 10 mm Hg fall in B.P., or 10 beat rise in resting heart rate.)

Application of ointment: Squeeze prescribed dose onto special measuring application supplied by manufacturer and use it, *not fingers,* to spread ointment. Apply thin layer to premarked 6 by 6 inch square nonhairy skin surface. Areas commonly used: chest, abdomen, anterior thigh, forearm. Do not massage or rub in ointment as this increases absorption and thus interferes with drug's sustained action.

Area may be covered with transparent kitchen wrap and secured with tape to protect clothing.

Rotate application sites to prevent dermal inflammation and sensitization. Remove ointment from previously used sites before reapplication.

To determine optimal dose, physician may initially prescribe ½ or 1 inch of ointment and increase dose ¼ or ½ inch at a time until headache (definitive sign of overdosage) occurs, then gradually reduce dose to that which does not cause headache. If treatment is to be terminated, dosage and frequency of application must be reduced gradually over period of 4 to 6 weeks to prevent withdrawal reactions (pain, severe myocardial ischemia).

Keep ointment container tightly closed and store in cool place.

General Points.

Advise patient to report blurred vision or dry mouth. Both reactions warrant discontinuation of nitroglycerin.

Pain of angina usually described as a squeezing, choking, tight or heavy substernal discomfort. Pain may radiate to arms, shoulders, neck, and lower jaw, and is short in duration, usually less than 10 minutes.

Dizziness, lightheadedness, and syncope (due to postural hypotension) occur most frequently in the elderly. Hasten recovery by head-low position, deep breathing, and movement of extremities. Advise patient to make position changes slowly and to avoid prolonged standing.

Inform patient that a shocklike syndrome (sharp drop in blood pressure, vertigo, flushing or pallor) may occur if alcohol is ingested too soon after taking nitroglycerin.

Tolerance to nitroglycerin rarely occurs with usual intermittent use, but is possible with repeated administration. May be prevented by using smallest effective dose. Temporary withdrawal (few days) usually restores original response to drug.

Advise patient to report to physician any evidence of refractoriness, ie, increase in frequency, duration, or severity of attacks.

Each patient must learn to identify stimuli that precipitate anginal pain in him, and pace his activities accordingly. Known factors that may provoke an attack include: emotional distress, heavy meals, smoking, temperature extremes, excessive use of coffee, tea, colas; sudden burst of physical activity; climbing stairs, especially while talking or carrying heavy bundles.

Regular program of graduated daily exercises is generally recommended as well as control or reduction of body weight, and low cholesterol diet.

Advise patient to carry medical information card or other suitable identification indicating that he is taking nitroglycerin. (May be purchased in drug store or through Medic Alert Foundation, Turlock, Ca. 95380).

LABORATORY TEST INTERFERENCES: Possibility that nitroglycerin may interfere with determinations of urinary catecholamines, and VMA.

DRUG INTERACTIONS: Combined use of nitroglycerin and **alcohol** may produce hypotension from additive vasodilation. Chronic administration of **pentaerythritol tetranitrate** or other long-acting **nitrites** may impair response to subsequently administered nitroglycerin, by producing tolerance.

NORETHINDRONE, U.S.P.
(MICRONOR, NORLUTIN, NOR-Q.D.)
NORETHINDRONE ACETATE, U.S.P.
(NORLUTATE)
NORETHISTERONE, B.P.

Progestogen

ACTIONS AND USES
Norethindrone is a synthetic progestational hormone with androgenic, anabolic, and antiestrogenic properties. Norethindrone acetate also has androgenic effects, but no antiestrogenic properties; it is the most potent anabolic agent available; it has approximately double the progestational potency of norethindrone and may produce excess estrogenic effect.
Both preparations are used in clinical conditions associated with progesterone deficiency. Also used as a contraceptive combined with an estrogen, or as progestin-only contraceptive (Micronor, Nor-Q.D.). See Dydrogesterone for absorption and fate and contraindications.
ADVERSE REACTIONS
Weight gain, acne, hirsutism, deepening of voice. Also see Dydrogesterone.
ROUTE AND DOSAGE
Oral: Norethindrone (Norlutin): Amenorrhea: 5 to 20 mg on day 5 through day 25 of menstrual cycle. Endometriosis: initially 10 mg daily for 2 weeks, with increments of 5 mg daily every 2 weeks up to 30 mg daily; therapy may remain at this level 6 to 9 months or until breakthrough bleeding demands temporary termination. Micronor or Nor-Q.D.: Contraception: 0.35 mg daily without interruption, even during menstruation. Norethindrone acetate: doses are approximately half those of norethindrone.

NURSING IMPLICATIONS
Failure rate of the "mini pill" (Micronor) is 2.54 pregnancies per 100 woman years, or about 3 times higher than the failure rate of the norethindrone-estrogen combinations.
See Dydrogesterone and Oral Contraceptives.

NORGESTREL, U.S.P.
(OVRETTE)

Progestin

ACTIONS AND USES
Potent antiestrogenic progestational hormone with little or no androgenic or anabolic properties. See Dydrogesterone for absorption, fate, contraindications, adverse reactions.
Used as a progestin-only contraceptive ("mini pill").
ROUTE AND DOSAGE
Oral: 0.075 mg (one tablet) daily every day of the year, beginning on first day of menstruation.

NURSING IMPLICATIONS
Reported average pregnancy rate with this contraceptive is 2.3 pregnancies per 100 woman years.
Pill is to be taken at same time each day, even if menstruating.
Amount and duration of flow, cycle length, breakthrough bleeding, spotting, and amenorrhea vary greatly with use of the mini pill.

Manufacturer supplies a patient information brochure that should be made available at time of purchase of norgestrel.
See Dydrogesterone and Oral Contraceptives.

NORTRIPTYLINE HYDROCHLORIDE, N.F., B.P.
(AVENTYL HYDROCHLORIDE)

Tricyclic antidepressant

ACTIONS AND USES
Dibenzocycloheptane derivative of amitriptyline, with actions, contraindications, and adverse reactions similar to those of imipramine (qv). Reportedly more likely to be effective in endogenous depressions than in other depressive states.

ABSORPTION AND FATE
Slowly absorbed from GI tract; peak serum levels occur within 7 to 8.5 hours. Metabolized in liver. Plasma half-life 16 hours to more than 90 hours. Up to 50% of daily dose is excreted in urine within 24 hours, largely as metabolites; small amounts eliminated in feces via bile. Crosses placenta.

CONTRAINDICATIONS AND PRECAUTIONS
Contraindicated in children under 12 years of age. Safe use during pregnancy and lactation not established. See Imipramine.

ADVERSE REACTIONS
High incidence of minor anticholinergic (atropinelike) effects. See Imipramine.

ROUTE AND DOSAGE
Oral: 10 mg twice daily on first day; increased to 3 times daily on second day, and 4 times daily thereafter. Usual dosage range: 75 to 100 mg daily, carefully individualized. Lower than average dosage recommended for adolescents, elderly patients, and outpatients (30 to 50 mg/daily in divided doses).

NURSING IMPLICATIONS
When administered 4 times daily, given after meals and at bedtime.
Since nortriptyline is long-acting, physician may prescribe entire daily dose at one time to improve patient compliance.
Advise patient to report persistent atropinelike effects: dry mouth, blurred vision, constipation, delayed micturition, drowsiness, or overstimulation.
Warn patient that drug may impair ability to perform potentially hazardous activities such as driving a car or operating machinery.
As with similar drugs, therapeutic response may not occur for 2 weeks or more.
Leukocyte and differential counts and liver function tests are advised prior to and during prolonged therapy.
To avoid possibility of precipitating withdrawal symptoms, nortriptyline should be withdrawn slowly in patients who have received high dosages for prolonged periods.
Preserved in tightly covered, light-resistant containers.
See Imipramine Hydrochloride.

DRUG INTERACTIONS: Nortriptyline may increase plasma levels of **dicumarol** and perhaps **other oral anticoagulants** (possibly by inhibiting its metabolism or by slowing GI motility). Also see Imipramine.

NOSCAPINE, N.F., B.P.
(TUSSCAPINE)

Antitussive (nonnarcotic)

ACTIONS AND USES
  Nonaddictive benzylisoquinoline alkaloid of opium, related to papaverine. Antitussive potency reportedly equivalent to that of codeine, but without side effects of codeine. Depresses activity of cough reflex, but does not act on higher centers. Used for temporary relief of nonproductive cough. Included in certain proprietary cough mixtures, eg, Conar.
CONTRAINDICATIONS AND PRECAUTIONS
  History of allergy to noscapine, children under 2 years of age.
ADVERSE REACTIONS
  Infrequently, with high dosage: nausea, drowsiness, slight dizziness, headache, skin rash.
ROUTE AND DOSAGE
  Oral: **Adults:** 15 to 30 mg 3 or 4 times daily; not to exceed 120 mg/24 hours. **Children:** 7.5 to 15 mg 3 or 4 times daily; not to exceed 60 mg/24 hours.

NURSING IMPLICATIONS
Effect of a single dose usually lasts up to 4 hours.
See Benzonatate for Nursing Implications.

NYLIDRIN HYDROCHLORIDE, N.F.
(ARLIDIN, CIRCLIDRIN, ROLIDRIN)

Vasodilator (peripheral)

ACTIONS AND USES
  Sympathomimetic amine (phenylisopropylamine) similar to ephedrine. Acts predominantly on β-adrenergic receptors. Increases blood flow to skeletal muscle by direct vasodilating action on arteries and arterioles; also causes slight increase in cerebral blood flow. Produces increase in cardiac output and some increase in heart rate; systolic blood pressure usually rises slightly, and diastolic may fall. Effect on cutaneous blood flow is negligible. Clinical value not established. Used in treatment of vasospastic disorders such as peripheral vascular disease, eg, acrocyanosis, Raynaud's syndrome, frostbite, night leg cramps, thromboangiitis obliterans, ischemic ulcer, diabetic vascular disease, and for circulatory disturbances of inner ear.
ABSORPTION AND FATE
  Readily absorbed from GI tract, but slowly metabolized; therefore, action is prolonged. Excreted slowly in urine.
CONTRAINDICATIONS AND PRECAUTIONS
  History of recent myocardial infarction, cardiac disease such as tachyarrhythmias, uncompensated heart failure, angina pectoris, thyrotoxicosis, peptic ulcer. Cautious use: hypertension.
ADVERSE REACTIONS
  Trembling, nervousness, weakness, dizziness, palpitation, nausea, vomiting, postural hypotension (not reported, but possible).
ROUTE AND DOSAGE
  Oral: 3 to 12 mg 3 or 4 times daily.

NURSING IMPLICATIONS
Palpitation is a prominent side effect that usually disappears with continued therapy; if it persists, reduction in dosage may be necessary.

Inform the patient that the benefits of nylidrin may not be apparent until after several weeks of therapy.

Observe for clinical response to therapy. For patients with peripheral vascular disease, note relief of rest pain or intermittent claudication and nail growth. For patients with circulatory disturbances of inner ear, note relief of dizziness, nausea, and nystagmus.

Hygienic care of extremities, properly fitting shoes and stockings, abstinence from smoking, avoidance of exposure to cold, and guidelines regarding acceptable activities are essential aspects of care in patients with peripheral vascular disease.

See Isoxsuprine Hydrochloride for other patient teaching points.

DRUG INTERACTIONS: Nylidrin may enhance the activity of **phenothiazines.**

NYSTATIN, U.S.P., B.P.
(KOROSTATIN, MYCOSTATIN, NILSTAT, O-V STATIN)

Antifungal

ACTIONS AND USES

Antifungal antibiotic produced by *Streptomyces noursei.* Has fungistatic and fungicidal activity against a variety of yeasts and fungi; not appreciably active against bacteria, viruses, or protozoa. Thought to act by binding to sterols in fungal cell membrane, thereby changing membrane potential and allowing leakage of intracellular components. Reportedly nontoxic, topical preparations are nonstaining even with prolonged administration.

Used to treat infections of skin and mucous membranes caused by *Candida (Monilia) albicans* and other *Candida* species, as in oral thrush, paronychia, and cutaneous, vulvovaginal, and intestinal candidiasis. Available commercially in combination with corticosteroids (eg, Myconef, Mycolog, Florotic) and tetracycline (eg, Achrostatin, Declostatin, Terrastatin).

ABSORPTION AND FATE

Poorly absorbed following oral administration; no detectable blood levels at recommended doses. Excreted in stool as unchanged drug. Not absorbed from intact skin or mucous membrane.

CONTRAINDICATIONS AND PRECAUTIONS

Hypersensitivity to nystatin or to any components in formulation.

ADVERSE REACTIONS

Usually mild: nausea, vomiting, epigastric distress, diarrhea (especially with high oral doses), hypersensitivity reactions (rare).

ROUTE AND DOSAGE

Oral tablet: **Adults:** 500,000 to 1,000,000 units 3 times daily. Oral suspension: **Adults and children:** 400,000 to 600,000 units 4 times daily; **infants:** 200,000 units 4 times daily; **premature and low-weight infants:** 100,000 units 4 times daily. Vaginal tablet: **Adults:** 1 or 2 tablets (100,000 units each) deposited high in vagina with supplied applicator. Topical: cream, ointment, powder containing 100,000 units/Gm.

NURSING IMPLICATIONS

Management of factors predisposing to candidiasis is equally as important as treatment in preventing reinfection and eliminating deep-seated infections.

Avoid contact of drug with hands. Hypersensitivity reactions occur rarely with nystatin alone; reportedly, preservatives used in some formulations are associated with a high incidence of contact dermatitis.

Advise patient to report onset of redness, swelling, or irritation. Drug should be discontinued if these symptoms occur.

Oral candidiasis (thrush): Divide prescribed dose of oral suspension so that one-half is placed in each side of mouth. Mouth should be clear of food debris before drug administration. Instruct patient to keep medication in contact with oral mucosa for at least several minutes, if possible, before swallowing. For infants, medication may be applied by means of swab.

Advise patient to brush teeth, or at least to rinse mouth thoroughly after each meal, and to floss teeth daily (patients with dentures should remove and clean them also after each meal). Overuse of commercial mouth washes tends to change oral flora and therefore should be avoided.

In elderly patients, oral candidiasis has been associated with poorly fitting dentures. If this is a problem, advise patient to contact dentist.

Treatment of oral candidiasis should be continued for at least 48 hours after symptoms have subsided and mouth cultures are normal. Pending laboratory confirmation, articles contaminated by mouth contact should be kept isolated for the patient's use or concurrently disinfected.

Candidiasis of feet, skin, and nails: for candidal infection of feet, instruct patient to dust shoes and stockings, as well as feet, with nystatin dusting powder.

Proper hygiene and skin care to prevent spread of infection and reinfection are essential aspects of therapy. Advise patient to change stockings and underclothing daily and to use his own linen and towels.

Occlusive dressings (including tight-fitting underclothing) or applications of ointment preparation to moist, dark areas of body favor growth of yeast and therefore should be avoided.

Cream formulation is preferred to the ointment for intertriginous areas. For very moist lesions, powder formulation is usually prescribed. Consult physician.

Infested areas should be cleaned gently before each application. Use of harsh soaps and vigorous scrubbing are contraindicated. Some physicians prescribe moist compresses with cool water for 15 minutes prior to application of medication (for soothing and drying action). Consult physician for specific guidelines.

Treatment of cutaneous candidal infections is usually continued for at least 2 weeks; discontinue only after two negative tests for *Candida.*

Paronychia: Advise patient to keep hands out of water as much as possible. Medication should be applied to nails and paronychial folds. Chronic paronychia may require several months of therapy to achieve clinical and mycologic cure. Relapses may be due to reinfection from *Candida* in intestinal tract.

Intestinal candidiasis: To prevent relapse, therapy is continued for at least 48 hours after symptoms have disappeared (vomiting, diarrhea, abdominal cramps, esophagitis).

Vulvovaginal candidiasis: Inform patient that medication should be continued during menstruation. In most cases 2 weeks of therapy are sufficient; however, some patients may require longer treatment.

In pregnant patients, vaginal tablets may be continued for 3 to 6 weeks before term in order to prevent thrush in newborns.

Cleansing douches may be used by nonpregnant patients if desired for aesthetic purposes (therapeutic douches, ie, with antiinfective medication, are not necessary and may be inadvisable).

Possible predisposing factors should be considered, eg, diabetes, pregnancy, infection by sexual partner, use of birth control pills, history of antibiotic therapy (candidal infections have occurred 6 to 8 weeks after therapy), corticosteroid therapy, use of tight-fitting nylon pantyhose.

Nystatin is preserved in tightly covered, light-resistant containers, away from heat. Expiration dates vary with manufacturer.

O

OPIUM TINCTURE, B.P.
(DEODORIZED OPIUM TINCTURE, LAUDANUM)

Antiperistaltic

ACTIONS AND USES

Hydroalcoholic solution containing 1% morphine (or 10% opium). Contains 25 times more morphine than does paregoric. General pharmacologic properties are like those of morphine (qv). Increases tone and spasticity of the large bowel, but decreases propulsive peristalsis, causing constipation. Used in symptomatic relief of diarrhea.

ROUTE AND DOSAGE

Oral: 0.3 to 1 ml (equivalent to 3 to 10 mg of morphine) up to 4 times daily.

NURSING IMPLICATIONS

Not to be confused with paregoric (camphorated tincture of opium), which is given in much larger dosages than opium tincture.

If respirations are 12 per minute or below or have changed in character and rate, report to physician before administering medication.

Give drug diluted with about one-third glass of water to assure passage into stomach.

Note character and frequency of stools; drug should be discontinued as soon as diarrhea is controlled.

Addiction is possible with prolonged use.

Classified as schedule II drug under federal Controlled Substances Act.

Preserved in tight, light-resistant containers. See nursing implications for paregoric.

ORAL CONTRACEPTIVES
(Estrogen-Progestin Combinations)

ACTIONS AND USES

Fixed combination of estrogen and progestin produces contraception by preventing ovulation and rendering reproductive tract structures hostile to sperm penetration and implantation. Estrogen suppresses release of gonadotropins follicle-stimulating hormone (FSH) and luteinizing hormone (LH); progestins cause structural and secretory changes in endometrium and inhibit ferning of cervical secretions, thus supporting an impenetrable mucoid network. Efficacy and many adverse reactions of oral contraceptives are due largely to estrogen component (see Estradiol, prototype for estrogens), while differences between combinations are due to relative potency and predominance of either progestational or estrogenic activity. All combination products incorporate an estrogen (ethinyl estradiol or mestranol) with one of 5 progestins (norethynodrel, norethindrone, norethindrone acetate, ethynodiol diacetate, norgestrel). Positive evidence associates thromboembolic and vascular disease with the dose of estrogens in oral contraceptives; reportedly the risk is reversed by drug withdrawal. Users over 40 years of age appear to incur greater risk of fatal or nonfatal myocardial infarction. Potential carcinogenicity of estrogens or progestins for users is neither refuted nor confirmed. Reportedly, risk of gallbladder disease increases after 6 months of contraceptive use.

Used to prevent conception and to treat hypermenorrhea and endometriosis. See Estradiol and Dydrogesterone (prototype for progestins).

ABSORPTION AND FATE

All preparations well absorbed from GI tract. Metabolism of individual components apparently not changed by simultaneous administration. Information about half-life and excretion of combinations is incomplete. Small amounts of estrogen and progestin are detected in breast milk.

CONTRAINDICATIONS AND PRECAUTIONS

Pregnancy, lactation, missed abortion. Familial or personal history of or existence of cancer of breast or genital tract; recurrent chronic cystic mastitis; history of or existence of thrombophlebitis or thromboembolic disorders, cerebrovascular or coronary artery disease, or severe hepatic dysfunction; family history of hepatic porphyria; known or suspected hormone-dependent neoplasm; undiagnosed abnormal genital bleeding; women age 40 and over (debatable); adolescents with incomplete epiphyseal closure. Cautious use: history of depression, preexisting hypertension, or cardiac or renal disease; impaired liver function; history of migraine, convulsive disorders, or asthma; multiparous women with grossly irregular menses, diabetes, or familial history of diabetes; gallbladder disease; lupus erythematosus; rheumatic disease; varicosities. Also see Estradiol and Dydrogesterone.

ADVERSE REACTIONS

Dose-related: **Estrogen excess:** nausea (common), bloating, menstrual tension, cervical mucorrhea, polyposis, chloasma (melasma), hypertension, headache, migraine, breast fullness or tenderness, edema. **Estrogen deficiency:** hypomenorrhea, early or midcycle breakthrough bleeding, increased spotting. **Progestin excess:** hypomenorrhea, breast regression, vaginal candidiasis, mental depression, fatigue, persistent weight gain, increased appetite, acne, oily scalp, hair loss, hirsutism. **Progestin deficiency:** late-cycle breakthrough bleeding, amenorrhea. **Other reported reactions: Cardiovascular:** thrombotic and thromboembolic disorders, increase in size of varicosities. **GI:** abdominal cramps, jaundice, cholelithiasis, diarrhea, constipation. **Genitourinary:** ureteral dilation, increased incidence of urinary tract infection. **Ophthalmic:** visual disturbances, optic neuritis, retinal thrombosis, papilledema. **Reproductive:** increased risk of congenital anomalies, decreased quality and quantity of breast milk, increased size of fibromyomata. **Also:** rash (allergic), porphyria, pyridoxine deficiency, increased incidence of chicken pox and other viral diseases. **Altered laboratory values:** increased BSP retention; increased prothrombin and factors VII, VIII, IX, and X; increased norepinephrine-induced platelet aggregability; altered thyroid function tests; increased triglycerides and phospholipids; depressed serum folate level; elevated blood glucose (mestranol compounds).

ROUTE AND DOSAGE

Oral (see product package insert and patient information brochure): The number 20, 21, or 28 following the trade name indicates number of tablets per package. Other numbers following trade name indicate dose of progestin/estrogen. Regimens are usually from day 5 through day 24 or 25 of cycle (day 1 is first day of menstruation), or 21 days of treatment followed by 7 to 8 days without pill. Progestin-only (mini pill) tablet: every day of year without interruption.

NURSING IMPLICATIONS

Complete medical and family history should be taken prior to initiating oral contraceptive therapy. Baseline and periodic physical examination should include blood pressure, breasts, abdomen, pelvis, Pap smear, and other relevant tests.

Urge patient not to skip scheduled visits for physical checkups while on oral contraceptive therapy. Teach breast self-examination and emphasize importance of doing this every month.

Tablets should be taken regularly at same time of day to assure intervals of

24 hours (eg, with a meal or at bedtime). Stress that strict adherence to dosage schedule is essential for efficacy of medication.

Nausea with or without vomiting occurs in approximately 10% of patients during the first cycle and is reportedly one of the major reasons for voluntary discontinuation of therapy. Most side effects tend to disappear in third or fourth cycle of use. Instruct user to report symptoms that persist after fourth cycle. Dose adjustment or a different product may be indicated.

In the first week of the initial cycle of oral contraceptive use, patient should also use an additional method of birth control.

If user forgets to take a pill, she should take it as soon as she remembers or should take 2 pills the next day. If 2 consecutive pills are omitted, she should begin using another method of contraception for the next 7 days, then take 2 tablets daily for 2 days, then resume regular schedule. If 3 consecutive doses are missed, cycle should be resumed 7 days after last tablet was taken; another method of contraception should be used while not taking tablet and for 7 days into new schedule.

Ovulation is unlikely with omission of one daily dose; however, the possibility of escape ovulation, spotting, or breakthrough bleeding increases with each missed dose.

Normally, withdrawal bleeding occurs 2 to 5 days after last tablet, but regardless of when bleeding occurs, the user should adhere to the dosage schedule.

If intracycle bleeding resembling menstruation occurs, patient should discontinue medication, then begin taking tablets from a new compact on day 5. If bleeding persists, advise patient to see physician to rule out nonfunctional cause. Amount, duration of flow, and placement in drug regimen are important diagnostic parameters to be reported.

If prescribed regimen has been followed, and two consecutive periods are missed, user should see physician to rule out pregnancy before continuing hormone contraception. If schedule has not been followed, the possibility of pregnancy should be considered at time of first missed period, and pills should be withheld until pregnancy has been ruled out.

Generally, it is advised to discontinue use of oral contraceptive temporarily every 18 months. Advise patient to consult physician regarding continuation of pill.

When pregnancy is desired, hormone contraception is discontinued, and patient is advised to use alternate method for at least 3 months to avoid risk of breakthrough pregnancy and congenital defects in fetus.

If possible, contraceptive pill should not be taken until infant is weaned; alternate method of birth control should be used during this period. Pill can be started immediately after delivery in the nonnursing mother, if desired.

Oral contraception may mask onset of climacteric. To determine if it has started, physician may advise patient to discontinue pill and to use alternate method of contraception. If menstruation occurs, the pill is indicated.

Anovulation or amenorrhea following termination of oral contraceptive regimen may persist more than 6 months. The user with pretreatment oligomenorrhea or secondary amenorrhea is most apt to have oversuppression syndrome.

The heavy smoker runs a higher risk of developing venous thromboembolitis than user who does not smoke.

Hirsutism and loss of hair are reversible with discontinuation of pill or by change of selected combination.

Acne may improve, worsen, or develop for first time. In women on the pill for at least a year, postcontraceptive acne sometimes occurs 3 to 4 months after stopping drug and may continue for 6 to 12 months.

Menstrual tension, bloating, and tender breasts may be relieved by diuretics, sedation, and low salt intake.

If feasible, the pill should be discontinued at least 1 cycle prior to surgery, which is associated with increased risk of thromboembolism or prolonged immobilization, and prior to diagnostic oral glucose tolerance test.

The Pathologist should be informed that the pill is being taken when relevant tissues are to be examined. Also inform dentist if oral surgery is anticipated.

To avoid later fertility and menstrual problems, hormone contraception is not advised for the adolescent until after at least 2 years of well-established menstrual cycles and completion of physiologic maturation.

An estrogen-dominant agent is the best choice for the adolescent with scanty menses, moderate or severe acne, or candidiasis. A progestin-dominant agent is the best choice for the adolescent with dysmenorrhea, hypermenorrhea, fibrocystic disease of breast, or cyclic premenstrual weight gain.

Teach patient how to elicit Homans' sign and to be alert to other manifestations of thrombotic or thromboembolic disorders: severe headache (especially if persistent and recurrent), dizziness, blurred vision, leg or chest pain, respiratory distress, unexplained cough. Advise patient to withhold pill if any of these symptoms appear and to report promptly to physician.

Sudden abdominal pain should be reported immediately to rule out hepatic adenoma or ectopic pregnancy. The pill is more effective in preventing intrauterine than ectopic pregnancy.

Users with clinical conditions worsened by fluid retention should report exacerbation of symptoms promptly; a preparation with less estrogen may be substituted. Frequent weight checks should be recorded to permit early recognition of fluid retention.

Ophthalmic sequelae can occur as soon as 24 hours after initiation of oral contraception. Advise patient to stop pill and contact physician if unexplained partial or complete sudden or gradual loss of vision, protrusion of eyeballs (proptosis), or diplopia occurs.

Astigmatic error and myopic refractive error may be increased twofold to threefold, usually after 6 months of oral contraceptive therapy. Changes in ocular contour and lubricant quality of tears may necessitate change in size and shape of contact lenses.

Chloasma (more marked in dark-skinned women) seems to be aggravated by sunlight and may persist beyond period of pill use. With anticipated exposure (as in summer), taking pill at bedtime will reduce circulating hormone level in daytime.

Leukorrhea is an expected physical reaction to the oral contraceptive; however, if accompanied by vaginal itching and irritation, candidiasis should be ruled out. Caution patient to report discomfort promptly.

Check blood pressure periodically. In some women changes in blood pressure occur within each cycle; in others slow ascension of pressure, particularly diastolic, over several months is significant. Drug-induced hypertension is usually reversible with discontinuation of the pill.

Instruct the diabetic user to report positive urine test to physician. Adjustment of antidiabetic medication may be necessary. The potential diabetic (family history) should also be closely observed for onset of diabetes and probably should not use mestranol combinations.

Advise user with history of premenstrual and other kinds of depression to report to physician if symptoms recur. A responsible family member should also be alerted to observe carefully.

Selecting the optimum combination oral contraceptive should take into account user's response to the estrogen/progestin ratio. Estrogen-dominant preparations: norethynodrel with mestranol (Enovid, Enovid-E), ethynodiol diacetate with mestranol (Ovulen), norethindrone with mestranol (Ortho-Novum 2 mg, Norinyl 2 mg). Progestin-dominant preparations: norethindrone acetate with ethinyl estradiol (Zorane 1.5/30, Zorane 1/20, Loestrin 1.5/30, Loestrin 1/20, Norlestrin 2.5/50), norgestrel with ethinyl estradiol (Lo Ovral, Ovral), norethindrone with mestranol (Ortho-Novum 10 mg). Other marketed products are intermediate with respect to estrogen/progestin ratio.

DRUG INTERACTIONS: See Estradiol and Dydrogesterone.

OUABAIN, U.S.P., B.P.
(G-STROPHANTHIN)

Cardiotonic

ACTIONS AND USES
Rapid-acting, potent cardiac glycoside derived from *Strophanthus gratus*. Capable of producing same therapeutic and toxic effects as digitalis (qv). Acts more rapidly, and duration of effect is shorter than that of digitalis glycosides; therefore cumulation less likely to occur.
Used for rapid digitalization as in emergency treatment of atrial flutter, paroxysmal atrial or nodal tachycardia, or acute congestive heart failure.
ABSORPTION AND FATE
Action starts within 3 to 10 minutes after IV administration. Effects peak in 30 minutes to 2 hours, regress in 8 to 12 hours, and end in 24 hours to 3 days. Plasma half-life about 21 hours. Degraded by liver and excreted in urine.
CONTRAINDICATIONS AND PRECAUTIONS
Cautious use: patients who have received any digitalis preparation during preceding 3 weeks, patients with frequent ventricular beats, patients with history of impaired renal function.
ROUTE AND DOSAGE
Intravenous: 0.25 to 0.5 mg; additional doses of 0.1 mg may be given hourly until desired results are obtained or until total reaches 1 mg/24 hours. Administered slowly, and carefully adjusted to patient's requirements and response.

NURSING IMPLICATIONS
ECG monitoring and close observation of patient are essential.
Drug administration should be discontinued if nausea, vomiting, or extreme bradycardia occurs or if arrhythmias develop in patient whose heart beat has been regular.
Oral therapy with a digitalis glycoside is instituted as soon as emergency has passed.
Preserved in tight, light-resistant containers.
See nursing implications and drug interactions for Digitalis (Leaf, Powdered).

OXACILLIN, SODIUM, U.S.P.
(BACTOCILL, PROSTAPHLIN)

Antibacterial

ACTIONS AND USES
Semisynthetic, penicillinase-resistant isoxazolyl penicillin. Effective against penicillinase-producing staphylococci, pneumococci, and β-hemolytic strep-

tococci. Mechanism of antibacterial action as for penicillin G potassium. **515**
Used primarily in treatment of infections caused by penicillinase-producing staphylococci, but may also be used to initiate therapy in suspected staphylococcal infection pending culture and sensitivity results.

ABSORPTION AND FATE
Peak serum levels in 30 minutes to 1 hour following oral and IM injection and in 5 minutes following IV injection. Oral solution produces slightly higher levels than do capsules. About 90% to 95% protein-bound. Distributed to bile, pleural and amniotic fluid, and milk. Penetrates cerebrospinal fluid only when meninges are inflamed. Half-life 30 to 60 minutes. Excreted rapidly by kidney as intact drug and metabolite; also eliminated in bile. Crosses placenta.

CONTRAINDICATIONS AND PRECAUTIONS
Hypersensitivity to penicillins or cephalosporins. Safe use during pregnancy not established. Cautious use: premature infants and neonates; history of allergies or asthma.

ADVERSE REACTIONS
Nausea, vomiting, flatulence, and diarrhea; hypersensitivity (pruritus, urticaria, rash, wheezing, anaphylaxis); superinfections; hepatocellular dysfunction; elevated SGOT or SGPT; leukopenia (rare); neutropenia (reported in children); transient hematuria, albuminuria, and azotemia (newborns and infants on high doses); thrombophlebitis (with IV therapy). Also see Penicillin G, Potassium.

ROUTE AND DOSAGE
Adults: Oral, intramuscular, intravenous: 250 mg to 1 Gm every 4 to 6 hours. Direct IV administration made slowly over 10-minute period. **Children:** Oral: 50 to 100 mg/kg/day in equally divided doses at 4- to 6-hour intervals; parenteral: 50 to 100 mg/kg/day divided into 4 doses. **Premature infants and neonates:** 25 mg/kg/day in divided doses.

NURSING IMPLICATIONS
Careful inquiry should be made concerning previous hypersensitivity reactions to penicillins, cephalosporins, and other allergens.
Administer oral drug 1 to 2 hours before meals, preferably, or 2 hours after meals. Food reduces absorption.
If oral solution is prescribed, note expiration date on label (reconstituted oral solution remains stable 14 days if refrigerated and 3 days at room temperature).
For IM administration, reconstitute with sterile water for injection (as directed in product monograph), and indicate date and time of reconstitution on vial. Shake vial vigorously until drug is completely dissolved. Discard unused solutions after 3 days at room temperature or 7 days under refrigeration. *Do not use undated vials.*
Administer IM by deep intragluteal injection (follow agency policy for appropriate IM site in young children and infants). Select site carefully. Injection into or near a major peripheral nerve or blood vessel can result in neurovascular damage. Rotate injection sites.
For IV administration, reconstitute with sterile water for injection or isotonic sodium chloride (as directed in product monograph). For IV infusion, reconstituted solution is added to compatible IV solution (eg, isotonic sodium chloride, 5% dextrose in water or in normal saline, lactated Ringer's, or others recommended by manufacturer).
Rate of IV infusion should be adjusted to administer drug over a 6-hour period (loss of drug activity increases after that time).
Periodic assessments of renal, hepatic, and hematopoietic functions should be made in patients on prolonged therapy. Close monitoring of kidney function is especially important in newborns and infants receiving high doses.
Hepatic dysfunction (possibly a hypersensitivity reaction) resembling chole-

static jaundice or viral hepatitis has been reported following IV oxacillin therapy; reversible with discontinuation of drug. Immediately report onset of nausea, vomiting, fever, or malaise.

Drug therapy is continued a minimum of 5 days for mild to moderate infections. For severe infections therapy is continued at least 1 to 2 weeks after patient is afebrile and cultures are negative. Treatment of osteomyelitis may require several months of therapy.

See Penicillin G, Potassium.

DRUG INTERACTIONS: Some **sulfonamides** (eg, **sulfaethidole** and **sulfamethoxypyridazine**) appear to inhibit GI absorption of oxacillin. Also see Penicillin G Potassium.

OXANDROLONE, N.F.
(ANAVAR, LONOVAR)

Anabolic agent

ACTIONS AND USES

Synthetic steroid with strong anabolic and low androgenic activity.

Used to promote weight gain in patients who have lost weight after extensive surgery, chronic infections, or severe trauma; used to reduce bone pain associated with osteoporosis and to offset protein catabolism accompanying prolonged corticosteroid administration.

ROUTE AND DOSAGE

Oral: **Adult:** 2.5 mg 2 to 4 times daily for 2 to 4 weeks (dosage may range from 2.5 to 20 mg daily), repeated intermittently if necessary; **Children:** 0.25 mg/kg/day.

NURSING IMPLICATIONS

A course of therapy of 2 to 4 weeks is usually adequate. Therapy for adults and children should not exceed 3 months.

See Ethylestrenol.

OXAZEPAM, N.F.
(SERAX)

Antianxiety agent (minor tranquilizer)

ACTIONS AND USES

Benzodiazepine derivative related to chlordiazepoxide and diazepam, with which it shares actions, uses, contraindications, and adverse reactions. Has shorter duration of action, but reportedly causes fewer side effects than do chlordiazepoxide and diazepam.

Used in management of anxiety, tension, agitation, irritability, and related symptoms associated with a wide range of emotional disturbances; used to control acute withdrawal symptoms in chronic alcoholism.

ABSORPTION AND FATE

Following absorption from GI tract, peak plasma concentrations occur in 1 to 2 hours. Metabolized in liver. Excreted slowly in urine, primarily as glucuronide metabolite, and in feces as unchanged drug. Most of a given dose is excreted within 2 days.

History of hypersensitivity to oxazepam; psychoses. Safe use during pregnancy and in women of childbearing potential and in children under age 12 not established. Cautious use: elderly patients. See Chlordiazepoxide.

ADVERSE REACTIONS

Usually infrequent and mild: drowsiness, dizziness, vertigo, headache, nausea, syncope, hypotension, stomatitis, skin rash, edema, lethargy, slurred speech, paradoxic excitement, tremor, ataxia, altered libido, leukopenia, hepatic dysfunction including jaundice. Also see Chlordiazepoxide.

ROUTE AND DOSAGE

Oral: 10 to 30 mg 3 or 4 times a day. For older patients, initial recommended dose is 10 mg 3 or 4 times daily, increased cautiously to 15 mg 3 or 4 times daily, if necessary.

NURSING IMPLICATIONS

Elderly patients should be observed closely for signs of CNS reactions associated with benzodiazepine derivatives.

Following prolonged therapy, drug should be withdrawn slowly to avoid precipitating withdrawal symptoms (including epileptiform seizures).

Caution patient against driving a car or operating dangerous machinery.

Warn patient that tolerance to alcohol may be lowered.

Mild paradoxic stimulation of affect and excitement, with sleep disturbances, may occur within the first 2 weeks of therapy. Report immediately.

Liver function tests and blood counts should be performed regularly.

Excessive and prolonged use may cause physical dependence.

Classified as schedule IV drug under federal Controlled Substances Act.

Also see Chlordiazepoxide.

OXIDIZED CELLULOSE, U.S.P., B.P.
(HEMO-PAK, OXYCEL, SURGICEL)

Hemostatic (local)

ACTIONS AND USES

Sterile, absorbable hemostatic material prepared from cellulose. On contact with blood, it swells into a brownish or black gelatinous mass that acts as artificial clot. Gradually absorbed from tissue bed, usually within 2 to 7 days; complete absorption of large amounts may require up to 6 weeks or more.

Used to control capillary, venous, and small arterial hemorrage when suture or ligation is impractical or ineffective.

CONTRAINDICATIONS AND PRECAUTIONS

Use as wadding or packing; use for implantation in bone defects, including fractures and laminectomy procedures (interferes with callus formation, and may cause cysts and nerve damage); hemorrhage from large arteries or non-hemorrhagic oozing surfaces; impregnation with anti-infective materials or other hemostatic substances.

ADVERSE REACTIONS

Foreign-body reactions, burning, stinging sensations, sneezing (when used for rhinologic procedures), necroses due to tight packing.

NURSING IMPLICATIONS

Hemostatic effect is greater when material is applied dry.

Hemostatic effect is not enhanced by thrombin (activity of thrombin is destroyed by low pH of oxidized cellulose). Absorption may be prevented by previous applications of silver nitrate or other escharotic materials. Only as much as necessary for hemostasis should be used; material is applied to bleeding site or held firmly in place until bleeding stops.

Once hemostasis is achieved, oxidized cellulose is usually removed from site of application. Removal is facilitated by irrigation with sterile water or saline. Observe wound site for bleeding following removal.

Oxidized cellulose is off-white or dusty yellow in color, but it may darken in its sealed container with age. Reportedly this does not affect its hemostatic action.

Material is supplied as a sterile preparation and cannot be resterilized. Autoclaving or other forms of heat sterilization cause physical breakdown. Discard unused portions.

OXTRIPHYLLINE, N.F.
(CHOLEDYL, THEOPHYLLINE CHOLINATE)
CHOLINE THEOPHYLLINATE, B.P.

Bronchodilator (xanthine)

ACTIONS AND USES

Choline salt of theophylline, with similar actions, uses, and limitations as other theophylline derivatives. Contains 64% theophylline. Compared to aminophylline, reportedly more stable, more soluble, and more uniformly and predictably absorbed, and produces less gastric irritation. Development of tolerance reported infrequently; therefore, useful in long-term therapy.

CONTRAINDICATIONS AND PRECAUTIONS

Safe use in women of childbearing potential and during pregnancy and lactation not established.

ROUTE AND DOSAGE

Oral: **Adults:** 100 to 200 mg 4 times a day. **Children** *2 to 12 years:* 15 mg/kg/24 hours divided into 4 doses.

NURSING IMPLICATIONS

Preferably administered after meals and at bedtime.

Advise patient to report gastric distress, palpitation, and CNS stimulation (irritability, restlessness, nervousness, insomnia). Reduction in dosage may be indicated.

Preserved in well-closed containers, away from heat. Elixir should be protected from light.

See Aminophylline.

OXYCODONE HYDROCHLORIDE
OXYCODONE TEREPHTHALATE
(PERCOBARB, PERCOCET, PERCODAN include oxycodone and other ingredients)

Narcotic analgesic

ACTIONS AND USES

Oxycodone is a semisynthetic phenanthrene derivative with actions qualitatively similar to those of morphine (qv). Appears to be more effective in relief of acute rather than long-standing pain. Analgesic potency and dependence

liability reportedly greater than those of codeine. Produces mild sedation, and
has little or no effect on cough reflex.
Used for relief of moderate to moderately severe pain such as may occur with
bursitis, dislocations, simple fractures and other injuries, neuralgia; used for
postoperative, postextractional, and postpartum pain. Available in U.S. only in
combination with other agents, eg, Percodan, Percobarb, Percocet.

ABSORPTION AND FATE
Analgesic effects of oxycodone occur within 10 to 15 minutes, peak in 30 to 60
minutes, and persist 3 to 6 hours. Detoxified by liver and kidney. Excreted
primarily in urine. Crosses placenta.

ADVERSE REACTIONS
Lightheadedness, dizziness, sedation, nausea, vomiting, euphoria, dysphoria,
constipation, pruritus.

ROUTE AND DOSAGE
Oral: Percodan contains 4.5 mg oxycodone hydrochloride, 0.38 mg oxycodone
terephthalate, 224 mg aspirin, 160 mg phenacetin, and 32 mg caffeine: 1 tablet
every 6 hours, as needed. Percobarb (same ingredients as Percodan with addition
of 100 mg hexobarbital): 1 capsule every 6 hours as needed. Percocet (contains
5 mg oxycodone hydrochloride and 325 mg acetaminophen): 1 tablet every 6
hours, as needed.

NURSING IMPLICATIONS
Administer after meals or with milk.
Caution patient to avoid potentially hazardous activities such as driving a car
or operating machinery.
Adverse effects (lightheadedness, dizziness, sedation, nausea, and vomiting)
seem to be more prominent in ambulatory than in nonambulatory pa-
tients and may be alleviated if patient lies down.
In evaluating adverse reactions and drug interactions of combination drugs,
each ingredient must be considered.
Evaluate patient's continued need for narcotic analgesic.
Psychic and physical dependence and tolerance may develop with repeated
use of oxycodone (addiction liability is reportedly about the same as that
of morphine).
Classified as schedule II drug under federal Controlled Substances Act.

OXYMETAZOLINE HYDROCHLORIDE, U.S.P. (AFRIN)

Adrenergic (vasoconstrictor)

ACTIONS AND USES
Imidazoline-derivative sympathomimetic agent structurally and pharmacologically related to naphazoline. Direct action on alpha receptors of sympathetic
nervous system produces constriction of smaller arterioles in nasal passages and
prolonged decongestant effect. Has no effect on beta receptors.
Used for relief of nasal congestion in a variety of allergic and infectious disorders of upper respiratory tract; used on nasal tampon to facilitate intranasal
examination or before nasal surgery. Also used as adjunct in treatment and
prevention of middle ear infection by decreasing congestion of eustachian ostia.

CONTRAINDICATIONS AND PRECAUTIONS
Hypersensitivity to drug components; use in children under 6 years of age. Safe
use in women of childbearing potential and during pregnancy not established.
Cautious use: patients receiving MAO inhibitors; coronary artery disease, hypertension, hyperthyroidism, diabetes mellitus.

Burning, stinging, dryness of nasal mucosa, sneezing. With excessive use: headache, lightheadedness, drowsiness, insomnia, palpitation, rebound congestion.

ROUTE AND DOSAGE

Topical (nasal spray 0.05%): 2 or 3 squeezes in each nostril 2 times a day; (nose drops 0.05%): 2 to 4 drops in each nostril 2 times a day.

NURSING IMPLICATIONS

Usually administered in the morning and at bedtime. Effects appear within 30 minutes and last about 6 to 7 hours.

If necessary, patient should blow nose gently to clear nasal passages before administration of medication.

Deliver spray with patient in upright position. Place spray nozzle in nostril without occluding it, and have patient bend head slightly forward and sniff briskly during administration.

Lateral, head-low position is recommended for instillation of nose drops.

Rinse dropper or spray tip in hot water after each use to prevent contamination of solution by nasal secretions.

Caution patient not to exceed prescribed or recommended dosage. Rebound congestion (chemical rhinitis) may occur with prolonged or excessive use. Systemic effects can result from swallowing excessive medication.

OXYMETHOLONE, N.F.
(ADROYD, ANADROL)

Androgen

ACTIONS AND USES

Potent steroid with androgenic/anabolic activity ratio approximately 1:3. Actions are similar to those of ethylestrenol (qv).

ROUTE AND DOSAGE

Osteoporosis: Oral: **Adults:** 2.5 mg 3 times daily; doses up to 15 mg/day may be employed; **Children** *up to 12 years:* 2.5 to 5 mg/day for 4 to 6 weeks followed by 1 month without anabolic steroid. X-rays should be taken to evaluate bone growth before starting drug regimen anew. *Aplastic anemia:* **Adults and children:** 1 to 5 mg/kg body weight per day. Highly individualized.

NURSING IMPLICATIONS

Periodic liver function tests are especially important for the geriatric patient. Drug should be stopped with first sign of liver toxicity (jaundice).

Oxymetholone does not replace supportive measures for treatment of anemia (such as transfusions and correction of iron, folic acid, vitamin B_{12}, or pyridoxine deficiency).

For treatment of anemias, a minimum trial period of 3 to 6 months is recommended, since response tends to be slow.

Optimal effects in treatment of osteoporosis are usually experienced in 4 to 6 weeks.

See Ethylestrenol.

Narcotic analgesic

ACTIONS AND USES
Semisynthetic phenanthrene derivative structurally and pharmacologically related to morphine (qv). Analgesic action of 1 mg is reportedly equivalent to that of 10 mg of morphine. Produces mild sedation, and unlike morphine, it has little antitussive action. In equianalgesic doses, may cause less constipation than does morphine, but more nausea, vomiting, and euphoria.

Used for relief of moderate to severe pain, preoperative medication, obstetric analgesia, support of anesthesia, and relief of anxiety in patients with dyspnea associated with acute ventricular failure and pulmonary edema.

ABSORPTION AND FATE
Onset of analgesic action usually occurs in 10 to 15 minutes after subcutaneous or IM, 5 to 10 minutes after IV, and 15 to 30 minutes after rectal administration. Peak action in about 1 to 1.5 hours; duration 3 to 6 hours. Metabolized primarily in liver; excreted in urine. Crosses placenta.

CONTRAINDICATIONS AND PRECAUTIONS
Use for pulmonary edema resulting from chemical respiratory irritants. Safe use during pregnancy (other than labor) and in children under 12 years of age not established. Also see Morphine.

ADVERSE REACTIONS
Nausea, vomiting, euphoria, dizziness. Also see Morphine.

ROUTE AND DOSAGE
Subcutaneous, intramuscular: initially 1 to 1.5 mg every 4 to 6 hours, as needed; for obstetric analgesia 0.5 to 1 mg IM recommended. Intravenous: initially 0.5 mg. Rectal suppository: 5 mg every 4 to 6 hours, as needed.

NURSING IMPLICATIONS
Evaluate patient's continued need for narcotic analgesic. Prolonged use can lead to dependence of morphine type.

Classified as schedule II drug under federal Controlled Substances Act.

Protect drug from light. Store suppositories in refrigerator (2 C to 15 C).

See Morphine Sulfate.

OXYPHENBUTAZONE, N.F., B.P. (OXALID, TANDEARIL)

Antiinflammatory, antirheumatic

ACTIONS AND USES
Pyrazolone derivative and metabolite of phenylbutazone. Shares actions, uses, absorption, fate, contraindications, precautions, and adverse reactions of phenylbutazone (qv).

ROUTE AND DOSAGE
Oral: 200 to 400 mg daily in 3 or 4 divided doses (usual range 100 to 400 mg daily).

NURSING IMPLICATIONS
Administer immediately before or after meals or with glass of milk. Physician may prescribe concurrent sodium-free antacid to reduce incidence of gastric upset.

Also see Phenylbutazone.

DRUG INTERACTIONS: **Methandrostenolone** may increase oxyphenbutazone plasma levels, possibly by displacing it from plasma protein binding. Also see Phenylbutazone.

OXYPHENCYCLIMINE HYDROCHLORIDE, N.F.
(DARICON, GASTRIX)

Anticholinergic

ACTIONS AND USES
Synthetic tertiary amine with clinical effects qualitatively similar to those of atropine. As with most tertiary amines, exerts direct spasmolytic action on smooth muscle, but has little effect on skeletal neuromuscular or ganglionic transmission.
Used as adjunct in management of peptic ulcer, spastic and inflammatory conditions of GI tract, spasms of ureter or bladder, biliary tract disease.
ABSORPTION AND FATE
Onset of effects in 1 to 2 hours; duration 8 to 12 hours.
CONTRAINDICATIONS AND PRECAUTIONS
Glaucoma, obstructive uropathy, obstructive diseases of GI tract, severe ulcerative colitis, myasthenia gravis, unstable cardiovascular status. Safe use in children not established. Cautious use: debilitated patients with chronic lung disease; elderly patients; renal, hepatic, or biliary disease; autonomic neuropathy. Also see Atropine.
ADVERSE REACTIONS
Atropinelike effects. High doses: CNS stimulation. See Atropine.
ROUTE AND DOSAGE
Oral: 5 to 10 mg twice daily. Maximum dosage 50 mg daily in divided doses.

NURSING IMPLICATIONS
Administered preferably in morning and at night before retiring.
Elderly patients are particularly sensitive to even small doses of anticholinergic drugs. Observe closely for excitement, drowsiness, or other untoward effects.
Incidence and severity of side effects are generally dose-related.
Onset of diarrhea in patients who have had ileostomy or colostomy may be an early sign of intestinal obstruction. Report immediately.
Caution patient not to perform activities requiring mental alertness or skill while taking oxyphencyclimine.
In presence of high environmental temperature, heat prostration can occur with use of oxyphencyclimine.
See Atropine Sulfate.

OXYPHENONIUM BROMIDE
(ANTRENYL BROMIDE)

Anticholinergic

ACTIONS AND USES
Potent synthetic quaternary ammonium compound. Pharmacologic effects qualitatively similar to those of atropine, but produces somewhat greater incidence of side effects. CNS activity is generally lacking. Toxic doses may block neuromuscular transmission (curarelike action).
Used in adjunctive management of peptic ulcer and other GI disorders as-

sociated with hyperacidity, hypermotility, and spasm. Also has been used as preanesthetic antisecretory agent in patients hypersensitive to atropine; used to relieve smooth-muscle spasm in bronchial asthma and to control excessive perspiration.

ABSORPTION AND FATE

Usually acts within 30 minutes, with peak action in about 2 hours; duration of action 4 to 6 hours.

CONTRAINDICATIONS AND PRECAUTIONS

Glaucoma, obstructive uropathy, obstructive diseases of GI tract, biliary tract disease, ulcerative colitis, unstable cardiovascular status, myasthenia gravis. Safe use during pregnancy and lactation and in children not established. Cautious use: debilitated patients with chronic lung disease, elderly patients, renal or hepatic disease, autonomic neuropathy. Also see Atropine.

ADVERSE REACTIONS

Atropinelike side effects. Toxic dose: respiratory depression, muscle weakness, cardiac disturbances. See Atropine.

ROUTE AND DOSAGE

Oral: **Adults:** initially 10 mg 4 times daily for several days; dosage then reduced according to patient's response. **Children:** 0.8 mg/kg/24 hours divided into 4 doses.

NURSING IMPLICATIONS

Preferably administered before meals and at bedtime.

Elderly patients are particularly sensitive to even small doses of anticholinergic drugs. Be alert to complaints of nausea, dizziness, constipation, urinary retention, weakness, or other unusual symptoms.

Onset of diarrhea in patients who have had ileostomy or colostomy may be an early sign of intestinal obstruction. Report promptly.

In presence of high environmental temperature, heat prostration can occur with use of this drug.

Caution patient not to engage in activities requiring mental alertness and skill while taking oxyphenonium.

Have on hand the antidote neostigmine in the event of severe toxic reactions.

See Atropine Sulfate.

OXYTETRACYCLINE CALCIUM, N.F.
(TERRAMYCIN CALCIUM)
OXYTETRACYCLINE HYDROCHLORIDE, U.S.P.
(DALIMYCIN, OXLOPAR, OXYBIOTIC, OXY-KESSO-TETRA, OXY-TETRACHEL, TERRAMYCIN, TETRAMINE, URI-TET)

Antibacterial

ACTIONS AND USES

Broad-spectrum antibiotic with actions, uses, contraindications, precautions, and adverse reactions similar to those of tetracycline (qv).

ABSORPTION AND FATE

Adequately but incompletely absorbed from GI tract; peak plasma concentrations in 2 to 4 hours. Appears to concentrate in hepatic system. Half-life 6 to 9 hours. Excreted in bile, feces, and urine in active form. Crosses placenta.

CONTRAINDICATIONS AND PRECAUTIONS

Hypersensitivity to tetracyclines; during tooth development (last half of pregnancy, infancy, childhood to age 8). Cautious use: impaired renal function. See Tetracycline.

Nausea, vomiting, diarrhea, stomatitis, skin rash, superinfections, renal toxicity. See Tetracycline.

ROUTE AND DOSAGE

Adults: Oral: 250 to 500 mg every 6 to 12 hours. Intramuscular: 100 mg every 8 to 12 hours; for severe infections up to 250 mg every 12 hours. Intravenous: 250 to 500 mg every 12 hours, not to exceed 500 mg every 6 hours. **Children:** Oral: 25 to 50 mg/kg daily in divided doses. Intramuscular: 15 to 25 mg/kg daily in 2 or 3 divided doses. No single injection should exceed 250 mg. Intravenous: 10 to 20 mg/kg daily in 2 divided doses.

NURSING IMPLICATIONS

Check expiration date. Degradation products of outdated tetracyclines can be highly nephrotoxic. Instruct patient to discard unused drug when course of therapy has ended.

Food may interfere with rate and extent of absorption of oral drug. Administer at least 1 hour before or 2 hours following meals. Do not give with antacids, milk, milk products, or other calcium-containing foods.

Caution patient to avoid excessive exposure to sunlight.

Dosage will require readjustment in the presence of renal dysfunction.

Dry powder for parenteral use is stable at room temperature. Reconstituted solutions are stable for 48 hours at refrigerated temperatures (2 C to 8 C).

The commercially available solution for IM use only contains 2% lidocaine.

Syrup formulation (oxytetracycline calcium) should be stored in a cool place protected from light.

See Tetracycline Hydrochloride.

OXYTOCIN INJECTION, U.S.P.
(PITOCIN, SYNTOCINON, UTERACON)
OXYTOCIN CITRATE
(PITOCIN CITRATE)

Hormone, posterior pituitary, oxytocic

ACTIONS AND USES

Synthetic, water-soluble polypeptide consisting of 8 amino acids, identical pharmacologically to the oxytocic principle of posterior pituitary. Oxytocic activity: 10 U.S.P. posterior pituitary units per milliliter. By direct action on myofibrils, produces phasic contractions characteristic of normal delivery. Promotes milk ejection (letdown) reflex in nursing mother, thereby increasing flow (not volume) of milk; also facilitates flow of milk during period of breast engorgement. Uterine sensitivity to oxytocin increases during gestation period and peaks sharply before parturition. Exerts slight intrinsic ADH-like effect in large doses.

Used to initiate or improve uterine contraction at term only in carefully selected patients and only after cervix is dilated and presentation of fetus has occurred; used to stimulate letdown reflex in nursing mother and to relieve pain from breast. Uses include: management of inevitable, incomplete, or missed abortion; stimulation of uterine contractions during third stage of labor; stimulation to overcome uterine inertia; control of postpartum hemorrhage and promotion of postpartum uterine involution. Also used to induce labor in cases of maternal diabetes, preeclampsia, eclampsia, and erythroblastosis fetalis.

ABSORPTION AND FATE

Uterine response following IM injection is evidenced in 3 to 7 minutes, with duration of 30 to 60 minutes; after IV injection, response occurs within 1 minute, with shorter duration; after buccal administration, response occurs in 30 minutes, with duration of 30 to 60 minutes. Plasma half-life is 1 minute to several minutes (shorter during late pregnancy and lactation). Rapidly removed from plasma by mammary gland, kidney, and liver and inactivated, perhaps by oxytocinase, an enzyme produced in placenta and uterine tissue during pregnancy. Small portion of dose is excreted in active form by kidney.

CONTRAINDICATIONS AND PRECAUTIONS

Hypersensitivity to oxytocin, significant cephalopelvic disproportion, unfavorable fetal position or presentation, obstetric emergencies where benefit-to-risk ratio for mother or fetus favors surgical intervention, fetal distress where delivery is not imminent, prematurity, placenta previa, prolonged use in severe toxemia or uterine inertia, hypertonic uterine patterns, previous surgery of cervix and cesarean section, conditions predisposing to thromboplastin or amniotic fluid embolism (dead fetus, abruptio placentae), grand multiparity, primipara over 35 years of age, past history of uterine sepsis or of traumatic delivery, intranasal route during labor, simultaneous administration of drug by two routes, use of buccal tablets in unconscious patient, use in management and control of third stage, use in postpartum bleeding, use to expel placenta or in management of abortion. Cautious use: concomitant use with cyclopropane anesthesia or vasoconstrictive drugs.

ADVERSE REACTIONS

Fetus: bradycardia and other arrhythmias, hypoxia, intracranial hemorrhage, trauma from too rapid propulsion through pelvis, death. **Mother:** hypersensitivity leading to uterine hypertonicity, tetanic contractions, uterine rupture, anaphylactic reactions, postpartum hemorrhage, cardiac arrhythmias, pelvic hematoma, nausea, vomiting, hypertensive episodes, subarachnoid hemorrhage, increased blood flow and afibrinogenemia, severe water intoxication, hypotension, ECG changes, anxiety, dyspnea, precordial pain, edema, cyanosis or redness of skin, cardiovascular spasm and collapse. Citrate: parabuccal irritation.

ROUTE AND DOSAGE

Induction or stimulation of labor: Intravenous infusion: 10 U (1 ml) in 1 liter of 5% dextrose; flow rate 14 drops/minute. As soon as labor begins, rate adjusted according to uterine contractions and fetal response. Buccal: initially 1 tablet (200 U); then 1 tablet every 30 minutes in alternate cheek pouch until desired response is experienced; note the number of tablets in cheeks and maintain that number until delivery or until total of 15 tablets (3000 U) have been given. *Postpartum hemorrhage:* Intramuscular: 3 to 10 units (0.3 to 1 ml). Intravenous infusion: 10 to 40 units in 1 liter of 5% dextrose. Intranasal: single spray (as a whiff) into one or both nostrils 2 or 3 minutes before nursing or pumping of breasts.

NURSING IMPLICATIONS

When diluting oxytocin for IV infusion, rotate bottle gently to distribute medicine throughout solution.

Refrigerate oxytocin for long-term storage.

Before instituting treatment, start flow charts to record maternal blood pressure and other vital signs, intake–output ratio, weight, and strength, duration, and frequency of contractions, as well as fetal heart tone and rate.

Oxytocin administration should be supervised by persons having thorough knowledge of the drug and the skill to identify complications. A qualified physician should be immediately available to manage complications.

Time of administration of oxytocin in relation to delivery of baby or placenta varies with physician's preference. The nurse should have a clear understanding of when drug is to be administered with respect to progress of labor.

Infusion flow rates (established by physician) should not exceed 14 drops/minute. Accurate control by infusion pump (or other device) is critical.

Use of a Y connection to infusion tubing is advised to allow oxytocin solution to be discontinued if necessary while vein is kept open.

Knowledge of time factors related to onset and duration of effects (see Absorption and Fate) is essential for prevention of fetal and maternal crises.

Oxytocin dosage for stimulation of labor may be less than that required for induction.

Incidence of hypersensitivity or allergic reactions is higher when oxytocin is given by IM or IV injection rather than by IV infusion (diluted solution).

Instruct patient to place buccal tablet in parabuccal space and not to disturb tablet by eating, smoking, tonguing, or drinking. If oxytocic activity must be stopped, or if patient complains of dry mouth, he may remove the tablet and rinse mouth with cold water. Tablet releases oxytocin at a regular rate, except during first few minutes before vasoconstriction in parabuccal contact area (a local response) has occurred.

Buccal tablets should be used only when adequate supervision is available.

Administration of tablet is continued until desired response is experienced (regular, firm uterine contractions not exceeding 40 to 60 seconds duration and not occurring more frequently than every 3 minutes).

Accidental swallowing of a buccal tablet causes no harm, but oxytocic action is destroyed in digestive tract. Warn patient to report swallowed tablet to physician.

During delivery, IM oxytocin is most easily injected deep into deltoid muscle (using needle at least 2.5 cm in length). Massage injection site to assist quick absorption.

If IM oxytocin is used, magnesium sulfate (10 ml of 20%) solution should be available for relaxation of the myometrium.

Intranasal preparation: Instruct patient to clear nasal passages well before administration. Hold squeeze bottle upright, and apply solution into nostril with patient's head in a vertical position.

If local or regional (caudal, spinal) anesthesia is being given to the patient receiving oxytocin, be alert to the possibility of hypertensive crisis: intense occipital headache, palpitation, marked hypertension, stiff neck, nausea, vomiting, sweating, fever, photophobia, dilated pupils, bradycardia or tachycardia, constricting chest pain.

When oxytocin is given to stimulate the letdown reflex, provide measures that support a beneficial response: quiet nonstressful environment, maternal confidence through knowledge and freedom from worry and pain.

Monitor intake and output during labor. If patient is receiving drug by prolonged IV infusion, watch for symptoms of water intoxication (drowsiness, listlessness, headache, confusion, anuria, weight gain). Report changes in alertness and orientation and changes in intake–output ratio.

During infusion period, monitor fetal heart rate and maternal blood pressure and pulse at least every 15 minutes; evaluate tone of myometrium during and between contractions and record on flow chart. Report change in rate and rhythm immediately.

If contractions are prolonged (occurring at less than 2-minute intervals) and if electric monitor records contractions above 50 mm Hg, stop infusion to prevent fetal anoxia, turn patient on her side, and notify physician. Stimulation will wane rapidly within 2 to 3 minutes. Oxygen administration may be necessary.

Oxytocin is incompatible with infusions of fibrinolysin, levarterenol bitartrate, prochlorperazine edisylate, protein hydrolysate, and warfarin sodium.

DRUG INTERACTIONS: **Ephedrine, methoxamine, and other vasopressors** can cause severe hypertension when administered at same time as oxytocin.

PANCREATIN, N.F., B.P.
(ELZYME 303, PANTERIC, VIOKASE)

Enzyme (digestive aid)

ACTIONS AND USES
Pancreatic enzyme concentrate of bovine or porcine origin containing principally lipase, protease, and amylase in standardized amounts. Assists in digestion of starch, protein, and fats; decreases nitrogen and fat content of stool.
Used as digestive aid in cystic fibrosis and other conditions associated with exocrine pancreatic deficiencies.
CONTRAINDICATIONS AND PRECAUTIONS
Cautious use: history of hypersensitivity reactions to beef or pig products.
ADVERSE REACTIONS
With large doses: anorexia, nausea, vomiting, diarrhea, buccal and anal soreness (particularly in infants), hypersensitivity reactions (sneezing, lacrimation, skin rashes).
ROUTE AND DOSAGE
Oral: **Adults:** 500 mg to 1 Gm (as high as 12 Gm daily may be prescribed in divided doses at 1- or 2-hour intervals or before and after meals, with an extra dose being taken with any food eaten between meals. **Pediatric:** 0.3 to 0.6 Gm 3 times daily.

NURSING IMPLICATIONS
Avoid inhalation of powder formulation.
Enteric-coated tablets are to be swallowed whole, not crushed or chewed.
  Milk or antacid should not be taken within 1 hour of taking tablets.
Monitor intake and output and weight. Note appetite, quality of stools weight loss, abdominal bloating (pancreatic insufficiency may present as diabetes mellitus, steatorrhea, bulky stools).
For pancreatic insufficiency, a special diet high in protein and low in fat is recommended. Multivitamin supplements in water-soluble form may also be prescribed.
Periodic measurement of fecal fat and nitrogen, serum carotene and calcium, and prothrombin activity may be made to evaluate response to drug therapy.
Stored in tight containers at room temperature (not exceeding 30 C).

PANCRELIPASE, N.F.
(COTAZYM, ILOZYME, KU-ZYME-HP)

Enzyme (digestive aid)

ACTIONS AND USES
Pancreatic enzyme concentrate of porcine origin standardized for lipase content. On a weight basis, has 12 times the lipolytic activity and at least 4 times the trypsin and amylase content of pancreatin.
Used as replacement therapy in symptomatic treatment of malabsorption syndrome due to cystic fibrosis and other conditions associated with exocrine pancreatic insufficiency.

Cautious use: history of allergy to hog protein or enzymes.

ADVERSE REACTIONS

High doses: anorexia, nausea, vomiting, diarrhea.

ROUTE AND DOSAGE

Oral: **Adults:** 1 to 3 capsules or tablets or 1 or 2 packets just prior to or with each meal or snack as prescribed: **Pediatric:** 1 or 2 capsules or tablets with each meal. In severe deficiencies, frequency may be increased to hourly intervals.

NURSING IMPLICATIONS

Dosage is usually determined by fat content in diet (suggested ratio: 300 mg pancrelipase for each 17 Gm dietary fat).

Proper balance between fat, protein, and starch intake must be maintained to avoid temporary indigestion.

Contents of capsule may be sprinkled on food or dispersed in liquid.

See Pancreatin.

PANCURONIUM BROMIDE
(PAVULON)

Skeletal muscle relaxant

ACTIONS AND USES

Synthetic curariform nondepolarizing neuromuscular blocking agent. Similar to tubocurarine chloride in actions, uses, and limitations. Reported to be approximately 5 times as potent as tubocurarine, but produces little or no histamine release or ganglionic blockade, and thus does not cause bronchospasm or hypotension. In high doses, has direct blocking effect on acetylcholine receptors of heart, and may cause increased heart rate, cardiac output, and arterial pressure.

ABSORPTION AND FATE

Onset of action within 45 seconds, with peak effect in about 5 minutes, and 90% recovery within 1 hour. Small amount metabolized and eliminated in bile. Excreted primarily unchanged by kidneys.

CONTRAINDICATIONS AND PRECAUTIONS

Hypersensitivity to the drug or bromides; tachycardia; children under 10 years of age; women of childbearing potential; pregnancy. Also see Tubocurarine.

ADVERSE REACTIONS

Increased pulse rate and blood pressure, transient acneiform rash, burning sensation along course of vein. Also see Tubocurarine.

ROUTE AND DOSAGE

Intravenous: 0.04 to 0.1 mg/kg body weight. Additional doses may be administered at 30 to 60 minute intervals, if necessary.

NURSING IMPLICATIONS

Plastic syringe may be used for administration, but drug may adsorb to plastic with prolonged storage.

Observe patient for residual muscle weakness and signs of respiratory distress during recovery period.

See Tubocurarine Chloride.

Proteolytic enzyme

ACTIONS AND USES
Combination of proteolytic enzymes extracted from *Carica papaya*. At recommended doses, does not affect uninjured cells or tissues.
Used topically for enzymatic debridement, promotion of normal healing, and deodorization of surface lesions. Tablet formulation is used for relief of symptoms related to episiotomy.

CONTRAINDICATIONS AND PRECAUTIONS
History of allergy to papain. Tablet formulation: systemic infection or severe blood clotting disorders; concomitant use of anticoagulants. Safe use during pregnancy not established. Cautious use: severe renal or hepatic disease. Topical preparation not to be used in eyes.

ADVERSE REACTIONS
Topical use: occasional stinging or itching. Tablet formulation: nausea, vomiting, diarrhea, dizziness, pruritus, rash, urticaria, mild local tingling at site of buccal absorption.

ROUTE AND DOSAGE
Oral (prophylactic): 2 tablets 1 or 2 hours before episiotomy; (therapeutic): 2 tablets 4 times a day for at least 5 days. Topical (ointment 10%): apply locally to lesion once or twice daily; at each redressing, irrigate lesion with mild (prescribed) cleansing solution to remove accumulated debris.

NURSING IMPLICATIONS
Tablets (Papase) may be administered buccally or orally, swallowed with water or chewed.
Mild local tingling at buccal site is usually relieved when tablet is moved.
Topical preparations may be covered with gauze.
Hydrogen peroxide inactivates topical papain and therefore should not be used as irrigating solution.
Itching or stinging sensation sometimes occurs when papain is first applied.
If symptoms persist, report to physician.

PAPAVERINE HYDROCHLORIDE, N.F., B.P.

(BLUEPAV, CEREBID, CERESPAN, DIPAV, DYLATE, J-PAV, LEMPAV, MYOBID, PAPACON, PAP-KAPS-150, P-A-V, PAVABID, PAVACEN, PAVADEL, PAVADUR, PAVADYL, PAVAGRANT, PAVAKEY, PAVASED, PAVATRAN, SUSTAVERINE, VASAL, VASOSPAN)

Smooth muscle relaxant

ACTIONS AND USES
Benzylisoquinoline alkaloid prepared synthetically or from opium. Lacks pharmacologic properties of narcotics; reportedly does not promote tolerance or habituation, and has little if any analgesic effect. Exerts direct spasmolytic effect on smooth muscles unrelated to innervation. Action is especially pronounced on coronary, cerebral, pulmonary, and peripheral arteries when spasm is present. Like quinidine, acts directly on myocardium, depresses conduction and irritability, and prolongs refractory period. Relaxes smooth muscles of bronchi, GI tract, ureters, and biliary system.
Used primarily for relief of cerebral and peripheral ischemia associated with

arterial spasm and myocardial ischemia complicated by arrhythmias. Also has been used for visceral spasm as in ureteral, biliary, and GI colic.

ABSORPTION AND FATE

Readily absorbed following oral administration. Peak plasma levels in 1 to 2 hours, falling to low levels after 6 hours with regular tablets and 12 hours after extended-release forms. About 90% bound to plasma proteins. Half-life approximately 90 minutes. Rapidly metabolized in liver; excreted in urine chiefly as metabolites.

CONTRAINDICATIONS AND PRECAUTIONS

Parenteral use in complete A-V block. Cautious use: glaucoma, myocardial depression.

ADVERSE REACTIONS

Parenteral use (low incidence): general discomfort, facial flushing, sweating, dry mouth and throat, pruritus, skin rash, dizziness, headache, excessive sedation (large doses), slight rise in blood pressure, increased depth of respiration, tachycardia, transient ventricular ectopic rhythms, hepatotoxicity (jaundice, eosinophilia, abnormal liver function tests); with rapid IV administration: respiratory depression, A-V block arrhythmias, fatal apnea. **Oral use:** nausea, anorexia, constipation, diarrhea, abdominal distress, dizziness, drowsiness, headache.

ROUTE AND DOSAGE

Oral: **Adult:** 100 to 300 mg 3 to 5 times daily; timed-release forms: 150 mg every 12 hours. Intramuscular, intravenous: 30 to 120 mg, repeated every 3 hours, as indicated. For treatment of cardiac extrasystoles, two doses may be administered 10 minutes apart. IV administered slowly over 1- to 2-minute period. **Pediatric:** Intramuscular, intravenous: 6 mg/kg/24 hours divided into 4 doses.

NURSING IMPLICATIONS

Aspirate carefully before injecting IM, to avoid inadvertent entry into blood vessel, and administer slowly.

Monitor pulse, respiration, and blood pressure in patients receiving drug parenterally.

Hepatic function and blood tests should be performed periodically. Hepatotoxicity (thought to be a hypersensitivity reaction) is reversible with prompt drug withdrawal.

Instruct patient to notify physician of any minor side effects.

Advise patient to avoid strenuous tasks immediately following drug ingestion because of possibility of dizziness.

Preserved in tightly covered, light-resistant containers.

Parenteral papaverine is incompatible with lactated Ringer's injection (forms precipitate).

PARALDEHYDE, U.S.P., B.P.
(Paracetaldehyde, PARAL)

Sedative, hypnotic

ACTIONS AND USES

Cyclic ether formed by polymerization of acetaldehyde. Potent CNS depressant with sedative and hypnotic actions similar to those of alcohol, barbiturates, and chloral hydrate.

Used as sedative and hypnotic in acute agitation due to alcohol withdrawal; used to control convulsions arising from tetanus eclampsia, status epilepticus, and drug poisoning. Has been used rectally to induce basal anesthesia, particularly in children.

Absorbed well from all routes. Acts within 30 minutes; effects last 6 to 8 hours or more. Average half-life 7.5 hours. Approximately 80% to 90% of dose is metabolized by liver. Significant amounts excreted unchanged through lungs; traces eliminated unchanged in urine. Readily crosses placenta.

CONTRAINDICATIONS AND PRECAUTIONS

Severe hepatic insufficiency, respiratory disease, GI inflammation or ulceration.

ADVERSE REACTIONS

Irritation of mucous membrane (oral and rectal routes), nausea, vomiting, erythematous skin rash. IM injection: pain, sterile abscess, necrosis, muscle irritation. Prolonged use: toxic hepatitis, nephrosis, metabolic acidosis. Overdosage: rapid labored breathing, pulmonary hemorrhage and edema, hypotension, bleeding gastritis, renal and liver damage, acidosis, dilation of right heart, cardiovascular collapse.

ROUTE AND DOSAGE

Each 1 ml contains approximately 1 Gm paraldehyde. **Adults:** Oral, rectal (*sedative*): 5 to 10 ml; (*hypnotic*): 10 to 30 ml. Intramuscular, intravenous (*sedative*): 5 ml; (*hypnotic*): 10 ml. For IV injection, drug should be diluted with several volumes of 0.9% sodium chloride injection and administered slowly and with caution. **Children:** Oral, intramuscular (*sedative*): 0.15 ml/kg body weight; (*hypnotic*): twice the sedative dose.

NURSING IMPLICATIONS

Paraldehyde is a colorless clear liquid with a strong characteristic odor and a burning, disagreeable taste.

On exposure to light, air, and heat, drug liberates acetaldehyde, which oxidizes to acetic acid. Do not use solution if it is colored in any way or smells of acetic acid (vinegar odor).

Decomposed paraldehyde is extremely corrosive to tissues and can cause fatal poisoning. Discard unused contents of any container that has been opened for more than 24 hours.

Paraldehyde is not an analgesic; therefore, it should not be given to relieve pain. The drug may produce excitement or delirium in the presence of pain.

Give oral drug well diluted in chilled fruit juice or milk to reduce irritation of GI tract and mask odor and taste. Oral capsules are available.

When given rectally, drug should be diluted with at least two volumes of olive oil or cottonseed oil or dissolved in 200 ml of 0.9% sodium chloride solution to prevent rectal irritation.

Parenteral preparation should be drawn into a glass syringe. Paraldehyde is not compatible with most plastics.

IM injection should be made deep into upper outer quadrant of buttock well away from nerve trunks. Aspirate carefully before injecting drug, and massage injection site well. Rotate injection sites.

In some hospitals, physicians administer parenteral paraldehyde because of danger of circulatory collapse or pulmonary edema, sterile abscesses, nerve injury, and paralysis.

Bronchial secretions may be increased. Keep the patient turned on side to prevent aspiration. Suctioning may be necessary.

Advise bed rest and no smoking. Bedsides are indicated.

Keep patient's room well ventilated to control the strong, pungent odor of exhaled drug. Patient's breath will have a characteristic odor for several hours.

Tolerance and physical and/or psychologic dependence can occur with prolonged use. Paraldehyde addiction resembles alcoholism.

Classified as schedule IV drug under federal Controlled Substances Act.

Rapid withdrawal after prolonged use may produce delirium tremens and hallucinations.

Treatment of overdosage: gastric lavage for oral ingestion (if endotracheal tube with cuff is in place to prevent aspiration of vomitus) or rectal lavage for rectal overdosage, followed by demulcent such as mineral oil (orally or by nasogastric tube). Have phenylenetetrazol on hand.

Preserved in tight, light-resistant containers in amounts not exceeding 30 ml and at temperatures not over 25 C (77 F).

Stock drug should be checked periodically for purity as defined by U.S.P.

LABORATORY TEST INTERFERENCES: Paraldehyde may cause false positive serum ketones (nitroprusside tube dilution method) and urine ketones (Acetest) and may interfere with urinary steroid determinations (by modification of Reddy, Jenkins, Thorn procedure).

DRUG INTERACTIONS: Theoretically, **disulfiram** may increase blood levels of paraldehyde by inhibiting its metabolism. Paraldehyde may increase the possibility of **sulfonamide** crystalluria. Additive CNS depression may occur when administered concomitantly with other **CNS depressant drugs.**

PARAMETHADIONE, U.S.P., B.P.
(PARADIONE)

Anticonvulsant

ACTIONS AND USES

Oxazolidinedione derivative with pharmacologic actions, uses, contraindications, precautions, and adverse reactions similar to those of trimethadione (qv). Unlike trimethadione, chronic administration is not associated with myasthenia-gravis-like syndrome, and incidence of other toxic reactions is lower, but it is reportedly less effective.

Used to control petit mal seizures refractory to other drugs.

ROUTE AND DOSAGE

Oral: **Adults:** 300 to 600 mg 3 or 4 times daily; therapy generally started at 900 mg daily; dosage then increased by 300 mg/day at weekly intervals until seizures are controlled or toxic symptoms intervene. **Children:** 300 to 900 mg in 3 or 4 equally divided doses (depending on age and weight). Highly individualized.

NURSING IMPLICATIONS

Oral solution contains alcohol 65% and must be diluted before administration.

See Trimethadione.

PARAMETHASONE ACETATE, N.F.
(HALDRONE, STEMEX)

Adrenocortical steroid (glucocorticoid)

ACTIONS AND USES

Synthetic steroid with antiinflammatory action, but very little sodium-retaining potency. On weight basis, 2 mg paramethasone is equivalent to 20 mg hydrocortisone. Has no particular advantages over other corticosteroids. Similar to hydrocortisone (qv) in actions, uses, absorption, and fate.

CONTRAINDICATIONS AND PRECAUTIONS

Systemic fungal infections, in presence of ocular herpes simplex. Also see Hydrocortisone.

ADVERSE REACTIONS

Increase in appetite, psychic derangement. Also see Hydrocortisone.

ROUTE AND DOSAGE

Oral: **Adults**: initially 2 to 24 mg daily until satisfactory response is achieved; dose is then decreased by small amounts to lowest therapeutic level for maintenance (1 to 8 mg daily, highly individualized).

NURSING IMPLICATIONS

At high dosage (above 15 mg daily), urinary excretion of calcium and nitrogen increases significantly.

If drug is to be stopped after long-term therapy, it should be withdrawn gradually rather than abruptly.

See Hydrocortisone.

PARATHYROID INJECTION, U.S.P.
(PAROIDIN)

Antihypocalcemic

ACTIONS AND USES

Protein hormone extracted from bovine parathyroid glands standardized to potency not less than 100 U.S.P. units per milliliter; regulates calcium (Ca) metabolism and Ca ion plasma concentration. Increases renal clearance of phosphates, stimulates Ca reabsorption from renal tubules, and (by promoting bone resorption) fosters Ca and phosphate release to serum. Conserves body magnesium, but increases excretion of water, sodium, and bicarbonate. By facilitating renal conversion of vitamin D to its active form, dihydroxycholecalciferol, provides the catalyst required for Ca absorption from small intestine. In deficiency states the hormone raises plasma Ca levels, thereby restoring normal threshold of excitability in polarized membranes. Recent research is directing effective use of dihydrotachysterol or other vitamin D_2 metabolites as pharmacologic substitutes for parathyroid hormone in persistent hypoparathyroidism.

Used as short-term treatment of acute hypoparathyroidism with tetany, as diagnostic tool for pseudoparathyroidism, and investigationally in conjunction with radioactive phosphorus as palliative treatment of prostatic cancer when other treatments have failed. Also used as treatment of oxalic acid and radiophosphorus poisoning.

ABSORPTION AND FATE

Well absorbed after parenteral administration. Phosphatemic response follows IV injection within 15 minutes, and serum Ca rises in about 1 hour. After IM or subcutaneous dose, serum Ca level rises in 4 hours, peaks in 12 to 18 hours, and returns to pretreatment levels after 20 to 24 hours. Binds to plasma proteins; plasma half-life about 20 minutes. Degradation sites not clear, but possibly in kidney and liver. Only 1% of dose is excreted in urine.

CONTRAINDICATIONS AND PRECAUTIONS

Hypercalcemia, hypercalciuria, tetany unrelated to parathyroid failure, IV administration when serum Ca levels are above normal. Cautious use: sarcoidosis, renal or cardiac disease, digitalized patients. Information about use during pregnancy not available.

Hypercalcemia (overdosage): muscular weakness, deep bone and flank pain, lethargy, headache, anorexia, nausea, vomiting, diarrhea, abdominal cramps, vertigo, tinnitus, ataxia, exanthema. **Hypercalcemic crisis:** dehydration, stupor, coma, azotemia. **Other:** subcutaneous site inflammation, vasodilation, decreased blood pressure, bradycardia, cardiac arrhythmias, syncope, cardiac arrest.

ROUTE AND DOSAGE

Subcutaneous, intramuscular, intravenous: **Adults:** 20 to 40 U every 12 hours, if necessary, for acute tetany secondary to hypoparathyroidism. **Infants:** 25 to 50 U every 12 hours for 1 to 3 days.

NURSING IMPLICATIONS

Before hormone is given IV, sensitivity should be tested by injecting a small amount subcutaneously or by instilling it into conjunctival sac.

IV flow rate should be slow in case of sensitivity, even though preliminary test may have been negative. Check with physician. Have epinephrine available for emergency treatment when adding parathyroid to another IV fluid; it is recommended that 2.5% to 5% dextrose be used rather than saline in order to prevent precipitation.

Calcium gluconate IV and by mouth is usually ordered with parathyroid injection, particularly during interim before parathyroid effect is established.

IM route is preferable to subcutaneous because there is less irritation at injection site.

Frequent determinations of serum Ca and phosphorus levels should be performed during therapy. Most physicians prefer to maintain serum Ca levels at 9 to 11 mg/dl, with 12 mg/dl the outside limit. Normal serum phosphorus level is 3 to 4.5 mg/dl.

Therapy of the deficiency state relieves latent tetany (muscular fatigue) and manifest tetany (paresthesias of extremities, carpopedal spasm, laryngospasm with dyspnea and cyanosis, and spasm of eye muscles, bronchi, stomach, intestines, or urinary bladder, as well as grand mal convulsions).

Until dosage has effectively restored Ca level, prepare for possibility of convulsions: padded bedrails, padded tongue blade, quiet and non-stimulating environment (reduced noise and lights, even temperature levels).

Calcium deficiency is tested by two signs:

Chvostek's sign: Tap seventh cranial nerve (facial) anterior to parotid. Muscle contraction of ipsilateral orbicularis oculi, or orbicularis oris, occurs if latent tetany exists.

Trousseau's sign: grasp patient's wrist so as to constrict circulation for a few minutes, or inflate sphygmomanometer cuff on upper arm to systolic reading. Resulting ischemia of peripheral nerves increases excitability and causes spasm of muscles of lower arm and hand. Carpal spasm occurs in presence of latent tetany.

Be alert for symptoms of drug-induced hypercalcemia. Should it present (may be due to adrenal insufficiency), discontinue parathyroid injection, Ca salts, and vitamin D. A low-calcium diet, forced fluids, and administration of a phosphate or sulfate laxative may give relief if hypercalcemia is mild.

Monitor intake–output ratio. Increased fluid intake may be ordered to prevent formation of renal stones.

If high-Ca, low-phosphorus diet is prescribed, the patient will be given a drug that blocks absorption of dietary phosphorus (eg, calcium carbonate or lactate, or aluminum hydroxide suspension) because most foods high in calcium are also high in phosphorus. See Index for foods high in calcium.

Store ampules at 2 C to 8 C (36 F to 46 F); avoid freezing.

DRUG INTERACTIONS: Hypercalcemia is promoted when parathyroid hormone is given with a **thiazide** (inhibits Ca secretion in proximal tubules and enhances hormone's bone resorption activity). **Dactinomycin** competitively inhibits bone resorption activity, and **anticonvulsants** decrease phosphatemic effect of parathyroid. **Cortisol** may antagonize parathyroid effect on Ca absorption from the gut. **Androgens** decrease bone resorption activity.

PAREGORIC, U.S.P.
Camphorated opium tincture

Antiperistaltic

ACTIONS AND USES
Contains 0.04% anhydrous morphine, alcohol, benzoic acid, camphor, and anise oil. Pharmacologic activity is due to morphine content. Increases smooth-muscle tone of GI tract, but decreases motility and propulsive peristalsis, and diminishes digestive secretions. Delayed passage of intestinal contents results in desiccation of feces and constipation.

Used as short-term treatment for symptomatic relief of acute diarrhea.

ROUTE AND DOSAGE
Oral: **Adults:** 5 to 10 ml after bowel movement (may be administered every 2 hours if necessary, up to but not exceeding 4 times daily until diarrhea is controlled). **Children:** 0.25 to 0.5 ml/kg body weight.

NURSING IMPLICATIONS
Not to be confused with opium tincture, which contains 25 times more anhydrous morphine.

Instruct patient to adhere strictly to prescribed dosage schedule.

Administer paregoric in sufficient water to assure its passage into the stomach (mixture will appear milky).

Possible cause of diarrhea and its duration and accompanying symptoms such as fever, abdominal pain, and passage of mucus or blood should be investigated (potential etiologic factors: acute food or chemical poisons; viral, parasitic, or bacterial contamination of food or water; dietary indiscretion; inflammatory disease of GI tract).

Advise bed rest until diarrhea is controlled.

Replacement of fluids and electrolytes is a vital part of therapy for diarrhea. Instruct patient to drink warm clear liquids until diarrhea stops. Physicians generally recommend a bland diet for 2 or 3 days (potato, rice, cooked cereals, eggs, custard, fluid), progressing gradually to normal diet.

Advise patient to observe character and frequency of stools. Drug should be discontinued as soon as diarrhea is controlled. Urge patient to report promptly to physician if diarrhea persists more than 3 days, if fever or abdominal pain develops, or if mucus or blood is passed.

Inform patient that constipation is often a consequence of antidiarrheal treatment and that normal habit pattern is usually established as dietary intake increases.

Although the volume of morphine in paregoric is small (0.4 mg/ml), prolonged use or excessive amounts can lead to psychic dependence.

Paregoric is classified as a schedule III drug under the federal Controlled Substances Act. Commercial preparations containing small amounts of paregoric are classified under schedule V (in certain circumstances they may be dispensed without prescription unless additional state regulations apply), eg, Diabismul, Kaoparin with paregoric, Ka-Pek with paregoric, Pabizol with paregoric, Parepectolin.

Preserved in tight, light-resistant container, away from heat.

See Morphine Sulfate.

PARGYLINE HYDROCHLORIDE
(EUTONYL)

Antihypertensive

ACTIONS AND USES

Nonhydrazine MAO inhibitor with pharmacologic actions similar to those of other MAO inhibitors (see Phenelzine). Exerts hypotensive effect and reportedly produces mood elevation. Mechanism of hypotensive activity not known, but thought to be related in part to modification of ganglionic transmission. Most prominent effect is on orthostatic blood pressure.

Used in treatment of moderate to severe hypertension. May be used concurrently with other antihypertensive agents such as thiazides and/or rauwolfia alkaloids.

ABSORPTION AND FATE

Excreted primarily in urine as unchanged drug.

CONTRAINDICATIONS AND PRECAUTIONS

Mild, labile, or malignant hypertension; hyperactive or excitable individuals; paranoid schizophrenia; hyperthyroidism; pheochromocytoma; advanced renal failure. Safe use during pregnancy and lactation and in women of childbearing potential and in children under 12 years of age not established. Cautious use: liver disease, arteriosclerosis, coronary artery disease, parkinsonism, diabetes mellitus.

ADVERSE REACTIONS

Orthostatic hypotension, sweating, dry mouth, fluid retention, congestive heart failure, increased appetite, weight gain, nausea, vomiting, mild constipation, headache, arthralgia, difficulty in micturition, impotence or delayed ejaculation, rash, purpura, nightmares, hyperexcitability, muscle twitching and other extrapyramidal symptoms, drug fever (rare), hypoglycemia (optic atrophy not reported, although it is associated with use of other MAO inhibitors). Overdosage: agitation, confusion, hallucinations, mania, hyperreflexia, convulsions, hyperextension or hypotension.

ROUTE AND DOSAGE

Oral: initially 25 mg once daily; may be increased once a week by 10-mg increments until desired response is obtained. Total daily dose not to exceed 200 mg. *Elderly or sympathectomized patients:* initially 10 to 25 mg daily for first 2 weeks. *Addition to established antihypertensive regimen:* initial dose should not exceed 25 mg (less in elderly or sympathectomized patients); maintenance 50 to 75 mg daily.

NURSING IMPLICATIONS

Dosage adjustments are based on blood pressure in standing position.

Instruct patient to report symptoms of orthostatic hypotension (dizziness, weakness, palpitation, fainting); dosage adjustment is indicated.

Warn patient to make position changes slowly, especially when getting out of bed, and to lie or sit down immediately if feeling dizzy or faint.

Actions of pargyline are cumulative. Maximal therapeutic effect may occur in 4 days, but it may not appear for 3 weeks or more; action may persist for 3 weeks after therapy is discontinued.

Instruct patient to keep daily record of weight and to check ankles and tibias for edema. Pargyline tends to promote weight gain from fluid retention as well as nonfluid retention (increased appetite).

Patients with impaired renal function should be closely observed for signs of cumulative drug effects. Monitor intake and output and BUN in these patients.

Although optic damage has not been reported with pargyline, patients on prolonged therapy should be checked periodically for changes in color perception, visual fields, fundi, and visual acuity.

Patients with diabetes may require adjustment in antidiabetic medication. Severe drug-induced hypoglycemia can occur.

Since drug may suppress anginal pain, patient should be warned not to increase physical activity in response to drug-induced sense of well-being.

Urinalyses, liver function tests, and complete blood counts should be performed periodically during therapy.

Tolerance to pargyline develops rapidly. Urge patient to keep scheduled follow-up appointments.

Drug may augment hypotensive effects of anesthetic agents, and therefore should be discontinued at least 2 weeks prior to elective surgery.

If drug therapy is temporarily interrupted for any reason, it should be reinstituted at a lower dosage level.

Caution patient not to add any medication to drug regimen without consulting physician. OTC preparations containing dextromethorphan or sympathomimetic amines can precipitate hypertensive crisis (eg, appetite suppressants, nasal decongestants, cold and hay fever remedies).

Acute hypertensive reaction (severe headache, marked hypertension, chest pain, palpitation, tachycardia, bradycardia) can result from ingestion of foods or liquids high in tyramine or tryptophan. Provide family or responsible family member with list of foods to avoid (see Phenelzine).

See Phenelzine.

PAROMOMYCIN SULFATE, N.F., B.P.
(HUMATIN)

Antibiotic

ACTIONS AND USES

Antibiotic produced by certain strains of *Streptomyces rimosus* with spectrum of antibacterial activity closely parallelling that of kanamycin and neomycin (qv). Exerts direct antibacterial and antiamebic action, primarily in lumen of GI tract. Ineffective against extraintestinal amebiasis. Reportedly produces significant reduction in serum cholesterol.

Used for treatment of acute and chronic intestinal amebiasis and to rid bowel of nitrogen-forming bacteria in patients with hepatic coma. Also has been used for tapeworm infestation.

ABSORPTION AND FATE

Poorly absorbed from intact GI tract; almost 100% of dose is recoverable in feces.

CONTRAINDICATIONS AND PRECAUTIONS

History of hypersensitivity to paromomycin; intestinal obstruction. Cautious use: GI ulceration.

ADVERSE REACTIONS
Diarrhea, abdominal cramps, nausea; (occasionally): headache, vomiting, vertigo, skin rash, pruritus ani, heartburn. Overgrowth of nonsusceptible organisms including fungi.

ROUTE AND DOSAGE
Oral (intestinal amebiasis): 25 to 35 mg/kg divided in 3 doses, for 5 to 10 days; (hepatic coma): 4 Gm daily in divided doses, given at regular intervals for 5 or 6 days.

NURSING IMPLICATIONS

Administer drug with meals.

Be alert for appearance of any new infection (superinfection) during therapy.

Patients receiving drug for intestinal amebiasis should be excluded from preparing, processing, and serving food until treatment is complete. Isolation is not required.

Emphasize personal hygeine, particularly handwashing after defecation and before eating food, and sanitary disposal of feces.

Criterion of cure is absence of amebae in stool specimens examined at weekly intervals for 6 weeks after completion of treatment, and thereafter at monthly intervals for 2 years.

Possible sources of contamination (eg, water, food, infected persons) should be investigated.

Household members and other suspected contacts should have microscopic examination of feces for amebae.

PEMOLINE
(CYLERT, PIOXOL)

CNS stimulant

ACTIONS AND USES
Oxazolidinone derivative with pharmacologic actions qualitatively similar to those of amphetamine and methylphenidate, but with weak sympathomimetic activity. Capable of producing increased motor activity, mental alertness, diminished sense of fatigue, and mild euphoria. Also thought to have anorexigenic effect.

Used as adjunctive therapy to other remedial measures (psychologic, educational, social) in minimal brain dysfunction (hyperkinetic behavior disorders) in children.

ABSORPTION AND FATE
Absorbed from GI tract. Peak serum levels within 2 to 4 hours. CNS stimulation effect peaks within 4 hours and lasts at least 8 hours. Serum half-life about 12 hours. Approximately 50% bound to plasma proteins. Distribution unknown. Probably metabolized in part by liver to active and inactive metabolites; 75% excreted in urine (43% unchanged, 22% as conjugates) within 24 hours.

CONTRAINDICATIONS AND PRECAUTIONS
Known hypersensitivity to pemoline; children younger than 6 years of age. Safe use during pregnancy and lactation not established. Cautious use: impaired renal function, history of drug abuse.

ADVERSE REACTIONS
Insomnia, anorexia, abdominal discomfort, malaise, nausea, diarrhea, skin rash, irritability, fatigue, mild depression, dizziness, headache, drowsiness. Overdosage: nervousness, tachycardia, hallucinations, excitement, agitation, restlessness. Also reported: elevated SGOT, SGPT, and alkaline phosphatase (after several months of therapy); reversible hepatic damage (rare).

Oral: **Children** *6 years of age and older:* initially 37.5 mg daily; may be increased by 18.75 mg at weekly intervals until desired clinical response is obtained. Effective dose range: 56.25 mg to 75 mg daily. Maximum recommended daily dose 112.5 mg.

NURSING IMPLICATIONS

Administer drug in morning to provide maximal effectiveness during waking hours and to avoid insomnia.

Insomnia and anorexia (most frequent side effects) appear to be dose-related.

Monitor weight and height throughout therapy. Anorexia is often accompanied by weight loss, particularly during first few weeks of therapy. Although growth suppression has not been reported with pemoline, it has been associated with other CNS stimulants used in children.

Significant benefits of drug therapy may not be evident until third or fourth week of drug administration.

Careful clinical evaluation and supervision of patient are essential. Patients receiving long-term therapy should have periodic liver function studies.

Occasional interruption of drug therapy is advised to determine if behavioral symptoms recur.

Pemoline can produce tolerance and physical and psychologic dependence. Classified as schedule IV drug under federal Controlled Substances Act.

PENICILLIN G BENZATHINE, U.S.P

(BICILLIN, BICILLIN L-A, Dibenzyl Penicillin, PERMAPEN)

Antibacterial

ACTIONS AND USES

Prepared by reaction of dibenzylethylenediamine with penicillin G. Has actions, contraindications, and adverse reactions similar to those of penicillin G potassium (qv), but produces lower and more prolonged blood levles.

Used in treatment of infections highly susceptible to penicillin G, such as mild to moderate streptococcal infections of upper respiratory tract and spirochetal infections such as syphilis, yaws, bejel, and pinta. Also used in follow-up prophylaxis of rheumatic fever and glomerulonephritis.

ABSORPTION AND FATE

Absorbed slowly following intramuscular injection, and converted by hydrolysis to penicillin G. Blood concentrations of 0.03 to 0.05 units/ml maintained for 4 or 5 days following IM administration of 300,000 units; blood levels persist 10 to 14 days following larger doses. Blood concentrations following oral administration may persist 6 or 7 hours, but absorption rate is not reliable. Approximately 60% bound to serum proteins. Distributed throughout body tissues and spinal fluids with highest levels in kidneys. Urinary excretion is considerably delayed in patients with impaired renal function and in young infants.

ADVERSE REACTIONS

Local pain, tenderness, and fever (associated with intramuscular injection); Jarisch-Herxheimer reaction in patients with seropositive primary and secondary syphilis; hypersensitivity reactions. Also see Penicillin G Potassium.

ROUTE AND DOSAGE

Adults Oral: 400,000 to 600,000 units every 4 to 6 hours; (rheumatic fever prophylaxis): 200,000 units twice daily. Intramuscular (therapy): 1.2 to 2.4 million units; (rheumatic fever prophylaxis): 1.2 million units once a month or 600,000 units every 2 weeks. **Children** *under 12 years*: Oral: 25,000 to 90,000 units/kg in 3 to 6 divided doses. Intramuscular: 300,000 to 1.2 million units. Highly individualized according to severity of infection.

NURSING IMPLICATIONS

Not to be confused with preparations containing penicillin G benzathine in combination with procaine penicillin G suspension.

As with other penicillins, therapy should be guided by bacteriologic studies, susceptibility tests, and clinical response.

Shake vial vigorously before withdrawing desired dose.

IM injection should be made deep into upper outer quadrant of the buttock (in infants and small children the midlateral aspect of the thigh is preferable). Rotate injection sites.

Carefully aspirate before injecting drug to make sure needle is not in blood vessel. If blood appears, remove needle and select another site. Inadvertent intravascular administration has resulted in arterial occulusion and cardiac arrest. Injection into or near major peripheral nerves has caused nerve damage.

Injections should be made at a slow steady rate to prevent needle blockage.

Allergic reactions develop slowly and persist for long periods of time following intramuscular use because of slow rate of absorption.

Oral preparations are not significantly affected by food.

Benzathine penicillin G suspensions for injection should be refrigerated (at 2 C to 8 C).

See Penicillin G Potassium.

PENICILLIN G POTASSIUM, U.S.P.

(CRYSPEN, DELTAPEN, GENECILLIN 400, G-RECILLIN, K-CILLIN, K-PEN, PENTIDS, PFIZERPEN G, SK-PENICILLIN G, SUGRACILLIN)

PENICILLIN G SODIUM, N.F.

Antibacterial

ACTIONS AND USES

A bactericidal and bacteriostatic preparation derived from the mutant *Penicillium chrysogenum* or *P. notatum.* Acts by interfering with synthesis of mucopeptides essential to formation and integrity of bacterial cell wall. Effective only on growing cells; ineffective on resting or intracellular microorganisms not in active growth phase. Drug of choice for treatment of infections caused by hemolytic streptococci, pneumococci, gonococci, *Treponema pallidum,* and many other spirochetes, clostridia, *B. anthracis* and other Gram-positive rods, *C. diphtheriae,* and *Actinomyces* species.

Used orally for treatment of mild to moderately severe infections, as prophylaxis for rheumatic fever, and for patients undergoing minor surgery in presence of history of rheumatic fever and rheumatic and congenital heart diseases. Used parenterally in treatment of severe infections caused by sensitive organisms. Buffered preparations may be used for intraarticular, intrapleural, or other local instillations.

ABSORPTION AND FATE

Oral preparation susceptible to destruction by gastric juices and by penicillinase produced by *E. coli* in large intestine; therefore, absorption is irregular and incomplete. Widely distributed following intramuscular injection. Peak serum levels following oral ingestion reached within 1 hour; therapeutic blood levels maintained for about 5 hours. Serum levels peak within 15 to 30 minutes following IM and decline within 3 to 5 hours. Enters ascitic, prostatic, and pleural fluids. Absorption into spinal fluid is poor unless meninges are inflamed and massive doses are administered. About 50% to 60% bound to plasma proteins. Half-life 30 minutes. Rapid excretion by renal tubules as free drug (antibacterial) or as conjugates; small amounts excreted in bile (feces) and saliva. Crosses placenta; enters breast milk.

Hypersensitivity to penicillin or to cephalosporins. Cautious use: patients with history of allergies, bronchial asthma, hepatic and renal insufficiency.

ADVERSE REACTIONS

Most common: allergic reactions. Anaphylactic reactions (rare with oral preparations) may be fatal. Pruritus, urticaria, exfoliative dermatitis, fever, serum sickness, ulcerated mucous membranes, pain at injection site, eosinophilia, phlebitis, polyarthritis, anorexia, nausea, vomiting, diarrhea, abdominal cramps, superinfection by overgrowth of penicillin-resistant organisms (especially *Pseudomonas, Candida, Proteus* species), Jarisch-Herxheimer reaction.

ROUTE AND DOSAGE

Oral: 200,000 to 800,000 units divided into 3 or 4 doses. Intramuscular, intravenous, 300,000 to 1.5 million units, up to 80 million units daily. Dosage varies according to age and severity of infection.

NURSING IMPLICATIONS

Note expiration date on container label or package label.

Incidence of hypersensitivity to penicillin is estimated to be 5% to 10% among adults in the United States. Careful medical history should be taken before treatment is initiated.

Oral preparation is given 1 to 2 hours before meals or at least 2 to 3 hours after meals to reduce gastric destruction of drug.

Before injecting IM dose, aspirate to be sure needle is not in a blood vessel. Inject deep into body of a large muscle.

Rapid appearance of red flare or a wheal at parenteral site is a sign of sensitivity and may indicate that drug should be discontinued. Consult physician.

A patient with sensitivity to penicillin G is likely to be sensitive to all penicillin products. All penicillins are cross-reacting and cross-sensitizing.

Inspect the patient's tongue periodically. "Black tongue" or black furry overgrowth indicates mucocutaneous superinfection with nonsensitive organisms. If this symptom or oral lesions or skin rash develop, report to physician. Appropriate measures (usually change in antibacterial) should be initiated. Inquire about patient's use of mouthwashes. Overuse can change mouth flora and contribute to oral superinfections.

Large doses of oral penicillin tend to promote luxuriant overgrowth of bacteria and yeasts in lower gastrointestinal tract, as evidenced by enteritis. Loose, foul-smelling stools and nausea should be reported to physician.

Observe the response to oral penicillin (monitor temperature, note subjective symptoms, etc). If a desired clinical response is not evident in 24 hours, parenteral preparation may be substituted or added. Small, ineffective doses of oral penicillin promote emergence of resistant strains of microorganisms.

In prolonged treatment with this drug, and especially when large doses are ordered, renal, hepatic, and hematologic systems should be evaluated frequently.

Minor changes in the results of liver function tests (such as SGOT levels and cephalin flocculation) have been reported. The significance is unknown.

Treatment is usually continued for at least 48 hours after the patient has become afebrile and asymptomatic and cultures are negative. For β-hemolytic streptococci, at least 10 days of treatment are recommended.

Be guided by the product information folder or by the pharmacist concerning mixing other drugs with intramuscular penicillin solution.

Advise the patient to discard remaining penicillin tablets after therapy is terminated. Self-medication with leftover tablets has a high potential for promoting later sensitivity to penicillin.

If a patient is allergic to penicillin, clearly note this on his chart and kardex and at his bedside. Suggest that he wear a tag certifying to this fact or carry wallet card. Warn him to tell the attending physician whenever he is to receive medical treatment.

LABORATORY TEST INTERFERENCES: In massive doses, potassium or sodium penicillin G may produce false positive urinary glucose test using Benedict's solution, but not with other cupric sulfate test (eg, Clinitest) or glucose oxidase reagent (eg, Clinistix, Tes-Tape). Large penicillin G (sodium or potassium) doses may also produce false positive urinary protein determinations (Ames reagent reportedly not affected).

PENICILLIN G, PROCAINE, U.S.P.
(CRYSTICILLIN A.S., DIURNAL-PENICILLIN, DURACILLIN A.S., PENTIDS-P, PFIZERPEN-AS, TU-CILLIN, WYCILLIN)

Antibacterial

ACTIONS AND USES

Long-acting repository form of penicillin G. Contains procaine which creates a tissue depot from which penicillin is slowly released and absorbed; also has slight anesthetic effect. Same antibacterial activity as that of penicillin G and is similarly inactivated by penicillinase, and destroyed by gastric acids. Produces lower serum concentrations than equivalent doses of penicillin G, but has longer duration of action. Therefore, used in moderately severe infections susceptible to low, but persisting serum concentrations of penicillin. Aqueous suspension produces higher blood levels than that achieved by preparation with aluminum stearate in sesame oil. May be used concomitantly with penicillin G or probenicid when higher plasma levels required.

ABSORPTION AND FATE

Slowly released following IM injection. Hydrolyzed to penicillin G in body. Peak blood levels in 4 hours. Widely distributed in body with highest concentrations in kidneys. Duration of action: aqueous suspension, 15 to 20 or more hours; preparation with aluminum stearate in oil, 96 to 120 hours. Approximately 60% bound to plasma proteins. Excreted rapidly by kidneys (60 to 90% of aqueous suspension dose excreted within 24 to 36 hours); excretion delayed in neonates, young infants and patients with impaired renal function.

CONTRAINDICATIONS AND PRECAUTIONS

History of sensitivity to any penicillin compound, cephalosporins, procaine, or other allergens. Also see Penicillin G Potassium.

ADVERSE REACTIONS

Hypersensitivity reactions; procaine toxicity (mental disturbances, seizures); superinfection.

ROUTE AND DOSAGE

Intramuscular (only): 600,000 to 1,200,000 units every 1 to 3 days. Up to 4.8 million units/day have been used.

NURSING IMPLICATIONS

Usually, intervals between doses of preparation with aluminum stearate in sesame oil longer than for aqueous suspension form.

Multiple dose vial should be shaken thoroughly to insure uniform suspension, before withdrawing medication.

Administer IM deeply into upper outer quadrant of buttock; in small children midlateral thigh is preferred. Subcutaneous injection is contraindicated. Aspirate carefully before injecting drug to avoid inadvertent entry into a blood vessel. Inadvertent IV administration has resulted in pulmonary infarcts and death. Inject drug at slow, steady rate to prevent needle blockage. Accidental injection into or near major peripheral nerves or blood vessels has resulted in neurovascular damage. Rotate injection sites.

If nondisposable syringe is used, remove needle and plunger soon after injection to prevent "freezing" of any remaining medication and rinse with water as soon as possible.

Immediate toxic reaction to procaine has occurred, particularly when large single dose is administered. Manifested by acute psychosis, weakness, fear of impending death, seizures, and usually lasts 15 to 30 minutes. May be treated by antihistamines.

Therapy is guided by culture and sensitivity tests and clinical response.

Report to physician onset of an allergic reaction or signs of superinfection.

Periodic evaluations of renal and hematopoietic systems recommended in patients on prolonged therapy, particularly with high dosage schedules.

Note expiration date and manufacturer's directions for storage. (Generally, aqueous suspensions of penicillin G procaine are refrigerated; preparations in sesame oil with stearate are stored at room temperature.)

See Penicillin G Potassium.

PENICILLIN V, U.S.P.

(PEN-VEE, Phenoxymethyl, Penicillin, V-CILLIN)

PENICILLIN V BENZATHINE, N.F.

(PEN-VEE SUSPENSION)

PENICILLIN V HYDRABAMINE, N.F.

(COMPOCILLIN-V)

PENICILLIN V POTASSIUM, U.S.P.

(BETAPEN VK, COMPOCILLIN-VK, DOWPEN-VK, KESSO-PEN VK, LEDERCILLIN VK, PENAPAR VK, PENICILLIN VK, PEN-VEE K, PFIZERPEN VK, REPEN-VK, ROBICILLIN VK, RO-CILLIN VK, SAROPEN-VK, SK-PENICILLIN VK, UTICILLIN VK, V-CILLIN K, VEETIDS)

Antibacterial

ACTIONS AND USES

Semisynthetic phenoxymethyl analog of penicillin G (qv) with similar range of antimicrobial activity. More resistant to inactivation by gastric acid and therefore more completely absorbed. Produces 2 to 5 times higher blood levels than equal doses of penicillin G. Like penicillin G, inactivated by penicillinase. Penicillin V benzathine, hydrabamine, and potassium are the salts of penicillin V. Penicillin V potassium is reportedly more readily absorbed and produces higher blood levels than parent compound and its other salts.

Used in treatment of mild to moderate streptococcal infections of upper respiratory tract, scarlet fever and erysipelas; pneumococcal infections of respiratory tract including otitis media, staphylococcal infections of skin and soft tissue; Vincent's infection; prophylaxis of rheumatic fever, chorea, and bacterial endocarditis.

ABSORPTION AND FATE

Rapidly absorbed from GI tract. Peak serum concentrations in 30 to 60 minutes; maintained for 6 or more hours. Approximately 80% bound to plasma proteins.

Highest levels in kidneys. Half-life: 30 minutes. Excreted in urine as rapidly as absorbed (excretion delayed in neonates, young infants, and patients with impaired renal function).

CONTRAINDICATIONS AND PRECAUTIONS

History of sensitivity to any penicillin compound, cephalosporins, or to multiple allergens. Also see Penicillin G Potassium.

ADVERSE REACTIONS

Nausea, vomiting, diarrhea, epigastric distress, black hairy tongue, hypersensitivity reactions. Also see Penicillin G Potassium.

ROUTE AND DOSAGE

Oral: **Adults and children** *over 12 years:* 125 to 300 mg every 6 to 8 hours. **Children** *under 12 years:* 15 to 50 mg/kg in 3 to 6 divided doses.

NURSING IMPLICATIONS

May be administered with food, but blood levels are reportedly higher when given on an empty stomach.

In staphylococcal infections, it is particularly important to determine continued sensitivity of infecting organism, by culture and sensitivity tests, since an increasing number of resistant staphylococcal strains have been reported.

Patients with Vincent's infection (trench mouth) should receive concomitant dental care to remove ulcerated tissue. Underlying cause (eg, poor oral hygiene, blood dyscrasia or other systemic disease) should be investigated. Usually treated adjunctively with mouth rinses of aqueous hydrogen peroxide (3% in an equal volume of warm water) and applications of carbamide peroxide (eg, Gly-Oxide, Proxigel) to ulcers to help debride devitalized tissue and to inhibit growth of infecting anaerobic organisms. Consult physician for specific guidelines.

Shake oral solutions well before pouring. Note expiration date and manufacturer's directions for storage.

As with other penicillin preparations, advise patient to withhold medication and report to physician at the onset of rash, pruritus, chills, fever, or signs of superinfection.

Periodic renal and hematopoietic studies are recommended in patients receiving prolonged therapy.

See Penicillin G Potassium Nursing Implications and Drug Interactions.

PENTAERYTHRITOL TETRANITRATE, N.F.

(ANGITRATE, ANTIME, ANTORA, CORODYL, DESATRATE, DILAVAS, DIVASO, DUOTRATE, EL-PETN, KAYTRATE, KORTRATE, METRANIL, NEO-COROVAS, PENTAFIN, PENTANITROL, PENTRASPAN, PENTRITOL, PENTRYATE, PENTYLAN, PERISPAN, PERITRATE, P.E.T.N., QUINTRATE, RATE, SK-PETN, TRANITE, VASITOL, VASO-80)

Vasodilator (coronary)

ACTIONS AND USES

Nitric acid ester of a tetrahydric alcohol. Actions, contraindications, precautions, and adverse reactions as for nitroglycerin (qv). Slower acting than nitroglycerin, but has more prolonged action. Not effective for control of acute attacks. Available in combination with nitroglycerin (for rapid action), also in combination with a barbiturate or meprobamate. Tolerance can occur, and cross-tolerance with other nitrites and nitrates is possible.

Used prophylactically to reduce frequency and severity of attacks of angina
pectoris.

ABSORPTION AND FATE

Onset of action in 30 minutes to 1 hour; duration 4 to 5 hours. Action of extended-release forms may persist up to 12 hours. Largely metabolized in liver prior to entering general circulation.

ROUTE AND DOSAGE

Oral: Dosage may be initiated at 10 or 20 mg 4 times daily and titrated upward to 40 mg 4 times daily. Sustained-action form: 80 mg 2 times daily.

NURSING IMPLICATIONS

Administered at least 30 minutes before or 1 hour after meals and at bedtime. Sustained-action form is also administered on an empty stomach (one dose on arising and second dose 12 hours later).

Advise patient to report onset of skin rash or persistent headaches to physician. Discontinuation of therapy may be required.

Inform patient that alcohol may enhance drug hypotensive effect.

Chronic administration may produce tolerance and may impair response to nitroglycerin or other concomitantly administered nitrites or nitrates. Advise patient to report signs of decreasing therapeutic effect.

Store at temperature between 15 C and 30 C (59 F and 86 F).

See Nitroglycerin.

DRUG INTERACTIONS: Pentaerythritol tetranitrate can act as a physiologic antagonist to acetylcholine, histamine, norepinephrine, and many other agents.

PENTAZOCINE HYDROCHLORIDE, N.F.
(TALWIN HYDROCHLORIDE)
PENTAZOCINE LACTATE, N.F.
(TALWIN LACTATE)

Narcotic analgesic

ACTIONS AND USES

Synthetic benzomorphan analgesic structurally related to phenazocine. On a weight basis, analgesic potency approximately one-third to one-fourth that of morphine, and somewhat greater than that of codeine. In general, adverse reactions are qualitatively similar to those of morphine (qv). Unlike morphine, large doses may cause increase in blood pressure and heart rate. Also, acts as weak narcotic antagonist (activity about 1/50 that of nalorphine) of meperidine and morphine, and has sedative properties. Available in combination with aspirin; eg, Talwin compound.

Used for relief of moderate to severe pain; also used in obstetrics and for preoperative analgesia or sedation.

ABSORPTION AND FATE

Onset of action 10 to 20 minutes following IM or subcutaneous administration, 2 to 3 minutes after IV administration, and 15 to 30 minutes after oral administration. Duration of action for parenteral preparations: 2 to 3 hours (about 4 to 5 hours or longer for oral form). Extensively metabolized in liver. About 60% of dose is eliminated in urine within 24 hours; small amounts excreted unchanged in urine and feces. (Individual variability in rate of drug metabolism.) Crosses placenta.

Head injury, increased intracranial pressure, emotionally unstable patients, or history of drug abuse. Safe use during pregnancy (other than labor) and in children under 12 years of age not established. Cautious use: impaired renal or hepatic function, respiratory depression, biliary surgery, patients with myocardial infarction who have nausea and vomiting.

ADVERSE REACTIONS

Drowsiness, sweating, flushing, dizziness, lightheadedness, nausea, vomiting, constipation (infrequent), dry mouth, alterations of taste, urinary retention, visual disturbances, allergic reactions, injection-site reactions (induration, nodule formation, sloughing, sclerosis, cutaneous depression). High doses: respiratory depression, hypertension, palpitation, tachycardia, psychotomimetic effects, confusion, anxiety, hallucinations, disturbed dreams, bizarre thoughts, euphoria and other mood alterations.

ROUTE AND DOSAGE

Oral: initially 50 mg every 3 to 4 hours. Total daily oral dosage not to exceed 600 mg. Intramuscular, subcutaneous, intravenous (excluding patients in labor); 30 mg every 3 to 4 hours as needed. Doses exceeding 60 mg IM or subcutaneously or 30 mg IV not recommended. Total daily parenteral dosage not to exceed 360 mg. Patients in labor: 20 to 30 mg IM; 20 mg may be repeated 2 or 3 times at 2- to 3-hour intervals as needed.

NURSING IMPLICATIONS

IM administration is preferable to subcutaneous route when frequent injections over an extended period are required. Rotation of injection sites (upper outer quadrant, mid-lateral thighs, deltoid) are recommended. Observe injection sites daily for signs of irritation or inflammation.

Pentazocine may produce acute withdrawal symptoms in some patients who have been receiving opioids on a regular basis.

Caution ambulatory patients to avoid potentially hazardous activities such as driving a car or operating machinery.

Tolerance to analgesic effect sometimes occurs. Psychologic dependence and physical dependence have been reported in patients with history of drug abuse, but rarely in patients without such history.

Abrupt discontinuation of drug following extended use may result in fever, chills, abdominal and muscle cramps, yawning, rhinorrhea, lacrimation, itching, restlessness, anxiety, drug-seeking behavior.

Overdosage is treated by supportive measures such as oxygen, IV fluids, vasopressors, assisted or controlled ventilation as necessary, and narcotic antagonist naloxone (levallorphan and nalorphine are not effective for respiratory depression).

Do not mix pentazocine in same syringe with soluble barbiturates, because precipitation will occur.

Preserved in tight, light-resistant containers.

PENTOBARBITAL, N.F.
(NEBRALIN, NEMBUTAL, PENTOBARBITONE)
PENTOBARBITAL SODIUM, U.S.P.
(MASO-PENT, NEMBUTAL SODIUM, NAPENTAL, NIGHT-CAPS, PALAPENT, PENITAL, PENTAL, SODITAL)

Sedative, hypnotic

ACTIONS AND USES
Short-acting barbiturate with actions, contraindications, precautions, and adverse reactions as for other barbiturates (see Phenobarbital).
Used as sedative or hypnotic for preanesthetic medication, induction of general anesthesia, adjunct in manipulative or diagnostic procedures, and emergency control of acute convulsions.

ABSORPTION AND FATE
Following oral administration, onset of action in 15 to 30 minutes; peak plasma levels in 30 to 60 minutes; duration of action 3 to 6 hours. Onset of action within 10 to 15 minutes after IM injection, and within 1 minute after IV administration. Approximately 35% to 45% bound to plasma proteins. Metabolized primarily in liver to inactive metabolites. Excreted in urine. Crosses placenta.

ADVERSE REACTIONS
With rapid IV: respiratory depression, laryngospasm, bronchospasm, apnea, hypotension. Also see Phenobarbital.

ROUTE AND DOSAGE
Adults: *Sedative:* Oral, 20 to 30 mg 3 or 4 times daily; timed-release form, 100 mg in morning. *Hypnotic:* oral, rectal, intramuscular, intravenous: 100 to 200 mg. After interval of at least 1 minute, additional small increments up to total of 200 to 500 mg IV may be given, if necessary. **Children:** *Sedative:* Oral, rectal suppository: 6 mg/kg/24 hours divided into 3 doses. *Hypnotic:* intramuscular, 3 to 5 mg/kg. Rectal suppository: **children** *12 to 14 years,* 60 to 120 mg; *5 to 12 years,* 60 mg; *1 to 4 years,* 30 to 60 mg; *2 months to 1 year,* 30 mg.

NURSING IMPLICATIONS
Do not use parenteral solutions that appear cloudy or in which a precipitate has formed.
Parenteral solution is highly alkaline. Extreme care should be taken to avoid extravasation and intraarterial injection. Necrosis may result.
When administered IV, monitor blood pressure, pulse, and respiration every 3 to 5 minutes. Observe patient closely; maintain airway. Equipment for artificial respiration should be immediately available.
Caution ambulatory patients against operating a motor vehicle or machinery for the remainder of day, after taking drug.
IM injections should be made deep into large muscle mass, preferably upper outer quadrant of buttock. Aspirate carefully before injecting to prevent inadvertent entry into blood vessel. No more than 5 ml (250 mg) should be injected in any one site because of possible tissue irritation.
After IM administration of hypnotic dose, observe patient closely for adverse effects for at least 30 minutes.
Classified as schedule II drug under federal Controlled Substances Act.
See Phenobarbital.

(TRILAFON)

Antipsychotic (major tranquilizer), antiemetic

ACTIONS AND USES

Piperazine phenothiazine derivative similar to chlorpromazine in actions, contraindications, precautions, and adverse reactions. Produces less sedation and hypotension, greater antiemetic effect, higher incidence of extrapyramidal reactions, and lower levels of anticholinergic side effects than chlorpromazine. Used in management of acute and chronic schizophrenia; in senile, involutional, organic, and toxic psychoses; in manic phase of manic–depressive psychosis; for anxiety and tension accompanying severe neuroses and for control of nausea and vomiting.

ABSORPTION AND FATE

Onset of action in 10 minutes following IM injection, with maximal effect in 1 to 2 hours; average duration of effective action is 6 hours, occasionally 12 to 24 hours. Excreted slowly through kidneys.

ROUTE AND DOSAGE

Oral: 4 to 16 mg 2 to 4 times daily; repeat-action form: 8 to 32 mg 2 times daily; doses in excess of 64 mg daily not advised. Intramuscular: 5 to 10 mg repeated every 6 hours if necessary. Intravenous: not to exceed 5 mg. Children over 12 years of age, ambulatory patients, and the elderly receive lowest-limit dosages.

NURSING IMPLICATIONS

Each 5 ml (16 mg) of oral concentrate should be diluted with 60 mg of water, orange juice, milk, or carbonated beverage. Color changes and precipitate may occur with cola drinks, black coffee, tea, grape juice, or apple juice.

Patient should be recumbent when receiving drug parenterally. Transient dizziness and hypotension may occur. Observe patient closely for a short period after injection.

Blood pressure and pulse should be monitored continuously during IV administration. Keep patient supine until assured that vital signs are stable. Have on hand levarterenol (epinephrine is contraindicated).

There is a high incidence of extrapyramidal effects, particularly with high doses and IV administration. Observe for and report restlessness, weakness of extremities, dystonia of neck and shoulder muscles, abnormal positioning, salivation, and other unusual symptoms.

Caution the patient to avoid potentially hazardous activities such as driving a car or operating machinery, since drug may produce drowsiness or dizziness.

Avoid contact of perphenazine solutions with hands and clothing. Contact dermatitis has been reported.

Protect solutions from light. Do not use parenteral solution if it is darker than light amber or discolored in any other way.

See Chlorpromazine Hydrochloride.

Anticonvulsant

ACTIONS AND USES
   Potent acetylurea antiepileptic agent.
   Used alone or with other anticonvulsants, particularly for mixed forms of psy-
   chomotor seizures refractory to other drugs.
ABSORPTION AND FATE
   Well absorbed from GI tract. Duration of action about 5 hours. Metabolized by
   liver. Excreted by kidneys as inactive metabolites.
CONTRAINDICATIONS AND PRECAUTIONS
   Safe use in women of childbearing potential or during pregnancy not estab-
   lished. Cautious use: history of personality disorders, liver dysfunction, allergies.
ADVERSE REACTIONS
   Nausea, anorexia, weight loss, headache, drowsiness, insomnia, dizziness, skin
   rash, paresthesias, personality changes, toxic psychoses, leukopenia, aplastic
   anemia, agranulocytosis, hepatitis, nephritis. **Overdosage:** mania followed by
   drowsiness, ataxia, coma.
ROUTE AND DOSAGE
   Oral: **Adults:** initially 250 to 500 mg 3 times daily; after first week, additional
   500 mg on arising may be added if necessary to control seizures; in third week,
   additional 500 mg at bedtime may be added, if necessary (dosage may range
   from 1.5 to 3 Gm daily). **Children** *5 to 10 years:* approximately one-half adult
   dosage.

NURSING IMPLICATIONS
Administration of drug with food may minimize GI side effects.
Complete blood counts, liver function tests, and urine tests should be per-
   formed before and at monthly intervals during therapy. If no abnormali-
   ties appear after 12 months, intervals may be widened.
Patient and responsible family members should be advised of need for close
   medical supervision, because drug has high potential for serious toxicity.
Personality changes, including attempts at suicide, are possible drug effects.
   Instruct patient and family to report changes in behavior, eg, depression,
   apathy, aggressiveness, paranoia, and severe headaches. All are indications for drug withdrawal.
Advise patient and family to report immediately the onset of fever, sore
   mouth or throat, and malaise (symptoms of developing blood dyscrasia),
   skin rash or other allergic manifestations, and any other unusual or new
   symptoms.
Teach patient and family to observe for and report evidence of jaundice:
   yellow skin and sclerae, petechiae, pruritus, dark amber urine with yellow
   froth.
Treatment of overdosage: emesis, gastric lavage as alternative or adjunct,
   general supportive measures. Follow-up evaluation of liver and kidney
   function, mental state, and blood-forming organs should be made.
Physician may prescribe vitamin K for infants born to mothers treated with
   anticonvulsants (anticonvulsants appear to reduce levels of vitamin-K-
   dependent clotting factors in newborns).

(Acetophenetidin)

Analgesic, antipyretic

ACTIONS AND USES
p-Aminophenol (aniline) derivative with analgesic and antipyretic actions approximately equivalent to those of aspirin. Actions, contraindications, and precautions similar to those of acetaminophen (qv). Analgesic and antipyretic effects may be due to conversion to acetaminophen, but reportedly phenacetin also has activity of its own. Appears to cause more central depression than does acetaminophen, produces higher methemoglobin blood levels and somewhat greater overall toxicity, and may increase occult blood loss.
Used primarily in combination with other drugs such as aspirin, caffeine, codeine, salicylamide, and phenobarbital in commercial analgesic mixtures.

ABSORPTION AND FATE
Completely absorbed from GI tract and rapidly distributed to most body tissues, especially liver. Peak plasma levels in 1 to 2 hours; duration of effect about 4 hours. Plasma half-life 45 to 90 minutes. Metabolized by liver microsomes, mainly to acetaldehyde and acetaminophen. Approximately two-thirds of dose is excreted as free and conjugated acetaminophen within 24 hours; 1% excreted unchanged.

ADVERSE REACTIONS
Slight euphoria, drowsiness, stimulation, lightheadedness, dizziness, sense of detachment; (large doses or chronic use): methemoglobinemia, sulfhemoglobinemia, hemolytic anemia, hypoglycemia, hepatic and renal damage. Also see Acetaminophen.

ROUTE AND DOSAGE
Oral: 300 to 600 mg repeated every 4 hours, if necessary. Total daily dosage not to exceed 2.4 Gm.

NURSING IMPLICATIONS
All phenacetin-containing compounds must carry warning that medication may damage kidneys when used in large amounts or for long periods of time and that phenacetin must not be taken regularly for longer than 10 days without consulting physician.

Some individuals experience slight drowsiness, euphoria, and relaxation—effects believed to be the result of pain relief and not tranquilizing action.

Habituation may occur in some patients, but physical dependence has not been reported. Abrupt withdrawal after prolonged use may precipitate symptoms of restlessness and excitement that may persist for 3 or 4 days.

Recent reports suggest that phenacetin combinations with aspirin, caffeine, and codeine may cause greater percentage of methemoglobinemia and nephrotoxicity than occurs with phenacetin alone.

Methemoglobinemia usually disappears spontaneously within 24 to 72 hours after drug discontinuation; however, methemoglobin blood levels exceeding 40% usually require therapy with methylene blue and oxygen.

Children are more susceptible to methemoglobinemia than are adults.

Metabolites of phenacetin may impart a dark brown or wine color to urine, especially on long standing.

Phenacetin is a common ingredient in many OTC headache and analgesic remedies, eg, Fiorinal (contains butalbital, caffeine, aspirin, and phenacetin) and compounds containing phenacetin in combination with aspirin and caffeine: A.S.A. compound, Capron, Duradyne, Empirin compound, P-A-C, Sal-Fayne, and others.

The official (N.F.) aspirin compound Aspirin, Phenacetin, and Caffeine contains aspirin 300 to 600 mg, phenacetin 300 mg, and caffeine 200 mg. No claims can be made that the analgesic effect of the compound is superior to that attained by either aspirin or phenacetin alone.

Caution patient to store medication out of reach of children.

Also see Acetaminophen.

LABORATORY TEST INTERFERENCES: Phenacetin may cause false positive test results for urinary 5-hydroxyindoleacetic acid and urine glucose using Benedict's solution and may produce interfering color in ferric chloride test for acetoacetic acid.

PHENAZOPYRIDINE HYDROCHLORIDE, N.F.
(AZODINE, AZO-STANDARD, AZO-STAT, AQUA TON, BARIDIUM, MALLOPHENE, PHENYLAZO, PHENYL-IDIUM, PIRID, PYRIDIUM, PYRODINE, URODINE)

Analgesic (urinary tract)

ACTIONS AND USES

Azo dye with local anesthetic action on urinary tract mucosa. Precise mechanism of action not known. Imparts little or no antibacterial activity.

Used for symptomatic relief of pain, burning, frequency, and urgency arising from irritation of urinary tract mucosa, as from infection, trauma, surgery, or instrumentation.

ABSORPTION AND FATE

Partly metabolized, probably in liver and other tissues. Excreted by kidney within 20 hours; about 65% excreted unchanged. Small amount eliminated in feces. Trace amounts believed to cross placenta.

CONTRAINDICATIONS AND PRECAUTIONS

Renal insufficiency, glomerulonephritis, pyelonephritis during pregnancy, severe hepatitis. Cautious use: GI disturbances, glucose-6-phosphate dehydrogenase deficiency.

ADVERSE REACTIONS

Infrequent: headache, vertigo, mild GI disturbances; (in patients with impaired renal function or with high dosage or prolonged therapy): methemoglobinemia, hemolytic anemia, skin pigmentation, renal stones, transient acute renal failure.

ROUTE AND DOSAGE

Oral: **Adults:** 200 mg 3 times daily; **Children:** 12 mg/kg/24 hours in 3 divided doses.

NURSING IMPLICATIONS

Administer phenazopyridine after meals.

Inform patient that drug will impart an orange to red color to urine and may stain fabric. Fabric stains may be removed by soaking in 0.25% solution of sodium dithionate or sodium hydrosulfite. Consult pharmacist.

Appearance of yellowish tinge to skin or sclerae may indicate drug accumulation due to renal impairment. Advise patient to report immediately. Drug should be discontinued.

Phenazopyridine should be discontinued when pain and discomfort are relieved (usually 3 to 15 days). Instruct patient to keep physician informed.

LABORATORY TEST INTERFERENCES: Phenazopyridine may interfere with any urinary test that is based on color reactions or spectrometry: *Bromsulphalein* and *phenolsulfonphthalein* excretion tests; urinary *glucose* test using Clinistix or Tes-Tape (copper-reduction methods such as Clinitest and Benedict's test reportedly not affected); *bilirubin* using "foam test" or Ictotest; *ketones* using nitroprusside (eg, Acetest, Ketostix, or Gerhardt ferric chloride); urinary *protein* using Albustix, Albutest, or nitric acid ring test; urinary *steroids; urobilinogen;* assays for *porphyrins.*

PHENDIMETRAZINE TARTRATE
(ADPHEN, BACARATE, BOF, BONTRIL PDM, ELPHEMET, LIMIT, LIMITITE, MELFIAT, MINUS, OBALAN, OBEPAR, OBE-TITE, OBEZINE, PHENZINE, PLEGINE, SLIM-TABS, STATOBEX, TRIMSTAT)

Anorexic

ACTIONS AND USES
Sympathomimetic amine with actions similar to those of other amphetamine-like compounds.
Used as adjunct to control endogenous obesity.
ABSORPTION AND FATE
Peak blood levels within 1 hour after regular tablet; effects persist about 4 hours, approximately 12 hours after sustained-release form.
CONTRAINDICATIONS AND PRECAUTIONS
Hypersensitivity to sympathomimetic amines, pregnancy, children under 12 years of age, severe coronary artery disease, moderate to severe hypertension, cardiac decompensation, hyperthyroidism, glaucoma, agitated persons, history of drug abuse, concomitant use with MAO inhibitors, CNS stimulants.
ADVERSE REACTIONS
Occasional: nervousness, insomnia, dizziness, mouth dryness, glossitis, stomatitis, nausea, mydriasis, blurring of vision, difficulty in starting urination, cystitis, constipation, abdominal cramps, palpitation, tachycardia, elevation of blood pressure. Also see Amphetamine.
ROUTE AND DOSAGE
Oral: 35 mg 2 or 3 times daily, or one sustained-release capsule once daily.

NURSING IMPLICATIONS
Administer 1 hour before meals. Sustained-release form is administered in the morning. Give last dose at least 6 hours before patient retires in order to avoid insomnia.
Psychogenic dependence is a possibility, as with all amphetaminelike compounds.
Classified as schedule III drug under federal Controlled Substances Act.
See Amphetamine Sulfate.

Antidepressant (MAO inhibitor)

ACTIONS AND USES

Potent hydrazide MAO inhibitor with amphetaminelike pharmacologic proper-ties. Precise mode of action not known. Antidepressant and diverse effects believed to be due to irreversible inhibition of MAO (mitochondrial enzyme involved in degradation and excretion of sympathomimetic amines), thereby permitting increased concentrations of endogenous epinephrine, norepineph-rine, serotonin, and dopamine within presynaptic neurons and at receptor sites. Also thought to inhibit hepatic microsomal drug-metabolizing enzymes; thus may intensify and prolong the effects of many drugs. Termination of drug action depends on regeneration of MAO, which occurs 2 to 3 weeks after discontinuation of therapy. Exerts paradoxic hypotensive effect (apparently by ganglionic blocking action), suppresses REM sleep, and reportedly may decrease serum cholinesterase. MAO inhibition has unpredictable effect on convulsive threshold in epilepsy.

Used in management of endogenous depression, depressive phase of manic–depressive psychosis, and severe exogenous (reactive) depression not responsive to more commonly used therapy.

ABSORPTION AND FATE

Readily absorbed from GI tract and rapidly metabolized. Excreted in urine as metabolites and unchanged drug.

CONTRAINDICATIONS AND PRECAUTIONS

Hypersensitivity to MAO inhibitors, pheochromocytoma, hyperthyroidism, congestive heart failure, cardiovascular or cerebrovascular disease, impaired renal function, hypernatremia, atonic colitis, glaucoma, history of frequent or severe headaches, history of liver disease, abnormal liver function tests, elderly or debilitated patients, paranoid schizophrenia. Safe use during pregnancy and lactation and in women of childbearing potential and children under 16 years of age not established. Cautious use: epilepsy, pyloric stenosis, diabetes, depres-sion accompanying alcoholism or drug addiction, manic–depressive states, agi-tated patients, suicidal tendencies, chronic brain syndromes, history of angina pectoris.

ADVERSE REACTIONS

Constipation, dry mouth, dizziness or vertigo, headache, orthostatic hypoten-sion, drowsiness or insomnia, weakness, fatigue, nausea, vomiting, anorexia, appetite stimulation, weight gain, edema, irritability, tremors, twitching, over-activity, hyperreflexia, mania, hypomania, confusion, memory impairment, blurred vision, hyperhidrosis, skin rash. Less common: glaucoma, nystagmus, incontinence, dysuria, urinary frequency or retention, transient impotence, galactorrhea, gynecomastia, black tongue, hypernatremia, edema of glottis, transient respiratory and cardiovascular depression, jaundice, hepatocellular damage, delirium, hallucinations, palilalia, euphoria, acute anxiety reaction, akathisia, ataxia, toxic precipitation of schizophrenia, convulsions, possibility of optic damage, peripheral neuropathy, spider telangiectasis, photosensitivity, hypoglycemia, decreased 5-hydroxyindoleacetic acid and vanillylmandelic acid, normocytic and normochromic anemia, leukopenia. **Hypertensive crisis:** in-tense occipital headache, palpitation, marked hypertension, stiff neck, nausea, vomiting, sweating, fever, photophobia, dilated pupils, bradycardia or tachy-cardia, constricting chest pain, intracranial bleeding. **Severe overdosage:** faint-ness, hypotension or hypertension, hyperactivity, marked agitation, anxiety, seizures, trismus, opisthotonos, respiratory depression, coma, circulatory col-lapse.

Oral: initially 15 mg 3 times a day. Increased gradually until after maximum benefit is achieved, dosage reduced slowly over several weeks to maintenance level: 15 mg daily or every other day, as long as required. Maximum recommended daily dose 75 mg.

NURSING IMPLICATIONS

Before initiation of phenelzine treatment, it is advisable to evaluate patient's blood pressure in standing and recumbent positions. Baseline blood cell counts and liver function tests should also be performed.

Many adverse reactions associated with MAO inhibitors are dose-related. Physician will rely on accurate observations and prompt reporting of patient's response to therapy to determine spacing and lowest effective dosage.

In titrating initial dosages, blood pressure and pulse should be monitored between doses, and patient should be closely observed for evidence of adverse drug effects. Thereafter, monitor at regular intervals throughout therapy.

Elastic stockings and elevation of legs when sitting may minimize hypotensive effects of drug (discuss with physician).

Instruct patient to make position changes slowly, especially from recumbent to upright posture, and to dangle legs over bed a few minutes before ambulating. Also caution against standing still for prolonged periods. Patient should avoid hot showers and baths (resulting vasodilatation may potentiate hypotension) and should lie down immediately if feeling lightheaded or faint. Supervise ambulation.

Headache and palpitation, prodromal symptoms of hypertensive crisis, indicate need to discontinue drug therapy. Instruct patient to report immediately the onset of these symptoms or any other unusual effects.

Ingestion of foods and beverages containing tyramine or tryptophan (form pressor amines in body) or drugs containing pressor agents can result in severe hypertensive reactions. Provide patient and responsible family members with a list of foods and beverages that may cause reactions (see below). These substances should be avoided during drug therapy and for at least 2 or 3 weeks after therapy has been discontinued.

Food and beverages to avoid: avocado, bananas, canned figs, raisins, licorice, chocolate, cheeses (particularly cheddar and other strong and aged varieties), yogurt, cream, sour cream, broad bean pods, liver (especially chicken liver), aged meats, pickled or kippered herring, yeast and meat extracts, soy sauce, meat tenderizers, game. Alcoholic beverages in general should be avoided (since tyramine content is difficult to determine), especially Chianti, other wines, and beer. Also advise against excessive amounts of caffeine beverages (eg, coffee, tea, cocoa, or cola) and cyclamates (believed to be converted in body in part to a pressor amine).

Treatment of hypertensive crisis: Have on hand short-acting α-adrenergic blocking agent (eg, phentolamine) to lower blood pressure; external cooling for hyperpyrexia.

Treatment of overdosage: Gastric lavage if performed early; maintain airway, hydration, and electrolyte balance. Have on hand phenothiazine tranquilizers (for agitation). Toxic effects may be delayed and prolonged; therefore, patient must be closely observed for at least 1 week after overdosage.

Advise patient to avoid self-medication. OTC preparations containing dextromethorphan, sympathomimetic agents, or antihistamines (eg, cough, cold, and hay fever remedies, appetite suppressants) can precipitate severe hypertensive reactions if taken during therapy or within 2 to 3 weeks after discontinuation of an MAO inhibitor.

Monitor intake–output ratio and pattern until dosage is stabilized to identify indirect indices of edema and urinary dysfunction. Report changes and abnormalities; impaired renal function increases the possibility of toxicity from cumulative effects.

Instruct patient to check weight two or three times weekly and report unusual gain.

Dry mouth may be relieved by sugarless candy or gum or by rinsing mouth with clear water.

Attempt at suicide by the depressed person is particularly possible when the response to drug therapy begins (ie, near end of depressive cycle). Careful observation of patient should be maintained until depression is controlled. Watch to see that drug is swallowed, not cheeked or hoarded.

In manic–depressive states, observe closely for rapid swing to manic phase. Patients with schizophrenia may present with excessive stimulation.

Hypomania (exaggeration of motility, feelings, and ideas) may occur as depression improves, particularly in patients with hyperkinetic symptoms obscured by a depressive affect. This reaction may also appear at higher than recommended doses or with long-term therapy. Report immediately.

Observe for and report therapeutic effectiveness of drug: improvement in sleep pattern, appetite, physical activity, interest in self and surroundings, as well as lessening of anxiety and bodily complaints.

If no therapeutic response occurs after 3 or 4 weeks, drug is usually discontinued. Maximum antidepressant effects generally appear in 2 to 6 weeks and persist several weeks after drug withdrawal.

Patient with diabetes should be closely observed for signs of hypoglycemia. Reduced dosage of insulin or oral antidiabetic drug may be necessary (see Drug Interactions).

MAO inhibitors should be discontinued at least 10 days before elective surgery to allow time for recovery of MAO before anesthetics are given.

Patients on prolonged therapy should be checked periodically for altered color perception, visual fields, and fundi. Changes in red–green vision may be the first indication of eye damage.

Instruct patient to report jaundice. Hepatotoxicity is believed to be a hypersensitivity reaction unrelated to dosage or duration of therapy.

Periodic hematologic studies and liver function tests are recommended during prolonged therapy and high dosage.

MAO inhibitors may suppress anginal pain that would otherwise serve as a warning sign of myocardial ischemia. Caution patient to avoid overexertion while receiving drug therapy.

Rapid withdrawal of MAO inhibitors should be avoided, particularly after high dosage, since a rebound effect may occur (headache, excitability, hallucinations, and possibly depression).

Preserved in tightly covered containers away from heat and light.

LABORATORY TEST INTERFERENCES: Phenelzine may cause a slight false increase in serum bilirubin.

DRUG INTERACTIONS: Hypertensive reaction and related symptoms may result from use (concurrently or within 2 weeks) of MAO inhibitors with amines having indirect sympathomimetic action: **amphetamines, cyclopentamine, ephedrine, metaraminol, methylphenidate, phenylephrine, phenylpropanolamine, pseudoephedrine.** Similar interactions are reportedly possible with **cyclamates, dextromethorphan, levodopa, methyldopa, methotrimeprazine, reserpine, tricyclic antidepressants, tryptamine,** and **tyramine**-rich foods and beverages.

With the exception of **dopamine** (contraindicated), direct-acting sympathomimetic amines (**epinephrine, isoproterenol, levarterenol, methoxamine**) reportedly are not significantly affected by MAO inhibitors; however, cautious administration is advised.

MAO inhibitors may potentiate the effects of **barbiturates;** potentiate adverse cardiovascular effects of **doxapram** (theoretical possibility); antagonize antihypertensive effects of **guanethidine** (concurrent use avoided); enhance or prolong hypoglycemic action of **insulin** and **oral antidiabetic agents;** cause severe CNS excitation and depression leading to coma and death with **meperidine**—thus concurrent use is to be avoided (other **narcotic analgesics** used only with extreme caution and in small doses); increase extrapyramidal reactions of **phenothiazines;** enhance the effect of **succinylcholine** by reducing its breakdown by plasma pseudocholinesterase; produce hypotension when used with **thiazide diuretics.**

PHENETHICILLIN POTASSIUM, N.F., B.P.
(CHEMIPEN, DARCIL, MAXIPEN, SYNCILLIN)

Antibacterial

ACTIONS AND USES

Semisynthetic penicillin reportedly more acid-resistant and better absorbed than penicillin G potassium. Does not resist degradation by penicillinase. Active against streptococci, *Diplococcus pneumoniae, Neisseria,* and *Staphylococcus aureus.*

Used in treatment of mild to moderately severe infections of respiratory tract; otitis media, erysipelas, skin and soft tissue infections, Vincent's infection, and for prophylaxis of rheumatic fever and chorea.

ABSORPTION AND FATE

Peak serum levels within 1 hour; negligible concentrations after 4 to 6 hours. Approximately 80% bound to plasma proteins. Rapidly excreted by kidneys (excretion delayed in neonates, young infants, and patients with impaired renal function).

CONTRAINDICATIONS AND PRECAUTIONS

History of sensitivity to any penicillin compound, cephalosporins, or other allergens. Also see Penicillin G Potassium.

ADVERSE REACTIONS

Nausea, vomiting, diarrhea, allergic reactions. Also see Penicillin G Potassium.

ROUTE AND DOSAGE

Oral: **Adults and children** *over 12 years:* 125 to 250 mg (200,000 to 400,000 units) every 4 to 8 hours, depending on severity of infection. **Children** *under 12 years:* 12.5 to 50 mg/kg divided into 3 to 6 doses.

NURSING IMPLICATIONS

Although drug may be given without regard to meals, slightly higher peak serum levels are achieved when administered on an empty stomach, ie, 1 hour before or 2 hours after meals.

Advise patient to discontinue drug and notify physican if skin eruption or other signs of allergic reaction (eg, chills, fever, joint pains), or superinfection develops.

When administered for group A beta-hemolytic streptococcal infection, therapy should be continued for at least 10 days to prevent development of rheumatic fever and/or chorea. Cultures are advised following completion of therapy to determine eradication of infection.

Periodic evaluations of renal, hepatic, and hematologic function recommended in patients receiving prolonged therapy.

See Penicillin G Potassium Nursing Implications and Drug Interaction.

(ERIDIONE, HEDULIN, INDON)

Anticoagulant

ACTIONS AND USES
  Indandione derivative similar to coumarin anticoagulants in actions, uses, con-
  traindications, precautions, and adverse effects, but potentially more toxic.
  Use generally limited to patients who cannot tolerate coumarin anticoagulants.
  See Warfarin.
ABSORPTION AND FATE
  Peak prothrombin effect in 24 to 48 hours; duration of effect 1 to 4 days.
  Considerable individual differences in absorption and metabolism rates. Almost
  completely bound to plasma proteins. Metabolized in liver. Excreted primarily
  in urine, as metabolites. Crosses placenta, and may appear in breast milk.
ADVERSE REACTIONS
  Sensitivity reactions, agranulocytosis, leukopenia, leukocytosis, eosinophilia,
  jaundice, hepatitis, nephropathy with renal tubular necrosis, proteinuria, massive generalized edema, fever, rash including severe exfoliative dermatitis,
  headache, diarrhea, oral ulcers, conjunctivitis, blurred vision, paralysis of ocular
  accommodation. Also see Warfarin.
ROUTE AND DOSAGE
  Oral: initially 200 mg (for patients 70 kg or less) or 300 mg (for patients over
  70 kg), given in 2 divided doses at 12-hour intervals (usually in morning and
  at bedtime). Maintenance 50 to 100 mg daily in 2 divided doses. Dosage carefully individualized according to prothrombin time determinations, other laboratory findings, and clinical response.

NURSING IMPLICATIONS
During period of dosage adjustment, prothrombin time results should be
  checked daily by physician and dosage order should be obtained.
When patient is controlled on maintenance dose, prothrombin time determinations may be prescribed biweekly, weekly, or at 2- to 4-week intervals,
  depending on uniformity of patient's response.
Periodic blood tests and liver function studies are advised for patients in
  prolonged therapy. Urine should be checked regularly for albumin and
  blood.
Instruct patient to report immediately the onset of fever, chills, sore throat or
  mouth, marked fatigue, jaundice, or any other unusual sign or symptom.
Metabolites of phenindione may impart a harmless red-orange color to alkaline urine. Alert patient to this possibility. Acidification of urine causes
  color to disappear (preliminary test for differentiating it from hematuria).
Orange or brownish yellow discoloration of fingernails, fingers, and palms
  has been reported in persons handling phenindione.
See Warfarin.

PHENMETRAZINE HYDROCHLORIDE, N.F., B.P.
(PRELUDIN, PRELUDIN ENDURETS)

Anorexic

ACTIONS AND USES
  Sympathomimetic agent chemically and pharmacologically related to the am-
  phetamines (qv), but reportedly produces less CNS stimulation.
  Used solely for short-term management of endogenous obesity.

ABSORPTION AND FATE

Peak serum concentration occurs about 2 hours after oral administration of conventional tablet; duration of action about 4 hours. Duration of action for sustained-release form approximately 12 hours.

CONTRAINDICATIONS AND PRECAUTIONS

History of hypersensitivity to sympathomimetic amines, hypertension, advanced arteriosclerosis, symptomatic cardiovascular disease, hyperthyroidism, hyperexcitable or psychotic states, concomitant use of CNS stimulants, during or within 2 weeks of MAO inhibitors. Safe use in women of childbearing potential, during pregnancy, and in children under 12 years of age not established.

ADVERSE REACTIONS

Headache, abdominal cramps, blurred vision, sweating, dry mouth, frequent urination, insomnia, urticaria, nervousness, dizziness, nausea, palpitation, tachycardia, elevated blood pressure. Large doses for prolonged periods: marked insomnia, irritability, severe dermatoses, hyperactivity, severe mental depression, personality changes, psychosis.

ROUTE AND DOSAGE

Oral: 25 mg 2 or 3 times daily; maximum dosage 75 mg/day. Sustained-release form: 50- or 75-mg tablet once daily.

NURSING IMPLICATIONS

Blood pressure checks before and periodically during treatment are advised.

Conventional tablet is administered at least 1 hour before meals. Schedule last dose of day at an appropriate time so that insomnia is avoided (see Absorption and Fate). Sustained-release form may be taken in the morning; administration time should be determined by period of day anorectic effect is needed (action lasts about 12 hours).

For maximal results, drug therapy should be used as part of a plan that includes reeducation of patient with respect to eating habits and attention to possible underlying psychologic factors.

Since drug may cause blurred vision and dizziness, caution patient to avoid potentially hazardous activities such as driving a car or operating machinery until reaction to drug is known.

Advise patient against excessive use of CNS stimulants such as coffee, tea, and cola drinks.

Instruct patient not to exceed recommended dosage. Tolerance to drug effects usually develops in a few weeks; drug should be discontinued when this occurs.

As with other amphetamines, physical and psychic dependence and tolerance may develop with prolonged use.

Classified as schedule II drug under federal Controlled Substances Act.

See nursing implications and drug interactions for amphetamine sulfate.

(BARBIPIL, BARBITA, ESKABARB, HENOMINT, HYPNETTE,
LUMINAL OVOIDS, PBR/12, PHENO-SQUAR, SK-PHENOBARBITAL,
SOLFOTON, SOLU-BARB, STENTAL)
PHENOBARBITAL SODIUM
(SODIUM LUMINAL)

Anticonvulsant, sedative, hypnotic

ACTIONS AND USES
Long-acting barbiturate. Sedative and hypnotic effects of barbiturates appear to be due primarily to interference with impulse transmission to cerebral cortex by inhibition of reticular activating system (concerned with both sleep and arousal mechanisms). Initially, sleep induced by barbiturates reduces REM sleep, but with chronic therapy REM sleep returns to normal. Has no analgesic properties, and small doses may increase reaction to painful stimuli. CNS dpression may range from mild sedation to coma, depending on dosage, route of administration, degree of nervous system excitability, and drug tolerance. Phenobarbital limits spread of seizure activity by increasing threshold for motor cortex stimuli. Anticonvulsant action of phenobarbital is shared by mephobarbital, but not other barbiturates, and is reportedly unrelated to sedative effect. Phenobarbital has a bilirubin lowering effect, by inducing production of glucuronyl transferase; also increases excretion and flow of bile salts.
Used as anticonvulsant in management of grand mal and cortical focal seizures, status epilepticus, eclampsia, and febrile convulsions in young children. Used when long-acting sedative or hypnotic is needed, as in insomnia, tension and anxiety states, and preoperative and postoperative management. Also used in treatment of neonatal hyperbilirubinemia.

ABSORPTION AND FATE
Well absorbed following all routes of administration, and widely distributed in tissues and body fluids. Hypnotic doses produce sleep within 10 minutes; duration varies from 6 to 10 hours. About 40% to 60% bound to plasma proteins and also to tissues, including brain. Half-life 2 to 5 days (somewhat shorter and more variable in children). Small amount metabolized in liver; excreted in urine largely as unchanged drug. Alkalinization of urine and hydration enhance renal excretion. Readily crosses placenta; enters breast milk. Barbiturates induce hepatic microsomal enzyme activity and thus may decrease effects of many drugs.

CONTRAINDICATIONS AND PRECAUTIONS
Sensitivity to barbiturates, manifest porphyria or familial history of porphyria, severe respiratory or cardiac or renal disease, history of previous addiction to sedative-hypnotics, uncontrolled pain, women of childbearing potential, pregnancy (particularly early pregnancy), nursing mothers. Cautious use: impaired hepatic, renal, cardiac, or respiratory function, history of allergies, elderly and debilitated patients, patients with fever, hyperthyroidism, diabetes mellitus, or severe anemia.

ADVERSE REACTIONS
Drowsiness, "hangover," headache, nausea, vomiting, diarrhea, dizziness, nystagmus, irritability, paradoxic excitement and exacerbation of hyperkinetic behavior (in children), confusion or depression or marked excitement (elderly patients), ataxia (large doses), hypersensitivity reactions, agranulocytosis, thrombocytopenia. **With prolonged therapy:** osteomalacia, elevated serum alkaline phosphatase, folic acid deficiency (mental dysfunction, neuropathy, psychiatric disorders, megaloblastic anemia). **Intravenous use:** coughing, hiccuping, laryngospasm, postoperative atelectasis, embolism. Extravascular injection: pain, swelling, thrombophlebitis, necrosis, nerve injury. **Overdosage:** respira-

tory depression, pupillary constriction (dilation with severe poisoning), oliguria, hypothermia (then hyperpyrexia), circulatory collapse, pulmonary edema.

ROUTE AND DOSAGE

Adults: *Sedative:* Oral: 16 to 32 mg 2 to 4 times/day. *Hypnotic:* Oral, parenteral (subcutaneous, IM, IV): 100 to 320 mg/day; not to exceed 600 mg/24 hours; IV rate not greater than 60 mg/minute. *Anticonvulsant:* Oral, parenteral: 100 to 320 mg/day. **Children:** *Sedative:* Oral, rectal suppository: 6 mg/kg/24 hours in 3 equally divided doses. *Hypnotic:* 3 to 6 mg/kg. *Anticonvulsant:* 1 to 6 mg/kg divided into 3 doses.

NURSING IMPLICATIONS

Solutions for injection (sodium phenobarbital) should not be used if a precipitate is present or if they are not absolutely clear.

Administer IM deep into large muscle mass; volume should not exceed 5 ml at any one site. Patients receiving large doses should be closely observed for at least 30 minutes to assure that narcosis is not excessive.

Keep patient under constant observation when drug is administered IV, and record vital signs at least every hour or more often if indicated. Maintain patient's airway. Resuscitation equipment and drugs should be immediately available.

Bedsides may be advisable for elderly patients and children, particularly when parenteral doses are administered, since they frequently manifest excitement and confusion with barbiturates.

When administering oral barbiturates, observe that patient actually swallows the pill and does not "cheek" it.

Barbiturates do not have analgesic action, and they may produce restlessness when given to patients in pain.

Patients receiving anticonvulsant therapy may experience drowsiness during first few weeks of treatment, but this usually diminishes with continued use of drugs.

Caution patient to avoid potentially hazardous activities such as driving a car or operating machinery until reaction to drug is known. Warn patient that alcohol in any amount may further impair judgment and psychomotor abilities.

Desired phenobarbital blood levels for epilepsy control are reportedly 10 to 25 µg/ml. Blood levels are particularly useful in children to assure that dosage is sufficient.

Phenobarbital and other long-acting barbiturates may be cumulative in action. Be alert for adverse reactions in patients who apparently have tolerated drug in the past.

Mental dullness, nystagmus, and staggering gait are useful indicators of excessive dosage.

It is important that pregnancy be avoided in patients receiving barbiturates. Patients on prolonged therapy who are also using oral contraceptives should be advised to consider alternative methods of contraception in addition to or instead of oral contraceptives (see Drug Interactions).

Sudden discontinuation of barbiturate therapy after chronic use may precipitate withdrawal symptoms: anxiety, insomnia, weakness, delirium, convulsions, status epilepticus (in patients with epilepsy).

Blood and liver tests and determinations of serum folate levels are advised during prolonged therapy.

Instruct patients on prolonged therapy to report to physician the onset of fever, sore throat or mouth, malaise, easy bruising or bleeding, petechiae, jaundice, rash.

Advise patients taking barbiturates at home not to keep drug on bedside table or in a readily accessible place. Patients have been known to forget having taken the drug, and in half-wakened conditions they have accidentally overdosed themselves.

Tolerance and physical and psychic dependence may develop with prolonged use.

Classified as schedule IV drug under federal Controlled Substances Act.

Treatment of overdosage: gastric lavage with cuffed endotracheal tube in place (for orally ingested barbiturate); maintenance of respiration, body temperature, supportive care as needed with vasopressors, oxygen, artificial respiration; monitoring of intake–output ratio. Dialysis may be required. Urinary alkalinization and hydration are sometimes used in treatment of phenobarbital overdosage.

Slang names for barbiturates include "barbs," "sleepers," "downs," "phennies," "peanuts," among many others. Addicts frequently use barbiturates to boost the effects of weak heroin.

LABORATORY TEST INTERFERENCES: There is the possibility that barbiturates may affect Bromsulphalein retention tests (by enhancing hepatic uptake and excretion of dye).

DRUG INTERACTIONS: Enhancement of CNS depression may result from concomitant use of barbiturates and other CNS depressants, eg, **alcohol, anesthetics, antianxiety agents, antihistamines, narcotic analgesics, sedative-hypnotics, phenothiazines,** and **rauwolfia alkaloids.** By increasing synthesis and activity of liver microsomal enzymes (involved in metabolism of many drugs), barbiturates may decrease the effects of: **oral anticoagulants, tricyclic antidepressants, antipyrine, carbamazepine, corticosteroids, digitoxin** and possibly other **digitalis glycosides** (effect is not marked), **doxycycline** (and possibly other tetracyclines), **estrogens (oral contraceptives), griseofulvin, lidocaine,** and **phenothiazines.** Barbiturates may enhance the toxicity of **cyclophosphamide. Disulfiram** and **MAO inhibitors** may inhibit metabolism of barbiturates (enhance and prolong these effects). **Sulfonamides** may increase the effects of barbiturates (by competing for plasma binding sites). Barbiturates may increase, decrease, or cause no change in **phenytoin** (and possibly other hydantoins); determinations of serum phenytoin levels advised prior to and periodically during concomitant therapy until stabilized.

PHENOLPHTHALEIN, N.F., B.P.
(CHOCOLAX, EVAC-U-GEN, EVAC-U-LAX, EX-LAX, FEEN-A-MINT, PHENOLAX)

Stimulant cathartic

ACTIONS AND USES

Diphenylmethane cathartic similar to bisacodyl in pharmacologic properties. Common ingredient in several OTC laxative preparations.

Used for temporary relief of simple constipation.

ABSORPTION AND FATE

Acts in 6 to 8 hours. Excreted in feces. Up to 15% of dose absorbed and eliminated primarily by kidney in conjugated form; some is excreted through bile and reabsorbed. Enterohepatic cycle may prolong drug action.

CONTRAINDICATIONS AND PRECAUTIONS

Hypersensitivity to phenolphthalein; abdominal pain, nausea, vomiting, fecal impaction, intestinal obstruction or perforation.

ADVERSE REACTIONS
Allergic reactions: skin eruptions, urticaria, Stevens-Johnson syndrome, lupus-erythematosus-like syndrome. Large doses or chronic use: electrolyte imbalance, impaired glucose tolerance from potassium loss.

ROUTE AND DOSAGE
Oral: 60 to 200 mg.

NURSING IMPLICATIONS

Usually administered at bedtime to produce effect the next morning (approximately 6 to 8 hours later).

Since drug enters enterohepatic circulation, inform patient that cathartic effect may persist for several days.

Advise patient to avoid prolonged or frequent use. Dependence on drug action, as well as electrolyte imbalance, can occur.

Drug may impart reddish or purplish pink discoloration to alkaline urine or feces (made alkaline by soapsuds enema). Inform patient of this possibility.

Instruct patient to discontinue drug immediately if skin rash appears.

Skin lesions resulting from allergic reaction may persist for months or years and may leave residual pigmentation.

Caution patient to store drug out of reach of children; fatalities have occurred when drug was eaten as candy.

See Bisacodyl.

LABORATORY TEST INTERFERENCES: Phenolphthalein may interfere with BSP excretion test.

PHENOXYBENZAMINE HYDROCHLORIDE, N.F., B.P. (DIBENZYLINE)

Antihypertensive (α-adrenergic blocking agent)

ACTIONS AND USES
Long-acting adrenergic blocking agent structurally related to azapetine. Apparently produces noncompetitive blockade of α-adrenergic receptor sites at postganglionic synapse. Alpha receptor sites are thus unable to react to endogenous or exogenous sympathomimetic agents. Blocks excitatory (alpha) effects of epinephrine, including vasoconstriction, but does not affect adrenergic cardiac inhibitory (beta) actions. Produces dilatation of muscular, cutaneous, and pulmonary vascular systems, but does not significantly alter cardiac output or renal, hepatic, and cerebral blood flow.

Used in management of pheochromocytoma and to improve circulation in peripheral vasospastic conditions such as Raynaud's acrocyanosis and frostbite sequelae.

ABSORPTION AND FATE
About 30% of oral dose is absorbed. Onset of action in 2 hours. Half-life approximately 24 hours. Excreted in urine and bile.

CONTRAINDICATIONS AND PRECAUTIONS
When fall in blood pressure would be dangerous; compensated congestive failure. Cautious use: marked cerebral or coronary arteriosclerosis, renal insufficiency, respiratory infections.

ADVERSE REACTIONS
Nasal congestion, dry mouth, miosis, drooping of eyelids, postural hypotension, tachycardia, palpitation, dizziness, fainting, inhibition of ejaculation, drowsi-

ness, GI irritation, vomiting, weakness, lethargy, shock, CNS stimulation (large
doses).
ROUTE AND DOSAGE
Oral: initially 10 mg daily in a single dose; dosage may be increased by increments of 10 mg daily at 4-day intervals. Maintenance: 20 to 60 mg daily in single or divided doses.

NURSING IMPLICATIONS

Administration with milk or food may reduce possibility of gastric irritation.

During period of dosage adjustment, monitor blood pressure and note pulse quality, rate, and rhythm in recumbent and standing positions. (Hypotension and tachycardia are most likely to occur in standing position.) Patient should be closely observed for at least 4 days from one dosage increment to the next.

Instruct patient to make position changes slowly, particularly from recumbent to upright posture, and to dangle legs for a few minutes before standing. Advise patient to lie down immediately at the onset of faintness or weakness.

Inform patient that postural hypotension and palpitation usually disappear with continued therapy, but they may reappear under conditions that promote vasodilation, such as exercise or ingestion of a large meal or alcohol.

Since phenoxybenzamine has cumulative action, onset of therapeutic effects may not occur until 2 weeks of therapy, and full therapeutic effects may not be apparent for several more weeks. (Drug action lasts several days after discontinuation of therapy.)

Therapeutic effectiveness in patients with pheochromocytoma is indicated by decreases in blood pressure, pulse, and sweating. In patients with peripheral vasospastic problems, observe for improvement in skin color, temperature, and quality of peripheral pulses, as well as less sensitivity to cold.

Treatment of overdosage: recumbent position with legs elevated (keep patient flat for 24 hours or more if necessary), application of leg bandages and abdominal binder. For severe hypotensive reaction, IV infusion of levarterenol may be given (epinephrine may cause further drop in blood pressure and therefore is contraindicated).

Preserved in air-tight containers, protected from light.

PHENPROCOUMON, N.F.
(LIQUAMAR)

Anticoagulant

ACTIONS AND USES
Long-acting coumarin derivative. Similar to other drugs of this class in actions, uses, contraindications, precautions, and adverse reactions. See Warfarin.
ABSORPTION AND FATE
Peak prothrombin time effect in 48 to 72 hours; normal values return in 7 to 14 days after cessation of treatment.
ROUTE AND DOSAGE
Oral: initially 24 mg; maintenance 0.75 to 6 mg daily. Dosage highly individualized on basis of prothrombin time determinations and clinical findings.

NURSING IMPLICATIONS

During period of dosage adjustment, prothrombin time results should be checked daily by physician and dosage order should be obtained. Follow hospital policies for administration of anticoagulants.

Prothrombin time should be determined prior to and 24 hours after administration of initial dose. Thereafter, prothrombin time is usually measured every 24 to 48 hours for first week, once or twice weekly for the next 3 or 4 weeks, and at 2- to 4-week intervals for patients on long-term therapy.

Prolonged duration of drug action may add to danger of anticoagulant therapy, since hemorrhage will be more difficult to control if it occurs.

Advise patient to report diarrhea. Dosage adjustment or drug withdrawal may be indicated.

Also see Warfarin.

PHENSUXIMIDE, N.F.
(MILONTIN)

Anticonvulsant (succinimide type)

ACTIONS AND USES

Succinimide derivative reportedly less potent but less effective than other drugs of this class. See Ethosuximide for actions, contraindications, precautions, and adverse reactions.

Used in management of petit mal epilepsy and with other anticonvulsants when other forms of epilepsy coexist with petit mal.

ABSORPTION AND FATE

Absorbed promptly; peak plasma levels in 1 to 4 hours. Not bound to plasma proteins. Half-life about 4 hours. Metabolized in liver; excreted in urine as active and inactive metabolites.

ADVERSE REACTIONS

Drowsiness, dizziness, ataxia, alopecia, muscle weakness, anorexia, nausea, flushing, periorbital edema, skin rash, reversible nephropathy. Also see Ethosuximide.

ROUTE AND DOSAGE

Oral: **Adults and children:** 0.5 to 1 Gm 2 or 3 times daily. Highly individualized. Total dosage, regardless of age, may vary between 1 and 3 Gm/day.

NURSING IMPLICATIONS

Shake oral suspension well before pouring to assure uniform dosage.

Caution against potentially hazardous tasks such as driving a car or operating machinery.

Advise patient to report onset of skin rash or other unusual symptoms to physician.

Stress importance of keeping scheduled appointments for blood, urine, and liver function studies.

Inform patient that phensuximide may color urine pink to red or red brown.

See Ethosuximide.

(ADIPEX-P, FASTIN, PARMINE, PHENTROL, ROLAPHENT, TORA, WILPO)
PHENTERMINE RESIN
(IONAMIN)

Anorexic

ACTIONS AND USES
Sympathomimetic amine related chemically and pharmacologically to amphetamine (qv). Cardiovascular actions and CNS stimulant effects are less prominent than those of amphetamine. Available as the hydrochloride salt and as a complex with a cationic-exchange resin of sulfonated polystyrene. Resin complex reacts with cations in GI tract and is designed to give controlled release of drug over 10- to 14-hour period. Effects of conventional oral tablet (hydrochloride) persist about 4 hours.
Used as short-term (a few weeks) adjunct in management of exogenous obesity.

CONTRAINDICATIONS AND PRECAUTIONS
History of hypersensitivity to sympathomimetic amines, advanced arteriosclerosis, symptomatic cardiovascular disease, moderate to severe hypertension, hyperthyroidism, glaucoma, agitated states, history of drug abuse, during or within 14 days of MAO inhibitors. Safe use during pregnancy or in children under 12 years of age not established.

ADVERSE REACTIONS
Nervousness, dizziness, insomnia, dry mouth, nausea, constipation, palpitation, tachycardia. Chronic intoxication: severe dermatoses, marked insomnia, irritability, hyperactivity, psychoses. Abrupt cessation following prolonged high dosage: extreme fatigue, depression, changes in sleep EEG patterns.

ROUTE AND DOSAGE
Oral (hydrochloride): 8 mg 2 or 3 times daily 30 minutes before meals; (timed-release form): 15 to 30 mg as single dose before breakfast; (resin): 15 to 30 mg before breakfast or 10 to 14 hours before retiring.

NURSING IMPLICATIONS
Not to be confused with chlorphentermine, also an anorexic, but given at much higher dosages.
To prevent insomnia, late evening medication should be avoided.
The resin preparation is ineffective if patient has diarrhea.
Caution patient to avoid potentially hazardous activities such as driving a car or operating machinery.
Tolerance to anorexigenic effect usually occurs within a few weeks. Drug should be discontinued when this occurs.
Classified as schedule IV drug under federal Controlled Substances Act.
Severe psychologic dependence has occurred in patients who have exceeded recommended dosage.
Also see Amphetamine.

PHENTOLAMINE HYDROCHLORIDE, N.F., B.P.
(REGITINE HYDROCHLORIDE)
PHENTOLAMINE MESYLATE, U.S.P., B.P.
(REGITINE MESYLATE)

Antiadrenergic (α-adrenergic blocking agent)

ACTIONS AND USES

Imidazoline α-adrenergic blocking agent structurally related to tolazoline, but has more potent blocking effects. Competetively blocks α-adrenergic receptors, but action is transient and incomplete. Inhibits hypertension resulting from elevated levels of circulating epinephrine and/or norepinephrine. Causes vasodilation, and decreases general vascular resistance and pulmonary arterial pressure, primarily by direct action on vascular smooth muscle. Through stimulation of β-adrenergic receptors, produces positive inotropic and chronotropic cardiac effects, and increases cardiac output. Also has histaminelike action that stimulates gastric secretions.

Used in diagnosis of pheochromocytoma and to prevent or control hypertensive episodes prior to or during pheochromocytomectomy. Also used to prevent dermal necrosis and sloughing following IV administration or extravasation of levarterenol.

ABSORPTION AND FATE

Maximum effect on blood pressure following IV administration in 2 minutes (persists 10 to 15 minutes), and in 15 to 20 minutes after IM (blood pressure returns to preinjection level in 3 to 4 hours).

CONTRAINDICATIONS AND PRECAUTIONS

Hypersensitivity to phentolamine or related drugs; myocardial infarction (previous or present). Safe use during pregnancy and lactation not established. Cautious use: gastritis, peptic ulcer, coronary artery disease.

ADVERSE REACTIONS

Weakness, dizziness, orthostatic hypotension, flushing, nasal stuffiness, conjunctival infection. GI side effects (common): abdominal pain, nausea, vomiting, diarrhea, exacerbation of peptic ulcer. With parenteral administration especially: acute and prolonged hypotension, tachycardia, anginal pain, cardiac arrhythmias, myocardial infarction, cerebrovascular spasm, shocklike state.

ROUTE AND DOSAGE

Oral: **Adults:** 50 mg 4 to 6 times daily. **Children:** 25 mg 4 to 6 times daily; alternatively, 5 mg/kg body weight, divided into 4 to 6 doses. Intravenous, intramuscular: **Adults:** 5 mg. **Children:** 1 mg; alternatively, 0.1 mg/kg. To prevent necrosis: 10 mg to each liter of IV fluid containing levarterenol. To treat extravasation: 5 to 10 mg in 10 ml of 0.9% sodium chloride injection infiltrated into affected area, within 12 hours after extravasation.

NURSING IMPLICATIONS

Patient should be in supine position when receiving drug parenterally. Monitor blood pressure and pulse every 2 minutes until stabilized.

Test for pheochromocytoma: (1) Medications not deemed absolutely essential should be withheld at least 24 hours, preferably 48 to 72 hours; antihypertensive agents withheld until blood pressure returns to pretreatment level (rauwolfia drugs withdrawn at least 4 weeks prior to testing). (2) Keep patient at rest in supine position throughout test, preferably in quiet darkened room. (3) Take blood pressure every 10 minutes for at least 30 minutes; when blood pressure stabilizes, injection should be administered by physician. (4) IV administration: record blood pressure immediately after injection and at 30-second intervals for first 3 minutes, then at 1-minute intervals for next 7 minutes. IM administration: blood pressure determinations at 5-minute intervals for 30 to 45 minutes.

Test results: Positive response (indicated by drop in systolic pressure of at least 35 mm Hg and 25 mm Hg diastolic) suggests pheochromocytoma. Presumptive negative response: blood pressure is unchanged, elevated, or reduced less than 35 mm Hg systolic and 25 mm Hg diastolic.

Treatment of overdosage: Keep patient recumbent with head lowered; supportive measures; IV fluids. Severe drop in blood pressure may be treated with IV infusion of levarterenol, carefully titrated. *Epinephrine is contraindicated,* since paradoxic fall in blood pressure may result.

Phentolamine hydrochloride is preserved in well-closed, light-resistant containers.

PHENYLBUTAZONE, U.S.P., B.P.
(AZOLID, BUTAZOLIDIN)

Antiinflammatory, antirheumatic

ACTIONS AND USES

Pyrazolone derivative with antiinflammatory, antipyretic, and mild uricosuric properties.

Used for short-term symptomatic relief of pain and disability when ordinary therapeutic measures have failed; used in patients with rheumatoid arthritis, ankylosing spondylitis, osteoarthritis, psoriatic arthritis, painful shoulder, and acute superficial thrombophlebitis.

ABSORPTION AND FATE

Readily absorbed from GI tract, with onset of action in 30 to 60 minutes. Peak plasma levels in 2 hours; duration of action 3 to 5 days. Repeated constant daily doses produce plateau in plasma levels in 3 to 5 days. Almost entirely bound to plasma proteins. Half-life 2.5 to 4 days. Distributed to most body tissues. Metabolized slowly in liver to two active metabolites: oxyphenbutazone and hydroxyphenylbutazone. Excreted slowly in urine. Crosses placenta; enters breast milk.

CONTRAINDICATIONS AND PRECAUTIONS

History of peptic ulcer, GI inflammatory disease or recurrent dyspepsia, drug allergy, blood dyscrasias, renal disease, hepatic or cardiac dysfunction, severe hypertension, edema, polymyalgia rheumatica, temporal arteritis, patients receiving other potent chemotherapeutic agents, patients on long-term anticoagulant therapy, children under age 14. Safe use during pregnancy not established. Cautious use: glaucoma, patients over age 40.

ADVERSE REACTIONS

GI: nausea, vomiting, diarrhea, epigastric pain, abdominal distension, ulcerative esophagitis, ulceration of bowel, peptic ulcer with bleeding and perforation. **Renal:** hematuria, proteinuria, glomerulonephritis, renal failure, renal stones. **Cardiovascular:** hypertension, palpitation, pericarditis, myocarditis, cardiac decompensation. **Hematologic:** thrombocytopenia, agranulocytosis, hemolytic or aplastic anemia, leukopenia, leukemia (causal relationship not established). **Endocrine/metabolic:** hyperglycemia, alkalosis, acidosis, hepatic damage, thyroid hyperplasia, toxic goiter (causal relationship not established). **CNS:** peripheral neuropathy, lethargy, confusion, nervousness, agitation, dizziness; toxic doses: headache, insomnia, euphoria, depression, psychosis, convulsions, coma. **Ophthalmic:** blurred vision, diplopia, optic neuritis, optic atrophy, retinal hemorrhage and detachment, toxic amblyopia. **Other:** hearing loss, ulcerative stomatitis, dry mouth, salivary gland enlargement.

ROUTE AND DOSAGE

Oral: 200 to 400 mg daily in 3 or 4 divided doses (usual range 100 to 600 mg daily). Maintenance: should not exceed 400 mg/day.

NURSING IMPLICATIONS

Administered immediately before, during, or immediately after meals or with full glass of milk. Physician may prescribe concurrent sodium-free antacid or commercially available preparation with aluminum hydroxide gel and aluminum trisilicate, eg, Azolid-A, Butazolidin alka.

Careful, detailed history and complete physical and laboratory examinations are advised prior to therapy.

Physical and laboratory examinations should be repeated at regular intervals during therapy (blood studies are advised every week in patients over age 40 and every 2 weeks in other patients). Follow-up blood studies are recommended because blood dyscrasias may occur days or weeks after termination of therapy.

Patients should be closely followed during therapy and carefully instructed to report adverse reactions. Symptoms of phenylbutazone toxicity are insidious in onset.

Keep physician informed of patient's response to medication. If no beneficial response is noted in 1 week, drug is discontinued. If improvement occurs, physician may make repeated attempts to reduce dosage to minimum effective level.

For patients over age 60, short-term treatment of 1 week is recommended because of high risk of potentially fatal reactions in this group (incidence of adverse effects increases in patients over 40 years of age).

Warn patient not to exceed prescribed dosage and to discontinue drug and report promptly to physician at the onset of fever, sore throat, mouth lesions, salivary gland enlargement, epigastric pain, dyspepsia, tarry stools, skin rashes, significant weight gain or edema, blurred vision, pruritus, jaundice, or other unusual symptoms.

Blurred vision is a significant toxic symptom. Complete ophthalmoscopic examination is indicated.

Consult physician regarding salt intake. Salt restriction is often prescribed because drug tends to induce sodium retention.

Monitor intake and output. Instruct home patients to note ratio of intake and output and to report oliguria. Also advise patients to examine stools and urine for blood (tarry stools, cloudy or pink urine). Inform patients that compensatory diuresis sometimes follows discontinuation of drug (due to retained sodium).

Instruct patients to keep a record of daily weights and to check legs and face for evidence of edema.

DRUG INTERACTIONS: Phenylbutazone enhances hypoprothrombinemic effect of **oral anticoagulants** (by displacing them from protein binding sites); it may enhance hypoglycemic activity of oral antidiabetic drugs (possibly by interfering with their renal excretion) and insulin. **Cholestyramine** may delay intestinal absorption of phenylbutazone (administer phenylbutazone at least 1 hour before or 4 to 6 hours after cholestyramine). **Desipramine** decreases phenylbutazone levels (by inhibiting its GI absorption). Phenylbutazone appears to enhance metabolism of **digitalis glycosides,** with resulting underdigitalization, and it may increase the half-life of **phenytoin.** Uricosuric activity of large doses of **salicylates** may be antagonized by phenylbutazone (possibly by competing for common binding sites).

(ALCONEFRIN, BIOMYDRIN, CORICIDIN NASAL MIST, CORYBAN-D
NASAL, DEGEST, EFRICEL, ISOPHRIN NASAL, MISTURA D,
NEO-SYNEPHRINE, PREFRIN, SYNASAL, TEAR-EFRIN)

Adrenergic

ACTIONS AND USES
Potent, noncatecholamine, direct-acting sympathomimetic with strong α-
adrenergic and weak β-adrenergic cardiac stimulant actions. Produces little or
no CNS stimulation. Elevates systolic and diastolic pressures through arteriolar
constriction; also constricts capacitance vessels and increases venous return to
heart. Rise in blood pressure causes reflex slowing of heart. Topical applications
to eye produce vasoconstriction and prompt mydriasis of short duration, usually
without causing cycloplegia. Reduces intraocular pressure by increasing outflow
and decreasing rate of aqueous humor secretion. Nasal decongestant action
qualitatively similar to that of epinephrine, but more potent and has longer
duration of action.
Used parenterally to maintain blood pressure during anesthesia and for treatment of vascular failure in shock; used to overcome paroxysmal supraventricular tachycardia. Used topically for rhinitis of common cold, allergic rhinitis, and
sinusitis; used in selected patients with open-angle glaucoma; used as mydriatic
for ophthalmoscopic examination or surgery and for temporary relief of eye
irritation.

ABSORPTION AND FATE
Duration of effect on blood pressure about 20 minutes following direct IV
injection and about 50 minutes or more after subcutaneous or IM administration. Mydriatic effect begins in 15 to 30 minutes and lasts 1 to 3 hours.

CONTRAINDICATIONS AND PRECAUTIONS
Severe coronary disease, severe hypertension, narrow-angle glaucoma. Cautious
use: hyperthyroidism, diabetes, myocardial disease, cerebral arteriosclerosis,
bradycardia, elderly patients, halothane anesthesia, tricyclic antidepressants,
MAO inhibitors, oxytocic drugs.

ADVERSE REACTIONS
Systemic effects: palpitation, tachycardia, extrasystoles, hypertension, trembling, sweating, pallor, sense of fullness in head, tingling of extremities, sleeplessness, dizziness, lightheadedness, weakness. **Nasal use:** burning, stinging,
dryness, sneezing. **Ophthalmic use:** transient stinging, browache, headache,
blurred vision, conjunctival allergy (pigmentary deposits on lids, conjunctiva,
and cornea with prolonged use).

ROUTE AND DOSAGE
Adults: Subcutaneous, intramuscular: 1 to 10 mg (initial dose not to exceed 5
mg). Intravenous: 0.1 to 0.5 mg (initial dose not to exceed 0.5 mg); not repeated
before 10 to 15 minutes. Continuous IV infusion: 10 mg added to 500 ml of 5%
dextrose in water or sodium chloride injection (provides 1:50,000 solution).
Children: 0.1 mg/kg subcutaneously or IM. Topical (nasal): 0.125% to 1%
solution, 0.5% jelly; (ophthalmic): 0.12% to 10% solution.

NURSING IMPLICATIONS
Do not use solutions that are discolored or that contain a precipitate.
IV infusion flow rate is prescribed by physician (initial flow rate for treat-
ment of shock may be 100 to 180 drops/minute, decreasing to mainte-
nance rate of 40 to 60 drops/minute as blood pressure stabilizes).
Monitor blood pressure and pulse. Be alert to abnormalities in cardiac rate

and rhythm and complaints of fullness in head and tingling of extremities (symptoms of overdosage).

Have on hand phentolamine (α-adrenergic blocking agent) for excessive blood pressure elevation.

Before administration of nasal preparations, instruct patient to blow nose gently to clear nasal passages.

Nasal drops are generally instilled in lateral, head-low position.

Rinse nasal spray tip or dropper with hot water after each use to prevent contamination of solution.

Physician may prescribe application of a topical anesthetic before eyedrops instillation to prevent stinging and discomfort.

Caution patient not to exceed recommended dosage. Systemic effects can follow topical application.

Preserved in tight, light-resistant containers, away from heat.

DRUG INTERACTIONS: Phenylephrine is potentiated by **guanethidine, MAO inhibitors,** and **tricyclic antidepressants.** Concurrent administration of **furazolidone** may result in hypertensive crisis. **Levodopa** reduces mydriatic effect of topical phenylephrine.

PHENYLPROPANOLAMINE HYDROCHLORIDE, N.F. (PROPADRINE)

Adrenergic (vasoconstrictor)

ACTIONS AND USES

Indirect-acting sympathomimetic amine with prominent peripheral adrenergic effects similar to those of ephedrine (qv), but its action is more prolonged and it causes less CNS stimulation. Acts by stimulating α-adrenergic (excitatory) receptors of vascular smooth muscles, with resulting constriction.

Used in symptomatic relief of nasal congestion associated with allergies, hay fever, common cold, sinusitis, nasopharyngitis. Used parenterally as vasopressor during surgery, particularly during spinal anesthesia.

CONTRAINDICATIONS AND PRECAUTIONS

MAO inhibitors. Cautious use: hypertension, cardiovascular disease, hyperthyroidism, diabetes, postatic enlargement, tricyclic antidepressants.

ADVERSE REACTIONS

High doses: hypertension, tachycardia, palpitation, nervousness, restlessness, insomnia, dilated pupils, headache, CNS stimulation, nausea, vomiting, anorexia. Also see Ephedrine.

ROUTE AND DOSAGE

Oral: **Adults:** 25 mg at 4-hour intervals or 50 mg at 8-hour intervals, as indicated. **Children** *6 to 12 years:* 12.5 mg at 4-hour intervals or 25 mg at 8-hour intervals; *2 to 6 years:* 6.25 mg at 4-hour intervals or 12.5 mg at 8-hour intervals, as indicated. Intramuscular: **Adults:** 37.5 to 75 mg (0.5 to 1 ml).

NURSING IMPLICATIONS

Caution patient not to exceed recommended dosage. Preserved in tight, light-resistant containers.

See Ephedrine.

DRUG INTERACTIONS: Phenylpropanolamine antagonizes effects of **bethanidine** and **guanethidine.** Concurrent use with **MAO inhibitor** may produce

hypertensive crisis. **Reserpine** may antagonize action of phenylpropanolamine. **571**
Tricyclic antidepressants may enhance pressor effects of phenylpropanolamine.
Also see Ephedrine.

PHENYTOIN, U.S.P. (formerly DIPHENYLHYDANTOIN)
(DIHYCON, DILANTIN, DI-PHENYL, DPH, EKKO)
PHENYTOIN SODIUM, U.S.P., B.P.
(DENYL SODIUM, DILANTIN SODIUM, DI-PHEN,
DIPHENYLHYDANTOIN SODIUM, KESSODANTEN, SDPH)

Anticonvulsant

ACTIONS AND USES
Hydantoin derivative chemically related to phenobarbital. Precise mechanism of anticonvulsant action not known. In motor cortex, inhibits spread of seizure activity along nerve pathways and stabilizes threshold against excessive stimuli possibly by promoting Na loss from neurons. Reduces posttetanic potentiation (PTP) of synaptic transmission and prevents firing of adjacent cortical areas. Unlike phenobarbital, has little hypnotic action, is ineffective for control of drug-induced seizures, and has limited ability to modify threshold in electroconvulsive seizures. Antiarrhythmic properties similar to those of procainamide and quinidine. Decreases force of myocardial contractions, suppresses ectopic pacemaker activity, improves A-V conduction depressed by digitalis glycosides, and prolongs effective refractory period relative to duration of action potential. Membrane stabilizing effect on pancreas may inhibit effective insulin release. Induces hepatic microsomal enzymes and therefore may affect metabolism of other drugs. Like other hydantoin derivatives, increases metabolic inactivation of vitamin D.
Used to control grand mal and psychomotor seizures, and in combination with phenobarbital or other anticonvulsant drugs may be used to control mixed grand mal-petit mal seizures. Used parenterally for status epilepticus and to control seizures occurring during neurosurgery. Investigational use: to treat cardiac arrhythmias associated with digitalis toxicity, acute myocardial infarction and open-heart surgery; and for treatment of migraine and tic douloureux.
ABSORPTION AND FATE
Slowly absorbed following oral administration (rate of absorption may vary with patient and product used). Peak plasma concentrations: 3 to 12 hours. Onset of action: 3 to 5 minutes following IV injection. Drug precipitates at IM injection site and is slowly and erratically absorbed. Wide distribution to all tissues with highest concentrations in liver and fat; 70 to 95% bound to plasma proteins (mainly albumin). Half-life generally ranges 18 to 24 hours (may be longer in black patients). Biotransformation in liver primarily, with excretion in bile as inactive metabolites which are reabsorbed from G.I. tract and excreted in urine as glucuronides. Less than 5% excreted unchanged. Crosses placenta; enters breast milk.
CONTRAINDICATIONS AND PRECAUTIONS
History of hypersensitivity to hydantoin products; seizures due to hypoglycemia; sinus bradycardia, complete or incomplete heart block. Cautious use: impaired hepatic or renal function, hypotension, severe myocardial insufficiency, impending or frank heart failure, elderly or gravely ill patients.
ADVERSE REACTIONS
CNS (most common): nystagmus, diplopia, blurred or dimmed vision, lethargy, drowsiness, ataxia, dizziness, slurred speech, mental confusion, silliness, hallucinations, insomnia, transient nervousness, headache; extrapyramidal disturbances (unusual movements of face, tongue, extremities; salivation); periph-

eral neuropathy, encephalopathy with increased seizure activity. Circumoral tingling, flapping tremors, extreme lethargy (associated with IV use). **GI:** nausea, vomiting, constipation, epigastric pain, dysphagia, loss of taste, weight loss. **Cardiovascular:** depressed atrial and ventricular conduction, ventricular fibrillation. **With rapid IV injection:** bradycardia, hypotension, cardiovascular collapse, cardiac (and respiratory) arrest. **Hypersensitivity:** pruritus, fever, arthralgia, morbilliform (measles-like) rash, exfoliative, purpuric or bullous dermatitis, Stevens-Johnson syndrome, lymphadenopathy, acute renal failure, hepatitis, liver necrosis. **Hematologic:** thrombocytopenia, leukopenia, leukocytosis, agranulocytosis, pancytopenia, eosinophilia macrocytosis, anemias. **Other:** gingival hyperplasia, hirsutism (especially young females), keratosis, facial coarsening (especially young patients); edema, photophobia, conjunctivitis, hyperglycemia, glycosuria, osteomalacia or rickets associated with hypocalcemia and elevated alkaline phosphatase activity; pulmonary fibrosis, periarteritis nodosum; acute systemic lupus erythematosus; injection site pain, phlebitis, tissue necrosis.

ROUTE AND DOSAGE

Epilepsy: Oral: **Adults:** initial, 100 mg 3 times daily; increased if necessary at 1- to 2- week intervals according to individual response. Maintenance: 100 to 200 mg 3 times daily. **Pediatric:** initial, 5 mg/kg/day in 2 or 3 equally divided doses; subsequent dosage individualized to maximum of 300 mg/day. Maintenance: 4 to 8 mg/kg/day. *Status epilepticus:* Direct IV: **Adults:** initial, 150 to 250 mg, at rate not exceeding 50 mg/min; subsequent doses of 100 to 150 mg, 30 minutes later if necessary. **Pediatric:** 250 mg/m^2 of body surface area. Each IV injection should be followed by injection of sterile normal saline through same needle or IV catheter, to avoid venous irritation. *Neurosurgery:* Intramuscular: **Adults:** 100 to 200 mg at approximately 4-hour intervals, continued during surgery and postoperative period. *Cardiac Arrhythmias:* Direct IV: **Adults:** 100 mg at 5-minute intervals until arrhythmia is abolished, or undesirable side effects intervene, or until 1 Gm is given. Oral: 100 mg 2 to 4 times daily.

NURSING IMPLICATIONS

Administer oral preparation with at least ½ glass of water immediately before, with, or immediately after meals, to minimize gastric irritation. Drug is strongly alkaline.

Shake suspension vigorously before pouring to ensure uniform distribution of drug, and use same measure for consistency in dosage.

Metabolic breakdown rate may differ among products. Some patients do not completely digest capsule form, thus blood levels may be lower than with tablet or suspension. Advise patient not to accept different formulation when having prescription refilled, unless otherwise advised by physician.

Inform patient that drug may impart a harmless pink or red to red-brown coloration to urine.

For parenteral administration, use only special diluent supplied by manufacturer. Store reconstituted solution temporarily, at room temperature; discard solution within 4 to 6 hours of preparation or if haziness or precipitation develops.

IM injections (infrequently prescribed) should be made deeply into large muscle mass. Carefully aspirate before injecting drug to avoid intravascular injection. Perivascular and subcutaneous injections should be avoided as drug is highly irritating to tissue.

Margin between toxic and therapeutic IV dose is relatively small. Monitor blood pressure, pulse, and respiration. Observe patient closely for CNS side effects. Have on hand oxygen, vasopressor, assisted ventilation, seizure precaution equipment (padded side rails, mouth gag, nonmetal airway, suction apparatus).

Solubility of phenytoin is pH dependent; therefore, avoid mixing with other drugs or adding to any infusion solution, because a fine precipitate may result.

Elderly patients (over 60 years of age) are more likely to show evidence of toxicity than younger patients. Monitor closely during dosage adjustment period and during any illness.

Instruct responsible family member how to take care of patient during a seizure, what to observe and record. Advise to call for emergency help if patient has one seizure after another, has trouble breathing, or has sustained an injury. General instructions: Do not attempt to restrain patient, but protect him from injury eg, pillow, blanket, or clothing under head, loosen constricting clothing. Place padded tongue depressor, or anything firm and soft between teeth. If teeth are clenched, do not force them open because they could be broken and aspirated. After convulsion is over, turn patient on side to facilitate drainage of oropharyngeal secretions. Record sequence of various phenomena during seizure (describe location and type movements; position of head, eyes, extremities; pupil size; duration of seizure, behavior following seizure to help physician to localize area of brain involved). Notify physician that patient had a seizure.

During dosage adjustment period, patient is usually advised to return in 3 weeks for serum drug level measurement, then at monthly intervals for 2 to 3 months, depending on values obtained. (Steady-state serum levels generally reached 7 to 12 days after start of therapy.)

Since drug levels do not always reflect toxicity, close clinical observation is essential. For example, some patients only partially metabolize phenytoin (possibly a genetic enzyme deficiency) and thus may manifest toxicity even when blood levels are normal.

Liver function tests, blood counts, and urinalyses are recommended prior to therapy and at monthly intervals during prolonged therapy. Reportedly hydantoin derivatives may interfere with folic acid metabolism with resulting megaloblastic anemia. Folic acid therapy may be required.

Instruct patient to report onset of CNS symptoms (see Adverse Reactions). Serum drug level determination may be indicated. Nystagmus generally appears when serum phenytoin level reaches 20 μg/ml or higher, gait ataxia when levels are around 30 μg/ml, and constant lethargy at 40 μg/ml. (Therapeutic serum levels are usually between 10 and 20 μg/ml, depending on assay method used.)

Caution patient not to alter prescribed drug regimen. Abrupt drug discontinuation may precipitate seizures and status epilepticus. Withdrawal must be done gradually, over a period of 1 to 3 or more months and in relation to serum drug levels and EEGs.

Gingival hyperplasia appears most commonly in children and adolescents; never occurs in edentulous patients. Condition can be minimized by daily brushing with multifaceted, soft toothbrush, careful flossing to remove dental plaque, and gum massage. Parents must brush and floss teeth for children once daily up to at least 6 to 8 years of age when child should be able to do it himself. Advise patient/parent to inform dentist that he is taking phenytoin; gingivectomy is sometimes necessary.

Use of electric toothbrush may assure better compliance in young children. For babies with erupting teeth, mechanical stimulation and relief of discomfort may be provided by nonimported, approved teething ring with frozen liquid.

Caution patient to avoid hazardous activities particularly during early therapy, and not to drive a car until approval is given by physician. Many states now permit patients with epilepsy to obtain a driver's license provided he has physician's certificate stating he has been seizure-free for a period of time (usually 1 to 2 years).

Hypoprothrombinemia has occurred in newborns whose mothers received hydantoin derivatives during pregnancy. Physician may prescribe doses of vitamin K.

Patients with diabetes should be monitored regularly for symptoms of hyperglycemia (polydipsia, polyuria, lethargy, drowsiness, psychotic manifestations, glycosuria). Adjustment of phenytoin dosage (for patients on insulin) or adjustment of oral hypoglycemic dosage may be necessary.

Hydration may be a significant factor in seizure control. Mild dehydration has been associated with decline in number of seizures. Discuss with physician.

A well balanced diet is an important adjunct to effective anticonvulsant therapy. Collaborate with dietician, patient/family in diet planning. Urge patient to eat regularly and to avoid overeating.

Patients on prolonged therapy should have adequate intake of vitamin D containing foods (eg, fortified milk, margarine, butter, liver, egg yolk), and sufficient exposure to sunlight. Periodic checks are indicated for decrease in serum Ca levels (sign of bone demineralization and potential rickets or osteomalacia). Particularly susceptible: black children, patients receiving other anticonvulsants concurrently, patients who are inactive, have limited exposure to sunlight, or whose dietary intake is inadequate.

Hydantoin derivatives may interfere with folic acid metabolism with consequent development of megaloblastic anemia. Observe patient for symptoms of folic acid deficiency (neuropathy, mental dysfunction, psychiatric disorders). Serum folate levels should be determined at onset of symptoms. Physician may prescribe folic acid (0.1 to 1 mg/day) as supplemental therapy. (See Drug Interactions.)

After patient has been well stabilized on divided dosage schedule, physician may prescribe single daily phenytoin dose of same amount. Clinical studies have indicated that single dose regimen demonstrates similar absorption rate and equilibrium levels as divided dosage schedule. However, individual differences in drug plasma half-life and GI side effects may preclude this change in some patients.

Duration of phenytoin treatment is extremely variable. In some patients, a lifetime of drug therapy is necessary; in others, physician may attempt to withdraw drug after a seizure-free period (including auras) of 2 to 5 years.

Patient/family may require help with emotional reaction to epilepsy, problems of stigmatized discrimination that may occur, and required life style adjustments.

Most states have local chapters or state associations concerned with special problems of the epileptic; e.g., Epilepsy Foundation of America (EFA), one among other nonprofit organizations provides information and services related to life insurance, legal problems, training and placement, school children, low-cost prescriptions, educational literature. Contact local chapter if available, or national headquarters: 1828 L Street, N.S., Washington, D.C., 20036.

Patient/family teaching plan (construct plan in collaboration with physician, dietitian, and other relevant health team members): (1) Reason for taking medication. (2) Take drug precisely as prescribed and keep check off record or calendar. (3) Adverse reactions. (4) What to do in the event of a seizure. (5) Avoid colds, infections: if they occur, notify physician. (6) Importance of regularity and moderation in life style. (7) Well-balanced diet; avoid overeating and overhydration. (8) Avoid OTC drugs. (9) Alcohol restriction (consult physician regarding allowable amount). (10) Moderation in physical activity; avoid high risk sports. (11) Avoid emotional stress; talk problems out with physician, nurse, or significant other. (12) Keep follow-up appointments. (13) Carry identification card, or jewelry with pertinent medical data (may be procured from local pharmacy, Medic Alert Foundation, or AMA).

pone, dexamethasone suppression, and thyroid function tests; may result in decreased urinary steroid determinations.

DRUG INTERACTIONS: Drugs that inhibit hepatic breakdown of phenytoin may raise serum phenytoin levels, thereby potentiating its effects: **aminosalicylic acid** (PAS): **oral anticoagulants; benzodiazepines; chloramphenicol; oral contraceptives** (also, these drugs may increase seizure activity by inducing fluid retention); **disulfiram; halothane** (by producing hepatotoxicity); **isoniazid** (phenytoin toxicity is likely); **methylphenidate; phenothiazines; phenylbutazone, oxyphenbutazone; phenyramidol; salicylates** (in large doses may displace phenytoin from plasma binding sites); **sulfonamides.** Seizure activity may be increased by drugs that enhance hepatic breakdown of phenytoin: **alcohol; barbiturates** (variable effect); **carbamazepine; folic acid** may directly antagonize anticonvulsant effect. **Tricyclic antidepressants** (especially in high doses) may induce epileptic seizures. Phenytoin may decrease effects of **corticosteroids, digitalis glycosides,** and **tetracyclines** by increasing their hepatic breakdown. Phenytoin may generate relatively high levels of phenobarbital in patients receiving **primidone** (converted to phenobarbital in body), and may increase effects of **methotrexate,** and **thyroid hormones** by displacing these drugs from plasma binding sites.

PHTHALYLSULFATHIAZOLE, N.F., B.P,
(SULFATHALIDINE)

Intestinal antibacterial (sulfonamide)

ACTIONS AND USES

Hydrolyzes to sulfathiazole in intestinal tract. Antibacterial action restricted to lumen of large intestine. Action is reflected in reduction of intestinal microorganisms and production of gelatinous, stringy, tenacious stool within 3 to 5 days.

Used in preoperative preparation and postoperative management of patients requiring intestinal surgery and as adjunctive therapy in treatment of nonspecific, acute ulcerative colitis.

ABSORPTION AND FATE

Poorly absorbed from GI tract. Excreted in feces; approximately 4% eliminated in urine as intact drug.

ADVERSE REACTIONS

Headache, malaise, anorexia, nausea, vomiting, drug fever, allergic reactions, excessive intestinal bleeding. Also see Sulfadiazine.

ROUTE AND DOSAGE

Oral: Preoperative and postoperative treatment: 125 mg/kg daily in 3, 4, or 6 divided doses; not to exceed 8 Gm daily. Ulcerative colitis: 50 to 100 mg/kg daily in 3 to 6 divided doses. Initial course: 2 to 4 weeks followed by rest period of 5 to 10 days.

NURSING IMPLICATIONS

Drug should be administered in conjunction with low-residue diet.

When administered to prepare bowel for surgery, therapy should begin 3 to 5 days preoperatively. If cleansing enema is required, physician may prescribe phthalylsulfathiazole enema (6 Gm/liter).

Drug therapy is resumed postoperatively as soon as patient's condition allows, and usually continues for 1 to 2 weeks.

Record number and character of stools. Stool should appear gelatinous and formed. Hard stools at onset of or continuation of diarrhea indicate need for dosage adjustment.

Advise patient to avoid preparations containing mineral oil, because it interferes with drug action.

Instruct patient to report any evidence of bleeding. Physician may prescribe vitamin K prophylactically, since phthalylsulfathiazole may interfere with intestinal bacterial synthesis of vitamin K.

Preserved in well-closed, light-resistant containers.

See Sulfisoxazole.

PHYSOSTIGMINE SALICYLATE, U.S.P., B.P.
(ANTILIRIUM, Eserine Salicylate, ISOPTO ESERINE)
PHYSOSTIGMINE SULFATE, U.S.P.
(Eserine Sulfate)

Cholinergic (cholinesterase inhibitor) (Ophthalmic)

ACTIONS AND USES

Reversible anticholinesterase, tertiary ammonium alkaloid of West African calabar or ordeal bean, *Physostigma venenosum*. Similar to neostigmine (qv) in actions and adverse effects, but produces greater secretion of glands, constriction of pupil, and effect on blood pressure, and less action on skeletal muscle. Also has direct blocking action on autonomic ganglia. Recent clinical evidence suggests that parenteral physostigmine can produce transient decrease in manic symptoms as well as precipitate mental depression. Topical application to conjunctiva produces constriction of ciliary muscle (spasm of accommodation) and iris sphincter (miosis) as result of which the iris is pulled away from anterior chamber angle, thus facilitating drainage of aqueous humor, with lowering of intraocular pressure.

Used to reverse CNS and cardiac effects of tricyclic antidepressant overdose, to reverse CNS toxic effects of atropine, scopolamine, and similar anticholinergic drugs, and to stimulate peristalsis in patients with postoperative intestinal atony. Applied topically to eye to reduce intraocular tension in certain types of glaucoma. Also has been used to counteract atropine mydriasis.

ABSORPTION AND FATE

Readily absorbed from mucous membranes, muscle, and subcutaneous tissue. Onset of action following parenteral administration occurs in 3 to 8 minutes; duration is 30 minutes to 5 hours. Readily passes blood–brain barrier; widely distributed throughout body. Largely hydrolyzed and inactivated by cholinesterases. Excretion not fully understood; only small amounts found in urine. Onset of action following topical application to conjunctiva occurs within 2 minutes; peak occurs within 1 to 2 hours, and action may persist 12 to 36 hours.

CONTRAINDICATIONS AND PRECAUTIONS

Asthma, diabetes mellitus, gangrene, cardiovascular disease, mechanical obstruction of intestinal or urogenital tract or any vagotonic state, secondary glaucoma, inflammatory diseases of iris or ciliary body, concomitant use with choline esters (eg, methacholine, bethanechol) or depolarizing neuromuscular blocking agents (eg, decamethonium, succinylcholine). Safe use during pregnancy not established. Cautious use: epilepsy, parkinsonism, bradycardia.

ADVERSE REACTIONS

Ophthalmic: headache, eye and brow pain, marked miosis, twitching of eyelids, conjunctival congestion, lacrimation, dimness and blurring of vision; prolonged use: changes in pigment epithelium of iris, chronic conjunctivitis, follicular cysts, contact allergic dermatitis. **Systemic absorption:** nausea, vomiting, epigastric pain, diarrhea, involuntary urination or defecation, miosis, salivation, sweating, lacrimation, rhinorrhea, dyspnea, bronchospasm, irregular pulse, palpitation, bradycardia, rise in blood pressure. **CNS:** restlessness, hallucinations, twitching, tremors, fasciculations, weakness, ataxia, convulsions, collapse, respiratory paralysis, pulmonary edema. With rapid IV: bradycardia, hyperactivity, respiratory distress, convulsions. **Acute toxicity:** cholinergic crisis (see Neostigmine).

ROUTE AND DOSAGE

Intramuscular, intravenous (physostigmine salicylate): 0.5 to 4 mg. Topical (instilled in conjunctival sac): ophthalmic ointment 0.25%; ophthalmic solution 0.25% to 0.5%, 1 or 2 drops, repeat as necessary to obtain miosis.

NURSING IMPLICATIONS

Physostigmine ophthalmic ointment may be prescribed at bedtime for patients with glaucoma to prevent nocturnal rise in ocular tension.

To reduce the possibility of systemic effects, apply gentle pressure just below inner angle of eye, against nose (nasolacrimal canaliculus), during and for 1 or 2 minutes following instillation. Instruct patient to avoid squeezing lids together. Blot excess medication with clean tissue.

Inform patient that physostigmine ophthalmic preparations may produce annoying lid twitching, temporary blurring of vision, and difficulty in seeing in dimmed light; therefore necessary safety precautions should be taken. Hospitalized patients will require supervised ambulation.

Emphasize the need for following prescribed drug regimen for glaucoma, and urge patient to remain under medical supervision. Untreated glaucoma can cause blindness.

Teaching plan for patients with glaucoma should include the following: proper administration of eyedrops; adverse symptoms to be reported; caution about not wearing constricting clothing, such as tight collar, belt, or girdle; activities to avoid that could provoke increase in intraocular pressure, such as heavy exertion, forceful nose blowing or coughing, straining at stool, crying, and emotionally upsetting situations.

Patient should be advised to wear identification tag indicating the presence of glaucoma and the medication being taken.

Closely monitor vital signs and state of consciousness in patients receiving drug for atropine poisoning. Since physostigmine is usually rapidly destroyed, patient can lapse into delirium and coma within 1 to 2 hours; repeat doses may be required.

Report immediately the onset of systemic symptoms (see Adverse Reactions). Dosage should be reduced or drug discontinued.

Because sensitivity to physostigmine may develop in some patients, the antidote atropine sulfate injection should always be readily available.

Preserved in tightly covered, light-resistant containers. Use only clear, colorless solutions. Red-tinted solution indicates oxidation, and such solutions should be discarded.

Also see Neostigmine.

PHYTONADIONE, U.S.P.

(AQUAMEPHYTON, KONAKION, MEPHYTON, Phylloquinone, Vitamin K_1)

PHYTOMENADIONE, B.P.

Prothrombogenic vitamin, vitamin K supplement

ACTIONS AND USES

Fat-soluble naphthoquinone derivative chemically identical to, and with similar degree of activity as naturally occurring vitamin K, which is necessary for hepatic biosynthesis of blood clotting factors II (prothrombin), VII (proconvertin), IX (plasma thromboplastin component), and X (Stuart factor). Promotes liver synthesis of clotting factors by unknown mechanism. Antagonizes inhibitory effects of coumarin and indandione anticoagulants on hepatic synthesis of clotting factors; does not reverse anticoagulant action of heparin. Use in newborns is reported to demonstrate a wide margin of safety.

Used to reverse prothrombin deficiency induced by anticoagulants and hypoprothrombinemia secondary to inadequate absorption or synthesis of vitamin K (eg, obstructive jaundice, biliary fistula, ulcerative colitis, intestinal resection) or secondary to administration of oral antibiotics, quinidine, quinine, salicylates, or sulfonamides. Also used in prophylaxis and therapy of hemorrhagic disease of newborn.

ABSORPTION AND FATE

Adequate absorption from intestinal lymph after oral administration occurs only if bile is present; effects occur within 6 to 12 hours. Drug response following oral intake appears in 6 to 12 hours; after IM injection, 1 to 2 hours; and after IV administration, 15 minutes. Hemorrhage is usually controlled within 3 to 8 hours. Normal prothrombin level may be obtained in 12 to 14 hours after parenteral administration. Concentrates in liver briefly after absorption; only small amounts accumulate in body tissues. Little is known about metabolic fate. Crosses placenta.

CONTRAINDICATIONS AND PRECAUTIONS

Hypersensitivity to phytonadione or its components; severe liver disease. Effect on fertility and teratogenic potential not known.

ADVERSE REACTIONS

Gastric upset, headache (after oral dose). **Following IV:** flushing sensation, constriction of chest, cramplike pains, convulsive movements, chills, fever, diaphoresis, weakness, dizziness, peculiar taste sensation, weak and rapid pulse, bronchospasm, dyspnea, hypersensitivity reactions or anaphylaxis. Also, swelling, pain, and nodule formation at injection site, erythematous skin eruptions (with repeated injections); paradoxic hypoprothrombinemia (patients with liver disease); (newborns, following large doses): hyperbilirubinemia, severe hemolytic anemia.

ROUTE AND DOSAGE

Adult: Oral, subcutaneous, intramuscular, intravenous: 0.5 to 25 mg; rarely, up to 50 mg daily. Oral dose may be repeated after 12 to 24 hours and parenteral dose after 6 to 8 hours if prothrombin time has not shortened satisfactorily. IV injection rate not to exceed 1 mg/minute. Hemorrhagic disease of newborn (prophylaxis): 0.5 to 1 mg IM (although less desirable, 1 to 5 mg subcutaneously or IM may be given to mother 12 to 24 hours before delivery); (treatment): 1 to 2 mg subcutaneously or IM.

NURSING IMPLICATIONS

Frequency, dose, and therapy duration are determined by prothrombin times and clinical response. Commonly used tests: one-stage prothrombin time and prothrombin and proconvertin (P and P) test.

Patients with bile deficiency receiving oral phytonadione will require concomitant administration of bile salts to assure absorption.

If possible, drugs that inhibit or interfere with vitamin K activity (eg, oral antibiotics, salicylates) may be discontinued or given at reduced dosages as an alternative or addition to phytonadione therapy.

In adults and older children, IM injection should be given in upper outer quadrant of buttocks. For infants and young children, anterolateral aspect of thigh or deltoid region is recommended. Carefully aspirate to avoid intravascular injection. Apply gentle pressure to site following injection. Swelling (internal bleeding) and pain sometimes occur with subcutaneous or IM administration.

Note that Konakion (which contains a phenol preservative) is intended for

IM use only. AquaMEPHYTON may be given subcutaneously, IM, or IV (as prescribed).

For IV infusion, dilution may be made with 0.9% sodium chloride, 5% dextrose, or 5% dextrose in 0.9% sodium chloride injection. *Other diluents should not be used.* Administer solution immediately after dilution. Discard unused solution and contents in open ampul.

Protect infusion solution from light by wrapping container with aluminum foil or other opaque material.

Severe reactions, including fatalities, have occurred during and immediately after IV injection (see Adverse Reactions). Patient should be under constant surveillance. Monitor vital signs.

Severe blood loss or lack of response to phytonadione may necessitate supplementary therapy with fresh whole blood or plasma.

Therapeutic responses to phytonadione: shortened prothrombin, bleeding, and clotting times, as well as decreased hemorrhagic tendencies.

Normal prothrombin time: 12 to 14 seconds; bleeding time (Ivy): 1 to 6 minutes; clotting time: 5 to 15 minutes.

Use of phytonadione to correct anticoagulant-induced prothrombin deficiency may promote same clotting hazards that existed prior to anticoagulant therapy.

Patients on large doses may develop temporary resistance to coumarin- or indandione-type anticoagulants. When anticoagulant therapy is reinstituted, larger than former doses of anticoagulant may be needed. Some patients may require change to heparin, which acts on a different principle.

Estimated minimum daily requirement of vitamin K for adults is 0.03 μg/kg body weight and up to 10 μg/kg for infants. Since vitamin K is synthesized by intestinal bacteria and is present in a wide variety of foods, deficiency in normal individuals is improbable.

Advise patient stabilized on phytondione to maintain well-balanced diet, and to avoid significant increases in daily intake of vitamin K-rich foods (especially green leafy vegetables). Other vitamin K-rich foods: tomatoes, vegetable oils, egg yolk, meats, dairy products, fruits, and cereals.

The American Academy of Pediatrics recommends routine administration of phytonadione to infants at birth to prevent the decline in concentration of clotting factors that occurs a few days following birth.

Stored in tight, light-resistant containers. Protect from light at all times.

PILOCARPINE HYDROCHLORIDE, U.S.P.
(ADSORBOCARPINE, ALMOCARPINE, ISOPTO-CARPINE, MI-PILO, MISTURA P, PILOCAR, PILOCEL, PILOMIOTIN)
PILOCARPINE NITRATE, U.S.P., B.P.
(P.V. CARPINE LIQUIFILM)

Cholinergic (ophthalmic)

ACTIONS AND USES

Tertiary amine derived from chief alkaloid of *Pilocarpus jaborandi.* Acts directly on cholinergic receptor sites, thus mimicking acetylcholine. Produces miosis, spasm of accommodation, and fall in intraocular pressure that may be preceded by a transitory rise. Decrease in intraocular pressure results from stimulation of ciliary muscle and pupillary sphincter muscle which pulls iris away from filtration angle and thus facilitates outflow of aqueous humor.

Used in initial and maintenance therapy for primary open-angle glaucoma, to relieve intraocular tension prior to emergency surgery of acute (closed-angle) galucoma and congenital galucoma, to counteract effects of mydriatics and cycloplegics following surgery or ophthalmoscopic examination. May be alternated with a mydriatic agent to break adhesions between iris and lens. Available in combination with epinephrine, e.g., E-Carpine.

ABSORPTION AND FATE

Penetrates cornea rapidly; miosis begins in 15 to 30 minutes. Peak action in about 75 minutes; duration 4 to 8 hours. Spasm of accommodation begins in 15 minutes and lasts 2 to 3 hours.

CONTRAINDICATIONS AND PRECAUTIONS

Hypersensitivity to drug components, secondary glaucoma, acute iritis, acute inflammatory disease of anterior segment of eye. Cautious use: bronchial asthma, hypertension.

ADVERSE REACTIONS

Generally well tolerated. Ciliary spasm with brow ache, pain with change in eye focus, miosis, diminished vision in poorly illuminated areas, blurred vision, sensitivity; (infrequent): contact allergy, follicular conjunctivitis, conjunctival irritation. Systemic absorption: nausea, vomiting, abdominal cramps, diarrhea, epigastric distress, salivation, lacrimation, bronchial constriction, hypertension, tachycardia.

ROUTE AND DOSAGE

Topical: 0.5% to 4% (concentrations above 4% used less frequently). 1 or 2 drops instilled into conjunctival sac. Choice of concentration and frequency of administration determined by severity of condition and patient response.

NURSING IMPLICATIONS

During acute phases, physician may prescribe instillation of drug into unaffected eye to prevent bilateral attack.

Apply gentle pressure to nasolacrimal canal for 1 to 2 minutes immediately following instillation to prevent access of drug to nasal mucosa and general circulation.

Hourly tonometric tests may be done during early treatment because drug may cause an initial transitory increase in intraocular pressure.

Since drug causes blurred vision and difficulty in focusing, caution patient to avoid hazardous activities such as driving a car or operating machinery until vision clears.

Brow pain and myopia tend to be more prominent in younger patients and generally disappear with continued use of drug.

Inform patient to withhold medication if symptoms of irritation or sensitization develop and to report to physician.

Advise patient to keep follow-up appointments.

Preserved in tight, light-resistant containers.

PIPERACETAZINE, N.F.
(QUIDE)

Antipsychotic agent (major tranquilizer)

ACTIONS AND USES

Potent piperidyl derivative of phenothiazine. Possesses tranquilizing, sedative, and antiemetic properties. Therapeutic effect similar to that of chlorpromazine (qv), but reportedly produces less toxic reactions.

Used to control hyperactivity, agitation, and anxiety states associated with acute and chronic schizophrenia.

Hypersensitivity to phenothiazines, thrombocytopenia and/or other blood dyscrasias, bone marrow depression, hepatic disease, pregnancy, children under 12 years of age. Cautious use: history of epilepsy or peptic ulcer; respiratory disorders; cardiovascular disease; patients receiving atropine or related drugs, barbiturates, or narcotics; patients exposed to extreme heat or to organophosphorous insecticides. See Chlorpromazine.

ADVERSE REACTIONS

Most common: drowsiness, sedation, dizziness, orthostatic hypotension, gastritis, syncope, edema, erythematous dermatitis, extrapyramidal reactions. Rarely: urinary retention, convulsions, nausea, vomiting, bradycardia. Also see Chlorpromazine.

ROUTE AND DOSAGE

Oral: initially 10 mg 2 to 4 times daily. Dosage may be increased gradually over a 3- to 5-day period until desired psychotherapeutic response is obtained. Maintenance: up to 160 mg daily in divided doses.

NURSING IMPLICATIONS

Drowsiness may occur, especially during first or second week; it generally disappears with continuation of therapy. Report to physician if it persists; dosage adjustment may be indicated.

Caution patient not to engage in potentially hazardous tasks such as driving a car or operating machinery until reaction to the drug is known. Mental and/or physical abilities may be impaired, particularly during first few days of therapy.

Advise patient to avoid undue exposure to sunlight because of possible drug-associated photosensitivity.

Concomitant use with alcohol should be avoided because of possible additive effect.

Stored in light-resistant containers.

Also see Chlorpromazine.

PIPERAZINE CITRATE, U.S.P.
(ANTEPAR CITRATE, BRYREL, MULTIFUGE, PARAZINE, PIN-TEGA, PIPRIL, TA-VERM, VERMAGO, VERMIDOL)
PIPERAZINE PHOSPHATE, N.F.
(ANTEPAR PHOSPHATE)

Anthelmintic

ACTIONS AND USES

Appears to act by producing muscle paralysis in parasite, thus promoting their elimination. Piperazine salts form piperazine hexahydrate in solution; dosages are usually expressed in terms of hexahydrate equivalent.

Used in pinworm disease or oxyuriasis *(Enterobius vermicularis)* and roundworm or ascariasis *(Ascaris lumbricoides)* infestations.

ABSORPTION AND FATE

Variable GI absorption. Excreted essentially unchanged in urine.

CONTRAINDICATIONS AND PRECAUTIONS

History of hypersensitivity to piperazine, impaired renal or hepatic function, convulsive disorders. Safe use during pregnancy not established.

ADVERSE REACTIONS

Low toxicity. Usually with excessive dosage: **GI:** nausea, vomiting, diarrhea. **CNS:** headache, vertigo, ataxia, tremors, choreiform movements, muscular weakness, hyporeflexia, paresthesias, blurred vision, paralytic strabismus, sense of detachment, memory defect, EEG abnormalities, convulsions. **Hypersensitivity:** urticaria, erythema multiforme, purpura, fever, arthralgia.

ROUTE AND DOSAGE

Roundworms: **Adults:** 3.5 Gm once daily for 2 consecutive days. **Children:** 75 mg/kg/day for 2 consecutive days; maximum daily dose 3.5 Gm. When repeated therapy is not practical, single dose of 70 mg/lb of body weight up to maximum of 3 Gm may be given. *Pinworms:* **Adults and children:** 65 mg/kg/day, with maximum daily dose of 2.5 Gm for 7 consecutive days. (Dosages are expressed in terms of hexahydrate equivalent.)

NURSING IMPLICATIONS

Use of laxatives or enema and dietary restrictions are usually not necessary.

Caution patient or parent not to exceed recommended schedule because of danger of neurotoxicity with high dosages.

Instruct patient to withhold medication if CNS, GI, or hypersensitivity reactions occur and report to physician.

In severe infections, course of therapy may be repeated after 1-week interval.

It is not unusual for an entire family to be infested with pinworms. Positive diagnosis in one family member warrants stool examination of other members to prevent reinfestation.

Specimens for pinworms are best obtained immediately on arising in the morning (female worm lays eggs at night around anal region). Obtain specimen by applying cellulose tape swab to perianal region; eggs can then be transferred to glass slide and examined microscopically.

Roundworm ova are examined in routine stool specimens.

Pinworms and roundworms are transmitted by direct and indirect transfer of ova, eg, by hands, food, and contaminated articles. Instruct patient and family in personal hygiene: washing hands after defecation and before touching food; sanitary disposal of feces; daily change of underwear and bedding (for pinworms). Ova are destroyed by household washing machine.

DRUG INTERACTIONS: There is a possibility that piperazine may exaggerate extrapyramidal effects of **phenothiazines.**

PIPOBROMAN, N.F.
(VERCYTE)

Antineoplastic (alkylating agent)

ACTIONS AND USES

Dicarboxylic acid amide of piperazine with toxic hematopoietic depressant properties. Exact mechanism of action unknown, but classified as a polyfunctional alkylating agent. Blocks DNA, RNA, and protein synthesis in rapidly proliferating cells.

Used primarily to treat polycythemia. Also used to produce remissions in chronic myelocytic leukemia.

ABSORPTION AND FATE

Readily absorbed from GI tract. Metabolic fate and excretion unknown.

CONTRAINDICATIONS AND PRECAUTIONS

Children under 15 years of age, myelosuppression from radiation or previous cytotoxic chemotherapy, pregnancy, women in childbearing years.

Leukemia, thrombocytopenia, anemia, cytopenia, skin rash, nausea, vomiting, abdominal cramps, diarrhea, anorexia (transient).

ROUTE AND DOSAGE

Oral: *Polycythemia:* initially 1 mg/kg daily for at least 30 days, after which dose may be increased to 1.5 to 3 mg/kg if no previous response; maintenance dose 0.1 to 0.2 mg/kg/day. *Chronic myelocytic leukemia:* initially 1.5 to 2.5 mg/kg daily until optimal therapeutic response occurs; maintenance dose 7 to 175 mg daily (highly individualized).

NURSING IMPLICATIONS

Since patient requires close observation, therapy is initiated in the hospital.

Bone marrow studies should be performed prior to therapy and repeated at time of maximum hematologic response. Liver and kidney function tests should also be performed before and during therapy.

Leukocyte and thrombocyte counts are advised every other day and complete blood counts weekly until desired response is obtained or toxic effects intervene.

Therapy is interrupted when platelet count falls to 150,000/mm^3 and leukocyte count to 3,000/mm^3.

Anemia (dose-related) is treated with blood replacement without interrupting therapy, but therapy is discontinued if rapid drop in hemoglobin, increased bilirubin levels, and reticulocytosis occur.

Monitor laboratory values for indicators of specific nursing actions.

Observe carefully for ecchymoses, petechiae, purpura, melena, and hemoptysis and report to physician promptly.

If nausea, vomiting, diarrhea, and skin rash persist, therapy will be interrupted.

Myelosuppression may not appear for 4 weeks or more after treatment begins.

Maintenance therapy is usually started when hematocrit is reduced to 50% to 55% in polycythemia vera, or when leukocyte count approaches 10,000/mm^3 in chronic myelocytic leukemia.

Therapy is continued for as long as needed to maintain a satisfactory clinical response.

PLASMA PROTEIN FRACTION (HUMAN), U.S.P.
(PLASMANATE, PLASMA-PLEX, PLASMATEIN, PROTENATE)

Blood volume supporter

ACTIONS AND USES

Five percent solution of stabilized human plasma proteins in NaCl containing approximately 88% albumin, 7% α-globulins, and 5% β-globulins. Each liter contains about 110 mEq sodium, 50 mEq chloride, and up to 0.25 mEq potassium. Oncotic action approximately equivalent to that of human plasma; does not provide coagulation factors or γ-globulins. Heat-treated to minimize hazard of transmitting serum hepatitis; risk of sensitization is reduced since it lacks cellular elements. Does not require cross-matching.

Used in emergency treatment of hypovolemic shock due to burns, trauma, surgery, and infections; used as temporary measure in treatment of blood loss when whole blood is not available; used to replenish plasma protein in patients with hypoproteinemia (if sodium restriction is not a problem).

CONTRAINDICATIONS AND PRECAUTIONS

Severe anemia, cardiac failure. Cautious use: patients with low cardiac reserve; absence of albumin deficiency; hepatic or renal failure.

Low incidence: nausea, vomiting, hypersalivation. With rapid IV infusion: circulatory overload, pulmonary edema.

ROUTE AND DOSAGE

Intravenous: *Hypovolemic shock* **Adults:** 250 to 500 ml, administered at rate up to 16 ml/minute; **Infants and children:** 10 to 15 ml/lb, at rate of 5 to 10 ml/minute. *Hypoproteinemia:* 1 to 1.5 liters (50 to 75 Gm protein) daily; rate not to exceed 5 to 8 ml/minute.

NURSING IMPLICATIONS

Check expiration date on label. Solutions that show a sediment or appear turbid should not be used.

Once container is opened, solution should be used promptly, because it contains no preservatives. Discard unused portions.

Rate of infusion and volume of total dose will depend on patient's age, diagnosis, and general condition. Specific flow rate should be prescribed by physician.

As with any oncotically active solution, infusion rate should be relatively slow. Range may vary from 1 to 16 ml/minute (see Route and Dosage).

Monitor blood pressure and pulse. Frequency of readings will depend on patient's condition. Flow rate adjustments are made according to clinical response and rising blood pressure.

Observe patient closely during and after infusion for signs of circulatory overload (distended neck veins, shortness of breath, cyanosis, persistent cough with or without frothy sputum, abnormal rises in blood pressure and pulse, sense of chest pressure, edema). Report these symptoms immediately to physician.

Make careful observations of patient who has had either injury or surgery in order to detect bleeding points that failed to bleed at lower blood pressure.

Report changes in input–output ratio and pattern.

Hypersensitivity reactions, serum hepatitis, and interference with blood typing or cross-matching procedures have not been reported.

Solution in unopened container remains stable under refrigeration (storage temperature and duration indicated on label).

POLDINE METHYLSULFATE, N.F., B.P.
(NACTON)

Anticholinergic

ACTIONS AND USES

Synthetic anticholinergic quaternary ammonium compound qualitatively similar to atropine in actions, contraindications, precautions, and adverse reactions. Used as adjunct in management of peptic ulcer and other GI disorders associated with hyperacidity, hypermotility, and spasm.

ABSORPTION AND FATE

Poorly absorbed from GI tract. Onset of effect in 1 to 2 hours, persisting about 6 to 8 hours. Excreted primarily in urine and bile; 70% excreted in feces as unchanged drug and metabolites.

ROUTE AND DOSAGE

Oral: 4 mg 3 or 4 times daily. Dosage gradually increased until mild side effects appear, then decreases of about 2 mg daily are made to optimum levels.

NURSING IMPLICATIONS

Administered before meals and at bedtime.

Incidence and severity of side effects are usually dose-related.

See nursing implications and drug interactions for atropine sulfate.

POLOXALKOL
(MAGCYL, POLYKOL, Poloxamer 188)

Cathartic (fecal softener)

ACTIONS AND USES

Nonionic surfactant with emulsifying and wetting properties similar to those of dioctyl sodium sulfosuccinate. Lowers surface tension of intestinal fluids, thereby softening feces.

Used for treatment of constipation associated with dry, hard stools.

ROUTE AND DOSAGE

Oral: **Adults:** 500 to 750 mg daily for not more than 5 days; total daily dose may be taken at once or in divided doses. **Children** *3 to 12 years:* 250 to 600 mg daily; *under 3 years and infants:* 100 to 400 mg daily.

NURSING IMPLICATIONS

Poloxalkol may increase absorption of mineral oil and other fat-soluble substances.

Several days of drug therapy may be required for full stool-softening effect.

Drug should be discontinued after desired effects are obtained.

See patient teaching points for Bisacodyl.

POLYESTRADIOL PHOSPHATE
(ESTRADURIN)

Estrogen

ACTIONS AND USES

Derivative of estradiol. Stimulates physiologic secretion of estrogen and provides exogenous estradiol supply over prolonged period. Principal use: palliation of prostatic carcinoma. See Estradiol.

ABSORPTION AND FATE

Injected solution leaves bloodstream within 24 hours; passively stored in reticuloendothelial system. As circulating estradiol levels drop, more enters bloodstream from storage site to furnish continuous, even therapeutic effect. For contraindications, precautions, and adverse reactions, see Estradiol.

ROUTE AND DOSAGE

Intramuscular: 40 to 80 mg every 2 to 4 weeks or less frequently, depending on clinical response.

NURSING IMPLICATIONS

Reconstitute solution using 20-gauge needle affixed to a 5-cc syringe. Swirl gently to produce clear solution.

Solution stored at room temperature and protected from direct light will remain stable for about 10 days.

Discard cloudy or precipitated solution.

Inject solution deep into gluteal muscle.

Burning sensation at site of injection is usually transitory. Persistent discomfort with injections may require concomitant administration of local anesthetic.

Clinical response will be apparent within 3 months. Hormone should be continued until disease is again progressive, then stopped; 30% of patients may have another period of improvement (rebound regression). See Estradiol.

POLYMYXIN B SULFATE, U.S.P., B.P.
(AEROSPORIN SULFATE)

Antibacterial (polymyxin)

ACTIONS AND USES

Basic polypeptide antibiotic of the polymyxin group derived from strains of *Bacillus polymyxa.* Bactericidal against susceptible Gram-negative organisms, particularly most strains of *Pseudomonas aeruginosa, Escherichia coli, Haemophilus influenzae, Enterobacter aerogenes,* and *Klebsiella pneumoniae.* Most species of *Proteus* and *Neisseria* are resistant, as are all Gram-positive organisms and fungi. Spectrum of antibacterial activity is similar to that of colistin derivatives; complete cross-resistance and cross-sensitivity reported. Binds to lipid phosphates in bacterial membranes, and through cationic detergent action changes permeability to permit leakage of cytoplasm. Neuromuscular blocking action usually associated with high serum levels, intracellular potassium deficit, or low serum calcium concentration.

Used primarily in hospitalized patients for treatment of acute infections of urinary tract, bloodstream, and meninges; used in treatment of serious infections resistant to other antibiotics. Used topically and subconjunctivally in superficial eye infections and in combination with other antiinfectives and/or corticosteroids for various superficial infections of eye, ear, mucous membrane, and skin.

ABSORPTION AND FATE

Not absorbed from GI tract (except in infants), and does not appear to be significantly absorbed from mucous membranes or skin. Plasma concentrations of 1 to 8 μg/ml reached in about 2 hours following IM injection of 20,000 to 40,000 units/kg body weight. Serum half-life 4.3 to 6 hours. Serum levels higher in patients with renal impairment and in infants and children. Widely distributed to most body tissues, but not evident in cerebrospinal fluid, synovial fluid, or aqueous humor. Not highly bound to plasma proteins, but possibly bound to phospholipids of cell membranes in various tissues. About 60% of dose is excreted unchanged in urine; excretion continues 1 to 3 days after single dose.

CONTRAINDICATIONS AND PRECAUTIONS

Hypersensitivity to polymyxin antibiotics; concurrent and sequential use of nephrotoxic and neurotoxic drugs; concurrent use of curariform muscle relaxants, ether, or sodium citrate (see Drug Interactions). Safe use during pregnancy not established. Cautious use: impaired renal function, myasthenia gravis.

ADVERSE REACTIONS

Neurotoxicity: irritability; facial flushing; drowsiness; dizziness; vertigo; ataxia; circumoral, lingual, and peripheral paresthesias (stocking-glove distribution); blurred vision; nystagmus; slurred speech; convulsions; coma; neuromuscular blockade (generalized muscle weakness, respiratory depression or arrest); meningeal irritation (intrathecal use); increased protein and cell count in cerebrospinal fluid; fever; headache; stiff neck. **Nephrotoxicity** (reversible): rising drug blood levels without increase in dosage; albuminuria; cylinduria; azotemia; hematuria. **Hypersensitivity:** drug fever, dermatoses, pruritus, urticaria, local irritation and burning (topical use), eosinophilia, anaphylactoid reaction (rarely). Other: GI disturbances, severe pain (IM site), thrombophlebitis (IV site), superinfections, electrolyte disturbances (prolonged use).

ROUTE AND DOSAGE

Dosages reduced for patients with renal impairment. Intramuscular: **Adults and children:** 25,000 to 30,000 units/kg/day; may be divided and given at 4- to 6-hour intervals; **infants:** up to 40,000 units/kg/day. Intravenous: **Adults and children:** 15,000 to 25,000 units/kg/day; **infants:** up to 40,000 units/kg/day. Intrathecal: **Adults and children** *over 2 years of age:* 50,000 units daily for 3 or 4 days, then every other day for at least 2 weeks after negative cerebrospinal fluid cultures; *under 2 years of age:* 20,000 units daily for 3 or 4 days followed by 25,000 units every other day. Topical (ophthalmic drops): 1 to 3 drops of 0.1% to 0.25% (10,000 to 25,000 units) /ml every hour; intervals increased as response indicates. Subjunctival injection: up to 10,000 units/day.

NURSING IMPLICATIONS

Follow manufacturer's directions for dilution and storage.

Baseline renal function tests should be performed prior to parenteral therapy. Frequent monitoring of renal function and serum drug levels is advised during therapy.

Culture and sensitivity tests are essential to determine susceptibility of causative organisms.

Routine administration by IM route not recommended because it causes intense discomfort, particularly in infants and children. Pain described as "aching" or "drawing" radiates along peripheral nerve distribution and reportedly is not relieved appreciably by addition of procaine.

In adults, IM injection should be made deep into upper outer quadrant of buttock. Select IM site carefully to avoid injection into nerves or blood vessels. Rotate injection sites. Follow agency policy for IM site used in children.

Renal toxicity usually occurs within first 3 or 4 days of therapy. Monitor intake and output. Fluid intake should be sufficient to maintain daily urinary output of at least 1500 ml. Consult physician.

Decreases in urine output (change in intake–output ratio) or increases in BUN, serum creatinine, or serum drug levels (not associated with dosage increase) can be interpreted as signs of nephrotoxicity. If any of these signs occurs, withhold drug and report findings to physician.

Nephrotoxicity is generally reversible, but it may progress even after drug is discontinued. Therefore, close monitoring of kidney function is essential, even following termination of therapy.

Neurotoxic reactions, including neuromuscular blockade (see Adverse Reactions), are usually associated with high serum drug levels and/or nephrotoxicity.

Report immediately signs of muscle weakness, shortness of breath, dyspnea, depressed respiration. These are rapidly reversible if drug is withdrawn and symptoms are treated promptly. Resuscitative equipment, oxygen, and intravenous calcium chloride should be available at all times.

Transient neurologic disturbances (paresthesias, numbness, formication, dizziness) occur commonly and usually respond to dosage reduction. Report promptly. Supervise ambulation.

Store parenteral solutions in refrigerator; discard unused portions after 72 hours.

DRUG INTERACTIONS: Additive effects may result from concurrent or sequential use of other nephrotoxic and neurotoxic drugs, particularly aminoglycoside antibiotics **(gentamicin, kanamycin, neomycin, streptomycin)** and polymyxin E (colistin). Increased and prolonged neuromuscular blockade (respiratory paralysis) may be produced by concurrent use of curariform muscle relaxants and other neurotoxic drugs such as **decamethonium, ether, gallamine, sodium citrate, succinylcholine,** and **tubocurarine.**

POLYTHIAZIDE, N.F.
(RENESE)

Diuretic (thiazide), antihypertensive

ACTIONS AND USES

Benzothiadiazine (thiazide) derivative. Similar to chlorothiazide in actions, uses, contraindications, precautions, and adverse reactions, but more potent and has longer diuretic action.

ABSORPTION AND FATE

Onset of diuretic effect in 2 hours; peak in 6 hours; duration 24 to 48 hours. Highly bound to plasma proteins. Excreted unchanged in urine. See Chlorothiazide.

ROUTE AND DOSAGE

Oral: **Adult:** (diuretic): 1 to 4 mg daily; (antihypertensive): 2 to 4 mg daily. **Pediatric:** 0.02 to 0.08 mg/kg/day.

NURSING IMPLICATIONS

Preserved in tightly covered, light-resistant containers. See Chlorothiazide.

POTASSIUM CHLORIDE, U.S.P.
(CENA-K, K-10, KAOCHLOR, KAON-CL, KAY CIEL, KATO, KLOR 10%, KLOR-CON, K-LOR, KLORIDE, KLORVESS, K-LYTE/CL, PAN-KLORIDE, PFIKLOR, RUM-K, SLOW-K, TASIDE)
POTASSIUM GLUCONATE, N.F.
(KALINATE, KAON)

Replenisher (electrolyte)

ACTIONS AND USES

Major cation of intracellular fluid. Essential for intracellular tonicity, conduction of nerve impulses, contraction of cardiac, skeletal, and smooth muscles, maintenance of normal renal function, and enzyme action.

Used to prevent and treat potassium depletions, as may occur in severe vomiting, diarrhea, diabetic ketoacidosis, intestinal drainage or malabsorption, prolonged diuresis; used for cardiac arrhythmias (especially those due to digitalis glycosides) and for Meniere's disease.

ABSORPTION AND FATE

Distributed to extracellular and intracellular compartments. Principally excreted via kidneys. Tubular excretion is influenced by acid–base balance and adrenal function.

CONTRAINDICATIONS AND PRECAUTIONS

Severe renal impairment with oliguria, anuria, azotemia, severe hemolytic reactions, untreated Addison's disease, crush syndrome, early postoperative oliguria (except during GI drainage), adynamia episodica hereditaria, acute dehydration, heat cramps, hyperkalemia, patients receiving aldosterone antagonists or triamterene, digitalis intoxication in presence of conduction disturbances. Cautious use: cardiac or renal disease, systemic acidosis.

Nausea, vomiting, diarrhea, abdominal discomfort, GI bleeding, GI distension and pain (with enteric- and sugar-coated tablets). **Hyperkalemia:** mental confusion, irritability, listlessness, paresthesias of extremities, muscle weakness and heaviness of limbs, flaccid paralysis, respiratory distress, fall in blood pressure, heart block, cardiac arrest, cardiac arrhythmias (with rapid IV administration of concentrated solutions), altered sensitivity to digitalis glycosides.

ROUTE AND DOSAGE

Highly individualized. Oral (prevention): 20 mEq/day; (treatment): 40 to 100 mEq/day or more. Intravenous: if serum potassium level is greater than 2.5 mEq/liter, total 24-hour dose not to exceed 200 mEq; if less than 2 mEq/liter, total 24-hour dose may be as high as 400 mEq. Usually not more than 3 mEq/kg of body weight/day.

NURSING IMPLICATIONS

Note that oral and parenteral preparations come in various strengths.

Advise patient to follow instructions regarding dilution. As a general rule, oral liquids, powders, and effervescent tablets should be diluted (and completely dissolved) before administration and should be sipped slowly, with meals or immediately after meals. Usual dilution is about one-half tumblerful (3 to 4 ounces) of cold water or citrus juice. Higher doses (eg, 40 mEq) should be given in a full glass of liquid (6 ounces) to minimize the possibility of a saline cathartic effect.

IV infusion should be administered slowly to prevent fatal hyperkalemia. Physician will prescribe specific flow rate according to patient's individual requirements (rate of administration is generally 10 to 20 mEq/hour).

Physicians generally prescribe oral forms that can be diluted, because the use of tablets (particularly enteric-coated) has been associated with intestinal ulceration and perforation.

When adding parenteral drug to infusion solution, mix thoroughly to prevent locally high potassium concentrations, and indicate on label that potassium chloride was added. Extreme care should be taken to avoid extravasation.

Serum potassium levels are not accurate indicators of intracellular potassium concentrations. Intracellular potassium deficit can occur without a decrease in serum potassium level, and vice versa. Therefore, close observation of patient, in addition to monitoring of ECG, serum potassium levels, and other electrolytes (particularly chloride, sodium, and calcium), is essential during therapy.

Normals: Serum chloride 95 to 103 mEq/L, plasma sodium: 136 to 142 mEq/L, serum calcium (total): 9–10.6 mg/dl; plasma potassium, 3.8–5.0 mEq/L; urine potassium excretion: 40–80 mEq/24 hours.

Monitor intake–output ratio and pattern (in patients receiving parenteral drug). Report to physician immediately if oliguria or change in ratio occurs.

For treatment of hypokalemia, observe for resolution or improvement of the following signs of potassium deficiency: weakness, fatigue, disturbances in cardiac rhythm (especially ectopic beats), flaccid paralysis, impaired ability to concentrate urine.

Potassium-rich foods and liquids: bananas, oranges and other citrus fruits, apricots, dates, prunes, raisins, cantaloupe, watermelon, tomato, beef, fowl. Usual dietary intake of potassium by the average adult is 40 to 80 mEq/day.

Salt substitutes (eg, Co-Salt, Diasal, Neocurtasal) contain potassium chloride and therefore carry the same contraindications and precautions as given above.

For treatment of potassium overdosage (hyperkalemia): Eliminate all potassium-containing foods and medications. Have on hand IV calcium gluconate 10% to overcome cardiac toxicity (not used in patients receiving digitalis), sodium bicarbonate and/or 10% dextrose, regular insulin (facilitates shift of potassium into cell), sodium polystyrene resin (hastens potassium elimination). Hemodialysis and peritoneal dialysis may be required for some patients.

DRUG INTERACTIONS: Severe hyperkalemia may result from concomitant administration of potassium chloride and **aldosterone antagonists,** eg, **spironolactone,** and potassium-sparing agents such as **triamterene.**

POTASSIUM IODIDE, U.S.P., B.P.
(KI-N, KISOL, PIMA)
POTASSIUM IODIDE SOLUTION, U.S.P.
(SSKI)

Expectorant, supplement (iodine)

ACTIONS AND USES

Pharmacologic use primarily related to iodide portion of molecule. By direct action on bronchial tissue, potassium iodide (KI) increases secretion of respiratory fluids, thereby decreasing mucus viscosity. If patient is euthyroid, excess iodide (ie, beyond dietary intake) causes minimal change in thyroid gland mass. Conversely, when thyroid is hyperplastic, excess iodide temporarily inhibits secretion of thyroid hormone, fosters colloid accumulation in thyroid follicles, and decreases vascularity of gland. "Escape" from temporary effects (ie, return of thyrotoxic symptoms) may occur after 10 to 14 days continuous treatment; consequently iodide administration for hyperthyroidism is limited to short-term therapy.

Used to facilitate bronchial drainage and cough in emphysema, asthma, chronic bronchitis, bronchiectasis, and respiratory tract allergies characterized by difficult-to-raise sputum. May be employed alone for treatment of hyperthyroidism or in conjunction with antithyroid drugs and propranolol in treatment of thyrotoxic crisis. Used in immediate preoperative period for thyroidectomy to decrease vascularity, fragility, and size of thyroid gland.

ABSORPTION AND FATE

Following adequate absorption from GI tract, iodide enters circulation and is cleared from plasma by renal excretion or by thyroid uptake. If patient is euthyroid, renal clearance rate is two times that of the thyroid. Also see Strong Iodine Solution.

CONTRAINDICATIONS AND PRECAUTIONS

Hypersensitivity or idiosyncrasy to iodine, tuberculosis, hyperkalemia, acute bronchitis. Cautious use: pregnancy.

ADVERSE REACTIONS

Nonspecific small bowel lesions (stenosis with or without ulceration), hyperthyroid adenoma, goiter, hypothyroidism, collagen-disease-like syndromes. **Hypersensitivity:** angioneurotic edema, cutaneous and mucosal hemorrhage, fever, arthralgias, lymph node enlargement, eosinophilia. **Iodine poisoning** (iodism): metallic taste, stomatitis, ptyalism, coryza, sneezing; swollen and tender salivary glands, frontal headache, vomiting (blue vomitus if stomach contained starches, otherwise yellow vomitus), bloody diarrhea. **Other:** productive cough, pulmonary edema, periorbital edema. **Altered laboratory values:** elevation in protein-bound iodine; interference with urinary 17-hydroxycorticosteroid determinations.

Oral (tablets, solution, syrup): expectorant: **Adult:** 300 or 600 mg 3 or 4 times daily unless symptoms of excess occur; interval and dose then individualized to level of desired clinical response; **Pediatric** 0.015 to 0.3 GM 3 or 4 times daily. Presurgical thyroid gland preparation: 0.3 ml (5 drops) SSKI 3 or 4 times daily for 10 to 14 days before surgery.

NURSING IMPLICATIONS

To disguise salty taste and decrease gastric distress, administer KI well diluted in full glass of water, milk, or fruit juice after meals and at bedtime.

Enteric-coated KI, used only when dietary supplementation of potassium is impractical, reportedly causes small bowel lesions. Advise patient to report promptly the occurrence of GI bleeding, abdominal pain, distension, nausea, or vomiting.

Instruct patient starting on KI as an expectorant to report clinical signs of iodism (see Adverse Reactions). Usually symptoms will subside with dose reduction and lengthened intervals between doses.

SSKI solution: 0.3 ml contains KI 300 mg.

When iodide is administered to prepare thyroid gland for surgery, strict adherence to schedule and accurate dose measurement are essential, particularly at end of treatment period when possibility of "escape" (from iodide) effect on thyroid gland increases.

Warn patient to avoid use of over-the-counter drugs without consulting physician. Many preparations contain iodides and could augment prescribed dose, eg, cough syrups, gargles, asthma medication, salt substitutes, cod liver oil, multiple vitamins (often suspended in iodide solutions).

Foods rich in iodine to be avoided if patient develops iodism: vegetables growing near seacoast, seafoods, fish liver oils.

Impress on the patient taking KI as an expectorant that optimum hydration is the best expectorant. Encourage increased daily fluid intake.

Consult physician about use of iodized salt during therapy with iodides.

Solutions may become slightly yellow on standing, especially if exposed to light, because of liberated trace of free iodine. Store in airtight, light-resistant container.

DRUG INTERACTIONS: **Lithium** may act synergistically with iodides, thereby increasing the potential for hypothyroidism.

POVIDONE-IODINE, U.S.P.
(AERODINE, BETADINE, EFO-DINE, FEMIDINE, ISODINE, MALLISOL)

Antiinfective, Topical

ACTIONS AND USES

Water-soluble iodine complex with microbiocidal spectrum that includes Gram-positive, Gram-negative, and antibiotic-resistant organisms, fungi, viruses, protozoa, and yeast. Maintains germicidal action in presence of blood, serum, and pus. Unlike iodine, it is virtually nonstinging and nonirritating to skin and mucous membrane and nonstaining to skin and clothing. Used for prevention and treatment of surface infections, as antiseptic for burns, lacerations, abrasions, and other minor wounds, and in management of vaginitis (monilial, trichomonas vaginalis, and nonspecific forms).

Sensitivity to iodine.

ROUTE AND DOSAGE

Topical: aerosol, antiseptic gauze pads, gargle, ointment, perineal wash, shampoo, skin cleanser, solution, surgical scrub, treated applicators, gauze pads, swabsticks, vaginal douche, vaginal gel.

NURSING IMPLICATIONS

Avoid contact with eyes.

Treated areas can be bandaged.

Use should be discontinued if irritation, redness, or swelling develops.

Available OTC.

PRALIDOXIME CHLORIDE, U.S.P.
(PROTOPAM CHLORIDE)

Cholinesterase reactivator

ACTIONS AND USES

Reactivates cholinesterase inhibited by phosphate esters (eg, organophosphorus insecticides and related compounds) by displacing the enzyme from its receptor sites; the free enzyme then can resume its function of degrading accumulated acetylcholine thereby restoring normal neuromuscular transmission. Less effective against carbamate anticholinesterases (ambenonium, neostigmine, pyridostigmine). More active against effects of anticholinesterases at skeletal neuromuscular junction than at autonomic effector sites or in CNS respiratory center; therefore, atropine must be given concomitantly to block effects of acetylcholine accumulation in these sites.

Used as antidote in treatment of poisoning by organophosphate insecticides and pesticides with anticholinesterase activity (eg, parathion, TEPP, sarin) and to control overdosage by anticholinesterase drugs used in treatment of myasthenia gravis (cholinergic crisis).

ABSORPTION AND FATE

Distributed throughout extracellular fluids; crosses blood–brain barrier only very slowly, if at all. Not bound to plasma proteins. Plasma half-life approximately 1.7 hours. Metabolized chiefly by liver. Rapidly excreted in urine, partly as unchanged drug.

CONTRAINDICATIONS AND PRECAUTIONS

Use in poisoning by carbamate insecticide Sevin, inorganic phosphates, or organophosphates having no anticholinesterase activity; asthma, peptic ulcer, severe cardiac disease, patients receiving aminophylline, theophylline, morphine, succinylcholine, reserpine, or phenothiazines. Cautious use: myasthenia gravis, renal insufficiency, concomitant use of barbiturates in organophosphorus poisoning.

ADVERSE REACTIONS

Most commonly following IV use (usually mild and transient): dizziness, nausea, blurred vision, diplopia, impaired accommodation, tachycardia, hyperventilation, headache, drowsiness, muscular weakness. With rapid IV: tachycardia, laryngospasm, muscle rigidity.

ROUTE AND DOSAGE

Adults: Organophosphorus poisoning: Intravenous infusion (preferred): 1 or 2 Gm in 100 ml isotonic NaCl injection, infused over 15 to 30 minutes. Direct intravenous injection: administered as 5% solution in sterile water for injection (without preservative) over not less than 5 minutes; second dose of 1 to 2 Gm repeated after 1 hour if muscle weakness not relieved; additional doses given cautiously, if indicated. Subcutaneous, intramuscular: when IV administration is not feasible. Oral: 1 to 3 Gm every 5 hours. Anticholinesterase overdosage in myasthenia gravis: Intravenous: 1 or 2 Gm followed by increments of 250 mg every 5 minutes, as indicated. **Children:** 20 to 40 mg/kg repeated every 10 to 12 hours if needed.

NURSING IMPLICATIONS

Generally used only in hospitalized patients. Have on hand respirator suction apparatus, tracheostomy set, oxygen, IV sodium thiopental (2.5% solution) for control of convulsions, atropine, gastric lavage equipment for ingested poison. ECG monitoring may be required in severe poisoning.

Treatment is most effective if started within a few hours after organophosphate poisoning has occurred. If exposure to poison was through skin, initial measures should include removal of contaminated clothing and washing skin thoroughly with sodium bicarbonate solution or alcohol.

Pralidoxime is started with or immediately after atropine IV or IM, 2 to 4 mg (adult) or 0.5 to 1 mg (pediatric), or after patient's response to atropine has been assessed. Some degree of atropinization is usually maintained for at least 48 hours.

Monitor vital signs and intake and output. Report oliguria or changes in intake–output ratio.

It is difficult to differentiate toxic effects of organophosphates or atropine from toxic effects of pralidoxime. Be alert for these signs and report them immediately: reduction in muscle strength, onset of muscle twitching, changes in respiratory pattern, altered level of consciousness, increases or changes in heart rate and rhythm.

Excitement and manic behavior reportedly may occur following recovery of consciousness. Observe necessary safety precautions.

Patient should be kept under close observation for 48 to 72 hours, particularly when poison was ingested, because of likelihood of continued absorption of organophosphate from lower bowel.

Pralidoxime is relatively short-acting. In patients with myasthenia gravis, overdosage with pralidoxime may convert cholinergic crisis into myasthenic crisis (see Index).

PRAZOSIN HYDROCHLORIDE
(MINIPRESS)

Antihypertensive

ACTIONS AND USES

Quinazoline derivative structurally unrelated to other antihypertensive drugs. Mode of action not fully understood. Appears to cause peripheral vasodilation by direct relaxant effect on arterial smooth muscle, with reduction in total peripheral vascular resistance. Reduces orthostatic and supine blood pressures, with more pronounced effect on diastolic. Reportedly does not significantly change cardiac output, heart rate, renal blood flow, or glomerular filtration. Used in treatment of hypertension as initial agent or in conjunction with a diuretic and/or another antihypertensive drug.

ABSORPTION AND FATE

Peak plasma levels in 2 to 3 hours in fasting patients (plasma levels usually do not correlate with therapeutic effect). Plasma half-life 2 to 3 hours. Approximately 97% bound to plasma proteins. Blood pressure begins to decrease within 2 hours, with maximum reduction in 2 to 4 hours; antihypertensive effect lasts less than 24 hours. Widely distributed to body tissues. Probably metabolized in liver and excreted mainly in bile and feces; about 6% to 10% excreted in urine.

CONTRAINDICATIONS AND PRECAUTIONS

Hypersensitivity to prazosin. Cautious use: chronic renal failure. Safe use in women of childbearing potential, during pregnancy and lactation, and in children not established.

ADVERSE REACTIONS

Most common: dizziness, lightheadedness, headache, drowsiness, fatigue, weakness, palpitation, nausea. **GI:** vomiting, diarrhea, constipation, abdominal discomfort, and/or pain. **Cardiovascular:** edema, dyspnea, syncope, tachycardia, angina. **CNS** (rare): nervousness, vertigo, depression, paresthesia, insomnia. **Dermatologic:** rash, pruritus. **Genitourinary:** urinary frequency, impotence. **EENT:** blurred vision, epistaxis, tinnitus, reddened sclerae, dry mouth, nasal congestion. Other: diaphoresis, arthralgia, transient leukopenia, increased serum uric acid and BUN.

ROUTE AND DOSAGE

Oral: initially 1 mg 3 times daily. Dosage may be increased slowly to total daily dosage of 20 mg in divided doses. Up to 40 mg daily in divided doses may be required. Highly individualized according to blood pressure response and tolerance. When diuretic or other antihypertensive drug is added, dosage should be reduced to 1 or 2 mg 3 times per day, and then retitration should be carried out.

NURSING IMPLICATIONS

Reportedly, food may delay absorption, but does not affect degree of absorption. It has been suggested that the frequency of hypotension and dizziness may be reduced by taking drug with food (based on single study).

Syncope with sudden loss of consciousness may occur within 30 minutes to 2 hours after initial dose is given; this is thought to be due to excessive postural hypotensive effect or to tachycardia. Caution patient to avoid situations that would result in injury should syncope occur. In most cases, effect does not recur after initial period of therapy.

Syncope is also associated with rapid dosage increase or addition of another antihypertensive drug to regimen.

Instruct patient to make position changes slowly, particularly from recumbent to upright posture, and to dangle legs a few minutes before standing. Advise patient to lie down immediately if feeling weak or faint and to avoid potentially hazardous activities such as driving a car or operating machinery until reaction to drug is known. Side effects usually disappear with continuation of therapy, but they may require dosage reduction.

Full therapeutic effect of prazosin may not be achieved until 4 to 6 weeks of therapy.

DRUG INTERACTIONS. Hypotensive effect of prazosin is increased when given concomitantly with other **antihypertensive agents,** particularly **propranolol** (may be used therapeutically; permits reduction in dosage of each drug).

PREDNISOLONE, U.S.P., B.P. **595**

(DELTA-CORTEF, DELTA-CORTRIL, FERNISOLONE, PREDNICEN, STERANE, ULACORT, and others)

PREDNISOLONE ACETATE, U.S.P., B.P.

(METICORTELONE, NISOLONE, PREDICORT, SAVACORT, and others)

PREDNISOLONE SODIUM PHOSPHATE, U.S.P., B.P.

(HYDELTRASOL, HYDELTRONE, METRETON, PSP-IV)

PREDNISOLONE SODIUM SUCCINATE, U.S.P.

(METICORTELONE SOLUBLE)

PREDNISOLONE TEBUTATE, U.S.P.

(HYDELTRA-T.B.A., METALONE T.B.A.)

Adrenocortical steroid (glucocorticoid)

ACTIONS AND USES

Synthetic dehydrogenated analog of hydrocortisone (qv) with 3 to 5 times greater potency; thus moderate dosage is effective, and potential for sodium and water retention and potassium loss is reduced. Plasma half-life about 3 hours. Side effects minimal, but insomnia sometimes occurs during first few days of treatment. Compared with hydrocortisone, prednisolone and its esters have greater tendency to produce gastric irritation, gastroduodenal ulceration, ecchymotic skin lesions, vasomotor symptoms.

Used in management of bursitis, diseases of joints and nonarticular structures, and dermatological, nasal, opthalmologic, and otic disorders.

ADVERSE REACTIONS

Hirsutism (occasional), perforation of cornea (with topical drug), sensitivity to heat, fat embolism, adverse effects on growth and development of the individual and on spermatozoa; hypotension and shocklike reactions. Also see Hydrocortisone.

ROUTE AND DOSAGE

Oral: **Adults:** (prednisolone), intramuscular (acetate, phosphate, succinate): initially 5 to 60 mg daily in 4 doses until response occurs; then dosage gradually reduced to lowest effective maintenance level (usually 5 to 20 mg daily). Intraarticular, intralesional (acetate, phosphate, succinate, tebutate): 10 to 30 mg. Intravenous (phosphate, succinate): 25 to 50 mg; repeated in 3 to 4 hours if necessary; may also be given (100 mg every 12 hours) by continuous IV drip. Topical: ophthalmic solutions (0.125% to 1%) may be applied to eye and ear. Also available: suspensions, cream, aerosol, usually applied 3 or 4 times daily.

NURSING IMPLICATIONS

Administer with meals to reduce gastric irritation. If distress continues, consult physician about possible adjunctive antacid therapy.

Since topical corticosteroid treatment may increase intraocular pressure in susceptible individuals, it is usual to have frequent tonometric exams during prolonged therapy.

In diseases caused by microorganisms, infection may be masked, activated, or enhanced by corticoids. Be alert to subclinical signs of lack of improvement such as continued drainage, low-grade fever, and interrupted healing. Observe and report exacerbation of symptoms after short period of therapeutic response.

If patient on long-term treatment, alternate day therapy (ADT) may be employed to reduce adverse reactions.

Temporary local discomfort may follow injection of corticoid into bursa or joint.

Preserved in airtight containers; protect from light. Follow manufacturer's directions for reconstitution and storage.
See Hydrocortisone.

PREDNISONE U.S.P., B.P.

(DELTA-DOME, DELTASONE, FERNISONE BUFFERED, KEYSONE, LISACORT, MASO-PRED, METICORTEN, ORASONE, PARACORT, PRED-5, ROPRED, SERVISONE, STERAPRED)

Adrenocortical steroid (glucocorticoid)

ACTIONS AND USES
Synthetic analog of hydrocortisone. Effect depends on biotransformation to prednisolone, a conversion that may be impaired in patient with liver dysfunction. Has less mineralocoid activity than hydrocortisone but Na (therefore fluid) retention and K depletion can occur. Shares actions uses, absorption and fate, contraindications, adverse reactions with hydrocortisone (qv). On weight basis 5 mg prednisone is equivalent to 5 mg prednisolone, 20 mg hydrocortisone and 25 mg cortisone.

ROUTE AND DOSAGE
Oral: **Adult:** Initial: 30 to 60 mg/24 hours in 2 to 4 divided doses until desired clinical response; then gradual decremental dose (5 to 10 mg) adjustment every 4 to 5 days to lowest effective maintenance level: usually 5 to 20 mg/24 hours. Dosage highly individualized. **Pediatric** (about 1/5 cortisone dose): 2 mg/kg/24 hours divided into 4 doses usually reduced gradually to 1.5 mg/kg/24 hours after 2 to 3 weeks.

NURSING IMPLICATIONS
Administer prednisone after meals and at bedtime.

Alternate-day drug administration may be advised to keep daily dose at minimal levels and to reduce degree of "steroid rebound" with withdrawal.

Periodic blood K levels are recommended. Urge patient to keep scheduled appointments for medical supervision.

Monitor weight to detect onset of fluid accumulation, especially if patient is on unrestricted salt intake and does not receive K supplement. Report if weight gain is more than 5 pounds/week.

Advise patient to report symptoms of K deficit (anorexia, paresthesias, drowsiness, muscle weakness, nausea, polyuria, postural hypotension, mental depression).

Protect drug from light and air in tightly closed dark container.

One member of the BACOP, CHOP, CMFOP, COAP, COP, MOPP, POMP combination chemotherapeutic regimens.

See Hydrocortisone.

PRIMAQUINE PHOSPHATE, U.S.P., B.P.

Antimalarial

ACTIONS AND USES
Synthetic 8-aminoquinoline that acts on primary exoerythrocytic forms of *Plasmodium vivax* and *P. falciparum* by an incompletely known mechanism. Destroys late tissue forms of *P. vivax* and thus effects radical cure (prevents relapse). Also

has gametocidal activity against all species of plasmodia that infect man, and thus can interrupt transmission of malaria. Not effective alone in acute attack, but may be used concurrently with chloroquine, which destroys erythrocytic parasites.

Used widely for radical cure of vivax malaria and following termination of chloroquine suppressive therapy in areas where vivax malaria is endemic.

ABSORPTION AND FATE

Absorbed well from intestine. Peak plasma levels in about 6 hours; only trace amounts detectable after 24 hours. Biodegradation products of primaquine are the active antimalarial and hemolytic agents. Concentrates in liver, lungs, heart, brain, and skeletal muscle. About 1% excreted unchanged in urine.

CONTRAINDICATIONS AND PRECAUTIONS

Rheumatoid arthritis, lupus erythematosus, hemolytic drugs, agents capable of bone marrow depression, quinacrine, pregnancy.

ADVERSE REACTIONS

Hematologic reactions including granulocytopenia and acute hemolytic anemia in patients with glucose-6-phosphate dehydrogenase deficiency. Overdosage: nausea, vomiting, epigastric distress, abdominal cramps, pruritus, methemoglobinemia (cyanosis), CNS and cardiovascular disturbances, moderate leukocytosis or leukopenia, anemia, granulocytopenia, agranulocytosis, disturbances of visual accommodation.

ROUTE AND DOSAGE

Oral: 26.3 mg (equivalent to 15 mg base) daily for 14 days.

NURSING IMPLICATIONS

Administration of drug at mealtime or with an antacid (prescribed) may prevent or relieve gastric irritation.

Primaquine may precipitate acute hemolytic anemia (sensitivity reaction) in persons with glucose-6-phosphate dehydrogenase deficiency, an inherited error of metabolism carried on the X chromosome, present in about 10% of American black males and certain Caucasian ethnic groups: Sardinians, Sephardic Jews, Greeks, and Iranians (Caucasians manifest more intense expression of hemolytic reaction than do blacks).

Advise all patients to examine urine after each voiding and to report reddening or darkening of urine and decrease in urine volume; also report chills, fever, precordial pain, cyanosis (all are suggestive signs of hemolytic reaction). Sudden reductions in hemoglobin or erythrocyte count suggest impending hemolytic reaction.

Repeated hematologic studies (particularly blood cell counts and hemoglobin) should be performed during therapy.

Preserved in well-closed, light-resistant containers.

DRUG INTERACTIONS: Primaquine is contraindicated in patients receiving other potentially **hemolytic drugs** or **bone marrow depressants** and in patients receiving or patients who have received **quinacrine,** because of possible additive toxic effects.

Anticonvulsant

ACTIONS AND USES
Not a true barbiturate, but closely related chemically and with similar mechanism of action. Converted in body to phenobarbital (qv) metabolite.

Used alone or concomitantly with other anticonvulsant agents to control cortical, focal, psychomotor (temporal lobe), and grand mal seizures.

ABSORPTION AND FATE
Approximately 60% to 80% of dose absorbed from GI tract. Peak serum levels reached in 4 hours. Plasma half-life varies from 3 to 24 hours. Not significantly bound to plasma proteins. Slowly metabolized in liver to two active metabolites: phenobarbital and phenylethylmalonamide (PEMA). Excreted in urine, approximately 15% to 25% as unchanged drug. Appears in breast milk.

CONTRAINDICATIONS AND PRECAUTIONS
Safe use in women of childbearing potential and during pregnancy not established. Cautious use: nursing mothers.

ADVERSE REACTIONS
Drowsiness, vertigo, ataxia, nausea, vomiting, diplopia, nystagmus, fatigue, hyperirritability, emotional disturbances, acute psychotic reactions (usually in patients with psychomotor epilepsy), impotence, alopecia, maculopapular or moribilliform rash, edema of eyelids and legs, leukopenia, thrombocytopenia, eosinophilia, decreased serum folate levels, megaloblastic anemia (rare), lupus-erythematosus-like syndrome, lymphadenopathy, osteomalacia.

ROUTE AND DOSAGE
Oral: **Adults and Children** *over 8 years:* initially 250 mg daily at bedtime; increased by 250 mg, usually at weekly intervals, to tolerance or therapeutic effect, up to maximum of 2 Gm daily. **Children** *under 8 years:* one-half adult dose on a similar schedule.

NURSING IMPLICATIONS
Caution patient that side effects, especially drowsiness, dizziness, and ataxia may be severe at beginning of treatment; therefore patient should avoid driving and other potentially hazardous activities. Symptoms tend to disappear with continued therapy; if they persist, dosage reduction or drug withdrawal may be necessary.

Transition of patient from another anticonvulsant to primidone should not be completed in less than 2 months.

Dosage may be adjusted with reference to primidone or phenobarbital metabolite plasma levels (concentrations of primidone greater than 10 mg/ml are usually associated with significant ataxia and lethargy).

Neonatal hemorrhage has been reported in newborns whose mothers were taking primidone. Monitor closely for bleeding.

Presence of unusual drowsiness in nursing newborns of primidone-treated mothers is an indication to discontinue nursing.

Pregnant women should receive prophylactic vitamin K therapy for 1 month prior to and during delivery to prevent neonatal hemorrhage.

Observe for signs and symptoms of folic acid deficiency: mental dysfunction, psychiatric disorders, neuropathy, megaloblastic anemia. When indicated, serum folate levels should be determined.

Megaloblastic anemia responds to folic acid 15 mg daily, without necessity of interrupting primidone therapy.

PROBENECID, U.S.P., B.P.
(BENACEN, BENEMID, BENN, PROBALAN, ROBENECID)

Uricosuric

ACTIONS AND USES

Sulfonamide-derivative renal tubular blocking agent. In sufficiently high doses, competitively inhibits renal tubular reabsorption of uric acid, thereby promoting its excretion and reducing serum urate levels (subtherapeutic doses may depress uric acid excretion). Prevents formation of new tophaceous deposits, and causes gradual shrinking of old tophi. Since it has no analgesic or antiinflammatory activity, it is of no value in acute gout, and may exacerbate and prolong acute phase. Increases plasma levels of weak organic acids, including penicillin and cephalosporin antibiotics, by competitively inhibiting their renal tubular secretion.

Used for treatment of hyperuricemia in chronic gouty arthritis and tophaceous gout, and as adjuvant to therapy with penicillin G and penicillin analogs when elevated and prolonged levels are indicated.

ABSORPTION AND FATE

Rapidly and completely absorbed from GI tract. Maximal renal clearance of uric acid in 30 minutes; effect on penicillin levels after about 2 hours. Plasma levels peak in 2 to 4 hours and persist for 8 hours. Plasma half-life 6 to 12 hours. About 75% to 95% bound to plasma proteins. Metabolized by liver. Excreted in urine after 2 days as metabolites and unchanged drug. Urine alkalinization decreases reabsorption of probenecid and increases uric acid solubility. Crosses placenta.

CONTRAINDICATIONS AND PRECAUTIONS

Hypersensitivity to probenecid, blood dyscrasias, uric acid kidney stones, during or within 2 to 3 weeks of acute gouty attack, overexcretion of uric acid (over 1000 mg/day), patients with creatinine clearance less than 50 mg/minute, use with penicillin in presence of known renal impairment, use for hyperuricemia secondary to cancer chemotherapy, children under 2 years of age. Cautious use: history of peptic ulcer.

ADVERSE REACTIONS

Headache, nausea, vomiting, anorexia, sore gums, urinary frequency, flushing, dizziness, anemia, hemolytic anemia (possibly related to glucose-6-phosphate dehydrogenase deficiency). **Hypersensitivity reactions:** dermatitis, pruritus, fever, anaphylaxis. Nephrotic syndrome, hepatic necrosis, and aplastic anemia (rare). Exacerbations of gout, uric acid kidney stones. **Overdosage:** CNS stimulation, convulsions, respiratory depression.

ROUTE AND DOSAGE

Oral: *Gout therapy:* first week 250 mg twice daily, followed by 500 mg twice daily; daily dosage increased in 500-mg increments every 4 weeks (usually not above 2 Gm/day) if symptoms are not controlled or 24-hour urate excretion is not above 700 mg. *Penicillin therapy:* **Adults:** 500 mg 4 times daily. **Children** *2 to 14 years:* initially 25 mg/kg; maintenance 40 mg/kg/day divided into 4 doses; children weighing over 50 kg may receive adult dosage.

NURSING IMPLICATIONS

GI side effects minimized by taking drug after meals, with food, or with antacid (prescribed). If symptoms persist, dosage reduction may be required.

During early therapy, high fluid intake (approximately 3 liters/day) to maintain daily urinary output of at least 2 liters or more as well as oral sodium bicarbonate or potassium citrate to alkalinize urine are recommended until uric acid levels return to normal range (males about 6 mg/100 ml, females about 5 mg/100 ml). Some physicians prescribe acetazolamide at bedtime to keep urine alkaline and dilute throughout night. Increased uric acid excretion is promoted by probenecid predisposes to renal calculi.

High-purine foods may be restricted during early therapy until uric acid level stabilizes. Foods high in purine: sweetbreads, anchovies, sardines, liver, kidney, meat extracts, dried beans, peas, lentils, meat soups and broth. Alcohol may increase serum urate levels and therefore should be avoided.

Caution patient not to stop taking drug without consulting physician. Irregular dosage schedule may cause sharp elevation of serum urate level and precipitation of acute gout.

Urate tophaceous deposits should decrease in size with probenecid therapy. Classic locations are in cartilage of ear pinna and big toe, but they can occur in bursae, tendons, skin, kidneys, and other tissues.

Since frequency of acute gouty attacks may increase during first 6 to 12 months of therapy, physician may prescribe concurrent prophylactic doses of colchicine for first 3 to 6 months of probenecid therapy (probenecid alone aggravates acute gout). Probenecid is available in combination with colchicine, eg, ColBENEMID.

When gouty attacks have been absent for 6 months or more and serum urate levels are controlled, daily dosage may be cautiously decreased by 0.5 Gm every 6 months to lowest effective dosage that maintains stable serum urate levels.

Lifelong therapy is usually required in patients with symptomatic hyperuricemia. Advise patient to keep scheduled appointments with physician and appointments for studies of renal function and hematology.

Instruct patient to report symptoms of hypersensitivity to physician. Discontinuation of drug is indicated.

Patients taking oral hypoglycemics may require dosage adjustment. Probenecid enhances hypoglycemic actions of these drugs. Also, see Laboratory Test Interferences below.

Inform patient not to take aspirin or other over-the-counter medication without consulting physician (if a mild analgesic is required, acetaminophen is usually allowed).

LABORATORY TEST INTERFERENCES: Probenecid may decrease urinary excretion of 17-ketosteroids and may interfere with hepatic excretion of Bromsulphalein and affect results of urinary phenolsulfonphthalein excretion test. False positive results are possible with Benedict's solution or Clinitest (glucose oxidase methods not affected, eg, Clinistix, Tes-Tape).

DRUG INTERACTIONS: By inhibiting renal excretion, probenecid may elevate plasma levels and potentiate effects and toxicity of **aminosalicylic acid, cephalosporins, chlorpropamide** and other **oral (antidiabetic) sulfonylureas, dapsone, indomethacin, nitrofurantoin** (probenecid may also decrease urinary tract antiinfective action), **penicillin** (used therapeutically), **rifampin, sulfinpyrazone,** and **sulfonamides. Salicylates** inhibit uricosuric action of probenecid. Drugs that tend to increase serum urate levels may change probenecid dosage requirements: **alcohol, diazoxide,** most **diuretics, mecamylamine, pyrazinamide. Antineoplastics** also increase serum urate levels, but they are contraindicated because of risk of uric acid nephropathy.

Cardiac depressant, antiarrhythmic

ACTIONS AND USES

Antiarrhythmic and antifibrillatory drug with pharmacologic actions qualitatively similar to those of quinidine. Depresses excitability of myocardium to electrical stimulation and produces conduction delay in atria, ventricles, and special conduction systems. Prolongs atrial refractory period but has insignificant effect on that of the ventricles. Has little effect on cardiac contractility or output unless myocardial damage is present. In absence of arrhythmia may cause accelerated heart rate indicating that this drug, like quinidine, has anticholinergic properties. Large doses can induce A.V. block and ventricular extrasystoles that may proceed to ventricular fibrillation. Has peripheral vasodilatation action; when administered intravenously, causes hypotension (may be precipitous) with greater drop in systolic than in diastolic pressure.

Used to treat ventricular extrasystoles and ventricular tachycardia. Also useful therapy for atrial flutter, fibrillation, and paroxysmal atrial tachycardia. Parenteral form given as therapy for cardiac arrhythmias associated with surgery and anesthesia, and to patients who fail to respond to maximally tolerated doses of quinidine.

ABSORPTION AND FATE

Rapid, nearly complete absorption from GI tract. Plasma levels peak within 15 to 60 minutes after IM and IV injections and within 30 to 90 minutes after oral administration. Protein binding about 15% and plasma half-life about 1.5 to 3 hours. Approximately one-quarter of dose converted to metabolite NAPA (N-acetylprocainamide) with 6 hour half-life. Metabolized by hydrolysis in liver and plasma; 50 to 60% drug excreted in urine unchanged.

CONTRAINDICATIONS AND PRECAUTIONS

Myesthenia gravis, hypersensitivity, A.V. block (unless pacemaker is operative), cross sensitivity to procaine and related drugs. Cautious use: patient who has undergone electrical reversion to sinus rhythm; partial A.V. block, hypotension, cardiac enlargement, myocardial infarction, coronary occlusion, congestive heart failure, ventricular dysrhythmia from digitalis intoxication, hepatic or renal insufficiency, acid-base abnormalities, electrolyte imbalance. Safe use during pregnancy or lactation not established.

ADVERSE REACTIONS

With IV doses: hypotension, flushing, giddiness, widened QRS interval, mild to serious hypotension, ventricular conduction disturbances. **Also:** anorexia, nausea, vomiting, urticaria, pruritus, systemic lupus erythematosus like (SLE-like) reaction (eg, polyarthralgias, pleuritic pain, pleural effusion, myalgia, fever, skin rashes, pericarditis); thrombocytopenia, Coombs positive hemolytic anemia (may be related to SLE-like reaction); reactions consisting of fever and chills, plus abdominal pain and acute hepatomegaly; bitter taste, diarrhea, weakness, mental depression, psychosis with hallucinations, hypersensitivity reactions (eg, muscle and joint pain, angioneurotic edema, maculopapular rash); agranulocytosis; elevated SGOT.

ROUTE AND DOSAGE

(Oral route preferred; intravenous use generally limited to extreme emergencies). Oral: initial bolus dose, 1 Gm. Maintenance: 50 mg/kg/day every 3 hours. Intramuscular (in preparation for oral maintenance): 0.5 to 1 Gm repeated every 4 to 6 hours until oral therapy is possible. (Cardiac arrhythmia associated with anesthesia and surgery): 0.1 to 0.5 Gm. Intravenous infusion (atrial fibrillation, paroxysmal atrial tachycardia): 25 to 50 mg/minute up to total dose of 1 Gm.

NURSING IMPLICATIONS

Administer oral preparation with food to decrease GI distress.

Ventricular dysrhythmias are usually abolished within a few minutes after IV dose and within an hour after p.o. or IM administration.

IV procainamide should be diluted to permit better control of flow rate; usually given no faster than 25 to 50 mg/minute.

When procainamide infusion is given to treat atrial dysrhythmia be alert to potential onset of ventricular tachycardia (a lethal arrhythmia). Procainamide sometimes slows atrial rate in flutter to such a level that 1:1 A.V. transmission becomes possible and the ventricle responds with catastrophically high rates (as high as 200 or more beats/minute).

If symptoms of ventricular dysrhythmia develop, talk with patient to assess level of consciousness. Be prepared to defibrillate immediately if he loses consciousness. Check carotid or femoral pulse to determine whether cardiac output is adequate to perfuse.

During IV infusion keep patient in supine position, observe oscilloscope and alert physician immediately to the following: excessive QRS widening (more than 25%) or prolongation of P-R interval; interruption of arrhythmia, change in consciousness, precipitous fall in blood pressure. If the latter drops more than 15 mm Hg, procainamide will be discontinued. Levarterenol or dopamine should be available to combat hypotension.

Constant cardiac monitoring and hourly determinations of blood pressure, pulse, and respiration are essential to avoid potential of overdosage and toxicity. Check temperature every 4 hours and monitor intake and output until condition stabilizes.

When IV administration is required more than several hours, plasma levels may be calculated. Effective procainamide plasma concentration: 4 to 8 μg/ml; levels higher than 16 μg/ml associated with symptoms of toxicity.

Procainamide treatment of atrial arrhythmias is usually preceded by digitalization.

Cardiotonic glycosides may induce sufficient increase in atrial contraction to cause dislodgment of atrial mural emboli with subsequent pulmonary embolism.

Be alert to symptoms of pleuritic chest pain, tachypnea, tachycardia, marked hypotension, cough.

Antinuclear antibody (ANA) titers are evaluated regularly when patient is on maintenance dosage or if SLE-like reaction appears. Not all patients who have the reaction will have elevated titers, but in most cases it is accompanied by ANA titers of 1:256 or higher within 6 months.

Advise patient to report promptly if symptoms of SLE-like reaction occur (see Adverse Reactions). Drug will be discontinued (quinidine may be substituted); steroid therapy may be used if symptoms are severe. Reversion to normal may require months or as long as 2 years.

Periodic blood counts and ECG studies are a part of long-term procainamide therapy.

Instruct patient on maintenance doses to record and report date, time, and duration of fibrillation episodes (lightheadedness, giddiness, weakness, or syncope); such symptoms suggest changed ventricular rhythm. Evaluation of ECG tracings and procainamide plasma levels will be necessary.

Tell patient to avoid driving his car until risk of lightheadedness and fainting has been eliminated.

Renal pathology increases chance of drug toxicity (may cause three-fold increase in biologic half-life of procainamide). Advise patient to report immediately symptoms of renal dysfunction (eg, dysuria, oliguria, hematuria).

Sore mouth, throat or gums; unexplained fever, respiratory tract infection, all symptoms associated with agranulocytosis, should be reported. If decreased leukocyte count is also present physician will discontinue therapy and institute appropriate treatment.

Instruct patient to report unexplained bleeding from any part of body (eg, ecchymoses, petechiae, hematemesis, melena, epistaxis).

Advise patient to avoid iced drinks.

Consult physician about whether patient should discontinue drinking caffeine beverages (tea, coffee, cola, hot chocolate).

Check patient's self-medication habits. If he has freely taken OTC medications for nasal congestion, allergy, pain, or obesity, instruct him to discuss with physician continued need and safe substitutes if necessary.

Store drug in light-proof, airtight container at room temperature. Discard solutions darker than amber color.

DRUG INTERACTIONS: Most drug interactions reported for quinidine (qv) may be applied to procainamide although documentation regarding the latter is sparse. Exception: procainamide does not appear to enhance hypoprothrombinemia effects of **oral anticoagulants:** therefore, it can be used as a substitute for quinidine in patient receiving concurrent anticoagulant therapy.

PROCARBAZINE HYDROCHLORIDE, U.S.P.
(MATULANE)

Antineoplastic

ACTIONS AND USES

Hydrazine derivative with antimetabolite properties. Precise mechanism of action unknown. Suppresses mitosis at interphase, and causes chromatin derangement. Highly toxic to rapidly proliferating tissue. Has immunosuppressive properties, and exhibits MAO inhibitory activity. May cause delayed myelosuppression. No cross-resistances with radiotherapy, steroids, or other antineoplastics have been demonstrated. Reportedly, does not affect survival time, but may produce remissions of at least 1 month's duration. One member of the MOPP combination chemotherapeutic regimens.

Used as adjunct in palliative treatment of Hodgkin's disease (MOPP regimen) and in patients nonresponsive to other forms of therapy. Also used experimentally for treatment of solid tumors.

ABSORPTION AND FATE

Readily absorbed from GI tract. Wide distribution through body fluids, with concentrations in liver, kidneys, intestinal wall, and skin. Half-life in plasma and cerebrospinal fluid about 1 hour. Metabolized in liver; excreted in urine (25% to 42% appearing during first 24 hours after administration) as unchanged drug and metabolites.

CONTRAINDICATIONS AND PRECAUTIONS

Hypersensitivity to procarbazine; myelosuppression; alcohol ingestion; foods high in tyramine content; sympathomimetic drugs; tricyclic antidepressants. Safe use during pregnancy and lactation and in women of childbearing potential not established. Cautious use: concomitant administration of CNS depressants; hepatic or kidney impairment; following radiation or chemotherapy before at least 1 month elapses.

ADVERSE REACTIONS

Hematologic: bone marrow suppression (leukopenia, anemia, thrombocytopenia), hemolysis, bleeding tendencies. **GI:** severe nausea and vomiting (common), anorexia, stomatitis, dry mouth, dysphagia, diarrhea, constipation, jaundice. **CNS:** myalgia, arthralgia, paresthesias, weakness, fatigue, lethargy, drowsiness. Infrequent: confusion, neuropathies, headache, dizziness, depression, apprehension, insomnia, nightmares, hallucinations, psychosis, slurred speech, ataxia, footdrop, decreased reflexes, tremors, coma, convulsions, **Dermatologic:** dermatitis, pruritus, herpes, hyperpigmentation, flushing, alopecia. **Other:** ascites, pleural effusion, cough, hoarseness, hypotension, tachycardia, chills, fever, sweating, gynecomastia, depressed spermatogenesis, atrophy of testes; (rare): edema, nystagmus, photophobia, retinal hemorrhage, diplopia, papilledema; altered hearing; photosensitivity; intercurrent infections.

ROUTE AND DOSAGE

Oral: **Adults:** during first week, 100 to 200 mg daily in single or divided doses, then 300 mg daily until WBC count falls below 4000/mm^3 or platelets below 100,000/mm^3 or maximum response obtained; maintenance 50 to 100 mg daily. **Children:** highly individualized dosage; during first week, 50 mg daily; then maintained at 100 mg/m^2 body surface (to nearest 50 mg) until leukopenia or thrombocytopenia or maximum response occurs; maintenance 50 mg daily.

NURSING IMPLICATIONS

Toxicity is a serious problem and demands that patient be hospitalized and under close medical and nursing supervision during treatment induction period.

Hematologic status (hemoglobin, hematocrit, WBC, differential, reticulocyte, and platelet counts) should be determined initially and at least every 3 or 4 days. Hepatic and renal studies (transaminase, alkaline phosphatase, BUN, urinalysis) are also indicated initially and at least weekly during therapy.

Start flow sheet, and record baseline blood pressure, weight, temperature, pulse, and intake–output ratio and pattern.

Since procarbazine has MAO inhibitory activity, nose drops, cough medicines, and antiobesity preparations containing sympathomimetic drugs (eg, ephedrine, amphetamine, epinephrine) should be avoided because they may cause hypertensive crises. Warn patient not to use over-the-counter preparations without physician's approval.

Intake of foods high in tyramine content should also be avoided (see Index). Warn patient that ingestion of any form of alcohol may precipitate a disulfiramlike (Antabuse) reaction.

Be alert to signs of hepatic dysfunction: jaundice (yellow skin, sclerae, and soft palate), frothy or dark urine, clay-colored stools.

Patient's hematologic status should be monitored carefully for indicators that suggest special nursing interventions and need for dosage adjustment or drug withdrawal.

As patient approaches nadir of leukopenia (below 4000/mm^3), protect patient from exposure to infection and trauma. Visitors and personnel with common colds should not visit. Alert patient to report any sign of impending infection. Note and report changes in voiding pattern, hematuria, and dysuria (possible signs of urinary tract infection). Intake–output ratio and temperature should be closely monitored.

Tolerance to nausea and vomiting (most common side effects) usually develops by end of first week of treatment. Doses are kept at a minimum during this time. If vomiting persists, therapy will be interrupted.

Instruct patient to report immediately signs of hemorrhagic tendencies: bleeding into skin and mucosa (epistaxis, hemoptysis, hematemesis, hematuria, melena, ecchymoses, petechiae). Bone marrow depression often occurs 2 to 8 weeks after start of therapy.

Prompt cessation of therapy is usual with appearance of CNS signs and symptoms (paresthesias, neuropathies, confusion), leukopenia (WBC count under 4000/mm^3), thrombocytopenia (platelet count under

100,000/mm³), hypersensitivity, the first small ulceration or persistent spot soreness of oral cavity, diarrhea, and bleeding. Patient should be warned to report promptly any signs and symptoms of toxicity.

DRUG INTERACTIONS. Procarbazine may enhance the effects of **CNS depressants.** A disulfiramlike reaction may occur following ingestion of **alcohol,** in addition to additive CNS depression.

PROCHLORPERAZINE, U.S.P.
(COMPAZINE)
PROCHLORPERAZINE, EDISYLATE, U.S.P.
(COMPAZINE EDISYLATE)
PROCHLORPERAZINE, MALEATE, U.S.P., B.P.
(COMPAZINE MALEATE)

Antipsychotic (major tranquilizer), antiemetic

ACTIONS AND USES
Piperazine phenothiazine derivative with similar actions, contraindications, and toxicity as chlorpromazine (qv). Reported to have greater antiemetic potency and to produce less sedative, hypotensive, and atropinelike effects than chlorpromazine, but has higher incidence of extrapyramidal reactions, motor restlessness, dystonias, and abnormal lactation. Available as prochlorperazine base (rectal suppository), edisylate (syrup, oral concentrate, aqueous solution for injection), maleate (oral tablet, and sustained-release form).
Used in management of psychotic disorders and to control nausea and vomiting. Possibly effective in management of excessive anxiety, tension, and agitation.
ABSORPTION AND FATE
Onset of action: oral tablet 30 to 40 minutes (duration 3 to 4 hours), extended-release form 30 to 40 minutes (duration 10 to 12 hours), rectal suppository 60 minutes (duration 3 to 4 hours), IM 10 to 20 minutes (duration 3 to 4 hours).
CONTRAINDICATIONS AND PRECAUTIONS
Hypersensitivity to phenothiazines, bone marrow depression, comatose or severely depressed states, children weighing less than 20 lb (9 kg) or children younger than 2 years of age, pediatric surgery, short-term vomiting in children or vomiting of unknown etiology, Reye's syndrome or other encephalopathies, history of dyskinetic reactions or epilepsy. See Chlorpromazine.
ADVERSE REACTIONS
Drowsiness, dizziness, hypotension, diuresis, skin reactions, contact dermatitis, galactorrhea, amenorrhea, blurred vision, cholestatic jaundice, leukopenia, agranulocytosis, extrapyramidal reactions (akathesia, dystonia or parkinsonism), persistent tardive dyskinesia, acute catatonia. Also see Chlorpromazine.
ROUTE AND DOSAGE
Adults: Oral tablet: 5 to 10 mg 3 or 4 times daily. Sustained-release capsule: 15 mg on arising or 10 mg every 12 hours. In adult psychiatry, oral dosage may range from 15 to 150 mg daily, depending on severity of condition. Rectal suppository: 25 mg twice daily. Intramuscular: 5 to 10 mg repeated every 2 or 4 hours depending on condition being treated. Total IM dosage not to exceed 40 mg/day. May be repeated once in 30 minutes if necessary. Intravenous infusion: 20 mg/liter of isotonic solution (added to IV infusion 15 to 30 minutes before induction of anesthesia). **Children:** Oral, rectal: 0.4 mg/kg body weight daily, divided into 3 or 4 doses. Intramuscular: 0.13 mg/kg body weight.

NURSING IMPLICATIONS

Minimum effective dosage is advised. Keep physician informed of patient's response to drug therapy.

Most elderly and emaciated patients and children with dehydration or acute illness appear to be particularly susceptible to extrapyramidal reactions. Observe these patients closely.

Avoid contact of oral concentrate or injection solution with hands or clothes because of possibility of contact dermatitis.

Oral concentrate is intended for institutional use only and is not to be administered to children.

To ensure stability and palatability of oral concentrate, add prescribed dose to 60 ml or more of diluent just prior to administration. Suggested diluents: tomato or fruit juice, orange or other simple syrup, carbonated drinks, tea, coffee, water, semisolid foods, eg, puddings, soups, etc.

IM injection in adults should be made deep into upper outer quadrant of buttock (subcutaneous administration is not advised, as it causes local irritation). Do not mix IM solution in same syringe with other agents. Follow hospital policy regarding IM injection site for children.

Postoperative patients who have received prochlorperazine should be carefully positioned to prevent aspiration of vomitus (reported in a few patients, although causal relationship not established).

Hypotension is a possibility in the elderly and in patients receiving the drug IV. Monitor blood pressure and supervise ambulation.

Since drug may impair mental and physical abilities, especially during first few days of therapy, caution patient to avoid hazardous activities such as operating a motor vehicle or machinery.

Patients on long-term antipsychotic therapy should be evaluated periodically for possibility of lowering dosage or discontinuing therapy.

Treatment of overdosage: early gastric lavage, airway maintenance, general supportive measures. Have on hand antiparkinson drugs, barbiturates, and diphenhydramine. Emesis should not be induced because it may precipitate dystonic reactions of head and neck, with possible aspiration of vomitus.

Slight yellow discoloration of ingestable form reportedly does not alter potency. However, discard markedly discolored solution.

Stored in tightly covered, light-resistant containers.

See Chlorpromazine.

PROCYCLIDINE HYDROCHLORIDE, N.F., B.P.
(KEMADRIN)

Antiparkinsonian, skeletal-muscle relaxant

ACTIONS AND USES

Centrally acting synthetic anticholinergic agent with actions similar to those of atropine (qv); closely related to trihexyphenidyl.

Used to relieve parkinsonism, including postencephalitic, arteriosclerotic, and idiopathic types, and extrapyramidal symptoms associated with use of phenothiazines and rauwolfia alkaloids.

ABSORPTION AND FATE

Onset of action in 30 to 45 minutes; duration 4 to 6 hours.

CONTRAINDICATIONS AND PRECAUTIONS

Angle-closure glaucoma. Safe use during pregnancy and use in women of childbearing potential, in nursing mothers, and in children not established. Cautious use: hypotension, mental disorders, tachycardia, prostatic hypertrophy.

Dry mouth, blurred vision, mydriasis, palpitation, flushing of skin, headache, dizziness, urinary retention, constipation, acute suppurative parotitis, skin eruptions; (occasionally): mental confusion, psychotic-like symptoms.

ROUTE AND DOSAGE
Oral: initially 2 to 2.5 mg 3 times daily after meals; if tolerated, dosage gradually increased to 4 to 5 mg 3 times daily; additional 4 to 5 mg at bedtime may be prescribed for some patients.

NURSING IMPLICATIONS

Side effects may be minimized by administration of drug after meals.

Drug-induced dryness of mouth may be relieved by sugarless gum or hard candy and by frequent sips of water.

If urinary hesitancy or retention is a problem, advise the patient to void before taking drug.

Drug occasionally causes mental confusion, disorientation, agitation, and psychoticlike symptoms, particularly in elderly patients who have low blood pressure.

Since procyclidine may cause blurred vision and dizziness, caution the patient to avoid potentially hazardous activities until reaction to drug is known.

Report palpitation, tachycardia, or decreasing blood pressure. Dosage adjustment or discontinuation of drug may be indicated.

Since dosage is guided by clinical response, observe and record improvement (or lack of it) that accompanies therapy.

Procyclidine is usually more effective in controlling rigidity than tremors. Tremors may temporarily appear to be exaggerated as rigidity is relieved, especially in patients with severe spasticity.

See Atropine for nursing implications and drug interactions.

DRUG INTERACTIONS: Procyclidine may partially inhibit the therapeutic effects of **haloperidol** (possibly by delaying gastric emptying time and increasing metabolism in GI tract) and **phenothiazines** (possibly by interfering with their absorption).

PROGESTERONE, U.S.P., N.F., B.P.
(FEMOTRONE, GESTEROL, LIPO-LUTIN, PROFAC, PROGELAN, PROGESTIN, PROLUTON, PRORONE)

Hormone, progestin

ACTIONS AND USES
Natural steroid compound with antiestrogenic properties; essential for normal maturation of female and maintenance of pregnancy. Synthesized in corpus luteum, in adrenal cortex, and in large amounts in placenta during pregnancy. Transforms endometrium from proliferative to secretory state; suppresses pituitary gonadotropin secretion, thereby blocking follicular maturation and ovulation (indirectly menstruation). Stimulates endocervical secretion of glycogen and thick mucus. Promotes mammary gland development without causing lactation, and increases body temperature about 1 F at time of ovulation. Relaxes myometrium; decreases glucose tolerance. Effectiveness depends on estrogen-primed endometrium.

Use largely supplanted by new progestins, which have longer action and oral effectiveness. See Dydrogesterone.

Used in habitual and threatened abortion, postpartum breast engorgement, functional uterine bleeding, endometriosis, dysmenorrhea, premenstrual tension, amenorrhea, female hypogonadism. Also used as diagnostic test for endogenous production of estrogen and progesterone and as a contraceptive, alone or combined with estrogen.

ABSORPTION AND FATE

Rapid absorption follows injection. Plasma half-life approximately 5 minutes; duration of action about 24 hours. Biotransformation takes place during one pass through liver; after enterohepatic circulation, portion of metabolites excreted in feces. Urinary excretion of remainder as pregnanediol glucuronide provides indirect partial index of progesterone metabolism and secretion. Small amounts detected in breast milk.

CONTRAINDICATIONS AND PRECAUTIONS

See Dydrogesterone.

ADVERSE REACTIONS

Masculinization of female fetus (slight risk), leg and abdominal cramps, greasy hair, rash with or without pruritus, urticaria, changes in appetite, GI disturbances, ulcerative stomatitis, pruritus vulvae, mastalgia, premenstrual depression, change in libido, leukorrhea or dry vagina, reduced menstrual loss, pain at injection site, weight change (gain or loss), fluid retention.

ROUTE AND DOSAGE

Intramuscular; (oil or aqueous suspension) *menstrual dysfunction:* 10 to 25 mg on alternate days during last 8 to 10 days before patient is expected to menstruate. *Habitual, threatened, or premature abortion:* 5 to 50 mg daily; dosage varies widely with indication for use. *Diagnostic test:* 100 mg.

NURSING IMPLICATIONS

Protect medication vial from light.

Immerse vial in warm water momentarily to facilitate aspiration of drug into syringe and to redissolve crystals.

Injection site is irritated by drug, whether in oil or water; the latter is particularly painful.

Normal 24 hour excretion values of pregnanediol in urine: males, 0–1 mg; females, 1–8 mg, pregnancy, 60–100 mg; children, negative.

Progesterone withdrawal is followed by a more complete endometrial deciduation than that following estrogen withdrawal.

Diagnostic use (note that withdrawal bleeding occurs from an estrogen-primed endothelium): Test for estrogen production in patient with amenorrhea: Failure to menstruate after administration of progesterone (negative response) signifies minimal estrogen production; bleeding 1 week or so after withdrawal (positive response) indicates sufficient estrogen to produce a proliferative endometrium. Test for pregnancy (progesterone production) in patient who is producing estrogen: Failure to menstruate following administration, then withdrawal, of progesterone indicates continued progesterone production (by a chorionic-gonadotropin-stimulated corpus luteum); thus pregnancy is confirmed.

Pathologist should be informed of progesterone therapy when relevant specimens are submitted.

See Dydrogesterone.

Antipsychotic (major tranquilizer), antiemetic

ACTIONS AND USES
   Dimethylaminopropyl derivative of phenothiazine with similar actions, contraindications, and toxicity as chlorpromazine (qv). Reportedly less potent in
   antipsychotic activity than chlorpromazine; produces less sedation and has
   more marked taming effect.
   Used in management of psychotic manifestations and for reducing agitation and
   tension associated with alcohol withdrawal. Occasionally used as antiemetic
CONTRAINDICATIONS AND PRECAUTIONS
   Hypersensitivity to phenothiazines, bone marrow depression, CNS depression,
   children under 12 years of age. Cautious use: convulsive disorders. See Chlorpromazine.
ADVERSE REACTIONS
   (Common): drowsiness, hypotensive effects; epileptic seizures in susceptible
   individuals, leukopenia, agranulocytosis (infrequent). See Chlorpromazine.
ROUTE AND DOSAGE
   Adults: Oral, intramuscular: 10 to 20 mg at 4- to 6-hour intervals. Total daily
   dose not to exceed 1 Gm. If administration is absolutely essential in inebriated
   patients, initial dose should not exceed 50 mg. Intravenous: 50 mg injected
   slowly; concentration should not exceed 25 mg/ml.

NURSING IMPLICATIONS
Oral route should be used whenever possible. Parenteral administration is
   reserved for patients who are acutely disturbed or uncooperative or who
   cannot tolerate oral preparation. Keep physician informed of patient's
   progress.
Syrup or oral concentrate may be prescribed when tablet is unsuitable or
   refused. Dilute concentrate in fruit juice, chocolate-flavored drinks, or
   other suitable vehicles.
Advise patient that dizziness or faintness may occur on arising. Caution
   patient to make all position changes slowly, particularly from recumbent
   to upright position.
Incidence of postural hypotension and drowsiness is particularly high after
   parenteral administration. Monitor blood pressure and pulse before administration and between doses. It is advisable to keep patient recumbent
   for about 1 hour after parenteral dose is given.
IM injection is made deep into upper outer quadrant of buttock. Tissue
   irritation can occur if given subcutaneously. Carefully aspirate before
   injecting drug; intraarterial injection can cause arterial or arteriolar spasm
   and consequent impairment of local circulation. Rotate injection sites.
IV route is reserved only for hospitalized patients; routine use not recommended. Localized cellulitis, thrombophlebitis, and gangrene have occurred because of improper drug dilution, extravasation, or injections
   made into previously damaged blood vessels. Observe IV injection site.
Although contact dermatitis occurs infrequently with promazine, it is advisable to avoid contact of oral concentrate or parenteral solution with skin
   and clothing.
Stored in tight, light-resistant containers.
See Chlorpromazine.

PROMETHAZINE HYDROCHLORIDE, U.S.P., B.P.
(FELLOZINE, GANPHEN, K-PHEN, LEMPROMETH, PHENCEN,
PHENERGAN, PROMINE, PROREX, PROVIGAN, QUADNITE,
REMSED, V-GAN, ZIPAN)

Antihistaminic, antiemetic

ACTIONS AND USES

Long-acting ethylamino derivative of phenothiazine with marked antihistaminic activity and prominent sedative, amnesic, antiemetic, and anti-motion-sickness actions. Unlike other phenothiazine derivatives, it is relatively free of extrapyramidal side efects; however, in high doses it carries same potential for toxicity. In common with other antihistamines, exerts antiserotonin, anticholinergic, and local anesthetic action. Reported to have slight antitussive activity, but this may be due to anticholinergic and CNS depressant effects.

Used for symptomatic relief of various allergic conditions, to ameliorate and prevent reactions to blood and plasma, and in prophylaxis and treatment of motion sickness, nausea, and vomiting. Used for preoperative, postoperative, and obstetric sedation, and as adjunct to analgesics for control of pain.

ABSORPTION AND FATE

Well absorbed from GI tract and parenteral routes. Antihistaminic effects occur within 20 minutes following oral, rectal, and IM and within 3 to 5 minutes after IV administration. Duration of action generally 4 to 6 hours; antihistaminic activity sometimes persists for 12 hours. Widely distributed in body tissues. Metabolized by liver; excreted slowly in urine and feces, primarily as inactive metabolites.

CONTRAINDICATIONS AND PRECAUTIONS

Hypersensitivity to phenothiazines, narrow-angle glaucoma, stenosing peptic ulcer, pyloroduodenal obstruction, prostatic hypertrophy, bladder neck obstruction, epilepsy, bone marrow depression, comatose or severely depressed states, pregnancy (except labor), nursing mothers, newborn or premature infants, acutely ill or dehydrated children. Cautious use: impaired hepatic function, cardiovascular disease, asthma, acute or chronic respiratory impairment (particularly in children), hypertension, elderly or debilitated patients.

ADVERSE REACTIONS

Pronounced sedative effect (drowsiness, confusion, dizziness, disturbed coordination), anticholinergic (atropinelike) actions (dry mouth, blurred vision, constipation, urinary retention, transient mild hypotension or hypertension), leukopenia, agranulocytosis, jaundice (rare), photosensitivity, restlessness, irregular respiration. With prolonged administration or high doses, toxic potential as for other phenothiazines (see Chlorpromazine). Acute toxicity: deep sleep, coma, convulsions, cardiorespiratory symptoms, extrapyramidal reactions, nightmares (in children), CNS stimulation, abnormal movements, respiratory depression.

ROUTE AND DOSAGE

Adults: Oral, rectal suppository, intramuscular, intravenous: 12.5 to 50 mg in a single dose, or repeated at 4- to 6-hour intervals if necessary. Highly individualized. For motion sickness, initial dose (usually 25 mg) should be taken 30 minutes to 1 hour before anticipated travel and repeated at 8 to 12 hours if necessary. For duration of journey: 25 mg on arising and again at evening meal. **Children:** Oral, rectal, parenteral: 0.25 to 0.5 mg/kg. Intravenous concentration should not be greater than 25 mg/ml; administration rate not to exceed 25 mg/minute.

NURSING IMPLICATIONS

Inspect parenteral drug before preparation. Discard if it is darkened or contains precipitate.

IM injection is made deep into large muscle mass. Aspirate carefully before injecting drug. Intraarterial injection can cause arterial or arteriolar spasm, with resultant gangrene. Subcutaneous injection (also contraindicated) can cause chemical irritation and necrosis. Rotate injection sites and observe daily.

When administered by IV infusion, wrap IV bottle with aluminum foil to protect drug from light.

Promethazine injection is reportedly incompatible with several drugs, especially those with alkaline pH. Consult pharmacist for specific information.

Oral doses for allergy are generally prescribed before meals and on retiring or as single dose at bedtime.

Promethazine sometimes produces marked sedation and dizziness. Bedsides and supervision of ambulation may be advisable.

Advise ambulatory patient to avoid driving a car or engaging in other activities requiring mental alertness and normal reaction time until reaction to drug is known.

Bear in mind that antiemetic action may mask symptoms of unrecognized disease and signs of overdosage of other drugs.

Patients in pain may develop involuntary (athetoid) movements of upper extremities following parenteral administration. These symptoms usually disappear after pain is controlled.

Respiratory function should be monitored in patients with respiratory problems, particularly children. Promethazine may suppress cough reflex and cause thickening of bronchial secretions.

Advise patient not to take OTC medications without physician's approval.

Treatment of overdosage: early gastric lavage (endotracheal tube with cuff in place to prevent aspiration of vomitus). Emesis should not be induced because dystonic reactions of head and neck may result in aspiration. Have on hand: antiparkinson drugs, barbiturates, diazepam, diphenhydramine, levarterenol, phenylephrine.

LABORATORY TEST INTERFERENCES: Promethazine may interfere with blood grouping in ABO system and may produce false results with urinary pregnancy tests (Gravindex, false positive; Prepurex and Dap tests, false negative). Promethazine can cause significant alterations of flare response in intradermal allergen tests.

DRUG INTERACTIONS: There is a possibility of additive sedative action when promethazine is given concurrently with drugs that have CNS depressant effect, eg, **alcohol,** other **antihistamines, barbiturates, narcotic analgesics,** and **tranquilizers** (if used, dose of barbiturates should be reduced by at least one-half and that of narcotic analgesic by one-fourth to one-half). Promethazine reverses vasopressor effect of **epinephrine** and may cause further lowering of blood pressure in patients with hypotension. **MAO inhibitors** intensify and prolong the anticholinergic effects of promethazine.

(GIQUEL, NORPANTH, PRO-BANTHINE, ROBANTALINE, ROPANTH, SPASTIL)

Anticholinergic

ACTIONS AND USES

Synthetic quaternary ammonium compound closely related chemically to methantheline. Similar to atropine (qv) in peripheral effects, contraindications, precautions, and adverse reactions. Potent in antimuscarinic activity and in nondepolarizing ganglionic blocking action. Very high doses block neurotransmission at myoneural junction.

Used as adjunct in treatment of peptic ulcer, irritable bowel syndrome, pancreatitis, ureteral and urinary bladder spasm; effectively controls excessive salivation and hyperhidrosis.

ABSORPTION AND FATE

Incompletely absorbed from GI tract. Onset of effects following oral administration in 30 to 45 minutes, persisting 4 to 6 hours. Excreted through all body fluids, but chiefly in urine and bile.

CONTRAINDICATIONS AND PRECAUTIONS, ADVERSE REACTIONS

See Atropine.

ROUTE AND DOSAGE

Adult: Oral: 15 mg with meals and 30 mg at bedtime. For geriatric patients or patients of small stature: 7.5 mg 3 times daily. Prolonged-action form: 30 mg every 8 hours. Intramuscular, intravenous: 30 mg or more every 6 hours. **Pediatric:** Oral: 1.5 mg/kg/24 hours, divided into 4 doses.

NURSING IMPLICATIONS

Oral preparation is generally administered 10 minutes before or with meals and at bedtime. Advise the patient not to chew tablet; drug is very bitter.

Liquid diet is recommended during initiation of therapy in patients with duodenal ulcers to prevent nausea.

Urinary hesitancy or retention (especially likely to occur in elderly patients) may be avoided by advising patient to void just prior to each dose. Instruct the patient to note daily urinary volume and to report voiding problems to physician.

Parenteral drug should be prepared immediately before administration.

When drug is administered parenterally, observe the patient closely for curarelike distress or paralysis. Equipment for artificial respiration should be readily available.

Patients with cardiac disease should have periodic checks of vital signs, especially heart sounds and rhythm.

Postural hypotension and tachycardia may occur during early therapy. Instruct the patient to make all position changes slowly and to lie down immediately if faintness, weakness, or palpitation occurs. Advise the patient to report these symptoms to the physician.

Caution the patient to avoid potentially hazardous activities such as driving a car or operating machinery. Drowsiness, dizziness, and blurred vision are common side effects.

Dryness of mouth may be relieved by sugarless hard candy or gum, rinsing mouth with cool tap water, and mouth care after meals. If symptom persists, dosage reduction may be indicated.

See Atropine Sulfate.

Sedative

ACTIONS AND USES
Ethylamino derivative of phenothiazines with prominent sedative effects. General properties similar to those of other phenothiazines. See Chlorpromazine. Action relieves apprehension and promotes sleep, from which patient can be easily aroused.
Used for sedative and antiemetic effects preoperatively and postoperatively and during labor. May be used alone or concomitantly with other CNS depressants.
ABSORPTION AND FATE
Peak sedative effect within 15 to 30 minutes following IV infusion and in 40 to 60 minutes after IM injection; duration of effect 4 to 5 hours.
CONTRAINDICATIONS AND PRECAUTIONS
Hypersensitivity to phenothiazines. See Chlorpromazine.
ADVERSE REACTIONS
Dry mouth, tachycardia, GI upsets, skin rash, dizziness, confusion, amnesia; restlessness, akathisia, respiratory depression (high doses); elevated blood pressure, hypotension; (with rapid IV): irritation, thrombophlebitis (IV injection site).
ROUTE AND DOSAGE
Intramuscular, intravenous: **Adults:** 10 to 40 mg, repeated in 4 hours as indicated. **Children** *under 60 lb:* 0.25 to 0.5 mg/lb body weight.

NURSING IMPLICATIONS
Do not use solution if it is cloudy or if it contains a precipitate.
Administer IM deep into large muscle mass, preferably upper quadrant of buttock. Aspirate carefully before injecting drug; intraarterial injection is specifically contraindicated because it may cause vascular spasm with resultant gangrene. Tissue irritation can occur if given subcutaneously. Rotate injection sites.
Check blood pressure and pulse before drug administration, and monitor between doses.
Elderly patients may experience dizziness, confusion, and amnesia. Bedsides and supervision of ambulation may be indicated.
Restlessness or akathisia is usually dose-related. Report to physician. Symptoms may last 30 minutes to 4 hours.
Caution ambulatory patients to avoid driving or operating machinery, because drug tends to impair mental alertness and physical coordination.
If patient requires a vasopressor agent, levarterenol may be used. Epinephrine is contraindicated, because it may augment the hypotensive effect of propiomazine.
See Chlorpromazine for other nursing implications and drug interactions.
Stored at room temperature away from heat. Protect drug from light.

614 PROPOXYPHENE HYDROCHLORIDE, U.S.P.
(DARVON, DOLENE, HARMAR, PARGESIC 65, PROGESIC-65
PROPOXYCHEL, PROXAGESIC, ROPOXY, SK-65, S-PAIN-65)
DEXTROPROPOXYPHENE, B.P.
PROPOXYPHENE NAPSYLATE
(DARVON-N)

Analgesic

ACTIONS AND USES
Structurally related to methadone, but similar to codeine in analgesic potency and duration of action. Unlike codeine, has little or no antitussive effect or narcotic activity, and somewhat lower abuse liability. Frequently combined with aspirin (hydrochloride reportedly accelerates aspirin degradation) and phenacetin, eg, Darvon compound, Poxy Compound-65, Procomp-65.
Used for relief of mild to moderate pain. Also has been used in combination with other drugs to relieve narcotic withdrawal state.

ABSORPTION AND FATE
Peak serum levels within 2 hours following the hydrochloride and within 3 hours after napsylate. Onset of analgesic effect within 15 minutes; persists 4 to 6 hours. Half-life approximately 3.5 hours. Degraded primarily in liver. Excreted in urine, within 6 to 48 hours, as metabolites and traces of unchanged drug.

CONTRAINDICATIONS AND PRECAUTIONS
Hypersensitivity to drug. Safe use during pregnancy and in children not established. Cautious use: history of drug dependence.

ADVERSE REACTIONS
Dizziness, headache, sedation, drowsiness, insomnia, nausea, vomiting, abdominal pain, constipation, minor visual disturbances, skin eruptions, euphoria, dysphoria, paradoxic excitement, hypoglycemia (patients with impaired renal function). **Overdosage:** toxic psychoses, coma, respiratory depression, circulatory collapse, pulmonary edema, convulsions, ECG changes, nephrogenic diabetes insipidus.

ROUTE AND DOSAGE
Oral (hydrochloride): 65 mg every 4 hours, as needed (available in capsule form); (napsylate): 100 mg every 4 hours as needed (available in tablet and suspension forms); 100 mg of napsylate are equivalent to 65 mg of hydrochloride.

NURSING IMPLICATIONS
Evaluate the patient's need for continued use of drug. Propoxyphene is commonly abused.

Tremulousness, restlessness ("speeding"), and mild euphoria frequently occur (effects desired by many addicts).

Dizziness, drowsiness, nausea, and vomiting appear to be prominent in ambulatory patients. Symptoms may be relieved if patient lies down.

Caution the ambulatory patient not to drive a car and to avoid other potentially hazardous activities.

Treatment of overdosage: emesis or gastric lavage; activated charcoal slurry. Have on hand narcotic antagonist (naloxone) to combat respiratory depression; assisted ventilation, oxygen, and IV therapy as indicated. Analeptic drugs (eg, amphetamines) are not used because of their tendency to precipitate fatal convulsions.

Tolerance and physical and psychic dependence can occur with excessive use.

Classified as schedule IV drug under federal Controlled Substances Act. When propoxyphene is included in combination products, cautions relative to each drug ingredient must be considered.

LABORATORY TEST INTERFERENCES: There is the possibility of false decreases in urinary steroid excretion tests: 17-hydroxycorticosteroids (Porter-Silber method) and 17-ketosteroids (Zimmermann reaction).

DRUG INTERACTIONS: Additive CNS depression may occur with concomitant use of CNS depressants: eg, **alcohol, antianxiety agents, antipsychotic agents, narcotics, sedatives, hypnotics. Amphetamines** may contribute to convulsions induced by toxic doses of propoxyphene.

PROPRANOLOL HYDROCHLORIDE, U.S.P., B.P.
(INDERAL)

Cardiac depressant (antiarrhythmic)

ACTIONS AND USES
Beta-adrenergic blocking agent which competes with epinephrine and norepinephrine for available beta-receptor sites. Selectively blocks cardiac effects of beta-adrenergic stimulation without abolishing cardiotonic action of nonadrenergic drugs such as digitalis. Reduces heart rate, myocardial irritability and force of contraction, depresses automaticity of sinus node and ectopic pacemaker, and decreases A-V and intraventricular conduction velocity. In higher doses, exerts direct quinidinelike membrane effects which together with decreased reflex sympathetic drive is associated with depression of cardiac function. Also blocks bronchodilator effect of catecholamines, reduces plasma levels of free fatty acids, and may interfere with carbohydrate metabolism by inhibiting glycogenolysis, and insulin release from pancreas. Lowers both supine and standing blood pressures in hypertensive patients possibly by decreasing cardiac output, suppressing renin activity, or by blocking sympathetic outflow from vasomotor centers in brain. Increases exercise tolerance by blocking sympathetic effects of exertion and emotions, and usually decreases myocardial oxygen requirements in patients with frequent anginal attacks.
Used in management of paroxysmal atrial tachycardias particularly those induced by catecholamines or digitalis, or associated with Wolff-Parkinson-White syndrome; sinus tachycardia; persistent atrial or premature ventricular extrasystoles; atrial flutter and fibrillation not controlled by digitalis alone; tachyarrhythmias associated with digitalis intoxication, anesthesia, and thyrotoxicosis. Not drug of first choice for ventricular arrhythmias with exception of those induced by catecholamines or digitalis. Effective in management of hypertrophic subaortic stenosis, angina pectoris not controlled by conventional measures; as adjunct with alpha-adrenergic agent in pheochromocytoma; and in treatment of essential hypertension alone, but generally with a thiazide or other antihypertensive. Also has been used in anxiety states, migraine prophylaxis, causalgia, and essential tremors.
ABSORPTION AND FATE
Almost completely absorbed from GI tract following oral administration. Onset of action within 30 minutes, peak plasma levels in 1 to 1½ hours (marked individual variations in plasma levels); duration about 6 hours. Following IV administration, action begins within 2 minutes, peaks within 15 minutes, with duration of 3 to 6 hours; plasma levels more consistent. Plasma half-life varies from 3.4 to 6 hours. Widely distributed in body tissues; more than 90% bound

to plasma proteins. Largely metabolized by liver. Excreted in urine as free and conjugated propranolol, and metabolites; 1 to 4% excreted in feces. Crosses placenta and blood-brain barrier; may appear in breast milk.

CONTRAINDICATIONS AND PRECAUTIONS

Greater than 1st degree heart block, congestive heart failure, right ventricular failure secondary to pulmonary hypertension; sinus bradycardia, cardiogenic shock, significant aortic or mitral valvular disease, bronchial asthma, allergic rhinitis during pollen season; concurrent use or within 2 weeks of adrenergic-augmenting psychotropic drugs (including MAO inhibitors). Safe use in women of childbearing potential, during pregnancy, and lactation not established. Cautious use: peripheral arterial insufficiency, history of allergy; patients prone to nonallergenic bronchospasm (chronic bronchitis, emphysema); renal or hepatic impairment, diabetes mellitus, hypoglycemic episodes, myasthenia gravis.

ADVERSE REACTIONS

GI: nausea, vomiting, diarrhea, constipation, flatulence, abdominal cramps, xerostomia. **Cardiovascular:** palpitation, profound bradycardia, A-V heart block, cardiac standstill, hypotension, angina pectoris, tachyarrhythmia, acute congestive heart failure, peripheral arterial insufficiency resembling Raynaud's, paresthesia of hands. **Respiratory:** dyspnea, laryngospasm, bronchospasm. **CNS:** confusion, agitation, giddiness, lightheadedness, fatigue, vertigo, syncope, tinnitus, hearing loss, visual disturbances, vivid dreams, hallucinations, delusions, mental depression, reversible organic brain syndrome. **Allergic:** erythematous, psoriasis-like eruptions, fever, pharyngitis, respiratory distress. **Hematologic:** transient eosinophilia, thrombocytopenia, nonthrombocytopenic purpura, agranulocytosis, hypoglycemia, hyperglycemia (rare); hypocalcemia (patients with hyperthyroidism); elevated BUN, serum transaminase, alkaline phosphatase, lactic dehydrogenase. **Other reported:** brown discoloration of tongue (rare), pancreatitis, reversible alopecia.

ROUTE AND DOSAGE.

Oral: *Hypertension:* 20 mg 4 times daily; increased by 20 mg increments (usual effective dose range is 160 to 480 mg/day). *Angina:* initially, 10 to 20 mg 3 or 4 times daily; dosage gradually increased at 3- to 7-day intervals until optimum response obtained (average optimum dosage appears to be 160 mg/day). *Arrhythmias:* 10 to 30 mg 3 or 4 times daily. *Hypertrophic subaortic stenosis:* 20 to 40 mg 3 or 4 times daily. *Pheochromocytoma:* 20 mg 3 times daily, 3 days prior to surgery (concomitantly with alpha adrenergic blocking agent); inoperable pheochromocytoma: 10 mg 3 times daily. Intravenous (for life-threatening arrhythmias): 1 to 3 mg at rate not exceeding 1 mg/minute; may be repeated after 2 minutes, if necessary. Thereafter, additional drug not given in less than 4 hours.

NURSING IMPLICATIONS

Oral propranolol is given preferably before meals and at bedtime. Administration with food delays peak plasma level time.

Careful medical history and physical examination are essential to rule out allergies, asthma, and other obstructive pulmonary diseases. Propranolol can cause bronchiolar constriction even in normal subjects.

Take apical-radial pulse before administering drug; if blood pressure is not stabilized, also take this reading before drug is given. Report to physician any change in pulse rate, rhythm, or amplitude pattern, or variation in blood pressure.

Apical pulse, respiration, blood pressure, and circulation of extremities should be closely monitored throughout period of dosage adjustment. Consult physician regarding acceptable parameters.

Response to propranolol is reported to be associated with a high degree of individual variability. Therefore, sensitive observations are critically essential for establishing the patient's optimal dosage level.

When administered IV careful monitoring must be made of ECG, blood pressure, and central venous pressure.

Adverse reactions generally occur most frequently following IV administration; however, incidence is also high following oral use in the elderly and in patients with impaired renal function. Reactions may or may not be dose-related and commonly occur soon after therapy is initiated.

Bradycardia is the most common adverse cardiac effect especially in patients with digitalis intoxication and Wolff-Parkinson-White syndrome.

Have on hand atropine (for excessive bradycardia), vasopressors (eg, epinephrine for hypotension), isoproterenol, and aminophylline (for bronchospasm). Cardiac failure is treated by digitalization and diuresis.

Intake-output ratio and daily weight are significant indices of fluid retention and developing heart failure. Consult physician regarding allowable salt intake.

Propranolol may mask typical signs of insulin overdosage (eg, nervousness, tremors, sweating, hunger, increased pulse rate, etc.) and may prolong hypoglycemic effects. Reduction in dosage of insulin or other hypoglycemic agents may be necessary. Instruct patient to report any symptom regardless of how minor it may seem to him.

Fasting for more than 12 hours may induce hypoglycemic effects produced by propranolol.

Since propranolol decreases adaptive response to exercise and stress, patient may experience lightheadedness, weakness, fatigue, and dyspnea with physical exertion or psychological stresses. Observe and record patient's response to stresses and individualize his activity program. Advise patient to avoid potentially hazardous activities such as driving a car until his reaction to drug is known.

In patients taking propranolol for angina pectoris, exercise performance studies and ECG's are recommended before therapy to establish baseline data, and during therapy to determine response to drug therapy. Therapy is not continued unless there is reduced pain and increased work capacity.

When propranolol is to be discontinued in patients who have received prolonged therapy, dosage should be reduced gradually over period of several weeks and patient closely monitored. Abrupt withdrawal in patients with angina pectoris has resulted in myocardial infarction and threatening arrhythmias.

Because propranolol impairs reflex response of the heart, manufacturer recommends that it be withdrawn gradually 48 hours prior to major surgery, with exception of patients with pheochromocytoma (however, physicians vary on this point).

Patients on prolonged therapy should be cautioned that propranolol may cause mild hypotension in some normotensive patients (experienced as dizziness or lightheadedness). Advise patient to make position changes slowly and to avoid prolonged standing.

When given for prolonged periods, periodic determinations should be made of hematologic, renal, and hepatic function.

Counsel patient to avoid excesses of alcohol, coffee, and food, and not to smoke. It is reported that smoking may cause elevation in blood pressure in some patients taking propranolol.

It may be helpful to construct a flow chart of significant parameters for the particular medical problem for which the drug is ordered.

Preserve in tightly-closed, light-resistant containers.

DRUG INTERACTIONS. Possibility that propranolol and **aminophylline** are mutually antagonistic. Propranolol may prolong hypoglycemic effects of **antidiabetic agents.** Possibility of additive hypotensive effects with **antihyper-**

tensive agents. **Atropine (and other anticholinergics)** counteract bradycardic effect of propranolol (used therapeutically). Propranolol potentiates bradycardic effect of **digitalis glycosides;** may block stimulating effects of **epinephrine** on heart (with resulting reflex bradycardia). In some patients, concurrent use with **ergot alkaloids** may produce excessive vasoconstriction. **Isoproterenol** and **levarterenol** reverse effects of propranolol, but may subject patient to severe hypotension. Propranolol may enhance therapeutic effects of **levodopa,** but also may elevate levodopa-induced plasma growth hormone levels. Theoretical possibility of interaction with **MAO inhibitors.** Additive hypotensive effect possible with **phenothiazines.** Possibility of additive cardiac depressant effect with **phenytoin** (theoretical), and with **quinidine.** Propranolol may prolong neuromuscular blockade (respiratory depression) produced by **tubocurarine** and other **muscle relaxants.**

PROPYLHEXEDRINE, N.F.
(BENZEDREX)

Adrenergic (vasoconstrictor)

ACTIONS AND USES
Volatile, indirect-acting sympathomimetic amine with vasoconstrictor and decongestant effects. Reportedly has wide margin of safety. Actions similar to those of amphetamine, but less potent as a vasoconstrictor, and has less CNS stimulant activity.
Used to relieve congestion of head cold and hay fever and for ear block and pressure pain in air travelers.
ADVERSE REACTIONS
Infrequent: stinging, irritation of nasal mucosa, temporary enlargement of nasal turbinates, rebound congestion, headache, elevation of blood pressure, insomnia (rare).
ROUTE AND DOSAGE
Topical (nasal inhalation): 2 inhalations through each nostril (approximately 0.5 mg).

NURSING IMPLICATIONS
Have patient blow nose gently before treatment to clear nasal passages.
    Instruct patient to sit upright and insert inhaler tip in one nostril, block opposite nostril, and inhale. Repeat for other nostril.
Advise not to exceed recommended dosage.

PROPYLTHIOURACIL, U.S.P.
(PTU)

Thyroid inhibitor

ACTIONS AND USES
Relatively nontoxic thioamide. Interferes with organification of iodine and blocks synthesis of thyroxine (T_4) and triiodothyronine (T_3). Does not interfere with release and utilization of stored thyroid; thus antithyroid action is delayed days and weeks until preformed T_3 and T_4 are degraded. Drug-induced hormone reduction results in compensatory release of thyrotropin (TSH), which causes marked hyperplasia and vascularization of thyroid gland. Concurrent administration of propranolol or iodine (Lugol's solution or SSKI) with propylthiouracil before surgery reduces thyroid size, friability, and vascularization.

With good adherence to drug regimen, chemical euthyroidism can be achieved 6 to 12 weeks after start of thioamide therapy. Used in medical treatment of hyperthyroidism; used to establish euthyroidism prior to surgery or radioactive treatment; used for palliative control of toxic nodular goiter. Also used to treat iodine-induced thyrotoxicosis and hyperthyroidism associated with thyroiditis.

ABSORPTION AND FATE

Absorption of effective amounts within 30 minutes after oral dose. Duration of action 2 or 3 hours; plasma half-life approximately 2 hours. 30% to 35% of drug is excreted in urine within 24 hours. Crosses placenta, inhibits fetal thyroid function, and is excreted in breast milk.

CONTRAINDICATIONS AND PRECAUTIONS

Hypersensitivity or idiosyncrasy to propylthiouracil, last trimester of pregnancy, lactation, concurrent administration of sulfonamides or coal tar derivatives such as aminopyrine or antipyrine. Cautious use: concomitant administration of anticoagulants or other drugs known to cause agranulocytosis.

ADVERSE REACTIONS

Three percent incidence: skin rash, urticaria, pruritus, nausea, vomiting, dyspepsia, arthralgia, myalgia, paresthesia, loss of taste, hyperpigmentation, abnormal hair loss, headache, vertigo, drowsiness, neuritis, edema, jaundice, sialoadenitis, lymphadenopathy, drug fever; (less frequent): myelosuppression, cholestatic jaundice, hepatitis, periarteritis, lupuslike syndrome, neuritis, hypoprothrombinemia, bleeding. **Goitrogenic hypothyroidism:** enlarged thyroid, reduced GI motility, periorbital edema, puffy hands and feet, bradycardia, cool and pale skin, worsening of ophthalmopathy, fatigue, dizziness, vertigo, sensitivity to cold, paresthesias, nocturnal muscle cramps. Altered laboratory values: protein-bound iodine decreased; radioactive iodine uptake decreased; prothrombin time increased.

ROUTE AND DOSAGE

Oral: **Adults:** initially 300 to 600 mg daily in divided doses, every 6 to 8 hours; maintenance 100 to 150 mg daily. **Pediatric** *6 to 10 years:* initially 50 to 150 mg daily; *10 years and over:* initially 150 to 300 mg daily; maintenance dose individualized.

NURSING IMPLICATIONS

Administer PTU with meals to reduce incidence of gastric distress.

Objective signs of clinical response to PTU (usually within 2 or 3 weeks): significant weight gain, reduced pulse rate, reduced serum T_4.

When thyroid gland is greatly enlarged, satisfactory euthyroid state may be delayed for several months.

Generally initial therapy covers a period of 1 or 2 years, followed by remission in 25% of patients. Medication is then stopped in the hope that natural remission will occur.

Long-term thioamide therapy is usually monitored by follow-up examinations and hematologic studies every 2 to 3 months. As soon as patient is euthyroid, thyroid hormone (especially T_3) may be added to regimen to prevent goitrogenic-induced hypothyroidism and to suppress TSH production.

If surgery fails to render patient euthyroid, PTU treatment may be reinstituted.

PTU given during pregnancy may be withdrawn 2 or 3 weeks before delivery to prevent excess drug passage across the placenta and the accompanying danger of cretinism and goiter in fetus. To prevent hypothyroidism in mother and fetus, thyroid may be given concomitantly with PTU throughout pregnancy and after delivery.

Postpartum patients receiving PTU should not nurse their babies. Exacerbation of hyperthyroidism 3 to 4 months postpartum in the mother is common; PTU therapy can be reinstituted.

The goitrogenic hypothyroid state (excess dosage) develops insidiously, and in some cases it may be noted only after an infrequent observer calls attention to changes such as periorbital edema.

Important diagnostic signs of excess dosage: contraction of a muscle bundle when pricked, mental depression, hard and nonpitting edema, and need for high thermostat setting and extra blankets in winter (cold intolerance).

Urticaria may occur (3% to 7% of patients) during period from second to eighth week of treatment. If mild, symptomatic treatment with an antihistamine may be started; switching to another thioamide is usual if rash is severe.

Warn patient to report sore throat, fever, and rash immediately (most apt to occur in first few months of treatment). Drug will be discontinued and hematologic studies initiated. If agranulocytosis is diagnosed, patient may be given broad-spectrum antibiotics and placed on reverse isolation.

Be alert to signs of hypoprothrombinemia: ecchymoses, purpura, petechiae, unexplained bleeding. Warn ambulatory patients to report these signs promptly.

Advise patients to avoid use of over-the-counter drugs for asthma, coryza, or cough treatment without checking with the physician. Iodides sometimes included in such preparations are contraindicated.

Teach patients how to take their own pulses accurately.

Clinical response is monitored through changes in weight and pulse. Advise patients to chart their weights 2 or 3 times weekly. Either the patient or a responsible other person should also record daily pulse rate. Sudden weight gain (onset of edema) and continued tachycardia should be reported as signs of inadequate clinical response.

Instruct patient in remission to continue monitoring and recording weight and pulse rate. Patient should report onset of tremor, anxiety state, gradual ascending pulse rate, and loss of weight to the physician (signs of hormone deficiency).

Some young females may have been "outeating" their hyperthyroidism and gaining weight prior to seeking treatment. Restoration of euthyroid state may be accompanied by further obesity; reduced caloric intake may be prescribed for these patients. Consult physician.

Check with physician about use of iodized salt and inclusion of seafood in the diet.

Store drug in light-resistant container.

DRUG INTERACTIONS: PTU may antagonize the action of **oral anticoagulants** (slows metabolic rate of vitamin-K-dependent clotting factors).

PROTAMINE SULFATE, U.S.P.

Antidote (to heparin)

ACTIONS AND USES

Purified mixture of simple proteins obtained from sperm or testes of suitable fish species. When used alone, has anticoagulant effect. Since it is strongly basic, protamine combines with strongly acidic heparin to produce a stable salt, thus neutralizing anticoagulant effects of both drugs. Each 1 mg of protamine neutralizes the activity of approximately 90 U.S.P. units of heparin derived from lung tissue or the activity of about 115 U.S.P. units of heparin derived from intestinal mucosa.

Used as antidote for heparin overdosage.

ABSORPTION AND FATE
Onset of heparin neutralization occurs within 5 minutes. Duration of action is about 2 hours.

CONTRAINDICATIONS AND PRECAUTIONS
Hemorrhage not induced by heparin overdosage. Reproductive studies have not been performed. Cautious use: cardiovascular disease, history of allergy to fish.

ADVERSE REACTIONS
Abrupt drop in blood pressure, bradycardia, dyspnea, transitory flushing and feeling of warmth, "heparin rebound" (hyperheparinemia), bleeding after cardiopulmonary bypass procedures or in patients undergoing extracorporeal dialysis.

ROUTE AND DOSAGE
Intravenous: administered slowly over 1- to 3-minute period. Dosage not to exceed 50 mg in any 10-minute period.

NURSING IMPLICATIONS

Monitor blood pressure and pulse every 15 to 30 minutes, or more often if indicated. Continue for at least 2 to 3 hours after each dose, or longer as dictated by patient's condition.

Patients undergoing extracorporeal dialysis or patients who have had cardiac surgery must be carefully observed for bleeding (heparin rebound). Even with apparent adequate neutralization of heparin by protamine, bleeding may occur 30 minutes to 18 hours after surgery. Monitor vital signs closely. Additional protamine may be required.

Dosage is guided by blood coagulation studies, such as the heparin titration test with protamine and the plasma thrombin time.

Drug should be stored in refrigerator, above freezing and below 50 F (10 C).

PROTEIN HYDROLYSATE (INJECTION), U.S.P.
(AMIGEN, AMINOSOL, C.P.H., HYPROTIGEN, TRAVAMIN)
PROTEIN HYDROLYSATES (ORAL)
(DELCOTABS, P.D.P. LIQUID PROTEIN)

Replenisher (fluid, nutrient)

ACTIONS AND USES
Contains amino acids and short-chain peptides derived from hydrolysis of protein (casein or fibrin). Commercial preparations differ in composition of essential and nonessential amino acids and electrolytes. Sufficient nonprotein caloric source (in the form of dextrose) must be maintained during therapy to prevent utilization of protein hydrolysate for energy rather than for protein synthesis (nitrogen-sparing effect).

Used parenterally as adjunct to prevent or reverse negative nitrogen balance when oral or tube feeding of dietary proteins is inadequate, impossible, or contraindicated. Oral formulation is used as dietary supplement to correct or prevent protein deficiency.

CONTRAINDICATIONS AND PRECAUTIONS
Hypersensitivity to any component, anuria, oliguria, severe liver disease or symptoms of impending hepatic coma, acidosis. Cautious use: hepatic and renal dysfunction, heart disease.

ADVERSE REACTIONS
With rapid IV administration: nausea, vomiting, headache, dizziness, tachycardia, hypotension, hyperglycemia, glycosuria, osmotic diuresis with dehydration. **Hypersensitivity:** fever, chills, myalgia, vasodilation, headache, abdominal pain, nausea, vomiting, urticarial rash, convulsions. **Other:** hyperammonemia (especially in infants), electrolyte imbalance, local phlebitis and

thrombosis at venipuncture site, hyperglycemia, glycosuria, osmotic diuresis with dehydration (with hyperosmolar solutions).

ROUTE AND DOSAGE

Intravenous: **Adults:** 1 to 1.5 Gm/kg daily. **Children:** 2 to 3 Gm/kg daily. Higher doses may be required in severe catabolic states. Highly individualized. Oral: 15 Gm daily.

NURSING IMPLICATIONS

Strongly hypertonic solutions should not be administered by peripheral infusion.

Hyperalimentation or total parenteral nutrition consists of infusing hypertonic solution of dextrose and protein hydrolysate into superior vena cava via subclavian or internal jugular vein. Solution is hypertonic in an amount that provides nutrients without exceeding daily fluid requirement.

Hyperalimentation requires specialized knowledge of fluid and electrolyte balance and nutritional and clinical expertise to recognize potential complications.

Because of constant risk of sepsis, mixing of dextrose with protein hydrolysate should be done in pharmacy under a laminar-flow filtered air hood or other closed system. Bottle should be labeled: time, expiration date (not to exceed 24 hours), components added, and patient's name. Sample of each solution lot should be sent to bacteriology laboratory for cultures.

Solutions should be used promptly after mixing. Any storage should be under refrigeration and limited to less than 24 hours. If solution has been refrigerated, it should be allowed to warm to room temperature before administration.

In-line bacterial filter is recommended to trap particulate matter, microorganisms, and air.

Check flow rate at least every 30 minutes, and reset to rate ordered when necessary. If administration rate falls behind schedule, no attempt should be made to catch up to planned intake. Solution must be administered at a constant rate.

Monitor vital signs. If patient suddenly develops fever or other significant adverse reaction, IV infusion should be terminated. Cultures should be taken of solution, tubing, and filter for bacterial and fungal studies.

Close observation of patient and frequent laboratory determinations are necessary during therapy (blood sugar, serum proteins, electrolytes, CBC, CO_2 combining power or content, serum and urine osmolarities, blood cultures, blood ammonia levels, kidney and liver function tests).

Accurate measurements of intake and output and daily weights (under standard conditions) provide important data for determining individual caloric and protein requirements.

In patients receiving protein hydrolysate–dextrose mixture, urine tests for glucose and acetone are done at regular intervals throughout the day, especially during first few days of therapy. Use reagents that test specifically for glucose, eg, Clinistix, Tes-Tape. Copper-reduction reagents (eg, Clinitest) may produce false positive test. Results are confirmed by blood glucose determinations as indicated. (Hyperglycemia may be controlled by decrease in flow rate or insulin administration.)

Abrupt discontinuation of protein hydrolysate–dextrose mixtures may result in rebound hypoglycemia. To prevent this possibility, dextrose 5% infusion is recommended if therapy must be stopped suddenly.

Procedure for maintenance of hyperalimentation system and catheter should be done according to hospital protocol and only by those qualified and approved following special training. Dressings are usually changed every 48 hours.

It is recommended that all IV apparatus, including filter and solution, be changed every 24 hours. Date and time of change should be indicated on record and on equipment.

Hyperalimentation system should not be used to administer drugs, withdraw blood, or measure central venous pressure because of possible danger of clotting and contamination.

Patients receiving hyperalimentation therapy require thoughtful and meticulous care, emotional support, reassurance, and explanatory answers to questions. Informed collaboration among pharmacy, medicine, and nursing personnel is critically essential.

Mouth care is an important nursing responsibility. Dryness of tongue, throat, glossitis, and parotitis are possible complications of NPO therapy. Such measures as crushed ice flavored with juice, mouth rinsing with plain or flavored tap water, brushing teeth and tongue with soft tooth brush, and daily flossing may help. Excessive use of mouth washes can change mouth flora and therefore should be discouraged.

Inform patients that stools will be reduced in size and frequency while receiving hyperalimentation therapy.

PROTOKYLOL HYDROCHLORIDE (VENTAIRE)

Adrenergic (bronchodilator)

ACTIONS AND USES
Long-acting derivative of isoproterenol, with which it shares same selective β-receptor stimulating activity, but reportedly is more stable. Contraindications, precautions, and adverse reactions similar to those of isoproterenol (qv).

Used for treatment of reversible bronchospasm associated with acute and chronic bronchial asthma, pulmonary emphysema, bronchitis, and bronchiectasis.

ABSORPTION AND FATE
Onset of action within 30 to 90 minutes; effects persist 3 to 4 hours.

CONTRAINDICATIONS AND PRECAUTIONS
Cardiac arrhythmias, coronary insufficiency. Safe use in women of childbearing potential or during pregnancy not established. Cautious use: cardiovascular disorders, diabetes mellitus, hyperthyroidism, prostatic hypertrophy, glaucoma.

ADVERSE REACTIONS
Tachycardia, palpitation, CNS stimulation (tremulousness, tenseness, insomnia, dizziness), weakness, gastric irritation, nausea, difficulty in voiding, skin rash (rare).

ROUTE AND DOSAGE
Oral: **Adult:** 2 to 4 mg 4 times a day. **Pediatric:** 1 to 2 mg 3 or 4 times/day.

NURSING IMPLICATIONS
Most side effects, principally tachycardia and palpitation, are dose-related.

Advise patient to stop medication if angina, precordial distress, or palpitation occurs and to notify the physician.

Gastric irritation may be minimized by administering drug with or after meals.

To prevent insomnia, patient should take drug at least 4 hours before bedtime.

See Isoproterenol Sulfate.

Tricyclic antidepressant

ACTIONS AND USES

Long-acting dibenzocycloheptene derivative. Shares pharmacologic actions, uses, contraindications, and toxic potential of other tricyclic antidepressants (see Imipramine). Reported to produce less sedation, to cause more cardiovascular and anticholinergic reactions, and to have more stimulatory properties than other tricyclics. Because it increases psychomotor activity, tension and anxiety may be aggravated in anxious, depressed patients.

Used to treat symptoms of mental depression in patients under close medical supervision. Particularly suitable for withdrawn and anergic patients.

ABSORPTION AND FATE

Completely absorbed from GI tract. Significant plasma levels occur within 2 hours; peak levels achieved in 24 to 30 hours, then gradually decline. Slow rate of urinary excretion; approximately 50% of dose excreted as metabolites during 16-day period. Fecal excretion negligible.

CONTRAINDICATIONS AND PRECAUTIONS

Safe use in pediatric age group not established. Cautious use: myocardial insufficiency. See Imipramine.

ROUTE AND DOSAGE

Oral: 5 to 10 mg 3 or 4 times daily. Highly individualized. As much as 60 mg/day may be required, depending on severity of symptoms. For adolescents and elderly patients: initially 5 mg 3 times daily, increased gradually, if necessary.

NURSING IMPLICATIONS

Reported to have fairly rapid onset of initial effect, characterized by increased activity and energy, usually within 1 week after therapy is initiated. Observe necessary safety precautions.

It is recommended that dosage increases, if required, be added to morning dose.

For patients with insomnia, last dose of day should be taken no later than midafternoon.

Protriptyline is associated with a relatively high incidence of palpitation, tachycardia, postural hypotension, and arrhythmias. Vital signs should be observed closely during early therapy, particularly in patients with cardiovascular disorders and in elderly patients receiving daily doses in excess of 20 mg.

Anticholinergic effects are prominent (dry mouth, blurred vision, constipation, paralytic ileus, urinary retention, delayed micturition).

Caution patient to avoid hazardous activities requiring alertness and skill, such as driving a car or operating machinery.

Maximum antidepressant effect may not occur for 2 weeks or more after therapy begins.

To reduce possibility of relapse, maintenance therapy is generally continued at least 3 months after satisfactory improvement is noted.

Patients receiving large doses for prolonged periods or in combination with other drugs should have periodic determinations of liver function and blood cell counts.

Photosensitization reactions have been reported. Caution patient to avoid direct exposure to sunlight.

See Imipramine Hydrochloride.

(BESAN, D-FEDA, NEOFED, NOVAFED, PSEUDO-BID, SUDADRINE, SUDAFED, SUDECON)

Adrenergic

ACTIONS AND USES
Sympathomimetic amine that, like ephedrine, produces decongestion of respiratory tract mucosa by action on sympathetic nerve endings. Unlike ephedrine, also acts directly on smooth muscle and constricts renal and vertebral arteries; reportedly produces fewer side effects and has less pressor action and longer duration of effects. Since it can be given orally, congestive rebound and irritation that occur with nasal sprays and solutions are obviated.

Used for symptomatic relief of nasal congestion associated with rhinitis, coryza, and sinusitis and for eustachian tube congestion.

ABSORPTION AND FATE
Onset of action within 15 to 30 minutes; peak activity in 30 to 60 minutes.

CONTRAINDICATIONS AND PRECAUTIONS
Hypersensitivity to sympathomimetic amines. Cautious use: hypertension, heart disease, glaucoma, hyperthyroidism, prostatic hypertrophy.

ADVERSE REACTIONS
Transient stimulation, tremulousness, transient increase in voiding. Sensitivity: palpitation, tachycardia, nervousness, dizziness, headache, sleeplessness, numbness of extremities, anorexia.

ROUTE AND DOSAGE
Oral: **Adults and children** *12 years and older:* 60 mg 3 or 4 times daily; *6 to 12 years:* 30 mg 3 or 4 times daily; *2 to 6 years:* 15 mg 3 or 4 times daily.

NURSING IMPLICATIONS
Since drug may act as a stimulant, advise patient to avoid taking it within 2 hours of bedtime.

Warn patient against concomitant use of over-the-counter medications containing ephedrine or other sympathomimetic amines.

Advise patient to withhold medication if extreme restlessness or signs of sensitivity occur and to consult physician.

See Ephedrine Sulfate.

PSYLLIUM HYDROPHILIC MUCILLOID
(EFFERSYLLIUM, KONSYL, L.A. FORMULA, METAMUCIL, MODANE BULK, MUCILLIUM, MUCILOSE, PLANTAMUCIN, REGACILIUM, TESTARR)

Cathartic (bulk-forming)

ACTIONS AND USES
Highly refined colloid of blond psyllium seed *(Plantago ovata)* with equal amount of dextrose added as dispersing agent. On contact with water, produces bland, lubricating, gelatinous bulk, which promotes peristalsis and natural elimination. Contains negligible amounts of sodium and about 14 calories/dose (instant-mix effervescent form is flavored and contains 0.25 Gm sodium and 43 calories/dose). Reportedly, chronic use may reduce plasma cholesterol, possibly by interfering with reabsorption of bile acids.

Used in treatment of chronic atonic or spastic constipation and in constipation associated with rectal disorders or anorectal surgery.

CONTRAINDICATIONS AND PRECAUTIONS
Intestinal obstruction, fecal impaction, abdominal pain.
ROUTE AND DOSAGE
Oral: **Adults:** 1 rounded teaspoonful or 1 packet (instant mix) 1 to 3 times a day.
Children *6 years and over:* 1 level teaspoonful a day.

NURSING IMPLICATIONS

Instruct patient to fill an ordinary water glass with cool water, milk, fruit juice, or other liquid, sprinkle powder into liquid, stir briskly, and drink immediately (if effervescent form is used, add liquid to powder).
Best results are obtained if each dose is followed by an additional glass of liquid.
Laxative effect usually occurs within 12 to 24 hours. Administration for 2 or 3 days may be needed to establish regularity.
Inform patient that drug may reduce appetite if taken before meals.
See Bisacodyl for patient teaching points.

PYRANTEL PAMOATE, U.S.P.
(ANTIMINTH)

Anthelmintic

ACTIONS AND USES
Exerts selective depolarizing neuromuscular blocking action, which results in spastic paralysis of worm.
Used in *Enterobius vermicularis* (pinworm) and *Ascaris lumbricoides* (roundworm) infestations.
ABSORPTION AND FATE
Partially absorbed from GI tract. Plasma levels of unchanged drug, which are low, peak in 1 to 3 hours. Metabolized in liver. Over 50% excreted in feces unchanged within 24 hours; about 7% eliminated in urine as free drug and metabolites.
CONTRAINDICATIONS AND PRECAUTIONS
Safe use during pregnancy and in children under 2 years of age not established. Cautious use: liver dysfunction.
ADVERSE REACTIONS
Anorexia, nausea, vomiting, abdominal cramps, diarrhea, tenesmus, transient elevation of SGOT, dizziness, headache, drowsiness, insomnia, skin rashes.
ROUTE AND DOSAGE
Oral: **Adults and children:** 11 mg pyrantel base/kg body weight administered in a single dose. Maximum total dose 1 Gm.

NURSING IMPLICATIONS

Shake suspension well before pouring to assure accurate dosage.
May be taken with milk or fruit juices and without regard to prior ingestion of food or time of day.
Purging is not necessary before, during, or after therapy.
See Piperazine for patient teaching points.

DRUG INTERACTIONS: There is a possibility that pyrantel and **piperazine** are mutually antagonistic.

(Aldinamide, PZA, Zinamide)

Antibacterial (tuberculostatic)

ACTIONS AND USES
Pyrazinoic acid amide, chemically similar to niacin. When employed alone, resistance may develop in 6 to 7 weeks; therefore, administration with other effective agents is recommended. Appears to interfere with renal capacity to concentrate and excrete uric acid; thus may cause hyperuricemia.
Used with other effective antituberculosis drugs for all forms of active tuberculosis when treatment with primary agents (eg, isoniazid, streptomycin, ethambutol) has failed.

ABSORPTION AND FATE
Readily absorbed from GI tract. Peak serum concentrations in about 2 hours, declining thereafter; half-life approximately 9 hours. Metabolized in liver. Slowly excreted in urine; 30% eliminated as metabolites and 4% as unchanged drug within 24 hours.

CONTRAINDICATIONS AND PRECAUTIONS
Severe hepatic damage. Safe use in children not established. Cautious use: presence or family history of gout or diabetes mellitus, impaired renal function, history of peptic ulcer.

ADVERSE REACTIONS
Arthralgia, active gout, difficulty in urination, headache, photosensitivity, urticaria, skin rash (rare), sideroblastic or hemolytic anemia, splenomegaly, lymphadenopathy, fatal hemoptysis, aggravation of peptic ulcer, rise in serum uric acid, hepatotoxicity, abnormal liver function tests, acute yellow atrophy of liver, decreased plasma prothrombin.

ROUTE AND DOSAGE:
Oral: 20 to 35 mg/kg/day in 3 or 4 divided doses; maximal dosage of 3 Gm/day is not to be exceeded.

NURSING IMPLICATIONS
Patients receiving pyrazinamide require close observation and medical supervision.
Drug should be discontinued if hepatic reactions or hyperuricemia with acute gout occur. (Normal serum uric acid: males, 2.1–7.8 mg/dl; females, 2.0 to 6.4 mg/dl).
Patients should be examined at regular intervals and questioned about possible signs of toxicity: liver enlargement or tenderness, jaundice, fever, anorexia, malaise, impaired vascular integrity (ecchymoses, petechiae, abnormal bleeding).
Hepatic reactions appear to occur more frequently in patients receiving high doses.
Liver function tests (especially SGOT, SGPT, serum bilirubin) should be done prior to and at 2- to 4-week intervals during therapy. Blood uric acid determinations are advised before, during, and following therapy.
Report to physician the onset of joint pains or difficulty in voiding.
Aspirin in large doses (eg, 3 to 5 Gm/day) or other uricosuric agents may be prescribed to control hyperuricemia.
Patients with diabetes should be closely monitored for possible loss of control.

LABORATORY TEST INTERFERENCES: Pyrazinamide may produce a temporary decrease in 17-ketosteroids and an increase in protein-bound iodine.

Cholinergic

ACTIONS AND USES

Synthetic quaternary ammonium compound similar to neostigmine (qv) in actions, contraindications, precautions, and adverse reactions. Has longer duration of action than does neostigmine, and reportedly produces less GI and other muscarinic side effects.

Used in treatment of myasthenia gravis. Has been used with ephedrine and/or potassium chloride to increase patient response. Used parenterally as antagonist to nondepolarizing muscle relaxants.

ABSORPTION AND FATE

Poorly absorbed from GI tract; onset of action in 30 to 45 minutes, with duration of 3 to 6 hours. Action begins within 15 minutes following IM and 2 to 5 minutes after IV injection. Metabolized in liver. Excreted in urine as metabolites and free drug up to 72 hours after a single IV dose. Reportedly metabolized and excreted more rapidly in patients with severe myasthenia. Crosses placenta.

CONTRAINDICATIONS AND PRECAUTIONS

Hypersensitivity to anticholinesterase agents or to bromides. Safe use in women of childbearing potential and use during pregnancy or lactation not established. Cautious use: bronchial asthma, cardiac dysrhythmias. See Neostigmine.

ADVERSE REACTIONS

Acneiform (bromide) rash, thrombophlebitis (following IV administration). With large doses: headache, increased peristaltic activity, diarrhea, abdominal cramps, increased bronchial secretions, bronchoconstriction, muscle weakness. Also see Neostigmine.

ROUTE AND DOSAGE

Oral (myasthenia gravis): **Adults**: dosage range 60 mg to 1.5 Gm daily, spaced according to requirements and response of patient. Timespan tablets: one to three 180-mg tablets once or twice daily, at intervals of at least 6 hours. **Children**: 7 mg/kg/24 hours divided into 5 or 6 doses. Intramuscular, intravenous: **Adults:** approximately 1/30 of usual (myasthenic) oral dose; (for reversal of muscle relaxants): IV 10 to 20 mg, followed shortly by IV atropine. **Neonates:** IM 0.05–0.15 mg/kg.

NURSING IMPLICATIONS

Failure of patient to show improvement may reflect either underdosage or overdosage. Report increasing muscular weakness, cramps, or fasciculations. See neostigmine for differentiation between myasthenic and cholinergic crises.

Observe for cholinergic reactions, particularly when drug is administered IV.

Duration of drug action reportedly may vary with physical and emotional stress, as well as with severity of disease.

Timespan tablets are generally prescribed only at bedtime for patients who complain of weakness on awakening.

Neonates of myasthenic mothers who have received pyridostigmine should be closely observed for difficulty in breathing, swallowing, or sucking.

When used as muscle relaxant antagonist, patient should be continuously observed. Airway and repiratory assistance must be maintained until full recovery of voluntary respiration and neuromuscular transmission is assured. Complete recovery usually occurs within 30 minutes.

Report onset of rash. Drug discontinuation may be indicated.

Timespan tablets may become mottled in appearance; this does not affect their potency.

Pyridostigmine syrup should be protected from light.

See Neostigmine.

DRUG INTERACTIONS: There is the possibility that **methocarbamol** may impair pyridostigmine effects. Also see neostigmine.

PYRIDOXINE HYDROCHLORIDE, U.S.P., B.P.
(BEESIX, HEXA-BETALIN, HEXAVIBEX, HYDOXIN, VITAMIN B$_6$)

Vitamin (enzyme cofactor)

ACTIONS AND USES

Water-soluble complex of three closely related compounds (pyridoxine and its active derivatives pyridoxamine and pyridoxal). Considered essential to human nutrition, although a deficiency syndrome is not well defined. Apparently converted in body to pyridoxal, a coenzyme important in protein, fat, and carbohydrate metabolism and in facilitating release of glycogen from liver and muscle. In protein metabolism, participates in many enzymatic transformations of amino acids and conversion of tryptophan to niacin and serotonin. Aids in energy transformation in brain and nerve cells, and is thought to stimulate heme production.

Used in prophylaxis and treatment of pyridoxine deficiency, as seen with inadequate dietary intake, drug-induced deficiency (eg, isoniazid, oral contraceptives), and inborn errors of metabolism (vitamin-B$_6$-dependent convulsions or anemia). Also has been used to prevent chloramphenicol-induced optic neuritis, toxic CNS effects of cycloserine, and alcoholic polyneuritis, as well as to control nausea and vomiting in radiation sickness and pregnancy.

ABSORPTION AND FATE

Readily absorbed following oral and parenteral administration. Half-life 15 to 20 days. Degraded in liver and excreted in urine primarily as 4-pyridoxic acid.

CONTRAINDICATIONS AND PRECAUTIONS

History of hypersensitivity to pyridoxine.

ADVERSE REACTIONS

Rarely: paresthesias, somnolence (particularly following large parenteral doses), slight flushing or feeling of warmth, low folic acid levels, temporary burning or stinging pain in injection site.

ROUTE AND DOSAGE

Oral, intramuscular, intravenous: *dietary deficiency:* 10 to 20 mg daily for 3 weeks; follow-up treatment with oral therapeutic multivitamin preparation containing 2 to 5 mg pyridoxine for several weeks. *Vitamin B$_6$ deficiency syndrome:* 600 mg/day may be required; maintenance 30 mg for life. *Isoniazid-induced deficiency:* 100 mg daily for 3 weeks; maintenance 50 mg daily. In isoniazid poisoning (ingestion of more than 10 Gm), an equal amount of pyridoxine should be given: 4 Gm IV followed by 1 Gm IM every 30 minutes.

NURSING IMPLICATIONS

Therapeutic effectiveness of vitamin B$_6$ therapy is evaluated by improvement of deficiency manifestations: nausea, vomiting, skin lesions resembling those of riboflavin and niacin deficiency (seborrhealike lesions about eyes, nose, and mouth, glossitis, stomatitis), edema, CNS symptoms (depression, irritability, peripheral neuritis, convulsions), hypochromic microcytic anemia.

Collaborate with physician, dietitian, patient, and a responsible family member in planning for diet teaching. A complete dietary history should be recorded so that poor eating habits can be identified and corrected (a single vitamin deficiency is rare; patient can be expected to have multiple vitamin deficiencies).

Recommended dietary allowance (RDA) of pyridoxine: 2 mg for adults; 2.5 mg during pregnancy and lactation. Need for pyridoxine increases with amount of protein in diet.

Rich dietary sources of vitamin B_6 include yeast, wheat germ, whole grain cereals, muscle and glandular meats (especially liver), legumes, green vegetables, bananas.

Preserved in tight, light-resistant containers.

DRUG INTERACTIONS: Pyridoxine (in doses of 5 mg or more daily) appears to enhance the peripheral metabolism of **levodopa** and thus may greatly reduce or abolish its therapeutic effects.

PYRILAMINE MALEATE, N.F.
(ALLERTOC, NISAVAL, PARAMINYL, PYRA-MALEATE, ZEM-HISTINE)
MEPYRAMINE MALEATE, B.P.

Antihistaminic

ACTIONS AND USES

Ethylenediamine derivative similar to tripelennamine (qv) in actions.

Used for allergic rhinitis and conjunctivitis, vasomotor rhinitis, mild urticaria, and angioedema. Included in a number of OTC antitussive formulations.

CONTRAINDICATIONS AND PRECAUTIONS

History of hypersensitivity to pyrilamine. Cautious use: children under 6 years of age.

ADVERSE REACTIONS

GI distress: anorexia, nausea, vomiting, dry mouth. Excessive dosage in children: convulsions. Also see Tripelennamine.

ROUTE AND DOSAGE

Oral: **Adults**: 25 to 50 mg every 6 to 8 hours; **children** *6 to 12 years:* 12.5 to 25 mg every 6 to 8 hours.

NURSING IMPLICATIONS

GI side effects may be minimized by taking drug with meals or with milk.

Although the incidence of drowsiness is low, caution the patient to avoid hazardous activities such as driving a car or operating machinery until reaction to drug is known.

See Tripelennamine.

PYRIMETHAMINE, U.S.P., B.P.
(DARAPRIM)

Antimalarial

ACTIONS AND USES

Long-acting folic acid antagonist chemically related to metabolite of chloroguanide. Selectively inhibits dehydrofolic reductase in parasite and thereby interferes with its ability to metabolize folic acid. Has no gametocidal activity, but prevents development of fertilized gametes in mosquito and thus helps to pre-vent transmission of malaria. Since action against blood-borne schizonts is slow in onset, has little value as single agent in treatment of acute primary malarial attack. Cross-resistance with chloroguanide may occur.

Used for prophylaxis of malaria due to susceptible strains of plasmodia. May be used conjointly with fast-acting schizonticide (eg, chloroquine, quinine) to initiate transmission control and suppressive cure. Used with a sulfonamide to provide synergistic action in treatment of toxoplasmosis.

ABSORPTION AND FATE

Well absorbed from GI tract; peak plasma concentrations in about 2 hours. Concentrates mainly in kidneys, lungs, liver, spleen. Slowly excreted in urine; excretion may extend over 30 days or longer. Appears in breast milk.

CONTRAINDICATIONS AND PRECAUTIONS

Chloroguanide-resistant malaria. Safe use during pregnancy not established. Cautious use: high doses in patients with convulsive disorders.

ADVERSE REACTIONS

With large doses or prolonged therapy: anorexia, vomiting, atrophic glossitis, skin rashes, folic acid deficiency (megaloblastic anemia, leukopenia, throm-bocytopenia, pancytopenia, diarrhea). Acute toxicity: CNS stimulation, includ-ing convulsions, respiratory failure.

ROUTE AND DOSAGE

Oral: *Malaria chemoprophylaxis:* **Adults and children** *over 10 years:* 25 mg once weekly; **Children** *4 through 10 years:* 12.5 mg once weekly; **Infants and children** *under 4 years:* 6.25 mg once weekly. *Toxoplasmosis:* **Adults:** initially 50 to 75 mg daily (together with a sulfonamide) for 1 to 3 weeks, depending on patient's tolerance and response; dosage may then be reduced by one-half for each drug and continued an additional 4 or 5 weeks. **Children:** 1 mg/kg/day divided into 2 equal daily doses (used together with sulfonamide); similar regimen as for adults.

NURSING IMPLICATIONS

GI distress may be minimized by taking drug with meals. If symptoms persist, dosage reduction may be necessary.

For malaria prophylaxis, drug should be taken on same day each week. Administration should begin when individual enters malarious area and should continue for 10 weeks after leaving the area.

Dosages required for treatment of toxoplasmosis approach toxic levels. Blood counts, including platelets, should be performed twice weekly dur-ing therapy. If hematologic abnormalities appear, dosage should be re-duced or drug discontinued; parenteral leucovorin (folinic acid) will be administered until blood counts return to normal.

Some physicians prescribe leucovorin concurrently to patients on high-dos-age therapy to prevent hematologic complications.

Advise patient to report immediately to physician the appearance of diar-rhea, fever, sore tongue, or rash.

Caution patient to keep drug out of reach of children. Fatalities from acci-dental poisoning have been reported.

Treatment of overdosage: gastric lavage; have on hand parenteral short-acting barbiturate, leucovorin (folinic acid), and facilities for artificial respiration.

DRUG INTERACTIONS: Antitoxoplasmic effects of pyrimethamine may be de-creased by **folic acid** and **para-aminobenzoic acid.** Pyrimethamine may in-crease **quinine** blood levels (displaces quinine from plasma binding sites).

(PYRONIL)

Antihistaminic

ACTIONS AND USES
Long-acting propylamine (alkylamine) antihistamine with low incidence of side effects. Has slow onset of action, but effects may last 9 to 11 hours. Shares actions, uses, contraindications, and precautions of other antihistamines. See Chlorpheniramine.

ROUTE AND DOSAGE
Oral: **Adults:** 15 to 30 mg 2 or 3 times daily. **Children:** 0.6 mg/kg body weight daily in 2 or 3 divided doses.

NURSING IMPLICATIONS
Commercially available tablets may be crushed and administered with food.
Preserved in tight, light-resistant containers.
See Chlorpheniramine Maleate.

PYRVINIUM PAMOATE, U.S.P.
(POVAN)
VIPRYNIUM EMBONATE, B.P.

Anthelmintic

ACTIONS AND USES
Cyanine dye. Appears to kill parasite by depleting carbohydrate stores; prevents parasite from using exogenous carbohydrate.
Used to control pinworm *(Enterobius vermicularis)* infestations (enterobiasis).

ABSORPTION AND FATE
Not appreciably absorbed from GI tract. Approximately 60% of dose is excreted in feces; small amounts appear in urine, blood, bile.

CONTRAINDICATIONS AND PRECAUTIONS
Inflammatory conditions of GI tract, intestinal obstruction. Safe use during pregnancy not established. Cautious use: children weighing less than 10 kg, renal or hepatic disease.

ROUTE AND DOSAGE
Oral (**Adults and children**): 5 mg/kg body weight, as a single dose (maximum adult dosage 350 mg). If necessary, dose may be repeated in 2 to 3 weeks.

NURSING IMPLICATIONS
Administer drug before or after a meal.
Caution patient to swallow tablets whole to avoid staining teeth (bright red).
GI side effects appear to occur more frequently with emulsion than with tablets, as well as in older children and in adults receiving high dosages.
Inform the patient that drug will cause a harmless bright red staining of stools and vomitus and that suspension form will stain clothing if spilled.
Pyrvinium (Povan) tablets should not be used in individuals sensitive to aspirin because of possible cross-sensitivity between tartrazine contained in tablet coating and aspirin. Suspension may be used.
When pinworm infection is found in a single member of a family or institution group, treatment of all members should be considered.
Pinworms are transmitted by direct transfer of infective eggs on hands (from

anus) to mouth, or indirectly by clothing, bedding, food, or other contaminated articles. Dustborne infection by inhalation is also possible in heavily contaminated households.

Instruct patient and family in personal hygiene: wash hands after defecation and before eating or preparing foods; keep nails short and avoid biting nails; daily bathing (showers preferable to tub baths); change bed linen and underwear daily (eggs are destroyed by household washing solutions).

Follow-up examination for pinworm ova should be done at least 5 weeks after end of treatment. Specimens are best procured on arising in the morning, before bathing, breakfast, or defecation. Female worms lay eggs at night in perianal region. Specimen is obtained by applying cellulose tape swab to contaminated areas; they are then transferred to glass slide for microscopic examination.

Protect suspension form from light.

Q

QUINACRINE HYDROCHLORIDE, U.S.P.
(ATABRINE)
MEPACRINE HYDROCHLORIDE, B.P.

Anthelmintic, antimalarial

ACTIONS AND USES

Acridine dye derivative. Eradicates beef, pork, dwarf, and fish tapeworm and *Giardia lamblia* by causing worm scolex to detach from intestinal tract. In neoplastic disease, intracavitary instillations appear to inhibit effusions by inducing inflammatory reaction of serosa, with subsequent production of local fibrotic adhesions. Acts as suppressive agent and controls clinical attacks of malaria, but is not a true causal prophylactic agent, nor does it produce radical cure. Also exerts anticonvulsant effect by unknown mechanism.

Used in treatment of tapeworm infestations and giardiasis. Use as antimalarial has been largely superseded by more effective and less toxic drugs. Also used in management of recurrent pleural and peritoneal effusions secondary to metastatic carcinoma and to control petit mal seizures in patients unresponsive to other drugs.

ABSORPTION AND FATE

Readily absorbed from GI tract. Widely distributed in tissues, and accumulates when administered chronically. Concentrates in liver, lungs, pancreas, erythrocytes. Excreted slowly, primarily in urine; small amounts eliminated in sweat, saliva, bile, milk. Significant amounts still detectable in urine for at least 2 months after discontinuation of oral drug. Crosses placenta.

CONTRAINDICATIONS AND PRECAUTIONS

Psoriasis, porphyria, pregnancy, concomitant use of primaquine, intracavitary use in patients with pneumothorax. Cautious use: patients over age 60, young children, history of psychosis, hepatic disease, alcoholism, concomitant use with hepatotoxic drugs, patients with glucose-6-phosphate dehydrogenase deficiency.

ADVERSE REACTIONS

Oral use: **GI:** nausea, vomiting, anorexia, abdominal cramps. **Dermatologic:** yellow pigmentation, urticaria, exfoliative dermatitis, contact dermatitis, lichen-planus-like eruptions. **Neuropsychiatric:** headache, dizziness; CNS stimulation: restlessness, confusion, irritability, emotional changes, insomnia, nightmares, psychotic reactions, convulsions (large doses). **Other** (usually with prolonged therapy): aplastic anemia, agranulocytosis, hepatitis, corneal edema or deposits (reversible), retinopathy (rare). *Intracavitary use* (in addition to those associated with oral use): fever, pleural or peritoneal pain, paralytic ileus, dyspnea.

ROUTE AND DOSAGE

Oral: *Beef, pork, or fish tapeworm:* **Adults**: 200 mg given 10 minutes apart for 4 doses; sodium bicarbonate 600 mg with each dose. **Children** *5 to 10 years:* total dose 400 mg; *11 to 14 years:* total dose 600 mg, divided into 3 or 4 doses administered 10 minutes apart; sodium bicarbonate 300 mg may be given with each dose. *Dwarf tapeworm:* **Adults**: 900 mg in 3 portions 20 minutes apart, then 100 mg 3 times daily for 3 days. **Children** *4 to 8 years:* initially 200 mg, then 100 mg after breakfast for 3 days; *8 to 10 years:* initially 300 mg, then 100 mg twice daily for 3 days; *11 to 14 years:* initially 400 mg, then 100 mg 3 times daily for 3 days. *Giardiasis:* **Adults**: 100 mg 3 times daily for 7 days. **Children**: 7 mg/kg/day in 3 divided doses (maximum 300 mg/day) for 5 days. *Neoplastic effusions (intrapleural, intraperitoneal:* 200 mg to 1 Gm. Powder may be dissolved in 10 ml effusion fluid

or sterile water for injection. *Malaria suppression:* **Adults**: 100 mg once daily.
Children: 50 mg daily.

NURSING IMPLICATIONS
General Information:
Inform patients that drug imparts a reversible yellow coloration to skin (not jaundice) and urine and sometimes may cause a grayish blue tinge to ears, nasal cartilage, and fingernail beds resembling cyanosis. Skin discoloration usually disappears in about 2 weeks after drug is discontinued.

Complete blood counts and ophthalmoscopic examinations should be done periodically in patients on prolonged drug therapy.

Advise patients to report immediately the onset of skin eruptions or visual disturbances; eg, halos of light, focusing difficulties, blurred vision.

Be alert for symptoms of drug-induced behavioral changes and psychosis. Psychotic reactions may last 2 to 4 weeks after drug is stopped.

Caution patients to keep drug out of reach of children.

Tapeworm infestations:
Patient is given a bland liquid or no-residue semisolid, nonfat diet for 24 to 48 hours before start of drug therapy, with fasting after evening meal before and on morning of treatment.

Generally, a saline purge and cleansing enema are given before treatment to reduce amount of stool that must be examined for scolex. Saline purge is repeated 1 to 2 hours after quinacrine is administered. Sodium bicarbonate is prescribed with each dose of quinacrine to reduce tendency to nausea and vomiting.

Entire stool specimen is collected for 48 hours and passed through sieve or cheesecloth to find the scolex (worm head). Provide receptacle for toilet paper, which should not be put in bedpan. Search for scolex is facilitated by using ultraviolet light (worm becomes fluorescent when it absorbs quinacrine). Worm is usually passed within 4 to 10 hours, alive, stained yellow, in one piece or segmented. Cure is presumed if scolex of beef, pork, or fish tapeworm is found; dwarf tapeworm infestations are usually multiple and require more persistent treatment.

If scolex is not found, stools should be examined periodically; they must be free of worm eggs or segments for 3 to 6 months to be certain of cure.

For pork tapeworm *(Taenia solium),* drug is administered by duodenal tube to prevent vomiting. Vomiting may cause passage of worm segments (proglottids) into stomach, with subsequent release of ova and invasion of tissue (cysticercosis).

Giardiasis:
Administer quinacrine after meals; stools are examined 2 weeks after last dose. Repeat course may be given, if indicated.

Neoplastic effusions:
Consult physician regarding posttreatment positions of patient to enhance drug distribution.

Most patients complain of pain shortly after intracavitary administration. Analgesia may be necessary.

Monitor vital signs. Fever may occur 4 to 8 hours after drug is given and usually lasts only a few hours; however, in some patients it may persist up to 10 days (degree and duration of fever appear to be dose-related). Observe patient for dyspnea, especially after intrapleural administration.

Antimalarial use:
Quinacrine should be taken after meals with a full glass of water, tea, or fruit juice.

For suppression of malaria, medication should be taken for 1 to 3 months.

LABORATORY TEST INTERFERENCES: Possibility of false positive adrenal function tests using Mattingly method (quinacrine is fluorescent in aqueous media).

DRUG INTERACTIONS: Concurrent use of **alcohol** with quinacrine may result in disulfiramlike reaction (due to accumulation of acetaldehyde). Quinacrine enhances toxicity of **primaquine.**

QUINETHAZONE, N.F.
(HYDROMOX)

Diuretic, antihypertensive

ACTIONS AND USES
Sulfonamide derivative chemically different from but pharmacologically similar to thiazides in actions, uses, contraindications, precautions, and adverse reactions. Has mild antihypertensive actions when used alone, and enhances effects of other antihypertensive agents when given in combination. See Chlorothiazide.
ABSORPTION AND FATE
Rapidly absorbed from GI tract. Onset of diuretic effect within 2 hours; peak effect at 6 hours; duration 18 to 24 hours. Excreted unchanged in kidneys. Crosses placenta.
ROUTE AND DOSAGE
Oral: 50 to 100 mg daily. Dose range: 50 to 200 mg daily.

NURSING IMPLICATIONS
Because diuretic action is relatively prolonged, a single daily dose administered in the morning is generally sufficient.
Be alert to complaints of joint pain. Drug may precipitate gout attack.
See Chlorothiazide.

QUINIDINE GLUCONATE, U.S.P.
(QUINAGLUTE)

Cardiac depressant (antiarrhythmic)

ACTIONS AND USES
Dextro isomer of quinine. Similar to quinidine sulfate in actions, uses, contraindications, and adverse reactions. Parenteral form used when oral therapy not feasible or when rapid effects are required. Contains 62.3% anhydrous quinidine alkaloid.
ABSORPTION AND FATE
Onset of action in 15 minutes following IM injection; peak effect in 30 to 90 minutes; duration of action 4 to 6 hours. Peak effect in 4 to 6 minutes following IV administration.
ADVERSE REACTIONS
Particularly with IV use: nausea, vomiting, abdominal cramps, urge to defecate or urinate, cold sweat, apprehension, severe hypotension. See Quinidine Sulfate.
ROUTE AND DOSAGE
Highly individualized. Oral (maintenance and prophylaxis): extended-release form, 1 or 2 tablets every 12 hours, or every 8 hours. Each tablet contains 324 mg quinidine gluconate. Intramuscular (acute tachycardia): initially 600 mg;

subsequently 400 mg may be repeated as often as every 2 hours, depending on need and response of patient. Intravenous: 200 to 750 mg. Suggested rate of administration: 1 ml (16 mg)/minute.

NURSING IMPLICATIONS

Examine parenteral solution before preparation; use only if clear and colorless.

An initial test dose (200 mg IM) is advised to determine idiosyncrasy, particularly if patient has not received quinidine before and if time permits.

Continuous monitoring of ECG and blood pressure and frequent determinations of plasma quinidine levels are advised when drug is administered intravenously.

Observe monitor before administration of each parenteral dose.

The following are indications to stop quinidine; report their onset immediately to physician: (1) worsening of minor side effects; (2) restoration of sinus rhythm; (3) prolongation of QRS complex (beyond 25%); (4) changes in Q-T or refractory period; (5) disappearance of P waves; (6) sudden onset of or increase in PVCs; (7) decrease in heart rate to 120 beats/minute.

When administering drug IM, aspirate carefully before injection to avoid inadvertent entry into blood vessel.

Severe hypotension is most likely to occur in patients receiving drug IV. Supine position during drug administration is advisable.

Observe patient closely following each parenteral dose. Amount of subsequent dose is gauged by response to preceding dose.

Extended-action tablet is used only for maintenance and prophylactic therapy.

GI distress may be minimized by administration of oral drug with food.

Oral quinidine gluconate is considerably more expensive than quinidine sulfate.

Protect solutions from light and heat to prevent brownish discoloration and possible precipitation.

Also see Quinidine Sulfate.

QUINIDINE POLYGALACTURONATE
(CARDIOQUIN)

Cardiac depressant (antiarrhythmic)

ACTIONS AND USES

Reported to have lower incidence of GI irritation than quinidine sulfate.

ROUTE AND DOSAGE

Oral: initially 1 to 3 tablets every 3 or 4 hours for 4 or more doses. (Each 275-mg tablet equivalent to 200 mg of quinidine sulfate); maintenance: 1 tablet 2 or 3 times a day.

NURSING IMPLICATIONS

See Quinidine Sulfate.

(CIN-QUIN, MASO-QUIN, QUINIDEX, QUINORA, SK-QUINIDINE SULFATE)

Cardiac depressant (antiarrhythmic)

ACTIONS AND USES

Dextro isomer of quinine and alkaloid of *Cinchona.* Like quinine, exhibits some antimalarial, antipyretic, and oxytocic properties. Contains 82.86% anhydrous quinidine alkaloid. Cardiac actions similar to those of procainamide. At the cellular level, decreases sodium influx during depolarization and potassium efflux in repolarization; also reduces calcium transport across cell membrane. Depresses myocardial excitability, contractility, automaticity, and conduction velocity, and prolongs effective refractory period. Anticholinergic action blocks vagal stimulation of A-V node, thus tending to increase ventricular rate, particularly in larger doses. Also exerts muscle relaxant action by decreasing effective transmission across neuromuscular junction. Hypotensive effect is produced primarily by peripheral vasodilation and in part by α-adrenergic blockade.

Used in treatment of atrial fibrillation, atrial flutter, paroxysmal supraventricular and ventricular tachycardia, and premature systoles. Has been used in treatment of intractable hiccups and as diagnostic measure in Wolff-Parkinson-White syndrome.

ABSORPTION AND FATE

Almost completely absorbed following oral administration. Maximal effects within 1 to 3 hours, persisting 6 to 8 hours or more. Widely distributed in body tissues, except brain. At therapeutic blood levels, about 60% strongly bound to plasma albumin. Plasma half-life 4 to 6 hours. Largely metabolized in liver. Approximately 10% to 50% excreted in urine within 24 hours as unchanged drug, and remainder as metabolites. Urinary pH influences excretion rate (alkalinization decreases and acidification increases excretion).

CONTRAINDICATIONS AND PRECAUTIONS

Hypersensitivity or idiosyncrasy to quinidine or *Cinchona* derivatives, thrombocytopenic purpura resulting from prior use of quinidine, intraventricular conduction defects, complete A-V block, digitalis intoxication, ectopic impulses and rhythms due to escape mechanisms, thyrotoxicosis, acute rheumatic fever, subacute bacterial endocarditis, extensive myocardial damage, frank congestive heart failure, hypotensive states. Cautious use: incomplete heart block, impaired renal or hepatic function, bronchial asthma or other respiratory disorders, myasthenia gravis, potassium imbalance.

ADVERSE REACTIONS

Cinchonism: diarrhea, abdominal cramps, nausea, vomiting, cutaneous flushing, intense pruritus, sweating, palpitation, headache, lightheadedness, vertigo, tinnitus, impaired hearing, visual disturbances, skin eruptions. **CNS:** restlessness, tremors, apprehension, excitement, confusion, delirium. **Cardiovascular:** hypotension, congestive failure, bradycardia, heart block, atrial flutter, ventricular flutter, fibrillation or tachycardia, "quinidine syncope," extrasystoles, embolization, cardiac standstill. **Hypersensitivity or idiosyncrasy:** may include symptoms of cinchonism plus fever, urticaria, angioedema, dizziness, polyarthralgia, bitter taste, salivation, dyspnea, asthma, respiratory depression or arrest, vascular collapse. **Hematologic:** acute hemolytic anemia, hypoprothrombinemia, thrombocytopenic purpura (rare), leukopenia, agranulocytosis (rare).

ROUTE AND DOSAGE

Dosages individualized according to patient's requirements and responses. Oral: **Adults:** *Test dose:* 200 mg. *Ectopic beats:* 200 to 300 mg 3 or 4 times daily. *Ventricular tachycardia:* 400 to 600 mg every 2 or 3 hours until paroxysms terminate. *Atrial flutter:* patient digitalized before receiving quinidine. Highly individualized dosage. *Atrial fibrillation* (various schedules): 200 mg every 2 or 3 hours for 5 to 8 doses; subsequent daily increase of individual dose until sinus rhythm restored or toxic effects intervene (ventricular rate and/or congestive failure controlled by digitalis prior to quinidine therapy). Total daily dose not to exceed 3 to 4 Gm. Maintenance: 200 to 300 mg 3 or 4 times daily at 6-hour intervals. Extended-action tablet: 300 mg every 8 to 12 hours. **Children:** Test dose: 2 mg/kg. Therapeutic dose: 6 mg/kg 5 times daily.

NURSING IMPLICATIONS

Test dose is advised to determine idiosyncrasy before establishing full dosage schedule.

GI symptoms (nausea, vomiting, diarrhea are most common) due to local drug irritant effect may be minimized by administering drug with food.

Extended-action tablet is usually reserved for maintenance and prophylactic therapy.

Continuous monitoring of ECG and blood pressure is required. Close observation of patient (check sensorium and be alert for any sign of toxicity) and frequent determinations of plasma quinidine levels are indicated when large doses (more than 2 Gm/day) are used or when quinidine is given parenterally (eg, quinidine gluconate).

Observe cardiac monitor and report immediately the following: (1) restoration of sinus rhythm; (2) widening QRS complex in excess of 25% (ie, greater than 0.12 seconds); (3) changes in Q-T or refractory period; (4) disappearance of P waves; (5) sudden onset of or increase in ectopic ventricular beats (extrasystoles, PVCs); (6) decrease in heart rate to 120 beats/minute. Also report immediately any worsening of minor side effects. All are indications for stopping quinidine, at least temporarily.

Dosage is adjusted to maintain drug concentration between 3 and 6 mg/liter of plasma. Levels of 8 mg/liter or more are associated with myocardial toxicity.

During acute treatment, monitor vital signs every 1 to 2 hours (frequency depends on individual patient requirements and dosage used). Count apical pulse for a full minute. Report any change in pulse rate, rhythm, or quality or any fall in blood pressure.

Severe hypotension is most likely to occur in patients receiving high oral doses (or parenteral quinidine).

Reversion to sinus rhythm in long-standing fibrillation, or when complicated by congestive failure, involves some risk of embolization from dislodgement of atrial mural emboli.

Bear in mind that quinidine can cause unpredictable rhythm abnormalities in the digitalized heart. Patients with atrial flutter or fibrillation may be pretreated with digitalis to increase A-V nodal block and thus reduce possibility of paradoxic tachycardia.

Monitor intake and output. Diarrhea occurs commonly during early therapy; most patients become tolerant to this side effect. If symptoms become severe, serum electrolytes and acid–base and fluid balance should be evaluated. Dosage adjustment may be required.

During long-term therapy, periodic blood counts, serum electrolyte determinations, and kidney and liver function tests are advised.

Hypersensitivity reactions usually appear 3 to 20 days after drug is started. Fever occurs commonly and may or may not be accompanied by other symptoms.

Instruct patient to report feeling of faintness ("quinidine syncope"). Symptom is caused by quinidine-induced changes in ventricular rhythm (eg, tachycardia, fibrillation) with resulting decrease in cardiac output and loss of consciousness (syncope).

Also advise patient to notify physician immediately of disturbances in vision, ringing in ears, sense of breathlessness, onset of palpitation, and unpleasant sensation in chest and to note time of occurrence and duration of chest symptoms.

The following pertinent teaching points should be included in the discharge plan (consult physician): (1) reason for taking drug; (2) specific dosage schedule; (3) use of calendar check-off sheet when dose is taken; (4) symptoms to report; (5) allowable planned physical activities; (6) importance of spaced rest periods; (7) diet and weight control; (8) things to avoid, eg, fatigue, excessive caffeine (coffee, tea, cola), alcohol, smoking, heavy meals, stressful situations, OTC medications (unless approved by physician).

Treatment of overdosage: Have on hand molar sodium lactate (for cardiotoxicity), vasoconstrictors and catecholamines (for hypotension), and equipment for cardiopulmonary resuscitation.

Preserved in tight, light-resistant containers away from excessive heat.

LABORATORY TEST INTERFERENCES: Possibility of false increases in urinary catecholamines (using Sobel and Henry modification of trihydroxyindole method), and the drug may interfere with urinary steroid (17-OHCS) determinations made with the Reddy, Jenkins, Thorn procedure.

DRUG INTERACTIONS: There is the possibility of elevated blood quinidine levels with drugs that alkalinize urine (increase renal tubular reabsorption of quinidine), eg, **acetazolamide** and other **carbonic anhydrase inhibitors, magnesium hydroxide, sodium bicarbonate, thiazide diuretics.** Conversely, drugs that acidify urine may increase quinidine excretion, eg, **ascorbic acid** in high doses. With **anticholinergic agents** there may be additive vagolytic actions; **anticoagulants** (coumarin and indanedione derivatives) may cause additive hypoprothrombinemic effects; **cholinergic agents** may be antagonized by quinidine; **phenothiazines** or **propranolol** may introduce the possibility of additive cardiodepressant effects; **rauwolfia alkaloids** and possibly other **antihypertensive agents** may cause additive hypotensive effects. Quinidine may potentiate the action (increased respiratory depression) of depolarizing and nondepolarizing (surgical) muscle relaxants (if given concurrently or shortly after these agents) and possibly antibiotics with neuromuscular action, eg, **aminoglycoside antibiotics.**

QUININE SULFATE, U.S.P.
(COCO-QUININE)

Antimalarial

ACTIONS AND USES

Chief alkaloid from bark of cinchoma tree. Exact mechanism of antimalarial action uncertain. Inhibits protein synthesis, and depresses many enzyme systems in malaria parasite. Has schizonticidal action and is gametocidal with *Plasmodium vivax* and *P. malariae,* but not *P. falciparum.* Resembles salicylates in analgesic and antipyretic properties, and exerts curarelike skeletal-muscle relaxant effect. Also has oxytocic action and hypoprothrombinemic effect. Qualitatively similar to quinidine in cardiovascular effects. Generally replaced by less toxic and more effective agents in treatment of malaria.

Used primarily for treatment of chloroquine-resistant falciparum malaria and in combination with other antimalarials for radical cure of relapsing vivax malaria. Also has been used for relief of nocturnal leg cramps.

Rapidly and completely absorbed from GI tract. Peak plasma concentrations in 1 to 3 hours. Approximately 70% bound to plasma proteins. Metabolized primarily in liver. Excreted in urine in about 24 hours, mostly as inactive metabolites; small amount eliminated in saliva, gastric juice, bile, and feces. Renal excretion is decreased when urine is alkaline. Crosses placenta.

CONTRAINDICATIONS AND PRECAUTIONS

Hypersensitivity or idiosyncrasy to quinine, patients with tinnitus, optic neuritis, myasthenia gravis, glucose-6-phosphate dehydrogenase deficiency, pregnancy. Same precautions as for quinidine when used in patients with cardiovascular conditions.

ADVERSE REACTIONS

Cinchonism (hypersensitivity): tinnitus, decreased auditory acuity, dizziness, headache, visual impairment, nausea, vomiting, diarrhea, fever, skin rash, urticaria, pruritus, flushing, asthma, hemoglobinemia. **CNS:** confusion, excitement, apprehension, syncope, delirium. **Hematologic:** leukopenia, thrombocytopenia, agranulocytosis, hypoprothrombinemia, hemolytic anemia. **Toxicity:** decrease in blood pressure and respiration, tachycardia, hypothermia, convulsions, cardiovascular collapse, coma, blackwater fever (extensive intravascular hemolysis with renal failure), death.

ROUTE AND DOSAGE

Oral: **Adults**: 325 mg 4 times daily for 7 consecutive days. **Children**: not to exceed 15 mg/kg/24 hours.

NURSING IMPLICATIONS

Administer drug after meals to minimize gastric irritation. Quinine has potent local irritant effect on gastric mucosa. Advise patients not to crush capsule; drug is not only irritating but also extremely bitter.

Patients should be informed about possible adverse reactions and advised to report promptly the onset of any unusual symptom.

Preserved in tight, light-resistant containers.

Treatment of overdosage: prompt emesis or gastric lavage is imperative because drug is rapidly absorbed; oxygen, support of respiration, and blood pressure.

LABORATORY TEST INTERFERENCES: Quinine may interfere with determinations of urinary catecholamines (Sobel and Henry modification procedure) and urinary steroids (17-hydroxycorticosteroids) (modification of Reddy, Jenkins, Thorn method).

DRUG INTERACTIONS: GI absorption of quinine may be delayed by **aluminum hydroxide.** Quinine enhances hypoprothrombinemic action of **oral anticoagulants** and may decrease anticoagulant action of **heparin.** Excessive quinine blood levels may result from concomitant use of **pyrimethamine.** Use of quinine with **skeletal-muscle relaxants** may prolong respiratory depression and apnea.

R

RAUWOLFIA SERPENTINA, N.F.
(HYPER-RAUW, RAUDIXIN, RAUPENA, RAUSERPA, RAUSERPIN, RAUTINA, RAUVAL, SERFIA, SERFOLIA, WOLFINA)

Antihypertensive, antipsychotic

ACTIONS AND USES

Powdered whole root of *Rauwolfia serpentina*. Contains reserpine (among other alkaloids), which is responsible for about half of its total activity. Actions, uses, contraindications, precautions, and adverse reactions are the same as for reserpine (qv).

ROUTE AND DOSAGE

Oral: initially 200 to 400 mg daily in divided doses, morning and evening; maintenance 50 to 300 mg daily as single dose or in 2 divided doses.

NURSING IMPLICATIONS

Administered after meals or with food or milk to minimize possibility of gastric irritation.

Preserved in tightly covered containers in a cool dry place.

See Reserpine for nursing implications and drug interactions.

RESCINNAMINE, N.F.
(ANAPREL, CINNASIL, MODERIL)

Antihypertensive, antipsychotic

ACTIONS AND USES

Extracted from *Rauwolfia serpentina* and other *Rauwolfia* alkaloids. Actions, uses, contraindications, precautions, and adverse reactions as for reserpine (qv). Reportedly, sedation and bradycardia may occur less frequently and in milder form than with reserpine.

ROUTE AND DOSAGE

Oral: initially 0.5 mg twice daily up to 2 weeks; increased gradually if necessary; maintenance may vary from 0.25 to 0.5 mg daily.

NURSING IMPLICATIONS

Administered after meals or with food or milk to minimize gastric irritation.

Preserved in tight, light-resistant containers.

See Reserpine for nursing implications and drug interactions.

(ALKARAU, ELSERPINE, LEMISERP, RAURINE, RAU-SED,
RESERCEN, RESERPOID, ROLSERP, SANDRIL, SERPALAN,
SERPALOID, SERPANRAY, SERPASIL, SERPATE, SERTINA,
VIO-SERPINE)

Antihypertensive, antipsychotic

ACTIONS AND USES

Principal alkaloid of *Rauwolfia serpentina* (Indian snakeroot). Interferes with binding of 5-hydroxytryptophan at receptor sites, decreases synthesis of norepinephrine and epinephrine by depleting dopamine (their precursor), and competitively inhibits their reuptake in storage granules. Causes intraneuronal depletion of these biogenic amines from brain, peripheral nervous system, heart, and other organs and tissues. Sympathetic inhibitory influence is reflected in small but persistent decrease in blood pressure, frequently associated with bradycardia and reduced cardiac output. Usually does not cause orthostatic hypotension, and has no marked effect on renal blood flow. Central effect results in tranquilization and sedation similar to that produced by chlorpromazine.

Used orally in treatment of mild essential hypertension and as adjunctive therapy with other antihypertensive agents in more severe forms of hypertension. Also used in agitated psychotic states, primarily in patients intolerant to phenothiazines or patients who also require antihypertensive medication. Used parenterally for treatment of hypertensive emergencies such as acute hypertensive encephalopathy and occasionally to initiate treatment in psychiatric emergencies.

ABSORPTION AND FATE

Slow onset of action after oral administration. Action begins within 1 hour following IV injection and persists 6 to 8 hours. Slower onset following IM, and action persists for 10 to 12 hours. Well distributed in body. Tightly bound to catecholamine storage sites. Slowly excreted in urine, mainly as metabolites.

CONTRAINDICATIONS AND PRECAUTIONS

History of mental depression, acute peptic ulcer, acute ulcerative colitis, patients receiving electroconvulsive therapy. Safe use during pregnancy and in women of childbearing potential and nursing mothers not established. Cautious use: renal insufficiency, cardiac arrhythmias, cardiac damage, cerebrovascular accident, epilepsy, bronchitis, asthma, elderly patients, debilitated patients, gallstones, obesity, chronic sinusitis.

ADVERSE REACTIONS

Drowsiness, lethargy, mental depression, nasal congestion, changes in sleep pattern, nightmares, bradycardia, excessive salivation, dry mouth, nausea, abdominal cramps, diarrhea, reactivation of peptic ulcer, cutaneous flushing, increased appetite, weight gain, edema, congestive heart failure (rare), epistaxis, blurred vision, miosis, dysuria, muscle aches, menstrual irregularities, impairment of sexual function, feminization in males, risk of breast cancer, orthostatic hypotension (parenteral doses), allergic reactions (rare), thrombocytopenia. Prolonged use of high doses: CNS stimulation (excitement, insomnia, extrapyramidal symptoms, convulsions), respiratory depression, hypothermia.

ROUTE AND DOSAGE

Oral (hypertension): initially 0.5 mg daily for 1 or 2 weeks; maintenance reduced to 0.1 to 0.25 mg daily; (psychiatric disorders): initially 0.5 mg; dosage adjusted upward or downward according to patient's response (range 0.1 to 1 mg daily). Intramuscular (hypertensive crisis): initially 0.5 to 1 mg, followed by doses of 2 and 4 mg at 3-hour intervals, if necessary; (psychiatric emergencies): 2.5 to 5 mg. **Pediatric:** (hypertension): 0.07 mg/kg/24 hours divided into 2 doses.

NURSING IMPLICATIONS

Reserpine is administered after meals or with food or milk to minimize possibility of gastric irritation (drug increases gastric secretions).

Take blood pressure and pulse at intervals prescribed by physician. Both should be taken before each parenteral dose. Compare readings with baseline determinations and keep physician informed. (Note: drop in blood pressure may be accompanied by bradycardia.)

Counsel patient regarding possible side effects and importance of prompt reporting. Untoward effects are usually minimal with proper dosage and adequate supervision.

Rauwolfia alkaloids are cumulative in action. Full therapeutic effect of oral drug for hypertension may not occur until 3 weeks of therapy, and effects may persist for as long as 4 weeks after drug is discontinued. Special precautions should be observed when reserpine is prescribed for the elderly.

Mental depression is a serious side effect and may be sufficiently severe to lead to suicide. It may not appear until 6 to 7 months of therapy and may last for several months after drug is withdrawn. Instruct patient and responsible family members to report altered sleep pattern, anorexia, self-deprecation, attitude of detachment, mood changes, or sexual impotence, all of which are early signs of depression. Hospitalization may be required.

Postural hypotension is not a usual side effect, but it may occur in patients receiving large doses parenterally. Supervise ambulation as indicated.

Advise patient to check for edema and to record weight daily. Distinction must be made between weight gain from edema and weight gain from increased appetite. Consult physician for weight gain of 3 to 5 lb in 1 week.

Consult physician regarding diet regimen, allowable salt intake, and physical activity program.

If vasopressor is needed for treatment of hypotension, levarterenol (or other direct-acting sympathomimetic amine) is preferred to ephedrine, which is indirect-acting (depends on release of catecholamines for action).

Rauwolfia alkaloids tend to lower the threshold for convulsions. Patients with epilepsy should be monitored for possible need of adjustment in anticonvulsant dosage.

Rauwolfia alkaloids should be discontinued 2 weeks prior to elective surgery and 1 week before electroconvulsive therapy.

Preserved in tight, light-resistant containers.

DRUG INTERACTIONS: Rauwolfia alkaloids may alter the effects of **oral anticoagulants;** they may enhance the CNS depression of **barbiturates,** with resulting increase in hypotension and bradycardia. Taken with **digitalis glycosides,** they increase the risk of cardiac arrhythmias. They may decrease the effects of **amphetamines, ephedrine,** and other indirect-acting amines. The response to **levodopa** may be inhibited by rauwolfia alkaloids. Additive hypotension may occur with **methotrimeprazine,** excitation and hypertension with **MAO inhibitors,** excessive sympathetic blockade with **propranolol,** and additive hypotensive effects with **thiazide diuretics.** There is potential hazard of excessive CNS stimulation (hyperactivity, mania) with **tricyclic antidepressants** and the possibility of additive cardiodepressant effects with **procainamide** and **quinidine.**

RIBOFLAVIN, U.S.P.
(HYRYE, Lactoflavin, Vitamin B$_2$, Vitamin G)
RIBOFLAVINE, B.P.

Vitamin (enzyme cofactor)

ACTIONS AND USES
Water-soluble vitamin and component of the flavoprotein enzymes that work together with a wide variety of proteins to catalyze many cellular respiratory reactions by which the body derives its energy.
Used in treatment and prevention of riboflavin deficiency (ariboflavinosis) and as supplement to other B vitamins in treatment of pellagra and beriberi.

ABSORPTION AND FATE
Readily absorbed from upper GI tract and from parenteral sites. Distributed to all tissues, with highest concentrations in liver, kidney, and heart. Little is stored. Bound to plasma proteins. Amounts in excess of body needs excreted unchanged in urine. In amounts approaching minimal daily requirements, approximately 9% excreted in urine; metabolic fate of remainder unknown.

CONTRAINDICATIONS AND PRECAUTIONS
None known.

ADVERSE REACTIONS
Apparently nontoxic.

ROUTE AND DOSAGE
Oral, parenteral (prophylaxis): 2 mg daily; (therapeutic): 10 mg or more daily. Usual dose range 5 to 50 mg daily.

NURSING IMPLICATIONS
Inform patient receiving large doses that an intense yellow discoloration of urine may occur.
Therapeutic effectiveness of vitamin B$_2$ therapy is evaluated by improvement of clinical manifestations of deficiency: digestive disturbances, headache, burning sensation of skin (especially "burning" feet), cracking at corners of mouth (cheilosis), glossitis, seborrheic dermatitis (often at angle of nose and anogenital region) and other skin lesions, mental depression, corneal vascularization (with photophobia, burning and itchy eyes, lacrimation, roughness of eyelids), anemia, neuropathy.
Recommended daily allowances of riboflavin: infants, 0.4 to 0.6 mg; children, 1.1 to 1.2 mg; adult males, 1.6 mg; adult females, 1.2 mg; pregnancy and lactation, 1.5 and 1.7 mg, respectively.
Rich dietary sources of riboflavin: liver, kidney, heart, eggs, milk and milk products, yeast, whole-grain cereals, and green vegetables.
Collaborate with physician, dietitian, patient, and responsible family member in planning for diet teaching. A complete dietary history is an essential part of vitamin replacement so that poor eating habits can be identified and corrected. Additionally, deficiency in one vitamin is usually associated with other vitamin deficiencies.
Preserved in airtight containers protected from light.

LABORATORY TEST INTERFERENCES: In large doses, riboflavin may produce yellow green fluorescence in urine and thus cause false elevations in certain fluorometric determinations of urinary catecholamines.

DRUG INTERACTIONS: Riboflavin decreases activity of **tetracyclines.**

(RIFADIN, RIFAMYCIN, RIMACTANE)

Antibacterial

ACTIONS AND USES

Semisynthetic derivative of rifamycin B, an antibiotic derived from *Streptococcus mediterranei,* with bacteriostatic and bactericidal actions. Inhibits DNA-dependent RNA polymerase activity in susceptible bacterial cells, thereby suppressing RNA synthesis. Active against *Mycobacterium tuberculosis, Neisseria meningitidis,* and a wide range of Gram-negative and Gram-positive organisms. Since resistant strains emerge rapidly when it is employed alone, it is used in conjunction with other antitubercular agents in treatment of tuberculosis.

Used primarily as adjuvant with other antitubercular drugs in initial treatment and retreatment of pulmonary tuberculosis and as short-term therapy to eliminate meningococci from nasopharynx of asymptomatic carriers when risk of meningococcal menigitis is high.

ABSORPTION AND FATE

Peak plasma concentrations (variability in levels) in 2 to 4 hours following 600-mg dose; still detectable for 24 hours. Widely distributed in body tissues and fluids, including cerebrospinal fluid, with highest concentrations in liver, gallbladder wall, and kidneys. Half-life about 1.5 to 5 hours (higher and more prolonged in hepatic dysfunction, and may be decreased in patients receiving isoniazid concomitantly). Rapidly deacetylated in liver to active and inactive metabolites; enters bile via enterohepatic circulation. Up to 30% of dose is excreted in urine, about half as free drug. Rifampin induces microsomal enzymes and thus may inactivate certain drugs. Crosses placenta and diffuses certain drugs into breast milk.

CONTRAINDICATIONS AND PRECAUTIONS

Hypersensitivity to rifamycin derivatives; obstructive biliary disease, intermittent rifampin therapy. Safe use during pregnancy and in children under 5 years of age not established. Cautious use: hepatic disease, history of alcoholism, concomitant use of other hepatotoxic agents.

ADVERSE REACTIONS

GI: heartburn, epigastric distress, nausea, vomiting, anorexia, flatulence, cramps, diarrhea. **CNS:** fatigue, drowsiness, headache, ataxia, confusion, dizziness, inability to concentrate, generalized numbness, pain in extremities, muscular weakness, visual disturbances, transient low-frequency hearing loss (infrequent). **Hypersensitivity:** fever, pruritus, urticaria, skin eruptions, soreness of mouth and tongue, eosinophilia, hemolysis, hemoglobinuria, hematuria, renal insufficiency, acute renal failure (reversible). **Hematologic:** thrombocytopenia, transient leukopenia, anemia, including hemolytic anemia. **Other:** hemoptysis, light-chain proteinuria, menstrual disorders, hepatorenal syndrome (with intermittent therapy), transient elevations in liver function tests (bilirubin, BSP, alkaline phosphatase, SGOT, SGPT), pancreatitis (infrequent). **Overdosage:** GI symptoms, increasing lethargy, liver enlargement and tenderness, jaundice.

ROUTE AND DOSAGE

Oral: *Pulmonary tuberculosis:* **Adults:** 600 mg once daily; used in conjunction with other antibacterial agent(s). **Children:** 10 to 20 mg/kg/day, not to exceed 600 mg/day. *Meningococcal carriers:* **Adults:** 600 mg daily for 4 consecutive days. **Children:** 10 to 20 mg/kg daily for 4 consecutive days, not to exceed 600 mg/day.

NURSING IMPLICATIONS

Administered 1 hour before or 2 hours after a meal. Peak serum levels are delayed and may be slightly lower when given with food.

A desiccant should be kept in bottle containing capsules; they become unstable with moisture.

Caution patient not to interrupt prescribed dosage regimen. Hepatorenal reaction with flulike syndrome has occurred when therapy has been resumed following interruption.

Serology and susceptibility testing should be performed prior to and in the event of positive cultures.

Inform patients that drug may impart a harmless red-orange color to urine, feces, sputum, sweat, and tears.

Periodic hepatic function tests are advised. Patients with hepatic disease must be closely monitored.

Instruct patients to report onset of jaundice (yellow skin, sclerae, and posterior portion of hard palate; dark urine, pruritus, light-colored stools), hypersensitivity reactions, and persistence of GI adverse effects.

Patients taking oral contraceptives should consider alternative methods of contraception (see Drug Interactions).

Caution patient to keep drug out of reach of children.

Treatment of overdosage: gastric lavage in absence of vomiting, followed by activated charcoal slurry; antiemetic to control severe nausea and vomiting. Forced diuresis, with measurement of intake–output ratio, to promote drug excretion. Extracorporeal hemodialysis may be required.

LABORATORY TEST INTERFERENCES: Possible interference with contrast media used for gallbladder study; may also cause retention of BSP.

DRUG INTERACTIONS: **Aminosalicylic acid** impairs GI absorption of rifampin and thus may cause lower rifampin serum levels (space doses 8 to 12 hours apart). Rifampin appears to stimulate metabolism of **oral anticoagulants** (with resulting increase in anticoagulant requirement) and **estrogens,** thus reducing the effectiveness of **oral contraceptives.** Rifampin may augment hepatotoxicity of **halothane.** Combined use of rifampin and **isoniazid** (INH) may result in hepatotoxicity (especially in patients with hepatic impairment and slow INH inactivators). By competing with rifampin for hepatic uptake, **probenecid** may produce higher rifampin blood levels. Rifampin, in combination with other antitubercular drugs, may affect blood concentrations of **corticosteroids, digitalis derivatives, methadone,** and **oral hypoglycemic agents** (dosage adjustment of interacting drugs is recommended).

SALICYLAMIDE, N.F.
(SALRIN)

Analgesic, antipyretic

ACTIONS AND USES
Salicylic amide with analgesic, antiinflammatory, and antipyretic properties similar to those of aspirin, but much milder. Significantly metabolized before entering systemic circulation. Overall toxicity appears to be less than that of aspirin (qv), and has shorter duration of action.

Used for temporary relief of moderate aches and pain due to arthritis, rehumatic conditions, and neuralgia and to relieve fever and discomfort of cold.

ROUTE AND DOSAGE
Oral **Adults:** 325 to 650 mg every 4 hours. **Children:** 65 mg/kg/24 hours divided into 6 doses.

NURSING IMPLICATIONS
Administered with food, milk, or full glass of water to minimize possibility of GI irritation.

Some patients experience drowsiness and dizziness with repeated doses. Caution the patient against potentially hazardous activities such as driving a car or operating machinery if these symptoms persist.

Advise patients to keep drug out of reach of children.

See Aspirin for nursing implications and drug interactions.

SALICYLIC ACID, U.S.P., B.P.

Keratolytic

ACTIONS AND USES
Aids in removal of horny skin layers, thereby facilitating penetration. Causes swelling and softening of keratin and cornified epithelium and scales, thereby facilitating their removal. Has weak bacteriostatic and fungistatic action. Destructive to tissues in concentrations above 6%.

Used as topical dermatologic aid in hyperkeratotic skin disorders such as psoriasis and various ichthyoses, and produces exfoliation in fungal infections. Available in plaster form or as ether-alcohol solution with about 20% salicylic acid and collodion for removal of warts, corns, and calluses.

CONTRAINDICATIONS AND PRECAUTIONS
Sensitivity to salicylates or to any ingredient in preparation; applications over large areas for prolonged periods. Cautious use: children under 12 years of age.

ADVERSE REACTIONS
Irritation, burning of skin. Systemic salicylate poisoning (prolonged applications to large areas). See Aspirin.

ROUTE AND DOSAGE
Topical: cream, gel, liquid, lotion, ointment, powder, 2% to 6%, collodion base, 10% to 20%.

NURSING IMPLICATIONS
Avoid contact of medication with eyes and mucous membranes.

Advise patients to rinse hands thoroughly following use of cream, gel, lotion, or ointment forms unless hands are also being treated.

Collodion preparation (for corns and warts) should not be used by patients with diabetes or peripheral vascular disease.

Caution patients to use drug as directed. Systemic absorption is possible. Application to normal skin can cause irritation and burning.

Hydration of part (wet packs, soaks, or baths) before or after application, as directed, enhances drug effect.

Advise patients to keep medication out of reach of children.

See Aspirin.

SCOPOLAMINE HYDROBROMIDE, U.S.P.
HYOSCINE HYDROBROMIDE, B.P.

Anticholinergic

ACTIONS AND USES

Alkaloid of belladonna with peripheral actions resembling those of atropine. In contrast to atropine, produces CNS depression, with marked sedative and tranquilizing effects, and is less effective in preventing reflex bradycardia during anesthesia (tends to slow heart even in large doses). More potent in mydriatic and cycloplegic actions and in inhibiting secretions of salivary, bronchial, and sweat glands, but has less prominent effect on heart, intestines, and bronchial muscles.

Used in obstetrics with morphine to produce amnesia and sedation ("twilight sleep"), and as preanesthetic medication. Used to control spasticity (and drooling) in postencephalitic parkinsonism, paralysis agitans, and other spastic states, as prophylactic agent for motion sickness and as mydriatic and cycloplegic in ophthalmology.

ABSORPTION AND FATE

Well absorbed from GI tract. Bound to plasma proteins. Peak mydriatic effect in 20 to 30 minutes, lasting 3 to 7 days; peak cycloplegic effect in 30 minutes to 1 hour, lasting 5 to 7 days.

CONTRAINDICATIONS AND PRECAUTIONS

Asthma, hepatitis, toxemia of pregnancy. Cautious use: cardiac disease, patients over 40 years of age. Also see Atropine.

ADVERSE REACTIONS

Sense of fatigue, dizziness, drowsiness, dry mouth and throat, disorientation, decreased heart rate, dilated pupils, depressed respiration. Also see Atropine.

ROUTE AND DOSAGE

Adults: Oral: 0.5 to 1 mg. Subcutaneous, intramuscular, intravenous (with suitable dilution): 0.3 to 0.6 mg. Topical (ophthalmic): 1 or 2 drops of 0.2% to 0.25% solution. **Children:** 0.006 mg/kg orally or subcutaneously.

NURSING IMPLICATIONS

Some patients manifest excitement, delirium, disorientation, and garrulousness shortly after drug is administered, until sedative effect takes hold. Observe patient closely for these effects.

Bedsides are advisable, particularly for the elderly, because of amnesic effect of scopolamine.

In the presence of pain, scopolamine may cause delirium, restlessness, and excitement unless given with an analgesic.

Tolerance may develop with prolonged use.

When used as mydriatic or cycloplegic, caution the patient that vision will be blurred; the patient should avoid potentially hazardous activities such as driving a car or operating machinery until vision clears.

Many OTC "sleep aids" contain scopolamine in small doses, eg, Compoz, Devarex, Nite Rest, San-man, Sominex, Sure-Sleep.

Preserved in tight, light-resistant containers.

See Atropine Sulfate for nursing implications and drug interactions.

SECOBARBITAL
(SECO-8, SECONAL)
SECOBARBITAL SODIUM, U.S.P.
(SECONAL SODIUM)

Sedative, hypnotic

ACTIONS AND USES

Short-acting barbiturate with CNS depressant effects and anticonvulsant action similar to that of phenobarbital (qv).

Used as hypnotic for simple insomnia, and preoperatively to provide basal hypnosis for general, spinal, or regional anesthesia. Effective in the emergency control of acute convulsive conditions (eg, tetanus, toxic reactions to poisons) and in the management of acute agitated behavior.

ABSORPTION AND FATE

Approximately 90% absorbed from GI tract following oral ingestion. Full hypnotic effect in 15 to 30 minutes after oral or rectal administration, 7 to 10 minutes after IM, and 1 to 3 minutes after IV injection. About 30% to 45% bound to plasma proteins. Half-life 20 to 28 hours. Metabolized by liver; excreted in urine as inactive metabolites and small amounts of unchanged drug. Crosses placenta.

CONTRAINDICATIONS AND PRECAUTIONS

History of sensitivity to barbiturates, use during parturition, fetal immaturity, uncontrolled pain. Use of sterile injection containing polyethylene glycol vehicle in patients with renal insufficiency. Cautious use: pregnant women with toxemia or history of bleeding. Also see Phenobarbital.

ADVERSE REACTIONS

Respiratory depression, laryngospasm, fall in blood pressure (with rapid IV). Also see Phenobarbital.

ROUTE AND DOSAGE

Adults: Oral (sedative): 30 to 50 mg 3 times per day; (preoperative sedative): 100 to 300 mg 1 or 2 hours before surgery; (hypnotic): 100 to 200 mg orally or IM. Intramuscular, intravenous (acute convulsive episodes): 5.5 mg/kg repeated every 3 to 4 hours if needed. **Children:** Oral, rectal (sedative): 6 mg/kg/24 hours, divided into 3 doses; (hypnotic): 3 to 5 mg/kg. Intramuscular (acute convulsive episodes): 3 to 5 mg/kg.

NURSING IMPLICATIONS

Discard parenteral solutions that are not clear or that contain a precipitate.

Aqueous solutions of secobarbital sodium for injection are not stable; they must be freshly prepared and used within 30 minutes after container is opened. Reconstitute secobarbital sodium powder with sterile water for injection (incompatible with bacteriostatic water for injection or lactated Ringer's injection). Following addition of water, rotate ampul; do not shake it. Several minutes are required to dissolve drug completely. If solution is not completely clear within 5 minutes, do not use. Consult package literature for details.

Secobarbital sodium injection in aqueous–polyethylene glycol vehicle is more stable than aqueous solution. It should be refrigerated (2 C to 8 C). May be diluted with sterile water for injection, 0.9% sodium chloride, or Ringer's injection (*not* lactated). Consult package literature for details.

Administer IM injection deep into large muscle mass. Carefully aspirate before injecting drug to avoid inadvertent entry into blood vessel.

Following IM injection of large hypnotic dose, observe patient closely for 20 to 30 minutes to assure that hypnosis is not excessive.

An occasional patient may become irritable, uncooperative, and restive after a subhypnotic dose of a short-acting barbiturate.

Patients receiving drug IV must be kept under constant observation. Monitor blood pressure, pulse, and respiration every 3 to 5 minutes. Maintain patient airway. Equipment for artificial respiration should be immediately available.

When administered to pregnant patient, fetal heart beat should be closely monitored. Report slowing or irregularities.

Following administration to a patient in ambulatory service or physician's office, the patient should not attempt to go home unescorted. Caution the patient to avoid driving a car for the remainder of day.

Classified as schedule II drug under federal Controlled Substances Act.

See Phenobarbital for nursing implications and drug interactions.

SENNA, N.F.
(BLACK DRAUGHT, CASAFRU, FLETCHER's CASTORIA, GLYSENNID, SENOKOT, X-PREP)

Cathartic (stimulant)

ACTIONS AND USES

Anthraquinone derivative prepared from dried leaflet of *Cassia acutifolia* or *Cassia angustifolia*. Similar to cascara sagrada, but with more potent action. Senna glycosides are converted in colon to active aglycones, which stimulate Auerbach's plexus to induce peristalsis. Available as crude drug (eg, Black Draught, Casafru), crystalline senna glycosides (sennosides A and B, eg, Glysennid), and as standardized senna concentrate (eg, Senokot, X-Prep). Standardized concentrate is purified and standardized for uniform action and is claimed to produce less colic than crude form.

Used for temporary relief of constipation and for preoperative and preradiographic bowel evacuation.

ABSORPTION AND FATE

Cathartic action usually occurs in 6 to 10 hours; may not act before 24 hours in some patients. Excreted in feces; some may be eliminated in urine.

CONTRAINDICATIONS AND PRECAUTIONS

Irritable colon, nausea, vomiting, abdominal pain, intestinal obstruction, nursing mothers.

ADVERSE REACTIONS

Abdominal cramps, flatulence. Prolonged use: watery diarrhea, excessive loss of water and electrolytes, weight loss, melanotic segmentation of colonic mucosa (reversible).

ROUTE AND DOSAGE

Oral: *Crude Senna leaf or fruit:* **Adults:** 0.5 to 2 Gm. **Children:** 4 mg/kg. *Senna fluid extract:* **Adults:** 2 ml. **Children:** 0.04 ml/kg. *Senna syrup:* **Adults:** 8 ml; **Children:** 0.15 mg/kg. *Sennocides A and B:* **Adults and children** *over 10 years:* 12 to 24 mg;

Children *6 to 10 years:* 12 mg. *Standardized senna concentrate:* **Adults:** 2 tablets (187 mg each); granules, 1 teaspoon (326 mg/tsp). Rectal suppository, 625 mg. **Children** *over 60 lb:* approximately one-half the usual adult dose.

NURSING IMPLICATIONS

Generally administered at bedtime for relief of constipation.

When given for preoperative or prediagnostic bowel preparation, usually prescribed to be taken between 2 and 4 P.M. on day prior to procedure. Diet is then confined to clear liquids.

Some patients may experience considerable griping; if medication is to be repeated, dose reduction may be indicated.

Inform patient that drug may impart yellowish brown color (in acid urine) or reddish brown color (in alkaline urine). Feces may be similarly colored.

Caution patient that continued use may lead to dependence. If constipation persists, consult physician.

Avoid exposure of drug to excessive heat; fluidextracts should be protected from light.

See Bisacodyl for patient teaching points.

SILVER NITRATE, U.S.P., B.P.
(AgNO₃)

Antiinfective (topical)

SILVER NITRATE, TOUGHENED, U.S.P.
(LUNAR CAUSTIC, SILVER NITRATE PENCIL)

Caustic

ACTIONS AND USES

Has bactericidal, astringent, and caustic properties. Contact of silver ion with chloride in tissue results in precipitation to silver chloride, which limits its effectiveness and penetrating ability. Therefore, debridement must accompany burn therapy. Bactericidal action thought to be due to ability to interfere with essential metabolic actions of microbial cells. Degree of action depends on concentration used and period of time drug is allowed to remain in contact with tissue.

Silver nitrate ophthalmic solution is used to prevent and treat ophthalmia neonatorum. Weak solutions are also used to irrigate bladder and urethra and for treatment of burns. Strong concentrations and toughened silver nitrate are used to cauterize mucous membranes, wounds, granulomatous tissue, and warts.

ADVERSE REACTIONS

Transient chemical irritation of eyes (redness, edema, discharge) following eye instillations. Argyria (silver discoloration of tissue with prolonged use), photosensitivity, methemoglobinemia, hypochloremia and loss of other electrolytes (following applications to extensive burns).

ROUTE AND DOSAGE

Topical (silver nitrate ophthalmic solution 1%): *Ophthalmia neonatorum:* 2 drops instilled into eye. Eyelids are first cleaned with sterile cotton and sterile water to remove blood, mucus, or meconium. Drug should remain in contact with whole conjunctival sac for 30 seconds or longer. (Irrigation of eyes following instillation of silver nitrate is not recommended by National Society for Preven-

nitrate applicators, toughened sticks. *Treatment of burns:* 0.5% solution.

NURSING IMPLICATIONS
Use only silver nitrate ophthalmic solution for the eyes.

Most states by law require instillation of silver nitrate for prophylaxis of ophthalmia neonatorum.

Follow agency policy or physician's directions for ophthalmic instillation in newborns.

Patients receiving silver nitrate treatment for burns should be closely observed for signs and symptoms of dehydration and electrolyte loss (particularly chloride, calcium, potassium, and sodium).

For wound cauterization, area to be treated should first be cleaned to remove organic matter (may interfere with drug action). If toughened silver nitrate (silver nitrate pencil) is used, it should be dipped in water and applied to area for period of time according to degree of action desired. Treated area will appear grayish black (silver stain).

Medication should be confined to specific area to be treated. If healthy skin is accidentally touched, it may be washed with physiologic salt solution (the chloride in salt solution forms insoluble precipitate with silver nitrate and thus cancels its action).

Handle silver nitrate with care. Solutions leave gray or black stain on skin, clothing, and utensils. Skin stains (argyria) usually persist indefinitely or disappear only very slowly. Argyria may be exaggerated by exposure to sunlight. Concentrations of silver nitrate 5% and higher are caustic.

Preserved in tight, light-resistant containers.

SILVER PROTEIN, MILD, N.F.
(ARGYROL S.S.)

Antiinfective (topical)

ACTIONS AND USES
Colloidal compound of silver and a protein derivative. Contains less concentration of ionized silver than silver nitrate, and consequently is less irritating to tissues. See Silver Nitrate for actions and adverse reactions.

Used preoperatively in eye surgery to stain and coagulate mucus, which can then be removed by irrigation; used in prevention and treatment of ophthalmia neonatorum and for mild inflammatory conditions of eye, nose, and throat.

ROUTE AND DOSAGE
Topical (ophthalmic solution 20%): *Ophthalmia neonatorum:* 1 or 2 drops instilled into each eye immediately after birth to remove blood, mucus, or meconium; drug should remain in contact with whole conjunctival sac for 30 seconds or longer. *Preoperatively in eye surgery:* 2 or 3 drops, then rinsed out with sterile irrigating solution. Available in 10% solution for mild inflammatory conditions.

NURSING IMPLICATIONS
Follow agency policy or physician's directions for instillation of eye drops for prevention of ophthalmia neonatorum.

See Silver Nitrate.

Antiinfective (topical)

ACTIONS AND USES
Produced by reaction of silver nitrate with sulfadiazine. Mechanism of action differs from that of either component. Silver salt is released slowly and exerts bactericidal effect only on bacterial cell membrane and wall, rather than by inhibiting folic acid synthesis; antibacterial activity is not inhibited by *p*-amino-benzoic acid (PABA). Contact with sodium chloride in body tissues and fluids results in slow release of sulfadiazine, which may be systemically absorbed from application site. Has broad antimicrobial activity including many Gram-negative and Gram-positive bacteria and yeast. Unlike silver nitrate solution, does not affect electrolyte balance, and reportedly does not alter acid–base balance. Used for prevention and treatment of sepsis in second- and third-degree burns.

CONTRAINDICATIONS AND PRECAUTIONS
Hypersensitivity to silver sulfadiazine and components (and possibly other sulfonamides), patients with glucose-6-phosphate dehydrogenase deficiency, women of childbearing potential, use during pregnancy, pregnant women at term, prematures and newborn infants under 2 months of age. Cautions use: impaired renal or hepatic function.

ADVERSE REACTIONS
Pain (occasionally), burning, itching, rash, reversible leukopenia. Potential for toxicity as for other sulfonamides. See Sulfisoxazole.

ROUTE AND DOSAGE
Topical (micronized) cream 1% applied once or twice daily to thickness of approximately 1/16 inch.

NURSING IMPLICATIONS

Silver sulfadiazine cream is water-soluble and white in color; if darkening occurs, do not use.

Applied with sterile, gloved hands to cleansed, debrided burned areas. Cream should be reapplied to areas where it has been removed by patient activity; burn wounds should be covered at all times.

Dressings are not required, but may be used if necessary. Silver sulfadiazine does not stain clothing.

Occasionally, pain is experienced on application; intensity and duration depend on depth of burn. Analgesic may be required.

When drug is applied to extensive areas, serum sulfa concentrations, urinalysis, and kidney function tests should be monitored, since significant quantities of drug may be absorbed. Observe patient for reactions attributed to sulfonamides.

Observe for and report hypersensitivity reaction manifested by rash, itching, or burning sensation in unburned areas.

If possible, patient should be bathed daily (in whirlpool or shower or in bed) as aid to debridement.

Unless adverse reactions occur, treatment should continue until satisfactory healing or until burn site is ready for grafting.

Preserved at room temperature away from heat.

See Nursing Implications, Laboratory Test Interferences, and Drug Interactions for Sulfisoxazole (applicable when silver sulfadiazine is applied to extensive areas).

DRUG INTERACTIONS: Silver sulfadiazine reacts with most heavy metals, with possible release of silver and darkening of cream. Topically applied **proteolytic enzymes** may be inactivated by the silver in silver sulfadiazine.

SITOSTEROLS, N.F.
(CYTELLIN)

Anticholesteremic

ACTIONS AND USES
Mixture of plant sterols. Exact mechanism of action unknown. Lowers elevated serum cholesterol, possibly by interfering with intestinal absorption and enterohepatic cycling of endogenous cholesterol. Serum levels of total lipids or triglycerides are less consistently reduced. Long-term effects not known.
Used as adjunctive therapy to diet and other measures in treatment of hypercholesterolemia and hyperbetalipoproteinemia.
ABSORPTION AND FATE
Poorly absorbed from GI tract. Excreted in feces unchanged.
CONTRAINDICATIONS AND PRECAUTIONS
Safe use during pregnancy not established. Cautious use: liver disease.
ADVERSE REACTIONS
Infrequent: anorexia, diarrhea, abdominal cramps.
ROUTE AND DOSAGE
Oral: 12 to 24 Gm daily divided so that some portion of total dose is given before each meal or snack. Daily dose not to exceed 24 to 36 Gm. Suggested dosage: 1 tablespoon (approximately 15 ml) before each meal; 1.5 to 2 tablespoons when large or high-fat meals are to be consumed; 1 tablespoon or fraction thereof before snacks.

NURSING IMPLICATIONS
Prior to treatment, three or more baseline serum cholesterol values are usually obtained while patient is on a controlled diet for 1 to 3 weeks.
Drug is administered immediately before meals or snacks. May be mixed with coffee, tea, fruit juice, or milk to increase palatability. Review dosage regimen prescribed by physician.
Consult physician regarding dietary control and weight regulation.
Inform patient that sitosterols may produce bulky, light-colored stools (from fecal excretion of cholesterol and other sterols). Also, since drug contains a methylcellulose derivative, stools may be loose. Restriction of foods containing roughage may be necessary.
Maximum therapeutic effect usually occurs during second or third month of therapy. When drug is discontinued, serum lipids return to pretreatment levels within 3 weeks.

SODIUM FLUORIDE, U.S.P., B.P.
(DENTA-FL, FLUORIDENT, FLUORITAB, FLURA, FLURA-LOZ, KARIDIUM, LURIDE, NUFLUOR, PEDIAFLOR, PHOS-FLUR, RESCUE SQUAD, SOLU-FLUR)

Dental caries prophylactic

ACTIONS AND USES
Incorporation of fluoride ion into tooth structure causes outer layers of enamel to be harder and more resistant to dental caries. Optimal benefits obtained

before permanent teeth erupt, but children of any age usually derive benefits from fluoride treatment.

CONTRAINDICATIONS AND PRECAUTIONS

When intake of fluoride from drinking water exceeds 0.7 parts per million (ppm) per day; low-sodium or sodium-free diets.

ADVERSE REACTIONS

Skin reactions: eczema, atopic dermatitis, urticaria. **Excessive intake:** dental fluorosis (brown or white mottling of tooth enamel). **Acute overdosage:** epigastric pain, nausea, vomiting, diarrhea, excessive salivation, decrease in serum protein-bound iodine, local paralysis in legs and face, convulsions, fall in blood pressure, respiratory depression.

ROUTE AND DOSAGE

Oral: **Children** *3 years old and under:* 0.5 mg daily; *over 3 years:* 1 mg daily. Water supplies with 0.2 parts per million (ppm) or less require supplementation of 0.5 mg/day for children under 3 years and 1 mg/day for children over 3 years. Water supplies with 0.2 to 0.6 ppm require supplementation of 0.25 mg/day for children under 3 years and 0.5 mg/day for children over 3 years.

NURSING IMPLICATIONS

To be effective, fluoride supplementation must be consistent and continuous, ie, from infancy until 12 to 14 years of age.

Advise parent not to exceed recommended dosage.

Parent should be informed that the fluoride preparation being used should be reviewed if family moves or if water supply is changed.

Stored in plastic or paraffin-lined glass containers (sodium fluoride reacts with ordinary glass at a slow but appreciable rate).

SODIUM IODIDE I 131, U.S.P.

(IODOTOPE, ORIODIDE, RADIOCAPS, Radio-iodide (I 131) Sodium, THERIODIDE, TRACERVIAL)

Diagnostic aid, antineoplastic, thyroid inhibitor

ACTIONS AND USES

Radiopharmaceutical with relatively long half-life (8.8 days). Processed in form of sodium iodide (NaI) from products of uranium fission or neutron bombardment of tellurium. Chemically and physiologically identical to stable, naturally occurring iodide. Affords relatively simple, effective, economic means of treating hyperthyroid Graves' disease by ablation without surgery. Therapeutic doses of radioactive iodine (RAI) deliver ionizing radiation to follicular cells, thereby damaging and destroying thyroid and neoplastic tissues. Comparatively, NaI (^{125}I) delivers relatively low radiation (no beta emissions); has half-life of 57 days. Required dose for imaging is less than that of ^{131}I. Antithyroid medication sometimes given to patient before and after RAI therapy.

Used therapeutically for subtotal ablation of thyroid, to suppress neoplastic disease of thyroid, and in management of euthyroid patients with angina pectoris or congestive heart failure refractory to other forms of therapy. As a diagnostic aid, tracer doses are used in thyroid function studies and imaging to evaluate suspected hyperthyroidism and to visualize thyroid malignancy and metastasis.

ABSORPTION AND FATE

Following oral administration, absorbed from GI tract; evident in blood within 3 to 6 minutes. Concentrates in thyroid gland and small amounts in salivary glands and stomach. Iodide secretion from these organs permits radioactivity detection in nasal secretion, oral cavity, trachea, female breast, gallbladder, liver, and intestines. Excreted primarily by kidneys, with small amounts in sweat and feces. Crosses placenta and appears in breast milk. Disintegrates primarily by beta particle emission (maximum range 2 to 3 mm of tissue). Radiation of therapeutic dose is expended within 56 days.

CONTRAINDICATIONS AND PRECAUTIONS
Acute hyperthyroidism, large nodular goiter, recent myocardial infarction, pregnancy, sensitivity to iodine, patients younger than 18 years of age unless indications are exceptional, lactation. Cautious use: patients in childbearing age, impaired renal and cardiac function.

ADVERSE REACTIONS
Permanent hypothyroidism, thyroid nodules, thyroid cancer (in children), angioedema, petechiae, transient thyroiditis (marked thyroid tenderness with swelling, fever, malaise, aching of teeth, headache, transient decrease in erythrocyte sedimentation rate, pain referred to ear, chest, or throat), alopecia (reversible), genetically transmissible chromosomal abnormalities, myelosuppression.

ROUTE AND DOSAGE
Oral (solution and capsules): Therapeutic: 2 to 25 mCi single dose; second dose, if necessary, 6 to 12 months later. Diagnostic tracer dose: 1 to 25 μCi or less (liquid or as prepared capsule).

NURSING IMPLICATIONS
Presence of food may delay absorption; therefore patient should fast overnight prior to RAI administration.

When administering oral liquid ^{131}I, rinse container 2 or 3 times to ensure delivery of total dose. Glass or plastic cups are preferable to wax cups or paper cups.

Urge patient to empty bladder frequently after therapeutic dosages of ^{131}I to reduce gonadal radiation.

Urinary excretion level of RAI (normal 40% to 70% in 24 hours) is inversely related to amount fixed by thyroid; thus it can be used as indirect measure of thyroid function. In hyperfunctioning organ, generally less than 30% of dose appears in urine in 24 hours; in hypofunctioning organ, over 80% usually appears.

Desirable clinical response (amelioration of thyrotoxicosis symptoms) is usually evident 3 to 6 weeks after treatment.

Expected pattern of response to therapy: first 2 weeks, minimal chemical or clinical change in thyrotoxicosis; next 4 to 8 weeks, decrease in thyroid function reaching nadir (acute effects of radiation) between 8 to 12 weeks post treatment.

If patient is hyperthyroid following treatment, RAI is repeated in 16 weeks and every 3 to 4 months thereafter until euthyroid state is achieved.

Emphasize need for rest following RAI therapy. Consult physician for activity guides.

Frequently, thyroxine replacement is instituted after patient achieves euthyroid state, as prophylaxis against myxedema. Patient should understand that this will be lifelong medication and that he will need to return to his physician at least once a year for medical surveillance. Consult physician about when to discuss this with the patient and family.

Teach the patient the symptoms of hypothyroidism (enlarged thyroid gland, reduced GI motility, periorbital edema, puffy hands and feet, cool and pale skin, fatigue, vertigo, nocturnal muscle cramps) and advise him to be sensitive to verbalized observations of friends who may see a change in his appearance. Myxedema develops insidiously over a period of years; objective and subjective symptoms are difficult to detect in oneself.

Transient thyroiditis (see Adverse Reactions) may occur 1 to 2 weeks after RAI treatment because of hormone leakage from damaged follicles into circulation. Patient should report symptoms promptly to permit treatment.

RAI uptake indicates status of thyroid hormone synthesis: an uptake at 6 hours that is higher than at 24 hours indicates rapid turnover of RAI; persistently high uptake at 48 hours or more suggests appreciable hormone stores.

The patient receiving 30 mCi or more of RAI is usually confined to a single room. A radiation survey is made of bedding, furnishings, and equipment when he is discharged. No special precautions are indicated when diagnostic tracer dose or dose less than 30 mCi is given.

Be fully knowledgeable about agency policies designed to protect patient and health personnel. Work in patient area and body contact with patient should be guided by the principle that radioactivity can be neither neutralized nor destroyed.

If patient is receiving therapeutic doses, plan patient-side activities so as to keep time spent at the bedside at a minimum. The nurse should wear gloves when handling urine or contaminated linen. The urine of the patient receiving therapeutic RAI is considered radioactive waste during the first day or two after treatment. Contaminated bed linens and clothing of patient should be monitored and handled separately. Disposable items, such as Kleenex, are also considered radioactive waste.

Decay time for ^{131}I is about 3 months. Radioactive contaminated articles may be stored for controlled decay for the 3-month RAI decay time. Liquid wastes may be disposed of in the sewer if certain AEC or state regulations are met.

Instruct visitors to remain several feet away during extended visits with the patient who is on therapeutic RAI.

Solution is clear and colorless; however, on standing, bottle and solution may darken (without interfering with efficacy).

Other iodine radionuclides and their diagnostic uses include the following: Iodinated I 125 Serum Albumen, U.S.P. and Iodinated I 131 Serum Albumen, U.S.P. (measurement of blood volume, cardiac output, cardiac blood pool scanning, placental localization); Iodinated I 131 Serum Albumen Aggregated (lung scanning); Liothyronine I 125 or I 131 (in vitro study of thyroid function); Iodohippurate Sodium I 131 Injection, U.S.P. (in conjunction with renogram; kidney scanning); Rose Bengal Sodium I 131 Injection, U.S.P. (liver function; liver scanning).

SODIUM NITROPRUSSIDE, U.S.P.
(NIPRIDE)

Antihypertensive

ACTIONS AND USES

Potent, rapid-acting hypotensive agent with effects similar to those of nitrite. Acts directly on vascular smooth muscle to produce peripheral vasodilation, with consequent marked lowering of arterial blood pressure, associated with slight increase in heart rate, mild decrease in cardiac output, and moderate lowering of peripheral vascular resistance. Thiocyanate metabolite may inhibit uptake and binding of iodine, with prolonged therapy.

Used for short-term, rapid reduction of blood pressure in hypertensive crises and for producing controlled hypotension during anesthesia to reduce bleeding.

ABSORPTION AND FATE

Onset of hypotensive effect usually occurs within 2 minutes; effect lasts 1 to 10 minutes after infusion is terminated. Rapidly converted to cyanogen (cyanides) in erythrocytes and tissue, which is metabolized to thiocyanate in liver. Excreted in urine, primarily as thiocyanate metabolite.

CONTRAINDICATIONS AND PRECAUTIONS

Use in treatment of compensatory hypertension, as in atriovenous shunt or coarctation of aorta, or for producing controlled hypotension in patients with inadequate cerebral circulation. Safe use during pregnancy and in women of childbearing potential and children not established. Cautious use: hepatic insufficiency, hypothyroidism, severe renal impairment, hyponatremia, elderly patients with low vitamin B_{12} plasma levels or with Leber's optic atrophy.

ADVERSE REACTIONS

Usually associated with too rapid reduction in blood pressure: nausea, retching, abdominal pain, nasal stuffiness, diaphoresis, headache, dizziness, apprehension, restlessness, muscle twitching, retrosternal discomfort, palpitation, increase or transient lowering of pulse rate. **Overdosage** (thiocyanate toxicity): profound hypotension, tinnitus, blurred vision, fatigue, metabolic acidosis, pink skin color, absence of reflexes, faint heart sounds, loss of consciousness. **Other:** irritation at infusion site, hypothyroidism with prolonged therapy (rare), increase in serum creatinine, fall or rise in total plasma cobalamins.

ROUTE AND DOSAGE

Intravenous infusion (only): average dose 3 μg/kg/minute, range 0.5 to 8 μg/kg/minute; usual infusion rate 20 to 400 μg/minute; rarely exceeds 800 μg/minute. 5% dextrose in water and reportedly, sterile water *without preservative* may be used preparing solutions.

NURSING IMPLICATIONS

Solutions must be freshly prepared and used no later than 4 hours after reconstitution.

Following reconstitution, solutions usually have faint brownish tint; if highly colored do not use. Promptly wrap container with aluminum foil or other opaque material to protect drug from light.

Administered by infusion pump, micro-drip regulator, or similar device that will allow precise measurement of flow rate.

Constant monitoring is required to titrate IV infusion rate to blood pressure response. If concomitant oral antihypertensive therapy is given, IV infusion rate will require further adjustment.

Adverse effects (see Adverse Reactions) are usually relieved by slowing IV rate or by stopping drug; they may be minimized by keeping patient supine.

Monitor intake and output.

Monitoring blood thiocyanate level is recommended in patients receiving prolonged treatment or in patients with severe renal dysfunction (levels usually are not allowed to exceed 10 mg/dl). Determination of plasma cyanogen level following 1 or 2 days of therapy is advised in patients with impaired hepatic function (see Fate and Absorption).

No other drug should be added to sodium nitroprusside infusion.

Treatment of overdosage: amyl nitrite inhalations for 15 to 30 seconds each minute pending preparation of 3% sodium nitrite solution (injection rate not to exceed 2.5 to 5 ml/minute, up to total dose of 10 to 15 ml, followed by IV sodium thiosulfate 12.5 Gm in 50 ml of 5% dextrose in water over 10-minute period; may be repeated at one-half the above doses, if necessary). Have on hand vasopressor agents. Patient must be closely observed for several hours, since signs of overdosage may reappear.

Protect drug from light, heat, and moisture.

Neoplastic suppressant, diagnostic aid

ACTIONS AND USES

Radiopharmaceutical with physical half-life of 14.3 days; processed in form of disodium phosphate from neutron bombardment of elemental sulfur. Disintegration by beta particle emissions having range of approximately 2 to 8 mm of tissue. Chemically and physiologically identical to stable, naturally occurring phosphorus (^{31}P). Delivers ionizing radiation to cells with high phosphate turnover; ultimately bone tissue becomes most radioactive. Reduces pain by preferential suppression of myelopoiesis, with no extrahematic reaction.

Used therapeutically both alone and in conjunction with alkylating antineoplastics in treatment of polycythemia vera; has been administered by local instillation after surgery of ovarian cancer. Has also been used diagnostically to detect and delineate eye tumors, prostatic metastases, and (12 to 24 hours preoperatively) brain tumor.

ABSORPTION AND FATE

Incompletely absorbed from intestinal tract; therefore oral route is rarely used. After IV administration, ^{32}P mixes with body pool of inorganic phosphates. Uniform distribution continues a few days, followed by preferential deposition in bone marrow, spleen, and liver to as much as 10 times concentrations in remaining tissues. Excreted in urine, 25% to 50% during first 4 to 6 days, slowing to 1% daily within 1 week. Small amounts excreted in feces.

CONTRAINDICATIONS AND PRECAUTIONS

Pregnancy, lactation, children younger than 18 years of age unless indications are exceptional, polycythemia vera when leukocyte count is less than 3000/μl or platelet count is less than 100,000/μl. Cautious use: women of childbearing age (given only during or after menstrual period).

ADVERSE REACTIONS

Myelosuppression [leukopenia (rare), thrombocytopenia, anemia], acute leukemia (10%), radiation sickness (rare), myelofibrosis.

ROUTE AND DOSAGE

Oral, intravenous (diagnostic): 250 μCi to 1 mCi; (therapeutic: chronic myelogenous leukemia, polycythemia suppressant): initially 3 to 4 mCi; decision to give additional doses is made at 4-week intervals; remission usually in 6 months to 1 year or several years following dose of 3 to 10 mCi; (neoplastic suppressant): 10 to 18 mCi (individualized).

NURSING IMPLICATIONS

Be aware of protective policies and procedures established by radioactive protection council of the institution and of radiation hazards to self and to patient.

Nurse should wear film badge or exposure meter on pocket while giving care to patient receiving P^{32}.

Avoid milk and milk products, iron, bismuth medications, and soft drinks if oral preparation is used.

Blood studies, including hemoglobin determinations and leukocyte, RBC, and platelet counts, are usually performed before therapy, at monthly intervals during treatment, and at regular intervals throughout life after therapy.

Before P^{32} therapy is instituted, hematocrit is usually reduced to below 50% by phlebotomy.

To minimize amount of radiation received from unabsorbed P^{32}, the patient fasts 2 hours before and 6 hours after administration of drug.

Follow established protocol for disposal of vomitus, wound seepage, feces, and equipment and linens they have contaminated.

If patient has dressings, remove them with long-handled forceps and carry them to established radioactive waste disposal unit in leaded container.

Transfer of P^{32} solution to syringe for injection should be done with gloved hands under a shielded hood.

The fraction of dose excreted in urine is small; thus no particular precautions are warranted.

The only external radiation from the patient is a small amount of continuous beta emission with short range that is insufficient to require patient isolation.

Clinical response to P^{32} treatment for polycythemia vera tends to occur within 3 to 4 weeks after start of treatment.

During remission (often lasting more than 1 or 2 years), visits for clinical evaluation are usually spaced at 3- to 4-month intervals. Urge patient to keep appointments.

P^{32}-induced remissions subsequent to hematologic relapses are successively shorter in duration.

Since P^{32} is excreted in urine, large urine volumes should be assured by high fluid intake. Monitor intake–output ratio during initial period of myelopoietic suppression with P^{32}. Symptoms of dysuria and oliguria should be reported.

Patient receiving P^{32} may develop radiation sickness: general malaise, nausea, and vomiting, followed by remission of symptoms; later there will be fever, hemorrhage, fluid loss, anemia, and CNS involvement.

Reinforce necessity of adhering to medical check-up schedule. Inform patient of symptoms that may indicate impending hematologic relapse (indicator for P^{32} injection): dizziness, fullness in head, itchy skin (especially after warm bath), ecchymoses, paresthesias, visual disturbances, suffusion of conjunctiva.

Solutions are clear and colorless; however, on standing, both solution and container may darken without interfering with efficacy.

SODIUM POLYSTYRENE SULFONATE, U.S.P. (KAYEXALATE)

Ion-exchange resin (potassium)

ACTIONS AND USES

Sulfonic cation-exchange resin. Removes potassium from body by exchanging sodium ion for potassium, particularly in large intestine; potassium-containing resin is then excreted. Small amounts of other cations such as calcium and magnesium may be lost during treatment.

Used as adjunct in treatment of hyperkalemia.

CONTRAINDICATIONS AND PRECAUTIONS

Cautious use: acute or chronic renal failure; patients receiving digitalis preparations; patients who cannot tolerate increase in sodium load, eg, actual or impending heart failure, hypertension, edema.

ADVERSE REACTIONS

Hypokalemia, hypocalcemia, sodium retention, anorexia, nausea, vomiting, constipation, fecal impaction, diarrhea (occasionally).

ROUTE AND DOSAGE

Oral: **Adults:** 15 Gm (4 *level* teaspoons) 1 to 4 times daily; **Infants and small children:** calculated on exchange rate of 1 mEq of potassium per gram of resin. Rectal: **Adults:** 30 Gm suspended in 100 to 200 ml of 1% methylcellulose solution or 10% dextrose solution or water (as prescribed) 1 or 2 times daily.

NURSING IMPLICATIONS

Oral dose should be given as a suspension in a small quantity of water or in syrup. Usual amount of fluid ranges from 20 to 100 ml or approximately 3 to 4 ml/Gm of drug.

Serum potassium levels should be determined daily throughout therapy. Acid–base balance, electrolytes, and minerals should also be monitored in patients receiving repeated doses.

Serum potassium levels do not always reflect intracellular potassium deficiency. Therefore, observe patient closely for early clinical signs of severe hypokalemia: irritability, confusion, delayed thought process, muscular pain and weakness. ECGs are also recommended.

Usually a mild laxative is prescribed to prevent constipation (common side effect) and fecal impaction. Check bowel function daily. Elderly patients are particularly prone to fecal impaction.

Since drug contains approximately 100 mg (4.1 mEq) of sodium per gram, sodium content from dietary and other sources may be restricted. Consult physician.

When administered by retention enema, use warm fluid (as prescribed) to prepare the emulsion. Do not heat sodium polystyrene sulfonate, since this may alter its exchange properties. Administer at body temperature.

An alternative method of rectal administration preferred by some physicians is to insert a sealed dialysis bag containing drug into the rectum.

Instruct patient to retain enema for prescribed period of time (varies from 4 to 10 hours) at which time colon is irrigated to remove resin.

DRUG INTERACTIONS: Potassium-exchange capability of sodium polystyrene sulfonate may be reduced by concomitant use of **antacids** or **laxatives** containing magnesium or calcium.

SODIUM SALICYLATE, N.F., B.P.
(SALBID, URACEL)

Analgesic

ACTIONS AND USES

A salicylate with properties and uses similar to those of aspirin (qv). About one-third as potent on a weight basis as aspirin. Liberates free salicylic acid in stomach, and therefore tends to cause gastric irritation.

Used primarily in treatment of acute rheumatic fever.

CONTRAINDICATIONS AND PRECAUTIONS

Severe renal disease; patients on low-sodium diet. Also see Aspirin.

ROUTE AND DOSAGE

Oral, intravenous: 325 to 650 mg every 4 to 6 hours as needed.

NURSING IMPLICATIONS

Physician may prescribe an equivalent amount of sodium bicarbonate to prevent gastric irritation. (Bicarbonate also increases rate of salicylate excretion, and thus may lower salicylate blood levels).

See Aspirin.

Anterior pituitary growth hormone

ACTIONS AND USES

Polypeptide hormone extracted from human pituitary gland at necropsy. Elicits all pharmacologic responses produced by endogenous human growth hormone (GH). Anabolic effect is equated with accelerated linear growth rate in children with GH deficiency and with increased body weight and muscle mass. Increases intracellular transport and utilization of amino acids and retention of potassium, nitrogen, phosphorus, sodium, magnesium, chloride, and calcium. With respect to calcium, increased urinary loss appears to be augmented by increased absorption from intestinal mucosa. Stimulates synthesis of chondroitin sulfate and collagen; increases serum concentration of alkaline phosphatase and urinary excretion of hydroxyproline. In large doses, may exert diabetogenic effect by causing hepatic gluconeogenesis, increased blood glucose levels, decreased glucose tolerance, and decreased sensitivity to exogenous insulin, particularly in diabetes. In some patients serum insulin concentration is increased. Promotes utilization of depot fat (increases circulating fatty acids), and appears to reduce serum cholesterol levels while increasing triglyceride concentrations. May induce bone marrow activity, increase hemoglobin synthesis, and elevate serum levels of immunoglobulin G and transferrin.

Used to treat hypopituitary dwarfism and as replacement therapy prior to epiphyseal closure in patients with idiopathic GH deficiency, GH deficiency secondary to intracranial tumors, or panhypopituitarism.

ABSORPTION AND FATE

Plasma half-life 15 to 50 minutes, but pharmacotherapeutic effects persist several days. More than 90% of drug metabolized in liver; approximately 0.1% of dose is excreted unchanged in urine. Does not cross placenta.

CONTRAINDICATIONS AND PRECAUTIONS

Patient with closed epiphyses; progression of underlying intracranial tumor. Cautious use: diabetes mellitus or family history of the disease, concomitant or prior use of thyroid and/or androgens in prepubertal male.

ADVERSE REACTIONS

Pain, swelling at injection site; myalgia, early morning headache (rare), hypercalciuria (frequent); oversaturation of bile with cholesterol, induction of hypothyroidism (rare), high circulating GH antibodies with resulting treatment failure, allergic reactions (rare), hyperglycemia, ketosis, accelerated growth of intracranial tumor.

ROUTE AND DOSAGE

Intramuscular: 1 ml (2 IU) or 0.05 to 0.1 IU/kg body weight 3 times weekly with a minimum of 48 hours between injections. If at any time during continuous administration growth rate does not exceed 2.5 cm (1 inch) in a 6-month period, dose may be doubled for next 6 months.

NURSING IMPLICATIONS

Reconstitute each vial (containing 10 IU of drug) with 5 ml bacteriostatic water for injection U.S.P. only. Record date of reconstitution on vial. Stored in refrigerator (at 2 C to 8 C); discard after 1 month.

Subcutaneous injection should be avoided because it may enhance development of neutralizing antibodies, with resulting treatment failure, and may cause local lipoatrophy (localized fat atrophy) or lipodystrophy (defective nutrition of subcutaneous tissue).

Rotate IM sites to prevent tissue damage.

Before initiating treatment, careful documentation is made of growth rate for at least 6 to 12 months. In addition, GH deficiency may be confirmed by demonstrating failure of plasma GH levels to exceed 5 to 7 ng/ml in response to two standard stimuli (eg, insulin, hypoglycemia, IV arginine, oral levodopa, or IM glucagon). Thyroid, adrenal, and gonadal functions are also evaluated to rule out multiple pituitary hormone deficiency.

Danger of premature epiphyseal closure with somatotropin therapy is usually minimal because acceleration of bone age progression is not as marked as that of linear growth rate. However, annual bone age assessments are advised in all patients and especially those also receiving concurrent thyroid and/or androgen treatment, since these drugs may precipitate early epiphyseal closure. Urge parent to take child for bone age assessment on appointed annual dates.

During first 6 months of successful treatment, linear growth rates may be increased 8 to 16 cm or more per year (average about 7 cm/year). Additionally, subcutaneous fat diminishes, but returns to pretreatment value later.

Instruct parent of child under treatment to record accurate height measurements at regular intervals and to report to physician if rate is less than expected.

In general, growth response to somatotropin is inversely proportional to duration of treatment. Somatotropin should be discontinued when patient has reached satisfactory adult height, when epiphyses have fused, or when patient fails to exhibit growth response.

Hypercalciuria, a frequent side effect in the first 2 to 3 months of therapy, may be symptomless; however, it may be accompanied by renal calculi, with these reportable symptoms: flank pain and colic, GI symptoms, urinary frequency, chills, fever, hematuria.

In patients who respond initially but who later fail to respond to somatotropin therapy, test for circulating GH antibodies (antisomatotropin antibodies) should be performed.

Diabetic patients or those with family history of diabetes should be observed closely. Regular testing of urine for glycosuria or fasting blood glucose levels is recommended.

Patient with GH deficiency secondary to intracranial lesion should be examined frequently for progression or recurrence of underlying disease process.

DRUG INTERACTIONS: Concomitant treatment with **thyroid hormone** and/or **androgens** may precipitate epiphyseal closure. **Corticosteroids** may diminish growth response to somatotropin and act synergistically with it in increasing blood glucose levels and decreasing sensitivity to exogenous insulin.

SPECTINOMYCIN HYDROCHLORIDE
(ACTINOSPECTOCIN, TROBICIN)

Antibiotic

ACTIONS AND USES

Aminocyclitol antibiotic (related to aminoglycosides) produced by *Streptomyces spectabilis*. Antibacterial action results from selective binding of 30S subunits of bacterial ribosomes, thereby inhibiting protein synthesis. Variable activity against a wide variety of Gram-negative and Gram-positive organisms. Inhibits majority of *Neisseria gonorrhoeae* strains. Not effective against syphilis.

Used only in acute genital and rectal gonorrhea, particularly in patients sensitized or resistant to penicillin or other effective drugs.

ABSORPTION AND FATE
Rapidly absorbed after IM injection. Plasma concentration peaks in 1 to 2 hours; appreciable levels persist 8 hours or more. Minimal binding to plasma proteins. Active form excreted in urine within 48 hours after injection.

CONTRAINDICATIONS AND PRECAUTIONS
Hypersensitivity to spectinomycin. Safe use during pregnancy and in infants and children not established. Cautious use: history of allergies.

ADVERSE REACTIONS
Soreness at injection site, urticaria, dizziness, nausea, chills, fever, insomnia. Following multiple doses: decrease in hemoglobin, hematocrit, or creatinine clearance; elevated alkaline phosphatase, SGPT, or BUN; decrease in urine output.

ROUTE AND DOSAGE
Intramuscular: 2 to 4 Gm (4-Gm dose should be divided and administered at two different gluteal sites). Reconstitute with accompanying diluent.

NURSING IMPLICATIONS

Shake vial vigorously immediately after adding diluent and before withdrawing drug. Following reconstitution, drug may be stored at room temperature, but it should be used within 24 hours.

Administer IM injection deep into upper outer quadrant of buttock. No more than 5 ml should be injected into single site (20-gauge needle is recommended). Injection may be painful.

All patients with gonorrhea should have serologic tests for syphilis at time of diagnosis and again after 3 months.

Clinical effectiveness of drug should be monitored to detect antibiotic resistance.

SPIRONOLACTONE, U.S.P., B.P.
(ALDACTONE)

Diuretic (aldosterone antagonist)

ACTIONS AND USES
Steroidal compound and specific pharmacologic antagonist of aldosterone. Presumably acts by competing with aldosterone for cellular receptor sites in distal renal tubule. Promotes sodium and chloride (and water) excretion without concomitant loss of potassium. Diuretic effect reportedly not associated with hyperuricemia or hyperglycemia. Activity depends on presence of endogenous or exogenous aldosterone. Lowers systolic and diastolic pressures in hypertensive patients by unknown mechanism.

Used in clinical conditions associated with augmented aldosterone production, as in essential hypertension, refractory edema due to congestive heart failure, hepatic cirrhosis, nephrotic syndrome, and idiopathic edema. May be used to potentiate actions of other diuretics and antihypertensive agents or for its potassium-sparing effect. Also used for treatment of (and as presumptive test for) primary aldosteronism. Commercially available in combination with hydrochlorothiazide (Aldactazide).

ABSORPTION AND FATE
Rapidly and extensively metabolized. Peak plasma levels of active metabolite (canrenone) within 2 to 4 hours, half-life following multiple doses between 13 and 24 hours. Maximal diuretic effect attained in about 3 days; activity persists 2 or 3 days after discontinuation of drug. Metabolites excreted slowly, primarily in urine, and also in bile.

Anuria, acute renal insufficiency, progressing impairment of renal function, hyperkalemia. Safe use in women of childbearing potential or during pregnancy not established. Cautious use: BUN of 40 mg/dl or greater, hepatic disease.

ADVERSE REACTIONS

Lethargy and fatigue (with rapid weight loss), headache, drowsiness, abdominal cramps, nausea, vomiting, anorexia, diarrhea, maculopapular or erythematous rash, urticaria, mental confusion, fever, ataxia, gynecomastia (males and females), inability to achieve or maintain erection, androgenic effects (hirsutism, irregular menses, deepening of voice), fluid and electrolyte imbalance (particularly hyperkalemia and hyponatremia), elevated BUN, mild acidosis.

ROUTE AND DOSAGE

Oral: Essential hypertension **(adults):** initially 50 to 100 mg daily in divided doses, continued for at least 2 weeks; subsequent dosage adjusted according to patient's response. Edema **(adults):** initially 25 to 200 mg daily in divided doses, continued for at least 5 days; dosage then adjusted to optimal therapeutic or maintenance level; if there is no response, a diuretic that acts on proximal renal tubule may be added; **(children):** 1.5 to 3.3 mg/kg body weight daily in 4 divided doses. Primary aldosteronism (therapy): 100 to 400 mg daily in divided doses; (long test): 400 mg daily for 3 to 4 weeks; (short test): 400 mg daily for 4 days.

NURSING IMPLICATIONS

Serum electrolytes should be monitored, especially during early therapy.

Potassium supplementation is not indicated in spironolactone therapy (unless patient is also receiving a corticosteroid). Patient is generally instructed to avoid excessive intake of high-potassium foods and salt substitutes (see Index). Consult physician regarding allowable potassium and sodium intake.

Inform patient that maximal diuretic effect may not occur until third day of therapy and that diuresis may continue for 2 or 3 days after drug is withdrawn.

Monitor daily intake and output and check for edema. Report lack of diuretic response or development of edema; both may indicate tolerance to drug action.

Weigh patient under standard conditions before therapy begins and daily throughout therapy. Weight is a useful index of need for dosage adjustment. For patients with ascites, physician may want measurements of abdominal girth.

Check blood pressure before initiation of therapy and at regular intervals throughout therapy.

Be alert for signs of fluid and electrolyte imbalance, and instruct patient to report dry mouth, thirst, abdominal cramps, lethargy, and drowsiness (symptoms of hyponatremia, most likely to occur in patients with severe cirrhosis), as well as paresthesias, confusion, weakness, or heaviness of legs (symptoms of hyperkalemia).

Observe for and report immediately the onset of mental changes, lethargy, or stupor in patients with hepatic disease.

Adverse reactions are generally reversible with discontinuation of drug. Gynecomastia appears to be related to dosage level and duration of therapy; it may persist in some patients even after drug is stopped.

Presumptive diagnosis of primary aldosteronism is made if short test produces serum potassium increase during spironolactone administration followed by decrease when it is discontinued or if long test results in correction of hypertension and hypokalemia with spironolactone.

Preserved in tight, light-resistant containers. Suspension formulation is stable for 1 month under refrigeration.

LABORATORY TEST INTERFERENCES: Spironolactone may produce marked increases in **plasma cortisol determinations** by Mattingly fluorometric method; these may persist for several days after termination of drug (spironolactone metabolite produces fluorescence). There is the possibility of false elevations in measurements of **digoxin serum levels** by radioimmunoassay procedures.

DRUG INTERACTIONS: Combinations of spironolactone and acidifying doses of **ammonium chloride** may produce systemic acidosis; use these combinations with caution. Diuretic effect of spironolactone may be antagonized by **aspirin** and other **salicylates** (possibly by competing for same receptor sites). Spironolactone potentiates the actions of other **antihypertensives,** particularly **ganglionic blocking agents** (dosage of these drugs should be reduced by at least 50% when spironolactone is added), and other **diuretics.** Patients receiving spironolactone and **digitoxin** or similar **cardiac glycosides** concurrently should be monitored for decreased effect of cardiac glycoside (spironolactone shortens its half-life, possibly by acting as enzyme inducing agent). Hyperkalemia may result with **potassium supplements** (spironolactone conserves potassium).

STANOZOLOL, N.F.
(WINSTROL)

Androgen

ACTIONS AND USES
Synthetic androgenic steroid with relatively strong anabolic and weak androgenic activity.
Used primarily as an anabolic agent. See Ethylestrenol for actions, indications, and limitations.
ROUTE AND DOSAGE
Oral: **Adults:** 2 mg 3 times daily; for young women, 2 mg once or twice daily. **Children:** *under 6 years of age,* 1 mg 2 times daily; *6 to 12 years of age,* 2 mg 3 times daily.

NURSING IMPLICATIONS
Administer just before or with meals to reduce incidence of gastric distress. See Ethylestrenol.

STREPTOKINASE-STREPTODORNASE
(VARIDASE)

Enzyme, aid in healing

ACTIONS AND USES
Combination of proteolytic enzymes cultivated from certain strains of hemolytic streptococci. Streptokinase functions indirectly by activating the transformation of plasminogen to plasmin, with resulting lysis of clots or fibrin-containing exudates. Streptodornase liquefies viscous nucleoprotein of dead cells and pus; it has no effect on living cells.
Used to aid in removal of fibrinous, purulent accumulation and edema resulting from trauma or inflammation. Also has been used as adjunct in treatment of hemothorax, hematoma, empyema, and chronic suppurative lesions and to dissolve clots in urinary bladder or in tubes and catheters.

CONTRAINDICATIONS AND PRECAUTIONS

Active hemorrhage, acute cellulitis without suppuration, active tuberculosis, bronchopleural fistulas, reduced plasminogen or fibrinogen levels, IM administration to patients with depressed liver function.

ADVERSE REACTIONS

Malaise, nausea, vomiting, diarrhea, pain at IM injection site, pyrogenic reaction (fever, increased drainage), hypersensitivity reactions, anaphylactic shock (rare).

ROUTE AND DOSAGE

Oral: 1 tablet 4 times daily (each tablet contains 10,000 units of streptokinase and at least 2500 units of streptodornase). Intramuscular: 0.5 ml (containing 5000 units of streptokinase and 1250 units of streptodornase). Topical jelly or solution (large cavities): 200,000 units streptokinase and 50,000 units streptodornase; (smaller spaces): 10,000 units streptokinase and 2500 units streptodornase. Highly individualized. Follow package insert for proper dilutions.

NURSING IMPLICATIONS

Enzymes may be destroyed by agitation. Add diluent slowly, and gently swirl vial until drug is dissolved (material is very soluble).

Date vial when drug is reconstituted. Stable up to 24 hours at room temperature after reconstitution; stable for 2 weeks if kept refrigerated at 2 C to 8 C (35 F to 45 F) when not in use.

IM injections are made preferably into upper outer quadrant of buttock. Aspirate carefully before injecting to avoid inadvertent entry into blood vessel. Injection may be painful.

When used for "chemical debridement" of chronically infected wounds, drug must be in intimate contact with suppurative material for maximum therapeutic effect.

Physician may prescribe addition of antibiotic to drug-jelly mixture (eg, tetracycline, penicillin, streptomycin, dehydrostreptomycin).

For topical applications to hand wounds, jelly formulation may be placed in a loose, sterile rubber glove and fastened at wrist.

Febrile reaction due to localized leukocytosis and accumulation of tissue fluid frequently occurs during first 24 hours of treatment. Reaction may be minimized by frequent removal or aspiration of exudate, particularly in closed areas.

Wound may require dressing reinforcement, as drainage on becoming liquefied will be more profuse.

Be alert for symptoms of hypersensitivity reaction (nausea, vomiting, chills, fever, tachycardia, dizziness, hypotension) that may occur with repeated administration.

STREPTOMYCIN SULFATE, U.S.P., B.P.

Antibiotic, tuberculostatic (aminoglycoside)

ACTIONS AND USES

Aminoglycoside antibiotic derived from *Streptomyces griseus,* with bactericidal and bacteriostatic actions. Appears to act by interfering with normal protein synthesis in susceptible bacteria by binding to 30S subunits of ribosomes. Active against a variety of Gram-positive, Gram-negative, and acid-fast organisms. Because of rapid emergence of resistant strains when used alone, most commonly used concurrently with other antimicrobial agents. Reportedly, the least nephrotoxic of aminoglycosides. In common with other aminoglycosides, has weak neuromuscular blocking effect.

Used only in combination with other antitubercular drugs in treatment of all forms of active tuberculosis caused by susceptible organisms. Used alone or in conjunction with tetracycline for tularemia, plaque, and brucellosis. Also used with other antibiotics in treatment of subacute bacterial endocarditis due to enterococci and streptococci (viridans group) and *H. influenzae* and in treatment of peritonitis, respiratory tract infections, granuloma inguinale, and chancroid when other drugs have failed. Used investigationally in treatment of bilateral Meniere's disease.

ABSORPTION AND FATE

Following IM administration, peak serum levels in 1 to 2 hours; levels slowly diminish by about 50% after 5 to 6 hours, but are still measurable up to 8 to 12 hours. About one-third of dose is bound to plasma proteins. Half-life about 2.5 hours for young adults (longer in newborns, in adults over age 40, and in impaired renal function). Diffuses rapidly into most body tissues and extracellular fluids and penetrates tuberculous cavities and caseous tissue. Does not diffuse into cerebrospinal fluid unless meninges are inflamed. Excreted rapidly, primarily by glomerular filtration; 30% to 90% of dose is excreted within 24 hours. Small amounts excreted in saliva, sweat, tears, bile, and milk. Crosses placenta.

CONTRAINDICATIONS AND PRECAUTIONS

History of toxic or hypersensitivity reaction to aminoglycosides, labyrinthine disease, myasthenia gravis, concurrent or sequential use of other neurotoxic and/or nephrotoxic agents. Cautious use: impaired renal function (given in reduced dosages), use during pregnancy, use in the elderly and in children.

ADVERSE REACTIONS

Ototoxicity: labyrinthine damage (most frequent), auditory damage. **Other neurotoxic effects:** paresthesias (peripheral, facial, and especially circumoral), headache, inability to concentrate, lassitude, muscular weakness, optic nerve toxicity (scotomata, dimmed or blurred vision), arachnoiditis, encephalopathy, CNS depression syndrome (infants): stupor, flaccidity, coma, respiratory depression. **Hypersensitivity:** skin rashes, pruritus, angioedema, fever, eosinophilia, exfoliative dermatitis, stomatitis, enlarged lymph nodes, anaphylactic shock, blood dyscrasias: leukopenia, thrombocytopenia (rare), neutropenia, pancytopenia, hemolytic or aplastic anemia, agranulocytosis (rare). **Other:** myocarditis (rare), nephrotoxicity (uncommon), hepatotoxicity, transient bleeding (due to inhibition of factor V), systemic lupus erythematosus, pain and irritation at IM site, superinfections, neuromuscular blockade (respiratory paralysis, cardiac arrest).

ROUTE AND DOSAGE

Intramuscular: **Adults:** Tuberculosis therapy (various regimens used): up to 1 Gm daily in conjunction with other antitubercular drugs; when sputum becomes negative, either streptomycin is discontinued or dosage is reduced to 1 Gm 1 to 3 times weekly for duration of therapy. For other disease conditions (highly individualized): 1 to 4 Gm daily in divided doses every 6 to 12 hours. **Pediatric:** *Prematures and newborns:* 10 to 30 mg/kg/day in divided doses.

NURSING IMPLICATIONS

Administer IM deep into large muscle mass to minimize possibility of irritation. Injections are painful.

Avoid direct contact with drug; sensitization can occur. Rubber or plastic gloves are advised when preparing drug.

Culture and sensitivity tests are done prior to and periodically during course of therapy.

Patient should be instructed to report any unusual symptom. Adverse reactions should be reviewed periodically, especially in patients on prolonged therapy.

Caloric stimulation and audiometric tests should be performed before, during, and 6 months after discontinuation of streptomycin. Periodic renal and hepatic function tests are also recommended.

Monitor intake and output. Report oliguria or changes in intake–output ratio (possible signs of diminishing renal function). Sufficient fluids to maintain urinary output of 1500 ml/24 hours are generally advised. Consult physician.

In patients with impaired renal function, drug accumulation reportedly occurs if administered more frequently than every 8 to 12 hours (intervals of 1 to 2 days are recommended if creatinine clearance is 10 ml/minute or greater, and 3 to 4 days if less than 10 ml/minute). Physician may prescribe an alkalinizing agent to reduce possibility of renal irritation. Frequent determinations of serum drug concentrations and periodic renal and hepatic function tests are advised (serum concentrations should not exceed 25 μg/ml in these patients).

Be alert for and report immediately symptoms suggestive of ototoxicity. Symptoms are most likely to occur in patients with impaired renal function, patients receiving high doses (1.8 to 2 Gm daily) or other ototoxic or neurotoxic drugs, and the elderly. If drug is not discontinued promptly, irreversible damage may occur.

Damage of vestibular portion of eighth cranial nerve (higher incidence than auditory toxicity) appears to occur in three stages: Acute stage may be preceded for 1 or 2 days by moderately severe headache, then followed by nausea, vomiting, vertigo in upright position, difficulty in reading, unsteadiness, and positive Romberg; lasts 1 to 2 weeks and ends abruptly. Chronic stage is characterized by difficulty in walking or in making sudden movements and ataxia; lasts approximately 2 months. Compensatory stage: symptoms are latent and appear only when eyes are closed. Full recovery may take 12 to 18 months; residual damage is permanent in some patients.

Auditory nerve damage is usually preceded by vestibular symptoms and high-pitched tinnitus, roaring noises, impaired hearing (especially to high-pitched sounds), sense of fullness in ears. Audiometric test should be done if these symptoms appear, and drug should be discontinued if indicated. Hearing loss can be permanent if damage is extensive. Tinnitus may persist several days to weeks after drug is stopped.

Refer patients receiving drug for tuberculosis to visiting nurse for home supervision and continued teaching, and encourage examination of contacts.

Except for tuberculosis and subacute bacterial endocarditis, streptomycin is rarely administered for more than 7 to 10 days.

Commercially prepared IM solution is intended *only* for intramuscular injection (contains a preservative, and therefore is not suitable for other routes). Stable at room temperature; expiration date 1 to 2 years depending on manufacturer.

Solutions made from streptomycin sulfate powder are preferably used immediately after reconstitution. If necessary, Lilly product may be stored up to 48 hours at room temperature or in refrigerator (2 C to 8 C) for 14 days; Pfizer states that reconstituted solutions may be stored up to 4 weeks without significant loss of potency.

Exposure to light may cause slight darkening of solution, with no apparent loss of potency.

LABORATORY TEST INTERFERENCES: Streptomycin reportedly produces false positive urinary glucose tests using copper sulfate methods (Benedict's solution, Clinitest), but not with glucose oxidase methods (eg, Clinistix, Tes-Tape). False increases in protein content in urine and cerebrospinal fluid using

Folin-Ciocalteau reaction and decreased BUN readings with Berthelot reaction may occur from test interferences. Culture and sensitivity tests may be affected if patient is taking salts such as sodium and potassium chloride, sodium sulfate and tartrate, ammonium acetate, calcium and magnesium ions.

DRUG INTERACTIONS: Streptomycin may produce additive anticoagulant effect in patients receiving **oral anticoagulants** (it is thought that streptomycin interferes with synthesis of intestinal vitamin K and stimulates production of factor V inhibitor). See Gentamicin for other drug interactions.

STRONG IODINE SOLUTION, U.S.P.
(COMPOUND IODINE SOLUTION, LUGOL'S SOLUTION)
AQUEOUS IODINE SOLUTION, B.P.

Supplement, iodine

ACTIONS AND USES
   Inorganic iodide solution; usually contains 5% elemental iodine dissolved in aqueous KI 10%. In the toxic thyroid gland, interferes with proteolysis of thyroglobin; thus blocks release of thyroid hormones (T_3 and T_4). Decreases size and vascularity of thyroid gland caused by previous thioamide medication. Suppresses mild hyperthyroidism completely, and partially suppresses more severe hyperthyroidism.
   Used to prepare thyroid gland for surgery; may be used with an antithyroid drug in the treatment of thyrotoxic crisis.
ABSORPTION AND FATE
   After absorption from GI tract, inorganic iodide enters circulation, from which it is cleared by renal excretion or thyroid uptake, to be utilized in hormone synthesis. Small amounts excreted in urine; more than 70% reabsorbed by renal tubules and distributed to tissues. Degradation principally in liver; glucuronide metabolites excreted in bile to feces. Fecal loss regulated by degree of absorption of oral iodide, liver function, intestinal motility, and fecal volume. Readily crosses placenta.
CONTRAINDICATIONS AND PRECAUTIONS
   Marked sensitivity to iodine, tuberculosis, hypothyroidism.
ADVERSE REACTIONS
   Iodism (see Index), goiter with hypothyroidism (rare).
ROUTE AND DOSAGE
   Oral: 0.1 to 0.3 ml 3 or 4 times daily for 10 to 14 days prior to thyroid surgery.

> **NURSING IMPLICATIONS**
> Administer solution well diluted in fruit juice, milk, or water after meals.
> Teach patients the symptoms of iodism and advise prompt reporting if they
>   appear. Symptoms usually subside rapidly with discontinuation of iodine
>   solution.
> Store in airtight container.
> See Potassium Iodide for nursing implications and drug interactions.

SUCCINYLCHOLINE CHLORIDE, U.S.P., B.P
(ANECTINE, QUELICIN, SUCOSTRIN, SUXAMETHONIUM CHLORIDE
[B.P.] SUX-CERT)

Skeletal Muscle Relaxant

ACTIONS AND USES

Synthetic, ultrashort-acting depolarizing neuromuscular blocking agent with high affinity for acetylcholine (ACh) receptor sites. Initial transient contractions and fasciculations are followed by sustained flaccid skeletal muscle paralysis produced by state of accommodation that develops in adjacent excitable muscle membranes. Rapidly hydrolyzed by plasma pseudocholinesterase. May increase vagal tone initially, particularly in children and with high doses, and subsequently produce mild sympathetic stimulation. Intraocular pressure may increase slightly and may persist after onset of complete paralysis. Reported to have histamine-releasing properties. Has no known effect on consciousness or pain threshold.

Used to produce skeletal muscle relaxation as adjunct to anesthesia, to facilitate intubation and endoscopy, to increase pulmonary compliance in assisted or controlled respiration, and to reduce intensity of muscle contractions in pharmacologically-induced or electroshock convulsions.

ABSORPTION AND FATE

Following IV administration, complete muscle relaxation occurs within 1 minute, persists 2 or 3 minutes, returns to normal in 6 to 10 minutes. Following IM injection, action begins in 2 to 3 minutes and last 10 to 30 minutes. Plasma level falls rapidly by redistribution. Rapidly hydrolyzed by plasma pseudocholinesterases to succinylmonocholine (a mildly active nondepolarizing muscle relaxant), and then more slowly to succinic acid and choline. Excreted in urine primarily as active and inactive metabolites; 10% excreted as unchanged drug. Does not readily cross placenta.

CONTRAINDICATIONS AND PRECAUTIONS

Hypersensitivity to succinylcholine; family history of malignant hyperthermia. Safe use in pregnancy and in women of childbearing potential not established. Cautious use: renal, hepatic, pulmonary, metabolic, or cardiovascular disorders; dehydration, electrolyte imbalance, digitalized patients, severe burns or trauma, fractures, spinal cord injuries, degenerative or dystrophic neuromuscular diseases, low plasma pseudocholinesterase levels (recessive genetic trait, but often associated with severe liver disease, severe anemia, dehydration, marked changes in body temperature, exposure to neurotoxic insecticides, certain drugs); collagen diseases, porphyria, intraocular surgery, glaucoma.

ADVERSE REACTIONS

Neuromuscular: muscle fasciculations, profound and prolonged muscle relaxation, muscle pain. **Respiratory:** respiratory depression, bronchospasm, hypoxia, apnea. **Cardiovascular:** bradycardia, tachycardia, hypotension, hypertension, arrhythmias, sinus arrest. **Other:** malignant hyperthermia, increased intraocular pressure, excessive salivation, enlarged salivary glands, myoglobinemia, hyperkalemia; hypersensitivity reactions (rare); decreased tone and motility of GI tract (large doses).

ROUTE AND DOSAGE

Intravenous: 10 to 30 mg administered over 10 to 30 seconds; continuous infusion (0.1 to 0.2% solution): 0.5 to 5 mg/minute. Intramuscular: 2.5 mg/kg body weight; single dose not to exceed 150 mg. Highly individualized.

NURSING IMPLICATIONS

Only freshly prepared solutions should be used; succinylcholine hydrolyzes rapidly with consequent loss of potency.

Primarily administered by anesthesiologist or under his direct observation. Some physicians order plasma pseudocholinesterase activity determinations before administering succinylcholine.

Initial small test dose may be given to determine individual drug sensitivity and recovery time.

IM injections are made deeply, preferably high into deltoid muscle. Baseline serum electrolyte determinations advised. Electrolyte imbalance (particularly potassium, calcium, magnesium) can potentiate effects of neuromuscular blocking agents.

Transient apnea usually occurs at time of maximal drug effect (1 to 2 minutes); spontaneous respiration should return in a few seconds, or at most, 3 or 4 minutes.

Facilities for emergency endotracheal intubation, artificial respiration, and assisted or controlled respiration with oxygen should be immediately available. A nerve stimulator may be used to assess nature and degree of neuromuscular blockade.

Selective muscle paralysis following drug administration develops in the following sequence: levator eyelid muscles, mastication, limbs, abdomen, glottis, intercostals, diaphragm. Recovery generally occurs in reverse order.

Adverse effects are primarily extensions of pharmacologic actions.

Patient may complain of postprocedural muscle stiffness and pain (caused by initial fasciculations following injection).

Monitor vital signs and keep airway clear of secretions. Observe for and report residual muscle weakness.

Tachyphylaxis (reduced response) may occur after repeated doses. Expiration date and storage before and after reconstitution varies with the manufacturer.

DRUG INTERACTIONS: Agents that may potentiate or prolong neuromuscular blockage of skeletal muscle relaxants: **acetylcholine, certain antibiotics** (gentamicin, kanamycin, neomycin, streptomycins); **benzodiazepines, cholinesterase inhibitors, colistin, cyclophosphamide, cyclopropane, echothiophate iodide, halothane, lidocaine, magnesium salts, methotrimeprazine, narcotic analgesics, organophosphamide insecticides, pantothenyl alcohol, phenelzine, phenothiazines, polymixins, procainamide** (possibly); **procaine, propranolol, quinidine, quinine, thio-tepa** (possibly). Succinylcholine may increase risk of cardiac arrhythmias in patients receiving **digitalis glycosides.**

SULFACHLORPYRIDAZINE
(NEFROSUL, SONILYN, VETISULID)

Antibacterial (sulfonamide)

ACTIONS AND USES

Short-acting sulfonamide slightly less soluble than sulfisoxazole. Shares actions, uses, contraindications, precautions, and adverse reactions of other sulfonamides (see Sulfisoxazole).

ABSORPTION AND FATE

Readily absorbed from GI tract. Peak blood levels within 3 to 4 hours. About 90% bound to plasma proteins. N_4 acetyl metabolite excreted 2.5 times faster than parent drug. About 85% of dose is excreted in urine within 24 hours as intact drug and 8% to 28% as N_4 acetylated form.

Oral: **Adults:** initially 2 to 4 Gm, then 2 to 4 Gm/24 hours in 3 to 6 divided doses (depending on severity of infection); **Children** *over 2 months of age:* initially 75 mg/kg, then 150 mg/kg/24 hours in 4 to 6 equally divided doses, with maximum of 6 Gm/24 hours.

NURSING IMPLICATIONS

Fluid intake should be adjusted to support urinary output of at least 1500 ml/day to prevent crystalluria and stone formation.

Treatment for urinary tract infection is generally continued for 5 to 7 days or until urinary cultures are sterile.

See nursing implications, laboratory test interferences, and drug interactions for sulfisoxazole.

SULFADIAZINE, U.S.P.
(COCO-DIAZINE, MICROSULFON)
SULFADIAZINE SODIUM, U.S.P.

Antibacterial (sulfonamide)

ACTIONS AND USES

Short-acting sulfonamide, slightly less soluble than sulfisoxazole. Shares actions, uses, contraindications, precautions, and adverse reactions of other sulfonamides (see Sulfisoxazole). Often used in combination with other antiinfective sulfonamides.

ABSORPTION AND FATE

Readily absorbed from GI tract. Detected in urine within 30 minutes following oral administration. Peak serum levels in 3 to 6 hours after oral ingestion and within 2 to 4 hours following subcutaneous administration. Distributed to most body tissues; readily diffuses into cerebrospinal fluid. About 32% to 56% bound to plasma proteins; 10% to 40% in plasma is acetylated. Approximately 50% of single dose is excreted in urine within 72 hours, 43% to 60% as intact drug and 15% to 40% as N_4 acetyl metabolite. Also see Sulfisoxazole.

ROUTE AND DOSAGE

Oral: **Adults:** initially 2 to 4 Gm, followed by 2 to 4 Gm daily in 3 to 6 equally divided doses. **Children:** *over 2 months of age:* initially 75 mg/kg, followed by 150 mg/kg in 4 to 6 equally divided doses; total daily dose not to exceed 6 Gm. Rheumatic fever prophylaxis: **Children** *under 30 kg:* 0.5 Gm every 24 hours; **Children:** *over 30 kg:* 1 Gm every 24 hours. Intravenous, subcutaneous **Adults, children** *over 2 months:* initially 50 mg/kg, followed by 100 mg/kg daily. Administrated slowly IV (over minimum of 10 to 30 minutes) in 4 equally divided doses, and in 3 equally divided doses subcutaneously (rarely given by this route). Parenteral solution must be diluted to concentration of 5% (50 mg/ml), preferably with sterile water for injection.

NURSING IMPLICATIONS

Incidence of renal complications is reportedly twice as high when drug is given IV than when given orally. Observe IV site for signs of inflammation; thrombosis occurs commonly.

Daily urinalysis is required during IV therapy.

Fluid intake must be sufficient to support urinary output of at least 1500 ml/day. If this cannot be accomplished, urinary alkalinizer such as sodium bicarbonate may be prescribed to reduce risk of crystalluria and stone formation.

Preserved in tight, light-resistant containers.
See Sulfisoxazole for nursing implications, laboratory test interferences, and
drug interactions.

SULFAMERAZINE, U.S.P.

Antibacterial (sulfonamide)

ACTIONS AND USES
Intermediate-acting sulfonamide with actions, uses, contraindications, precautions, and adverse reactions of other sulfonamides (see Sulfisoxazole). More
likely to cause crystalluria in acid urine than sulfisoxazole. Most frequently used
in conjunction with other sulfonamides.

ABSORPTION AND FATE
Readily absorbed from GI tract. Peak serum levels in about 4 hours. Approximately 10% to 40% in blood is present as N_4 acetyl derivative; 84% protein-bound; distributed to more body tissues and appears to cross cell membrane.
Penetrates cerebrospinal fluid, particularly when meninges are inflamed. Approximately 80% of dose is reabsorbed from renal tubules. Excreted primarily
in urine as intact drug and metabolites, over 3 days; about 55% in N_4 acetylated
form. Also see Sulfisoxazole.

ROUTE AND DOSAGE
Oral: **Adults:** initially 2 to 4 Gm, then 1 Gm every 8 hours. **Children:** *infants under
6 months:* initially 500 mg, then 250 mg every 12 hours; *older infants and young
children:* initially 1 Gm, then 500 mg every 12 hours; *children 3 to 10 years:* initially
1.5 Gm, then 1 Gm every 12 hours.

NURSING IMPLICATIONS
Fluid intake should be sufficient to support urinary output of at least 1500
mg/24 hours and should be continued for 24 to 48 hours after drug is
discontinued. Urinary alkalinizer may be prescribed during therapy to
reduce risk of crystalluria and stone formation.
Preserved in tight, light-resistant containers.
See Sulfisoxazole for nursing implications, laboratory test interferences, and
drug interactions.

SULFAMETER
(SULLA)
SULPHAMETHOXYDIAZINE, B.P.

Antibacterial (sulfonamide)

ACTIONS AND USES
Long-acting sulfonamide with actions, contraindications, precautions, and adverse reactions of other sulfonamides (see Sulfisoxazole). More effective against
Klebsiella-Aerobacter and species of *Paracolon, Streptococcus,* and *Staphyloccus* than
Pseudomonas or *Proteus.* Used only in treatment of acute and chronic urinary tract
infections.

ABSORPTION AND FATE
Readily absorbed from GI tract. Serum levels peak within 4 to 8 hours; measurable amounts still detectable 96 hours after single dose. Approximately 90% of
drug in plasma in nonacetylated form. Conflicting reports on degree of plasma
binding. Distributed to most body tissues; diffuses poorly into cerebrospinal

fluid. Metabolized by liver and kidney; significant amounts of intact drug undergo tubular reabsorption. Excreted slowly, principally in urine as intact drug (50%), N_4 acetyl derivative (20%), and other metabolites. Also see Sulfisoxazole.

CONTRAINDICATIONS AND PRECAUTIONS

Children under 12 years or those weighing less than 45 kg, during pregnancy, pregnant women near term, nursing mothers. Safe use in women of childbearing potential not established. Also see Sulfisoxazole.

ROUTE AND DOSAGE

Oral: **Patients** *over 45 kg or 12 years:* initially 1.5 Gm, then 500 mg at 24-hour intervals.

NURSING IMPLICATIONS

Administered preferably after breakfast.

Fluid intake should be sufficient to support urinary output of at least 1500 mg/24 hours and should be maintained for at least an additional 48 hours after drug is discontinued. Urinary alkalinizer may be prescribed during therapy to reduce risk of crystalluria or stone formation.

Early recognition of adverse effects is critically essential, because several days are required to eliminate drug from body. See Adverse Reactions for Sulfisoxazole.

Drug should be discontinued immediately if there is a reduction in urinary output, if abnormalities are noted in renal and hepatic function tests, urinalyses, or blood counts, or if a rash develops.

Diabetics receiving oral hypoglycemic agents should be observed closely for hypoglycemic reactions.

If bacteriologic or clinical response is not achieved within 14 days, drug is usually discontinued. If therapeutic response is apparent, drug is generally continued until patient is symptom-free for at least 48 hours.

Continuous drug therapy should not exceed 180 days.

Preserved in tight, light-resistant containers.

See Sulfisoxazole for nursing implications, laboratory test interferences, and drug interactions.

SULFAMETHIZOLE, N.F.
(MICROSUL, PROKLAR, SULFASOL, SULFSTAT, SULFURINE, THIOSULFIL, URIFON)
SULPHAMETHIZOLE, B.P.

Antibacterial (sulfonamide)

ACTIONS AND USES

Short-acting sulfonamide with actions, contraindications, precautions, and adverse reactions as for other sulfonamides. Like sulfisoxazole (qv), excreted in high antibacterial concentrations, mostly in active rather than acetylated form. Most effective against *E. coli, Klebsiella-Aerobacter, Staphylococcus aureus,* and *Proteus mirabilis.*

Used primarily in treatment of acute and chronic urinary tract infections. Also marketed in combination with phenazopyridine.

ABSORPTION AND FATE

Readily absorbed from GI tract. Peak blood levels within 2 hours. Approximately 2% to 11% in blood is in acetylated form. Distributed to most body tissues; does not appear to diffuse into cerebrospinal fluid. Almost 90% bound to plasma proteins. Excreted rapidly. About 60% of dose eliminated in 5 hours, only 5% to 7% as N_4 acetyl derivative. Also see Sulfisoxazole.

Oral: **Adults:** 0.5 to 1 Gm 3 or 4 times daily. **Children:** *over 2 months:* 35 to 45 mg/kg/24 hours divided into 4 doses.

NURSING IMPLICATIONS

Fluid intake sufficient to support urinary output of at least 1500 mg/day is usually prescribed. Urinary alkalinization generally is unecessary.

Preserved in tight, light-resistant containers.

See Sulfisoxazole for nursing implications, laboratory test interferences, and drug interactions.

SULFAMETHOXAZOLE, N.F.
(GANTANOL)

Antibacterial (sulfonamide)

ACTIONS AND USES

Intermediate-acting sulfonamide closely related chemically to sulfisoxazole and similar to it in actions, uses, contraindications, precautions, and adverse reactions. Intestinal absorption and urinary excretion are somewhat slower than those of sulfisoxazole, and thus it is given less frequently to avoid excessive blood levels. Marketed in fixed-dose combinations with trimethoprim to enhance antibacterial effect (Co-trimoxazole) and with phenazopyridine (Azo Gantanol) for relief of associated dysuria in urinary tract infections.

ABSORPTION AND FATE

Readily absorbed from GI tract. Peak serum levels in 3 to 4 hours; 12% to 20% in blood is in N_4 acetyl form. About 50% to 70% bound to plasma proteins. Half-life 9 to 12 hours. Metabolized primarily in liver. About 25% to 75% of dose is excreted in 24 hours as unchanged drug (20%), N_4 acetylated derivative (50% to 70%), and other metabolites.

ROUTE AND DOSAGE

Oral: **Adults:** initially 2 Gm, followed by 1 Gm 2 or 3 times daily (8- to 12-hour intervals), depending on severity of infection. **Children** *over 2 months:* initially 50 to 60 mg/kg, then 25 to 30 mg/kg morning and evening (12-hour intervals); not to exceed 75 mg/kg/24 hours.

NURSING IMPLICATIONS

Fluid intake must be sufficient to support urinary output of at least 1500 mg/24 hours. Concomitant administration of urinary alkalinizer may be prescribed to reduce possibility of crystalluria and stone formation.

Preserved in tight, light-resistant containers.

See Sulfisoxazole for nursing implications, laboratory test interferences, and drug interactions.

SULFAMETHOXYPYRIDAZINE
(MIDICEL)

Antibacterial (sulfonamide)

ACTIONS AND USES

Long-acting sulfonamide with actions, uses, contraindications, precautions, and adverse reactions as for other sulfonamides (see Sulfisoxazole).

Used primarily in urinary and upper respiratory tract infections, bacillary dysentery, surgical and soft-tissue infections. Also has been used in treatment of acne vulgaris, as prophylaxis against streptococcal infections in patients with rheumatic fever, and in meningococcal meningitis.

ABSORPTION AND FATE

Readily absorbed from GI tract. Blood levels peak in 1 to 2 hours and are maintained about 10 hours. Diffuses fully into intravascular fluids; little penetration into cerebrospinal fluid unless meninges are inflamed. Approximately 85% bound to plasma proteins. Free drug may be reabsorbed by renal tubules. About 45% of dose is excreted in urine in 48 hours as N_4 acetylated form (40% to 70%) and intact drug (30% to 60%). Also see Sulfisoxazole.

ROUTE AND DOSAGE

Oral: **Adults:** initially 1 Gm, followed by 0.5 Gm daily or 1 Gm every other day; **Children** *over 2 months:* first day, 30 mg/kg, followed by 15 mg/kg daily; not to exceed 1 Gm first day nor 0.5 Gm daily maintenance. Prophylactic for streptococcal infection: single weekly dose of 2 to 3 Gm, depending on weight; 110 lb (50 kg) may be used as arbitrary line between doses of 2 and 3 Gm.

NURSING IMPLICATIONS

Fluid intake must be adequate to support urinary output of at least 1500 mg/day during therapy and continued an additional 24 to 48 hours after drug is stopped.

High doses (over 1 Gm) may be associated with drowsiness; administration of drug at bedtime may be advisable. Consult physician.

Early recognition of adverse reactions is critically essential, since drug is slowly eliminated from body. Fatalities have occurred as result of Stevens-Johnson syndrome. See Sulfisoxazole.

Complete blood and platelet counts, urinalyses, and renal and hepatic function tests should be closely monitored.

Therapy should continue for 5 to 7 days or until patient is asymptomatic for 48 to 72 hours.

Preserved in tight, light-resistant containers.

See Sulfisoxazole for nursing implications, laboratory test interferences, and drug interactions.

SULFAPYRIDINE

Suppressant (dermatitis herpetiformis)

ACTIONS AND USES

Intermediate-acting sulfonamide with actions, contraindications, precautions, and adverse reactions as for other sulfonamides (see Sulfisoxazole). Mechanisms of action in ability to suppress dermatitis herpetiformis unknown.

Use largely restricted to treatment of dermatitis herpetiformis when sulfones are contraindicated.

ABSORPTION AND FATE

Irregularly and slowly absorbed from GI tract. Peak blood levels within 5 to 7 hours. Distributed to most body tissues; readily enters cerebrospinal fluid. Approximately 10% to 45% bound to plasma proteins; up to 75% in blood present as N_4 acetyl derivative. Urinary excretion rate irregular, but usually complete within 72 to 96 hours; up to 60% excreted in acetylated form, 18% to 59% as intact drug.

ROUTE AND DOSAGE

Oral: 500 mg 4 times per day until improvement is noted; daily dose then reduced by 500 mg at 3-day intervals until symptom-free maintenance is achieved. Minimum effective dose used for maintenance.

NURSING IMPLICATIONS

Fluid intake must be sufficient to support urinary output of at least 1500 ml/day. Urinary alkalinizer is usually prescribed to reduce risk of crystal-luria and stone formation.

Toxic effects occur commonly. Close observation of patient and early recognition and reporting of adverse reactions are critically essential.

Preserved in tight, light-resistant containers.

See nursing implications, laboratory test interferences, and adverse reactions for sulfisoxazole.

SULFASALAZINE, N.F.

(AZULFIDINE, Salazopyrin, Salicylazosulfapyridine, S.A.S.-500, S.A.S.P., SULCOLON)

Antibacterial (sulfonamide)

ACTIONS AND USES

Mechanism of action not completely known. Believed to be converted by intestinal microflora to sulfapyridine (which has antibacterial action) and 5-aminosalicylic acid (which may exert antiinflammatory effect). Contraindications, precautions, and adverse reactions are as for other sulfonamides (see Sulfisoxazole).

Used in treatment of ulcerative colitis, relatively mild regional enteritis, and granulomatous colitis. Used investigationally in scleroderma.

ABSORPTION AND FATE

About one-third of dose absorbed from small intestine. Remaining two-thirds absorbed from colon, where it is converted to sulfapyridine (SP), most of which is absorbed, and 5-aminosalicylic acid (5-ASA), 30% of which is absorbed, with remainder being excreted in urine. Peak serum levels in 1.5 to 6 hours for parent drug and 6 to 24 hours for SP (serum levels tend to be higher in slow acetylator phenotypes). Excreted in urine as unchanged drug, SP, 5-ASA, and acetyl derivatives.

ADVERSE REACTIONS

Frequent: nausea, vomiting, diarrhea, anorexia, arthralgia, rash. Also see Sulfisoxazole.

ROUTE AND DOSAGE

Oral: **Adults:** initially 1 to 2 Gm daily, then 3 to 4 Gm daily (up to 8 Gm daily) in equally divided doses; maintenance 1.5 to 2 Gm daily in 4 divided doses. **Children** *over 2 years:* 40 to 60 mg/kg/24 hours in 3 to 6 divided doses; maintenance 30 mg/kg/24 hours in 4 divided doses.

NURSING IMPLICATIONS

If possible, drug should be administered after food.

Sulfasalazine should be given in evenly divided doses over each 24-hour period. Intervals between nighttime doses should not exceed 8 hours.

If GI intolerance occurs after first few doses, symptoms are probably due to irritation of stomach mucosa. Symptoms may be relieved by spacing total daily dose more evenly over the day and by administration of enteric-coated tablets. Consult physician.

Some patients pass enteric-coated tablets intact in feces, possibly because they lack enzymes capable of dissolving them. Advise patient to examine stools.

GI symptoms that develop after a few days of therapy may indicate need for dosage adjustment. If symptoms persist, physician may withhold drug for 5 to 7 days and restart it at a lower dosage level.

Adverse reactions generally occur within a few days to 12 weeks after start of therapy and are most likely to occur in patients receiving high doses (4 Gm or more).

Forewarn patient that drug may impart an orange-yellow color to alkaline urine and to skin.

Advise patient to remain under close medical supervision. Relapses occur in about 40% of patients after initial satisfactory response. Response to therapy and duration of treatment are governed by endoscopic examinations.

Preserved in tight, light-resistant containers.

See nursing implications and laboratory test interferences for sulfisoxazole.

DRUG INTERACTIONS: **Antibiotics** may alter metabolism of sulfasalazine by altering intestinal flora. By chelating **iron,** sulfasalazine absorption may be inhibited, with resulting lower blood levels. Sulfasalazine inhibits **folic acid** absorption. **Phenobarbital** administered concomitantly may decrease urinary excretion of sulfasalazine. Also see drug interactions for sulfisoxazole.

SULFINPYRAZONE, U.S.P.
(ANTURANE)

Uricosuric (pyrazolone)

ACTIONS AND USES

Potent pyrazolone-derivative renal tubular blocking agent structurally related to phenylbutazone. At therapeutic doses, promotes urinary excretion of uric acid and reduces serum urate levels by competitively inhibiting tubular reabsorption of uric acid. Like all uricosurics, low doses may inhibit tubular secretion of uric acid and cause urate retention. Inhibits release of adenosine diphosphate and 5-hydroxytryptophan, and thus decreases platelet adhesiveness and increases platelet survival time; has no effect on prothrombin or blood clotting time. May cause slight but significant decrease in serum cholesterol. Since it has no apparent analgesic or antiinflammatory activity, it is not used for relief of acute gout. Reportedly not associated with cumulative effects, development of tolerance, or electrolyte imbalance.

Used for maintenance therapy in chronic gouty arthritis and tophaceous gout.

ABSORPTION AND FATE

Readily and completely absorbed from GI tract. Peak plasma levels in 1 to 2 hours. Duration of action 4 to 6 hours, but may persist to 10 hours. About 98% bound to plasma proteins. Average half-life 3 hours (range 1 to 9 hours). Rapidly metabolized by liver to active and inactive metabolites. After 2 days, 45% of single dose is excreted as unchanged drug and metabolites.

CONTRAINDICATIONS AND PRECAUTIONS

Known hypersensitivity to pyrazolone derivatives, active peptic ulcer, concurrent administration of salicylates, patients with creatinine clearance less than 50 mg/minute, treatment of hyperuricemia secondary to neoplastic disease or cancer chemotherapy. Cautious use: impaired renal function, pregnancy, history of healed peptic ulcer, use in conjunction with sulfonamides and sulfonylurea, hypoglycemic agents.

ADVERSE REACTIONS

GI disturbances (common): nausea, vomiting, diarrhea, epigastric pain, blood loss, reactivation or aggravation of peptic ulcer; ataxia, dizziness, vertigo, tinnitus; edema, labored respirations, convulsions, coma, hypersensitivity reactions (skin rashes, fever), blood dyscrasias (rare: anemia, leukopenia,

agranulocytosis, thrombocytopenia), jaundice, precipitation of acute gout,
urolithiasis, renal colic.
ROUTE AND DOSAGE
  Oral (first week of therapy): 100 to 200 mg initially twice daily, gradually
  increased as needed to full maintenance range of 200 to 400 mg twice daily; after
  serum urate levels are controlled, dosage may be reduced to 200 mg daily in
  divided doses. Patients previously controlled with other uricosuric agents may
  begin sulfinpyrazone at full maintenance dosage.

NURSING IMPLICATIONS
Administered with meals, milk, or antacid (prescribed) to prevent local drug
  irritant effect. Severity and frequency of symptoms increase with dosage.
  Persistence of GI symptoms may require discontinuation of drug.
During early therapy, fluid intake should be sufficient to support urinary
  output of at least 2000 to 3000 ml/day (consult physician), and urine
  should be alkalinized (eg, with sodium bicarbonate) to increase solubility
  of uric acid and minimize risk of uric acid stones.
Serum urate levels are used to monitor therapy. Aim of therapy is to lower
  serum urate levels to about 6 mg/dl and thus to reduce joint changes,
  tophi formation, and frequency of acute attacks and improve renal function.
Patient must remain under close medical supervision while taking sulfinpyrazone. Therapy is continued indefinitely.
Caution patient to avoid experimentation with dosage, since subtherapeutic
  doses may enhance urate retention, and large doses may increase risk of
  toxicity.
Periodic blood cell counts are advised during prolonged therapy. Patients
  with impaired renal function should have periodic assessments of renal
  function.
Sulfinpyrazone may increase the frequency of acute gouty attacks during
  first 6 to 12 months of therapy, even when serum urate levels appear to
  be controlled. Physician may prescribe prophylactic doses of colchicine
  concurrently during first 3 to 6 months of treatment to prevent or at least
  lessen severity of attacks.
Sulfinpyrazone therapy should be continued without interruption even
  when patient has an acute gouty attack, which may be treated with full
  therapeutic doses of colchicine or other antiinflammatory agent.
Caution patient to avoid aspirin-containing medications (see Drug Interactions). If an analgesic is required (in patients with normal renal function),
  generally acetaminophen is recommended.
Patients receiving oral hypoglycemic agents should be supervised closely (see
  Drug Interactions).

LABORATORY TEST INTERFERENCES: Sulfinpyrazone decreases urinary excretion of aminohippuric acid and phenolsulfonphthalein.

DRUG INTERACTIONS: Possibility of additive uricosuric effects with **allopurinol** (may be used therapeutically). The uricosuric action of sulfinpyrazone is antagonized by **aspirin** and other **salicylates.** Sulfinpyrazone may affect
urinary excretion of weak organic acids with resulting higher serum levels, eg,
**aminosalicylic acid, cephalosporins, dapsone, indomethacin, nitrofurantoin,
penicillins. Probenecid** may increase toxicity of sulfinpyrazone by inhibiting
its renal excretion. Sulfinpyrazone may potentiate hypoglycemia by interfering
with renal excretion of **sulfonylurea** hypoglycemic agents. There is the possibility that sulfinpyrazone may enhance hypoprothrombinemic effect of **warfarin** and **other coumarin-type anticoagulants.** Concomitant administration of

drugs that tend to increase serum urate levels may necessitate higher sulfinpyrazone dosage, eg, **alcohol, aluminum nicotinate, diazoxide,** most **diuretics, mecamylamine, pyrazinamide. Cholestyramine** may delay absorption of sulfinpyrazone (administer sulfinpyrazone at least 1 hour before or 4 to 6 hours after cholestyramine). There is the possibility of increased risk of blood dyscrasias with concomitant use of sulfinpyrazone and **colchicine.**

SULFISOXAZOLE, U.S.P.
(GANTRISIN, G-SOX, J-SUL, ROSOXOL, SK-SOXAZOLE, SOSOL, SOXA, SOXOMIDE, SULFAGAN, SULFALAR, SULFIZIN, URISOXIN, URIZOLE,. VELMATROL)
SULFISOXAZOLE ACETYL, U.S.P.
(GANTRISIN ACETYL, LIPO GANTRISIN)
SULFISOXAZOLE DIOLAMINE, N.F.
(GANTRISIN DIOLAMINE)

Antibacterial (sulfonamide)

ACTIONS AND USES

Short-acting derivative of sulfanilamide. In common with other sulfonamides, has broad antimicrobial spectrum against both Gram-positive and Gram-negative organisms. Bacteriostatic action believed to be by competitive inhibition of *p*-aminobenzoic acid (PABA), thereby interfering with folic acid biosynthesis required for bacterial growth. Increase in resistant organisms is a limitation to usefulness of sulfonamides; cross-resistance to other sulfonamides is possible. Since sulfisoxazole and its derivatives are highly soluble in alkaline urine and slightly acidic urine and are excreted rapidly, the risk of crystalluria is small. Used in treatment of acute, recurrent, and chronic urinary tract infections, chancroid, used as adjunctive therapy in trachoma, chloroquine-resistant strains of malaria, acute otitis media due to *H. influenzae,* and meningococcal and *H. influenzae* meningitis. Ophthalmic preparations used in treatment of conjunctivitis, corneal ulcer, and other superficial eye infections and as adjunct to systemic sulfonamide therapy for trachoma. Topical vaginal preparation used for *Hemophilus vaginalis* vaginitis.

ABSORPTION AND FATE

Sulfisoxazole and diolamine forms readily absorbed. Peak blood levels within 2 to 4 hours after oral and IM administration and within 30 minutes after IV injection; wide variations in blood levels. About 85% protein-bound (65% to 72% in nonacetylated form). Distributed only into extracellular fluids. Half-life 3 to 6 hours. Deacetylation of acetyl sulfisoxazole by enzymes in GI tract results in slower absorption and lower peak levels than equal oral doses of sulfisoxazole. Metabolized chiefly in liver. Major metabolite (N_4 acetyl) is less soluble in acid urine, has no antibacterial activity, and has same toxic potential as parent drug (concentrations in blood and urine approximately 30%). Up to 95% of single dose is excreted in urine within 24 hours (70% as free drug). Small amounts eliminated in feces, sweat, saliva, tears, breast milk, and intestinal and other secretions. Crosses placenta.

CONTRAINDICATIONS AND PRECAUTIONS

History of hypersensitivity to sulfonamides, salicylates, or chemically related drugs; use in treatment of group A β-hemolytic streptococcal infections; infants less than 2 months of age (except in treatment of congenital toxoplasmosis); pregnant women at term; nursing mothers, porphyria; advanced renal or hepatic disease; intestinal and urinary obstruction. Cautious use: impaired renal or liver function, severe allergy, bronchial asthma, blood dyscrasias, patients with glucose-6-phosphate dehydrogenase deficiency.

Low toxicity level, but may include the following: **Hypersensitivity:** headache, fever, chills, arthralgia, malaise, pruritus, urticaria, conjunctival or scleral infection, skin eruptions including Stevens-Johnson syndrome and exfoliative dermatitis, allergic myocarditis, serum sickness, anaphylactoid reactions, photosensitization, vascular lesions. **Blood dyscrasias:** acute hemolytic anemia (especially in patients with glucose-6-phosphate dehydrogenase deficiency), aplastic anemia, methemoglobinemia, agranulocytosis, thrombocytopenia, leukopenia, eosinophilia, hypoprothrombinemia. **GI:** nausea, vomiting, diarrhea, abdominal pains, hepatitis, jaundice, pancreatitis, stomatitis, impaired folic acid absorption. **CNS:** headache, peripheral neuritis, peripheral neuropathy, tinnitus, hearing loss, vertigo, insomnia, drowsiness, mental depression, acute psychosis, ataxia, convulsions, kernicterus (newborns). **Renal:** crystalluria, hematuria, proteinuria, anuria, toxic nephrosis. **Other:** conjunctivitis, goiter, hypoglycemia, diuresis, overgrowth of nonsusceptible organisms, lupus erythematosus phenomenon, retardation of corneal healing (ophthalmic ointment), alopecia, reduction in sperm count, lymphadenopathy, local reaction following IM injection.

ROUTE AND DOSAGE

Oral: **Adults:** initially 2 to 4 Gm, followed by 2 to 4 Gm divided into 3 to 6 doses per 24 hours; not to exceed 6 Gm/24 hours. **Children** *over 2 months of age:* initially 75 mg/kg/24 hours; maintenance 150 mg/kg/24 hours divided into 4 to 6 doses per 24 hours; not to exceed 6 Gm/24 hours. Extended-release preparation: total daily dosage given in 2 equally divided doses. Intravenous, intramuscular, subcutaneous: **Adults and children** *over 2 months:* initially 50 mg/kg/24 hours; maintenance 100 mg/kg/24 hours, divided into 4 doses per 24 hours for IV and given by slow injection or IV drip, divided into 2 or 3 doses per 24 hours for IM. No dilution required for IM, but subcutaneous and IV must be diluted (follow manufacturer's directions). Topical: *Vaginal cream:* 250 to 500 mg (0.5 to 1 applicator) into vagina twice daily (morning and on retiring) up to 2 weeks; course may be repeated. *Ophthalmic* (4% solution): 2 or 3 drops 3 or more times daily; (4% ointment): small amount into lower conjunctival sac 1 to 3 times a day and at bedtime.

NURSING IMPLICATIONS

Administration with food appears to delay, but reportedly does not reduce absorption.

Monitor intake and output. Report oliguria and changes in intake–output ratio. Fluid intake should be adequate to support urinary output of at least 1500 ml/day to prevent crystalluria and stone formation.

Since a fall in urinary pH (more acidic) may markedly affect solubility of sulfisoxazole, daily check of urine pH with Nitrazine paper or Labstix is advisable.

Report increasing acidity. If urine output is inadequate or urine is highly acidic, physician may prescribe a urinary alkalinizer, eg, sodium bicarbonate (routine alkalinization of urine not necessary with sulfisoxazole).

Monitor temperature. Sudden appearance of fever may signify sensitization (serum sickness) or hemolytic anemia (most frequent in patients with glucose-6-phosphate dehydrogenase deficiency, which is most common among black males and Mediterranean ethnic groups). These reactions generally develop within 10 days after start of drug. Agranulocytosis may develop after 10 days to 6 weeks of therapy.

Fever, sore throat or mouth, malaise, unusual fatigue, joint pains, pallor, bleeding tendencies, rash, and jaundice are possible early manifestations of blood dyscrasias or hypersensitivity reactions. Skin lesions of Stevens-Johnson syndrome (severe erythema multiforme) may be preceded by high fever, severe headache, stomatitis, conjunctivitis, rhinitis, urticaria, balanitis (inflammation of penis or clitoris). Termination of drug therapy is indicated.

Frequent kidney function tests and urinalyses (including microscopic examination) are recommended; complete blood tests and hepatic function tests are advised, especially in patients receiving sulfonamides for longer than 2 weeks.

Determinations of drug blood levels are advised, particularly in patients receiving high doses. Therapeutically effective blood levels range from 5 to 15 mg/dl; levels above 20 mg/dl are usually associated with adverse reactions.

Bacterial sensitivity tests are not always reliable and therefore must be closely correlated with bacteriologic studies and accurate assessments of clinical response.

Diabetic patients receiving oral hypoglycemic agents should be closely observed for hypoglycemic reactions (see Drug Interactions). Determinations of serum glucose levels are advised before and shortly after initiation of sulfonamide therapy.

Advise patients to avoid exposure to ultraviolet light and excessive sunlight to prevent photosensitivity reaction.

Caution patients not to take OTC medications without consulting physician. Many proprietary analgesic mixtures contain aspirin in combination with p-aminobenzoic acid (see Drug Interactions). Inform patients that large doses of vitamin C acidify urine and therefore should be avoided.

Advise patients using topical applications to stop treatment if local irritation or sensitivity reaction develops and to report to physician. Patient should be informed that sensitization to topical application precludes future systemic use of sulfonamides.

Topical applications are inactivated by pus, cellular debris, and blood.

Sulfonamides are incompatible with silver preparations.

Preserved in tight, light-resistant containers.

LABORATORY TEST INTERFERENCES: Sulfonamides may interfere with BSP retention and PSP excretion tests and may affect results of thyroid function tests (^{131} I uptake may be decreased for about 7 days). Large doses of sulfonamides reportedly may produce false positive urine glucose determinations with copper reduction methods (eg, Benedict's and Clinitest). Sulfonamides may produce false positive results for urinary protein (with sulfosalicylic acid test) and may interfere with urine urobilinogen determinations using Ehrlich's reagent or Urobilistix. Follow-up cultures are unreliable unless p-aminobenzoic acid is added to culture medium.

DRUG INTERACTIONS: Note: except when indicated, interactions are due to displacement of drug from plasma protein binding sites by sulfonamides. Sulfonamides may increase adverse effects of **alcohol.** Antibacterial activity of sulfonamides may be antagonized by **local anesthetics** derived from p-aminobenzoic acid, eg, **benzocaine, butacaine, procaine, tetracaine. Antacids** may decrease or delay absorption of sulfonamides. **Aspirin** and other **salicylates** may increase sulfonamide blood levels. Sulfisoxazole may reduce amount of **thiopental** required for anesthesia. Sulfonamides may enhance **methotrexate** toxicity. Risk of sulfonamide crystalluria may be increased by **paraldehyde. Probenecid** and **sulfinpyrazone** may result in higher sulfonamide serum levels (by displacing sulfonamides from plasma protein binding). Sulfonamides may increase the effects of **oral anticoagulants,** possibly by plasma binding displacement and by decreasing vitamin K synthesis by gut flora (unlikely). Sulfonamides may enhance hypoglycemic effects of **oral hypoglycemic agents,** particularly chlorpropamide and tolbutamide, and may cause excessive **phenytoin** effect (inhibits metabolism of phenytoin). Concurrent administration with **methenamine** may result in crystalluria. There is the possibility of decreased **oxacillin** blood levels (sulfonamides may inhibit GI absorption).

SULFOXONE, SODIUM, U.S.P.
(DIASONE)

Antibacterial (leprostatic)

ACTIONS AND USES
  Sulfone derived from dapsone (qv) and similar to parent drug in actions, uses, contraindications, precautions, and adverse reactions.
  Used in treatment of all forms of leprosy and also in dermatitis herpetiformis.
ABSORPTION AND FATE
  Approximately 50% absorbed from GI tract. Undergoes hydrolysis and is absorbed chiefly in form of dapsone. Distributed throughout body water; only small amount enters cerebrospinal fluid. About 48% of dose is excreted slowly in urine and 44% in feces. Some excretion in sweat, saliva, sputum, tears, breast milk.
ROUTE AND DOSAGE
  Oral: *Leprostatic:* **Adults:** 1st and 2nd weeks, 330 mg twice weekly (alternatively, 165 mg 4 times a week); 3rd and 4th weeks, 330 mg 4 times a week (alternatively, 165 mg daily); 5th week and succeeding weeks, 330 mg daily for 6 days, 1 day rest, and continue. **Children** *4 years and older:* one-half adult dosage. *Dermatitis herpetiformis:* **Adults:** first week, 330 mg daily, increased to 660 mg daily, if necessary; maintenance 330 mg daily.

NURSING IMPLICATIONS
Administer with meals to minimize GI side effects.
Inform patient that tablets are enteric coated to prevent gastric irritation and
  therefore should not be cut, chewed, or crushed.
Dosage increases are made only in the absence of serious side effects or
  intolerance.
Preserved in tightly covered, light-resistant containers.
See Dapsone.

SYROSINGOPINE, N.F.
(SINGOSERP)

Antihypertensive

ACTIONS AND USES
  Produced from reserpine, but less potent and reportedly causes less sedation. Similar actions, uses, contraindications, precautions, and adverse reactions as for reserpine. Commercially available in combination with hydrochlorothiazide (Singoserp-Esidrix).
ROUTE AND DOSAGE
  Oral: Syrosingopine: initially 1 to 2 mg daily in 1 or 2 doses; maintenance 0.5 to 3 mg daily. Syrosingopine with hydrochlorothiazide (Singoserp-Esidrix): 1 tablet #1 (0.5 mg/25 mg) or 1 tablet #2 (1 mg/25 mg) 3 times daily, depending on individual requirements and severity of hypertension.

NURSING IMPLICATIONS
Preserved in tight, light-resistant containers.

For the combination drug, refer to nursing implications and drug interactions for both reserpine and chlorothiazide.

TALBUTAL, N.F.
(LOTUSATE)

Sedative, hypnotic

ACTIONS AND USES
Short- to intermediate-acting barbiturate with actions, contraindications, precautions, and adverse reactions as for phenobarbital.
Used as hypnotic in patients with simple insomnia.
ABSORPTION AND FATE
Peak plasma levels within 2 hours following oral dose. Plasma half-life about 15 hours. Metabolized in liver. Excreted in urine as metabolites and traces of unchanged drug.
ROUTE AND DOSAGE
Oral (hypnotic): 120 mg administered 15 to 20 minutes before retiring.

NURSING IMPLICATIONS
Sleep usually occurs in 15 to 30 minutes and lasts 6 to 8 hours.
Classified as schedule III drug under federal Controlled Substances Act.
See Phenobarbital.

TERPIN HYDRATE ELIXIR, N.F.
TERPIN HYDRATE AND CODEINE ELIXIR, N.F.

Expectorant

ACTIONS AND USES
Terpin hydrate is a volatile oil derivative claimed to have direct action on bronchial secretory cells, thereby increasing respiratory tract fluid production and facilitating expectoration, but effect is doubtful in recommended doses. Commonly used as a vehicle for other cough medications, eg, terpin hydrate and codeine elixir contains 10 mg codeine in each 5 ml (added for antitussive effect).
CONTRAINDICATIONS AND PRECAUTIONS
Severe diabetes mellitus, peptic ulcer.
ROUTE AND DOSAGE
Oral (terpin hydrate elixir): 5 to 10 ml, repeated in 3 to 4 hours, if necessary; (terpin hydrate and codeine elixir): 5 to 10 ml 3 or 4 times a day.

NURSING IMPLICATIONS
Some patients experience epigastric pain following administration on an empty stomach.
Soothing, local effect of the syrup is enhanced if it is administered undiluted and not immediately followed by water.
Adequate fluid intake and humidification of air will help to liquefy sputum and relieve bronchial irritation.
Because of the high alcoholic content (42.5%) of terpin hydrate elixir, it is undesirable to administer larger doses than recommended.
Terpin hydrate and codeine elixir is classified as a schedule V drug under the federal Controlled Substances Act. Warn patient not to exceed recommended dose. See Codeine.

Antineoplastic

ACTIONS AND USES

Chemotherapeutic agent with chemical configuration similar to that of certain androgenic hormones, but devoid of androgenic activity in therapeutic doses. Exact mechanism of antineoplastic action unknown but has been found effective in approximately 15% of patients with advanced disseminated breast cancer.

Used as adjunctive treatment in palliation of breast carcinoma in postmenopausal women when hormone therapy is indicated. Also effective in women diagnosed before menopause in whom ovarian function has been subsequently terminated.

CONTRAINDICATIONS AND PRECAUTIONS

Pregnancy, breast cancer in males. Cautious use: hypercalcemia.

ADVERSE REACTIONS

Pain and inflammation at injection site (relationship to drug and/or disease not clarified). Maculopapular erythema; aches, paresthesias and pain in extremities; glossitis, anorexia, nausea, vomiting; increase in blood pressure. Rare and temporary: alopecia, nail growth disturbances.

ROUTE AND DOSAGE

Intramuscular: 100 mg three times weekly. Oral: 250 mg 4 times a day.

NURSING IMPLICATIONS

Shake vial vigorously and immediately administer IM dose to prevent drug settling out of suspension.

Inject IM dose deeply into upper outer quadrant area and aspirate with care to prevent inadvertent injection into blood vessel and a large nerve. Use 1½ inch needle for the average adult, and a longer one for an obese patient.

Avoid subcutaneous injection. If this does happen, pain and induration can be alleviated by applying ice.

Alternate sites of injection. Inspect site for signs of inflammation.

Testalactone treatment is usually continued for a minimum of three months (unless there is active progression of the disease) in order to evaluate response.

Clinical response is measured according to the following criteria; decrease in size of tumor, more than 50% of nonosseous lesions decrease in size even though all bone lesions remain static.

Plasma calcium levels are checked routinely and periodically.

Be alert to and report signs that may suggest impending hypercalcemia: hypotonicity of muscles, bone and flank pain, polyuria, thirst, anorexia, nausea, vomiting, constipation.

Note intake-output ratio.

Encourage patient mobility if feasible; if not, assist her with passive exercises.

Androgen

ACTIONS AND USES
Steroid compound isolated from testes of the bull or prepared synthetically, with both androgenic and anabolic activity (1:1). Controls development and maintenance of accessory male organs and sex characteristics. Restores and maintains positive nitrogen balance, and in males and some females it reduces excretion of phosphorus, nitrogen, potassium, sodium, and chloride. Stimulates skeletal muscle growth and bone, skin, and hair growth; accelerates epiphyseal line closure. Increases erythropoiesis, possibly by stimulating production of renal or extrarenal erythropoietin, and promotes vascularization and darkening of skin. Antagonizes effects of estrogen excess on female breast and endometrium. Large doses suppress male gonadotropic secretion, thereby causing testicular atrophy. Unlike other androgens, testosterone and its esters do not produce cholestatic hepatitis or creatinuria.

Used primarily as androgen replacement in male sex hormone deficiency states: eunuchism and eunuchoidism, hypopituitarism related to hypogonadism, male climacteric, cryptorchidism, impotence. In women, given to treat postpartum breast engorgement, menstrual disorders, and menopausal symptoms and for palliation of androgen-responsive inoperable breast cancer. Also employed to treat refractory anemias and osteoporosis; used to reverse protein loss after trauma, burns, extensive surgery, debilitating disease, and prolonged immobilization; used to stimulate growth in prepubertal males. Combined with estrogens in many preparations.

ABSORPTION AND FATE
Absorption following oral administration is rapid; more prolonged after IM injection. Less than one-sixth of dose is available for action; remainder inactivated by liver. Serum half-life about 2 hours. Metabolites (including androsterone and etiocholanolone) conjugated and excreted through enterohepatic route (about 10%) and urinary route (90%). Implanted pellets provide continued effects for 3 to 6 months. Crosses placenta and appears in breast milk.

CONTRAINDICATIONS AND PRECAUTIONS
Hypersensitivity to androgens; pregnancy, lactation, women of childbearing potential (possibility of virilization of female infant); hypercalcemia; cardiac, hepatic, or renal decompensation; prostatic or breast cancer in male; benign prostatic hypertrophy with obstruction; patients easily stimulated sexually; elderly, asthenic males who may react adversely to androgenic overstimulation; conditions aggravated by fluid retention; hypertension. Cautious use: history of myocardial infarction or coronary artery disease; prepubertal males.

ADVERSE REACTIONS
Both sexes: hypersensitivity, anaphylactoid reaction (rare), increased libido, skin flushing and vascularization, acne, excitation and sleeplessness, chills, leukopenia, sodium and water retention (especially in the elderly) with edema, nausea, vomiting, anorexia, diarrhea, gastric pain, bladder irritability, hypercalcemia, renal calculi in bedfast or partially immobilized patient, aggravation of disease being treated, site irritation and sloughing (pellet implantation), hepatocellular carcinoma (rare). Male (post pubertal): testicular atrophy, decreased ejaculatory volume, azoospermia, oligospermia (after prolonged administration or excessive dosage), impotence, epididymitis, priapism, gynecomastia; (prepubertal): phallic enlargement, priapism, premature epiphyseal closure. Female: suppression of ovulation, lactation, or menstruation; virilism manifested as hoarseness or deepening of voice (often irreversible); hirsutism; oily skin; acne; clitoral enlargement; regression of breasts; male-pattern baldness (in dis-

seminated breast cancer). Altered laboratory values: decreased glucose tolerance; decrease in protein-bound iodine; increased uptake of triiodothyronine by RBC; increase in clotting factors II, V, VII, and X; decreased creatinine and creatinine excretion (lasting up to 2 weeks after therapy is discontinued); increased 17-ketosteroid excretion; decreased response to metyrapone test; elevation or decrease in serum cholesterol.

ROUTE AND DOSAGE

Intramuscular (hypogonadism): 10 to 25 mg 2 or 3 times weekly; (postpartum breast engorgement): 25 to 50 mg for 3 or 4 days starting at time of delivery; (metastatic cancer of breast): 100 mg 3 times weekly, as long as improvement is maintained. Subcutaneous implantation (hypogonadism): 2 to 6 pellets (75 mg each) every 3 to 6 months (highly individualized).

NURSING IMPLICATIONS

IM injections should be made deep into gluteal musculature. A wet syringe or needle may cloud the solution, but potency of material reportedly is unaffected.

Store IM formulations prepared in oil at room temperature. Warming and shaking vial will redisperse precipitated crystals.

Check intake and output, and weigh patient daily during dose adjustment period. Weight gain suggests need for decreased dosage. When dosage is stabilized, urge patient to check weight at least twice weekly and to report increases, particularly if accompanied by edema in dependent areas. Dose adjustment and diuretic therapy may be started. Sodium and water retention respond to diuretic therapy; use of this effect differentiates skeletal growth weight gain from edema.

Restoration of positive nitrogen balance, as in patients with metastatic carcinoma, is supported by a diet high in protein and calories. Sodium restriction may be prescribed to control edema. Collaborate with physician and dietitian in developing a dietary teaching plan that includes patient and responsible family members.

Periodic serum cholesterol and calcium determinations and cardiac and liver function tests should be performed throughout testosterone therapy.

Improvement from testosterone therapy is slow. Therapeutic response in patients with breast cancer is usually apparent within 3 months after regimen begins. If signs of disease progression appear, therapy should be terminated.

In patients with metastatic breast cancer, hypercalcemia usually indicates progression of bone metastasis. Report immediately signs and symptoms of hypercalcemia (nausea, vomiting, constipation, lethargy, asthenia, loss of muscle tone, polydipsia, polyuria, dehydration, increased urine and serum calcium levels). Treatment consists of withdrawing testosterone, providing fluids to assure daily urinary output of 3 to 4 liters or more (to prevent urinary calculi), and appropriate drug therapy. Calcium, phosphate, and BUN levels should be checked daily.

Bedridden patients should be given range-of-motion exercises at least twice daily to prevent mobilization of calcium from bone. The immobilized patient is particularly prone to develop hypercalcemia. Consult physician about daily activity and dietary calcium intake.

Since testosterone-induced anabolic action enhances hypoglycemia, instruct diabetic patient to report symptoms of hyperinsulinism (sweating, tremor, anxiety, diplopia, vertigo). Dosage adjustment of antidiabetic agent may be required.

Be sensitive to the fact that the patient may find it embarrassing to initiate questions or report symptoms related to sexual organs and functions. Attention to such symptoms should not be delayed by hesitant reporting, since many signify overdosage.

Instruct male patient to report priapism (sustained and often painful erections occurring especially in early replacement therapy), reduced ejaculatory volume, and gynecomastia. These symptoms indicate necessity for temporary withdrawal or discontinuation of testosterone therapy.

Observe the patient who is on concomitant anticoagulant treatment for signs of overdosage (eg, ecchymoses, petechiae). Report promptly to physician; anticoagulant dose may need to be reduced.

Advise female patient to report increase in libido (early sign of toxicity), growth of facial hair, and voice changes. The onset of hoarseness can easily be overlooked unless its significance as an early and possibly irreversible sign of virilism is appreciated. Reevaluation of treatment plan is indicated.

With continued use of testosterone in doses required for mammary carcinoma, female patient may develop male-pattern baldness and virilism (possibly irreversible).

Prepubertal males should be monitored by radiology throughout therapy for rate of bone maturation. Skeletal stimulation may continue 6 months beyond termination of therapy.

Pellet implantation (an office procedure) follows dose stabilization by oral or parenteral administration (pellet is implanted subcutaneously into medial aspect of thigh, infrascapular region, or postaxillary line).

Warn patient to report tenderness and redness over implantation area. Sloughing followed by loss of a pellet requires prompt medical attention and reevaluation of dose regimen.

Alterations in clinical laboratory test values persist 2 to 3 weeks after drug discontinuation. Notify laboratory and pathologist that patient is on testosterone.

DRUG INTERACTIONS (androgenic action): concomitant use with **adrenal steroids** or **ACTH** may increase testosterone-induced edema; (anabolic action): **antidiabetic drugs** may require dosage adjustments because of additive hypoglycemic effect. Testosterone may increase the effects of **anticoagulants,** necessitating reduced dosage of the anticoagulant. **Oxyphenbutazone** and **phenylbutazone** effects may be increased by testosterone.

TESTOSTERONE CYPIONATE, U.S.P.
(DEPO-TESTOSTERONE, DURANDRO, MALOGEN CYP, TESTOJECT, T-IONATE P.A.)
TESTOSTERONE ENANTHATE INJECTION, U.S.P.
(ATLATEST, DELATESTRYL, DURA-TESTOSTERONE, MALOGEN L.A., TESTATE, TESTONE L.A., TESTOSTROVAL-P.A.)
TESTOSTERONE PROPIONATE, U.S.P., B.P.
(ANDRUSOL-P, NEO-HOMBREOL, ORETON PROPIONATE, SYNERONE, TESTODET, VULVAN)

Androgen

ACTIONS AND USES

Esters of testosterone with similar actions, androgenic/anabolic activity (1:1), and contraindications as parent compound (see Testosterone). Duration of action of cypionate and enanthate is longer than that of testosterone. The propionate is more intense in action, but has somewhat shorter duration than testosterone; parenteral route is not suited to long-term treatment.

Uses are indicated under Route and Dosage.

ADVERSE REACTIONS

Urticaria at injection site, postinjection induration, furunculosis. Also see Testosterone.

ROUTE AND DOSAGE

Testosterone cypionate or enanthate: Intramuscular (hypogonadism): initially 100 to 400 mg every 1 to 2 weeks, and every 1 to 5 weeks for maintenance once response occurs; (anabolic effects and osteoporosis): 200 to 400 mg every 3 to 4 weeks; (metastatic breast cancer): 200 to 400 mg every 2 weeks or at longer intervals. Testosterone propionate: Intramuscular (hypogonadism): 10 to 25 mg daily 2 to 4 times weekly; (postpartum breast engorgement): 25 to 50 mg daily for 3 or 4 days starting at delivery; (metastatic breast cancer): 50 to 100 mg 3 times weekly; (anabolic effect): 5 to 10 mg daily. Buccal (hypogonadism): 5 to 20 mg daily; (postpartum breast engorgement): 40 mg daily in divided doses for 3 to 5 days starting shortly after delivery; (metastatic breast cancer): 200 mg daily as long as improvement is maintained or for 3 months if no improvement.

NURSING IMPLICATIONS

Inject intramuscular preparation deep into gluteal muscle. Advise patient to report soreness at injection site, since postinjection furunculosis may be an associated adverse reaction.

Priapism (persistent erection) and virilization are signs of overdosage and indicate necessity for temporary drug withdrawal. Advise patient to report to physician.

Patients taking buccal form should be instructed to place tablet under tongue or in upper or lower buccal pouch between gum and cheek. Advise patient not to chew or swallow tablet and to avoid eating, drinking, or smoking until absorption is complete. Also advise patient to change location of tablet with each dose.

Good oral hygiene should be stressed in order to decrease possibility of irritation from buccal tablet.

Advise patient to report inflamed, painful buccal mucosa. In addition to physical discomfort, absorption rate is changed by altered mucosal surface.

See Testosterone.

TETRACYCLINE, U.S.P.

(ACHROMYCIN, CANCYCLINE, PANMYCIN, SK-TETRACYCLINE, SUMYCIN, T-125, T-150, TETRACYN)

TETRACYCLINE HYDROCHLORIDE, U.S.P., B.P.

(ACHROMYCIN-V, AMER-TET, AMTET, ANACEL, BRISTACYCLINE, CENTET, CYCLOPAR, PANMYCIN HCl, ROBITET, SUMYCIN, TETRACYN, and others)

Antiamebic, antibacterial, antirickettsial

ACTIONS AND USES

Broad-spectrum antimicrobial effective against a variety of Gram-positive and Gram-negative bacteria, certain mycoplasma, rickettsiae, protozoa. Believed to act by inhibiting phosphorylation and protein synthesis of susceptible microorganisms. Oral administration results in suppression of intestinal flora; used for this purpose in preoperative preparation of bowel for surgery.

Irregularly absorbed from GI tract. Peak levels reached in 2 to 4 hours; effective blood levels maintained for at least 6 hours. IM administration produces lower blood levels than oral administration. Half-life 6 to 9 hours. Well distributed in tissues and body fluids; lower levels in spinal and joint fluids, and higher than plasma concentrations in bile. Excreted mainly in feces and urine. Crosses placenta; enters breast milk.

CONTRAINDICATIONS AND PRECAUTIONS

Liver and renal impairment, hypersensitivity to tetracyclines, use during pregnancy, use in nursing mothers, use during period of tooth development (4th month of fetal life through 8th year), concomitant administration of potentially hepatotoxic drugs. Cautious use: undernourished patients.

ADVERSE REACTIONS

Nausea, anorexia, vomiting, diarrhea, dizziness, thrombophlebitis at site of injection, fever, hypersensitivity reactions, photosensitization, superimposed candidal growth (skin eruptions, gingivitis, stomatitis, pharyngitis, dysphagia, lingua nigra, anal pruritus, proctitis, vaginal discharge), hepatotoxicity, nephrotoxicity, blood dyscrasias, intracranial hypertension (pseudotumor cerebri): bulging fontanels, impaired vision, papilledema, severe headache, permanent discoloration and inadequate calcification of deciduous teeth, enamel hypoplasia, onycholysis and discoloration of nails.

ROUTE AND DOSAGE

Oral **(adults):** 250 mg every 6 hours; **(children):** 25 to 50 mg/kg divided into 2 to 4 equal doses. Intramuscular **(adults):** 250 mg once every 24 hours or 300 mg in divided doses at 8- to 12-hour intervals; **(children):** 15 to 25 mg/kg divided and given at 8- to 12-hour intervals. Intravenous **(adults):** 250 to 500 mg every 12 hours, not to exceed 500 mg every 6 hours; **(children):** 12 mg/kg/day divided into 2 doses.

NURSING IMPLICATIONS

Check expiration date before administering drug. Renal injury (Fanconi-like syndrome) has been attributed to administration of outdated tetracyclines.

To enhance drug absorption, administer oral preparation on an empty stomach (at least 1 hour before or 2 hours after eating). However, if nausea, anorexia, and diarrhea occur, they are usually controlled by administering drug with some food (exception: foods high in calcium, such as milk, interfere with absorption of tetracycline preparations) or by reducing drug dosage. Consult physician. If symptoms persist, drug should be discontinued.

Avoid concurrent use of antacids. See Drug Interactions.

Deep IM injection into body of a large muscle is recommended. Inadvertent injection into subcutaneous or fat layer may result in painful local irritation; may be relieved by an ice pack.

Solutions prepared for IM injection should be used within 24 hours. Initial reconstituted IV solutions are stable at room temperature for 12 hours, but when final dilution is made, they should be administered immediately.

Be alert for evidence of overgrowth of nonsensitive organisms. Inspect tongue regularly to note development of black, furry appearance. The incidence of infection by candida may be reduced by meticulous hygienic care of skin and mouth and by allowing patient to wash perineal area several times a day, particularly after each bowel movement.

It is important to distinguish between frequent stools resulting from local irritant effect of drug (usually occur early during therapy) and those due to superinfection, which require immediate discontinuation of therapy.

Monitor intake and output. Report oliguria or changes in intake–output ratio (patient can be taught to make rough estimates).

Advise patient to avoid exposure to direct or artificial sunlight during use of tetracyclines. Certain hypersensitive persons develop a phototoxic reaction (exaggerated sunburn) precipitated by exposure to sun or ultraviolet light. At the first sign of skin discomfort, drug should be discontinued.

Tetracycline may combine with calcium of developing teeth to cause yellow-gray-brownish discoloration. Its use during bone formation and tooth development periods (prenatally, neonatally, and in childhood) is generally avoided.

The drug is generally administered for 24 to 72 hours after fever and other symptoms have subsided. Warn patient to discard unused tetracycline after therapy is completed.

Tetracyclines decompose with age, with exposure to light, and when improperly stored under conditions of extreme humidity and heat. The resulting product may be toxic.

LABORATORY TEST INTERFERENCES: Possibility of false increases in urinary catecholamines (Hungert method) and false decreases in urinary urobilinogen. Parenteral tetracycline containing ascorbic acid may produce false positive urinary glucose determinations by copper reduction methods (eg, Benedict's and Clinitest) and false negative values with glucose oxidase methods (eg, Clinistix, Tes-Tape).

DRUG INTERACTIONS: Bacteriostatic drugs such as the tetracyclines may interfere with bactericidal action of **penicillin.** Concomitant administration of **iron preparations** and **antacids** containing aluminum, calcium, magnesium, or other divalent and trivalent cations results in chelate formation; do not administer tetracyclines within 1 or 2 hours of antacid; administer iron 3 hours before or 2 hours after tetracycline. Tetracyclines may enhance the hypoprothrombinemic effects of **oral anticoagulants** and antagonize the activity of **heparin.** There may be additive renal toxicity with **methoxyflurane. Sodium bicarbonate** and other alkalis may interfere with GI absorption of tetracycline.

TETRAHYDROZOLINE HYDROCHLORIDE, U.S.P.
(MURINE Z, TETRASINE, VISINE; TYZINE)

Adrenergic (vasoconstrictor)

ACTIONS AND USES

Imidazole derivative structurally and chemically related to naphazoline (qv). In common with naphazoline, has more marked α-adrenergic activity than β-adrenergic activity, and large doses cause CNS depression, rather than the stimulation produced by other sympathomimetic amines.

Used for symptomatic relief of minor eye irritation and allergies and nasopharyngeal congestion of allergic or inflammatory origin.

CONTRAINDICATIONS AND PRECAUTIONS

Hypersensitivity to any component, use of ophthalmic preparation in glaucoma or other serious eye diseases, use of drug in children under age 2, use of 0.1% or higher strengths in children under age 6, concomitant use of MAO inhibitors. Safe use during pregnancy not established. Cautious use: hypertension, cardiovascular disease, hyperthyroidism, diabetes mellitus, young children.

ADVERSE REACTIONS

Transient stinging, irritation, sneezing, dryness, headache, tremors, drowsiness, lightheadedness, insomnia, palpitation. Overdosage: CNS depression (marked drowsiness, sweating, coma, hypotension, shock, bradycardia).

Topical: Ophthalmic **(adults):** 1 or 2 drops of 0.05% solution in each eye 2 or 3 times a day. Nasal **(adults and children** *over 6 years):* 2 to 4 drops of 0.1% solution in each nostril as needed, never more often than every 3 hours; **(children** *2 to 6 years*): 2 or 3 drops of 0.05% solution in each nostril as needed, never more often than every 3 hours.

NURSING IMPLICATIONS

Since drug action lasts about 4 hours, interval between doses is usually 4 to 6 hours.

Instruct patient to discontinue medication and to consult physician if relief is not obtained within 48 hours or if symptoms for which drug was given persist or increase.

Caution patient not to exceed recommended dosage. Rebound congestion and rhinitis may occur with frequent or prolonged use of nasal preparation.

When using squeeze bottle, patient should be in upright position. When reclined, a stream rather than a spray may be ejected, with consequent overdosage.

Nasal drops are usually administered in lateral, head-low position.

THEOBROMINE CALCIUM SALICYLATE, N.F. (THEOCALCIN)

Diuretic, smooth-muscle relaxant

ACTIONS AND USES

Xanthine derivative with actions qualitatively similar to those of other xanthines (eg, caffeine, theophylline); diuretic and cardiovascular actions are less, but more sustained than those produced by theophylline (qv). Reportedly well tolerated, noncumulative, and not associated with dehydration or electrolyte imbalance even after prolonged use; therefore, suitable for maintenance diuresis in older patients.

Used for treatment of coronary insufficiency, convalescence after coronary occlusion, various conditions of decreased cardiac reserve, and congestive failure with edema. May be used concomitantly with mercurial diuretics, chlorothiazide, or digitalis to reduce requirements of these drugs.

CONTRAINDICATIONS AND PRECAUTIONS

Hypersensitivity to components. Cautious use: hyperthyroidism.

ADVERSE REACTIONS

Rarely: nausea, gastric upset, headache.

ROUTE AND DOSAGE

Oral: initially 500 mg to 1 Gm 3 times daily; dosage gradually reduced to optimum maintenance level.

NURSING IMPLICATIONS

Administer drug with or directly after meals.

See Theophylline.

(ATHEMOL)

Diuretic, smooth-muscle relaxant

ACTIONS AND USES
Xanthine derivative qualitatively similar to other xanthines (caffeine, theophylline). Relaxes vascular smooth muscle and thereby may help to relieve pain of angina pectoris and coronary insufficiency, peripheral vascular circulatory disease, and arteriosclerosis. In combination with magnesium nicotinate (Athemol-N), reportedly inhibits precipitation of cholesterol in vascular wall and helps to resolubilize already existing deposits.
CONTRAINDICATIONS AND PRECAUTIONS
Serious kidney disease, obstructive lesions of urinary tract.
ADVERSE REACTIONS
Rarely: gastric upset.
ROUTE AND DOSAGE
Oral: 200 to 400 mg 3 times daily.

NURSING IMPLICATIONS
Forewarn patients taking Athemol-N (theobromine magnesium oleate and magnesium nicotinate) that a transient tingly flushing sensation and pruritus may follow each dose.
See Theophylline.

THEOPHYLLINE, U.S.P., B.P.

(ADOPHYLLIN, AEROLATE, AQUALIN, BRONKODYL, ELIXOPHYLLIN, LANOPHYLLIN, SLO-PHYLLIN, SOMNOPHYLLIN, THEOBID, THEO-DUR, THEOLAIR, THEOLLINE, THEON, THEOPHYL)

Smooth-muscle relaxant (xanthine)

ACTIONS AND USES
Xanthine derivative with pharmacologic actions qualitatively similar to those of other xanthines (caffeine, theobromine). Relaxes smooth muscle by direct action, particularly of bronchi and pulmonary vessels, and stimulates medullary respiratory center with resulting increase in vital capacity. Also relaxes smooth muscles of biliary and GI tracts. Stimulates myocardium, thereby increasing force of contractions and cardiac output, and stimulates all levels of CNS, but to a lesser degree than caffeine. Produces mild diuresis by increasing renal blood flow and by inhibiting sodium and chloride reabsorption at proximal tubule. At cellular level, xanthines block phosphodiesterase, thereby promoting cyclic AMP accumulation. Cyclic AMP excess promotes catecholamine stimulation of lipolysis, glycogenolysis, and gluconeogenesis and induces release of epinephrine from adrenal medulla cells. Unlike sympathomimetic agents, tolerance to bronchodilator effects of theophylline derivatives rarely develops. Available in combination with ephedrine and phenobarbital (eg, Tedral, Thalfed, Lussmin). Used for prophylaxis and symptomatic relief of bronchial asthma, as well as bronchospasm associated with chronic bronchitis and emphysema; used for emergency treatment of paroxysmal cardiac dyspnea and edema of congestive heart failure.
ABSORPTION AND FATE
Rate of absorption depends on drug solubility. Oral solution and uncoated tablet are well absorbed from GI tract; peak blood levels in 1 to 2 hours. Absorption following sustained-release forms and rectal suppository is report-

edly variable and unreliable. Rectal suppository may be well absorbed by children. Peak plasma levels occur in about 5 hours for sustained-release form and 3 to 5 hours for rectal suppository, but this varies with manufacturer. Rapidly distributed throughout extracellular fluid and tissues. About 20% bound to plasma proteins. Plasma half-life approximately 5 hours in adults, 3.5 hours in children. Partially demethylated and oxidized in liver (individual variability in rate of metabolism). About 10% excreted unchanged in urine. Small amount excreted in feces. Readily crosses placenta; appears in breast milk in high concentrations.

CONTRAINDICATIONS AND PRECAUTIONS

Hypersensitivity to xanthines; coronary artery disease or angina pectoris when myocardial stimulation might be harmful; severe renal or liver impairment. Safe use during pregnancy and lactation and in women of childbearing potential not established. Cautious use: children, compromised cardiac or circulatory function, hypertension, hyperthyroidism, peptic ulcer, prostatic hypertrophy, glaucoma, diabetes mellitus.

ADVERSE REACTIONS

GI: nausea, vomiting, anorexia, epigastric or abdominal pain, diarrhea, activation of peptic ulcer. **CNS** (stimulation): irritability, restlessness, insomnia, dizziness, headache, hyperexcitability, muscle twitching, convulsions. **Cardiovascular:** palpitation, tachycardia, extrasystoles, flushing, marked hypotension, circulatory failure. **Respiratory:** tachypnea, respiratory arrest. **Renal:** transient urinary frequency, albuminuria, kidney irritation. **Other:** fever, dehydration, rectal irritation and strictures following rectal administration, increased urinary catecholamine excretion.

ROUTE AND DOSAGE

Oral: **Adults:** 100 to 200 mg every 6 hours; **Children:** 50 to 100 mg every 6 hours. Rectal: **Adults:** 250 to 500 mg every 8 to 12 hours; **children:** not to exceed 10 to 12 mg/kg/24 hours, in divided doses at 8- to 12-hour intervals. All dosages highly individualized.

NURSING IMPLICATIONS

Because individuals metabolize xanthines at different rates, dosage is determined by close monitoring of response, tolerance, pulmonary function, and theophylline plasma levels.

Therapeutic theophylline plasma level ranges from 10 to 20 μg/ml. Levels exceeding 20 μg/ml are associated with toxicity. Theophylline saliva levels (used when plasma levels cannot be obtained) are equal to approximately 60% of simultaneous plasma levels.

Oral preparations should preferably be administered with a full glass of water and may be given after meals to minimize gastric irritation. Food delays but does not reduce absorption. Physician may prescribe an antacid if GI symptoms continue. Dosage reduction may also be indicated.

Monitor vital signs and intake and output. Improvement in quality of pulse and respiration and diuresis are expected clinical effects.

Observe and report early signs of possible toxicity: anorexia, nausea, vomiting, dizziness, wakefulness, restlessness, irritability.

During early therapy, dizziness is a relatively common side effect in the elderly. Take necessary safety precautions and forewarn patient of this possibility.

Patients receiving rectal preparations should be instructed to report immediately the onset of rectal irritation.

Caution patient not to take OTC medications without approval of physician.

Reportedly, duration of drug action is reduced in cigarette smokers (smoking may decrease half-life as much as 40%).

Pertinent teaching points for patients with respiratory problems (consult physician): (1) drug action; reason for taking drug; (2) dosage schedule;

stress importance of taking drug precisely as prescribed; (3) adequate fluid intake to thin secretions; (4) humidification of environment, particularly in winter months; (5) postural drainage (for patients who have difficulty coughing up secretions) performed especially on arising and at bedtime; (6) breathing exercises; (7) physical reconditioning programs; (8) avoid exposure to infection, chilling, sprays, smoke, and other irritants; (9) do not smoke; (10) keep follow-up appointments.

LABORATORY TEST INTERFERENCES: False positive elevations of serum uric acid (Bittner or colorimetric method).

DRUG INTERACTIONS: Xanthine derivatives appear to increase excretion of **lithium** ions and thus may decrease its effectiveness; they enhance sensitivity to and toxic potential of **cardiac glycosides;** they may exhibit synergistic toxicity with **ephedrine** and other **sympathomimetic** amines (particularly in children); they have mutually antagonistic action with **propranolol.** In high doses, xanthines may increase plasma prothrombin and factor V and thus may antagonize effect of **oral anticoagulants.** Decreased hepatic clearance (increased theophylline plasma level) has been reported in patients receiving **clindamycin, erythromycin, lincomycin,** or **troleandomycin.**

THEOPHYLLINE OLAMINE
(FLEET THEOPHYLLINE, Theophylline Monoethanolamine)

Smooth-muscle relaxant

ACTIONS AND USES
Monoethanolamine salt of theophylline (qv), with similar actions, uses, adverse reactions, and precautions as other theophylline derivatives. Contains 73% to 75% theophylline.
ROUTE AND DOSAGE
Rectal (suppository, retention enema): 250 to 500 mg once daily or every 12 hours.

> **NURSING IMPLICATIONS**
> Not administered to children, since pediatric dose not established.
> See Theophylline.

THEOPHYLLINE SODIUM GLYCINATE, N.F.
(GLYNAZAN, SYNOPHYLATE, PANOPHYLLINE FORTE, THEOFORT)

Smooth-muscle relaxant (xanthine)

ACTIONS AND USES
Mixture of sodium theophylline and aminoacetic acid (glycine). Contains 45% to 47% theophylline. Similar actions, uses, adverse reactions, and precautions as other theophylline derivatives, but claimed to produce less gastric irritation. See Theophylline.
ROUTE AND DOSAGE
Oral: **Adults:** 330 to 660 mg every 6 to 8 hours. **Children** *over 12 years:* 220 to 330 mg; *3 to 6 years,* 110 to 165 mg; *1 to 3 years,* 55 to 110 mg.

NURSING IMPLICATIONS
Administered after meals with a full glass of liquid (if allowed) to minimize
GI irritation from local drug effect.
See Theophylline.

THIAMINE HYDROCHLORIDE, U.S.P., B.P.
(BETALIN S, BETAXIN, BEWON, THIA, THIAMINE CHLORIDE, VITAMIN B₁)

Vitamin (enzyme cofactor), antiberiberi and antineuritic vitamin

ACTIONS AND USES
Water-soluble vitamin and member of B-complex group. Functions as an essential coenzyme in carbohydrate metabolism. Also has role in conversion of tryptophan to nicotinamide.
Used in treatment and prophylaxis of beriberi, to correct anorexia due to thiamine deficiency states, and in treatment of neuritis associated with pregnancy, pellagrà, and alcoholism, including Wernicke-Korsakoff syndrome. Therapy generally includes other members of vitamin B complex, since thiamine deficiency rarely occurs alone.

ABSORPTION AND FATE
Limited absorption following oral administration, as compared with IM injection, which is rapid and complete. Wide distribution to most body tissues, with highest concentrations in liver, brain, kidney, and heart. Minimal body storage. Excreted in urine as pyrimidine and, with excessive intake, as unchanged drug.

ADVERSE REACTIONS
Slight fall in blood pressure following rapid IV administration; anaphylactic shock. Toxic doses: weakness, labored breathing, respiratory failure.

ROUTE AND DOSAGE
Oral: 5 to 100 mg daily. Intramuscular, intravenous (rarely used): 30 to 60 mg divided into 3 equal doses.

NURSING IMPLICATIONS
Intradermal test dose is recommended prior to administration in suspected thiamine sensitivity. Deaths have occurred following IV use.
IM injections may be painful. Rotate sites and apply cold compresses to area if necessary for relief of discomfort.
Careful recording of patient's dietary history is an essential part of vitamin replacement therapy. Collaborate with physician, dietitian, patient, and responsible family member in developing a diet teaching plan that can be sustained by patient.
Therapeutic effectiveness is evaluated by improvement of clinical manifestations of thiamine deficiency: anorexia, gastric distress, depression, irritability, insomnia, palpitation, tachycardia, loss of memory, paresthesias, muscle weakness and pain, elevated blood pyruvic acid level (diagnostic test for thiamine deficiency), elevated lactic acid level. Severe deficiency: ophthalmoplegia, polyneuropathy, muscle wasting ("dry" beriberi), edema, serous effusions, congestive heart failure ("wet" beriberi).
Body requirement of thiamine is directly proportional to carbohydrate intake and metabolic rate; thus, requirement increases when diet consists predominantly of carbohydrates. Total absence of dietary thiamine can produce a deficiency state in about 3 weeks.
Classic beriberi is uncommon in the United States, but it is endemic in Asia. Like deficiencies of other B vitamins, subclinical states often accompany poverty, chronic alcoholism, dietary fads, and pregnancy.

Recommended daily allowance: children 4 to 6 years of age, 0.9 mg; adult males, 1.4 mg; adult females, 1 mg; pregnancy and lactation, 1.3 mg.

Rich thiamine food sources: yeast, pork, beef, liver, wheat and other whole grains, fresh vegetables, especially peas and dried beans.

Preserved in tight, light-resistant, nonmetallic containers. Thiamine is unstable in alkaline solutions (eg, solutions of acetates, barbiturates, bicarbonates, carbonates, citrates) and neutral solutions.

THIETHYLPERAZINE MALEATE
(TORECAN)

Antiemetic

ACTIONS AND USES

Piperazine phenothiazine derivative with contraindications, precautions, and toxic effects similar to those of chlorpromazine (qv). Reported to have higher ratio of antiemetic action to tranquilizing action than other phenothiazines. Thought to act directly on chemoreceptor trigger zone and vomiting center. Used to control nausea and vomiting. Possibly effective for treatment of vertigo.

ABSORPTION AND FATE

Onset of effects in less than 1 hour following oral or rectal administration and within 30 minutes following IM injection. See Chlorpromazine.

CONTRAINDICATIONS AND PRECAUTIONS

Hypersensitivity to phenothiazines, CNS depression or comatose states, pregnancy, IV administration. Safe use in children under age 12, in nursing mothers, or following intracardiac or intracranial surgery not established. Cautious use: renal or hepatic disease. Also see Chlorpromazine.

ADVERSE REACTIONS

Drowsiness, dizziness, headache, dry mouth and nose, blurred vision, tinnitus, restlessness, fever, orthostatic hypotension. Occasionally: extrapyramidal symptoms including convulsions; sialorrhea with altered taste sensations, cholestatic jaundice. See Chlorpromazine.

ROUTE AND DOSAGE

Oral, rectal suppository, intramuscular: 10 mg 1 to 3 times a day.

NURSING IMPLICATIONS

Examine parenteral solution and administer only if it is clear and colorless.

Patient should be recumbent when administering drug IM. Postural hypotension (manifested by weakness, lightheadedness, faintness) and drowsiness may occur, particularly after initial injection. Advise patient to remain in bed for about 1 hour or longer, if indicated, and supervise ambulation. If vasopressor agent is required, levarterenol or phenylephrine is used. Epinephrine is contraindicated.

Administer IM deep into large muscle mass, and aspirate carefully before injecting drug in order to avoid inadvertent entry into a blood vessel. IV administration is specifically contraindicated because it can cause severe hypotension.

Patients who have received drug preoperatively may manifest restlessness or depression during anesthesia recovery.

Report immediately the onset of extrapyramidal effects: gait disturbances, difficulty in speaking, muscle spasms, torticollis, deviations in eye movements. Reduction in dosage or discontinuation of medication is indicated.

Caution patient to avoid potentially hazardous activities such as driving a car or operating machinery because of possibility of drowsiness and dizziness.

Stored at room temperature, away from heat, in light-resistant containers. Suppositories should be stored below 77 F.
See Chlorpromazine Hydrochloride.

THIMEROSAL, N.F.
(AEROAID, MERSOL, MERTHIOLATE)
THIOMERSAL, B.P.

Topical antiinfective, pharmaceutical aid (preservative)

ACTIONS AND USES
Organic mercurial with sustained bacteriostatic and fungistatic activity. Ineffective against spore-forming organisms. Used in first-aid treatment of wounds, in antisepsis of intact skin, and in pustular dermatoses; used as antifungal agent in athlete's foot. Ophthalmic preparation is used in treatment of conjunctivitis and corneal ulcer and for prevention of infection following removal of foreign bodies. Also used as preservative for biologic and pharmaceutical products.
CONTRAINDICATIONS AND PRECAUTIONS
History of sensitivity to thio or mercurial compounds, prolonged use.
ADVERSE REACTIONS
Hypersensitivity reaction: erythema, papular or vesicular eruptions. Prolonged use: mercury poisoning (metallic taste, salivation, stomatitis, lethargy, peripheral neuropathy).
ROUTE AND DOSAGE
Topical: 1:1000 cream, glycerite, solution, tincture; aerosol 0.33%; ophthalmic ointment 1:5000.

NURSING IMPLICATIONS
For first-aid treatment of wounds, appropriate cleansing should precede application of antiseptic.
To prevent skin irritation, do not apply bandage or other occlusive dressing until tincture application has completely dried.
Thimerosal is antagonized by whole blood and is incompatible when used concurrently or following applications of boric acid, iodine, strong acids, aluminum, silver, or other salts of heavy metals. It is compatible with sulfonamides.
Reportedly not inactivated by soaps or cotton materials, and action is not significantly diminished by nonsanguineous drainage (plasma, serum) or discharge.
Preserved in tightly covered, light-resistant containers. Avoid exposure to excessive heat.

THIOGUANINE, U.S.P., N.F.
(TG, 6-THIOGUANINE)

Antineoplastic (purine antagonist)

ACTIONS AND USES
Antimetabolite and purine antagonist qualitatively and quantitatively similar to mercaptopurine (qv). Produces delayed myelosuppression, and displays teratogenic properties. Cross-resistance exists between mercaptopurine and thioguanine. For contraindications and adverse reactions, see Mercaptopurine.
Used in treatment of chronic myelocytic leukemia and acute leukemia. Investi-

gational use in treatment of autoimmune diseases has produced unimpressive results. Has little advantage over mercaptopurine.

ABSORPTION AND FATE

Partially absorbed from GI tract, with maximum blood levels achieved in 10 to 12 hours. Partially detoxified in liver; excreted in feces and urine.

ROUTE AND DOSAGE

Oral (dosage depends on clinical and hematologic responses and is highly individualized): usual initial dose 2 mg/kg body weight daily; if no clinical improvement occurs after 4 weeks of treatment, dosage is cautiously increased to 3 mg/kg body weight daily administered at one time; usual maintenance dose 2 mg/kg daily.

NURSING IMPLICATIONS

Unlike mercaptopurine, thioguanine dose schedule may be maintained during concomitant administration of allopurinol.

Blood counts are determined weekly; monitor reports as indicators for adaptations in nursing and drug regimens.

Maintenance doses are continued throughout remissions.

Monitor intake–output ratio and report oliguria.

Observe patient's skin and sclera for jaundice. It is thought to be a reversible clinical sign, but it should be reported promptly as a symptom of toxicity.

Expected descent of leukocyte count may be slow over a period of 2 to 4 weeks. Treatment is interrupted if there is a rapid fall within a few days.

Since there is no known antagonist to thioguanine, prompt discontinuation of the drug is essential in avoiding irreversible myelosuppression when toxicity develops.

Store drug in airtight containers.

See Mercaptopurine.

THIOPENTAL, SODIUM, U.S.P.
(PENTOTHAL SODIUM)
THIOPENTONE SODIUM, B.P.

Anesthetic, anticonvulsant, hypnotic

ACTIONS AND USES

Ultra-short-acting barbiturate. CNS depressant action prolongs hypnosis and anesthesia, but without analgesia.

Used to induce hypnosis and anesthesia prior to or as supplement to other anesthetic agents, or as sole agent for brief (15-minute) procedures. Also used to control convulsive states and for narcoanalysis and narcosynthesis in psychiatric disorders.

ABSORPTION AND FATE

Hypnotic action within 30 to 40 seconds following IV administration. Rapidly absorbed by rectal route, with onset of action in 8 to 10 minutes and duration of about 1 hour. With repeated doses, fatty tissue acts as reservoir (concentrations 6 to 12 times that of plasma), with slow release of drug and prolonged anesthesia. Destroyed by liver. Crosses placenta.

CONTRAINDICATIONS AND PRECAUTIONS

Absolute contraindications: hypersensitivity to barbiturates, absence of suitable veins for IV administration, status asthmaticus, manifest or latent porphyria. Relative contraindications: severe cardiovascular disease, hypotension or shock, conditions that may potentiate or prolong hypnotic effect (excessive premedication, Addison's disease, hepatic or renal dysfunction, myxedema, increased BUN, severe anemia, increased intracranial pressure, asthma, myasthenia gravis).

Respiratory and myocardial depression, cardiac arrhythmias, prolonged somnolence and recovery, sneezing, coughing, bronchospasm, laryngospasm, shivering, hypersensitivity reactions, pain, neurosis, sloughing with IV extravasation. Also see Phenobarbital.

ROUTE AND DOSAGE

Intravenous, rectal suspension. Highly individualized by titration against patient's requirements as governed by age, sex, and body weight.

NURSING IMPLICATIONS

Solution should be freshly prepared and used promptly. If a precipitate is present, solution should not be used. Unused portions should be discarded within 24 hours.

Solutions should be prepared with one of the following diluents: sterile water, 0.9% sodium chloride, or 5% dextrose for injection. Sterile water for injection is not used for concentrations less than 2% because they cause hemolysis.

Resuscitation equipment, endotracheal tube, suction, and oxygen should be readily available for treatment of respiratory depression.

Test dose is advisable to determine unusual sensitivity to thiopental.

Physician may prescribe normal saline enema several hours before administration of rectal suspension (soap solution may interfere with drug effect).

If extravasation occurs, chemical irritant effects and pain can be reduced by local injections of 1% procaine and applications of heat to increase circulation and removal of drug.

Vital signs should be taken every 3 to 5 minutes after drug administration, and patient should be constantly observed.

Shivering or twitching of facial muscles sometimes progressing to localized or generalized tremors is a thermal reaction due to increased sensitivity to cold. It is most likely to occur if room environment is cold. Treatment: application of blankets; have on hand chlorpromazine or methylphenidate.

Classified as schedule III drug under federal Controlled Substances Act.

See Phenobarbital.

THIORIDAZINE HYDROCHLORIDE, U.S.P., B.P.
(MELLARIL)

Antipsychotic agent (major tranquilizer)

ACTIONS AND USES

Piperidyl phenothiazine derivative with actions, uses, contraindications, precautions, and adverse reactions similar to those of chlorpromazine. Compared with chlorpromazine, rarely produces extrapyramidal effects, has minimal antiemetic and hypothermic activity, and is less frequently associated with marked sedation and lethargy.

Used in management of psychotic manifestations and in selected patients with depressive neuroses. Also used to control moderate to severe agitation and hyperactivity in disturbed children and for alcohol withdrawal syndrome, intractable pain, and senility.

CONTRAINDICATIONS AND PRECAUTIONS

Severe CNS depression, children under age 2. Cautious use: patients with premature ventricular contractions.

Sedation, lethargy, orthostatic hypotension, nasal congestion, blurred vision, constipation, nausea, vomiting, diarrhea, pallor, galactorrhea, breast engorgement, amenorrhea, retrograde ejaculation, peripheral edema, ventricular dysrhythmias, pigmentary retinopathy. Infrequent: leukopenia, agranulocytosis, extrapyramidal symptoms. Also see Chlorpromazine.

ROUTE AND DOSAGE

Oral: **Adults**: Psychotic manifestations: initially 50 to 100 mg 3 times daily, gradually increased to maximum of 800 mg/day, if necessary; once symptoms are controlled, dosage is reduced gradually to lowest effective maintenance level. Neurosis, alcohol withdrawal, intractable pain, senility: initially 25 mg 3 times daily; total daily dosage range 20 to 200 mg. **Children** *over 2 years:* 0.5 to 3 mg/kg/day; *hospitalized psychotic children:* initially 25 mg 2 or 3 times daily; increased gradually until optimum therapeutic effect or maximum dosage is reached.

NURSING IMPLICATIONS

Liquid concentrate should be diluted just prior to administration with either distilled water, acidified tap water, or suitable juices. Preparation and storage of bulk dilutions are not recommended.

Faintness and vertigo associated with orthostatic hypotension may occur, especially at beginning of therapy. Female patients appear to be more susceptible to this drug effect than male patients.

Advise patient to make position changes slowly, particularly from recumbent to upright posture, and to dangle legs a few minutes before standing. Also inform patient that vasodilation produced by hot showers or baths may accentuate hypotensive drug effect.

Marked drowsiness may occur, especially when large doses are given early in treatment, but this generally subsides with continued therapy or reduction in dosage.

Caution patient to avoid potentially hazardous activities such as driving a car or operating machinery until his reaction to drug is known.

Instruct patient to report to physician the onset of any change in visual acuity, brownish coloring of vision, or impairment of night vision. These symptoms suggest pigmentary retinopathy (observed primarily in patients receiving extremely high doses).

Periodic blood and hepatic function tests are advised during therapy.

Preserved in tightly covered, light-resistant containers.

See Chlorpromazine Hydrochloride.

THIOTHIXENE, N.F.
(NAVANE)

Antipsychotic (major tranquilizer)

ACTIONS AND USES

Thioxanthene derivative with chemical and pharmacologic properties similar to those of chlorprothixene and phenothiazine derivatives (see Chlorpromazine). Has sedative, adrenolytic, antihistaminic, antiemetic, and anticholinergic activity. Used in management of acute and chronic schizophrenia.

ABSORPTION AND FATE

Well absorbed by oral and parenteral routes. Widely distributed to body tissues; may remain in body several weeks after administration. Metabolized in liver. Excreted in bile and feces as metabolites and unchanged drug.

Hypersensitivity to thioxanthene derivatives (and possibly phenothiazines), children under age 12, comatose patients, CNS depression, circulatory collapse, blood dyscrasias. Safe use in women of childbearing potential or during pregnancy not established. Cautious use: history of convulsive disorders, alcohol withdrawal, glaucoma, prostatic hypertrophy, impaired renal or hepatic function, cardiovascular disease, those who might be exposed to extreme heat or who are receiving atropine or related drugs. Also see Chlorpromazine.

ADVERSE REACTIONS

Drowsiness, weakness, fatigue, dizziness, dry mouth, polydipsia, blurred vision, constipation, hyperhidrosis, tachycardia, orthostatic hypotension, ECG alterations, impotence, galactorrhea, amenorrhea, rash, convulsions, leg cramps, photosensitivity, pigmentary retinopathy, lenticular pigmentation, extrapyramidal symptoms, insomnia (especially with large doses). Carries potential for same side effects and toxicity associated with phenothiazines (see Chlorpromazine).

ROUTE AND DOSAGE

Oral: 2 to 5 mg 2 or 3 times daily; if necessary, increased gradually to 60 mg maximum daily dose. Intramuscular: 4 mg 2 to 4 times daily; if necessary, increased gradually to maximum of 30 mg daily. Oral form substituted as soon as possible.

NURSING IMPLICATIONS

Avoid contact of drug with hands or clothing. Contact dermatitis has been reported with phenothiazines and may be possible with this drug.

Administer IM injection deep into large muscle mass, preferably upper outer quadrant of buttock or midlateral thigh. Aspirate carefully before injecting to avoid inadvertent entry into blood vessel. Rotate injection sites.

Because of the possibility of hypotension, patient should be recumbent when receiving drug IM. Advise patient to remain in bed for at least 1 hour following injection. Instruct patient to make position changes slowly, particularly from recumbent to upright, and to dangle legs a few minutes before ambulation.

Dosage adjustment may be necessary when patient is changed from IM to oral form.

Mild drowsiness is common during first few days after drug initiation and usually subsides with continuation of therapy.

Extrapyramidal effects, especially inability to sit still, pacing, restlessness (akathisia), and slow distorted movements (dystonia), occur commonly during early therapy and indicate need for dosage adjustment.

Since thiothixene has pharmacologic properties similar to those of the phenothiazines, patient may be prone to suicide, restlessness, aggression, anxiety, and depression, particularly during first few weeks of therapy.

Caution patient to avoid potentially hazardous activities such as driving a car or operating machinery until his response to drug is known.

Therapeutic effect may occur in 1 to 6 hours following IM administration and within a few days to several weeks after oral administration.

Periodic ophthalmologic examinations and blood and hepatic function tests are advisable in patients on prolonged therapy.

Advise patient to avoid excessive exposure to sunlight, concomitant use of alcohol or other depressants, and OTC medications unless approved by physician.

Drug withdrawal following prolonged use should be accomplished slowly. Abrupt withdrawal may result in severe delirium.

Preserved in tight, light-resistant containers.

See Chlorpromazine for nursing implications and drug interactions.

THIPHENAMIL HYDROCHLORIDE (TROCINATE)

Smooth-muscle relaxant

ACTIONS AND USES

Synthetic tertiary amine anticholinergic agent with actions similar to those of atropine. Considerably less potent than atropine in antisialogogue activity; unlike atropine, does not significantly reduce gastric secretions or produce mydriasis. Causes reduced GI motility by direct spasmolytic action on smooth muscle, resembling that of papaverine. Also has vasodilator and strong local anesthetic properties.

Used for relief of hypermotility and muscle spasm associated with a variety of GI disorders.

CONTRAINDICATIONS AND PRECAUTIONS

Safe use during pregnancy and in children not established.

ADVERSE REACTIONS

Uncommon: dry mouth, constipation. High doses: possibility of CNS stimulation. See Atropine.

ROUTE AND DOSAGE

Oral: initially 400 mg; may be repeated in 4 hours.

NURSING IMPLICATIONS

Contact of drug with oral mucosa may produce irritation and temporary numbness (local anesthetic effect). Advise patient not to chew tablet or allow it to dissolve in mouth.

For maximum therapeutic effect, dosage must be titrated to individual patient's needs. Once relief is obtained, physician may reduce dosage or increase intervals between doses.

See Atropine for drug interactions.

THROMBIN, U.S.P.

Hemostatic (local)

ACTIONS AND USES

Sterile plasma protein prepared from prothrombin of bovine origin. Clots fibrinogen of blood directly. Potency standardized and expressed in terms of NIH units (1 NIH unit is amount required to clot 1 ml of standardized fibrinogen solution in 15 seconds).

Used when oozing of blood from capillaries and small venules is accessible, as in dental extraction, plastic surgery, grafting procedures, and epistaxis.

CONTRAINDICATIONS AND PRECAUTIONS

Known hypersensitivity to any of drug components or to material of bovine origin, parenteral use, entry or infiltration into large blood vessels.

ADVERSE REACTIONS

Sensitivity, allergic and febrile reactions, intravascular clotting and death when thrombin is allowed to enter large blood vessels.

Topical: 100 to 2000 NIH units/ml, depending on extent of bleeding. May be used as solution, in dry form, or by mixing thrombin with blood plasma to form a fibrin "glue." Also used in conjunction with absorbable gelatin sponge: sponge strips of desired size are immersed in thrombin solution; sponge is kneaded vigorously to remove trapped air, then applied and held in place 10 to 15 seconds with dry sterile cotton pledget or gauze sponge. Oral (method 1): patient is given 60 ml milk to neutralize gastric acid; after 2 minutes, 10,000 to 20,000 NIH units thrombin are administered in 60 ml milk; repeated 3 times daily for 4 or 5 days or until bleeding is controlled; (method 2): 60 ml phosphate buffer solution are introduced via Levin tube; stomach contents are aspirated; 60 ml phosphate buffer are repeated; after 5 minutes additional 60 ml of buffer containing 10,000 NIH units thrombin are given; Levin tube is clamped off for 30 minutes, at the end of which time it is aspirated gently; if there is no fresh bleeding, patient is given buffer for 48 hours (15 ml every hour); entire procedure is repeated, if necessary.

NURSING IMPLICATIONS

Solutions may be prepared in sterile distilled water or isotonic saline.

Solutions should be used within a few hours of preparation. If several hours are to elapse between time of preparation and use, solution should be refrigerated, or preferably frozen, and used within 48 hours.

Thrombin activity is affected by dilute acids, alkalis, heat, and salts of heavy metals.

THYROGLOBULIN, N.F.
(PROLOID)

Hormone, thyroid

ACTIONS AND USES

Obtained from purified extract of hog thyroid; contains levothyroxine (T_4) and liothyronine (T_3) in approximate ratio of 2.5:1. Clinical effects similar to those of thyroid (qv). For absorption and fate, see Thyroid.

Used in thyroid replacement therapy of hypothyroidism.

CONTRAINDICATIONS AND PRECAUTIONS

Cautious use: myxedema (such patients are extremely sensitive to thyroid). Also see Thyroid.

ADVERSE REACTIONS

Signs and symptoms of hyperthyroidism such as menstrual irregularities, nervousness, angina pectoris, cardiac arrhythmias. Also see Thyroid.

ROUTE AND DOSAGE

Oral: start dosage in small amounts; increments at intervals of 1 or 2 weeks; usual maintenance 0.5 to 3.0 grains (approximately 32 to 200 mg) daily.

NURSING IMPLICATIONS

Dosage is adjusted to maintain protein-bound iodine at 4 to 8 μg/dl.

Transfer from thyroglobulin to liothyronine: thyroglobulin is discontinued and therapy initiated with low daily dose of liothyronine; in the reverse situation, thyroglobulin replacement precedes complete withdrawal of liothyronine by several days in order to prevent relapse.

Drug is stable when stored at room temperature.

Also see Thyroid.

(ARCO THYROID, ARMOUR THYROID, DELCOID, S-P-T,
THERMOLOID, THYROCRINE, THYROID STRONG, THYRO-TERIC,
THY-SPAN-3, TULOPAC)

Hormone, thyroid

ACTIONS AND USES

Preparation of desiccated animal thyroid gland containing active thyroid hormones, *l*-thyroxine (T_4) and *l*-triiodothyronine (T_3); total iodine content between 0.17% and 0.23%. Action mechanism unknown; reportedly T_4 largely converted to T_3, which exerts principal effects. Influences growth and maturation of various tissues (including skeletal and CNS) at critical periods. Promotes a generalized increase in metabolic rate of body tissues, producing increases in the following: rate of carbohydrate, protein, and fat metabolism, enzyme system activity, oxygen consumption, respiratory rate, body temperature, cardiac output, heart rate, blood volume. Thyroid affects water and ion transport and directly promotes synthesis and transcription of nuclear RNA. Potentiates actions of catecholamines; eg, many prominent features of hyperthyroidism (tachycardia, lid lag and tremor) represent increased catecholamine effects. Therapeutic actions are slow to develop and prolonged.

Used as replacement or substitution therapy in primary hypothyroidism (cretinism, myxedema, simple goiter, deficiency states in pregnancy and in the elderly) and secondary hypothyroidism caused by surgery, excess radiation, or antithyroid drug therapy. May be given as adjunct to thyroid inhibiting agents when it is desirable to limit release of thyrotropic hormones.

ABSORPTION AND FATE

Adequate absorption from GI tract. Binds competitively and reversibly to plasma transport proteins: thyroxine-binding globulin (TBG), thyroxine-binding prealbumin (TBPA), and albumin. Maximum effect of T_4 (half-life 6.9 days) not reached for several days; that of T_3 (half-life 2 days) reached in 12 to 24 hours; full effect usually achieved in 10 to 14 days. Excreted in urine and stool in both free and conjugated forms. Fecal excretion (10% to 15%) is variable, depending on hepatic function, luminal contents, and physical state of intestines. Minimal transport across placenta.

CONTRAINDICATIONS AND PRECAUTIONS

Thyrotoxicosis, acute myocardial infarction uncomplicated by hypothyroidism, hyperthyroidism, cardiovascular disease, morphologic hypogonadism, nephrosis, uncorrected hypoadrenalism. Cautious use: angina pectoris, hypertension, elderly patients who may have occult cardiac disease, renal insufficiency, pregnancy, concomitant administration of catecholamines.

ADVERSE REACTIONS

Overdosage (thyrotoxicosis): staring expression in eyes, cardiac arrhythmias, palpitation, tachycardia, weight loss, tremors, headache, nervousness, fever, diarrhea or abdominal cramps, insomnia, warm and moist skin, heat intolerance, congestive heart failure, angina pectoris, leg cramps, shock, changes in appetite, hyperglycemia (usually offset by increased tissue oxidation of sugar). **Massive overdosage:** thyroid storm; **chronic overdosage:** hyperthyroidism. **Altered laboratory values:** increased serum protein-bound iodine, lowered serum cholesterol level.

ROUTE AND DOSAGE

Oral (highly individualized): **Adults:** *Myxedema:* 15 mg/day for 2 weeks, followed by 30 mg/day for 2 weeks or more, then 60 mg/day; thereafter, dosage increased as clinically indicated; maintenance 60 to 180 mg/day; (hypothyroidism without myxedema): initially 60 mg/day; then increased by 60 mg every 30 days to maintenance dose. **Children** *Cretinism or severe hypothyroidism:* same dosage regimen as for adults; increments at 2-week intervals; final maintenance may be greater in growing child than in adult.

NURSING IMPLICATIONS

Administer as a single dose, preferably before breakfast.

Transfer from thyroid treatment to liothyronine: discontinue thyroid and initiate treatment with low daily dose of liothyronine; transfer in reverse direction: therapy initiated with replacement several days before complete withdrawal of liothyronine in order to avoid collapse.

During institution of treatment, observe patient carefully for untoward reactions such as angina, palpitation, cardiac pain.

Physical examination at monthly intervals and protein-bound iodine (PBI) levels every 3 months are usual during dose adjustment period.

Normal values of laboratory tests used to determine clinical response to thyroid: Basal metabolic rate: plus or minus 10 (imprecise as diagnostic tool). PBI: 4 to 8 $\mu g/dl$. ^{131}I uptake: 10% to 20% at 6 hours; 20% to 40% at 24 hours. Free thyroxine: 1.4 to 3.5 ng/dl. T_3 (radioimmunoassay) mean values (6-week infant): 163 ng/dl; (adult): 111 ng/dl. T_4 (radioimmunoassay) mean values (6-week infant): 10.3 $\mu g/dl$; (adult): 7.6 $\mu g/dl$. Thyroid stimulating hormone (TSH) level: up to 10 $\mu U/ml$.

Generally dosage is initiated at low level and systematically increased in small increments to desired maintenance dose.

Be alert for symptoms of overdosage (see Adverse Reactions) that may occur 1 to 3 weeks after therapy is started. If they develop, treatment should be interrupted for several days and restarted with reduced dosage.

Toxic effects of thyroid develop slowly and disappear gradually. T_4 effects require up to 3 to 6 weeks to dissipate; T_3 effects last 6 to 14 days after drug withdrawal.

If patient has taken hormone during pregnancy, dose is frequently discontinued in the postpartum period, with evaluation of thyroid function 6 weeks later.

Serial height measurement of the juvenile being treated with thyroid is an important means of monitoring influence of thyroid on growth. Too rapid growth rate results in premature epiphyseal closure. Urge parent to keep accurate record of height measurements for reporting to physician.

Useful guides of thyroid therapy in children include sleeping pulse and basal morning temperature.

Prepare parent and juvenile hypothyroid for a dramatic response to therapy: excessive shedding of hair, increased assertiveness of previously passive child, initial rapid weight loss and rapid catch-up growth. Symptoms usually disappear with continued therapy.

Earliest clinical response to thyroid (adult) is diuresis, accompanied by loss of weight and puffiness, followed by sense of well-being, increased pulse rate, increased pulse pressure, increased appetite, increased psychomotor activity, loss of constipation, normalization of skin texture and hair, and increased T_3 and T_4 serum levels.

In patient teaching, emphasize that replacement therapy for hypothyroidism is life-long; therefore, continued follow-up surveillance is important. Regular yearly appointments for evaluation are recommended.

Keep in mind that these patients tend to discontinue their medication when they begin to feel well.

Thyroid hormone is no longer used as a therapeutic agent for treatment of obesity, reproductive disorders (eg, habitual abortion), breast cancer, and depression. The patient should not be taking thyroid at home without medical supervision.

Inadequate dosage in infant hypothyroidism is manifested by bradycardia, circulatory mottling, inactivity, hoarse cry, constipation, delay in relaxation phase of deep-tendon reflexes.

Pulse rate is an important clue to drug effectiveness. Count pulse before each dose during period of dosage adjustment. Consult physician if rate is 100 or more, or if there has been a marked change in rate or rhythm.

When patient is euthyroid, teach him how to take his own pulse and to record it periodically. If rate begins to increase or if rhythm changes, patient should notify physician.

Adrenocortical insufficiency may occur with prolonged therapy (dehydration, hypotension, asthenia, hypoglycemia, increased pigmentation of skin and mucous membranes). The diabetic patient receiving thyroid hormone may require increased dosage of insulin or oral hypoglycemic agent. Conversely, decreasing the thyroid dose may cause a hypoglycemic reaction unless insulin dosage is also reduced. Reinforce the necessity of continuing regular testing of urine for sugar.

Thyroid hormones will alter the results of thyroid function tests.

If patient is receiving anticoagulant therapy, a decrease in the requirement usually develops within 1 to 4 weeks after starting treatment with thyroid. Close monitoring of prothrombin time (normal 12 to 14 seconds) is necessary. Warn patient to report evidence of excess anticoagulant, evidenced by ecchymoses, petechiae, purpura, unexplained bleeding.

Onset of chest pain or other signs of aggravated cardiovascular disease (dyspnea, tachycardia) should be reported promptly. The physician will decrease dosage.

Steatorrhea and other disease states that interfere with enterohepatic circulation may lead to excessive fecal loss of drug. Patient should be cautioned to report persistent diarrhea.

Teach the patient on periodic PBI determinations to avoid ingestion or exposure to even a small amount of iodine in order to assure accurate findings. Instruct him to avoid application of topical iodine, ingestion of OTC medications with iodides, dentifrices, intake of foods high in iodine (eg, turnip, cabbage, soy beans, some breads, kelp). Iodized salt and iodine-containing multivitamin preparations usually do not interfere with thyroid uptake test. The physician will want to know if he has had any procedure requiring radiopaque dyes (eg, bronchography, myelography, cisternography) during the past 4 to 6 weeks.

Store in dark bottle to minimize spontaneous deiodination. Keep desiccated thyroid dry. Potency in this form reportedly persists for as long as 17 years.

LABORATORY TEST INTERFERENCES: PBI level increases about 1 or 2 μg/dl for each 60 mg thyroid given daily. On maintenance dose, PBI should be about normal.

DRUG INTERACTIONS: Thyroid hormone may increase requirements for **insulin** and **oral hypoglycemics** (because of its own hypoglycemic activity). It may potentiate and be potentiated by **tricyclic antidepressants** (extensive confirmatory evidence is lacking). Therapeutic effects of **anticoagulants** are enhanced by thyroid hormone, as are the toxic effects of **digitalis** and **indomethacin** (especially cardiac arrythmias). Thyroid enhances cardiovascular effects of **epinephrine** and **levarterenol** and increases tissue demands for **corticosteroids. Cholestyramine** decreases thyroid action (reduces absorption from GI tract). **Estrogens** reduce bioavailability of thyroid, and **phenytoin** decreases protein binding of thyroid, thus increasing its effect.

Diagnostic aid (myxedema); Hormone, thyroid-stimulating

ACTIONS AND USES
   Highly purified thyrotropic hormone (TSH) isolated from bovine anterior pituitary. Increases iodine uptake by thyroid, and stimulates formation and secretion of thyroid hormone. May cause hyperplasia of thyroid cells, a rapidly reversible effect.
   Used as diagnostic tool to determine subclinical hypothyroidism or low thyroid reserve, to assess need for continued thyroid medication, to differentiate primary and secondary hypothyroidism, and to detect remnants and metastases of thyroid carcinoma. Also used therapeutically in management of selected types of thyroid carcinoma.

ABSORPTION AND FATE
   Following parenteral injection, rapidly cleared by kidney. Half-life 35 minutes in euthyroid; increased in hypothyroidism, and decreased in hyperthyroidism.

CONTRAINDICATIONS AND PRECAUTIONS
   Hypersensitivity to TSH, coronary thrombosis. Cautious use: in presence of angina pectoris, cardiac failure, hypopituitarism, adrenocortical suppression.

ADVERSE REACTIONS
   Menstrual irregularities, fever, headache, nausea, vomiting, urticaria, transitory hypotension, tachycardia, atrial fibrillation, thyroid swelling (especially with large doses), postinjection flare, anaphylactic reactions, induced or exaggerated angina pectoris or congestive heart failure.

ROUTE AND DOSAGE
   Subcutaneous, intramuscular (diagnosis): 10 international units (I.U.) for 1 to 3 days; (therapy of thyroid carcinoma): 10 I.U. daily for 3 to 8 days.

NURSING IMPLICATIONS
Ten I.U. lyophilized powder is dissolved in 2 ml sterile physiologic saline
   solution for injection.
Diagnostic tests may be made even though patient is receiving thyroid hormone therapy.
TSH is stable at room temperature when kept dry. Retains potency in solution at least 2 weeks if refrigerated.
Diagnostic use: in presence of normal thyroid tissue, stimulation provided by
   daily doses of 10 I.U. TSH for 1 to 3 days causes an elevated serum
   thyroxine level and increased radioactive iodine uptake (RAI) by thyroid
   gland. If hypothyroidism is primary, there will be no change in RAI
   uptake following several days of TSH stimulation. Conversely, there will
   be a significant increase in RAI uptake if hypothyroidism is secondary to
   hypopituitarism.
Treatment of overdosage: discontinue thyrotropin and supply supportive
   measures required by shock and potential adrenal insufficiency.

DRUG INTERACTIONS: **Levodopa** lowers TSH levels.

Antibacterial (aminoglycoside)

ACTIONS AND USES

Water-soluble aminoglycoside antibiotic derived from *Streptomyces tenebrarius.* Closely related to gentamicin (qv) in spectrum of antibacterial activity and pharmacologic properties. Crossed allergenicity and some cross-resistance among aminoglycosides have been demonstrated.

Used in treatment of severe infections caused by susceptible organisms.

ABSORPTION AND FATE

Following IM injection, peak serum concentrations in 30 to 90 minutes in adults and 1 to 2 hours in children. Measurable levels persist up to 8 hours. Serum concentrations higher and more prolonged in patients with reduced kidney function and infants. Widely distributed to body tissues and fluids; significant levels in cerebrospinal fluid usually not achieved. Almost no serum protein binding. Serum half-life about 2 hours. Not appreciably metabolized in body. Eliminated by glomerular filtration; up to 93% of dose is excreted in urine in 24 hours. Crosses placenta.

CONTRAINDICATIONS AND PRECAUTIONS

History of hypersensitivity to tobramycin and other aminoglycoside antibiotics, concurrent use with other neurotoxic and/or nephrotoxic agents or potent diuretics. Safe use during pregnancy and in nursing mothers not established. Cautious use: impaired renal function, premature and neonatal infants. Also see Gentamicin.

ADVERSE REACTIONS

Neurotoxicity (including ototoxicity), nephrotoxicity, increased SGOT and SGPT, increased serum bilirubin, anemia, agranulocytopenia, thrombocytopenia, fever, rash, pruritus, urticaria, nausea, vomiting, lethargy, superinfections. Also see Gentamicin.

ROUTE AND DOSAGE

Intramuscular, intravenous **(adults, children, and older infants** *with normal renal function*): 3 mg/kg/day in 3 equal doses every 8 hours; life-threatening infections: up to 5 mg/kg/day in 3 or 4 equal doses; dosage in **neonates** *1 week of age or younger* not to exceed 4 mg/kg/day in equally divided doses every 12 hours; *(patients with impaired renal function):* initially 1 mg/kg/day; subsequent dosage adjusted either with reduced doses at 8-hour intervals or usual doses at longer intervals. For IV injection, usual volume of diluent (0.9% sodium chloride injection or 5% dextrose injection) is 50 to 100 ml for adults and proportionately less for children, infused in not less than 20 minutes (range 20 to 60 minutes).

NURSING IMPLICATIONS

Weigh patient before treatment for calculation of dosage (by physician).

Culture and sensitivity tests are advised prior to and during tobramycin therapy.

As with other aminoglycosides, patient receiving tobramycin must remain under close clinical observation because these antibiotics carry potential for nephrotoxicity and neurotoxicity, including both vestibular and auditory damage, even in conventional doses.

Monitoring of serum drug concentrations is advised, if feasible, as well as urinalyses for protein cells and casts. Prolonged serum concentrations above 12 μg/ml are not advised.

Renal, auditory, and vestibular functions and serum drug levels should be closely monitored, particularly in patients with known or suspected renal impairment and patients receiving high doses.

Evidence of impaired renal function (increasing BUN or NPN, increasing creatinine, cylinduria, proteinuria, cells, oliguria), auditory toxicity (hearing impairment, tinnitus), or vestibular damage (dizziness, vertigo, nystagmus, ataxia) indicates need for discontinuation of drug or dosage adjustment.

Monitor intake and output. Report oliguria, changes in intake–output ratio, and cloudy or frothy urine (may indicate proteinuria). Patient is usually kept well hydrated to prevent chemical irritation in renal tubules. Consult physician.

Therapy is generally continued for 7 to 10 days. Complicated infection may require longer course of therapy, in which case close monitoring of renal, auditory, and vestibular function and serum drug concentrations is essential.

Solutions of tobramycin are clear and colorless and require no refrigeration. Tobramycin should not be mixed with other drugs.

See Gentamicin for nursing implications and drug interactions.

TOLAZAMIDE, U.S.P.
(TOLINASE)

Antidiabetic (oral)

ACTIONS AND USES

Orally effective sulfonylurea hypoglycemic structurally and pharmacologically related to tolbutamide (qv), but about 5 times more potent in action. Lowers blood sugar by stimulating beta cells of pancreas to secrete insulin. For contraindications, precautions, and adverse reactions, see Tolbutamide.

Used in management of maturity-onset diabetes mellitus. Reportedly effective in the patient who is a primary or secondary failure with other sulfonylurea agents or who has developed intolerance to similar drugs.

ABSORPTION AND FATE

More slowly absorbed than tolbutamide, but absorption is complete. Onset of action in 4 to 6 hours; peak blood levels in 4 to 8 hours; duration of maximum hypoglycemic effect 10 hours. Average half-life 7 hours; drug accumulates in blood for first 4 to 6 doses, then steady state is reached, after which peak and nadir values do not vary from day to day. Approximately 85% of drug is excreted in urine.

ROUTE AND DOSAGE

Oral (individualized): 100 to 500 mg once daily with breakfast; doses exceeding 500 mg should be given twice daily.

NURSING IMPLICATIONS

When patient is newly diagnosed, dosage is guided by fasting blood sugar values: if less than 200% (true), start with 100 mg daily (one dose); if greater than 200% (true), start with 250 mg daily (one dose). Subsequent adjustments are made according to urine and blood tests and physician's evaluations. Dose increments made at home for geriatric, debilitated, or underweight patients are on the order of 50 to 125 mg daily at weekly intervals.

Doses larger than 1000 mg/day rarely provide improvement in diabetic control; patient then usually is maintained on insulin alone.

Patient must be under medical supervision for first 6 weeks of treatment. He should see his physician at least once weekly and should check urine daily for sugar and acetone.

Transferral from another sulfonylurea drug usually does not require primary or initial dose or transitional period.

Reduction of dose frequently alleviates most of the mild to moderately severe hypoglycemic symptoms.

Unlike tolbutamide, tolazamide is effective in some patients with a history of ketoacidosis or coma; close observation of these patients is especially important during the early adjustment period.

No false positive tests for urinary albumin have been reported (these occasionally are noted with other sulfonylureas).

See Tolbutamide.

TOLAZOLINE HYDROCHLORIDE, N.F., B.P.
(PRISCOLINE, TAZOL, TOLOXAN, TOLZOL)

Peripheral vasodilator

ACTIONS AND USES

Imidazoline derivative chemically related to phentolamine. In addition to weak α-adrenergic blocking activity, sympathomimetic action causes cardiac stimulation, parasympathomimetic effect increases GI motility, and histaminelike activity stimulates gastric secretions. Produces vasodilation, primarily by direct relaxant effect on vascular smooth muscle.

Used to improve blood flow in Buerger's disease, diabetic arteriosclerosis gangrene, scleroderma, postthrombotic conditions, frostbite sequelae, and other vasospastic disorders.

ABSORPTION AND FATE

Absorbed well by all routes. Maximal effects in 45 minutes to 1.5 hours following oral administration and in 30 to 60 minutes after IM injection. Effects persist for several hours. Excreted in urine, largely as unchanged drug.

CONTRAINDICATIONS AND PRECAUTIONS

Following cerebrovascular accident; coronary artery disease. Cautious use: gastritis, peptic ulcer (previous or current).

ADVERSE REACTIONS

Nausea, vomiting, diarrhea, epigastric discomfort, flushing, increased pilomotor activity with tingling and chilliness, mydriasis, tachycardia, cardiac arrhythmias, anginal pain, postural hypotension, blood pressure changes, marked hypertension (particularly following parenteral use), exacerbation of peptic ulcer. Intraarterial administration: feeling of warmth or burning at injection site, transient weakness, postural vertigo, palpitation, formication, apprehension, paradoxic impairment of blood supply, gangrene. Severe overdosage: hypotension to shock levels.

ROUTE AND DOSAGE

Oral: 25 mg 4 to 6 times daily; may be gradually increased up to 50 mg 6 times daily; long-acting tablet: 80 mg every 12 hours. Subcutaneous, intramuscular, intravenous: 10 to 50 mg 4 times daily. Intraarterial: initially 25-mg test dose; depending on response, 50 to 75 mg 1 or 2 times daily, then 2 or 3 injections weekly for maintenance.

NURSING IMPLICATIONS

Side effects are generally mild and usually decrease with continued therapy. Gastric irritation may be relieved by giving drug after meals or with a glass of milk. Physicians sometimes prescribe concurrent administration of an antacid and an antispasmodic (for diarrhea). Persistence of GI symptoms may require dosage reduction.

During period of dosage adjustment in patients receiving drug orally, check blood pressure and pulse 3 or 4 times during the day, and more frequently if indicated.

Patients receiving drug by any parenteral route should be closely observed for blood pressure changes and excessive cardiac effects. Monitor blood pressure and pulse at 2- to 4-hour intervals as indicated and report changes to physician.

Observe affected limbs for changes in color and skin temperature, and keep physician informed.

Feelings of warmth, piloerection, crawling or chilly sensations in affected limb (or generalized) indicate that effective dosage has been reached. Report to physician immediately.

Since postural hypotension is a possibility, instruct patient to make position changes slowly, particularly from recumbent to upright posture, and to dangle legs for a few minutes before standing.

Caution patient that alcohol ingestion may cause a severe (disulfiramlike) reaction.

Drug effectiveness is enhanced by keeping patient comfortably warm. Avoid exposure and cold environment.

Treatment of overdosage: for ingested drug in absence of coma, induction of vomiting and/or gastric lavage. Hypotension is treated by head-low position and IV fluids. Ephedrine should be administered as needed. *Epinephrine is contraindicated,* since paradoxic fall in blood pressure may result.

Discuss the following possible teaching points with physician for specific patient instructions: hygienic care of affected parts (frequency and details of care); avoidance of hot-water bottles, heating pads, garters, as well as smoking and alcohol; importance of properly fitting shoes and hosiery; positioning (some physicians prescribe elevation of head of bed on 6-inch blocks to enhance circulation to legs).

TOLBUTAMIDE, U.S.P., B.P.
(ORINASE)
TOLBUTAMIDE SODIUM, U.S.P.
(ORINASE DIAGNOSTIC)

Antidiabetic (sulfonylurea)

ACTIONS AND USES

Short-acting sulfonylurea compound chemically related to sulfonamides, but without antibacterial activity. Lowers blood sugar by stimulating beta cells of pancreas to synthesize and release insulin. Precise mechanism unclear, but reportedly causes degranulation of beta cells, a cellular mechanism associated with increased rate of insulin secretion. No action demonstrated if functional beta cells are absent. With long-term use, may be mildly goitrogenic without producing clinical hypothyroidism or thyroid enlargement.

Used in management of mild uncomplicated maturity-onset diabetes mellitus not controlled by diet alone. Also used adjunctively to stabilize certain cases of labile diabetes and as diagnostic agent to rule out islet cell tumor.

ABSORPTION AND FATE

Following absorption from GI tract, tolbutamide is detected in blood within 30 minutes; maximum concentration reached in 3 to 5 hours; half-life 5 hours; duration of action 6 to 12 hours. Binds to plasma proteins; subsequently oxidized in liver to carboxytolbutamide, inactive metabolite excreted in urine within 24 hours.

Real or suspected sulfa drug allergy, juvenile or labile diabetes, pregnancy, history of repeated episodes of acidosis or coma, severe stress, infection or trauma, use prior to or during surgery, fever; severe renal, hepatic, or thyroid insufficiency. Cautious use: cardiac, pituitary, or adrenal dysfunction, women of childbearing age, debilitation, alcoholism, geriatric patients.

ADVERSE REACTIONS

Dose-related (usually transient): headache, GI disturbances (nausea, vomiting, anorexia, constipation, diarrhea). **Hypoglycemia** (vague symptoms, but require immediate attention): fatigue, headache, drowsiness, lassitude, tremulousness, nausea; (other): hunger, lightheadedness, profuse sweating, tachycardia, paresthesias, circumoral pallor, blurred vision, diplopia, mydriasis, irritability, negative tests for glycosuria (second voiding), inability to concentrate, delirium, convulsions, unconsciousness, coma. **Hematologic** (rare): leukopenia, thrombocytopenia, aplastic and hemolytic anemia, agranulocytosis, pancytopenia. **Dermatologic:** skin eruptions, pruritus, erythema; (rare): phototoxic reactions; hypersensitivity. **Other** (rare): cholestatic jaundice, purpura, fatigue, vertigo, dizziness, malaise, headache, edema associated with hyponatremia, hepatic porphyria, porphyria cutanea tarda; (uncommon): paradoxic severe hypoglycemia that may mimic acute neurologic disorders such as cerebral thrombosis. **Altered laboratory values:** reduced RAI uptake (after long-term administration), altered liver function tests (SGOT, SGPT, alkaline phosphatase, bilirubin).

ROUTE AND DOSAGE

Oral (individualized): initially 1 or 2 Gm daily, adjusted to minimal dosage for adequate control (range 0.25 to 3 Gm); maintenance dose of over 2 Gm daily seldom required; total dose may be taken before breakfast or in divided doses through the day. Intravenous (tolbutamide sodium): 1 Gm (given in sterile water) over period of 2 or 3 minutes.

NURSING IMPLICATIONS

Tolbutamide is neither oral insulin nor substitute for insulin; however, the same diagnostic and therapeutic measures required to insure optimum insulin control of diabetes are required for control by tolbutamide.

Because of danger of nocturnal hypoglycemia, tolbutamide should not be taken at bedtime unless specifically ordered.

Elderly patients may be hyperresponsive to oral antidiabetic therapy; thus initial dose should be low and given before breakfast. If blood and urine glucose tests are negative during first 24 hours of therapy, initial dose may be continued on a daily basis; if hypoglycemia occurs, dose is reduced to minimum level or discontinued.

In trial period, patient is under close medical supervision until dosage is established (using negative tests for glucosuria and ketonuria as criteria).

Transfer from one sulfonylurea compound to another can be effected without transitional period or priming dose.

Transfer from insulin to oral hypoglycemic agent (best controlled in hospital): Patient receiving 20 units or less insulin daily: start oral drug at time insulin is discontinued. Patient receiving 20 to 40 U daily: begin oral hypoglycemic at maintenance level, with concurrent 30% to 50% reduction in insulin dose; continue to decrease insulin gradually. Patient taking more than 40 U insulin daily: begin oral hypoglycemic at maintenance level, with concurrent 20% reduction in insulin on first day, followed by cautious decremental adjustments of insulin to omission. Absence of sugar in urine is criterion for reduction of insulin dose. During transfer, patient should test his urine for sugar and ketone bodies at least 3 times daily and report results to physician.

Be alert for possibility of hyperglycemia and ketoacidosis (flushed and dry skin, weight loss, fatigue, Kussmaul respiration, double or blurred vision, soft eyeballs, irritability, fruity-smelling breath, abdominal cramps, nausea, vomiting, diarrhea, dyspnea, polydipsia, polyphagia, polyuria, headache, hypotension, weak and rapid pulse, positive ketonuria and glucosuria). Report symptoms promptly so that emergency antidiabetic therapy can be instituted. Onset of ketoacidosis usually indicates "primary failure" (ie, diabetes cannot be controlled by tolbutamide) and the necessity of returning to insulin therapy.

Frequent causes of hypoglycemia include overdosage of hypoglycemic drug, too little food, delay in taking antidiabetic drug, vomiting, diarrhea, added exercise without caloric supplement or dose adjustment, emotional stress, or stress due to infection.

Hypoglycemia (exaggeration of expected therapeutic action) indicates need for immediate reevaluation of patient's diet, medication regimen, and compliance.

Early hypoglycemic reactions can be stemmed quickly by eating soluble glucose (such as Life-Savers, soft drinks, fruit juice, all with real sugar). If symptoms do not subside in 10 to 15 minutes, repeat glucose; if after another 10 to 15 minutes patient still has symptoms and urine test for sugar is negative, he should notify his physician.

When hypoglycemic reaction progresses to grogginess, the patient can be given a teaspoon of honey or corn syrup into his mouth; the sugar will be absorbed by oral membranes, and patient should revive enough to drink a glass of fruit juice. Unconsciousness should be treated in hospital, where IV dextrose in water and clinical supervision will be given until maintenance dose is reestablished.

Hypoglycemic symptoms may be especially vague in the elderly; therefore, check out nondefinitive expressions such as "I don't feel good today" to discover real meaning; observe patient carefully, especially 2 to 3 hours after eating, and check urine for sugar and ketone bodies.

Repetitive complaints of headache and weakness after eating may signal incipient hypoglycemia.

Urge patient to report promptly if he feels sick or has a fever or sore throat (common cold symptoms). The physician may want to evaluate quality of imposed stress or rule out agranulocytosis by blood studies.

Pruritus and rash, frequently reported side effects, may clear spontaneously, may be reversible, or may increase after drug has been discontinued.

Caution patient that moderate amounts of alcohol (equal to 50 ml of 100 proof whiskey) can precipitate a disulfiramlike reaction. He should also be informed that if he becomes hypoglycemic after ingesting alcohol, he may be thought to be inebriated and may be deprived of necessary emergency treatment.

The patient should understand that undereating is as hazardous as overeating; warn him that a self-directed weight-loss regimen, redistribution of dietary carbohydrate, or skipped meals interfere with drug control of diabetes.

Monitor weekly body weights, and report a progressive gain, especially if edema is present. These signs indicate the necessity of discontinuing tolbutamide.

Advise patient to report immediately signs of hepatic dysfunction (pruritus, jaundice, dark urine, light-colored stools) or renal insufficiency (dysuria, anuria, hematuria). Tolbutamide will be withdrawn by the physician. Either situation can lead to hypoglycemia: impaired hepatic degradation of drug extends action period, and renal insufficiency compromises glucose and sodium exchange in renal tubules.

Transient alterations in certain liver function tests during initial period of sulfonylurea therapy reportedly have little clinical significance because fluctuating abnormalities of liver function frequently occur in patients with diabetes.

Intercurrent complications such as infection, severe trauma, major surgery, and protracted vomiting or diarrhea are usually treated temporarily with insulin alone or in combination with the oral agent. The patient may need a review of insulin injection technique during this period so that he can give his own medication.

Tolbutamide sodium IV differentiates the nondiabetic (rapid, intense drop in blood sugar within 1 hour after dose) from the diabetic (slow response). If a pancreatic insulinoma is present, the response is rapid; the hypoglycemia produced lasts as long as 3 hours. Observe injection site carefully for signs of irritation and local pain, and report to physician.

Careless, casual attitudes toward tolbutamide regimen lead to noncompliance and lack of diabetic control. Encourage and support the patient in accepting responsibility for keeping his condition under control and maintaining schedule for periodic clinical evaluation.

The patients most prone to "secondary failure" (loss of response to tolbutamide after initial control by the drug) may be underweight, erratic in their meal schedules, or careless about dosage, or they may have developed drug resistance.

Impress on the patient and family that tolbutamide controls diabetes, but will never cure it.

Instruct the patient to carry identification card (available at most drug stores) with him at all times; the card will contain his and his physician's names and addresses and his diagnosis, medication, and dose being taken.

For teaching plan outline, see Insulin Injection.

DRUG INTERACTIONS: **Allopurinol, chloramphenicol, oral anticoagulants, MAO inhibitors, oxyphenbutazone, phenylbutazone,** and **phenyramidol** prolong the effects of oral hypoglycemics by decreasing or inhibiting hepatic biotransformation. Reduced plasma protein binding and consequent increase in oral hypoglycemic action are produced by **phenylbutazone, salicylates, sulfonamides,** and **oral anticoagulants. Alcohol** and **MAO inhibitors** enhance hypoglycemic response by suppressing gluconeogenesis. **Insulin** has additive action. **Phenylbutazone** may inhibit excretion of tolbutamide, thereby prolonging its hypoglycemic action.

TOLMETIN SODIUM
(TOLECTIN)

Antiinflammatory

ACTIONS AND USES

Pyrrole acid derivative, nonsteroidal agent structurally and pharmacologically related to indomethacin. Has analgesic, antiinflammatory, and antipyretic properties. Exact mode of antiinflammatory action not known, but believed to be related to reduction of prostaglandin synthesis. Provides symptomatic relief but does not alter basic rheumatoid process. Decreases platelet aggregation, and may prolong bleeding time, but changes in prothrombin and whole blood clotting times not reported. Comparable to aspirin and indomethacin in antirheumatic activity, but incidence of GI symptoms and tinnitus is less than in aspirin-treated patients, and CNS effects are less than in patients receiving indomethacin. Each tablet contains 18 mg (0.784 mEq) of sodium.

Used in treatment of acute flares and in management of chronic rheumatoid arthritis. May be used alone or in combination with gold or corticosteroids.

719

Rapidly and almost completely absorbed. Peak serum levels in 30 to 60 minutes. Approximately 99% bound to plasma protein. Half-life about 1 hour. Metabolized in liver; almost entirely excreted in urine within 24 hours, primarily as inactive metabolite, glucuronide, and unchanged drug (about 20%). Animal studies suggest that excretion is enhanced by alkalinization of urine.

CONTRAINDICATIONS AND PRECAUTIONS

History of intolerance or hypersensitivity to tolmetin, aspirin, and other non-steroidal antiinflammatory agents, active peptic ulcer. Safe use not established during pregnancy and lactation, in children under age 12, in patients severely incapacitated, bedridden, or confined to wheelchair. Cautious use: history of upper GI tract disease, impaired renal function, compromised cardiac function.

ADVERSE REACTIONS

GI: epigastric or abdominal pain or discomfort, nausea, vomiting, heartburn, constipation, peptic ulcer, GI bleeding. **CNS:** headache, dizziness, vertigo, light-headedness, mood elevation or depression, tension, nervousness, weakness, drowsiness, fever, tinnitus, hearing impairment (rare). **Dermatologic:** rash, urticaria, pruritus. **Cardiovascular:** mild edema (sodium and water retention), mild to moderate hypotension. **Hematologic:** transient and small decreases in hemoglobin and hematocrit, granulocytopenia, leukopenia, prolongation of bleeding time, elevations in BUN, alkaline phosphatase, and SGOT.

ROUTE AND DOSAGE

Oral: initially 400 mg 3 times daily, adjusted according to patient's response; daily dosage range 600 to 1800 mg in divided doses 3 or 4 times daily, not to exceed 2000 mg/day.

NURSING IMPLICATIONS

Dosage preferably scheduled to include a morning dose (on arising) and a bedtime dose.

Food delays absorption, but does not affect total amount absorbed. If GI disturbances occur, instruct patient to take drug with meals, milk, or antacid (prescribed). Sodium bicarbonate is not recommended, since it may enhance drug excretion. Advise patient to notify physician if symptoms persist; dosage reduction may be necessary.

Since tolmetin and other nonsteroidal antiinflammatory agents have produced eye changes and renal toxicity in laboratory animals, manufacturer recommends that extended therapy be guided by periodic eye examinations and frequent evaluations of kidney function.

Caution the patient to avoid potentially hazardous activities such as driving a car or operating machinery until his response to the drug is known.

Instruct patients with impaired renal or cardiac function to monitor weight and to check ankles and tibiae for edema.

Therapeutic response generally occurs within a few days to 1 week, with progressive improvement in succeeding week: reduced joint pain, reduced swelling, less morning stiffness, improved grip strength and functional capacity.

Overdosage: Stomach should be emptied by induced vomiting or gastric lavage, followed by administration of activated charcoal slurry; forced alkaline diuresis may be attempted to hasten drug excretion.

LABORATORY TEST INTERFERENCES: Metabolites of tolmetin may produce false positive results for proteinuria (with tests that rely on acid precipitation, eg, sulfosalicylic acid); dye-impregnated reagent strips (eg, Albustix, Uristix) not affected.

DRUG INTERACTIONS: Although they have not been reported, patients receiving tolmetin with other protein-bound drugs (eg, **dicumarol, warfarin, hydantoin, sulfonamides, sulfonylureas**) should be observed closely for signs of toxicity of either drug (tolmetin may be displaced by or may displace these drugs from binding sites). Tolmetin may potentiate ulcerogenic effects of **ibuprofen, indomethacin, phenylbutazone,** and **salicylates.**

TRANYLCYPROMINE SULFATE, N.F., B.P.
(PARNATE)

Antidepressant (MAO inhibitor)

ACTIONS AND USES

Potent nonhydrazine MAO inhibitor structurally related to amphetamine. Actions and toxicity similar to those of hydrazine MAO inhibitors, but also has rapid and direct amphetaminelike CNS stimulatory action, is less likely to cause hepatotoxicity, and does not produce prolonged MAO inhibition.

Owing to its toxic potential, use is reserved for treatment of severe mental depression in hospitalized patients who have not responded to other antidepressant therapy. See Phenelzine.

ROUTE AND DOSAGE

Oral: initially 10 mg in morning and 10 mg in afternoon. This dosage may be continued for 2 weeks. If no response, dosage may be adjusted to 20 mg in morning and 10 mg in afternoon for another week. Following improvement, dosage then is reduced to lowest effective maintenance level. Dosage not to exceed 30 mg daily.

NURSING IMPLICATIONS

Incidence of severe hypertensive reactions appears to be greater with tranylcypromine than with other MAO inhibitors.

Usually produces therapeutic response within 3 days, but full antidepressant effects may not be obtained until 2 or 3 weeks of drug therapy.

See Phenelzine Sulfate.

TRIAMCINOLONE, N.F.
(ARISTOCORT, KENACORT, SK-TRIAMCINOLONE)
TRIAMCINOLONE ACETONIDE, U.S.P., B.P.
(ARISTOCORT ACETONIDE, ARISTODERM FOAM, KENALOG)
TRIAMCINOLONE DIACETATE, N.F.
(ARISTOCORT, CENOCORTE FORTE, CINO-400, KENACORT)
TRIAMCINOLONE HEXACETONIDE, U.S.P.
(ARISTOSPAN INTRALESIONAL, ARISTOSPAN PARENTERAL)

Adrenocortical steroid (glucocorticoid)

ACTIONS AND USES

Synthetic fluorinated adrenal corticosteroid with glucocorticoid and antirheumatic activity 7 to 13 times more potent than that of hydrocortisone. Plasma half-life about 5 hours. Possesses minimal sodium and water retention properties in therapeutic doses. Administered orally, 4 mg triamcinolone is equivalent to 20 mg hydrocortisone on a weight basis. Acetonide formulation has longer duration of action than parent compound; when administered into joint or bursa, pharmacologic activity begins within few hours and may persist a number of weeks. Differs from other corticosteroids in that it does not increase appetite. Shares uses, absorption, fate, contraindications, and precautions with hydrocortisone (qv).

CONTRAINDICATIONS AND PRECAUTIONS

Renal dysfunction. Also see Hydrocortisone.

ADVERSE REACTIONS

Tissue atrophy at injection site, muscle weakness and loss of tissue mass. Also see Hydrocortisone.

ROUTE AND DOSAGE

Oral (triamcinolone and diacetate), intramuscular, intraarticular, intralesional (acetonide, hexacetonide, diacetate), topical (acetonide): creams, lotions, foam, opththalmic ointment; wide dose range dependent on condition being treated and response of patient. **Adults:** Usual initial dose is 4 to 60 mg daily in single or divided doses. Subsequent reduction of dose is gradual and consistent with patient response. **Children**: *acute leukemia:* 1 to 2 mg/kg.

NURSING IMPLICATIONS

This preparation may cause natriuresis, negative nitrogen balance, with weight loss in most patients (along with headache, fatigue, and dizziness) and sodium retention with weight gain and moon facies in others. Adequate diet to counter these effects should be designed. Plan with dietician, patient, and physician. High protein, high K diet is often needed.

Postural hypotension may accompany sodium and weight loss. It may be necessary to keep patient in supine position for 30 minutes after triamcinolone is given. Warn patient to keep this possibility in mind as he ambulates.

Protect drug from light.

See Hydrocortisone for nursing implications related to topical application.

TRIAMTERENE, U.S.P.
(DYRENIUM)

Diuretic (potassium-sparing)

ACTIONS AND USES

Pteridine derivative structurally related to folic acid. Like spironolactone, has weak diuretic action and a potassium-sparing effect. Promotes excretion of sodium, chloride (to lesser extent), and carbonate, with no excretion or slight excretion of potassium ion. Unlike spironolactone, acts directly on distal tubule, rather than by inhibiting aldosterone, and activity is independent of aldosterone levels. May cause decrease in alkali reserve and slight increase in urinary pH. Does not appear to inhibit excretion of uric acid, but serum uric acid levels may increase in predisposed individuals. Decreased glomerular filtration rate and elevated BUN are associated with daily administration, but seldom with intermittent (every other day) therapy. Has slight hypotensive effect.

Used in treatment of edema associated with congestive heart failure, hepatic cirrhosis, and nephrotic syndrome; used in idiopathic edema, steroid-induced edema, and edema due to secondary hyperaldosteronism.

ABSORPTION AND FATE

Rapidly and irregularly absorbed from GI tract (individual variability). Onset of diuretic action in 2 to 4 hours; usually tapers off 7 to 9 hours later. Duration of action may be 24 hours or longer. Approximately 67% bound to plasma proteins. Plasma half-life 100 to 200 minutes. Excreted by renal filtration and tubular secretion; 10% to 80% of dose is eliminated within 24 hours.

CONTRAINDICATIONS AND PRECAUTIONS

Hypersensitivity to drug, severe or progressive kidney disease or dysfunction, severe hepatic disease, elevated serum potassium. Safe use during pregnancy and in women of childbearing potential and nursing mothers not established. Cautious use: impaired renal or hepatic function, history of gouty arthritis, diabetes mellitus.

ADVERSE REACTIONS

Diarrhea, nausea, vomiting, and other GI disturbances; dizziness, headache, dry mouth, anaphylaxis, photosensitivity, rash, weakness and hypotension (large doses), muscle cramps, hyperkalemia and other electrolyte imbalances, elevated BUN, elevated uric acid (patients predisposed to gouty arthritis), hyperchloremic acidosis, blood dyscrasias: granulocytopenia, eosinophilia, megaloblastic anemia (patients with reduced folate stores).

ROUTE AND DOSAGE

Oral: initially 100 mg twice daily; titrated to needs of patient. Total daily dosage not to exceed 300 mg. When edema is controlled, patient usually is maintained on 100 mg/day or 100 mg every other day. When used with other diuretics, initial dose of each drug is reduced, then adjusted according to patient's response and tolerance.

NURSING IMPLICATIONS

Give drug after meals to prevent or minimize nausea. Note that nausea and vomiting are also symptoms of electrolyte imbalance and renal failure; therefore, they should be reported. Dosage reduction or discontinuation of drug may be indicated.

Weigh patient under standard conditions (preferably before breakfast, after voiding, same scale, same clothing) prior to drug initiation and daily during therapy.

Diuretic response usually occurs on first day of therapy, but maximum effect may not occur for several days.

Monitor intake and output. Report oliguria and unusual changes in intake–output ratio. Hyperkalemia is reportedly not as likely to occur in patients with adequate urinary output. Consult physician regarding allowable fluid intake.

Unlike most diuretics, triamterene promotes potassium retention. Therefore, potassium supplements, potassium-rich diet, and salt substitutes are usually discontinued when drug is used alone or when added to other diuretic therapy.

Generally salt restriction is not prescribed because of possibility of low-salt syndrome (hyponatremia). Consult physician.

Observe for signs and symptoms of hyperkalemia (see Index), particularly in patients with renal insufficiency, in patients on high-dose or prolonged therapy, in the elderly, and in patients with diabetes. Periodic serum potassium determinations are advised.

Periodic evaluations of renal function (BUN, serum creatinine) are advised in patients with known or suspected renal insufficiency. Fatigue, insomnia, decreased mental acuity, nausea, vomiting, stomatitis, and unpleasant taste are suggestive symptoms of advancing renal insufficiency.

Patients with cirrhosis are usually hospitalized during triamterene therapy because rapid alterations in fluid and electrolyte balance can precipitate hepatic coma or precoma: irritability, restlessness, confusion, stupor, liver flap (asterixis), coma.

Periodic blood studies are advised in patients with cirrhosis (who are susceptible to hematologic abnormalities) and in patients on prolonged therapy.

Monitor blood pressure during period of dosage adjustment. Hypotensive reactions, although rare, have been reported. Implications for ambulation should be noted, particularly for elderly patients.

Instruct patient to report overpowering fatigue or weakness, malaise, fever, sore throat or mouth (possible symptoms of granulocytopenia).

Drug should be withdrawn gradually in patients on prolonged therapy, or patients who have received high doses, in order to prevent rebound kaliuresis (increased urinary excretion of potassium).

Triamterene reportedly may increase blood glucose, primarily in patients with moderate diabetes. Patient should be closely monitored.

Preserved in tight, light-resistant containers.

LABORATORY TEST INTERFERENCES: Triamterene produces a pale blue fluorescence that interferes with fluorometric assay of quinidine and lactic dehydrogenase activity.

DRUG INTERACTIONS: Concomitant use with **antihypertensive agents** may produce some additive hypotensive effect.

TRICHLORMETHIAZIDE, N.F.
(AQUAZIDE, DIURESE, METAHYDRIN, NAQUA, ROCHLORMETHIAZIDE)

Diuretic (thiazide), antihypertensive

ACTIONS AND USES

Benzothiadiazine (thiazide) derivative. Similar to chlorothiazide (qv) in actions, uses, contraindications, precautions, and adverse reactions, but with longer duration of effects.

ABSORPTION AND FATE

Onset of diuretic effect in 2 hours; peak effect in 6 hours; duration 24 hours or longer. Believed to be excreted primarily as unchanged drug in urine.

ROUTE AND DOSAGE

Oral: initially 2 to 4 mg once daily after breakfast, or twice daily; maintenance 1 to 4 mg daily. Highly individualized according to patient's requirements and response. **Pediatric:** 0.07 mg/kg/day.

NURSING IMPLICATIONS

See Chlorothiazide.

TRICLOFOS SODIUM
(TRICLOS)

Sedative, hypnotic

ACTIONS AND USES

Rapidly hydrolyzed in body to trichloroethanol, the major active metabolite of chloral hydrate (qv). Actions, uses, contraindications, precautions, and adverse reactions as for chloral hydrate; reported to produce less gastric irritation.

CONTRAINDICATIONS AND PRECAUTIONS

Allergy to triclofos or chloral hydrate; marked renal or hepatic impairment; during labor; persons under 12 years of age. Safe use during pregnancy established. Also see Chloral Hydrate.

ADVERSE REACTIONS

Nausea, vomiting, flatulence, hangover, headache, malaise, ataxia, vertigo, lightheadedness, bad taste, urticaria, nightmares, ketonuria, leukopenia, relative eosinophilia, and possibly excitement and delirium. See Chloral Hydrate.

Oral (hypnotic): 1500 mg 15 to 30 minutes before bedtime.

NURSING IMPLICATIONS

Addiction liability probably similar to that of chloral hydrate. Periodic blood
cell counts recommended during prolonged use.

See Chloral Hydrate.

TRIETHYLENETHIOPHOSPHORAMIDE, N.F.
(THIOTEPA)

Antineoplastic (alkylating agent)

ACTIONS AND USES

Nitrogen-mustard-like alkylating agent that selectively reacts with DNA phosphate groups to produce chromosome cross-linkage and consequent blocking of
nucleoprotein synthesis. A nonvesicant, highly toxic hematopoietic agent with
a high therapeutic index. Myelosuppression is cumulative and unpredictable,
and it may be delayed.

Used to produce remissions in malignant lymphomas, including Hodgkin's disease and carcinoma of breast and ovary. Also used in treatment of chronic
granulocytic and lymphocytic leukemia; used for brief responses in bronchogenic carcinoma and for management of intracavitary effusions secondary to
diffuse or localized neoplastic disease of serosal cavities.

ABSORPTION AND FATE

Parenterally administered, including direct injection into tumor. Slow onset of
action, with therapeutic response becoming increasingly evident over period of
several weeks. Slowly bound to tissues; significant amounts remain in blood for
several hours. Excreted chiefly through kidneys.

CONTRAINDICATIONS AND PRECAUTIONS

Pregnancy (drug is actively teratogenic), acute leukemia, hypersensitivity to
drug, acute infection, myelosuppression produced by radiation, other antineoplastics, bone marrow invasion by tumor cells, impaired kidney or hepatic
function.

ADVERSE REACTIONS

Less than with other nitrogen-mustard-like drugs. Anorexia, decrease in spermatogenesis and ovarian function, slowed or lessened response in heavily irradiated area, hyperuricemia, leukopenia (predisposing to infections).

ROUTE AND DOSAGE

Local: intratumor and intraserosal (pleural, pericardial, peritoneal): 45 to 60 mg
initially. Intravenous: ½ the local dose. Topical (eg, solution introduced into
urinary bladder): Dosage and route carefully individualized according to clinical
and hematologic response. Maintenance doses are no more frequent than
weekly in order to preserve correlation between dose and blood counts.

NURSING IMPLICATIONS

Refrigerate drug in powder form in tight, light-resistant container.

Reconstituted solution may be stored at 2 C to 8 C (35 F to 46 F) for 5 days
after preparation; however, it is advisable to use solution immediately and
discard unused portion.

Reconstitute solution with sterile water for injection. Usual dilution: 1.5 ml
diluent (5 mg/0.5 ml solution). Larger volumes are used for IV drip or
intracavitary or perfusion therapy.

Avoid exposure of skin and respiratory tract to particles of Thiotepa during
solution preparation.

Discuss possibility of amenorrhea with patient (reversible in 6 to 8 months).

Because of cumulative effects, maximum myelosuppression may be delayed 3 or 4 weeks after termination of therapy. Warn patient to report onset of a cold or illness, no matter how mild; medical supervision may be necessary.

Hemoglobin level and leukocyte and thrombocyte counts are determined daily for the first 7 to 10 days of treatment, weekly through maintenance dosage, and for 4 weeks after therapy is discontinued.

Monitor leukocyte and thrombocyte counts as indicators for adaptations in nursing and drug regimens.

Treatment of bladder tumor: patient is dehydrated 8 to 12 hours prior to treatment; 60 mg in 30 to 60 ml distilled water are instilled into bladder by catheter to be retained for 2 hours (if patient cannot retain 60 ml solution, 30 ml dilution is used); if desired, patient is repositioned every 15 minutes for maximal area contact. Usual course of treatment is once a week for 4 weeks; repeated beyond this with caution, since bone marrow depression may increase.

See Mechlorethamine.

DRUG INTERACTIONS: Thiotepa increases pharmacologic and toxic effects of **succinylcholine** by decreasing pseudocholinesterase levels.

TRIFLUOPERAZINE HYDROCHLORIDE, N.F., B.P. (STELAZINE)

Antipsychotic agent (major tranquilizer)

ACTIONS AND USES
Piperazine-type phenothiazine similar to chlorpromazine in most actions, uses, contraindications, precautions, and adverse reactions. Compared with chlorpromazine, produces less sedative and hypotensive effects, less potentiation of CNS depressants, and more prominent extrapyramidal effects, and has more prolonged duration of action.

Used in management of acute and chronic psychosis and in selected patients with neuroses or somatic conditions characterized by excessive anxiety, tension, and agitation.

ABSORPTION AND FATE
Rapid onset of action; effects persist for more than 12 hours. Also see Chlorpromazine.

ADVERSE REACTIONS
Nasal congestion, dry mouth, sweating, blurred vision, drowsiness, insomnia, dizziness, agitation, fatigue, weakness, skin reactions, anorexia, extrapyramidal reactions, lactation; (occasionally): agranulocytosis, leukopenia, thrombocytopenia, jaundice, lenticular opacities. Also see Chlorpromazine.

ROUTE AND DOSAGE
Adults: Oral: Outpatients: 1 or 2 mg 2 times daily. Hospitalized or closely supervised patients: 2 to 5 mg 2 times daily. Usual dosage range 15 to 20 mg daily (40 mg or more may be required for some patients). Elderly patients: one-fourth to one-half the usual dosage. Intramuscular: 1 or 2 mg every 4 to 6 hours; rarely exceeds 10 mg/24 hours. **Children** *6 to 12 years:* Oral, intramuscular: initially 1 mg 1 or 2 times daily, gradually increased until symptoms are controlled or side effects intervene; rarely necessary to exceed 15 mg daily.

NURSING IMPLICATIONS

Not to be confused with triflupromazine hydrochloride.

Dilute the oral concentration just before administration by adding to 60 ml or more of suitable diluent (eg, water, fruit juice, tomato juice, carbonated beverage, milk, tea, coffee) or semisolid food such as soups, puddings, etc.

Liquid preparation prevents hoarding of tablet by patient and also provides for more rapid absorption.

Administer IM injection deep into large muscle mass (unlike other phenothiazines, apparently causes little if any pain and irritation at injection site). Intervals between injections should be no less than 4 hours because of possible cumulative effects. Oral therapy should be substituted for IM as soon as feasible.

Hypotension and extrapyramidal effects (especially akathisia and dystonia) are most likely to occur in patients receiving high doses or parenteral administration and in the elderly. Symptoms are usually reversible with reduction in dosage or temporary discontinuation of drug.

Caution patient to avoid potentially hazardous activities such as driving a car or operating machinery, especially during first days of therapy (drowsiness and dizziness may be prominent during this time).

Increase in mental and physical activity is an expected result of therapy. Caution patients with angina to avoid overexertion and to report increase in frequency of anginal pain.

Maximum therapeutic response generally occurs within 2 to 3 weeks after initiation of therapy.

Preserved in tight, light-resistant containers. Slight yellow discoloration of injectable drug reportedly does not alter potency. If markedly discolored, discard solution.

See Chlorpromazine

TRIFLUPROMAZINE HYDROCHLORIDE, N.F. (VESPRIN)

Antipsychotic agent (major tranquilizer)

ACTIONS AND USES

Propylamino derivative of phenothiazine similar to chlorpromazine in actions, uses, contraindications, precautions, and adverse reactions. Compared with chlorpromazine, extrapyramidal and antiemetic effects are more pronounced, but hypotensive and sedative effects are somewhat less, and incidence of dry mouth and blurred vision appears to be lower.

Used in management of psychotic disorders (excluding psychotic depressive reactions), especially when hallucinations and delirium are present; used in treatment and prophylaxis of severe vomiting and as adjunct in preoperative and postoperative management.

CONTRAINDICATIONS AND PRECAUTIONS

Use in children under 2.5 years of age, IV use in children of any age.

ROUTE AND DOSAGE

Optimum dosage level determined individually for each patient. *Psychotic disorders:* **Adults:** Oral: initially 30 mg up to 150 mg maximum total daily dose; when symptoms are controlled, dosage may be reduced to maintenance level. Intramuscular: 60 mg up to 150 mg maximum daily. **Children:** Oral: 2 mg/kg up to 150 mg maximum total daily dose. Intramuscular: 0.2 to 0.25 mg/kg up to 10 mg maximum total daily dose. *Nausea and vomiting:* **Adults:** Oral: 20 mg up to maximum of 30 mg daily. Intramuscular: 5 to 15 mg as single dose, repeated every 4 hours up to maximum of 60 mg daily; for elderly or debilitated patients,

2.5 mg up to maximum of 15 mg daily. Intravenous: 1 mg up to maximum of 3 mg daily. **Children:** Oral: 0.2 mg/kg up to maximum of 10 mg divided into 3 doses. Intramuscular: 0.2 to 0.25 mg up to maximum of 10 mg daily.

NURSING IMPLICATIONS

Not to be confused with trifluoperazine hydrochloride.

Transient hypotension may occur when drug is administered parenterally. Monitor blood pressure and pulse before administration and between doses. Advise patient to remain recumbent until assured that vital signs are stable. Have on hand vasopressors, eg, levarterenol and phenylephrine. Epinephrine should not be used with phenothiazines, since further lowering of blood pressure may result.

Extrapyramidal reactions and sedation are prominent in patients receiving high doses, particularly the elderly and debilitated.

In psychotic disorders, optimum clinical improvement may not occur until after prolonged therapy.

Preserved in tight, light-resistant containers at room temperature, away from excessive heat. Parenteral solution may vary from colorless to light amber; if solution is darker than this or otherwise discolored, it should not be used.

See Chlorpromazine.

TRIHEXYPHENIDYL HYDROCHLORIDE, U.S.P.
(ANTITREM, ARTANE, HEXYPHEN, PIPANOL, TREMIN)
BENZHEXOL HYDROCHLORIDE, B.P.

Anticholinergic (antiparkinsonian)

ACTIONS AND USES

Synthetic tertiary amine anticholinergic agent with actions, contraindications, precautions, and adverse reactions similar to those of atropine (qv). Thought to act by blocking acetylcholine at certain cerebral synaptic sites. Relaxes smooth muscle by direct effect and by atropinelike blocking action on parasympathetic nervous system. Antispasmodic action appears to be one-half that of atropine, and side effects are usually less frequent and less severe.

Used in symptomatic treatment of all forms of parkinsonism (arteriosclerotic, idiopathic, postencephalitic). Also used to prevent or control drug-induced extrapyramidal disorders.

ABSORPTION AND FATE

Rapidly absorbed from GI tract, with onset of action within 1 hour. Peak effects last 2 to 3 hours; duration of action 6 to 12 hours. Metabolic fate not determined. Excreted in urine.

CONTRAINDICATIONS AND PRECAUTIONS

Hypersensitivity to trihexyphenidyl, narrow-angle glaucoma. Safe use during pregnancy and in nursing mothers and children not established. Cautious use: history of drug hypersensitivities, arteriosclerosis, hypertension; cardiac disease, renal or hepatic disorders, obstructive diseases of GI or genitourinary tracts, elderly patients with prostatic hypertrophy. Also see Atropine.

ADVERSE REACTIONS

Common: dry mouth, dizziness, blurred vision, mydriasis, photophobia, nausea, nervousness. Insomnia, constipation, drowsiness, urinary hesitancy or retention. **CNS** (usually with high doses): confusion, agitation, delirium, psychotic manifestations, euphoria. Hypersensitivity reactions, angle-closure glaucoma, suppurative parotitis secondary to mouth dryness (infrequent). Also see Atropine.

Highly individualized. Oral: initially 1 mg; increased by 2-mg increments at 3- to 5-day intervals up to 6 to 10 mg daily in 3 or more divided doses; some patients may require 12 to 15 mg daily. Sustained-release capsule (5 mg each): 1 or 2 capsules daily in single or divided doses (maximum 4 capsules daily).

NURSING IMPLICATIONS

May be taken before or after meals, depending on how patient reacts. Elderly patients and patients prone to excessive salivation (eg, postencephalitic parkinsonism) may prefer to take drug after meals. If drug causes excessive mouth dryness, it may be better taken before meals, unless it causes nausea.

Drug-induced mouth dryness may be relieved by sugarless gum or hard candy and by frequent sips of water.

Incidence and severity of side effects are usually dose-related and may be minimized by dosage reduction.

CNS stimulation (see Adverse Reactions) may occur with high doses and in patients with arteriosclerosis or history of hypersensitivity to other drugs. If severe, drug may be discontinued for a few days and then resumed at lower dosage.

If patient develops urinary hesitancy or retention, voiding before taking drug may relieve problem.

In patients with severe rigidity, tremors may appear to be accentuated during therapy as rigidity diminishes.

Gonioscopic evaluations and close monitoring of intraocular pressure at regular intervals are advised.

Caution patient not to engage in activities requiring alertness and skill, as drug causes dizziness, drowsiness, and blurred vision. Supervision of ambulation may be indicated.

Close follow-up care is advisable. Tolerance may develop, necessitating dosage adjustment or use of combination therapy, and patients over age 60 frequently develop sensitivity to trihexyphenidyl action.

Also see Atropine Sulfate for nursing implications and drug interactions.

DRUG INTERACTIONS: Trihexyphenidyl may partially inhibit the therapeutic effects of **haloperidol** and **phenothiazines** (possibly by delaying gastric emptying time and increasing metabolism in GI tract). Trihexyphenidyl may be potentiated by **MAO inhibitors.**

TRIMEPRAZINE TARTRATE, U.S.P.
(TEMARIL)

Antihistaminic, antipruritic

ACTIONS AND USES

Phenothiazine derivative similar to chlorpromazine (qv), with prominent, antipruritic activity. Also shares sedative, antihistaminic effects of chlorpromazine, but to lesser degree. In common with antihistamines, exerts some anticholinergic and antiserotonin action.

Used primarily for symptomatic relief of pruritic symptoms in a variety of dermatologic and nondermatologic conditions.

CONTRAINDICATIONS AND PRECAUTIONS

Hypersensitivity to phenothiazines; pregnancy; infants under 6 months of age; use of extended-release form in children 6 years of age and younger. Cautious use: hepatic disease, history of convulsive disorders. See Chlorpromazine.

Drowsiness, dizziness, dry mucous membranes, GI upset, allergic skin reactions, cholestatic jaundice, extrapyramidal reactions, leukopenia, agranulocytosis. In some children: paradoxic hyperactivity, irritability, insomnia, hallucinations. Acute poisoning: CNS depression with hypotension, hypothermia. Toxic potential as for other phenothiazines. See Chlorpromazine.

ROUTE AND DOSAGE

Oral (**adults**): 2.5 mg 4 times daily; (**children**): *over 3 years,* 2.5 mg at bedtime or 3 times daily, if needed; *6 months to 3 years:* 1.25 mg at bedtime or 3 times daily, if needed. Sustained-release formulation (**adults**): 5 mg every 12 hours; (**children**): *over 6 years,* 5 mg daily. Dosages highly individualized according to severity of symptoms and patient response.

NURSING IMPLICATIONS

Usually administered after each meal and at bedtime.

Incidence and severity of adverse reactions are generally dose-related; however, in some patients individual sensitivity is involved.

Caution parents not to administer more than the prescribed dose to children.

Drowsiness occurs frequently, but it generally disappears after a few days of medication. If it persists, dosage adjustment is indicated. Bedsides and supervision of ambulation may be necessary for some patients.

Warn patient to avoid activities requiring mental alertness and normal reaction time, such as operating a car or other hazardous activities, until drug response is known.

Patient should know that sedative action of trimeprazine is additive to that of alcohol, barbiturates, narcotics, analgesics, and other CNS depressants.

Toxic manifestations of phenothiazine derivatives are most likely to occur between 4 and 10 weeks of therapy.

Preserved in tight, light-resistant containers.

See Chlorpromazine Hydrochloride.

TRIMETHADIONE, U.S.P.
(TRIDIONE)
TROXIDONE, B.P.

Anticonvulsant

ACTIONS AND USES

Oxazolidinedione derivative similar to paramethadione in pharmacologic properties. Elevates seizure threshold in cortex and basal ganglia and reduces synaptic response to repetitive low-frequency impulses.

Used for control of petit mal epilepsy refractory to other drugs. May be administered concomitantly with other anticonvulsants when other forms of epilepsy coexist with petit mal.

ABSORPTION AND FATE

Rapidly and completely absorbed. Peak plasma concentrations in 30 minutes to 2 hours. Uniformly distributed in tissues, including brain. Not significantly bound to plasma proteins. Largely demethylated to active metabolite (dimethadione) by hepatic microsomal enzymes. Metabolite has plasma half-life of 6 to 13 days; slowly excreted in urine (excretion rate increases with alkalinization of urine or increased urine volume).

CONTRAINDICATIONS AND PRECAUTIONS

Hypersensitivity to oxazolidinediones, severe hepatic or renal impairment, blood dyscrasias. Safe use in women of childbearing potential and during pregnancy not established. Cautious use: diseases of retina and optic nerve.

GI: hiccups, nausea, vomiting, abdominal pain, gastric distress, anorexia, weight loss. **CNS:** hemeralopia, photophobia, diplopia, vertigo, ataxia, drowsiness, insomnia, headache, fatigue, malaise, paresthesias, irritability, personality changes. **Hematopoietic:** blood dyscrasias (leukopenia, neutropenia, thrombocytopenia, pancytopenia, agranulocytosis, aplastic anemia). **Hypersensitivity:** lymphadenopathy with splenomegaly, hepatomegaly, pruritus, morbilliform rash, exfoliative dermatitis. **Other:** bleeding gums, epistaxis, retinal and petechial hemorrhages, vaginal bleeding, systemic lupus erythematosus syndrome, myasthenia-gravis-like syndrome, changes in blood pressure, albuminuria, nephrosis, hepatitis, precipitation of grand mal seizures, hair loss (rare), acneiform dermatitis.

ROUTE AND DOSAGE

Oral: **Adults:** 300 to 600 mg 3 or 4 times daily (therapy generally started at 900 mg daily; dosage then increased by 300 mg/day at weekly intervals until seizures are controlled or toxic symptoms intervene); **children:** 300 to 900 mg in 3 or 4 equally divided doses (depending on age and weight).

NURSING IMPLICATIONS

Because of potential for toxicity, close medical supervision, especially during first year of therapy, is essential.

A transitory increase in number of petit mal episodes may occur at beginning of therapy. Instruct patient and responsible family member to keep a record of number, duration, and time of attacks. Clinical improvement usually occurs 1 to 4 weeks after start of therapy.

Visual disturbances are usually controlled by reduction in dosage. Hemeralopia (glare effect or blurring of vision in bright light) is sometimes relieved by wearing dark glasses.

Drowsiness tends to diminish with continued therapy, or it can be controlled by dosage reduction or concurrent administration of an amphetamine. Caution patient to avoid potentially hazardous activities such as driving a car or operating machinery until this side effect is controlled.

Instruct patient to report immediately to physician the onset of fever, sore throat or mouth, muscle weakness, joint pains, skin rash, swollen lymph nodes, jaundice, scotomata, hair loss, or other unusual symptoms.

Complete blood and differential counts and urinalyses are recommended at monthly intervals or more frequently if indicated. Therapy should be discontinued if neutrophil count drops to 2500/mm^3 or below or if albuminuria persists or increases.

Plasma concentrations of dimethadione, active metabolite of trimethadione, may be used as guide to dosage adjustment (usually maintained at about 700 μg/ml for effective seizure control).

Advise patient to follow prescribed regimen precisely, and stress the importance of keeping follow-up appointments.

Advise patient to wear medical identification bracelet, necklace, or card at all times.

Following prolonged use, withdrawal should be accomplished gradually to avoid precipitating petit mal status or seizures.

Preserved in tightly closed containers in a dry place at temperatures not exceeding 25 C (77 F).

(ARFONAD)

Antihypertensive (ganglionic blocking agent)

ACTIONS AND USES

Potent, short-acting nondepolarizing ganglionic blocking agent. Blocks both sympathetic and parasympathetic ganglia; also has direct peripheral vasodilation action and thus can produce marked hypotension; causes histamine release. Used to produce controlled hypotension for certain surgical procedures (eg, neurologic, ophthalmic, and plastic surgery) and for treatment of hypertensive crises associated with pulmonary edema.

ABSORPTION AND FATE

Effects appear almost immediately following IV administration and may persist 10 to 20 minutes. Metabolic fate not completely known. Approximately 20% to 40% excreted in urine.

CONTRAINDICATIONS AND PRECAUTIONS

Anemia, hypovolemia, shock, asphyxia, respiratory insufficiency. Cautious use: history of allergy; elderly and debilitated patients; children; cardiac disease; arteriosclerosis; hepatic or renal disease; degenerative CNS disease; Addison's disease; patients receiving steroids, antihypertensive agents, anesthetics (especially spinal), diuretics.

ROUTE AND DOSAGE

Intravenous infusion: 500 mg of drug in 500 ml of 5% dextrose injection (1 mg/ml); rate of administration 1 to 4 mg/minute.

NURSING IMPLICATIONS

IV flow rate is prescribed by physician to maintain desired level of hypotension.

Patient must be observed continuously while receiving infusion. Blood pressure should be checked every 2 minutes until stabilized at desired level, then every 5 minutes for duration of treatment. Pulse and respiration should also be monitored closely.

Intensity of hypotensive effect is largely dependent on positioning. If blood pressure fails to drop with patient in supine position, physician may prescribe elevation of head of bed. Caution is necessary to avoid cerebral anoxia.

Bear in mind that pupillary dilatation may not necessarily indicate anoxia or depth of anesthesia, but may represent a specific effect of the drug.

Facilities for resuscitation and maintenance of oxygenation and ventilation should be immediately available. Have on hand vasopressor drugs to counteract undesirably low blood pressure, eg, phenylephrine, mephentermine, norepinephrine (used only if other vasopressors are not effective).

Infusion should be terminated gradually while blood pressure is closely monitored.

Some patients become refractory to trimethaphan within 48 hours after initiation of therapy, as evidenced by lack of blood pressure response.

Monitor intake and output. Ganglionic blockade may reduce voiding contractions and urge to void. Check lower abdomen for bladder distension.

Infusion solution should be freshly prepared, and unused portion should be discarded.

Do not use trimethaphan infusion as a vehicle for administration of other drugs.

Trimethaphan should be refrigerated, but freezing should be avoided.

(TIGAN)

Antiemetic

ACTIONS AND USES

Structurally related to ethanolamine antihistamines, but with weaker antihistaminic activity. Has sedative effect and antiemetic action. Less effective than phenothiazine antiemetics, but produces fewer side effects. Must be used with other agents when vomiting is severe. Primary locus of action is thought to be the chemoreceptor trigger zone.

Used for control of nausea and vomiting.

ABSORPTION AND FATE

Onset of antiemetic action within 20 to 40 minutes following oral administration, with duration of 3 to 4 hours. Action begins within 15 minutes following IM injection and persists 2 to 3 hours. Approximately 30% to 50% of dose is excreted intact in urine within 48 to 72 hours.

CONTRAINDICATIONS AND PRECAUTIONS

Hypersensitivity to drug, parenteral use in children, rectal administration in prematures and newborns, known sensitivity to benzocaine (in suppository) or to similar local anesthetics. Safe use during pregnancy and lactation not established. Cautious use: patients who have recently received other centrally acting drugs (eg, barbiturates, belladonna derivatives, phenothiazines).

ADVERSE REACTIONS

Infrequent: hypersensitivity reactions (including allergic skin eruptions), extrapyramidal symptoms (including parkinsonism), hypotension, blurred vision, dizziness, drowsiness, headache, depressed mood, disorientation, diarrhea, exaggeration of nausea, acute hepatitis, jaundice, muscle cramps. Rarely: convulsions, opisthotonos, coma (Reye's syndrome); causal relationship not established. Also reported: pain, stinging, burning, redness, irritation at IM site, local irritation following rectal administration.

ROUTE AND DOSAGE

Adults: Oral: 250 mg 3 or 4 times daily. Rectal: 200 mg 3 or 4 times daily. Intramuscular: **Adults only:** 200 mg 3 or 4 times daily. **Children** *30 to 90 lb:* Oral, rectal: 100 to 200 mg 3 or 4 times daily; *under 30 lb:* Rectal (not used in prematures and newborns): 100 mg 3 or 4 times daily.

NURSING IMPLICATIONS

Restoration of body fluids and electrolytes is important adjunct to therapy.

Administer IM deep into upper outer quadrant of buttock. To minimize possibility of irritation and pain, avoid escape of solution along needle track. If allowable by agency policy, this can be accomplished by drawing a small bubble of air into syringe after drug is measured; when medication is injected, air bubble will clear needle of drug.

Hypotension is reported, particularly in surgical patients receiving drug parenterally. Monitor blood pressure.

Abrupt onset of persistent vomiting, hyperpnea, lethargy, or confused or irrational behavior should be reported immediately. These are possible early signs of Reye's syndrome, characterized by convulsions, coma, opisthotonos, and fatty changes in liver, kidneys, and other organs; most likely to occur in children and elderly and debilitated patients following a mild upper respiratory illness or influenza.

Bear in mind that antiemetic effect of drug may obscure GI diagnoses.

Advise patient to report promptly to physician the onset of rash or other signs of hypersensitivity. Drug should be discontinued immediately.

Since drug may cause drowsiness and dizziness, caution patient to avoid driving a car or other potentially hazardous activities.

(Pyribenzamine Citrate)
TRIPELENNAMINE HYDROCHLORIDE, U.S.P., B.P.
(PBZ-SR, Pyribenzamine Hydrochloride, RO-HIST)

Antihistaminic

ACTIONS AND USES
Ethylenediamine antihistamine with mild CNS depressant effects and relatively high incidence of GI side effects. Like other antihistamines, competes for histamine receptor sites on effector cells. Antagonizes histamine action that leads to increased capillary permeability, edema formation, itching, and constriction of respiratory, GI, and vascular smooth muscle. Does not inhibit gastric secretion. Also has antiemetic, antitussive, anticholinergic, and local anesthetic action. Used to relieve symptoms of various allergic conditions, to ameliorate reactions to blood or plasma, and in anaphylaxis as adjunct to epinephrine and other standard measures after acute symptoms have been controlled. Used topically for temporary relief of itching due to minor skin problems, insect bites, stings, contact dermatitis, hives, and sunburn. Also has been used to provide oral mucous membrane analgesia in young children with herpetic gingivostomatitis.

ABSORPTION AND FATE
Onset of effects within 15 to 30 minutes; duration of action about 4 to 6 hours (generally, up to 8 hours with sustained-release formulation). Appears to be detoxified by liver. Most of drug excreted in urine.

CONTRAINDICATIONS AND PRECAUTIONS
Hypersensitivity to antihistamines of similar structure; narrow-angle glaucoma; symptomatic prostatic hypertrophy; bladder neck obstruction; GI obstruction or stenosis; lower respiratory tract symptoms, including asthma; pregnancy; nursing mothers; prematures and neonates; patients receiving MAO inhibitors. Cautious use: history of asthma; convulsive disorders; increased intraocular pressure; hyperthyroidism; cardiovascular disease; hypertension; diabetes mellitus.

ADVERSE REACTIONS
GI (common): epigastric distress, anorexia, nausea, vomiting, constipation or diarrhea. Low incidence of other side effects: **CNS:** drowsiness, dizziness, tinnitus, vertigo, fatigue, disturbed coordination, tingling, heaviness, weakness of hands, tremors, euphoria, nervousness, restlessness, insomnia. **Overdosage** (especially in children): hallucinations, excitement, fever, ataxia, athetosis, convulsions, coma, cardiovascular collapse. **Atropinelike effects:** dry mouth, nose, and throat; thickened bronchial secretions; wheezing; sensation of chest tightness; blurred vision; diplopia; headache; urinary frequency, hesitancy, or retention; dysuria; palpitation; tachycardia; mild hypotension or hypertension. **Hypersensitivity:** skin rash, urticaria, photosensitization, anaphylactic shock. **Hematologic:** leukopenia, agranulocytosis, hemolytic anemia.

ROUTE AND DOSAGE
Recommended doses are based on the hydrochloride. Oral: **Adults:** 25 to 50 mg every 4 to 6 hours (as much as 600 mg daily in divided doses, if necessary). Long-acting tablet and sustained-release form: 100 mg morning and evening or every 8 to 12 hours. **Children:** 5 mg/kg/24 hours divided into 4 to 6 doses. Not to exceed 300 mg/24 hours. Long-acting tablet (**children** *over 5 years of age*): 50 mg morning and evening. All dosages highly individualized. Each 1 ml of tripelennamine citrate (elixir) is equal to 5 mg of the hydrochloride. Topical: 2% cream or ointment applied gently to affected area 3 or 4 times daily.

NURSING IMPLICATIONS

In patients receiving antihistamines for allergic manifestations, a careful history should be taken that includes change from usual pattern of recently ingested foods and drugs, as well as social or emotional stress.

Urinary hesitancy can be reduced if patient voids just before taking drug. GI side effects may be lessened by administration of drug after meals.

Note that tripelennamine in long-acting tablet form (50 mg) may be prescribed for children over 5 years of age, but sustained-release formulation (100 mg) is not intended for use in children of any age.

Mild to moderate drowsiness, blurred vision, and dizziness occur in some patients. Caution against operating motor vehicle or engaging in hazardous activities until drug response has been determined.

Dizziness, sedation, and hypotension are more likely to occur in the elderly.

Patient should know that antihistamines have additive effects with one another and with alcohol and other CNS depressants. Caution patient not to take OTC preparations without consulting physician.

Prolonged use of topical preparations is not recommended, since irritation or sensitization may occur. Avoid contact with eyes.

Patients receiving long-term therapy with antihistamines should have periodic blood cell counts.

Antihistamines should be discontinued prior to skin testing procedure for allergy, since they may obscure otherwise positive reactions.

Caution patient to store antihistamines out of reach of children. Fatalities have been reported.

Preserved in tight, light-resistant containers.

DRUG INTERACTIONS: **MAO inhibitors** prolong and intensify anticholinergic (drying) effect of antihistamines. Mutual potentiation of CNS depression may occur with concurrent administration of an antihistamine and **alcohol, antianxiety agents, barbiturates, hypnotics, sedatives, tranquilizers,** or **other CNS depressants.** There is the theoretical possibility that antihistamines may decrease the effects of **propranolol** (by preventing β-adrenergic blocking action) and may increase its quinidinelike effect (myocardial depression).

TRIPROLIDINE HYDROCHLORIDE, N.F., B.P. (ACTIDIL)

Antihistaminic

ACTIONS AND USES

Long-acting, potent propylamine (alkylamine) antihistaminic, similar to chlorpheniramine (qv) in actions, uses, contraindications, precautions, and adverse reactions. Has rapid onset of action, with maximum effect in about 3.5 hours and duration up to 12 hours. Reported to entail low incidence of drowsiness and other side effects.

ROUTE AND DOSAGE

Oral: **Adults:** 2.5 mg 2 or 3 times daily; **children** *over 2 years of age:* 1.25 mg 2 or 3 times daily; *infants:* 0.6 mg 2 or 3 times daily.

NURSING IMPLICATIONS

The product Actifed combines the antihistaminic action of triprolidine and the decongestant effect of pseudoephedrine.

Preserved in tight, light-resistant containers.

See Chlorpheniramine Maleate.

TROLEANDOMYCIN, N.F.
(CYCLAMYCIN, TAO, TRIACETYLOLEANDOMYCIN)

Antibacterial

ACTIONS AND USES

Derivative of oleandomycin, a macrolide antibiotic prepared from cultures of *Streptomyces antibioticus.* Chemically related to streptomycin, and has similar range of antibacterial activity, but reportedly less effective and has higher potential for toxicity. Cross-sensitivity with erythromycin reported.

Used in treatment of acute, severe infections of upper respiratory tract caused by susceptible strains of pneumococci and α- and β-hemolytic streptococci.

ABSORPTION AND FATE

Readily absorbed from GI tract. Peak serum concentrations in 2 to 3 hours; still detectable in serum after 12 hours. Well distributed throughout body fluids, including cerebrospinal fluid. Metabolized in liver. Excreted in bile and urine.

CONTRAINDICATIONS AND PRECAUTIONS

Hypersensitivity to drug, use for prophylaxis or for minor infections. Safe use during pregnancy not established. Cautious use: impaired hepatic function.

ADVERSE REACTIONS

Abdominal cramps (frequent), nausea, vomiting, diarrhea, allergic reactions (urticaria, skin rash, anaphylaxis), cholestatic jaundice, superinfections.

ROUTE AND DOSAGE

Oral **(adults):** 250 to 500 mg every 6 hours; **(children):** 6.6 to 11 mg/kg every 6 hours.

NURSING IMPLICATIONS

Periodic liver function tests are advised in patients receiving drug longer than 10 days or in repeated courses. Some patients develop an allergic type of hepatitis with right upper quadrant pain, fever, nausea, vomiting, jaundice, eosinophilia, and leukocytosis. Liver changes are reversible if drug is discontinued immediately.

Generally, drug therapy does not exceed 10 days. For streptococcal infections, therapy should continue for 10 days to prevent development of rheumatic fever or glomerulonephritis.

Superinfections are most likely to occur in patients on prolonged or repeated therapy. Drug should be discontinued if infection develops, and appropriate therapy should be started.

LABORATORY TEST INTERFERENCES: Troleandomycin may cause false elevations of urinary 17-ketosteroids (Drekter), and 17-hydroxycorticosteroids (Porter-Silver method).

DRUG INTERACTIONS: Possibility that concomitant use with **ergotamine-containing drugs** may induce ischemic reaction.

(MYDRIACYL)

Anticholinergic (ophthalmic)

ACTIONS AND USES
  Derivative of tropic acid, with pharmacologic properties similar to those of atropine (qv). Mydriatic and cycloplegic effects occur more rapidly and are less prolonged than with atropine. Used to induce mydriasis and cycloplegia for ophthalmologic diagnostic procedures.
ABSORPTION AND FATE
  Maximal mydriatic and cycloplegic effects occur in 20 to 25 minutes and are maintained for 15 to 20 minutes; full recovery in 2 to 6 hours.
CONTRAINDICATIONS AND PRECAUTIONS
  Hypersensitivity to drug, known or suspected glaucoma.
ADVERSE REACTIONS
  Transient stinging, photophobia, blurred vision.
ROUTE AND DOSAGE
  Ophthalmic (for refraction): 1 or 2 drops of 1% solution in eye, repeated in 5 minutes; if patient is not seen within 20 to 30 minutes an additional drop may be instilled to prolong mydriatic effect; (examination of fundus): 1 or 2 drops of 0.5% solution 15 to 20 minutes prior to examination.

NURSING IMPLICATIONS
Forewarn patient that transient stinging may occur on instillation.
Possibility of systemic absorption may be minimized by applying pressure against lacrimal sac during and for 1 or 2 minutes following instillation.
Photophobia may disappear as early as 2 hours after application; if troublesome, advise patient to wear dark glasses.
Caution patient to avoid potentially hazardous activities such as driving a car if vision is blurred.

TUAMINOHEPTANE SULFATE, N.F.
(TUAMINE SULFATE)

Adrenergic

ACTIONS AND USES
  Indirect-acting sympathomimetic agent with marked α-adrenergic vasoconstrictor effects. Lacks central stimulant action of ephedrine (qv).
  Used in treatment of nasal congestion associated with infections and allergic rhinitis or sinusitis.
CONTRAINDICATIONS AND PRECAUTIONS
  Cautious use: cardiovascular disease, hypertension, arteriosclerosis.
ADVERSE REACTIONS
  Rebound congestion, rhinitis (frequent or prolonged use). Overdosage: increase in blood pressure, tachycardia, mydriasis, intestinal spasm.
ROUTE AND DOSAGE
  Not to be used for more than 4 or 5 times daily or for periods longer than 3 or 4 consecutive days. Instillations may be made at 3- to 4-hour intervals. Available as 1% solution and inhaler (325 mg). **Adults:** 4 or 5 drops in each nostril. **Children** *1 to 6 years:* 2 or 3 drops in each nostril. **Infants** *under 1 year:* 1 or 2 drops in each nostril.

NURSING IMPLICATIONS
Advise patient not to exceed prescribed dosage.
Tuaminoheptane is a volatile drug. Close container tightly after use.
See Ephedrine.

TUBOCURARINE CHLORIDE, U.S.P., B.P.
(TUBADIL, TUBARINE, D-TUBOCURARINE)

Skeletal-muscle relaxant

ACTIONS AND USES
Curare alkaloid, nondepolarizing neuromuscular blocking agent extracted from the plant *Chondodendron tomentosum.* Produces skeletal-muscle relaxation or paralysis by competing with acetylcholine at cholinergic receptor sites on skeletal-muscle endplate, and thus blocks nerve impulse transmission. Also has histamine-releasing and ganglionic blocking properties. Has no known effect on intellectual functions, consciousness, or pain threshold.
Used to induce skeletal-muscle relaxation as adjunct to general anesthesia, to facilitate management of mechanical ventilation, to reduce intensity of muscle contractions in tetanus and in pharmacologically or electrically induced convulsions, to treat spastic states in children, and for diagnosis of myasthenia gravis when conventional tests have been inconclusive.

ABSORPTION AND FATE
Following IV injection, muscle relaxation begins within seconds. Maximal effects in 2 to 3 minutes; effects usually last 25 to 90 minutes. IM injection is slowly and irregularly absorbed; action time unpredictable. Appreciably bound to plasma proteins. Minimally degraded in liver and kidney. Approximately 35% to 75% excreted unchanged in urine within 24 hours; about 10% excreted in bile. Crosses placenta.

CONTRAINDICATIONS AND PRECAUTIONS
Hypersensitivity to curare preparations; when histamine release is a hazard; hyperthermia; electrolyte imbalance; acidosis; neuromuscular disease; renal disease. Safe use in women of childbearing potential or during pregnancy not established. Cautious use: impaired cardiovascular, renal, hepatic, pulmonary, or endocrine function; hypotension; carcinomatosis; thyroid disorders; collagen diseases; porphyria; familial periodic paralysis; history of allergies; myasthenia gravis; elderly or debilitated patients.

ADVERSE REACTIONS
Slight dizziness, feeling of warmth, profound and prolonged muscle weakness and flaccidity, respiratory depression, hypoxia, apnea, increased bronchial and salivary secretions, bronchospasm, decreased GI motility, hypotension, circulatory collapse, malignant hyperthermia, hypersensitivity reactions.

ROUTE AND DOSAGE
Intravenous, intramuscular (adjunct to general anesthesia): 0.1 to 0.3 mg/kg body weight; (electroshock therapy): 0.1 to 0.2 mg/kg; (diagnosis of myasthenia gravis): 4.1 to 33 μg/kg (varies with manufacturer).

NURSING IMPLICATIONS
Primarily administered by anesthesiologist or under his direct observation.
Baseline tests of renal function and determinations of serum electrolytes are generally done before drug administration. Electrolyte imbalance (particularly potassium and magnesium) can potentiate the effects of nondepolarizing neuromuscular blocking agents.
Preparations should be made in advance for endotracheal intubation, suc-

tion, or assisted or controlled respiration with oxygen administration. Have on hand atropine and antagonists neostigmine or edrophonium (cholinesterase inhibitors). A nerve stimulator may be used to assess nature and degree of neuromuscular blockade.

Selective muscle paralysis following drug administration occurs in the following sequence: jaw muscles, levator eyelid muscles and other muscles of head and neck, limbs, intercostals and diaphragm, abdomen, trunk. Facial and diaphragm muscles are first to recover, followed in order by legs, arms, shoulder girdle, trunk, larynx, hands, feet, pharynx. Muscle function is usually restored within 90 minutes.

Monitor vital signs and airway until assured of patient's recovery from drug effects. Ganglionic blockade (hypotension) and histamine liberation (increased salivation, bronchospasm) are known effects of tubocurarine.

Tubocurarine is retained in the body long after effects of neuromuscular blockade appear to have dissipated. Observe for and report residual muscle weakness.

Patient may find oral communication difficult until muscles of head and neck recover.

Measure and record intake–output ratio during day of drug administration. Renal dysfunction will prolong drug action. Peristaltic action may be suppressed.

Test for myasthenia gravis is considered positive if muscle weakness is exaggerated.

Solutions of drug should not be used if more than faintly discolored.

DRUG INTERACTIONS: Drugs that may potentiate or prolong neuromuscular blocking action of curariform skeletal-muscle relaxants: **certain inhalation anesthetics** (cyclopropane, ether, halothane, methoxyflurane); **certain antibiotics** (aminoglycosides, ie, gentamicin, kanamycin, neomycin, streptomycin; amphotericin B; bacitracin; clindamycin; colistin; lincomycin; polymyxins; tetracyclines; viomycin); **diazepam; potassium-depleting diuretics** (eg, furosemide, thiazides); **magnesium salts; methotrimeprazine; narcotic analgesics; phenothiazines; procainamide; propranolol; quinidine.**

TYBAMATE, N.F.
(SOLACEN, TYBATRAN)

Tranquilizer (minor)

ACTIONS AND USES

Propanediol carbamate chemically and structurally related to meprobamate (qv). Reportedly produces less marked sedation than meprobamate and is associated with fewer adverse effects.

Used for symptomatic treatment of psychoneurotic anxiety and tension states and for controlling agitation in the elderly. Has been used as adjunctive therapy in some psychotic states.

ABSORPTION AND FATE

Readily absorbed from GI tract. Peak blood levels in 1 to 2 hours, persisting 4 to 6 hours. Half-life 4 to 4.5 hours. Metabolized in liver; excreted in urine, mainly as hydroxylated compounds.

CONTRAINDICATIONS AND PRECAUTIONS

History of convulsive disorders, drug allergies, blood dyscrasias, lactating patients. Safe use in children under 6 years of age not established. Cautious use: hepatic or renal dysfunction.

CNS: drowsiness, dizziness, fatigue, weakness, ataxia, depressive or panic reactions, paradoxic irritability, excitement, confusion, euphoria, feeling of unreality, insomnia, headache, paresthesias, petit mal and grand mal seizures (with large doses or when given concurrently with other psychotherapeutic agents). **GI:** nausea, anorexia, dry mouth, glossitis. **Allergic or idiosyncratic:** urticaria, pruritus, rash. **Cardiovascular:** flushing, lightheadedness, hypotension, palpitation, tachycardia, syncope. **Other:** blurred vision, pruritus ani. Blood dyscrasias not reported, but possible. See Meprobamate.

ROUTE AND DOSAGE

Oral: **Adults:** 250 to 500 mg 3 or 4 times daily, or 350 mg 3 times daily and 700 mg at bedtime; not to exceed 3 Gm/24 hours. **Children** *6 to 12 years:* 20 to 35 mg/kg in 3 or 4 equally divided doses.

NURSING IMPLICATIONS

Dryness of mouth may be relieved by frequent sips of water (if allowed) and sugarless gum or hard candy. Overuse of mouthwashes should be avoided, since they may produce change in oral flora.

Elderly and debilitated patients are particularly likely to manifest drowsiness, dizziness, and confusion. If symptoms persist, dosage reduction is indicated.

Since drug may cause drowsiness and dizziness, caution patient to avoid potentially hazardous tasks such as driving a car or operating machinery.

Inform patient that alcohol may potentiate drug action and therefore should be avoided.

Drug should be discontinued if signs of allergy or idiosyncratic reactions occur.

Regularly scheduled blood counts and renal and liver function tests are recommended in patients receiving high doses or prolonged therapy.

Possibility of psychic dependence should be borne in mind.

See Meprobamate for nursing implications and drug interactions.

U–Z

URACIL MUSTARD

Antineoplastic

ACTIONS AND USES

Nitrogen mustard alkylating agent thought to react selectively with phosphate groups of DNA causing chromosomal cross-linkage and interference with normal mitosis. Cytotoxic with a low therapeutic index. Has cumulative hematopoietic depressive properties at therapeutic dosage levels, with maximum bone marrow depression occurring 2 to 4 weeks after uracil termination. Primary use is in palliative treatment of neoplasms of hematopoietic and reticuloendothelial tissues. May be beneficial as adjunct to therapy of ovary or lung carcinoma.

ABSORPTION AND FATE

Well absorbed from GI tract. Plasma concentrations decrease rapidly, with no evidence after 2 hours; less than 1% recovered unchanged in urine.

CONTRAINDICATIONS AND PRECAUTIONS

Severe leukopenia, thrombocytopenia, aplastic anemia, pregnancy. See Mechlorethamine.

ADVERSE REACTIONS

Dose-related: bone marrow depression (sometimes irreversible), anorexia, epigastric distress, nausea, vomiting, diarrhea, oral ulcerations. Pruritus, dermatitis, partial alopecia (rare), pigmentation, irritability, nervousness, mental cloudiness, depression (rare).

ROUTE AND DOSAGE

Dose and schedule highly individualized. Oral: 1 or 2 mg daily for at least 3 months (unless clinical improvement or bone marrow depression occurs before that time); maintenance 1 mg daily for 3 out of 4 weeks until optimum response or relapse occurs. Alternatively, 3 to 5 mg for 7 days (total dose during this period not to exceed 0.5 mg/kg, followed by 1 mg daily).

NURSING IMPLICATIONS

Usually administered at bedtime to alleviate GI side effects.

Severe nausea and vomiting may require discontinuation of drug.

In some patients, drug appears to act slowly, and response may not be apparent for 2 to 3 months after drug therapy is initiated.

Frank alopecia is not a usual side effect as with other nitrogen mustards.

As total cumulative dose of uracil approaches 1 mg/kg body weight, irreversible bone marrow damage may occur.

Depression of platelets is apt to be more serious than that of leukocytes; watch carefully for beginning signs of bleeding into skin and mucosa. Report immediately.

Complete blood counts, including platelets, are advised 1 or 2 times weekly during and at least 1 month after end of therapy (maximum bone marrow depression may not occur until 2 to 4 weeks after discontinuation of therapy).

Unlike mechlorethamine (nitrogen mustard), uracil mustard is not a vesicant.

See Mechlorethamine.

(Carbamide, UREAPHIL, UREVERT, AQUACARE, CARMOL,
NUTRAPLUS, REA-LO, ULTRA-MIDE)

Diuretic (osmotic), topical keratolytic agent

ACTIONS AND USES

Diamide salt of carbonic acid. When present in high concentrations in blood,
induces diuresis by elevating osmotic pressure of glomerular filtrate, with subsequent decrease in sodium and water reabsorption and promotion of chloride
and (to a lesser extent) potassium excretion. Increased blood toxicity results in
transudation of fluid from tissue, including brain, cerebrospinal, and intraocular
fluid, into the blood.

Used to reduce or prevent intracranial pressure (cerebral edema) and intraocular
pressure and to prevent acute renal failure during prolonged surgery or trauma.
Topical preparation used to promote hydration and removal of excess keratin
in dry skin and hyperkeratotic conditions.

ABSORPTION AND FATE

Following IV administration, maximum reductions of intraocular and intracranial pressures occur in 1 or 2 hours and may persist 3 to 10 hours; diuretic
effect in 6 to 12 hours. Distributed in extracellular and intracellular fluids.
Excreted in urine essentially unchanged.

CONTRAINDICATIONS AND PRECAUTIONS

Severely impaired renal or hepatic function; congestive heart failure; active
intracranial bleeding; marked dehydration; IV injection into lower extremeties,
especially in elderly patients. Extreme caution if used at all during pregnancy
or lactation or in women of childbearing potential.

ADVERSE REACTIONS

Nausea, vomiting, somnolence (prolonged use in patients with renal dysfunction), headache, acute psychosis, confusion, disorientation, nervousness, fluid
and electrolyte imbalance, dehydration, hyperthermia, tachycardia, hypotension, syncope, intraocular hemorrhage (rapid IV in patients with glaucoma),
pain, irritation, sloughing, venous thrombosis, phlebitis at injection site (infrequent).

ROUTE AND DOSAGE

Intravenous infusion: **Adults** (30% solution): 1 to 1.5 Gm/kg body weight over
1 to 2.5 hours; maximum dose 120 Gm in 24 hours; rate not to exceed 4 ml (60
drops) per minute. **Children:** 0.5 to 1.5 Gm/kg; *up to 2 years of age,* 0.1 Gm/kg.
Topical cream, lotion: 2% to 25%.

NURSING IMPLICATIONS

Solution should be freshly prepared for each patient; discard unused portion.
May be reconstituted with 5% or 10% dextrose in water or 10% invert
sugar in water.

Reconstituted solution should be used within a few hours if stored at room
temperature. If refrigerated at 2 C to 8 C, solution should be used within
48 hours; prolonged storage leads to ammonia formation.

Infusion flow rate will be prescribed by physician. Rapid administration may
be associated with increased capillary bleeding and hemolysis.

Extreme care must be taken to avoid extravasation; thrombosis and tissue
necrosis can occur. Inspect injection sites for signs of inflammation: swelling, heat, arrested motion, redness, pain.

Dosage is individualized on basis of water and electrolyte balance, urinary
volume, clinical signs.

Determinations of serum and urinary sodium should be performed every 12
hours. Frequent BUN and kidney function studies are advised, particularly in patients suspected of having renal dysfunction.

Be alert for signs of hyponatremia, hypokalemia, dehydration, or transient overhydration.

Monitor vital signs and mental status; promptly report any changes.

Observe postoperative patients closely for signs of hemorrhage. Urea reportedly may increase prothrombin time.

Monitor intake and output. If diuresis does not occur within 6 to 12 hours following administration, or if BUN exceeds 75 mg/dl, drug should be withheld until renal function is evaluated.

Urea should not be administered by same IV set through which blood is being infused.

Comatose patients receiving urea should have an indwelling catheter to insure satisfactory bladder emptying.

Also see Mannitol. Urea may decrease effects of lithium.

VANCOMYCIN HYDROCHLORIDE, U.S.P., B.P.
(VANCOCIN HYDROCHLORIDE)

Antibacterial

ACTIONS AND USES

Glucopeptide antibiotic prepared from *Streptomyces orientalis,* with bactericidal and bacteriostatic actions. Active against many Gram-negative organisms, including group A β-hemolytic streptococci, staphylococci, pneumococci, enterococci, clostridia, and corynebacteria. Gram-negative organisms, mycobacteria, and fungi are highly resistant. Cross-resistance with other antibiotics, or resistance to vancomycin has not been reported.

Used parenterally for potentially life-threatening infections in patients allergic, nonsensitive, or resistant to other less toxic antimicrobial drugs. Used orally only in treatment of staphylococcal enterocolitis (not effective by oral route for treatment of systemic infections).

ABSORPTION AND FATE

Poorly absorbed from GI tract. Serum levels of 25 mg/ml achieved in 2 hours following IV injection of 1 Gm. Diffuses into pleural, ascitic, pericardial, and synovial fluids; does not readily penetrate cerebrospinal fluid. About 10% bound to plasma proteins. Half-life about 6 hours (longer in patients with impaired renal function). About 80% to 90% of IV dose excreted in urine within 24 hours. Oral dose eliminated primarily in urine. Readily crosses placenta.

CONTRAINDICATIONS AND PRECAUTIONS

History of hypersensitivity to vancomycin, impaired renal function, hearing loss, concurrent or sequential use of other ototoxic or nephrotoxic agents. Safe use during pregnancy not established. Cautious use: neonates.

ADVERSE REACTIONS

Ototoxicity (auditory portion of eighth cranial nerve), nephrotoxicity leading to uremia, hypersensitivity reactions, chills, fever, skin rash, urticaria, shocklike state, transient leukopenia, eosinophilia, anaphylactoid reaction, vascular collapse, superinfections, severe pain, thrombophlebitis at injection site, nausea, warmth, and generalized tingling following rapid IV infusion.

ROUTE AND DOSAGE

Oral, intravenous: **Adults:** 500 mg every 6 hours or 1 Gm every 12 hours. **Children:** 44 mg/kg body weight in divided doses.

NURSING IMPLICATIONS

For oral administration, contents of vial (500 mg) may be diluted in 30 ml of water. It may also be administered at this dilution via nasogastric tube.

Extravasation of IV infusion must be avoided; severe irritation and necrosis can result.

Periodic urinalyses, renal and hepatic function tests, and hematologic studies are advised in all patients.

Serial tests of vancomycin blood levels are recommended in patients with borderline renal function and in patients over age 60 (generally maintained at 10 to 20 mg/ml).

Vancomycin may cause damage to auditory branch (not vestibular branch) of eighth cranial nerve, with consequent deafness, which may be permanent. Elderly patients and patients receiving large doses or prolonged treatment are most susceptible. Tinnitus often precedes hearing loss and therefore is an indication to stop drug immediately. Deafness may progress even after drug is discontinued.

Monitor intake and output; report changes in intake–output ratio. Oliguria or cloudy or pink urine is a possible sign of nephrotoxicity (also manifested by transient elevations in BUN, albumin, and hyaline and granular casts in urine).

Following reconstitution, commercially available oral preparation is stable for 2 weeks in refrigerator. For IV solutions, manufacturer recommends refrigerator storage for 96 hours only.

DRUG INTERACTIONS: Possibility of additive toxicity with other ototoxic and/or nephrotoxic drugs (eg, **aminoglycoside antibiotics, cephaloridine, colistin, polymyxin B, viomycin**).

VASOPRESSIN INJECTION, U.S.P., B.P.
(PITRESSIN)
VASOPRESSIN TANNATE
(PITRESSIN TANNATE)

Hormone (antidiuretic)

ACTIONS AND USES

Polypeptide hormone extracted from animal posterior pituitaries. Contains pressor and antidiuretic (ADH) principles, but is relatively free of oxytocic properties. Produces concentrated urine by increasing tubular reabsorption of water (ADH activity), thus preserving up to 90% water. May increase Na and decrease K reabsorption, but plays no causative role in edema formation. In doses greater than those required for ADH effects, directly stimulates smooth-muscle contraction (especially in small arterioles and capillaries), thereby decreasing blood flow to splanchnic, coronary, GI, pancreatic, skin, and muscular systems. May precipitate myocardial infarction, decrease heart rate and cardiac output, and increase pulmonary arterial pressure and blood pressure. Pressor effects on GI system promote increased peristalsis (especially in large bowel), increased GI sphincter pressure, and decreased gastric secretion without effect on gastric acid concentration. Also contracts smooth muscle of gallbladder and urinary bladder; in large doses may stimulate uterine contraction. Causes release of growth hormone, FSH, and corticotropin. The tannate (in peanut oil) is preferred for chronic therapy; intranasal aqueous vasopressin is effective for daily maintenance of mild diabetes insipidus.

Used to treat diabetes insipidus, to dispel gas shadows in abdominal roentgenography, and as prevention and treatment of postoperative abdominal distension. Also given to treat transient polyuria due to ADH deficiency, and used investigationally as emergency and adjunct pressor agent in the control of massive GI hemorrhage.

ABSORPTION AND FATE

Following IM or subcutaneous injection of aqueous preparation, antidiuretic activity maintained 1 to 8 hours. Absorption of IM tannate is cumulative and cannot be determined for days; average duration of action 48 to 96 hours. Distributed throughout extracellular fluid, with little evidence of plasma protein binding; plasma half-life 10 to 20 minutes. Most of drug is destroyed in liver and kidneys. Approximately 5% of subcutaneous dose of aqueous vasopressin is excreted unchanged after 4 hours.

CONTRAINDICATIONS AND PRECAUTIONS

Intravenous injection, chronic nephritis accompanied by nitrogen retention, coronary artery disease, advanced arteriosclerosis, during first stage of labor. Cautious use: epilepsy, migraine, asthma, heart failure, any state in which rapid addition to extracellular fluid may be hazardous, vascular disease, angina pectoris, preoperative and postoperative polyuric patients, renal disease, goiter with cardiac complications, elderly patients, children, pregnancy.

ADVERSE REACTIONS

Infrequent with low doses. Hypersensitivity reactions, urticaria, anaphylaxis, tremor, sweating, vertigo, edema, circumoral and facial pallor, pounding in head, eructations, passage of gas, nausea, vomiting, bronchial constriction, anginal pain, cardiac arrest, uterine cramps, water intoxication (drowsiness, listlessness, headache, confusion, anuria, weight gain), elevated plasma cortisol levels. Large doses: blanching of skin, abdominal cramps, nausea (almost spontaneously reversible), hypertension, bradycardia, minor arrhythmias, premature atrial contraction, heart block, peripheral vascular collapse, coronary insufficiency, myocardial infarction. Nasal spray: nasal congestion, rhinorrhea, irritation, ulceration and pruritus of mucosa, headache, conjunctivitis, heartburn secondary to excessive use, postnasal drip, abdominal cramps, increased bowel movements.

ROUTE AND DOSAGE

Vasopressin, aqueous (20 pressor units/ml): subcutaneous, intramuscular, topical. Vasopressin tannate (5 pressor units/ml): intramuscular. Abdominal distention (aqueous) IM or SC: initially 5 U; increase if necessary to 10 U given at 3- to 4-hour intervals as required. Diabetes insipidus: (aqueous) IM or SC: 5 to 10 U 2 or 3 times daily as necessary; (tannate) IM: 1.5 to 5 U, repeated as necessary. Topical (intranasal): on cotton pledgets, by nasal spray or by dropper; individualized dosage and times daily. Pediatric doses proportionately less and individualized.

NURSING IMPLICATIONS

Refrigeration should preserve potency of drug for at least 2 years.

Vasopressin tannate should never be administered IV. Before withdrawal of drug for IM administration, shake ampul thoroughly to assure uniform suspension.

Warm the ampul of vasopressin tannate to body temperature and shake vigorously to disperse active principle before administration.

The tannate injection is often painful, and allergic reactions may develop.

The tannate is preferred for use in children and in patients with severe diabetes insipidus.

Administration of 1 or 2 glasses of water with a large dose of vasopressin tannate may reduce side effects.

Infants and children are more susceptible to volume disturbances (such as sudden reversal of polyuria) than are adults.

The use of vasopressin to stimulate peristalsis is being replaced largely by cholinergic drugs.

Following vasopressin injection given to relieve abdominal distension, a lubricated rectal tube (prescribed by physician) is inserted just past rectal sphincter and kept in place for about 1 hour. Auscultate abdomen at frequent intervals for peristaltic sounds. Record decrease in distension. Question patient about passage of flatus and return of normal pattern of bowel movements.

Some roentgenologists advise giving an enema before the first dose of vasopressin being used to clear abdomen of gas for x-rays.

Polyuria and thirst of diabetes insipidus are usually controlled for 36 to 48 hours with a single dose of the tannate.

At beginning of therapy, establish baseline data of blood pressure, weight, intake–output pattern and ratio. Monitor both blood pressure and weight throughout therapy. Report sudden changes in pattern to physician.

Patient with vascular disease and diabetes insipidus may receive small doses of vasopressin. He should be prepared for possibility of anginal attack and should have available a coronary vasodilator (eg, nitroglycerin). Such pain should be reported to the physician.

Be alert to the fact that even small doses of vasopressin may precipitate myocardial infarction or coronary insufficiency, especially in elderly patients.

Dose used to stimulate diuresis has little effect on blood pressure.

Check patient's alertness and orientation frequently during therapy. Lethargy and confusion associated with headache may signal onset of water intoxication. Although insidious in rate of development, symptoms can lead to convulsions and terminal coma.

If water intoxication occurs, vasopressin is withdrawn and fluid intake is restricted until specific gravity is at least 1.015 and polyuria occurs. With severe overhydration, osmotic diuresis is effected by drug therapy (eg, mannitol, alone or in conjunction with furosemide).

Urine output and osmolality and serum osmolality and specific gravity are monitored while patient is hospitalized. At home, patient must measure and record data related to polydipsia and polyuria. Teach him how to determine specific gravity and how to keep an accurate record of output. He should understand that intense thirst should diminish with treatment and undisturbed normal sleep should be restored.

Patient should avoid intake of hypertonic fluids (such as undiluted syrups), since these increase urine volume (increased sodium load).

Vasopressin test to determine functional ability of kidney to concentrate urine: give vasopressin 5 to 10 U intramuscularly; measure specific gravity 1 and 2 hours later (results are equivalent to that resulting from 18 hours of water deprivation). Normal response: urine osmolality 600 mOsm/kg or greater; specific gravity greater than 1.020. In diabetes-insipidus-like syndromes, urine remains hyposmotic relative to plasma.

DRUG INTERACTIONS: **Ganglionic blocking agents** cause increased sensitivity to pressor effects of vasopressin; **lithium,** large doses of **heparin, alcohol, demeclocycline,** and **epinephrine** block antidiuretic activity; **chlorpropamide, urea,** and **fludrocortisone** potentiate antidiuretic response to vasopressin; **cyclophosphamide** decreases and **acetaminophen** increases antidiuretic effects.

(VELBAN, VINCALEUKOBLASTINE SULFATE, VLB)

Antineoplastic

ACTIONS AND USES

Cell-cycle-specific vinca alkaloid; extracted from periwinkle plant *Vinca rosea.* Arrests mitosis in metaphase by combination with microtubular proteins; may also interfere with other microtubular functions such as phagocytosis and cell mobility. In contrast to vincristine, has potent myelosuppressive and immunosuppressive properties, but produces less neurotoxicity. Spectrum of activity not completely established. One member of the ABVD combination chemotherapeutic regimen.

Principal use is for palliative treatment of generalized Hodgkin's disease and other lymphomas, choriocarcinoma, and other malignancies resistant to other chemotherapy. Used singly or in combination with other chemotherapeutic drugs.

ABSORPTION AND FATE

Following IV administration, rapidly clears bloodstream; concentrates in liver. Poor penetration of blood–brain barrier. Excreted in bile to feces; less than 5% of dose excreted in urine.

CONTRAINDICATIONS AND PRECAUTIONS

Leukopenia, bacterial infection, pregnancy, men and women of childbearing potential, elderly patients with cachexia or skin ulcers. Cautious use: malignant cell infiltration of bone marrow, obstructive jaundice.

ADVERSE REACTIONS

Generally dose-related. **Hematologic:** leukopenia (most common), agranulocytosis, thrombocytopenia and anemia (infrequent). **GI:** stomatitis, pharyngitis, anorexia, nausea, vomiting, diarrhea, ileus, constipation, rectal bleeding, hemorrhagic enterocolitis, bleeding of old peptic ulcer. **Dermatologic:** alopecia (reversible), mouth and skin vesiculation. **Neurologic:** mental depression, neuritis, numbness and paresthesias of tongue and extremities, loss of deep tendon reflexes, headache, convulsions, psychoses (rare), odd behavior patterns, CNS damage (overdosage). **Other:** phlebitis, cellulitis (at injection site), fever, weight loss, muscular pains, weakness, urinary retention, parotid gland pain and tenderness, tumor site pain, aspermia.

ROUTE AND DOSAGE

Intravenous: 0.1 mg/kg body weight once every 7 days, with increments of 0.05 mg/kg up to no more than 0.5 mg/kg body weight. Individualized on basis of oncolytic activity and hematologic response. Maintenance dose is 0.05 mg/kg less than any dose that produces leukopenia (3000/mm^3) administered once every 7 to 14 days (usually 0.15 to 0.2 mg/kg). To prepare solution: add 10 ml sodium chloride injection (preserved with phenol or benzyl alcohol) to 10 mg of drug (yields 1 mg/ml). Other solutions not recommended.

NURSING IMPLICATIONS

Drug is usually injected into tubing of running infusion over period of 1 minute. If given directly into vein, fresh, dry needle is used (discard needle used to withdraw drug). To ensure no spillage into extravascular tissue, needle and syringe should be rinsed with venous blood before withdrawal from vein.

If extravasation occurs, stop infusion; applications of moderate heat and local injection of hyaluronidase are advised to help disperse extravasated drug. Infusion should be restarted in another vein. Observe injection site; sloughing may occur.

Avoid contact with eyes. Severe irritation and corneal ulcer may occur.

Copious amounts of water should be applied immediately and thoroughly.

Course of therapy may be continued 12 weeks or more for adequate clinical trail. Encourage community-based patient to keep all appointments.

Temporary mental depression sometimes occurs on second or third day after treatment begins.

Instruct patient to avoid exposure to infection, injury to skin or mucous membranes, and excessive physical stress.

For all dose levels, drug is not administered until WBC nadir (lowest point) has been passed and leukocyte count rises to at least 4000/mm^3.

WBC nadir may be expected between 4 and 11 days after initiation of treatment; recovery from leukopenia follows rapidly, usually within 7 to 14 days. With high doses, total leukocyte count may not return to normal until 3 weeks.

Alopecia is frequently not total; in some patients, regrowth begins during maintenance therapy period.

Signs of agranulocytosis (overpowering weakness, high fever, chills, rapid and weak pulse, sore throat, dysphagia, pharyngeal and buccal ulcerations) must be reported to facilitate immediate treatment.

See Mechlorethamine Hydrochloride for nursing care of stomatitis.

Instruct patient, or family provider of care, to give close attention to condition of skin. Ulcerations in the elderly patient necessitate termination of therapy because of high susceptibility to leukopenic effects of vinblastine.

Preserved in tight, light-resistant containers in refrigerator. Reconstituted solution may be refrigerated up to 30 days without loss of potency.

VINCRISTINE SULFATE, U.S.P.
(Leurocristine, LCR, ONCOVIN, VCR)

Antineoplastic

ACTIONS AND USES

Cell-cycle-specific vinca alkaloid (obtained from periwinkle plant *Vinca rosea*), and an analogue of vinblastine. Antineoplastic mechanism unclear; appears to arrest mitosis at metaphase, thereby inhibiting cell division. In contrast to vinblastine, has relatively low toxic effect on normal cells and thus produces minimal myelosuppression; however, neurologic and neuromuscular effects are more severe. One member of the BACOP, COMA, MOPP chemotherapeutic combination regimens.

Principal use: acute leukemia in children. Limited use: lymphomas, acute lymphocytic or undifferentiated stem cell leukemia, and some solid tumors. Adjunctive use in advanced stages of Hodgkin's disease with mechlorethamine, prednisone, and procarbazine (MOPP regimen) and in disseminated malignant melanoma with carmustine.

ABSORPTION AND FATE

Distribution and excretion not determined; appears to be excreted primarily by liver into bile. Does not cross blood–brain barrier.

CONTRAINDICATIONS AND PRECAUTIONS

Obstructive jaundice, pregnancy, men and women of childbearing age. Cautious use: leukopenia, preexisting neuromuscular disease, hypertension, infection, patients receiving drugs with neurotoxic potential.

ADVERSE REACTIONS

Usually dose-related and reversible. **Neuromuscular:** peripheral neuropathy, neuritic pain, paresthesias, sensory loss, ataxia, slapping gait, loss of deep tendon reflexes, muscle atrophy, dysphagia, weakness in larynx and extrinsic eye muscles, ptosis, diplopia, mental depression. **GI:** stomatitis, pharyngitis, anorexia, nausea, vomiting, diarrhea, abdominal pain, severe constipation, paralytic ileus, rectal bleeding. **Hematologic** (rare): leukopenia, thrombocytopenia, anemia. **Dermatologic:** urticaria, rash, alopecia, cellulitis and phlebitis at injection site. **Other:** hypertension, malaise, fever, convulsions, headache, pain in parotid gland area, hyperuricemia, hyperkalemia, weight loss, polyuria, dysuria, inappropriate ADH syndrome (high urinary sodium excretion, hyponatremia, dehydration, hypotension).

ROUTE AND DOSAGE

Various schedules have been used. Highly individualized. Intravenous: **Adults:** 1.4 mg/m² at weekly intervals; **children:** 2 mg/m² at weekly intervals. Solution may be injected either directly into vein or into tubing of running IV over 1 minute. Diluting solution bacteriostatic sodium chloride injection provided; may also be diluted with physiologic saline or sterile water for injection to concentrations of 0.01 to 1 mg/ml.

NURSING IMPLICATIONS

When given directly into vein, syringe and needle should be rinsed with blood before needle is withdrawn.

If extravasation occurs, drug should be discontinued immediately and injection restarted into another vein. Hyaluronidase should be injected locally into surrounding tissue. Moderate heat applications may be helpful (used with caution because of possible sensory loss).

Monitor intake–output ratio and pattern, blood pressure, and temperature daily. Record on flow chart as indicators for adaptations in nursing and drug regimen.

Regularly scheduled serum uric acid determinations, adequate hydration, and administration of a uricosuric agent may be prescribed to prevent uric acid nephropathy.

Weigh patient under standard conditions weekly or more often if ordered. In the presence of edema or ascites, patient's ideal weight is used to determine dosage. Report a steady gain or sudden weight change to physician.

A prophylactic regimen against constipation and paralytic ileus (adequate fluids, roughage in diet, cathartics) is usually recommended. Encourage patient to report changes in bowel habit as soon as manifested. Paralytic ileus is most likely to occur in young children.

Note that while fluid intake should be encouraged to prevent constipation, if hyponatremia is a problem, fluid deprivation may be necessary. Discuss with physician for guidelines.

An empty rectum with colicky pain may be misdiagnosed. Physician may order an abdominal flat plate to rule out high fecal impaction. If present, high enema or cathartic may be prescribed.

Complete bone marrow remission in leukemia varies widely and may not occur for as long as 100 days after therapy is started.

Toxicity with vincristine occasionally follows an irreversible sequence: sensory impairment and paresthesias, neuritic pain, motor difficulties.

Neuromuscular side effects are most apt to appear in the patient with preexisting neuromuscular disease and may persist for several months after therapy is discontinued.

Grasp hands of patient each day to detect onset of hand muscular weakness, and check deep tendon reflexes (depression of Achilles reflex is the earliest sign of neuropathy). Also observe for and report promptly: mental depression, ptosis, double vision, hoarseness, paresthesias, neuritic pain, and motor difficulties.

If patient is bedridden, provide prophylactic measures to prevent footdrop.

Walking may be impaired; check patient's ability to ambulate, and supply support if necessary.

Dental caries or periodontal disease should be treated since patient is highly susceptible to superimposed infection.

See Mechlorethamine for nursing care of stomatitis.

Partial alopecia (reversible) is reportedly the most common adverse reaction and may persist for the duration of therapy. Discuss with patient the possibility of its occurrence to permit plans for cosmetic substitution if desired.

To prevent injury to rectal mucosa, use of rectal thermometer or intrusive tubing should be avoided if possible.

Leukopenia occurs in a significant number of patients; leukocyte count in children usually reaches nadir on 4th day and begins to rise on 5th day after drug administration. Provide special protection during leukopenic days.

Reconstituted solution may be refrigerated up to 14 days. Label vial for concentration (mg/ml). Both dry form and solutions should be protected from light.

VIOMYCIN SULFATE, U.S.P., B.P.
(VIOCIN)

Antibacterial (tuberculostatic)

ACTIONS AND USES

Polypeptide antibiotic derived from *Streptomyces puniceus,* with bacteriostatic activity against *Mycobacterium tuberculosis.* Reportedly less active than streptomycin and more active than PAS. Has little effect in presence of extensive caseation or fibrosis. Viomycin-resistant strains are emerging rapidly. Some cross-resistance with streptomycin, kanamycin, and capreomycin is possible; therefore not used in combination with these drugs. Has neuromuscular blocking activity similar to that of the aminoglyosides.

Used in treatment of various forms of tuberculosis in conjunction with one or more antituberculous drugs to minimize emergence of resistant strains.

ABSORPTION AND FATE

Quickly absorbed following IM injection. Peak serum levels within 1 hour; still detectable after 8 hours. Poor penetration into cerebrospinal fluid and peritoneal and pleural cavities. Excreted mainly by kidneys.

CONTRAINDICATIONS AND PRECAUTIONS

History of hypersensitivity to viomycin; concomitant administration of other ototoxic drugs. Safe use in children not established. Cautious use: impaired renal function.

ADVERSE REACTIONS

Nephrotoxicity: hematuria, proteinuria, cylinduria, nitrogen retention, decreased creatinine clearance, renal loss of electrolytes. Ototoxicity: hypersensitivity (rash, fever, laryngeal edema, eosinophilia).

ROUTE AND DOSAGE

Intramuscular: 1 Gm at 12-hour intervals twice weekly, continued for at least 4 to 6 months, depending on nature of lesion. In special instances, same dosage may be given daily but for no longer than 1 month. Not to exceed 2 Gm daily.

NURSING IMPLICATIONS

Administer IM deep into body of large muscle mass, preferably upper outer quadrant of buttock or midlateral thigh. Deltoid should be used only if it is well developed and care is taken to avoid radial nerve (do not use lower or mid-third area of upper arm). Aspirate carefully to avoid inadvertent entry into blood vessel, and inject drug slowly. Keep record to assure rotation of injection sites.

Viomycin has a high potential for toxicity. Patient must remain under close medical supervision during therapy.

Audiometric and vestibular function tests should be conducted prior to and during therapy.

Monitor intake and output. Report oliguria or changes in intake–output ratio. Progressive renal insufficiency requires discontinuation of drug.

Determinations of renal function (including urinary electrolytes) are advised prior to and every 1 to 2 weeks during therapy. Tests of auditory and vestibular function are also advised prior to therapy.

Impairment of vestibular function occurs quite commonly; auditory impairment is also possible. Ototoxic symptoms usually develop within 1 month or more after drug is initiated. Vestibular function and audiometer tests should be done if patient experiences vertigo, tinnitus, loss of balance, nystagmus, or hearing loss.

Some patients require supplemental calcium, potassium, and other electrolytes because of excessive urinary loss. Be alert for signs of edema, hypocalcemic tetany, and hypokalemia (see Index).

Solutions for injection are prepared by adding sterile water for injection. May be stored at room temperature, under sterile conditions, without appreciable loss of potency, but manufacturer recommends refrigeration storage.

DRUG INTERACTIONS: Concomitant use of viomycin with other neuromuscular blocking agents (eg, **aminoglycoside antibiotics, tubocurarine,** and related drugs) may result in additive neuromuscular blockade (prolonged respiratory depression, apnea).

VITAMIN A, U.S.P.
(ACON, ALPHALIN, AQUASOL A, DISPATABS, Oleovitamin A, TESTAVOL S, VI-DOM-A)

Vitamin (antixerophthalmic)

ACTIONS AND USES

Fat-soluble vitamin obtained from seawater fish liver oils or prepared synthetically. Includes vitamin A as well as its precursors, alpha, beta, and gamma carotene, and crystoxanthin. Expressed in terms of international units (I.U.): 1 I.U. (equivalent to 1 U.S.P. unit) is equal to 0.3 μg of retinol (vitamin A alcohol), 0.34 μg of vitamin A acetate, or 0.6 μg of beta carotene (provitamin A). Vitamin A is essential for normal growth and development of bones and teeth, for integrity of epithelial cells, and for formation of rhodopsin (visual purple) necessary for visual dark adaptation. Also, thought to act as cofactor in biosynthesis of adrenal steroids, mucopolysaccharides, cholesterol, and RNA. Reportedly stimulates healing of cortisone-retarded wounds when applied topically. Used in treatment of vitamin A deficiency and as dietary supplement during periods of increased requirements, such as pregnancy, lactation, and infancy; used as replacement therapy in conditions that affect absorption, mobilization, or storage of vitamin A, eg, steatorrhea, severe biliary obstruction, hepatic cirrhosis, total gastrectomy.

Readily absorbed from GI tract (in presence of bile salts, pancreatic lipase, and dietary fat). Aqueous formulations produce more rapid and higher blood concentrations than oil form; absorption of emulsion is intermediate. Stored mainly in liver; small amounts also found in kidney and body fat. Metabolites excreted in feces and urine. Does not readily cross placenta, but passes into breast milk.

CONTRAINDICATIONS AND PRECAUTIONS

History of sensitivity to vitamin A or to any ingredient in formulation, hypervitaminosis A, oral administration to patients with malabsorption syndrome. Safe use in amounts exceeding 6000 I.U. during pregnancy not established. Cautious use: women on oral contraceptives, high doses in nursing mothers.

ADVERSE REACTIONS

Hypervitaminosis A syndrome. General manifestations: malaise, lethargy, abdominal discomfort, anorexia, vomiting. **Skeletal:** slow growth; deep tender hard lumps (subperiosteal thickening) over radius, tibia, occiput; migratory arthralgia; retarded growth; premature closure of epiphyses. **CNS:** irritability, headache, intracranial hypertension (pseudotumor cerebri), increased intracranial pressure, bulging fontanelles, papilledema, exophthalmos, miosis, nystagmus. **Dermatologic:** gingivitis, lip fissures, excessive sweating, drying or cracking of skin, pruritus, increase in skin pigmentation, massive desquamation, brittle nails, alopecia. **Other:** hypomenorrhea, hepatosplenomegaly, jaundice, leukopenia, hypoplastic anemias, vitamin A plasma levels over 1200 I.U./dl, elevations of sedimentation rate and prothrombin time.

ROUTE AND DOSAGE

Oral: Severe deficiency: **Adults and children** *over 8 years:* 100,000 I.U. daily for 3 days, followed by 50,000 I.U. daily for 2 weeks; follow-up therapy 10,000 to 20,000 I.U. daily for 2 months. Dietary supplement: **Children** *4 to 8 years:* 15,000 I.U. daily; *under 4 years:* 10,000 I.U. daily. Intramuscular: **Adults:** 100,000 I.U. daily for 3 days, followed by 50,000 I.U. daily for 2 weeks. **Children** *1 to 8 years:* 17,500 to 35,000 I.U. daily for 10 days; *(infants):* 7,500 to 15,000 I.U. daily for 10 days.

NURSING IMPLICATIONS

Evaluation of dosage is made with consideration of patient's average daily intake of vitamin A. Dietary and drug history is advisable, eg, intake of fortified foods, dietary supplements, self-administration or prescription drug sources. Women taking oral contraceptives tend to have significantly high plasma vitamin A levels.

Vitamin A deficiency is often associated with protein malnutrition as well as other vitamin deficiencies. May be manifested by night blindness, retardation of growth and development, epithelial alterations, susceptibility to infection, abnormal dryness of skin, mouth, and eyes (xerophthalmia) progressing to keratomalacia (ulceration and necrosis of cornea and conjunctiva), urinary tract calculi.

Recommended daily allowance (RDA)(for healthy individuals): adult males 5000 I.U., adult females 4000 I.U. lactating women 6000 I.U., children 4 to 6 years 2500 I.U., infants 1400 to 2000 I.U.

Cause of deficiency should be clearly identified for patient, and he and responsible family members should be included in dietary planning.

About half of vitamin A activity in the average American diet comes from carotene (provitamin A), found in yellow and green (leafy) vegetables and yellow fruits. Carotene and liver (1 μg is equivalent in biologic activity to 0.167 μg vitamin A). Sources of preformed vitamin A are supplied primarily from livers of cod, halibut, tuna, and shad, fat of dairy products, fortified margarine and milk, and egg yolk.

Patients receiving therapeutic doses should be closely supervised. Inform

patient and family that self-medication with vitamin A is potentially harmful.

For treatment of overdosage (hypervitaminosis A), drug should be discontinued immediately. Most signs and symptoms (see Adverse Reactions)
subside within a week, but tender, hard swellings in extremities and
occiput may remain for several months.

Caution patient to keep drug out of reach of children.

Preserved in tight, light-resistant containers.

DRUG INTERACTIONS: Concomitant administration of mineral oil may decrease absorption of vitamin A.

VITAMIN E, N.F.
(AQUASOL E, E-FEROL, EPROLIN, EPSILAN-M, SOLUCAP E, TEGA-E CREAM, TOCO-DERM CREAM, TOCOPHER, TOCOPHEREX, TOCOPHEROL, TOKOLS, WHEAT GERM OIL)

Vitamin E supplement

ACTIONS AND USES

Vitamin E refers to a group of naturally occurring fat-soluble substances known
as tocopherols (alpha, beta, gamma, and delta). Alpha tocopherol, comprising
90% of the tocopherols, is the most biologically potent and has been synthesized. Nutrient and therapeutic value of vitamin E is equivocal. Appears to
function as a tissue antioxidant, and is thought to facilitate vitamin A absorption, storage, and utilization. Also, seems to play a role in hemoglobin synthesis,
but precise mechanism not understood. Use in man is based largely on deficiency states in lower animals. Found to have some therapeutic value in macrocytic, megaloblastic anemia associated with protein-calorie malnutrition
(kwashiorkor), hemolytic anemia in premature infants, and malabsorption syndromes. Has been used investigationally in muscular dystrophy, sterility, habitual abortion, coronary, cerebral and peripheral vascular disorders, and a number
of other conditions, with no conclusive evidence of its value. Used topically for
dry or chapped skin and for temporary relief of minor skin disorders.

ABSORPTION AND FATE

Readily and almost completely absorbed from GI tract, if fat absorption is
normal, and enters blood via lymph. Distributed to all body tissues, and is
stored for long periods of time. Most excreted in bile and feces; remainder
excreted in urine as glucuronides and other metabolites. Crosses placenta only
to a limited extent.

ADVERSE REACTIONS

Appears to be nontoxic at therapeutic dosage range. With excessive doses for
prolonged periods, may cause skeletal-muscle weakness, fatigue, disturbances
of reproductive function, GI upset, creatinuria.

ROUTE AND DOSAGE

Prophylactic: 5 to 30 IU. Therapeutic: according to needs of patient. Usual: 30
to 100 mg orally or parenterally. Topical cream, lotion, oil, ointment, spray.

NURSING IMPLICATIONS

N.R.C. recommended daily dietary allowance of vitamin E for infants is 4 IU;
for children 4 to 6 years, 9 IU; adult males, 15 IU; adult females, 12 IU;
pregnant and lactating women, 15 IU.

Estimated daily requirement is usually provided by the normal adult diet, but
requirements are higher with increased intake of unsaturated fats.

Wheat germ is the richest source of vitamin E; also found in vegetable oils (sunflower, corn, soybean, cottonseed); green leafy vegetables, nuts, dairy products, eggs, cereals, meat, liver.
Preserved in tight containers, protected from light.

DRUG INTERACTIONS: Preliminary studies indicate that concomitant administration of vitamin E may impair hemolytic response to **iron** therapy in children with iron-deficiency anemia and may enhance **oral anticoagulant** activity.

WARFARIN, POTASSIUM, N.F.
(ATHROMBIN-K)
WARFARIN, SODIUM, U.S.P., B.P.
(COUMADIN, PANWARFIN)

Anticoagulant

ACTIONS AND USES
Intermediate-acting coumarin derivative. Indirectly interferes with blood clotting by blocking hepatic synthesis of vitamin-K-dependent clotting factors: II (prothrombin), VII (proconvertin), IX (Christmas factor or plasma thromboplastin component), and X (Stuart factor). Prevents further extension of formed clots and secondary thromboembolic complications but has no effect on circulating clotting factors, established thrombi, or ischemic tissue. Effects are cumulative and prolonged.
Used for prophylaxis and treatment of venous thrombosis and its extension, pulmonary embolism, treatment of atrial fibrillation with embolization, and as adjunct in treatment of coronary occlusion. May be given with heparin to accomplish immediate and long-term anticoagulant therapy simultaneously. Used extensively as rodenticide.

ABSORPTION AND FATE
Onset of action 2 to 12 hours following oral administration, peaks in 24 to 36 hours; onset of action 1 to 9 hours following parenteral injection, peaks in 36 to 72 hours. Duration of action: 4 to 5 days following single therapeutic dose. Half-life 2½ days. Approximately 97% of drug bound to plasma albumin. Accumulates mainly in liver where it is metabolized; also distributed to lungs, spleen, kidney. Excreted in urine largely as metabolites and traces of unchanged drug. Marked individual differences in metabolism and excretion rates. Crosses placenta and enters breast milk.

CONTRAINDICATIONS AND PRECAUTIONS
Hemorrhagic tendencies: vitamin C or K deficiency, thrombocytopenia, blood dyscrasias, hemophilia, purpura; active bleeding, open ulcerative, traumatic, or surgical wounds; GI ulcerations, visceral carcinoma, diverticulitis, colitis, continuous tube drainage of GI tract, severe hepatic or renal disease, subacute bacterial endocarditis, severe hypertension, aneurysms, recent surgery of brain, spinal cord, eye; regional and lumbar block anesthesia, threatened abortion, noncompliant patients. Safe use in women of childbearing potential, pregnancy, and nursing mothers not established. Cautious use: history of alcoholism, hypotension, active tuberculosis, history of ulcerative diseases of GI tract; severe diabetes, myxedema, congestive heart failure, allergic disorders, collagen diseases, cachexia, spinal puncture, mild liver or kidney dysfunction, during menstruation, postpartum period, patients in hazardous occupations.

Anorexia, nausea, vomiting, abdominal cramps, diarrhea, steatorrhea, bleeding from peptic ulcer or carcinoma, paralysis of accommodation, priapism (rare), nephropathy, hepatitis, jaundice. **Hematopoietic;** anemia, leukopenia, failure of myeloid maturation, atypical mononuclear cells, leukemoid reaction, agranulocytosis, aplastic anemia. **Allergic:** dermatitis, urticaria, alopecia, fever. **Overdosage:** hematuria; bleeding from skin, mucous membranes, wounds, GI tract; paralytic ileus, submucosal or intramural hemorrhage, excessive menstrual flow; necrosis of toes, female breast and other fat-rich areas.

ROUTE AND DOSAGE

Oral, intramuscular, intravenous: initial, 40 to 60 mg (half this for elderly or debilitated patients); maintenance: 2 to 10 mg daily. Dosages individualized according to prothrombin activity and clinical findings.

NURSING IMPLICATIONS

During period of dosage adjustment, prothrombin activity data should be checked daily by physician and dose order verified or changed.

Since so many drugs interfere with anticoagulant drug activity, a careful medication history should be obtained before initiation of therapy and when interpreting altered responses to therapy.

Question patient incisively as to previous bleeding responses: eg, did he previously develop abnormal bleeding after dental manipulations, surgery, or trauma? Were spontaneous hemorrhages in the skin or mucous membranes usual?

Start flow chart indicating prothrombin activity data, control values, and administered anticoagulant doses.

The one-stage prothrombin time test (PT or Quick) is widely used as a guide for anticoagulant dosage. Usual aim of therapy: maintain prothrombin time at 1 to 1½ times normal (eg, 21 to 35 seconds) with control of 14 seconds.

When heparin is given with warfarin (or other oral anticoagulants) a period of 4 to 5 hours after last IV heparin dose or 12 to 24 hours after last subcutaneous dose should intervene before a blood sample is drawn, since heparin may prolong the one-stage prothrombin time. (Warfarin is reportedly compatible in same syringe with sodium heparin.)

Prothrombin time determinations may be prescribed for patient on maintenance dosage at biweekly, weekly, or 2- to 4-week intervals depending upon response to drug. Periodic blood studies, urinalyses, and liver function tests are also usually recommended.

Impress upon patient/family the importance of adhering to drug regimen and of keeping all appointments made for laboratory tests. Advise patient to record daily dose taken on dosage calendar (available from some drug companies).

Continued anticoagulant therapy should not be ordered in the absence of laboratory facilities or if patient is noncompliant.

Studies suggest that patients who are elderly, psychotic, or alcholic present the greatest problems regarding compliance.

The 2½ day drug half-life presents the possibility that effects may become more pronounced as daily maintenance doses overlap. Observe carefully for signs of overdosage particularly during early phase of establishing pharmacologic control.

Warn patient that bleeding or signs of bleeding should be reported immediately to physician and drug withheld, eg, hematuria (red or dark brown urine), hematemesis, dark or tarry stools, bleeding gums or oral mucosa, ecchymoses, purpura, petechiae, epistaxis, bloody sputum, abdominal or lumbar pain (retroperitoneal bleeding) excessive menstrual flow, prolonged oozing from any minor injury.

Instruct patient to use a soft tooth brush and to floss teeth gently. Also advise use of electric razor for shaving to avoid scraping skin.

Anticoagulant effect usually reversed by omission of one or more doses of warfarin and by administration of phytonadione (vitamin K_1). Physician may advise patient to carry vitamin K with him at all times. Be certain he understands its use in treatment of spontaneous hemorrhage.

If bleeding is severe, parenteral vitamin K and fresh whole blood transfusion may be necessary.

Instruct patient/family to discontinue anticoagulant and report immediately: prodromal symptoms of agranulocytosis (marked fatigue, sore throat or mouth, chills, fever); hepatitis (dark urine, itchy skin, jaundice); or hypersensitivity reactions.

Alert patient to factors that may affect anticoagulant response. Prothrombin time may be lengthened by fever, alcoholism, prolonged hot weather, renal insufficiency, malnutrition, scurvy, exposure to x-ray, and shortened by diarrhea, edema (reduces drug absorption and distribution) high fat diet or diet unusually high in vitamin K-rich foods (cabbage, cauliflower, kale, spinach, fish, liver), exposure to DDT or chlordane.

Drug should be withdrawn prior to surgery of CNS or eye. Other surgical procedures may be carried out by maintaining patient on minimal therapeutic dosage and by providing close vigilance of possible bleeding sites.

Advise patient to inform his dentist or any new physician about anticoagulant therapy and duration of treatment.

Warn against taking OTC medications unless specifically ordered by physician. Anticoagulant action is affected by many drugs: eg, acetaminophen (Tylenol), antacids, antihistamines, aspirin, mineral oil, oral contraceptives, vitamin C and vitamin K in large doses.

Urge patient to maintain a well-balanced diet and to avoid excess intake of alcohol (consult physician regarding allowable amount).

Patient should carry, on his person, identification card or jewelry which notes medication being taken and physician's name, address, and telephone number.

When anticoagulant therapy is terminated, dose is withdrawn gradually over 3 to 4 weeks to prevent rebound thromboembolic complications. Prothrombin activity usually returns to normal in 2 to 10 days following total drug withdrawal.

Following reconstitution, parenteral solution is stable for several days at 4 C. Discard solution if precipitation occurs.

Preserved in tight, light-resistant containers. Protect oral drug from moisture.

LABORATORY TEST INTERFERENCES: Warfarin may cause increased serum T_3, decreased serum uric acid.

DRUG INTERACTIONS: The number of drugs implicated in producing clinically significant lengthening of prothrombin time (potentiation of anticoagulant effect) or shortening of prothrombin time (inhibition of anticoagulant effect) are too numerous to list. Consult pharmacist about particular drugs. Prothrombin time should be closely monitored whenever a drug is added to or withdrawn from patient's therapeutic regimen.

Adrenergic (topical vasoconstrictor)

ACTIONS AND USES
Imidazoline derivative with marked α-adrenergic activity on vascular smooth muscles. Structurally related to naphazoline. Produces decongestion of nasal mucosa by constricting smaller arterioles.
Used for relief of nasal congestion caused by rhinitis and sinusitis.

ABSORPTION AND FATE
Effects appear immediately and persist for about 4 hours.

CONTRAINDICATIONS AND PRECAUTIONS
Sensitivity to adrenergic substances, narrow-angle glaucoma, concurrent therapy with MAO inhibitors or tricyclic antidepressants. Safe use during pregnancy not established. Cautious use: hypertension; hyperthyroidism; heart disease, including angina; advanced arteriosclerosis; use in the elderly, infants, or children.

ADVERSE REACTIONS
Usually mild and infrequent: local stinging, burning, dryness, sneezing, headache, insomnia, drowsiness, palpitation. With excessive use: rebound congestion, tremulousness, increase in blood pressure, lightheadedness, tachycardia, arrhythmias, somnolence, sedation, coma.

ROUTE AND DOSAGE
Topical: **Adults:** (nasal spray 0.1%): 1 or 2 sprays in each nostril every 4 to 6 hours; (nasal solution 0.1%): 2 or 3 drops in each nostril every 4 to 6 hours. **Pediatrics** *under 12 years:* 2 or 3 drops of pediatric solution (0.05%) in each nostril every 4 to 6 hours; *under 6 months:* 1 drop (pediatric solution) every 6 hours.

NURSING IMPLICATIONS
Instruct patient to clear each nostril gently before administering drops or spray (see Naphazoline for technique of nose drop administration).
Do not shake nasal spray solution. To administer, patient should tilt head slightly forward and hold tube vertically (spray end up) so that solution is delivered in a fine spray.
Systemic effects are possible, particularly when excessive amounts introduced intranasally are swallowed.
To prevent contamination of nasal solution, rinse dropper and tip of nasal spray in hot water after use.
Prolonged use may cause rebound congestion and chemical rhinitis. Caution patient not to exceed prescribed dosage and to report to physician if drug fails to provide relief.
Xylometazoline solution should not be placed in atomizers made of aluminum parts.
Preserved in tight, light-resistant containers.

ZINC OXIDE, U.S.P.
(ZINCOFAX, ZnO)

Astringent, protectant (topical)

ACTIONS AND USES
Water-insoluble substance with mildly astringent, protective, antipruritic, and weakly antiseptic properties.
Used topically for minor skin wounds, chafing, eczema, and sunburn and to protect skin from wound drainage. Incorporated in many topical preparations.

Patients being x-rayed or receiving x-ray therapy (zinc, like other metals, may alter dosage of x-ray).
ROUTE AND DOSAGE
Topical: cream 15%, ointment 20%, paste 25%.

NURSING IMPLICATIONS
Repeated applications of an ointment can cause skin maceration by interfering with evaporation of perspiration. Folliculitis may result if applied to hairy areas.
Apply zinc oxide sparingly. Before reapplying, gently cleanse skin. Consult physician about appropriate solvent.

ABVD*	Adriamycin (Doxorubicin), Bleomycin, Vinblastine, Dactinomycin
ADH	antidiuretic hormone
AChE	acetylcholinesterase
ACTH	adrenocorticotrophic hormone
ADT	alternate-day therapy
APTT	activated partial prothrombin time
AV	atrioventricular
BACOP*	Bleomycin, Adriamycin (Doxorubicin), Cyclophosphamide, Oncovin (Vincristine), Prednisone
BAL	British Anti-Lewisite
BMR	basal metabolic rate
B.P.	British Pharmacopoeia
BSP	Bromsulphalein
BUN	blood urea nitrogen
cAMP	cyclic adenosine monophosphate
CHOP*	Cyclophosphamide, 14-Hydroxydaunorubicin (Doxorubicin), Oncovin (Vincristine), Prednisone
CMFOP*	Cyclophosphamide, Methotrexate, Fluorouracil, Oncovin (Vincristine), Prednisone
COAP*	Cyclophosphamide, Oncovin (Vincristine), Ara-C (Cytarabine), Prednisone
COMA*	Cyclosphosphamide, Oncovin (Vincristine), Methotrexate, Ara-C (Cytarabine)
COP*	Cyclophosphamide, Oncovin (Vincristine), Prednisone
CPK	creatine phosphokinase
CSF	cerebrospinal fluid
CTZ	chemoreceptor trigger zone
CVP	central venous pressure
1,25-DHCC	1, 25 dihydrocholecalciferol
DNA	deoxyribonucleic acid
FSH	follicle-stimulating hormone
GFR	glomerular filtration rate
GH	growth hormone
G-6-PD	glucose-6-phosphate dehydrogenase
HCG	human chorionic gonadotropin
HCT	hematocrit
Hgb	hemoglobin
5-HIAA	5-hydroxyindole acetic acid
17-OH	17-hydroxysteroids
5-HT	5-hydroxytryptamine, serotonin
I 131	radioactive iodine
IgG	immunoglobulin G
17-KGS	17-ketogenic steroids
17-KS	17-ketosteroids
LDH	lactic dehydrogenase

*Combination chemotherapeutic regimen.

LDL	low-density lipoprotein
LE	lupus erythematosus
LH	luteinizing hormone
MAO	monamine oxidase
MAOI	monamine oxidase inhibitor
MBD	minimal brain dysfunction
μCi	microcurie
mCi	millicurie
MDR	minimum daily requirement
MOPP*	Mechlorethamine, Oncovin (Vincristine), Prednisone, Procarbazine
N.F.	National Formulary
NPN	non-protein nitrogen
NRC	National Research Council
NSR	normal sinus rhythm
OTC	over-the-counter
P 32	radioactive phosphorus
PABA	para-aminobenzoic acid
PAH	para-aminohippuric acid
P and P	prothrombin and proconvertin
PBI	protein-bound iodine
PEMA	phenylethyl malonamide
POMP*	Prednisone, Oncovin (Vincristine), Mercaptopurine, Procarbazine
PSP	phenolsulfonphthalein
PVP	premature ventricular contraction
RAI	radioactive iodine
RDA	recommended daily allowance
REM	rapid eye movement
RNA	ribonucleic acid
SA	sinoatrial
SGOT	serum glutamic-oxaloacetic transaminase
SGPT	serum glutamic-pyruvic transaminase
SIADH	syndrome of inappropriate antidiuretic hormone
SRS-A	slow-reacting substance of anaphylaxis
TSH	thyrotropic stimulating hormone
U.S.P.	United States Pharmacopeia
VLDL	very low density lipoprotein
VMA	vanilmandelic acid

*Combination chemotherapeutic regimen

Schedule I	Substances in this group have no acceptable medical use in the United States; furthermore they have a high potential for abuse. Examples: heroin, marihuana, LSD, and mescaline.
Schedule II	Drugs in this group have a high abuse potential and high liability for severe psychic or physical dependence. Examples: morphine, meperidine, cocaine, and amphetamine. Prescription required.
Schedule III	These compounds contain limited quantities of certain narcotic and non-narcotic drugs. Potential for abuse is less than for drugs in Schedule II. Examples: paregoric, nalorphine, and chlorphentermine. Prescription required.
Schedule IV	Drugs under Schedule IV have lower potential for abuse than those in Schedule III. Examples: phenobarbital, chloral hydrate, and meprobamate. Prescription required.
Schedule V	The abuse potential for these drugs is less than for those in Schedule IV. Preparations contain limited quantities of certain narcotic drugs; generally intended for antitussive and antidiarrheal purposes and may be distributed without a prescription provided that

1. such distribution is made only by a pharmacist;
2. not more than 240 ml or not more than 48 solid dosage units of any substance containing opium, nor more than 120 ml or not more than 24 solid dosage units of any other controlled substance may be distributed at retail to the same purchaser in any given 48-hour period without a valid prescription order;
3. the purchaser is at least 18 years old;
4. the pharmacist knows the purchaser or requests suitable identification;
5. the pharmacist keeps an official written record of name and address of the purchaser, kind and quantity of controlled substance purchased, date of sale, and initials of dispensing pharmacist. This record is to be made available for inspection and copying by officers of the U.S., authorized by the Attorney General.

*Under jurisdiction of the federal Controlled Substances Act.

AMA Drug Evaluation, 3rd ed. Acton Mass., Publishing Sciences Group, Inc., 1977

American Hospital Formulary Service: American Society of Hospital Pharmacists, Washington, D.C. (Updated quarterly)

APhA Drug Names: American Pharmaceutical Association, Washington, D.C. 1976

Arndt KA: Manual of Dermatologic Therapeutics. Boston, Little, Brown, 1974

Assessing Vital Functions Accurately (Nursing 77 Books): Horsham, Penn. Intermed Communications, Inc., 1977

Beland IL, Passos JY: Clinical Nursing: Pathophysiological and Psychological Approaches, 3rd ed. New York, Macmillan, 1975

Benenson AS (ed): Control of Communicable Diseases in Man, 11th ed. Washington, D.C., The American Public Health Association, 1970

Billups NF: American Drug Index 1977, Philadelphia, Lippincott, 1977

Blahd WH: *Nuclear Medicine,* 2nd ed. New York, McGraw-Hill, 1971

Braude AI: Antimicrobial drug therapy. Vol. VIII. In Major Problems in Internal Medicine, Philadelphia, Saunders, 1976

Bushness SS: Respiratory Intensive Care Nursing. Boston, Little, Brown, 1973

Cluff LE, Caransos GJ, Stewart RB: Clinical problems with drugs. Vol. V. In Major Problems in Internal Medicine. Philadelphia, Saunders, 1975

Conn HF (ed): *Current Therapy 1977,* Philadelphia, W.B. Saunders Company, 1977.

Cooper P: Ward Procedures and Techniques. New York, Appleton-Century-Crofts, 1967

Drugs and the Elderly: University of Southern California, Los Angeles, Ca., Ethel Percy Andrus Gerontology Center, 1973

Evaluation of Drug Interactions, 2nd ed: American Pharmaceutical Association, Washington, D.C. 1976

Friedman, SA., Steinhuber FU (eds): Symposium on Geriatric Medicine, The Medical Clinics of North America, Philadelphia, Saunders, 1976

Goodman LS, Gilman A (eds): The Pharmacological Basis of Therapeutics, 5th ed. New York, Macmillan 1975

Goth A: Medical Pharmacology, 6th ed. St. Louis, Mosby, 1972

Griffiths MC (ed): *USAN and the USP Dictionary of Drug Names.* Maryland, United States Pharmaceutical Convention, Inc., 1976

Guyton AC: Textbook of Medical Physiology, 5th ed. Philadelphia, Saunders, 1976

Hansten, PD: Drug Interactions, 3rd ed. Philadelphia, Lea & Febiger, 1975

Handbook of Nonprescription Drugs, 5th ed. American Pharmaceutical Association, Washington, D.C. 1977.

Harvey AM et al., (eds): The Principles and Practice of Medicine, 19th ed. New York, Appleton-Century-Crofts, 1976

Hollister LE: Clinical Use of Psychotherapeutic Drugs. Springfield, Ill., Charles C Thomas, 1974

Howells JG (ed): Modern Perspectives in The Psychiatry of Old Age. New York, Brunner/Mazel, 1975

Kastrup EK (ed): Facts and Comparisons. Missouri, Facts and Comparisons, Inc. (updated monthly)

Lewis AJ (ed): Modern Drug Encyclopedia and Therapeutic Index. (MDE/14). New York, Yorke Medical Books, 1977

Luckmann J, Sorenson KC: Medical-Surgical Nursing: A Psychophysiologic Approach. Philadelphia, Saunders, 1974

764 Managing Diabetics Properly (Nursing 77 Books): Horsham, Penn., Intermed Communications, Inc., 1977

Martindale W: The Extra Pharmacopoeia, 26th ed. London, The Pharmaceutical Press, 1973

Meyers FH, Jawetz E, Goldfien A: Review of Medical Pharmacology, 5th ed. Los Altos, Ca., Lange Medical Publications, 1976

Oberfield RA (ed): Symposium on Malignant Disease. The Medical Clinics of North America. Philadelphia, Saunders, 1975

Physicians' Desk Reference, 32nd ed. New Jersey, Medical Economics Company, 1978

Pinneo R: Unit I: Congestive Heart Failure. New York, Appleton-Century-Crofts, 1978

Pritchard JA, MacDonald PC: Williams Obstetrics, 15th ed. New York, Appleton-Century-Crofts, 1976

Ravel R: Clinical Laboratory Medicine. Chicago, Year Book Medical Publishers, 1973

Reading A, Wise TN (eds); Symposium on Psychiatry in Internal Medicine. The Medical Clinics of North America. Philadelphia, Saunders, 1977.

Reidenberg MM (ed): Symposium on Individualization of Drug Therapy. The Medical Clinics of North America. Philadelphia, Saunders, 1974.

Remington's Pharmaceutical Sciences, 15th ed. Pennsylvania, Mack Publishing Company, 1975

Rossman I (ed): Clinical Geriatrics. Philadelphia, Lippincott, 1971

Rudolph AM (ed.): Pediatrics, 16th ed. New York, Appleton-Century-Crofts, 1977

Shirkey HC: Pediatric Dosage Handbook. Washington, D.C., American Pharmaceutical Association, 1973

Trissel, LA: Handbook on Injectable Drugs. Washington, D.C., American Society of Hospital Pharmacists, 1977

Stecher, PG: The Merck Index: An Encyclopedia of Chemicals and Drugs, 8th ed. New Jersey, Merck & Company Inc., 1968

Stroot VR, Lee CA, Schaper CA: Fluids and Electrolytes: A Practical Approach, 2nd ed. Philadelphia, F. A. Davis, 1977

Sutton AL: Bedside Nursing Techniques in Medicine and Surgery. Philadelphia, Saunders, 1969

Talso PJ (ed): Internal Medicine Based on Mechanisms of Disease. St. Louis, Mosby, 1968

Terry, WD (ed): Symposium on Immunotherapy in Malignant Disease. The Medical Clinics of North America. Philadelphia, Saunders, 1976

Wallach J: Interpretation of Diagnostic Tests. Boston, Little, Brown, 1970

Wasserman E, Slobody LB: Survey of Clinical Pediatrics, 6th ed. New York, McGraw-Hill, 1974

Whipple GH, Peterson MA, Haines VM, Learner E, McKinnon EL: Acute Coronary Care. Boston, Little, Brown, 1972

Widman, FK: Goodale's Clinical Interpretation of Laboratory Tests. Philadelphia, F.A. Davis, 1973

Wiernik PH (ed): Symposium on Advances in Treatment of Cancer. The Medical Clinics of North America. Philadelphia, Saunders, 1977

Youmans GP, Paterson PY, Sommers HM: The Biologic and Clinical Basis of Infectious Diseases. Philadelphia, Saunders, 1975

INDEX

Generic names of prototype drugs, major drug categories, and areas applicable to patient teaching are set in **boldface.**

A

Aarane, 156
Abbreviations, 759
A'cenol, 1
Aceta, 1
Acetaldehyde derivative, paraldehyde, 530
Acetaminophen, 1
Acetanilid metabolites
  acetaminophen, 1
  paracetamol, 1
Acetazide, 2
Acetazolamide, 2
Acetohexamide, 4
Acetophenetidin, 550
Acetosulfone sodium, 5
Acetylcholine chloride, 5
Acetylcysteine, 6
Acetyldigitoxin, 8
Acetylsalicylic acid, 44
Acetylurea derivative, phenacemide, 549
Achromycin, 692
Achrostatin, 507
Acidifiers, gastric
  glutamic acid hydrochloride, 311
  hydrochloride acid, 335
Acidifier, systemic, ammonium chloride, 26
Acidifier, urinary
  ascorbic acid, 43
  methenamine mandelate, 447
Acid Mantle, 14
Acidosis, metabolic, symptoms of, 407
Acidulin, 311
Acnestrol, 203
Acon, 750
Acridine dye derivatives
  mepacrine hydrochloride, 634
  quinacrine hydrochloride, 634
Acrisorcin, 8

ACTH, 153
Acthar, 153
Actidil, 734
Actifed, 734
Actinomycin D, 170
Actinospectocin, 664
Activated carbon, 110
Activated charcoal, 110
Activated charcoal, and ipecac, 370
Activated 7-dehydrocholesterol, 135
Acylanid, 8
Adapin, 230
Adenosine 5-monophosphate, 9
Adenosine phosphate, 9
Adenylic acid, muscle, 9
Adipex-P, 565
Adiphenine hydrochloride, 9
Adolescent and oral contraceptive use, 513
Adophyllin, 696
Adphen, 552
Adrenalin chloride, 248
Adrenergic blocking agents. *See* Blocking agents
Adrenergics (sympathomimetics)
  benzphetamine hydrochloride, 59
  diethylpropion hydrochloride, 202
  dopamine hydrochloride, 227
  ephedrine, 246
  epinephrine, 248
  fenfluramine hydrochloride, 280
  hydroxyamphetaminehydrobromide, 343
  isoproterenol, 378
  isoxsuprine hydrochloride, 381
  levarterenol bitartrate, 388
  mephentermine sulfate, 427
  metaproterenol sulfate, 435
  metaraminol, 436
  methoxamine hydrochloride, 456
  methoxyphenamine hydrochloride, 457
  naphazoline hydrochloride, 488

noradrenaline acid tartrate, 388
nylidrin hydrochloride, 506
orciprenaline sulfate, 435
oxymetazoline hydrochloride, 519
phendimetrazine tartrate, 552
phenmetrazine hydrochloride, 557
phentermine, 565
phenylephrine hydrochloride, 569
phenylpropanolamine hydrochloride, 570
propylhexedrine, 618
protokylol hydrochloride, 623
pseudoephedrine hydrochloride, 625
tetrahydrozoline hydrochloride, 694
tuaminoheptane sulfate, 736
xylometazoline hydrochloride, 756
Adrenochrome semicarbazone, carbazochrome salicylate, 94
Adrenocortical steroids
betamethasone, 64
cortisone acetate, 155
deoxycortone, 183
desoxycorticosterone, 183
dexamethasone, 185
fludrocortisone acetate, 290
flumethasone, 290
fluocinolone acetonide, 291
fluocinonide, 291
fluorometholone, 292
fluprednisolone, 297
hydrocortisone, 337
methylprednisolone, 466
paramethasone acetate, 532
prednisolone, 595
prednisone, 596
triamcinolone, 720
Adrenocorticotropic hormones
corticotropin, 153
cosyntropin, 155
somatotropin, 663
Adrenosem salicylate, 94
Adriamycin, 231
Adroyd, 520
Adsorbent charcoal, 110
Adsorbocarpine, 579
Aeroaid, 701
Aerocaine, 57
Aerodine, 591
Aerolate, 696

Aeroseb-D, 185
Aerosporin sulfate, 586
A5MP, 9
Afrin, 519
Agranulocytosis, symptoms of, 416
AHF, 40
AHG, 40
Airet, 239
Akineton, 66
Akrinol, 8
Al-Anon, 227
Alateen, 227
Albumin, normal human serum, 10
Albuminar, 10
Albumisol, 10
Albuspan, 10
Albutein, 10
Alcohol, unusual sources, 226
Alcohol deterrent, disulfiram, 225
Alcoholics Anonymous, 227
Alconefrin, 569
Alcopara, 63
Aldactazide, 665
Aldactone, 665
Aldinamide, 627
Aldoclor, 461
Aldomet, 461
Aldoril, 461
Aldosterone antagonist, spironolactone, 665
Alidase, 333
Alkalinizers, urinary
acetazolamide, 2
milk of magnesia, 472
Alidol-Pepsin, 311
Alkarau, 643
Alka-Seltzer, 46, 208
Alkeran, 419
Alkylating agents
busulfan, 75
carmustine, 100
chlorambucil, 113
cyclophosphamide, 162
dacarbazine, 169
lomustine, 403
mechlorethamine hydrochloride, 414
melphalan, 419
pipobroman, 582
triethylenethiophosphoramide, 724
uracil mustard, 740

C

G

Q

R

815

U–V